Equine Medicine and Surgery

Fourth Edition

Volume I

Editors

Patrick T. Colahan, DVM, Dip ACVS
Ian G. Mayhew, BVSc, PhD, MRCVS, Dip ACVIM
Alfred M. Merritt, AB, DVM, MS
James N. Moore, DVM, PhD, Dip ACVS

Book Editor: Paul W. Pratt, VMD
Associate Editor: Carolyn M. Richards, BS
Production Manager and Cover Design: Elisabeth S. Stein
Cover Concept: Francis Merritt

American Veterinary Publications, Inc.
5782 Thornwood Drive
Goleta, California 93117
© 1991

While every effort has been made to ensure the accuracy of information contained herein, the publisher and authors are not legally responsible for errors or omissions.

Reprinted, 1992.

Library of Congress Card Number: 90-081427
ISBN 0-939674-27-0

Printed in the United States of America

Chapter Editors

Stephen B. Adams, DVM, MS, Dip ACVS
Professor
Veterinary Teaching Hospital
School of Veterinary Medicine
Purdue University
West Lafayette, IN 47907

Jorg A. Auer, Dr Med Vet, Dip ACVS
Director
Veterinar-Chirurgischen Klinik
University of Zurich
Winterthurerstrasse 260
CH-8057 Zurich, Switzerland

J.L. Barbet, DVM
31 SW 21st Road
Archer, FL 32618

Gary M. Baxter, VMD, MS, Dip ACVS
Assistant Professor
Department of Large Animal Medicine
College of Veterinary Medicine
Colorado State University
Fort Collins, CO 80523

Jill Beech, VMD, Dip ACVIM
Associate Professor
New Bolton Center
Department of Clinical Studies
School of Veterinary Medicine
University of Pennsylvania
Kennett Square, PA 19348

Frederick J. Derksen, DVM, PhD, Dip ACVIM
Professor
Department of Small Animal Clinical Sciences
College of Veterinary Medicine
Michigan State University
East Lansing, MI 48824

Thomas J. Divers, DVM, Dip ACVIM
Associate Professor
New York State College of Veterinary Medicine
Cornell University
Ithaca, NY 14853

Michelle M. LeBlanc, DVM, Dip ACVT
Assistant Professor
Department of Large Animal Clinical Sciences
College of Veterinary Medicine
University of Florida
Gainesville, FL 32610

Robert J. MacKay, DVM, PhD, Dip ACVIM
Assistant Professor
Department of Large Animal Clinical Studies
College of Veterinary Medicine
University of Florida
Gainesville, FL 32610

Debra Deem Morris, DVM, MS, Dip ACVIM
Associate Professor
Department of Large Animal Medicine
College of Veterinary Medicine
University of Georgia
Athens, GA 30602

Peter W. Physick-Sheard, BVSc, MSc, MRCVS
Associate Professor
Department of Population Medicine
Ontario Veterinary College
University of Guelph
Guelph, Ontario, N1G 2W1 Canada

**William C. Rebhun, DVM, Dip ACVIM,
  Dip ACVO**
Professor
Department of Clinical Studies
New York State College of Veterinary Medicine
Cornell University
Ithaca, NY 14853

**Reuben J. Rose, BVSc, PhD, FRCVS, Dip VetAn,
  MACVSc, FACBS**
Professor
Equine Clinic and Exercise Physiology Unit
Department of Veterinary Clinical Sciences
University of Sydney
New South Wales 2006
Australia

Dickson D. Varner, DVM, Dip ACVT
Assistant Professor
Department of Large Animal Medicine & Surgery
College of Veterinary Medicine
Texas A&M University
College Station, TX 77843

Authors

Atwood C. Asbury, DVM, Dip ACT
Professor
Department of Large Animal Clinical Sciences
College of Veterinary Medicine
University of Florida
Gainesville, FL 32610

A.N. Baird, DVM, MS
Assistant Professor
Department of Large Animal Medicine & Surgery
College of Veterinary Medicine
Auburn University
Auburn, AL 36849

Gordon J. Baker, BVSc, Dip ACVS
Professor, Head of Equine Medicine & Surgery
Large Animal Clinic
College of Veterinary Medicine
University of Illinois
1008 W Hazelwood Drive
Urbana, IL 61801

Spencer M. Barber, DVM, Dip ACVS
Professor
Department of Veterinary Anesthesiology,
    Radiology & Surgery
Western College of Veterinary Medicine
University of Saskatchewan
Saskatoon, Saskatchewan S7N 0W0
Canada

Ralph E. Beadle, DVM, PhD
Professor
Department of Veterinary Clinical Sciences
School of Veterinary Medicine
Louisiana State University
Baton Rouge, LA 70803

William V. Bernard, DVM, Dip ACVIM
Rood and Riddle Equine Hospital
POB 12070
Lexington, KY 40580

Diane E. Bevier, DVM, Dip ACVD
Assistant Professor
Department of Companion Animal & Special
    Species Medicine
College of Veterinary Medicine
North Carolina State University
Raleigh, NC 27606

John C. Bloom, VMD, PhD
Eli Lilly & Co
POB 708
Greenfield, IN 46140

L.R. Bramlage, DVM, MS, Dip ACVS
Rood and Riddle Equine Hospital
POB 12070
Lexington, KY 40580

Barbara D. Brewer, DVM, MA, Dip ACVIM
Associate Professor
Department of Large Animal Clinical Studies
College of Veterinary Medicine
University of Florida
Gainesville, FL 32610

**Margaret A. Brownlow, BVSc, MVSc,
    MACVSc, Dip VA**
Senior Tutor
Department of Companion Animal Health
Rural Veterinary Centre
University of Sydney
Camden, New South Wales 2571
Australia

Claus D. Buergelt, DVM, PhD
Associate Professor
Department of Comparative &
    Experimental Pathology
College of Veterinary Medicine
University of Florida, J-145 JHMHC
Gainesville, FL 32610

Jenny I. Cahill, BVSc, PhD
Animal Hospital
519 Church Street
Palmerston North, New Zealand

**Martha Campbell-Thompson, DVM, PhD,
    Dip ACVS**
Research Instructor
Department of Medicine, Box J-214
University of Florida
Gainesville, FL 32610

John P. Caron, DVM, Dip ACVS
Assistant Professor
Department of Large Animal Medicine
College of Veterinary Medicine
Michigan State University
East Lansing, MI 48824

G. Kent Carter, DVM, MS, Dip ACVIM
Associate Professor
Department of Large Animal
    Medicine & Surgery
College of Veterinary Medicine
Texas A&M University
College Station, TX 77843

Leroy Coggins, DVM, PhD
Professor, Head of Department
Department of Microbiology, Pathology &
    Parasitology
College of Veterinary Medicine
North Carolina State University
Raleigh, NC 27606

Patrick T. Colahan, DVM, Dip ACVS
Associate Professor
Department of Large Animal Clinical Studies
College of Veterinary Medicine
University of Florida
Gainesville, FL 32610

Howard Dobson, BVM&S,DVSc, Cert EO, MRCVS
Assistant Professor
Division of Diagnostic Imaging
Department of Clinical Studies
Ontario Veterinary College
University of Guelph
Guelph, Ontario N1G 2W1
Canada

Sue J. Dyson, MA, Vet MB, DEO, FRCVS
Equine Clinical Unit
Animal Health Trust
Snailwell Rd
Newmarket, Suffolk CB8 7DW England

Susan Clark Eades, DVM, PhD, Dip ACVIM
Assistant Professor
Department of Large Animal Medicine
College of Veterinary Medicine
University of Georgia
Athens, GA 30602

G.E. Fackelman, DVM, Dr Med Vet, Dip ACVS
Professor
Department of Surgery
Tufts University
North Grafton, MA 01536

Charles S. Farrow, DVM, Dr Med Vet
Professor
Department of Anesthesia, Radiology & Surgery
Western College of Veterinary Medicine
University of Saskatchewan
Saskatoon, Saskatchewan S7N 0W0
Canada

David T. Galligan, DVM, MBA
Assistant Professor
New Bolton Center
Department of Clinical Studies
School of Veterinary Medicine
University of Pennsylvania
Kennett Square, PA 19348

Marolo C. Garcia, DVM, PhD
601 West State Street
Kennett Square, PA 19348

Harold E. Garner, DVM, PhD
Professor
Department of Veterinary Medicine & Surgery
College of Veterinary Medicine
University of Missouri
Columbia, MO 65211

Brian E. Goulden, BVSc, PhD, MRCVS, MACVSc
Reader
Department of Veterinary Clinical Sciences
Massey University
Palmerston North, New Zealand

Barrie D. Grant, DVM, MS, Dip ACVS
Professor
Department of Clinical Medicine & Surgery
Washington State University
Pullman, WA 99164-661

Eleanor M. Green, DVM, Dip ACVIM, Dip ABVP
Associate Professor
Department of Veterinary Medicine & Surgery
Equine Center at Middlebush Farm
College of Veterinary Medicine
University of Missouri
Columbia, MO 65211

Sherril L. Green, DVM
Staff Veterinarian
Department of Clinical Studies
Ontario Veterinary College
University of Guelph
Guelph, Ontario N1G 2W1 Canada

Dan Hawkins, DVM
Appleton Visiting Professor
Department of Large Animal Clinical Sciences
College of Veterinary Medicine
University of Florida
Gainesville, FL 32610

Michelle M. Henry, DVM, PhD
Merck Foundation Fellow
College of Veterinary Medicine
University of Georgia
Athens, GA 30602

David R. Hodgson, BVSc, PhD, Dip ACVIM
Associate Professor
Department of Veterinary
    Clinical Medicine & Surgery
Washington State University
Pullman, WA 99164-661

Clifford M. Honnas, DVM, Dip ACVS
Assistant Professor
Department of Large Animal Medicine & Surgery
College of Veterinary Medicine
Texas A&M University
College Station, TX 7784

David R. Hutchins, BVSc, MACVSc
124 Shirley Road
Roseville, New South Wales 2069
Australia

Leo B. Jeffcott, B Vet Med, PhD, FRCVS, DVSc
Professor and Head
Veterinary Clinical Centre
Princes Highway
Department of Veterinary Clinical Sciences
University of Melbourne
Werribee, Victoria 3030 Australia

Janet K. Johnston, DVM, Dip ACVIM
Clinical Associate
New Bolton Center
Department of Clinical Studies
School of Veterinary Medicine
University of Pennsylvania
Kennett Square, PA 19348

Ian B. Johnstone, DVM, MSc, PhD
Professor
Department of Biomedical Science
Ontario Veterinary College
University of Guelph
Guelph, Ontario N1G 2W1 Canada

Carl A. Kirker-Head, MA, VetMB, MRCVS
Assistant Professor
Department of Surgery
School of Veterinary Medicine
Tufts University
North Grafton, MA 01536

Ralph C. Knowles, DVM
Veterinary Consultant
27 Oak Avenue
Rehoboth, DE 19971

Catherine W. Kohn, VMD
Associate Professor
Department of Veterinary Clinical Sciences
The Ohio State University
Columbus, OH 43210

Anne M. Koterba, DVM, PhD, Dip ACVIM
Associate Professor
Department of Large Animal Clinical Studies
College of Veterinary Medicine
University of Florida
Gainesville, FL 32610

Ann E. Kraus-Hansen, DVM
LSU Alumni Association Fellow
Department of Veterinary Physiology, Pharmacology
    & Toxicology
School of Veterinary Medicine
Louisiana State University
Baton Rouge, LA 70803

Kenneth S. Latimer, DVM, PhD, Dip ACVP
Associate Professor
Department of Pathology
College of Veterinary Medicine
University of Georgia
Athens, GA 30602

Douglas Leach, BSc, MSc, PhD
Professor
Department of Veterinary Science
University of Kentucky
108 Gluck Equine Research Center
Lexington, KY 40546

Edward A. Mahaffey, DVM, PhD, Dip ACVP
Professor
Department of Veterinary Pathology
College of Veterinary Medicine
University of Georgia
Athens, GA 30602

Richard A. Mansmann, DVM, PhD
Santa Barbara Equine Practice
Rt. 1, Box 237-M
Goleta, CA 93117

Mark D. Markel, DVM, PhD, Dip ACVS
Research Fellow
Orthopedics Biomechanics Laboratory
Mayo Clinic/Mayo Foundation
Rochester, MN 55905

I.G. Mayhew, BVSc, PhD, MRCVS, Dip ACVIM
Chairman of Clinical Studies
Animal Health Trust
Snailwood Road
Newmarket, Suffolk CB8 7DW England

Angus O. McKinnon, BVSc, MSc, Dip ACT,
    Dip ABVP
Associate Professor
Animal Reproduction Laboratory
Colorado State University
Fort Collins, CO 80525

William C. McMullan, DVM, MS
Professor
Department of Large Animal Medicine & Surgery
College of Veterinary Medicine
Texas A&M University
College Station, TX 77843

Alfred M. Merritt, AB, DVM, MS
Professor
Department of Large Animal Clinical Sciences
College of Veterinary Medicine
University of Florida
Gainesville, FL 32610

James N. Moore, DVM, PhD, Dip ACVS
Professor
Department of Large Animal Medicine
College of Veterinary Medicine
University of Georgia
Athens, GA 30602

William A. Moyer, DVM
Associate Professor
New Bolton Center
Department of Sports Medicine
School of Veterinary Medicine
University of Pennsylvania
Kennett Square, PA 19348

Gillian D. Muir, DVM
Postdoctoral Fellow
Department of Zoology
University of British Columbia
6270 University Boulevard
Vancouver, BC V6T 2A9
Canada

Alan J. Nixon, DVM, Dip ACVS
Associate Professor
Department of Clinical Studies
New York State College of Veterinary Medicine
Cornell University
Ithaca, NY 14853

David M. Nunamaker, VMD, Dip ACVS
Jacques Jenny Professor
New Bolton Center
Department of Orthopedic Surgery
School of Veterinary Medicine
University of Pennsylvania
Kennett Square, PA 19348

Peter James O'Brien, DVM, MS, PhD, DVSc, BSc
Assistant Professor
Department of Pathology
Ontario Veterinary College
University of Guelph
Guelph, Ontario N1G 2W1 Canada

Jonathan E. Palmer, DVM
New Bolton Center
382 W. Street Road
Kennett Square, PA 19348

Mary Rose Paradis, DVM, Dip ACVIM
Chief of Staff, Hospital for Large Animals
Assistant Professor
School of Veterinary Medicine
Tufts University
North Grafton, MA 01536

Andrew H. Parks, MA, VetMB, MRCVS,
    Dip ACVS
Assistant Professor
Department of Large Animal Medicine
College of Veterinary Medicine
University of Georgia
Athens, GA 30602

John R. Pascoe, BVSc, PhD
Assistant Professor
Department of Surgery
School of Veterinary Medicine
University of California
Davis, CA 95616

Peter J. Pascoe, BVSc, DVA, Dip ACVA
Associate Professor
Department of Surgery
University of California
Davis, CA 95616

Lance E. Perryman, DVM, PhD, Dip ACVP
Professor
Department of Veterinary Microbiology & Pathology
Washington State University
Pullman, WA 99164

Mimi Porter, MS, Cert & Lic Athletic Trainer
Equine Therapist
Equine Therapy
4350 Harrodsburg Road
Lexington, KY 40513

Gary D. Potter, PhD, PAS
Professor/Equine Program Leader
Department of Animal Science
Texas A&M University
College Station, TX 77843

P.J. Provost, VMD, MS
Assistant Professor
Department of Surgery
School of Veterinary Medicine
Tufts University
North Grafton, MA 01536

N.W. Rantanen, DVM, MS, Dip ACVR
POB 11849
Lexington, KY 40578

Virginia B. Reef, DVM, Dip ACVIM
Assistant Professor
New Bolton Center
Department of Clinical Studies
School of Veterinary Medicine
University of Pennsylvania
Kennett Square, PA 19348

Dean W. Richardson, DVM, Dip ACVS
Assistant Professor
New Bolton Center
Department of Surgery
School of Veterinary Medicine
University of Pennsylvania
Kennett Square, PA 19348

Johanna Riemer, DVM
Instructor
New Bolton Center
Department of Clinical Studies
School of Veterinary Medicine
University of Pennsylvania
Kennett Square, PA 19348

James T. Robertson, DVM, Dip ACVS
Associate Professor
Department of Veterinary Medicine
The Ohio State University
Columbus, OH 43210

N. Edward Robinson, BVSc, PhD
Professor
Department of Large Animal Medicine
College of Veterinary Medicine
Michigan State University
East Lansing, MI 48824

Michael W. Ross, DVM, Dip ACVS
Lecturer
New Bolton Center
Department of Clinical Studies
School of Veterinary Medicine
University of Pennsylvania
Kennett Square, PA 19348

James Schumacher, DVM, MS, Dip ACVS
Associate Professor
Department of Large Animal
    Medicine & Surgery
College of Veterinary Medicine
Texas A&M University
College Station, TX 77843

Susan D. Semrad, VMD, PhD
Assistant Professor
Department of Medical Sciences
School of Veterinary Sciences
University of Wisconsin
Madison, WI 53706

G. Michael Shires, BVSc, MS, MRCVS, Dip ACVS
Professor
Department of Rural Practice
College of Veterinary Medicine
University of Tennessee
Knoxville, TN 37901

James L. Shupe, DVM, MS, Dip ATS
Lifetime Fellow, AACVT
Professor Emeritus
Utah State University
Logan, UT 84321

Janice E. Sojka, VMD, MS, Dip ACVIM
Assistant Professor
Department of Large Animal Medicine
School of Veterinary Medicine
Purdue University
West Lafayette, IN 47907

T.E. Specht, DVM
POB 37458
Raleigh, NC 27627

Ronald F. Sprouse, PhD
Professor
Department of Pathology
School of Medicine
University of Missouri
Columbia, MO 65211

Gareth H. Spurlock, DVM, MS, Dip ACVS
Assistant Professor
Marion duPont Scott Equine Medical Center
Virginia-Maryland Regional
     College of Veterinary Medicine
Leesburg, VA 22075

Ed Squires, PhD
Professor
Animal Reproduction Laboratory
Colorado State University
Fort Collins, CO 80525

John A. Stick, DVM, Dip ACVS
Professor
Department of Large Animal Clinical Sciences
College of Veterinary Medicine
Michigan State University
East Lansing, MI 48824

Kenneth E. Sullins, DVM, MS, Dip ACVS
Associate Professor
Marion duPont Scott Equine Medical Center
Virginia-Maryland Regional
     College of Veterinary Medicine
Leesburg, VA 22075

James R. Taylor, DVM, MS
Cedarcrest Equine Clinic
Rt 1, Box 1669
Palestine, TX 75801

Cynthia M. Trim, BVSc, MRCVS, Dip ACVA
Professor
Department of Large Animal Medicine
College of Veterinary Medicine
University of Georgia
Athens, GA 30602

Eric P. Tulleners, DVM, Dip ACVS
Assistant Professor
New Bolton Center
Department of Clinical Studies
School of Veterinary Medicine
University of Pennsylvania
Kennett Square, PA 19348

Tracy A. Turner, DVM, MS, Dip ACVS
Rochester Equine Clinic
Ten Rod Rd
POB 2071
Rochester, NH 03867

Pamela C. Wagner von Matthiesson, DVM, MS, Dip ACVS
Assistant Dean / Professor
Department of Large Animal Surgery
College of Veterinary Medicine
Oregon State University
Corvallis, OR 97331

Jeffrey P. Watkins, DVM, MS, Dip ACVS
Assistant Professor
Department of Large Animal Medicine & Surgery
College of Veterinary Medicine
Texas A&M University
College Station, TX 77843

Barbara Watrous, DVM, Dip ACVR
Associate Professor
Department of Radiology
College of Veterinary Medicine
Oregon State University
Corvallis, OR 97331

Robert D. Welch, DVM
Veterinary Clinical Associate
Department of Large Animal Medicine & Surgery
College of Veterinary Medicine
Texas A&M University
College Station, TX 77843

Nathaniel A. White II, DVM, MS, Dip ACVS
Professor
Marion duPont Scott Equine Center
Virginia-Maryland Regional
     College of Veterinary Medicine
Leesburg, VA 22075

R. David Whitley, DVM, MS, Dip ACVO
Professor
Department of Ophthalmology
College of Veterinary Medicine
Auburn University
Auburn, AL 36849

Robert H. Whitlock, DVM, PhD, Dip ACVIM
Professor
New Bolton Center
Department of Medicine
School of Veterinary Medicine
University of Pennsylvania
Kennett Square, PA 19348

J. Dick Wright, BVSc, MACVSc, MRCVS
Registrar in Equine Medicine and Surgery
Department of Companion Animal
     Medicine & Surgery
University of Queensland
St. Lucia, Queensland, Australia

Ellen L. Ziemer, DVM, MS, Dip ACVIM
Postdoctoral Fellow
Department of Animal Biology
School of Veterinary Medicine
University of Pennsylvania
Kennett Square, PA 19348

Contents

Volume I

Chapter   **Page**

PREFACE vii
USING THIS BOOK viii

1   DIAGNOSTIC APPROACHES TO COMMON PRESENTING COMPLAINTS
Abdominal Distention 1
Abortion 2
Back Problems 3
Behavioral Abnormalities 5
Bleeding 7
Blindness 9
Colic 10
Acute Collapse 11
Cough 13
Depression 14
Eating Difficulties 15
Examination for Purchase or Insurance 16
Eye Problems 19
Feces, Abnormal 21
Fever 22
Haircoat Abnormalities 23
Infertility in Mares 24
Infertility in Stallions 25
Lameness and Gait Abnormalities 26
Lumps and Bumps 27
Malformations and Genetic Defects 28
Nasal Discharge 29
Neonatal Foals, Abnormalities in 30
Performance Problems 33
Recumbency or Inability to Rise 35
Respiratory Noises and Difficulties 36
Salivation, Excessive 37
Scratching and Rubbing 38
Straining or Tenesmus 39
Sudden Death 40
Sweating Abnormalities 42
Swellings 43
Urine and Urination, Abnormal 45
Weight Loss 46
Wounds 48

2   PRINCIPLES OF PATIENT EVALUATION AND DIAGNOSIS
Handling the Emergency Call 51
Presenting Clinical Signs 52
The History 53
Referrals and Second Opinions 54
Physical Restraint 55

Record Keeping and the Problem-Oriented Medical Record 64
Physical Examination 64
Prepurchase Examination 70
Insurance Examination 78
Diagnostic Aids 79
Anesthesia and Chemical Restraint 81
Necropsy 123

3   PRINCIPLES OF THERAPY
Fluid and Electrolyte Therapy 139
Antibacterial Therapy 142
Antiinflammatory and Antipyretic Therapy 145
Principles of Nutrition 152

4   SYSTEMIC DISEASES INVOLVING MULTIPLE BODY SYSTEMS
Septicemia 159
Shock 161
Disseminated Intravascular Coagulation 162

5   DISEASES OF THE CARDIOVASCULAR SYSTEM
Detailed Examination of the Cardiovascular System 165
Ancillary Diagnostic Aids 187
Pathophysiology and Principles of Therapy 220
Diseases of Arteries 277
Diseases of Veins 291
Diseases of the Endocardium and Valves 295
Diseases of the Myocardium 314
Diseases of the Pericardium and Thoracic Cavity 330
Diseases of the Thoracic Cavity 334

6   DISEASES OF THE RESPIRATORY SYSTEM
Examination of the Respiratory System 353
Evaluating Foals for Respiratory Disease 356
Ancillary Diagnostic Aids 357
Pathophysiology of Upper Airway Disease 361
Pulmonary Physiology and Pathophysiology 362
Principles of Emergency Respiratory Therapy 372
Medical Respiratory Therapy 374
Principles of Therapy for Foals 377
Respiratory Diseases Affecting Multiple Sites 378
Diseases of the Nasal Cavity and Paranasal Sinuses 386
Diseases of the Pharynx 398
Diseases of the Guttural Pouch 402
Diseases of the Larynx 411
Diseases of the Trachea 424
Diseases of the Lung 429
Diseases of the Pleura, Mediastinum, Diaphragm and Thoracic Wall 456

7   DISEASES OF THE ALIMENTARY SYSTEM
Examination of the Alimentary System 473
Ancillary Diagnostic Aids 479
Pathophysiology and Principles of Therapy 490
Diseases Affecting Multiple Sites 532
Diseases of the Lips, Mouth, Tongue and Oropharynx 543
Diseases of the Hyoid Apparatus 548
Diseases of the Teeth 550
Diseases of the Salivary Glands 570
Diseases of the Esophagus 572

Diseases of the Stomach 593
Diseases of the Small Intestine 606
Diseases of the Cecum 627
Diseases of the Large Colon 633
Diseases of the Small Colon 659
Diseases of the Rectum 663
Diseases of the Peritoneum and Mesentery 667
Diseases of the Abdominal Wall 683
Diseases of the Liver 692

8   DISEASES OF THE NERVOUS SYSTEM
Examination of the Nervous System 723
Diseases of Multiple or Unknown Sites 743
Diseases of the Forebrain 770
Diseases of the Brainstem and Cranial Nerves 781
Diseases of Vestibular and Cerebellar Structures 792
Diseases of the Spinal Cord 797
Diseases of the Cauda Equina 823
Diseases of the Peripheral Nerves 826
Diseases of the Neuromuscular Junction 832

Volume II

9   DISEASES OF THE REPRODUCTIVE SYSTEM: THE STALLION
Examination of the Stallion 847
Pathophysiology and Principles Of Therapy 856
Diseases Affecting Multiple Sites 883
Diseases of the Scrotum 888
Diseases of the Testes 894
Diseases of the Epididymis 908
Diseases of the Tunica Vaginalis 910
Diseases of the Spermatic Cord 914
Diseases of the Accessory Genital Glands 916
Diseases of the Urethra 918
Diseases of the Penis 920
Diseases of the Prepuce 935
Diseases Affecting Semen 939

10   DISEASES OF THE REPRODUCTIVE SYSTEM: THE MARE
Examination of the Mare 949
Ancillary Diagnostic Aids 956
Pathophysiology and Principles of Therapy 982
Diseases Affecting Multiple Sites 1013
Diseases of the Ovary 1022
Diseases of the Oviduct 1028
Diseases of the Uterus 1029
Diseases of the Cervix 1037
Diseases of the Vagina, Vestibule and Vulva 1039
Diseases Involving the Placenta 1058
Diseases of the Embryo 1063
Abortion 1066

11   DISEASES OF THE OCULAR SYSTEM
Examination of the Eye 1083
Ancillary Diagnostic Aids 1085

Principles of Ocular Therapy 1087
Diseases of the Orbit And Globe 1094
Diseases of the Eyelids 1097
Diseases of the Conjunctiva and Nasolacrimal System 1105
Diseases of the Cornea 1109
Diseases of the Uvea 1119
Diseases of the Lens and Vitreous 1125
Diseases of the Choroid and Retina 1128
Diseases of the Optic Nerve 1132

12   DISEASES OF THE MUSCULOSKELETAL SYSTEM
Examination of the Musculoskeletal System 1143
Ancillary Diagnostic Aids 1163
Principles of Therapy 1200
Diseases of Multiple Bones and Joints 1281
Diseases of Muscle 1317
Diseases of the Hoof, Distal Phalanyx and Associated Structures 1331
Diseases of the Pastern Region 1372
Diseases of the Fetlock Region 1379
Diseases of the Metacarpus/Metatarsus 1405
Diseases of the Carpal Region 1421
Diseases of the Forearm and Elbow Region 1440
Diseases of the Proximal Forearm 1450
Diseases of the Shoulder 1451
Diseases of the Head and Neck 1460
Diseases of the Tarsus 1467
Diseases of the Tibia 1482
Diseases of the Stifle 1488
Diseases of the Thigh 1499
Diseases of the Hip and Pelvis 1502
Diseases of the Thoracolumbar Region 1506
Diseases of the Lumbosacral Region 1515

13   DISEASES OF THE URINARY SYSTEM
Examination of the Urinary System 1539
Ancillary Diagnostic Aids 1540
Pathophysiology and Principles of Therapy 1545
Diseases of the Kidney 1548
Diseases of the Ureter 1558
Diseases of the Bladder 1558
Diseases of the Urachus and Umbilicus 1563
Diseases of the Urethra 1565

14   DISEASES OF THE SKIN
Examination of the Skin 1569
Ancillary Diagnostic Aids 1574
Pathophysiology and Principles of Therapy 1581
Diseases Characterized by Wheals, Papules or Small Nodules 1648
Diseases Characterized by Nodules or Tumors 1654
Diseases Characterized by Granulomatous, Draining Nodules or Masses 1664
Diseases Characterized by Diffuse Swelling or Edema 1677
Diseases Characterized by Nonpruritic Alopecia and Scaling 1680
Diseases Characterized by Pruritus and Hair Loss 1685
Diseases Characterized by Multifocal to Diffuse Alopecia, Crusts and Papules . . . 1694
Diseases Characterized by Focal Erythema, Exudation,
    Crusting, Scaling and Alopecia 1702
Diseases Characterized by Ulceration and Crusting of Mucocutaneous Regions . . 1706

Diseases Characterized by Ulceration, Exudation and
   Crusting of the Distal Extremities 1709
Diseases Characterized by Focal or Diffuse Scaling, Crusting and Alopecia 1712
Diseases Characterized by Pigmentary Changes in the Skin or Hair 1716
Diseases Characterized by Abnormalities of the Haircoat 1718
Diseases of the External Ear 1719
Miscellaneous Dermatoses 1720

15   DISEASES OF THE ENDOCRINE SYSTEM
Examination for Endocrine Disorders 1737
Ancillary Diagnostic Aids 1738
Disorders in Glucose Metabolism 1739
Hyperlipemia Syndrome 1740
Diseases of the Pituitary Gland 1740
Diseases of the Thyroid Gland 1745
Diseases of the Adrenal Gland 1748
Diseases of the Pancreas 1749

16   DISEASES OF THE HEMOLYMPHATIC SYSTEM
Clinical Evaluation of the Hemolymphatic System 1753
Ancillary Diagnostic Aids 1755
Pathophysiology and Principles of Therapy 1774
Diseases Affecting Multiple Sites 1795
Diseases Affecting Erythrocytes 1802
Diseases Affecting Leukocytes 1809
Diseases of the Immune System 1819
Diseases Affecting Plasma Proteins 1826
Diseases Affecting the Hemostatic System 1831
Diseases Affecting the Glandular and Tubular Lymphatic System 1843
Diseases of the Spleen 1844

INDEX

This page is intentionally left blank.

Preface

The decision to organize this fourth edition of *Equine Medicine and Surgery* was made at a time when we were not aware of the magnitude of the changes that had occurred in all aspects of equine practice since the previous edition of the book. Once we got into the task, however, the immense number of changes became all too clear. It was our aim to put together a comprehensive text that would approach the diagnosis of clinical problems in much the same way as do most veterinarians.

The massive undertaking this book represents could not have been accomplished without the magnificent efforts of the section editors and contributors. We wish to express our extreme gratitude to all these colleagues for their effort, their patient endurance when we exercised our editorial prerogatives, and the professionalism with which they approached their tasks.

Deserving special consideration is our Associate Editor, Carolyn Richards, who put the conglomeration together and molded it into form for final editing. Her countless hours of labor have contributed tremendously to the completion and quality of this text.

Finally, we extend special thanks to Carlye, Rachel, Nancy and Cynthia for bearing with us while we struggled to bring this tome into being.

Patrick T. Colahan
Ian G. Mayhew
Alfred M. Merritt
James N. Moore

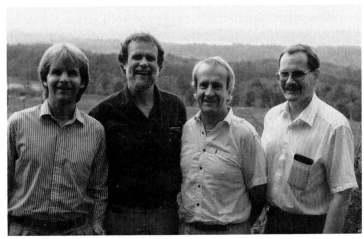

From left to right:
James N. Moore,
Alfred M. Merritt,
Ian G. Mayhew,
Patrick T. Colahan
(Photograph by Bruce A. Richards)

Using This Book

Every day, veterinarians must examine an animal, make a diagnosis, prescribe an appropriate regimen of treatment, and offer the client an accurate prognosis; texts should be written to help complete these tasks. Some textbooks are not of much help to the practitioner because it is *presumed* that the definitive diagnosis already has been made when the veterinarian turns to the book for information. This is not the way that clinical practice works.

Under more realistic circumstances, the client notices or suspects that something is wrong with a horse. Eventually, the veterinarian's office is contacted and arrangements are made for the animal to be examined. The veterinarian then compiles information from the animal's medical history, a general physical examination, and information arising from use of routine diagnostic aids to determine which organ systems are involved. To make a diagnosis and subsequently decide which methods of treatment should be used and to formulate a reasonable prognosis, the veterinarian must decide *how* the abnormality occurred. This may require a more detailed examination of the affected organ systems and use of more refined diagnostic aids. Once all the necessary data have been gathered, the veterinarian can make the diagnosis. Only at this point do classic books help the veterinarian decide what is the most appropriate method of treatment and what the client should be able to expect as an outcome.

We have organized this book to follow closely the steps that the veterinarian follows in making the diagnosis; this book facilitates this process from start to finish. The first part of this book presents logical approaches to the most common problems as perceived and related to the veterinarian's office by clients. These discussions were written to help the receptionist handling the initial telephone contact with the client, and to remind the veterinarian of important considerations. This section of the book describes the necropsy procedure and how it can be used in diagnosis of the problem when all else fails.

The second section of this book describes the methods used to gather information about the horse, perform a thorough general physical examination, and ensure that the horse's ration is adequate. This section also covers life-threatening conditions that affect several organ systems, common treatment modalities applicable to more than one organ system, and the appropriate methods to produce sedation, analgesia and anesthesia. This section should serve as a reference for the practitioner and veterinary student concerning these more general aspects of clinical practice.

The remainder of the book is organized according to individual organ systems. Because specialized diagnostic techniques, particular ancillary aids, pathophysiologic principles and methods of therapy exist for each system, this information has been included at the beginning of the discussion of each system. Diseases that characteristically affect multiple sites within that organ system are then discussed, followed by important diseases affecting the individual parts of the system. When appropriate, the authors have included a short discussion of specific diagnostic and therapeutic considerations relevant to that part of the system. Each disease is then considered according to its particular pathophysiology.

Thus, this book should follow the veterinarian's logical progression from identification of the problem, through determination of the organ system involved, to the most likely mechanism involved in development of the problem, and to diagnosis and management of diseases of the horse.

1 Diagnostic Approaches to Common Presenting Complaints

P.T. Colahan, I.G. Mayhew, A.M. Merritt, J.N. Moore

This section presents logical approaches to problems commonly encountered in equine practice. Because this text was designed with the practitioner in mind, each clinical problem is described as it would be presented to the veterinarian's office staff by the client. In the interval between the client's telephone call and examination of the animal, the practitioner naturally begins to plan how to identify and solve the problem. In this section, we have assembled a series of short discussions to assist the veterinarian in that planning process.

These discussions are entitled in lay terms because this is how problems are usually presented to the practitioner. When ap-plicable, these discussions include information the veterinarian's staff can give to the client about possible emergency treatments and safety advice for the animals and the handlers involved. Most of the discussion is a summary of the probable causes of the problem and a diagnostic plan. The remainder of the book contains detailed information of management of specific problems.

Abdominal Distention

A.M. Merritt

When a client calls with the complaint that a horse has abdominal distention or is "bloated," there are 2 important questions

Abdominal Distention	1
Abortion	2
Back Problems	3
Behavioral Abnormalities	5
Bleeding	7
Blindness	9
Colic	10
Collapse, Acute	11
Cough	13
Depression	14
Eating Difficulties	15
Examination for Purchase or Insurance	16
Eye Problems	19
Feces, Abnormal	21
Fever	22
Haircoat Abnormalities	23
Infertility in Mares	24
Infertility in Stallions	25
Lameness and Gait Abnormalities	26
Lumps and Bumps	27
Malformations and Genetic Defects	28
Nasal Discharge	29
Neonatal Foals, Abnormalities in	30
Performance Problems	33
Recumbency or Inability to Rise	35
Respiratory Noises and Difficulties	36
Salivation, Excessive	37
Scratching and Rubbing	38
Straining or Tenesmus	39
Sudden Death	40
Sweating Abnormalities	42
Swellings	43
Urine and Urination, Abnormalities of	45
Weight Loss, Progressive	46
Wounds	48

to address: Has the distention developed suddenly? Is the horse in pain? If the answer to either or both of these questions is "yes," the case should be regarded as an emergency. If the animal is colicky, the client should make every effort to prevent it from lying down and rolling, even if this involves continual walking until the veterinarian arrives.

The most common cause of acute abdominal distention with pain is a large intestinal obstruction due to displacement, blockage by intraluminal contents or primary stasis due to colitis. A less likely cause is grain engorgement. Unless emergency therapy is required first, a complete history should be obtained and a complete evaluation for an abdominal crisis performed. It is critical to learn what analgesics, if any, have been given to the horse, as these can influence the signs.

Additional information about the localization of the distention can be obtained from simultaneous auscultation and percussion of the abdomen. A thorough rectal examination must be performed to distinguish large colon problems from other causes of distention. If there is tachycardia, dark red or purple mucous membranes, prolonged capillary refill time and very tense abdominal musculature, then rupture of a viscus should be suspected. Abdominocentesis should be performed to determine if this is so. If a large gas-distended viscus can be identified by auscultation and rectal examination, if the horse is in severe abdominal pain, and if immediate surgical intervention is not an option, one should consider trocarization of the cecum via the right flank to relieve some of the excessive intraluminal pressure.

Abdominal distention with colic in adult horses usually implies an abnormality involving the large intestine or, much less commonly, an extensive small intestinal problem. However, in foals, abdominal distention frequently occurs with a small intestinal obstruction or a ruptured bladder.

Marked subcutaneous edema occasionally occurs along the entire ventral abdomen and thorax. This ventral edema may be misinterpreted by the client as abdominal distention. It is important to determine whether the swelling is inflammatory (warm and painful to the touch) or not. If so, the area should be examined for a localized wound or abscess. If the ventral abdomen is cool and "pitting," hypoproteinemia or, more rarely, cardiac failure are considerations.

Excluding pregnancy, the most frequent cause of progressive abdominal distention without pain in horses is ascites. No "pinging" is heard upon simultaneous auscultation and percussion of the abdomen. Unfortunately, it is difficult to establish a transabdominal fluid wave due to the natural tone of equine abdominal muscles. The impression that the abdominal contents are floating when palpated during rectal examination sometimes confirms the presence of ascites. Alternatively, masses or adhesions indicative of neoplasia or chronic peritonitis are palpated. When ascites is suspected, peritoneal fluid should be collected for cell count, protein determination and cytologic examination.

Horses that are malnourished or severely parasitized and eating large amounts of low-quality roughage in an attempt to meet their energy requirements frequently have an apparently enlarged abdomen due to loss of fat and muscle mass. Generally the underlying cause can be determined from the history and fecal examination. Finally, horses with pituitary adenoma and hyperadrenocorticism can develop a pendulous abdomen in addition to other, more distinctive signs.

Abortion

M.M. LeBlanc

Abortion, defined as the expulsion of a (nonviable) fetus between 120 and 320 days of gestation, causes considerable economic losses to the equine industry. Due to the mare's long gestation of 340 days and the January 1 "birth date" of foals, mares that abort after the fourth month of gestation usually lose 1 year of their reproductive lives. Consequently, clients are extremely concerned if a mare aborts or they suspect impending abortion.

Because the cause of abortion is less likely to be determined as the time from abortion to collection of samples increases, affected mares should be seen on an emergency basis. The client should be advised to save the fetus and placenta for examination by the veterinarian. The placental membranes should be spread flat and examined carefully. Swabs should be taken from the area of the cervical star and from other suspicious areas. Any tears or missing portions of the placenta should be noted. With methodic examination of the fetus and the placenta and collection of appropriate tissue samples, the cause may be identified in 50-60% of the cases. Complications associated with abortion may include retained placenta, metritis and laminitis.

The veterinarian should be aware that most abortions in mares are due to twins, equine herpesvirus-1 infection, and placentitis due to bacterial or fungal organisms. Signs of impending abortion (premature lactation, vulvar discharge) are common in mares that abort because of twins or placentitis. If the abortion is protracted and involves some degree of placental separation, the mare may drip milk for weeks before the abortion.

If the cause of abortion is twins, the placenta has a large avillous area and frequently 1 of the 2 fetuses is mummified. If equine herpesvirus-1 is the cause, no placental abnormalities are present and the aborted fetus is fresh and not autolyzed. In other cases, the autolyzed fetus may be found in the paddock, the fetal membranes may be seen hanging from the vulva, or the mare may simply be "empty" at the end of gestation. Characteristically, the lungs of a fetus aborted due to equine herpesvirus-1 infection are severely edematous and pit on digital pressure. Additional findings include excessive clear pleural fluid, slight jaundice and small focal areas of necrosis under the capsule of the liver.

If the cause of abortion is placentitis, the fetus usually is mummified, especially if it is aborted before 8 months of gestation. The infected chorionic surface is brown and covered with a fibrinonecrotic exudate. The inflamed placenta may be edematous and thickened. Because it is not possible to differentiate between bacterial and fungal causes of placentitis on gross examination alone, samples of the placenta must be submitted for culture.

Other less common causes for abortion include equine viral arteritis, severe stress (as from gastrointestinal diseases), torsion of the umbilicus, and nutritional imbalances or toxicities. Mares that abort due to equine viral arteritis show clinical signs of acute disease and subsequently abort 7-10 days later. Mares most likely to abort after a severe bout of colic are those that require intensive fluid therapy, nonsteroidal anti-inflammatory drugs and broad-spectrum antibiotics. Conversely, mares that undergo surgical intervention for an intestinal displacement generally fare better. In either case, the well-being of the fetus can be monitored by transabdominal ultrasonography or fetal electrocardiography. As a general rule, fetuses with a heart rate <60 beats/minute are likely to die.

Abortion also may occur if the umbilical cord is long and becomes twisted. When twisting of the cord is the cause for the abortion, the cord is longer than 90 cm, edematous and congested. Ingestion of various plants has been associated with fetal deaths. The most common of these include fescue grasses, Sudan grasses and sorghum. Because abortions have occurred after deworming of the mare with organophosphates, phenothiazine and carbon tetrachloride, these anthelmintics are generally avoided in pregnant mares.

Whether or not the cause of the abortion can be identified immediately, steps must be taken to prepare the mare for a subsequent pregnancy. Consequently, a complete reproductive examination should be performed and therapy instituted if there is evidence of endometritis. Appropriate cultures and tissue samples should be submitted and the client advised that additional information may be forthcoming.

Back Problems

S. Dyson and I.G. Mayhew

There are many reasons why a client presumes a horse has a back (thoracolumbar) problem. Some horses move stiffly and have a localized area or areas of pain identifiable by palpation during an acute episode of pain of muscular or ligamentous origin. Other horses have a so-called "cold back," tending to dip their backs excessively when tacked or mounted. Clients often attribute poor performance to back pain but actually may have several different specific concerns about a horse. These include persistently shortened stride, poor hind limb impulsion, refusal to work on the bit, reluctance to turn, difficulty in performing certain movements, and refusing or rushing jumps.

Difficult behavior, such as nipping, rearing or bucking, often is thought to be related to back pain. However, it seems somewhat incongruous that a horse with back pain would be willing to extend and flex its back to buck. Reluctance to walk downhill or a tendency to walk downhill sideways may be attributed to back pain, as may difficulty rising from recumbency. Because headshaking sometimes is seen when a horse is ridden but not during lunging, it is commonly assumed that the weight of the rider on the back is causing discomfort.

Finally, a horse may be presented for a suspected back problem because the animal has an abnormal conformation, either congenital or acquired, such as lordosis, kyphosis or scoliosis.

The signs demonstrated by a horse with back problems are often insidious in onset and of a chronic nature. It is important to establish when signs are noticed. Is the horse under tack or mounted? Are other problems like lameness present as well? Were the signs precipitated by a traumatic event, such as a fall? The veterinarian and client must realize that some horses are less athletically talented than others and thus sometimes are physically incapable of performing what is asked of them. Poor hind limb impulsion can reflect back pain, but not necessarily so. Many such horses, if ridden strongly forward on the bit, work with a correct outline (*ie,* the head and neck in the proper position) and have good hind limb impulsion and swing through the back. Likewise, for jumping horses, it must be remembered that reluctance to jump may be due to factors other than pain. Good jumping performance requires trust and confidence between horse and rider. If either is lacking, the horse may refuse.

It must be borne in mind that if the horse has been treated in any way or rested, the clinical signs of back pain may resolve, only to recur when regular work is resumed.

A horse with acute back pain should be subjected to a complete physical examination. Before and/or during the examination, the client should be prepared to lunge and ride the horse. Also, it may be useful to see the horse ridden by an expert. In some instances, this may need to be done for several weeks to differentiate rider/trainer problems from pain-related problems. The fitting of the tack should be checked, as a poorly fitted saddle or one with a broken tree can induce back pain.

Particular attention should be paid to the mouth and teeth. The neck should be examined carefully for evidence of pain, stiffness, muscle atrophy or patchy sweating. The limbs should be examined and a lameness evaluation performed. Bilateral hind limb lameness, such as that caused by degenerative joint disease of the distal joints of the hocks (bone spavin), can cause poor performance, unwillingness, stiffness or reduced stride length. Mild neurologic ataxia also may cause hind limb stiffness.

Marked asymmetry of the hindquarters can reflect previous damage of the sacroiliac joints, causing poor hind limb impulsion and a tendency to move closely behind. Skeletal asymmetry should be differentiated from asymmetry due to muscle atrophy.

Detection of chronic back pain is not easy. Often it is impossible unless the horse is in regular work, as the pain subsides with rest. Also, there is considerable variation in the ability of sound horses to flex and extend the thoracolumbar vertebral column. Some normal horses become agitated if repeatedly stimulated to flex and extend the back. A tendency to hold the back very stiffly, or to sink (especially on the hindquarters), rather than extend the back in response to manual pressure, may reflect back pain, especially if muscle spasm is induced.

Though the results frequently are equivocal, injection of local anaesthetic between the dorsal spinous processes to produce a change in gait can be attempted to locate the source of pain. Use of nonsteroidal anti-inflammatory drugs, such as phenylbutazone, sometimes helps establish if a performance problem is pain related. The horse must be treated for at least 7 days at relatively high dosages (3-5 mg/kg BID PO) for conclusive findings. A negative response does not preclude thoracolumbar pain. Radiographs of the thoracolumbar vertebrae must be interpreted cautiously and in conjunction with clinical signs.

It usually is relatively easy to identify spasm of the longissimus dorsi muscles. This may reflect primary back pain or develop secondary to hind limb lameness. Such spasms may occur unilaterally or bilaterally, and may be focal or diffuse. The

4

horse may hold the back stiffly, being unwilling to flex and extend the back, and may groan. Additionally, there may be localized muscle fasciculations. The horse may move in a resentful, stiff way with shortened strides.

If there is pain in the withers region, fracture of the dorsal spinous processes should be ruled out. Usually there is palpable distortion of the withers and occasionally palpable crepitus in such cases. The horse holds the neck very stiffly, often abnormally low, and may be reluctant to move, tending to plait the forelimbs. The diagnosis is confirmed radiographically. Fractures of the more caudal dorsal spinous processes are rare. Acute back pain should not be confused with exercise-associated rhabdomyolysis, colic, laminitis, pleuritis or peritonitis.

There is a poorly understood syndrome in horses thought to relate to back pain. The signs vary. The horse may become tense when saddled, especially as the girth is tightened, and may explode into a violent bucks and plunges, then become quiet and behave normally. Such a horse can then be mounted and will perform. Other horses become tense and do not react until led forward after saddling. A third group behaves violently when mounted, often dislodging the rider. Such a horse, if remounted, may behave quite normally. Sometimes there is a history of being difficult to break; in other instances, the problem is sudden with no predisposing factors. The problem can be avoided in some horses by tightening the girth very slowly, moving the horse forward before retightening the girth, lunging before riding, or mounting from a mounting block. Because many horses exhibiting this behavior have been high-level competitive horses, it is difficult to conclude that they have a significant lesion. In some it appears that pressure applied to the sternum or brisket area induces the behavior. A focus of pain should be sought by palpation, but rarely is one identified. In most horses with this behavior, clinical examination is unrewarding. Radiographic abnormalities of the sternum or ribs occasionally are identified and it is possible that neuroma of the lateral thoracic nerve or abnormal pressure in the lateral thoracic blood vessels induces this behavior. These possible causes remain to be confirmed.

Conformational abnormalities of the back may be congenital or acquired, and include lordosis, kyphosis and scoliosis. If they are congenital, radiographic examination sometimes reveals vertebral malformations, such as a wedge-shaped vertebral body. Frequently, when the condition is acquired, there are no abnormalities detectable radiographically. Horses with bilateral hind limb lameness, such as that caused by osteochondrosis of the lateral trochlear ridges of the stifles, may adopt a kyphotic stance. Bilateral hind limb lameness always should be excluded in a horse with kyphosis.

Behavioral Abnormalities

B.D. Brewer

Behavioral abnormalities can be the bane of the horse trainer's existence. Examining such a horse for a possible medical condition can be equally daunting to the veterinarian because the underlying cause usually is not determined. Many problems of behavior result from the artificial environments, constraints and behaviors required of horses that are so different from their phylogenetic history. The animals are placed under extreme stress that is manifested by behavioral or physiologic signs. It also must be borne in mind that inherited behavior plays a role in many instances, as certain breeds and families are deliberately bred for differences in personality and athletic ability.

Equine veterinarians need to understand normal behavioral patterns of horses as well as the common aberrations seen to aid the owner in behavioral conditioning or to diagnose a systemic disease. Veterinarians unfamiliar with the art of horse training and horsemanship, particular breed dispositions and the specific demands placed on horses undertaking different athletic pursuits are well advised to consult with experts in the area when good physical and neurologic examinations are unrewarding.

The aims of examining a horse with a behavioral abnormality are: to identify the nature of the problem, to establish a list of possible reasons for the behavior pattern, and to formulate an appropriate treatment plan. Therapy may include removing the underlying cause, such as relieving boredom or treating an existing medical problem, using behavior modification with positive reinforcement or aversive conditioning and, if all else fails, preventing expression of the problem by use of a neck cradle, provision of a companion animal, or changing the animal to a different athletic pursuit.

Behavioral abnormalities can be classified under 3 general categories: training, personality and husbandry problems; neurologic problems; and miscellaneous problems.

These are by far the most common cause of behavioral problems. Conditioned or learned responses such as bucking, rearing, shying, refusing jumps and kicking at individuals entering the stall, are typical annoyances and usually fit this category, assuming that the possibility of ill-fitting tack has been ruled out. A horse handler with patience and ability can use feed, touch and voice conditioning to solve such problems or resort to force, if necessary. Occasionally a rider is unable to do this and professional help is needed to terminate such behavior.

Improper socialization can be a major problem in orphan foals. These foals should be placed with herdmates as soon as possible; otherwise they can become quite unmanageable.

Common vices, such as pawing and stall-walking and fencewalking, often are due to a horse's frustration when it is restrained from running, eating and joining its herdmates. Cribbing, windsucking and weaving often are caused by boredom and can lead to chronic flatulent colic, weight loss, poor performance and exacerbation of orthopedic problems.

Coprophagy is normal in young foals but, in older animals, the possibility of nutritional imbalances should be investigated. The same is true for pica involving any natural or unnatural substance.

Horses apparently can develop "phobias," such as fear of buzzing insects, certain sounds and dark confinement areas but they usually respond to careful, patient, positive reinforcement. Owners may believe their horse has developed a deliberate "psychosomatic lameness," but this rarely is the case, and such horses should be examined for musculoskeletal abnormalities.

If a horse suddenly becomes depressed or excited, administration of stimulant or depressant drugs may be the cause, though this may have been done without the owner's or trainer's knowledge.

Forebrain diseases commonly cause behavior changes as do any other causes of depression and/or blindness. Early signs of problems include frequent yawning, lack of recognition of well-known people, places, objects or procedures, bizarre posturing, or leaving food in the mouth for long periods. At first, signs may wax and wane, and the horse behaves normally between episodes.

Rabies must be considered in any horse with any type of sudden personality change. Though no sign is typical of rabies, horses that suddenly become aggressive toward their owners or herdmates or begin biting at themselves, inanimate objects or people are suspects, and appropriate precautions should be taken immediately.

Horses that are partially or unilaterally blind or have impaired hearing may behave oddly and shy at objects or adopt unusual head postures. Such partial blindness can be difficult to identify with certainty (see Blindness).

Narcolepsy and seizures also should be considered. Prodromal or postictal phases of a seizure that has not been observed may leave the horse depressed or acting oddly. Minor seizures may be manifested as nothing more than the horse's suddenly acting lost or frightened when it is in a situation to which it should be well accustomed.

Peripheral neuropathies, including the time during which an injured nerve is repairing, can cause a horse to scratch or to shake a limb constantly. Stringhalt is a very unusual gait abnormality.

On rare occasions, a horse with a long-standing pituitary adenoma, massive cholesterol granuloma or any other brain tumor may behave strangely as the lesion compresses brain tissue.

Horses with chronic, painful conditions may adopt unusual behavior. For example, older horses with chronic, severe lumbar arthrosis have been observed to repeatedly flex and abduct one or both pelvic limbs. Horses experiencing back pain for various reasons may react violently to grooming or saddling, where previously the animal never objected to the procedure.

Four uncommon disorders for which no cause has been documented are head rubbing, tail wringing, head shaking and self-mutilation syndrome of stallions (see the chapter on Diseases of the Nervous System).

Behavior problems in horses frequently are difficult to resolve and may be medical or nonmedical in origin. A complete history, close observation of the interaction of the rider with the horse, a thorough physical examination and, occasionally, outside consultation with a skilled trainer may result in a satisfactory solution to the problem.

Bleeding

T.E. Specht

Bleeding requiring urgent assistance usually is the result of trauma from an accident. Even when a veterinarian is unavailable for immediate assistance or telephone advice, a veterinary technician or an informed receptionist can ask specific questions and give exact first-aid instructions pending veterinary consultation, attendance, examination, and treatment. Two critical questions are: From where is the horse bleeding? and Can you describe the wound? These questions are critical because bleeding from wounds near the jugular vein and carotid artery or from wounds high on the inside of a foreleg or rear leg require immediate application of pressure or clamping or ligating the vessel. Almost all telephone descriptions of bleeding can easily include the description of the location and size of the wound, and thereby help assess the urgency of the situation. Two exceptions are profuse nasal hemorrhage from head trauma, and erosion of the internal carotid artery wall by guttural pouch mycosis.

Other important questions are: Is a foreign body present? In what sort of surroundings is the horse? Does the horse limp? Are behavioral abnormalities present? How much blood has the horse lost?

To effectively stop bleeding with pressure, it is important to apply pressure directly to the bleeding vessels and maintain compression. The client should be instructed to apply direct pressure to the bleeding wounds, manually if possible. Any wound that still bleeds after 5 minutes of direct manual pressure with gauze sponges or clean cloths should have a pressure bandage applied. Bleeding wounds located between the elbow and foot, and gaskin and

foot, and bleeding head and neck wounds should be bandaged if direct pressure does not stop the bleeding. It may be difficult to apply a pressure bandage to bleeding wounds on other parts of the body. In no situation should a client be instructed to apply a tourniquet. Concerned owners and managers can be prepared for a bleeding emergency by having first-aid bandage material (rectangular gauze sponges, rolled gauze, leg wraps, elastic bandage) preassembled and available. Improvization may be necessary (*eg,* any clean fabric and electrical or duct tape).

The client should be instructed to leave any foreign body alone other than breaking or cutting the foreign body above skin level before bandaging. A pressure bandage can be fashioned by applying gauze squares directly on the bleeding site and securing them with any available rolled material such as rolled gauze, elastic wrap, elastic tape (Elastoplast, Vetwrap, Elastikon), derby bandage or tack bandage. After 1 wrap of the rolled material is placed around the limb, several folded gauze sponges, a roll of gauze, or a small piece of folded fabric is placed on the bandage over the bleeding site. The wrapping is continued snugly. If the wound is large and/or there is diffuse bleeding with no identifiable source, a quilted leg wrap, disposable diaper, clean cloth or sheet-cotton leg wrap should be applied and held tightly in place with rolled material, tape or rope.

A horse that can walk without an obvious gait deficit or weakness should be confined to a small pen or stall. If there is any question that the horse also incurred a fracture or lacerated tendon, no movement should be allowed and, if possible, a splint should be applied to the affected limb.

Tho·.gh it is difficult for a client to determine the quantity of blood lost and all lost blood may not have been observed, an inquiry should be made. This subjective determination may allow a more accurate telephone assessment of the severity of an injury, as the client may not be able to evaluate the horse objectively. Additional questions may help determine the severity of blood loss: Is the blood squirting out or only dripping slowly from the wound? How long ago did the wound occur? If the blood is squirting out, how large is the stream (*eg,* size of a pencil vs size of a pin)?

Behavioral abnormalities indicating profound shock from excessive blood loss; hypovolemic shock and acute collapse or coma can occur. Phenothiazine tranquilizers can potentiate shock. The client should be instructed not to administer a tranquilizer.

Upon arriving and before examining the horse, if it is still bleeding, identifiable bleeding vessels should be clamped or ligated. When no bleeding vessels are easily and quickly identifiable, a pressure bandage should be applied. If blood is coming through a previously applied pressure bandage, additional compression of the wound can be achieved by rewrapping or by adding focal padding and tightly wrapping the site with tape.

After achieving hemostasis, the cardiovascular system should be examined. Because hypovolemic shock can develop with acute loss of ≥30% (10-11 L) of a 450-kg horse's blood volume (36 L), the heart rate, mucous membrane color, capillary refill time, pulse strength from a palpable artery (digital, great metatarsal, facial, mandibular, proximal radial artery) should be determined and the quantity of blood in the pen or stall noted. Also, the horse should be examined for muscle weakness, reluctance to move and depression. An increase in heart rate (>70 bpm), pale mucous membranes (pale pink to white), increased capillary refill time (<5 seconds), poor pulse quality or a thready pulse, cold distal extremities and ears, depression, reluctance to move, and muscle weakness are the signs of hypovolemic shock.

After evaluating the entire horse and especially the cardiovascular system, emergency treatment should be administered if there are signs of hypovolemic shock or the possibility of hypovolemic shock. First, an adequate intravenous catheter should be placed and secured in an accessible vein (jugular, cephalic or lateral thoracic vein). Intravenous fluid therapy with balanced crystalloid solutions (eg, Plasmalyte A, lactated Ringer's solution, Normosol R) should be instituted. When a large volume of blood has been lost, a plasma or whole blood transfusion is indicated. If plasma or whole blood is not immediately available, crystalloid solution should be administered while they are being secured.

The decision to refer a horse to a hospital or clinic depends on the severity of the injury, need for additional medical therapy, available instrumentation, expected wound therapy, value of the horse, and insurance status of the horse. Before transporting an injured horse, an assessment should be made of the pressure bandage. If there is concern about additional bleeding, the bandage should be improved. When necessary, splints should be applied to prevent additional musculoskeletal system injury.

When a horse is not referred, adequate assistance, bandage material and instrumentation should be available before wound evaluation and treatment are attempted. If sedation is necessary, xylazine can be administered. In an adult horse, 150-200 mg of xylazine can be given IV; repeat doses can be administered as necessary.

Profuse arterial hemorrhage from the nostril and/or the mouth as a result of head trauma or erosion of a major vessel is only treatable rarely and usually is fatal or symptomatic of a fatal injury. Common causes for such hemorrhage are: rupture of the internal carotid artery secondary to mycotic lesions in the guttural pouch; laceration of the vessels at the base of the skull due to fracture of the basisphenoid bone secondary to a blow to the occipital crest; and penetrating wounds to the head that lacerate major vessels.

Bleeding from the vulva or anus is difficult to control and usually indicates severe wounds involving the peritoneal cavity. As such, the peritonitis secondary to peritoneal contamination and potentiated by hemoglobin in the peritoneal cavity usually is the life-threatening problem. If the hemorrhage is life threatening, packing the wound may help control bleeding. Surgical repair of the wound should be considered if the peritoneal cavity has been invaded.

Wounds can be packed with rolled gauze to control hemorrhage if they are not amenable to pressure bandaging. Even the nostrils can be packed if the airway is maintained through one nostril or tracheostomy. Bleeding from wounds into major muscle masses or on the body or head may not be manageable by any other means.

Packing simply involves pushing clean cloth into the wound until pressure on the vessels causes hemorrhage to cease and a clot to form in the fabric of the packing material. Clean, preferably sterile, packing material is desirable. Roll gauze (eg, Kling,

NuGauze) or long sheets of sterilized muslin (available at fabric stores) are best. Continuous gauze roll is far superior to gauze sponges because it is easier to account for complete removal of the packing using gauze roll. Frequently, when sheet or pound cotton has been used for packing material, portions are left in the wound when the packing material is removed.

Blindness

B.D. Brewer

When a client calls you about a horse that is blind, it is necessary first to ascertain if an emergency situation exists. When the onset is truly acute, the horse should be examined as soon as possible. Generally, in such situations an eye lesion is obvious or additional signs of neurologic disease are present. In either case, immediate treatment is warranted. In addition, acute blindness has been associated with chronic epistaxis or severe blood loss from any site, hypoxia from an anesthetic accident, and intracarotid injections. When injected into an artery, irritating and nonwater-soluble substances most often result in contralateral blindness.

While discussing the situation over the telephone, the veterinarian should try to elicit information on the duration of the problem as well as any of the aforementioned historical points. Other important queries should include whether one or both eyes seem to be involved, if the eyes look abnormal, whether any other signs accompany the problem, and whether the blindness is intermittent or constant. Any subtle clues that may have signalled a slowly progressive onset of the condition should be investigated. Also, any previous traumatic injury to the head should be noted, as optic nerve atrophy with subsequent blindness may become evident following a head injury, despite the fact that the horse had apparently recovered from the injury.

An owner may incorrectly report that a severely depressed horse is blind, believing that the abnormal behavior is the result of suspected blindness. Similarly, a horse that stumbles because of a neurologic problem may be perceived as blind. Conversely, unilateral blindness that has gone undetected by the owner or trainer can be noted on a neurologic examination being conducted for other reasons.

The purpose of an examination is to determine if indeed the horse is blind, and to determine whether the blindness is due to a lesion in the eye or in the nervous system. The presence of a lesion of the eye itself, and occasionally the optic nerve, can be confirmed by routine ophthalmologic examination. Lesions associated with hypoxia or severe blood loss usually appear as diffuse retinopathy with multifocal streaks and vermiform changes on fundic examination. Most cases of blindness not associated with an eye problem are neurologic in origin.

Unilateral and partial blindness can be difficult to confirm. This is best accomplished by placing a patch over one of the horse's eyes at a time and walking the animal through an obstacle course. The obstacles should not be aromatic and the patch must be quickly removable should the horse panic because it cannot see.

When an optic lesion has been ruled out, a complete neurologic examination must be performed. A detailed description of the examination protocol can be found in the chapter on Diseases of the Nervous System. When blindness is noted in conjunction with other neurologic abnormalities, particular attention must be directed toward examining cranial nerve function. If the horse is truly blind and the lesion is not in the eye, the veterinarian is likely to be directed to optic nerve disease or focal or diffuse forebrain disease. The prognosis with optic nerve atrophy is poor.

General signs of cerebral disease include frequent yawning, dementia, aimless wandering, severe depression that may wax and wane, head pressing, mild ataxia and circling. If only one side of the cerebrum is involved, the animal is blind on the contralateral side but usually circles toward the side of the lesion, and may have a sluggish gait, particularly in the limbs on the side opposite the lesion. The appropriate workup for forebrain disease relies especially on a complete history. This includes vaccination status for equine encephalitis, recent tetanus antitoxin administration with regard to Theiler's disease, exposure to plants, such as locoweed and plants containing pyrrolizidine that are toxic to the liver, as well as recent seizure or head trauma. A good physical examination is imperative to detect icterus, sepsis and injury.

Colic

J.N. Moore

A common reason for emergency calls received by an equine practitioner is colic. Fortunately, only a small percentage of horses that experience colic require surgical intervention. Because it is common knowledge, however, that many causes for colic necessitate emergency surgery, often the client is distraught and requires extra attention. The person dealing with the client over the telephone must remain calm and supportive, and persevere to obtain accurate answers to a few pertinent questions.

To provide the veterinarian with a minimum data base, it is important to learn the age and sex of the animal as well as the duration and severity of pain exhibited by the horse. Though answers to these questions may seem to be inconsequential at the moment, they allow the veterinarian to begin considering the most likely causes for the problem. For instance, several conditions causing colic occur far more often in horses of certain ages (cecal impaction, epiploic foramen entrapment, pedunculated lipoma, etc) or occur most often in mares (large colon volvulus) or in stallions (inguinal hernia).

To accurately gauge severity of pain, it is advisable to have the client describe the horse's actions rather than simply ask, "Is the horse in severe pain?" Finally, it is important to learn how long the horse has been showing signs of colic and whether any treatments have been given. Because some clients may prefer to conceal the fact that they have treated the horse themselves, this last question should be asked in a nonaccusatory manner. Consequently, a more truthful answer may be obtained if the question is posed as, "Has the horse responded to any treatment?", rather than as, "Have you treated the horse with anything?"

Invariably, the client asks the following question: "What should we do until the veterinarian arrives?" Though the immediate needs of a mare with a large colon volvulus are different from those of a horse with pelvic flexure impaction, it is vital that the person dealing with the client give well-founded advice that, above all, will cause no harm. Because this situation occurs often in a practice, the veterinarian and the person handling the telephone should discuss beforehand the specific pieces of advice that should be offered. Generally, the client should be advised to minimize any opportunities for the horse to traumatize itself or the people around it. Thus, if the horse is repeatedly lying down and rolling, it should be taken to an open space and walked. If, however, the horse prefers to lie down quietly, it should be allowed to do so. In any case, children and people with minimal horse experience should be kept away from the animal. The veterinarian should be contacted by the receptionist before any advice is given about treating the horse with analgesics or sedatives.

Once the veterinarian arrives at the farm, a quick physical examination should be performed while simultaneously listening to the client's recounting of the history. Particular attention should be paid to the color of the oral mucous membranes, capillary refill time, heart rate, presence or absence of abdominal distention, and presence or absence of borborygmi. This assessment takes a few minutes and, if the horse is showing signs of pain, should immediately precede passage of a stomach tube. Because of the propensity for the equine stomach to rupture during gastric dilatation, it is vital that care be taken to ensure that the tube has entered the stomach and that any gas or fluid is removed. This latter maneuver may require siphoning gastric contents.

Based on the findings of the initial physical examination, the immediate needs of the horse must be determined. These may include administration of analgesics and further diagnostic procedures. A thorough rectal examination should be performed to identify palpable reasons for the colic episode. Based on physical examination findings, the veterinarian also must decide if laboratory tests (packed cell volume, plasma protein concentration) and/or abdominocentesis are indicated. Further, the veterinarian must decide if intravenous administration of polyionic fluids or intragastric administration of mineral oil is indicated. The most difficult decision to be made, however, is whether the horse can be treated effectively on the client's premises or if the animal should be referred to a veterinary hospital for more intensive medical therapy and/or surgical intervention. The results of the rectal examination, color of the peritoneal fluid, and clinical signs exhibited by the animal may prove most useful in making this decision.

It is important that the veterinarian and client discuss various treatment possibilities early in the event that difficult or expensive decisions must be made; the decision to refer an animal for further workup, treatment or surgery be made as early as possible; and the client be informed of the animal's prognosis for survival. Though certain clients may cling to slim chances for success, it is vital that the veterinarian is certain that the client understands the gravity of a particular situation and the costs involved to the client and the horse.

Acute Collapse

I.G. Mayhew

To witness a horse or foal suddenly collapse or to be called urgently to evaluate a patient that has had one or more episodes of collapsing can be quite confusing for the clinician and certainly is distressing for the owner or manager. On most occasions, the situation quickly evolves to acute death, recovery with recumbency, a gait abnormality, other neurologic syndrome, intermittent collapse, or recovery with or without evidence of a nonneurologic problem.

A caring client deserves some urgent instructions by telephone, relayed expeditiously by an informed receptionist. However, poorly informed clients and children must be reminded of their own safety and advised to keep clear until the veterinarian arrives. In the former circumstance, the client may be directed to stop any massive bleeding or to roll a horse that might be cast. In addition, in the event that the horse might rise, the client can be reminded to guide the horse, if it is ambulatory, to soft ground away from potentially harmful objects.

Upon arriving at the scene of a collapsed horse, the "ABCs" of acute care must be attended to concurrently.

Airway: determine that the airway is patent and that the horse is breathing adequately. Institute oxygen and/or assisted ventilation if necessary. Remove any obstructing fluids or objects from the airway.

Give 10 ml of 50% ethanol intratracheally or another suitable nonirritant antifoment for pulmonary edema.

Bleeding: Stop any hemorrhage by packing, suturing, etc.

Cardiovascular: Briefly evaluate cardiovascular function and institute cardiac resuscitation with thoracic massage and intravenous or intracardiac epinephrine (0.5-1.0 ml of 1:1000 in 10 ml of water) if asystole and/or anaphylaxis is evident. Intravenous volume expansion with polyionic fluids, plasma, or blood is used as indicated and when available.

Any fractures that may mean a hopeless prognosis (femur), may be life threatening (ribs), or may require splinting (metacarpus) must be identified and appropriate measures taken.

A thrashing patient may require sedation and/or anticonvulsant therapy. If shock or respiratory depression is not a problem and there is no evidence of seizure activity, then xylazine, chloral hydrate or pentobarbital, can be given. Diazepam in doses of 5-10 mg (foal) to 25-100 mg (horse) should be given IV to control seizures. A horse recumbent for any reason can become terribly violent in its frantic attempt to rise and also in response to pain. It is impossible to differentiate such behavior from cerebral seizures. With the latter, the horse is in a state of unconsciousness and its attention cannot be attracted. Usually there are violent jaw and facial muscle spasms with eyeball movements, a tendency for opisthotonos and, sometimes, voiding of urine and feces.

Following these steps, an initial verbal history can be acquired while a brief physical examination is undertaken. Such aspects as the duration and frequency of the collapse episode, whether herdmates have been affected and the presence of other environmental, managerial and clinical factors (excessive heat, poisonous plants, injections, previous and prodromal illness, feed) all are noted.

The general aim, at this stage, is to determine in which basic category of acute collapse this horse best fits. These general categories include: syncope, seizures, sleep disorders, coma, motor paralysis and generalized and metabolic disorders.

A few horses suffering one or more episodes of acute collapse may be suspected of having syncope or fainting. Usually this is because of the presence of a cardiac arrhythmia and/or a cardiac murmur. In a few such cases, definitive cardiac disease is confirmed. Such documented disorders include atrial fibrillation, ruptured chordae tendineae, myocardial infarction, myocardial fibrosis, aortic endocarditis and pericarditis.

With syncopal attacks, usually there is little or no premonitory warning of collapse and, because of cerebral hypoxia, a temporary, quiet, comatose state ensues. Some struggling may occur during recovery before the horse regains its feet. Other overt signs of cardiac failure might become evident.

A seizure, convulsion or fit is the physical expression of bizarre electrical neuronal discharges in all or part of the cerebrum. Often, there is a pre-ictal aura of a few seconds to minutes, followed by the ictus or seizure, which lasts a few seconds to minutes, then a post-ictal phase of several minutes to hours. The aura may involve the horse's being distracted from its environment, having a blank expression and, occasionally, being restless. If the seizure becomes generalized, usually a horse becomes recumbent and lies rigidly in lateral recumbency for a while before paddling or thrashing for several seconds to minutes. With status epilepticus, the phase is repeated continually and is fatal unless anticonvulsant drugs are given. After a seizure, a horse usually regains its feet relatively easily; it then may pace about, act blind or drink or eat constantly, and may not recognize its handler. Depending on the underlying cause, other neurologic signs may be evident.

Anticonvulsant therapy, first with diazepam, then with phenobarbital or possibly dilantin, as outlined in the chapter Diseases of the Nervous System, is required if more than one seizure has occurred.

Narcolepsy is characterized by repeated uncontrolled episodes of sleep. Unlike seizures and many metabolic disorders, such as hyperkalemia, there are no warning signs, though with multiple attacks the horse may appear sleepy between attacks. Adult horses do not always drop to the ground and may catch themselves after the head suddenly lowers and the thoracic limb stay apparatus begins to fail. Most often

there is prominent cataplexy that entails sudden loss of all voluntary motor effort, with the horse collapsing to the ground. Petting about the head and neck, hosing down after exercise, beginning to eat or drink, and resting quietly in a barn at night all have been associated with episodes. Sleep episodes usually do not occur while a horse is exercising vigorously.

Coma is a state of recumbency with unconsciousness and total unresponsiveness. Mostly it is associated with profound changes in the forebrain or midbrain. Head trauma, birth asphyxia, bacterial meningoencephalitis, parasitic infarction/migration, spontaneous hemorrhage, moldy corn intoxication, liver disease, and intracarotid injections are some of the more frequent causes of acute coma. Consequently, a history or evidence of trauma and other premonitory neurologic signs are important facts to determine. Immediately following head trauma, a temporary period of coma often ensues; thus, such an animal should not be euthanized immediately, and appropriate diagnostic and therapeutic approaches should be instituted.

Collapse without loss of consciousness can be due to loss of motor function. These pathways may be interrupted at the level of the brainstem, vestibular apparatus, spinal cord, peripheral nerve, neuromuscular junction or muscle. A neurologic examination is paramount to identify the location of the lesions. Trauma is the most common mechanism at the first 3 of these sites. Other causes of acute collapse with no loss of consciousness are botulism (including the shaker foal syndrome), postanesthetic myasthenic syndrome, postanesthetic neuromyopathy, exercise-associated rhabdomyolysis, and hyperkalemia periodic paralysis.

This category of acute collapse includes such miscellaneous disorders as hyperthermia, shock, hypoglycemia, hypocalcemia, hyperkalemia, hypokalemia, endotoxemia, anaphylaxis, anaphylactoid reaction, acute exotoxemia and snakebite. Several systems usually are noted to be abnormal on physical examination, and subsequent appropriate system examinations and therapy should be undertaken.

Appropriate advice and warnings should be given immediately to a client who has a horse showing acute collapse. Several lifesaving procedures and treatment can be considered. A fairly quick physical examination allows the clinician to decide in which category the case belongs: syncope, seizures, sleep disorders, coma, motor paralysis or generalized and metabolic disorders. Following this, detailed examination of other systems, especially the cardiovascular, respiratory, nervous and musculoskeletal systems, allows formulation of an appropriate plan for diagnosis, treatment and client education.

Cough

A.M. Koterba

In many cases, the clinical approach to a horse or foal with a cough is very straightforward, with rapid response to treatment. Conversely, a coughing horse can present a diagnostic and therapeutic challenge to the veterinarian, and can be a frustrating problem for the client. Initial considerations include presenting clinical signs, the duration and severity of clinical signs and the environment where the horse is kept. A cough rarely requires emergency treatment unless it is accompanied by respiratory distress or dysphagia (as occurs with choke). Determining the cause of the cough and initiating appropriate treatment should be the main emphasis.

A complete history often is essential to pinpoint the cause of a cough. The age of the horse is very important, as certain viral upper respiratory diseases (equine herpesvirus or rhinovirus infection) and bacterial diseases (*Streptococcus equi* bronchopneumonia) are encountered more commonly in suckling and weanling foals and in young performing horses, respectively. Similarly, *Rhodococcus equi* infections are rarely observed in foals >6 months of age. Lymphoid hyperplasia is a common cause of coughing and decreased performance in young horses (2-3 years) but is rarely observed in older horses. Though such diseases as influenza and *Streptococcus equi* infection may cause outbreaks of respiratory disease and coughing in adult horses, particularly following long-distance shipping, such noninfectious factors as allergic reactions to the environment that cause chronic bronchitis are more common in adults. Lungworm infections (*Dictyocaulus arnfieldi*) may occur in horses of any age.

It is important to question the client about the duration of the cough and to try to determine if it is related to other problems, such as decreased exercise tolerance. The vaccination record and any history of previous medical or surgical treatment are important. Other questions to be addressed are: Has the horse been exposed to any potentially infected animals? Has the horse been shipped recently or been subjected to any other serious stresses?

In a horse with a chronic or intermittent cough, particular evaluation of the environment is warranted. For example, an occasional cough might be expected from a normal horse exercising in a dusty arena; however, a deep cough consistently noticed when the horse is exposed to hay suggests an allergic etiology. Other questions to consider include: Is the cough more noticeable in certain seasons? Is the cough less severe when the horse's environment is changed? Finally, are any other horses on the premises coughing or showing signs of respiratory disease? Most viral respiratory diseases have short incubation periods; therefore, susceptible horses begin to show clinical signs within a short time of exposure. Exposure to donkeys infected with lungworms can cause a coughing problem in a horse herd.

Any evaluation of a coughing horse or foal should include a complete physical examination to determine if the respiratory system is the source of the problem and which part of the system is involved. To be noted are the character of any nasal discharge and other signs accompanying the cough. Fever, anorexia, depression and painful or enlarged lymph nodes suggest an infectious process. An elevated heart rate, weak jugular pulse, ventral edema and ascites indicate cardiovascular compromise.

To more precisely define the location of the disease in the respiratory system, the horse's breathing pattern and rate must be assessed. Inspiratory dyspnea is observed more commonly in horses with upper airway obstruction. Increased abdominal effort on expiration suggests a lower airway obstruction due to chronic bronchitis or severe restrictive pulmonary disease, as occurs with pleural effusion. A rapid, shallow breathing pattern may accompany restrictive respiratory diseases, such as acute pleuropneumonia, interstitial pneumonia and pneumothorax, or a number of nonpulmonary conditions, such as fever, pain, anhidrosis and toxemia. A consistently elicitable cough on laryngeal or tracheal palpation should be considered abnormal but is not diagnostic of disease in any certain location.

Thorough auscultation and percussion of both sides of the chest wall is critical. To adequately auscult respiratory sounds in an adult horse, it often is necessary to augment the resting respiratory sounds by stimulating deeper breathing by placing a rebreathing bag over the nose, by transiently occluding the nostrils or by light exercise. Percussion detects areas of consolidation noted by lack of resonance, as well as pleural pain that commonly accompanies acute pleuritis.

Once a thorough history has been obtained and a complete physical examination completed, the veterinarian must decide whether to perform additional diagnostic tests or simply to institute therapy directed toward the most likely cause of the cough. Though a cough is considered a hallmark of respiratory disease, it is important to remember that the absence of a cough does not exclude respiratory disease. For example, large lung abscesses may be associated with virtually no localizing clinical signs. Neonatal foals typically do not cough, even in the face of severe pneumonia.

Depression

B.D. Brewer

In most cases of depression, clients report that their horse is exhibiting signs in addition to depression. A complaint of severe, acute depression even without other signs, however, is an emergency and the horse should be examined at once.

Depression is manifested to various degrees. A horse exhibiting mild depression is only lethargic in its performance. A moderately depressed horse is obviously abnormal and stands immobile in the stall or pasture. Often these horses are anorectic. A severely depressed horse appears unaware of its surroundings and is comatose and/or recumbent.

Depression with or without additional signs occurs under several circumstances.

Horses respond to hot days, changes in feed or, in mares, to estrus by appearing sluggish and depressed. Behavioral problems during training may be perceived as a medical problem by a client who prefers to imagine that the horse is ill rather than misbehaving.

Many mild and common infectious diseases (particularly viral respiratory diseases) are manifested initially as depression. Fever usually accompanies this stage of the disease. Mild colic also may be manifested only as depression. Generally, a thorough physical examination and careful observation for more serious signs of disease are all that is needed to identify the most likely underlying causes in these cases.

In these cases, depression is mild to moderate and is at least partially responsive to analgesic medication. Depression commonly accompanies and occurs as a sequel to many chronic diseases, including severe pulmonary disease, acute diarrhea, renal failure and occasionally anhidrosis. Horses suffering from chronically painful conditions appear depressed and recumbent horses become progressively more depressed as they become exhausted by their attempts to stand.

Two situations are common. In one instance, the horse has not been observed for some time (usually >8 hours) and then is found severely depressed. If the condition is life threatening, physical examination usually permits rapid identification of the problem. Examples of this include ruptured viscus, prolonged dystocia, severe endotoxemia, septicemia, acute blood loss due to a ruptured artery, severe trauma, or heat stroke. A neonatal foal that has not eaten or has developed diarrhea or septicemia becomes extremely acidotic, hypoglycemic and dehydrated. These metabolic conditions resulting in severe depression are not restricted to the neonate, however, and may also be seen in adult horses.

In the second instance, the horse has been observed frequently and either has a confirmed onset of acute depression or has a history of minimal depression that suddenly becomes extreme. The following possibilities should be considered:

Severe Pain: For example, a horse with an acute cervical vertebral fracture may have no external signs of trauma but appears very depressed and holds its head in a ventral position.

Toxicity: Toxins that induce depression as the sole clinical sign include pyrrolidine alkaloids, carbon tetrachloride, phenothiazine, vitamin D overdose, reserpine, urea and snake venom. Several other toxins that cause concurrent signs referable to specific organ systems also should be considered.

These diseases may or may not be accompanied by fever or other abnormalities evident on routine physical examination or neurologic examination. Mentation abnormalities are best identified by monitoring the horse's response to tactile, painful, auditory and visual stimuli. Many such affected horses exhibit signs of diffuse forebrain disease and are blind with normal pupillary light reflexes. One must consider rabies as a possible cause of the condition.

Documented or suspected head trauma is an emergency warranting immediate treatment. Signs of trauma may not be evident. Such vestibular signs as a head tilt, circling, ataxia, leaning, strabismus, nystagmus and violent rolling, with or without abnormalities in facial nerve function, typically are noted in addition to depression. Occasionally only cerebral edema occurs and signs other than those of forebrain disease are not seen. In either case, treatment may have to be instituted immediately to reduce the edema and prevent brain herniation. In horses, the most practical treatment includes administration of dexamethasone, but there is risk of subsequent side effects, including laminitis. For this reason, many practitioners prefer to give a 10% DMSO solution, in saline or 5% dextrose IV at 1 g/kg. This drug is not licensed for such use in horses. However, provided that it is diluted and only medical-grade DMSO is used, it is considered the best therapy. In many such cases, treatment is not undertaken because of the apparent severity of the situation. However, the horse may recover if treated early and sufficient convalescence is allowed. Improvement is noted within days, but full recovery takes weeks to months.

In summary, depression is a sign that accompanies a multitude of medical and occasionally nonmedical problems. An accurate history and a complete physical and neurologic examination are crucial to determining the cause and selecting appropriate therapy.

Eating Difficulties

S.L. Green

When a client calls because a horse is having difficulty eating, the client first should be instructed to remove food and water immediately and not return it until the horse has been evaluated by a veterinarian. This is especially critical to prevent aspiration pneumonia if feed material or gastric contents are evident at the horse's nares. Because regurgitation of gastric contents is uncommon, feed or fluid spilling from the mouth or nose is more likely due to a dysphagia. Chronic dysphagia often is associated with weight loss that may be noted by the client. Anorexia or an inadequate ration may contribute to weight loss and must be considered in the evaluation. Dysphagia can be due to inability to grasp food with the lips and teeth, inability to chew food or inability to swallow properly. Each of these functions should be evaluated to help identify the cause of the problem.

The receptionist should have the client describe the horse's appearance and estimate when the difficulty began, if possible. If drooling or excessive salivation is a predominant clinical sign and if there has been a sudden change in the horse's behavior, the client should be advised to avoid contact with the horse's mouth, as rabies must be a consideration.

Possible causes of eating difficulties to be considered in an adult horse include dysphagia due to dental problems, esophageal obstruction, head and face trauma, neuromuscular disorders and liver failure.

Eating difficulties commonly accompany dental problems that usually are chronic in nature and most frequently occur in horses >5 years of age. Though prehension and swallowing usually are not affected, chewing becomes painful. Dental problems cause weight loss, slow and deliberate chewing, excessive salivation, spilling of grain, selective preference for hay, "quidding" or spilling of hay or grass boluses, and tilting the head while eating. Additional signs of dental problems include halitosis, unilateral purulent nasal discharge, swellings or draining tracts over the jaw, a painful response to external palpation over the cheek teeth

15

or upon flotation of the teeth, and unwillingness to accept the bit. It is a good idea to offer the horse a small amount of grain or hay so as to observe the eating difficulty.

A thorough oral examination should be performed and usually requires a mouth speculum, flashlight and tranquilization. The examination may identify important abnormalities, such as excessively sharp wolf teeth, sharp enamel points on the molar teeth, mucosal lacerations, broken or missing cheek teeth with correspondingly long teeth in the opposite arcade, foreign bodies, gingivitis, receding gums, draining tracts in the gums and tooth infection. Because sinus empyema is a common sequel to tooth root infection, sinuses should be percussed. Deciduous premolars (dental caps) that have fragmented and caused oral lacerations or that are retained and impacted may be associated with facial swelling.

Choke is a common cause of dysphagia in horses and typically is acute in onset. Passage of feed or water down the esophagus is prevented by the obstruction, and excessive drooling and a nasal discharge containing feed material usually are present. Dehydration and aspiration pneumonia may be additional problems. Examination of the mouth for dental problems that may have prevented adequate mastication should not be overlooked. Changes in feed and feeding practices may be precipitating factors.

Neurologic disorders may affect prehension, mastication and the swallowing reflex. The onset of the clinical signs may be acute or slowly progressive. Pharyngeal paralysis causes food and water to exit the nares. A brainstem lesion affecting the pharyngeal branches of the glossopharyngeal (IX) and vagus (X) nerves produces neurologic defects paralyzing the larynx and pharynx, causing dysphagia. The severity of signs depends on whether the involvement is unilateral or bilateral.

Evidence of neurologic dysfunction can be assessed by testing the swallowing reflex during an endoscopic examination of the pharynx and by passing a nasogastric tube. Unilateral paralysis of the larynx also may be assessed by palpating the larynx for atrophy of the cricoarytenoideus dorsalis muscle and performing the laryngeal adductor response test ("slap test"). Because these cranial nerves are in close contact within the guttural pouches, endoscopic and radio-graphic examination of the guttural pouches is recommended. Multifocal diseases, such as protozoal myelitis, should be considered when such signs exist.

Bilateral lesions involving the motor trigeminal (V), facial (VII), or hypoglossal (XII) nerves also cause inability to grasp or chew food, and a limp, weak, protruding tongue, respectively, resulting in dysphagia. Other neurologic causes of dysphagia may be due to focal brainstem or peripheral cranial nerve disease. Horses with severe diffuse forebrain disease and marked depression also exhibit dysphagia without complete loss of the swallowing reflex. Dysphagia also can occur due to diffuse neuromuscular disease, such as botulism, or from tetanus, peripheral neuropathy or liver failure.

The onset of dysphagia may occur immediately or some time after head trauma. Chronic osteoarthrosis and fusion of the temporohyoid joint may be radiographically evident, as well as fractures of the basilar, temporal or hyoid bones. Dysphagia after head trauma also can be the result of fractures of the jaw bones or of the hyoid bones with loss of tongue function. If the onset of dysphagia has been associated with head trauma, other neurologic deficits, including peripheral vestibular deficits and facial paralysis, may be present.

In summary, dysphagic horses require a thorough oral examination, passage of a nasogastric tube and neurologic, radiographic and endoscopic evaluations. Secondary aspiration pneumonia and dehydration also may require treatment.

Examination for Purchase or Insurance

D. Hawkins

When a veterinarian is contacted by a client about examining a horse for purchase or insurance, the client should be asked: the age, breed, sex and intended use of the horse; whether the client is the buyer, seller or owner of the horse; who is paying for the examination; and the service the client expects. In turn, the client should be told the importance of knowing for whom the examination is being performed, the limitations of the examination, what can be reasonably expected from the examination, the procedures to be performed during the examination, and the value of knowing the intended use of the horse. Proper service can be rendered best when accurate information is provided and there is good communication among all parties involved. Time, expense and goodwill can be saved if the client clearly understands during the telephone conversation the examination process and its limitations before the veterinarian travels to examine the horse or conversely before the horse travels to the veterinarian.

The purchase examination has become increasingly complex in recent years, especially for private sales, as clients generally expect a secure investment when purchasing a horse. The procedures used in public sale purchases, while they have changed to some degree, still are constrained by the wishes of the consignors and sales company in the environment of the public sales barn. The thrust for this change in procedure and our attitudes toward purchase examinations comes from the large amount of money involved in these transactions and the willingness of disappointed buyers to sue the veterinarian that performed the examination.

To conduct the examination properly, the veterinarian should be familiar with the breed of horse to be examined, have a clear understanding of the buyer's intentions for the horse and an appreciation of the physical demands to be placed upon the horse. The veterinarian must determine if the horse has any infirmity precluding satisfactory performance. To do that, the veterinarian must understand what constitutes satisfactory performance.

Because the examiner's objectivity must be above question, it is not advisable for a veterinarian to conduct a purchase examination for the seller or accept compensation from the seller. Similarly, it is ill advised for a veterinarian to perform a purchase examination for a buyer on a horse owned by one of that veterinarian's clients or on a horse about which the veterinarian has prior knowledge. Each of these situations increases the likelihood of an apparent conflict of interest.

It is highly advisable to have the buyer present during the purchase examination for direct consultation. Though some buyers prefer to have an agent present to act as an intermediary instead, the examining veterinarian has no guarantee that the agent will convey the veterinarian's findings and opinions accurately. Because relationships between clients and their agents vary and because agents sometimes can make a personal gain from the transaction, it is advisable for the veterinarian to mail a written report that clearly explains the results of the examination directly to the purchaser. This standard practice helps reduce the chance for miscommunication if the purchaser is not present personally during the examination. In all purchase examinations, a copy of the written report should be kept by the examining veterinarian to certify the findings of the examination if the sale is questioned later.

Veterinarians most frequently are asked to perform an examination for athletic soundness. Horses subjected to this examination are performance horses, show horses and pleasure horses. To accurately interpret the results of such an examination, the level of experience or background of the horse must be established. This information is based on an accurate history, the buyer's personal knowledge of the horse, or any available performance records (race record, show circuit record, etc). It is important to know the amount and nature of exercise to which the horse has been subjected before the examination. The veterinarian can assess the suitability of the horse more accurately for the buyer knowing that a horse is in training and has been performing at the same level sought by the buyer. Under these circumstances, the horse should have been subjected to the same work intensity and level of stress that will be expected by the buyer.

Examination for athletic performance is more difficult if the horse has had limited experience in a sport or has been competing at a lower level than the buyer intends for the horse. The limitation of the examination becomes compounded if the horse has had no experience in the intended use. For instance, the buyer may want to change the animal's use by buying a racehorse and developing it into a show jumper. Conditions of soundness considered to be acceptable for a racehorse may not be acceptable for a show jumper. Often yearlings, weanlings and even foals may be purchased for racing or other athletic endeavors. Obviously evaluation of younger, inexperienced horses is less exact and involves more risk for the buyer. The details of conducting a complete examination for purchase evaluation in various situations is covered in the chapter on General Physical Examination.

The problem of evaluating horses that may have had drugs administered to mask unsoundness is inconsistently considered by veterinarians conducting purchase examinations. Some veterinarians routinely include drug screening as a part of their examination procedure. Others do so sporadically or allow the buyer to decide whether or not these screening procedures should be used. As laboratory services have become more economical and more readily available, and provide results quickly, it has become more common to determine serum concentrations of certain drugs.

Horses being purchased for breeding comprise another major category of animals for which purchase evaluations are requested. In addition to the general history, when possible, a detailed history of the horse's reproductive performance should be obtained. If the horse is in training or recently retired from athletic training, it is important to know if medications (*eg*, anabolic steroids) that may affect gonadal size, gonadal activity or spermatogenesis have been given previously. Interpretation of reproduction examination findings is always made in consideration of time of year.

If the horse may be required to travel abroad, evaluation of contagious equine metritis and equine viral arteritis status is imperative. Because mares and stallions are purchased to reproduce a breed, the animal's conformation as representative of the breed type should be evaluated. Basic to the breeding soundness examination is a complete general physical examination, including evaluation of the conformation of the external genitalia and careful inspection for musculoskeletal injuries, particularly laminitis, and neurologic, cardiac, respiratory and ophthalmic problems.

Mares: The history should indicate if the mare is nulliparous, primiparous or pluriparous. In some nulliparous fillies, the stress of training and racing may delay the onset of normal ovarian cyclic activity. Alternatively, a crippling injury may exclude a mare from breeding even if she has a functional reproductive tract. If a filly is still in training, the buyer may want to continue to

race or show her while she is being bred. If so, the filly also must be examined as to performance as an athlete. Fillies that have been bred but are not in foal should be examined as if they were a barren mare.

Primiparous and pluriparous mares are evaluated as pregnant or barren. The state of their reproductive cycle (*eg*, estrus, diestrus, seasonal anestrus, transitional phase, pregnancy) in which the examination is conducted has great impact on overall interpretation. Though the examination procedure is the same, evaluation of mares to be bred on nonrefundable season contracts causes added concern for everyone involved. Consequently, a critique of any available offspring is helpful when the veterinarian is asked to judge the mare on factors other than reproductive soundness. The scope of the examination performed at a public sale is far more limited. Under these circumstances, the evaluation is based on only rectal and speculum examinations and an evaluation of records provided in the sales catalog by the consignor.

Stallions: Evaluation of horses for purchase as breeding stallions can be more complex logistically. Stallions may be categorized as inexperienced or experienced. Inexperienced stallions frequently are in training or are competing at the time of the evaluation. Consequently, the stallion's schedule must be considered and time allowed to train him to mount a mare or a phantom for semen collection, in addition to evaluating the semen for fertility. An owner's concern about an injury occurring during semen collection may represent a special challenge to the examiner, especially if the stallion's value is dependent upon his continued performance as an athlete. For the retired horse, the situation is generally less complex except for stallions that are retired with injuries that could interfere with mounting or be worsened by the examination process. Experienced stallions generally do not require training to mount.

The following points must be clearly understood before the examination. The first is to know for whom you are doing the examination. It might be for a single potential owner, one of several potential owners, or a potential syndication group. Second, the proposed number of mares to be serviced and the intended method of service (natural service or artificial insemination) must be established. Finally, it must be ascertained if the routine stallion fertility evaluation protocol is adequate; there may be special requirements in the purchase agreement or fertility insurance contract.

The examination should be performed where the facilities are adequate to set up the necessary equipment, collect and examine semen. A docile mare in estrus or a phantom must be available. The stallion should be trained to mount and to serve an artificial vagina before the examination. In some instances, a designated number of mares must be selected and available for "test matings," in addition to semen evaluation. The chapter on Diseases of the Reproductive System contains more specific information regarding fertility evaluation.

All companies that write mortality insurance policies for horses use similar questionnaires that the examining veterinarian must complete. In almost all cases, a complete physical examination provides all the information required by the insurance company. One problematic aspect of the mortality insurance examination is that the veterinarian generally is asked to perform the examination for the insurance company but the owner of the horse must pay for the examination. Regardless, all questions should be answered to the best of one's knowledge. If there are omissions of pertinent data or inaccurate statements and a claim is filed later, the claim may be denied.

Stallion fertility insurance generally is purchased only on the first season a stallion is at stud. Because there is some variation in the requirements of these insurance contracts, the guidelines of the respective insurance company must be strictly followed.

Owners of valuable mares that conceive on expensive, nonrefundable breeding contracts most frequently want prospective foal insurance. The insurance contracts usually are made in advance, and consummation of the contract depends on obtaining specific data at precise times early during the mare's pregnancy. These data may include properly labeled ultrasonograms, results of assays for pregnant mare serum gonadotropin, and results of manual palpation for pregnancy. The insurance company's requirements should be clearly established in advance so they can be fulfilled at the designated times during pregnancy.

Eye Problems

R.D. Whitley

The most frequent complaint received from a client concerning an eye problem is that the horse is holding the eye closed and there is epiphora (excessive tearing), which indicates pain. Other complaints include cloudy eye, blood in the eye, red eye, an eye laceration, a growth on the eye, a swollen eye, ocular discharge, blindness, decreased vision in bright light, and decreased vision in dim light. The veterinarian or receptionist should try to ascertain exactly what type of eye problem the client has observed.

Of these complaints, the more pressing emergencies include corneal lacerations, deep corneal ulcers and uveitis. The client should be instructed to keep the horse in a quiet place, preferably a clean stall. The horse should be cross-tied or a protective helmet placed over the eye to prevent additional damage. The surrounding hair or forelock should be cut or braided to prevent its interfering with the eye. If hay is fed, it should be placed on the ground to prevent foreign material from entering the eye. Petroleum jelly may be placed on the skin of the face, ventral to the eye, to prevent tears from scalding the skin and causing excoriation. Ocular medications in general should be avoided until the eye can be assessed by a qualified veterinarian.

Squinting and epiphora are common with ocular pain caused by corneal trauma, ocular foreign body, keratitis, corneal ulceration, entropion and uveitis. Conjunctivitis and glaucoma also should be considered. Pain may be manifested by squinting (blepharospasm), holding the head to one side, or head tossing. If the owner can further evaluate the eye, cloudiness on the cornea or within the eye may be described. Corneal opacity may vary from simple edema to deep ulceration or laceration. Cloudiness within the eye and evidence of pain frequently indicate uveitis. Cloudiness may be due to aqueous flare, fibrin, hypopyon or corneal edema.

Cloudiness or opacities of the clear ocular media may occur in the cornea, anterior chamber, lens and vitreous body. Corneal clouding may be due to corneal ulcer, keratitis, corneal edema or glaucoma. Anterior chamber clouding usually is due to aqueous flare, hypopyon and the presence of fibrin, indicating uveitis. Uveitis and hypopyon may be associated with concurrent systemic illness, especially in foals. Therefore, a thorough physical examination is necessary, with emphasis on the respiratory and gastrointestinal systems. Opacities of the lens (cataracts) and vitreous humor (retinal detachment) usually are not associated with pain but may affect vision severely in that eye.

The complaint of "blood in the eye" must be divided into true blood within the globe (hyphema) and bloody discharge from the eyelid(s), conjunctiva or a lacerated cornea with uveal hemorrhage (see also Red Eye below). Hyphema and subconjunctival hemorrhage may be associated with trauma and inflammation. However, the animal should also be evaluated for bleeding tendencies and clotting abnormalities.

With red eye, the owner frequently is describing hyperemia of the conjunctiva or third eyelid, prolapse of the third eyelid or subconjunctival hemorrhage. Hemorrhage within the eye (hyphema) also should be considered.

Hyperemia of the conjunctiva and third eyelid may be due to conjunctivitis, uveitis, foreign body, insects, chemical or drug irritation, or trauma. Subconjunctival hemorrhage frequently is due to trauma or vasculitis; the latter sometimes indicates a systemic disorder. Hyphema may be due to trauma or inflammation. Systemic infections and bleeding disorders must also be considered in differential diagnosis of subconjunctival hemorrhage and hyphema.

The complaint of a cut eye usually entails an eyelid or third eyelid laceration and requires thorough evaluation of the globe, conjunctiva and cornea. Corneal, scleral and conjunctival lacerations, with or without iris prolapse, also must be considered.

Complaints of a growth on the eye usually imply a cancer or granuloma of the eyelids, third eyelid, conjunctiva or cornea. Corneal rupture with iris prolapse is an important differential consideration when an owner describes a growth on the cornea. In foals, congenital dermoids may be described as growths on the eye. Owners also may describe prolapse or protrusion of the third eyelid as a mass on the eye. Traction should *not* be applied to the mass if iris prolapse is suspected. Corneal and eyelid foreign bodies initially may be mistaken for growths on the eye. Owners may also mistake the corpora nigrans (granula iridica) at the dorsal or ventral pupillary border for abnormal masses.

The complaint of a swollen eye must further be delineated as periorbital swelling, exophthalmos, macrophthalmos (glaucoma) or chemosis. Swollen eyelids and blepharospasm may be seen in severe cases of uveitis.

Obstruction of the nasolacrimal duct usually results in an initial aqueous discharge, changing to a mucopurulent discharge with time. A mucopurulent or purulent discharge is a common complaint. Ocular discharge often occurs with conjunctivitis, corneal ulceration, uveitis, foreign bodies, dacryocystitis and corneal laceration. Conjunctivitis and dacryocystitis are not urgent conditions. However, the other causes of ocular discharge benefit from immediate care.

By most clients, excessive tearing (epiphora) is understood as a watery or clear discharge from the eyes. Epiphora frequently indicates nasolacrimal obstruction, early uveitis or ocular discomfort associated with foreign bodies, conjunctivitis or corneal ulceration. In foals, atresia of the lacrimal puncta or nasal meatus is a cause of epiphora. Acute corneal laceration with leakage of aqueous humor must also be considered in this category.

Blindness is covered earlier in this chapter. The owner may complain that the horse bumps into stationary objects, in which case visual impairment must be differentiated from dementia and ataxia. The owner may complain that the animal is clumsy and traumatizes its forelegs, chest, face and neck, when in fact the animal is blind. Vision should be evaluated in each eye in a lighted and a darkened environment.

Decreased vision in bright light (hemeralopia) may indicate that an axial opacity in the cornea, lens or vitreous humor causes decreased vision when the pupil constricts in bright light. Retinopathy involving the photoreceptors for light vision (cones) should also be considered as a cause of visual impairment in bright light.

Except for the congenital and possibly inherited night blindness that occurs in the Appaloosa breed, decreased vision at night (nyctalopia) is not a common complaint by clients. Decreased vision in dim light may also occur due to other abnormalities of the rod photoreceptors.

Abnormal Feces

A.M. Merritt

A client may contact the veterinarian because changes have occurred in the volume, consistency, frequency, odor, color or contents of a horse's feces. Usually clients are explicit about fecal abnormalities and can relate obvious accompanying signs, such as colic, quite well. What may not have been observed, however, was the precise onset of clinical signs or when subtle alterations in the feces began. Consequently, the duration of the problem may not be accurately identified and a novice horse owner may not be expected to note less obvious signs of dehydration and shock. Thus, depending on the expertise of the individual client the abnormalities may or may not be recognized until an emergency situation requires immediate attention. Presenting clinical signs are extremely important. For example, a naive owner may not know that a neonatal foal does not form fecal balls or that an adult horse on lush grass pasture may have a loose stool because of that diet.

Changes in the volume and consistency of the feces often occur simultaneously. Though an increase in the water content of feces (diarrhea) frequently is accompanied by an increase in volume, and *vice versa*, this is not always true. Consequently, distinctions about whether the volume or fluid content is increased can be difficult to make and may be critical to diagnosis. The cause of acute, profuse, watery diarrhea usually is infectious, whereas scant watery diarrhea may indicate a partial intestinal obstruction that allows only the fluid content of the ingesta to pass. Chronic diarrhea, whether watery or "cow-flop" consistency, is less commonly infectious in origin. Definitive diagnosis requires thorough and often repetitive microbiologic investigations.

Conversely, excessively dry feces, whether they are formed into fecal balls or not, often occur when the frequency and volume of defecations are reduced. This change in fecal consistency primarily occurs due to large colon obstruction by impaction or water deprivation. A thick mucous coating on the feces also indicates a reduced rate of passage through the descending colon and concurrent reduction in stool volume. If a colonic impaction is being eliminated, large volumes of relatively dry contents not formed into fecal balls may be passed. One should always keep the horse's breed in mind during evaluation of fecal consistency, as small firm fecal balls are common in Arabian horses.

It is abnormal for a horse to go a number of days without defecating unless it has been completely anorectic or deprived of food, or is recovering from a severe bout of infectious diarrhea. Further, it should be emphasized that, in contrast to carnivores and many omnivores with relatively simple large intestines, fecal consistency in adult horses is almost solely determined by colonic function. When diarrhea exists, qualitative fecal analysis always is indicated to learn the nature of the problem.

The slightly pungent odor of normal horse feces is probably due to the volatile fatty acid content. The most characteristic abnormal odor is the "septic-tank" odor of some *Salmonella*-induced diarrheic feces. The feces of some horses with chronic diarrhea have a very strong offensive odor. Though no cause for this odor has been identified, it most likely indicates colonic maldigestion.

The feces of adult horses normally vary from a light to a dark, drab olive color, depending upon the horse's diet. Sometimes bright green feces are passed if the horse has eaten lush grass. Melena and most other fecal discolorations of diagnostic value are rare in adult horses. When melena does occur, it indicates small intestinal obstruction with infarction. A blackish diarrheic stool suggests that the horse has been treated with bismuth subsalicylate. Postmeconium feces of neonatal foals are normally dark brown. Light-colored, soft feces are characteristic of small intestinal malabsorption in the foal.

Unlike melena, frank blood in the feces most likely originates in the distal colon and indicates severe colitis or trauma. If there is blood on the rectal sleeve following rectal examination, a rectal laceration and/or perforation is strongly suspect and must be investigated immediately. Hematochezia is rarely seen in adult horses otherwise, even in those with devastating colitis. This change in fecal color may occur occasionally in foals with salmonellosis and is a cardinal sign of *Clostridium perfringens* type-C infection of foals.

Sand sometimes is grossly evident in equine feces and occasionally is defecated in the form of balls. More commonly, sand is recognized on the surface of the rectal sleeve or diagnosed by swirling a fecal sample in water. Significant quantities of sand can collect in the colon of horses and cause diarrhea or colic.

Other abnormal contents of horse feces include adult *Strongylus vulgaris* nematodes (bloodworms), mineral oil, small pebbles and whole grain kernels. A history of a poor deworming program, recent colic or shipping, pica and dental problems, respectively, provide explanations for their presence.

Fever

J.N. Moore

It is not uncommon for a client to contact a veterinarian's office because a horse appears to have a fever. The client may have noticed that the horse is sweating or that it has a rapid respiratory rate. In some instances, the client may have taken the horse's temperature but was not aware that a horse's normal body temperature can exceed 100 F. Consequently, it is important for the receptionist to determine if the horse's rectal temperature has been measured. Because the horse's body temperature may be increased as a result of muscular exertion, the location and recent activity of the animal should be determined. If the client routinely records the body temperatures of their horses, it should be determined if this reading was taken at the usual time of day and whether this reading truly is out of line with the normal diurnal variations observed in most animals. It also must be remembered that the thermoregulatory systems of foals are incompletely developed; thus a foal's normal body temperature may reach 102 F.

If it can be determined that the animal indeed has a fever, several lines of questioning are pursued to determine if the animal must be seen on an emergency basis. Generally this decision is based on the presence of other clinical signs indicative of a serious systemic disease. Consequently, the client should be asked if the horse has been coughing or if there is any nasal discharge. It also should be determined if the horse has lost its appetite, if there is any change in the consistency of the feces, if the temperatures of other horses on the premises have been taken, and if there has been any noticeable change in the horse's demeanor. If there is no evidence of systemic disease other than mild depression and the animal's temperature is <104 F, the client should be advised to measure the horse's temperature again in a few hours and call back with the finding. Until that time, the veterinarian's schedule may be rearranged to examine the animal later in the day.

Generally it is not necessary for a horse with a fever to be seen on an emergency basis. In fact, the cause for low-grade fevers in many instances remains undetermined despite intensive examination and laboratory testing. Of course, this does not mean that all horses with fevers should be ignored or that a fever is not important. If the fever is high and the client reports signs that may be attributable to systemic disease, the horse should be seen quickly.

The aim of the physical examination should be to determine if systemic disease exists. Because viral respiratory diseases can cause relatively high fevers (*eg*, 106 F), the veterinarian should pay particular attention to the respiratory system during physical examination. If the clinical findings are consistent with influenza, rhinopneumonitis or other respiratory tract infections, the other horses in the stable should be watched closely. If the affected horse is young, the mandibular lymph nodes should be palpated, as infection with *Streptococcus equi* must be considered.

If there is no apparent involvement of the respiratory tract, the diagnostic approach then involves a detailed examination of each major body system. The central nervous system should be considered as a possible source of the fever if the horse is ataxic, depressed or unable to stand. In such instances, the horse's vaccination history should be determined, particularly in reference to the viral encephalitides including rabies. Because equine infectious anemia may cause recurring fever, the Coggins status of the horse should be assessed. Particular attention should be paid to the alimentary system, as abdominal abscesses, neoplasia, endotoxemia, impending colitis and peritonitis cause fever. Thus, a rectal examination, abdominocentesis and complete blood count may be performed if the horse is systemically ill.

The best therapeutic approach can be planned after affected body systems have been identified and the most likely cause determined. There may be an indication for antibiotics or intravenous fluids, or no treatment may be required. Generally fevers <106 F are not life threatening and affected animals do not require treatment with antipyretic drugs. Though nonsteroidal antiinflammatory drugs often are used to reduce fevers in horses with temperatures in this range, these drugs should not be used indiscriminately. The client should be advised of the potential ill effects of these drugs, and intravenous and/or oral fluids with electrolytes should be given if the horse is hypovolemic and not drinking.

Haircoat Abnormalities

D.E. Bevier

Clients usually contact a veterinarian for 1 of 4 typical problems concerning their horse's haircoat: hair is being lost; the horse has too much hair; hair quality is poor; or the haircoat has changed color. Haircoat problems are very rarely emergencies unless the client indicates the horse is mutilating itself. These problems do require a planned appointment, however, so the client can prepare the horse and facilitate diagnosis. The client should be requested not to bathe the horse for at least 1 week before the dermatologic evaluation and to brush the horse well 2-3 days before the examination. During the physical examination, it is important to look for evidence of systemic diseases that produce or contribute to obvious skin lesions.

While obtaining the history, careful attention must be paid to nutritional management of the horse, especially to changes of feed. The following questions should be asked: Is the horse removing hair by biting or rubbing, or is it falling out? Is the change in haircoat associated with underlying skin lesions? In that haircoat problems can be congenital, has the horse had a normal haircoat in the past? Is more than 1 horse having haircoat problems? Are the abnormalities occurring over the whole body or only over parts of the body? Are the alterations in the haircoat patchy or complete?

Alopecia is complete loss of hair, while hypotrichosis implies that less than the normal amount of hair is present (partial alopecia). Alopecia and hypotrichosis may have inflammatory, hormonal, neoplastic, developmental or idiopathic causes.

Scratching against fences, stalls, trees or other objects because of pruritic dermatitis causes alopecia. This typically is patchy alopecia and frequently is associated with secondary lesions, including crusts, erosions, excoriations, hyperpigmentation and lichenification. When crusts on the skin are removed, hairs often are lost. Conversely, an inflammatory nonpruritic cause of single or multiple areas of complete alopecia is alopecia areata.

Hormonal disorders cause generalized haircoat problems characterized by dry, dull, brittle, easily epilated hairs. Also, hair may fail to regrow after clipping. Endocrine disorders are classically nonpruritic. Secondary seborrheic skin disease and pyodermas may accompany chronic hormonal skin disease. One such hormonal cause, hypothyroidism, is rare in horses.

Large numbers of neoplastic cells in the dermis can prevent development of or destroy hair follicles, causing alopecia in affected areas. This can be localized due to a solitary tumor, or generalized as part of a diffuse neoplastic process.

Some causes of hair loss have no known cause and are idiopathic. These include mane and tail dystrophy, and black and white hair follicle dystrophy. In some horses, abnormal spring shedding causes excessive hair loss and areas of marked hypotrichia or alopecia. These horses recover in 1-3 months. Stressful circumstances, such as high fever, pregnancy, shock, severe illness, malnutrition, surgery or anesthesia, may cause hair loss in days (anagen defluxion) or hair loss 2-3 months after the stress (telogen defluxion). The resultant partial or complete alopecia spares the mane and tail. A dry, dull, rough haircoat and patchy to complete alopecia can be associated with some chemical and plant toxicities.

An increase in the number of hairs is called hypertrichosis or hirsutism. Pituitary adenoma is the only clinical condition causing this clinical appearance due to increase in hair length. This disease is associated with myriad clinical signs in aged horses.

Variable degrees of localized or generalized dryness, dullness, brittleness and ease of epilation may affect the haircoat. These signs may occur alone or precede or accompany alopecia. Inflammatory and hormonal dermatoses, plus a wide range of systemic illness, can be associated with a poor haircoat. Nutritional factors are important influences in the health of the hair and skin. Similarly, intestinal parasitism interferes with absorption of nutrients and can cause a dry, dull, seborrheic haircoat and skin.

Pigmentary disturbances of hair rarely involve increased pigmentation (melanotrichia). Usually the problem is decreased pigmentation (leukotrichia). Hypopigmentation of hairs may be associated with inflammatory disorders, most commonly trauma, or an idiopathic or congenital problem. Causes of hypopigmentation include onchocerciasis, herpes coital exanthema, lupus erythematosus, ventral midline dermatitis and regressing viral papillomatosis, and pressure sores, freezing and burns. Leukotrichia also has been reported in horses at the site of nerve blocks performed with local anesthetics containing epinephrine. Quarter Horses with a cross-hatched pattern of white hair over the rump have a condition called reticulated leukotrichia. A similar condition develops as white spots over the rump and sides in Arabians.

Infertility in Mares

M. LeBlanc

Infertility in mares is a problem of the mare or with her management. Clients would like each mare to produce 1 foal each year for at least 20 years. However, stud farm management systems include an arbitrary breeding season, do not select mares because of their fertility and do not cull mares of poor fertility. This frustrates veterinarians, aggravates stud managers, and worries owners.

Obtaining an accurate breeding history can be the most useful aspect of the entire evaluation procedure. Yet this is often overlooked because of the difficulties involved in obtaining the information. The owner or agent often does not have the specific information necessary to define the problem.

Written records often are sketchy or nonexistent. Obtaining information that identifies the management practices causing infertility in the absence of physical causes in mares requires careful and persistent observation and questioning.

Most infertility problems of mares can be identified by asking the following 3 questions: Does the mare cycle? Does the mare cycle but fail to conceive? Does the mare cycle, become pregnant and then lose the pregnancy during the first 90 days of gestation?

The answers to these questions allow the veterinarian to categorize an infertile mare and establish a logical process for diagnosis.

The general aim of physical examination and review of the mare's previous breeding history is to determine if infertility is caused by a problem of the mare or by poor management. The examination includes evaluation of the external genitalia, vaginoscopic examination, palpation of the internal genitalia per rectum, and bacterial, cytologic and histologic examination of the endometrium. Ultrasonography, hysteroscopy, endocrinologic analyses and leukocyte karyotyping may also be helpful.

The most probable and frustrating cause of infertility is bacterial or fungal endometritis due to incompetent uterine defense mechanisms. Mares in this category usually are over 12 years of age, frequently have negative bacterial cultures, have variable uterine cytologic results before breeding, and demonstrate signs of acute inflammation 4-7 days after breeding. Many mares in this category have shortened interestrus intervals following breeding. Anatomic defects, poor conformation, urine pooling or rectovaginal fistulae contribute to the problem and require correction.

Pyometra occasionally occurs in mares. Affected mares continue to cycle, though irregularities in cycle length are common.

Mares that ovulate but do not become pregnant and lack clinical signs of inflammation may have intraluminal uterine adhesions, oviductal adhesions, a uterine tumor or endometrial atrophy.

Some horses presented for infertility are actually pregnant. Pregnancy can be difficult to confirm by rectal palpation at 6-9 months of gestation, but transabdominal ultrasonography may help locate a fetus.

If the mare is not pregnant, the ovarian structures and uterine and cervical status should be thoroughly evaluated. Particular attention should be paid to the season and sexual behavior, as most mares do not cycle due to seasonal influences, behavioral abnormalities or cyclic irregularities.

Early embryonic death may be caused by infectious (endometritis) or noninfectious causes (uterine glandular failure, embryonic defects, cervical incompetence or progesterone deficiencies). A complete examination, including uterine culture, cytologic examination and biopsy, is performed on these mares. With suspected progesterone deficiency, genital examinations show no abnormalities. In older, previously fertile mares with normal reproductive tracts, early embryonic death may be due to embryonic defects.

In summary, an accurate, detailed history of the reproductive status of the mare and complete examination of the reproductive tract can provide answers to the physical causes of infertility. Many cases of infertility are due solely to poor management. By observing and improving teasing practices, breeding techniques and record keeping, many of these problems can be solved.

Infertility in Stallions

D.D. Varner

Clients often request evaluation of a stallion's reproductive capabilities because an injury occurred during breeding or a fertility determination must be made. Acute breeding injuries generally require prompt emergency therapy. Therefore, the duration and severity of injuries are critical pieces of information to be obtained when the client first contacts the veterinarian.

Clients usually request fertility evaluation because a stallion has failed to settle mares, because a young stallion is being considered for use as a sire, or because the stallion is being considered for purchase as a sire. Though economic considerations may make fertility evaluation urgent, such evaluations are not emergencies despite the concerns occasionally expressed by clients. Time and careful preparation are important to permit a thorough evaluation that will identify any problems. An explanation to the client of the nature of the examination to be performed and its goals and limitations helps ensure cooperation and ultimately satisfaction with the service given.

A thorough history often provides insight into underlying problems. The horse's physical condition is critical information and should not be ignored. The veterinarian is responsible for the accuracy of this information, and this is important if sale of the stallion is pending. Physical examination entails assessment of general body functions, in addition to inspection and evaluation of the genital tract, as systemic ailments may have deleterious effects on reproductive function.

Infertility in stallions has many causes, and diagnostic plans, prognostic considerations and remedial procedures vary. Consequently, some of the more common disorders of the stallion genital tract that can lead to infertility should be kept foremost in the veterinarian's mind.

The external genitalia are fairly unprotected against traumatic injury. Breeding accidents account for a large percentage of these traumatic incidents. Progressive edema, contusions, hematomas and lacerations are the most common lesions; these should be regarded as emergencies.

Differential diagnoses for scrotal swelling may include such ailments as scrotal dermatitis, infectious orchitis, testicular neoplasia, periorchitis, hydrocele or inguinal herniation and torsion of a spermatic cord. Swelling of the prepuce or penis often is attributed to space-occupying lesions, such as skin tumors, sarcoids or cutaneous habronemiasis. Systemic diseases (equine viral arteritis and equine infectious anemia) also can produce edematous swelling of the preputial and scrotal areas. The diagnostic approach and therapeutic considerations for each of these conditions are discussed in other chapters of this book.

One must be cautious when judging semen quality, as it is influenced by handling procedures in the laboratory as well as semen characteristics inherent to that stallion. Some abnormalities of semen, such as contamination with blood, urine or purulent material, can easily be detected by gross evaluation of the ejaculate. Less conspicuous contamination or other aberrations, such as abnormal spermatozoal motility or morphology and oligospermia or azoospermia, require microscopic techniques or other laboratory procedures for proper diagnosis.

Because underlying causes of abnormal semen often remain unidentified, even after exhaustive studies, it is important to communicate this difficulty to the client early on. The permanence of reduced semen quality can usually be determined only by serial collection of ejaculates at 2-month intervals for comparative analysis. An accurate account of any pertinent history also may disclose meaningful information regarding prognosis for attaining or restoring normal fertility. Any identifiable underlying abnormalities should be suitably treated, when applicable, to prevent progressive deterioration of semen quality. Idiopathic conditions are presently not considered treatable.

Abnormal sexual behavior can have many contributing factors, including inherent or induced libido deficiencies, excessive sexual aggression, erection failure, ejaculatory failure, or mounting or intromission difficulties. A detailed history and a systematic evaluation of the stallion before and during sexual stimulation are required to distinguish these abnormalities. Possible treatments for the various ailments are quite diverse and include use of psychotropic drugs, hormonal therapy or controlled exercise.

Several microorganisms, including bacteria, protozoa and viruses, can be transmitted venereally in horses. Some of these organisms produce overt clinical signs in affected stallions whereas others are transmitted venereally by stallions that remain asymptomatic carriers. Therapeutic and regulatory considerations for these diseases vary and may require involvement of state or federal agencies.

Lameness and Gait Abnormalities

G.D. Muir and P.T. Colahan

When a client seeks veterinary assistance because a horse is lame or has difficulty moving, the underlying cause of the problem can range from a minor sprain to a fractured bone. The site, severity and mechanisms of locomotor abnormalities are varied, and the clinical signs and the client's perception of the problem add to the diagnostic challenge. It is the veterinarian's task to identify the cause and to initiate therapy.

The task at hand is facilitated if the veterinarian uses a logical routine approach and uses all of the diagnostic tools available. A genuine desire to help the horse and the client, a willingness to communicate with the client, and the ability to handle the horse are prerequisites to successful management.

This ability to communicate begins with the initial telephone conversation. Emergency situations must be distinguished from routine problems. If the horse refuses to use the affected limb or limbs, the animal should be attended to immediately. Generally this situation arises if the horse has sustained a fracture to a weightbearing bone or has an infection involving a synovial structure. Because numerous problems can cause signs of severe pain, carefully considered questions should include: Why do you think the leg is broken? Is the limb deformed and, if so, what does it look like? Is the horse standing on the limb? How is the horse holding the limb? Is there any area of the limb that is particularly swollen? Is there blood loss?

Most horses with acute severe injuries of a limb require immobilization of the injured limb as soon as possible to reduce pain and prevent further injury. With simple instructions, many clients can apply a Robert Jones bandage to the affected limb, assuming bandage material is available and the horse will tolerate the bandage. The client also may be able to calm and restrain the animal. At a minimum, the client should be instructed to confine the animal to a stall. This will save the veterinarian time and prevent further delay in initiation of emergency treatment.

Lameness is not a disease in itself but rather is only a sign of underlying disease. It is best defined broadly as abnormal locomotion caused by pain originating in and/or dysfunction of the nervous, musculoskeletal or cardiovascular systems involved in locomotion. For example, lameness due to a fracture of a long bone involves both pain and loss of the mechanical ability to support weight on a limb. Conversely, a neuroma causes lameness due to pain.

Presumably, the normal locomotor patterns of a horse are those that require the least expenditure of energy. Consequently, when a horse moves, movement of its center of mass reflects this minimal expenditure of energy. However, when a mechanical abnormality affects a limb, such as fibrosis and contracture of muscles, arthrodesis of a joint and loss of proprioception or motor nerve function, movement of the horse's center of mass is less efficient. Lameness due to such mechanical factors is the result of attempts of the normally functioning portions of the locomotor system to maintain normal movement of the body's center of mass and thus minimize the energy expenditure, despite the mechanical restriction.

A focus of pain in a limb overrides the body's natural tendency to move efficiently. Lameness from pain is a manifestation of the body's attempt to minimize pain, rather than to minimize expenditure of energy. Thus, horses with locomotor pain do not move efficiently and may tire far more easily than a horse that is lame primarily due to a mechanical dysfunction.

Horses with locomotor pain may reduce or eliminate motion within the affected limb during either the stance phase or swing phase of the stride. Specific changes in limb motion depend upon the source and location of the pain. For example, a joint that is painful during flexion may be held in extension through as much of the limb cycle as is possible. It is this type of compensatory movement that accounts for the alterations in the length of the cranial and caudal phases of the stride and in the foot flight patterns discussed in the literature.

Alternatively, the horse can minimize the pain in a limb by reducing the impulse (total force in the limb during the periods of weightbearing) acting through the limb. This reduction in impulse can be achieved by reducing the velocity of movement. This reduction in velocity reduces the force acting through all of the limbs, including the painful limb. The horse also can reduce the time spent bearing weight on the painful limb and increase the weightbearing responsibilities of the other limbs. This is accomplished by shortening the stance phase of the painful limb and by altering the timing of the other limbs such that at least 1 sound limb shares the weightbearing duties with the painful limb.

The horse also may reduce the impulse of a painful limb by shifting the body's center of mass away from the limb during the stance phase. This reduces the force acting through the painful limb and increases the force acting through the sound limbs. This shift in the body's center of mass is accomplished by altering the normal movements of the head and neck. The weight of the head and neck, which represent approximately 10% of the total body mass, is a powerful lever that can alter the position of the center of mass. The familiar "head nod" of a trotting horse with a painful forelimb is an excellent example of this maneuver. Raising the head and neck during the stance phase of the painful forelimb shifts the center of mass caudally so that less force acts through that forelimb and more through the rear limb. Similarly, a trotting horse with a painful rear limb may drop the head during the stance phase of that limb to move the body's center of mass cranially. This increases the force acting through the forelimb and reduces the force acting through the painful rear limb.

Because some locomotor abnormalities are caused by both pain and dysfunction, horses with these problems use the above maneuvers simultaneously. Consequently, these horses move in a manner that minimizes the pain caused by movement and that also attempts to minimize the expenditure of energy. It must be realized, however, that these compensatory changes vary with different causes. With future locomotion and lameness research, we will be able to improve our understanding and diagnosis of lameness significantly over that possible with current clinical techniques.

Lumps and Bumps

D.E. Bevier

Lumps and bumps involving the skin can range from many small, transient papules or pustules that quickly become crusts, to a single nodule or tumor. As with most other dermatologic problems, it is seldom necessary for the horse to be seen on an emergency basis. In fact, in most cases, it is preferable that the client be instructed not to medicate the lesions for 5-7 days before the veterinarian's examination. If, however, there is a large amount of discharge associated with the lesions, the client may clean the area with warm water and mild soap. Clients should be advised to wear rubber gloves when cleaning the affected area and should be advised never to squeeze a lesion, as some infectious diseases, such as sporotrichosis, have zoonotic potential. It also is important to emphasize to the client that it is possible to spread the disease to other horses if tack and grooming equipment are shared among animals.

Because clients rarely are satisfied with a "nothing to worry about" answer regarding the cause of these lesions, historical information and characteristics of the lesions must be critically evaluated to develop a logical diagnostic and therapeutic plan. The most important questions to consider are: Are the lesions multiple or solitary? How long have the lesions been present? How quickly did the lesions become apparent? Are the lesions pruritic or painful? Is there discharge, crusting or hair loss associated with the lesions? Has this animal had a similar problem in the past? Are there any signs of systemic illness or lameness associated with the skin disease? Are any other animals affected?

Though the client may indicate that there is a single lesion, the horse should be examined thoroughly for other lesions and the findings of the physical examination compared with the information obtained previously from the client. Because certain nodular skin diseases of horses tend to affect specific sites, the size and distribution of any lesions should be noted.

Though visual inspection of the lesion usually is the most important step in the diagnostic approach, certain ancillary aids are useful. Consequently, the veterinarian may wish to consider microscopic examination of hairs plucked from the region and suspended in mineral oil or potassium hydroxide, impression smears or needle aspirates. Depending on the nature of the lesion, cultures of samples taken from a cut surface of an aseptically prepared lesion may provide important information if the lesion has a bacterial or fungal cause. Finally, microscopic examination of excised tissue taken with a punch biopsy or by excision of the entire nodule may be diagnostic. The veterinarian must remember that nodular lesions may develop secondary to mosquito and stable fly bites, especially during warm weather. In some geographic locations, nodular collagenolytic granulomas, otherwise known as nodular necrobiosis or eosino-philic granulomas, are common findings and presumably occur as a hypersensitivity to insect bites.

Several neoplasms can cause cutaneous swellings. For instance, small hairless lesions around the muzzle of young horses are characteristic of papillomatosis. This condition may be enzootic on some breeding farms. In contrast, pigmented nonulcerated nodules near the vulva, anus or base of the tail in older gray horses are characteristic of melanomas. Sarcoids may occur either singly or in groups, often on the head, neck and thoracic limbs. Diagnosis of these common neoplasms depends on close visual inspection of the lesion and use of ancillary aids, where appropriate.

Malformations and Genetic Defects

I.G. Mayhew

Generally, clients contact the veterinarian as soon as a malformation is suspected, often when an affected foal is born. These malformations may be present at birth (congenital) or acquired during life. Congenital malformations are the result of defective *in-utero* development. Some congenital malformations, particularly those involving the neuromuscular, reproductive and hemolymphatic systems, may not be manifested until a particular period of postnatal development but are considered congenital malformations because the original defect was present at birth. It is estimated that 3-4% of all Thoroughbred foals have congenital malformations. Because any form of abnormal development reduces viability, live birth of monsters is unusual.

The client must be informed that all malformations are caused by genetic or environmental factors and particularly by the interactions between the genetic makeup of the individual and the environment. Thus, the abnormal phenotype is the result of an abnormal genotype, environmental insult or interaction between the genotype and environment.

Two important etiologic factors in malformations in all species are toxins and viruses that can cross the placental barrier. In horses, very few if any infectious agents consistently cause congenital malformations. This is particularly evident when one considers the many viral agents that produce malformations in cattle. Only a few toxic plants have been proven to cause malformations in horses. Cyclops foals can be produced when mares ingest *Veratrum eschscholtizii*. Arthrogrypotic foals can develop following ingestion of *Sorghum, Astragalus* or *Oxytropus* spp by pregnant mares. When attempting to unravel the cause of a particular malformation, it is important to consider the timing of embryologic development of the malformed part and the exposure to environmental insults. Thus, the timing of exposure of pregnant mares to Sudan grass is paramount in production of contracted foals.

Some of the more common congenital malformations and genetic defects are listed in Table 1. It is interesting to note that only a few of these malformations have been proven to be genetically caused. This must be considered when counselling a client about a foal with a malformation. Though a nongenetic cause may be suspected for a malformation, the best advice may be to avoid breeding the dam and sire again in the same environment. In this way, recurrence of malformations associated with environmental factors is avoided.

Finally, when one malformation is identified in a patient, it is wise to examine the animal thoroughly for malformations involving other systems. If multisystem anomalies are found, karyotyping to detect chromosomal abnormalities is more likely to be productive.

Nasal Discharge

P.T. Colahan

A horse with a nasal discharge is a cause of concern to clients. Often their concern stems from the obvious nature of nasal discharge, from the fact that it is readily observed, and from the associations people make with the nasal discharge in themselves when they have a common cold. Discharge from the nose may originate from several sites. For instance, it may come from the mucous membranes of the respiratory tract, or the mucous membranes, exocrine glands, and ingesta of the gastrointestinal tract. Alternatively, the discharge may originate from the blood vessels of the head, guttural pouches or peripharyngeal lymphoid tissue. Though a nasal discharge

Table 1. Common congenital malformations and genetic defects in horses. Malformations printed in *italics* have known genetic causes. (From Noden DM and De Lahunta A: *The Embryology of Domestic Animals.* Williams & Wilkins, Baltimore, 1985)

Affected Body System	Malformation
Cardiovascular system	Cardiac defects Major vessel anomalies Portosystemic shunts
Gastrointestinal system	Stenosis and atresia
Hemolymphatic system	*Hemophilia* *Combined immunodeficiency*
Skin	*Albinism* *Lethal white foal*
Musculoskeletal system Cranium/head	Cleft palate Parrot mouth Choanal atresia Cyclopia Wry nose (cranial scoliosis) Entropion
Limbs	*Arthrogryposis* *Contracted digital flexor tendons* *Multiple exostosis* Amelia, micromelia, meromelia Contracted foal
Trunk	Torticollis, kyphosis, scoliosis, lordosis Occipitoatlantoaxial malformation Hernias Cervical vertebral malformation
Nervous system	*Cerebellar hypoplasia* Hydrocephalus
Eyes	Myelodysplasia Microophthalmia Optic nerve hypoplasia
Respiratory system, pharynx	Branchial cyst
Urogenital system	*Intersex animals* Cryptorchidism Gonadal dysgenesis Partial agenesis of urinary tract

rarely indicates a life-threatening emergency, concern is warranted because nasal discharge frequently is a sign of a serious problem.

To determine the severity of the underlying problem via a telephone conversation, the nature and quantity of the discharge and presence of any other accompanying signs must be determined. The quantity and nature of nasal discharges vary tremendously, from copious to scant and from serous to purulent or hemorrhagic. Though the quantities and types of discharge vary greatly, signifying any of a large number of problems of varying severity, generally if the discharge is copious, purulent, hemorrhagic or malodorous, the underlying condition usually is severe. Accompanying signs of respiratory distress, ataxia, collapse or massive swelling of the nose or head also are characteristic of a serious condition.

Discharges that indicate an immediate and severe threat to the horse's life usually contain saliva, feed or large amounts of blood and are accompanied by other signs. Regurgitation of feed through the nose in horses with gastric dilatation is a serious sign of pending gastrorrhexis and requires immediate attention. Esophageal choke and guttural pouch mycosis are 2 other conditions that cause such nasal discharge. These should be considered critical emergencies. When the nasal discharge includes saliva and feed, esophageal choke or dysphagia must be considered high on the list of differential diagnoses. Under such circumstances, the client should be instructed immediately to remove all feed and water from the horse pending veterinary evaluation. If the nasal discharge is hemorrhagic and in large quantities, the only action a client can take is to attempt to keep the horse calm. If the horse is bleeding severely, a firm, clear warning should be given to the client concerning the frantic, violent and dangerous behavior of exsanguinating horses. If the discharge is hemorrhagic but in small amounts, the veterinarian should recognize the likely need for endoscopic examination of the nasal passages and turbinate region.

Most nasal discharge does not indicate an emergency condition. A slight amount of clear discharge from the nose may indicate nothing more than irritation of the mucous membranes caused by breathing cold or dusty air. When accompanied by fever or inappetence, this type of discharge may indicate an early viral upper respiratory infection. A mucopurulent to purulent discharge may signify a generalized viral infection of the mucous membranes, or drainage of pus from an abscess, an infected paranasal sinus, the guttural pouches or bacterial pneumonic lesions. A hemorrhagic discharge indicates injury to the head or respiratory tract, exercise-induced pulmonary hemorrhage, guttural pouch mycosis, ethmoid hematoma, nasal polyp, tumor or mycotic granuloma of the nasal or pharyngeal airway, among other conditions. Diagnosing the origin and cause of the discharge requires a complete history, detailed physical examination and judicious use of ancillary aids, such as radiography and endoscopy.

Abnormalities in Neonatal Foals

A.M. Koterba

When a telephone call is received regarding a neonatal foal that is "not acting normally," such complaints usually should be considered a true emergency, and priority placed on examining and treating the foal as soon as possible. Depending on the condition, a time delay of as little as 2 hours can mean the difference between success and failure.

Before travelling to see the foal, the veterinarian or receptionist should direct the owner or foal attendant to address certain important concerns. Thus, if the foal is down and thrashing, it should be placed in a clean, warm environment and manually restrained as necessary. In particular, the eye nearer the ground should be protected from injury. If entropion is present, the lower eyelids should be everted to avoid continued corneal irritation. If the foal's body temperature is <100 F, efforts should be made to raise the body temperature, using a warm environment, heat lamps, blankets and heating pads. If the foal is wet, it should be dried off.

With a newborn foal, the placenta should be saved for examination and possible bacterial culture and histopathologic examination. If the foal is not nursing well and the mare still has colostrum, the colostrum should be collected and saved in a clean container. The mare's udder should also be stripped out if it is distended and painful. An assessment should be made by the attendant of how effectively the foal is nursing.

While examining the neonate, a few general principles should be kept in mind. First, the early signs of neonatal disease usually are quite vague and may be manifested as decreased nursing vigor or reduced activity, and may be missed entirely if the foal is not observed closely by an experienced person. At this stage, though the clinical signs are relatively mild, hematologic and metabolic derangements may be marked. Unfortunately, the first indication of a problem may be acute collapse. Sick neonatal foals with a variety of diseases closely resemble one another on the basis of physical examination alone. Therefore, a diagnostic approach that includes hematologic examination, clinical chemistry profiles, acid-base determination, radiographs, serum immunoglobulin assessment, and bacterial cultures is highly recommended to more accurately identify the foal's problems. In addition, the failure of many foals to adapt properly after birth may be directly related to an abnormal uteroplacental environment or to adverse events at the time of parturition. Therefore, a detailed history should be obtained for the mare and the mare examined to identify risk factors that could have contributed to the foal's problems.

As compared to adult horses, neonatal foals can have rapid changes in clinical status and viability. Thus, the time allotted for decision making, monitoring and institution of therapy must be adjusted to allow for this difference. Seizures should be controlled as quickly as possible. Xylazine should be avoided in compromised neonates, because of its depressive effects on cardiopulmonary function. If infection is suspected, broad-spectrum antibiotic therapy for Gram-negative and Gram-positive bacteria should be started immediately, after appropriate samples (blood, synovium, spinal fluid, tracheal aspirate) for bacterial cultures are obtained.

Body temperature, respiratory rate and effort of breathing, mucous membrane color, heart rate, and fluid balance should be assessed quickly to establish the need for immediate intervention and stabilization. Assess the state of hydration (eyeball placement, skin turgor, urine output) and state of circulating volume (pulse quality, capil-

lary refill time, temperature of limbs). A foal with moderately to severely sunken eyeballs can be estimated to be 8-10% dehydrated (4-5 L water deficit in a 45-kg foal). Maintenance fluid requirements alone are estimated at 80-100 ml/kg/day in the absence of fluid deficits and increased fluid losses.

Blood glucose and acid-base status are very difficult to assess from physical examination only. The main clinical signs of hypoglycemia are weakness and depression; seizures are much less common. Severely hypoglycemic foals (<40 mg/dl) can remain remarkably active until they collapse, and even then they may continue to struggle. Therefore, in any weak neonate, the blood glucose level should be determined as quickly as possible so that appropriate fluid therapy can be chosen. Response to glucose infusion should also be monitored carefully by blood and urine glucose determinations. Mild to moderate metabolic acidosis resulting from poor perfusion often can be corrected entirely by replacement therapy using isotonic fluids, such as lactated Ringer's solution. However, foals with severe metabolic acidosis secondary to severe diarrhea may need to be maintained on a considerable amount of sodium bicarbonate to keep blood pH within an acceptable range until diarrhea abates. In these foals, base deficit or total CO_2 levels should be monitored closely.

The status of the passive transfer of maternally derived antibodies is of critical importance, regardless of the neonate's primary problem, as infection secondary to failure of passive transfer of maternally derived antibodies is a common, often insidious secondary complication to many neonatal conditions. The quality of colostrum provided to the foal should be assessed by determination of its color, stickiness and, preferably, specific gravity, using a colostrometer. The owner should be asked if the mare lactated prematurely and if the foal nursed effectively during the first (particularly the first 6) hours of life.

In every abnormal foal, regardless of the nursing history, serum IgG levels should be checked at 18-24 hours of age. When testing for immunoglobulin levels in neonatal foals, remember there is a considerable difference between an "adequate" level (≥400 mg/dl or "positive" on many rapid field tests) and "normal" (>800 mg/dl, the level attained by most normal foals). Though a serum IgG level of <400 mg/dl is a definite risk factor for septicemia, many septicemic foals have serum IgG levels of ≥400 mg/dl.

Always suspect infection in a neonatal foal that "just isn't right." Many infected foals have a normal body temperature, a normal total WBC count, and no localizing signs of infection even when blood cultures are positive. The most common early sign has been diarrhea, often overlooked initially. As most neonatal infections are due to Gram-negative bacteria (including *E coli, Actinobacillus* spp, *Klebsiella* spp), antibiotics should be administered at the first suspicion of sepsis. Any delay in institution of therapy frequently results in a poor outcome, most commonly because of subsequent septic shock or osteomyelitis.

If the foal is small for its gestational age or "dysmature," placental insufficiency, maternal illness or congenital abnormalities may be responsible. Also, degree of laxity or contracture of all 4 legs, development of the haircoat, softness of the pinnae, and flexibility of the joints should all be assessed to determine the maturity of the foal. If there was a premature (<320 days gestation) or postterm delivery, efforts should be made to identify a reason for it. In particular, consider the possibility of placental insufficiency, infection or maternal illness. If placentitis was present, the foal should be monitored closely for signs of pneumonia, uveitis or other infections acquired *in utero*, and failure of passive transfer, as chronic placental dysfunction and premature lactation of colostrum are strongly associated. Long-term complications in growth-retarded, premature foals have included chronic infections, angular limb deformities and failure to grow at a normal rate.

Many diseases occur at a specific age. Clinical signs relating to asphyxial insults at birth usually occur during the first 24 hours of age, though such foals can look very normal in the first several hours after birth. Foals with a ruptured bladder usually are presented on days 3-6 of life. Meconium impaction usually is a problem in the first 1-2 days. Various forms of sepsis in foals can occur at any time. Some affected foals may be abnormal at birth from an infection acquired *in utero*, while others appear normal for the first 1-2 days and then become acutely ill at 2-3 days of age.

Though somewhat dependent on the projected use of the animal, foals with severe, irreversible structural abnormalities usually are not considered for salvage. Examples of such defects include multiple, severe musculoskeletal contractures (arthrogryposis, contracted foal syndrome), cardiac malformations (tetralogy of Fallot, large ventricular septal defect), and incompletely developed gastrointestinal tracts (atresia coli, lethal white foals). It should be remembered, however, that a loud systolic murmur alone is not diagnostic of a cardiac malformation. Some foals with very crooked legs at birth can improve dramatically with time and proper support. Also, many congenital malformations and deformities are not a result of genetic defects.

If the support staff on a farm is experienced and committed to providing good nursing care, and if appropriate diagnostic facilities are available, many mildly to moderately ill foals can be successfully treated on the farm. When the foal is more compromised and in need of considerable supportive care, including continuous intravenous fluid therapy and oxygen insufflation, a more rational decision is to refer the foal to a clinic or referral hospital. The more sick or immature the foal, the more complications it usually develops during the course of treatment. A neonatal intensive-care facility often is better equipped to handle these problems and provide longer-term support. The referral center should not be considered a place of last resort; it is preferable to refer a foal early in the clinical course.

If the foal is to be referred, the method of transportation is extremely important to the outcome of the case. Body temperature, blood glucose levels and oxygenation must be maintained during the trip. In a severely compromised foal, glucose-containing fluids and oxygen insufflation may be required during travel. If hypothermia (body temperature <100 F) is a problem or if the foal cannot stand, every effort must be made to provide adequate warmth and restraint and to protect the foal from trauma by the mare. A warm station wagon is often a far better transport vehicle than a cold horse trailer or van.

Several important points should be remembered when evaluating an abnormal neonatal foal:

- *Mucous membranes of foals can appear icteric for many different reasons.* Neonatal isoerythrolysis is only one possibility. If a foal appears mildly icteric and is very weak but has a PCV >20%, a disease other than neonatal isoerythrolysis (particularly sepsis) may be involved.

- *Foals strain to urinate or develop a distended abdomen for many reasons* in addition to a ruptured bladder. There is no pathognomonic sign of a ruptured bladder. A careful diagnostic plan should be formulated to confirm the various possibilities.

- *Clinical signs relating to asphyxia or prematurity can be mild at birth* and for the first hours following delivery, but they usually worsen at 12-24 hours of age.

- *There are many different causes of seizures,* only one of which is "neonatal maladjustment syndrome." Electrolyte abnormalities, septicemia, meningitis and malformations are other common causes. These should be ruled out, if possible, before neonatal maladjustment syndrome is diagnosed.

- *Meconium impactions may be secondary to other disease,* such as the effects of asphyxia and enteritis, which presumably alter gastrointestinal motility.

- *Certain normal aspects of foal behavior often are considered abnormal by the inexperienced observer.* These normal activities include avid consumption of the mare's feces, rapid eye movement sleep, which may be confused with seizures, and sudden collapse while being tightly restrained.

- *A lame foal,* with or without swollen joints, *should be considered infected* until proven otherwise, unless a traumatic episode was clearly observed and associated with the onset of lameness.

- *Absence of pulmonary lesions cannot be confirmed by physical examination alone,* as lung auscultation can be very misleading. Adequacy of oxygenation cannot be assessed from examination of mucous membrane color. Cyanosis usually is not observed until the PaO_2 is <40 mm Hg. Signs of hypoxia can be as vague as restlessness, irritability and colicky behavior.

- *Parturition should never be induced on the basis of gestational age or owner convenience alone* if there is any concern at all about the viability of the foal. Regardless of clinical appearance, serum IgG levels should be checked at 18-24 hours of age in every foal born by induced parturition.

- In deciding on therapy, *evaluate the whole animal* and not just one specific problem.

Performance Problems

R.J. Rose

Apart from musculoskeletal disorders, problems relating to poor performance in athletic horses are among the most common encountered by veterinarians in equine practice. In some cases, the history may indicate that the horse's performance has always been inadequate. Such cases are seldom worth extensive investigation. However, the most common presenting history is reduced performance with or without signs of slow recovery from exercise.

While a common approach can be taken to investigation of performance problems, the variety of equine competitive events makes such an approach to assessment more difficult. Because many of the abnormalities that produce poor performance are quite subtle, it is necessary to obtain a data base from a range of diagnostic tests. Thus, it is important to explain to the client that to reach a diagnosis, a process of elimination must be worked through. Depending on the value of the horse and complexity of the problem, one or more diagnostic tests are necessary. I have found the following sequence useful in investigating performance problems in endurance horses, 3-day event horses, and Thoroughbred and Standardbred racehorses.

Important questions in the history include: How recently have the performance problems occurred? Does the horse make a respiratory noise or cough during exercise? Is there any history of lameness? Are there signs of respiratory distress after exercise? Is poor performance consistent or intermittent? Is the problem evident during training or only during competition or racing?

The importance of a complete physical examination is obvious. When evaluating a horse with poor performance, a few body systems are particularly important.

Cardiovascular System: Congenital or acquired heart abnormalities are important causes of poor performance in athletic horses. With some congenital conditions, such as interventricular septal defects, the murmur may not be detected until the horse goes through its first training and shows reduced stamina. Therefore, auscultation of the heart is very important to detect murmurs and rhythm disturbances, which are found with such conditions as atrial fibrillation. However, second-degree atrioventricular block, which is manifested during auscultation as regular dropping of a beat, is of no clinical significance.

Respiratory System: Viral respiratory diseases are a common cause of poor racing performance. Additionally, subclinical respiratory disease associated with various environmental allergens and irritants can cause significant lower airway and lung lesions. Therefore, the lung fields should be carefully auscultated, with and without a rebreathing bag, and the chest percussed. It also is important to palpate the muscular processes of the arytenoid cartilages to detect atrophy of the dorsal cricoarytenoid muscle. Such a finding could indicate laryngeal hemiplegia.

Musculoskeletal System: Obvious musculoskeletal disorders resulting in lameness clearly impair performance. However, subtle lamenesses may not be obvious to the trainer or owner, and such problems as hind limb lameness and back abnormalities may be very difficult to diagnose without a very detailed examination. Back problems are a common cause of poor performance in Standardbred trotters and pacers, eventing horses and show jumpers. In such cases, no signs of lameness or gait abnormalities may be evident.

Unfortunately, in many horses with poor performance, even a very detailed clinical examination does not reveal any abnormalities. Use of various diagnostic aids then becomes important, depending on equipment and facilities available. The sequence of investigation should begin with the simplest tests available and work through to the more complex, such as treadmill exercise testing.

Blood Assays: A complete blood count (CBC) and plasma or serum biochemical estimations are useful as a screening process. However, the limitations of hematologic and biochemical assays must be kept in perspective. Because of splenic erythrocyte release in response to fear or excitement, little information can be gained from red cell indices. In particular, unless a very low PCV (<25%) is present, poor performance cannot be attributed to anemia. Additionally, there are no distinctive changes in the CBC and serum biochemical levels that permit evaluation of fitness in response to training. To be most useful for monitoring health during training, a series of CBCs should be performed over several months, with the blood collected at the same time of day each week. Small changes then may be of more significance, as the normal range of values for the individual is much smaller than for the species.

Various common abnormalities in the CBC and serum biochemistry can result in poor performance. Increased WBC counts and serum fibrinogen levels indicate a subclinical infection. Common biochemical abnormalities associated with poor performance include elevated serum activity of muscle-derived enzymes (CPK, AST), electrolyte disturbances and liver disorders.

Electrocardiography: Conduction abnormalities in the hearts of performance horses are quite common. Such problems as paroxysmal atrial fibrillation appear to affect a number of racehorses and it is important that the electrocardiogram (ECG) be recorded as soon after the event as possible. While there is some debate about the significance of alterations in T-wave direction and polarity, abnormal T waves are associated with poor racing performance in racehorses and inadequate heart rate recoveries in endurance horses.

The ECG also is useful for determining the heart score. The heart score is the mean QRS duration in milliseconds in leads I, II and III of the ECG. It provides an indirect assessment of heart size and is directly correlated with racing performance. I have found that heart score provides some indication of performance potential in Standardbred and Thoroughbred racehorses, endurance and 3-day event horses.

Endoscopy and Bronchoalveolar Lavage: Various upper respiratory tract abnormalities will result in reduced performance in horses performing high-speed exercise. These may be assessed using a fiberoptic endoscope. With a scope of sufficient length, it is possible to view as far down the respiratory tract as the main bronchi. This sometimes is very useful to obtain lower respiratory tract cytologic samples using bronchoalveolar lavage. Lavage also can be performed without an endoscope. Abnormal cytologic findings may indicate that performance could be reduced due to suboptimal gas exchange.

Exercise Testing: Because many performance problems occur during exercise, it is often difficult to determine the cause using tests performed at rest. Under standardized testing conditions, the heart rate, blood lactate level, blood volume and electrocardiographic abnormalities can be determined. This is most easily performed using high-speed treadmills, which allow blood to be collected during an incremental speed exercise test. Additionally, the relationship between heart rate and speed can be examined. This allows determination of derived values, such as speed at a heart rate of 200 bpm (V_{200}), speed at maximum heart rate (HRmax), and speed at which the blood lactate level reaches 4 mmol/L (V_{LA4}). The higher the speeds for each of these, the more fit the horse and more capable of good performance. Facilities for these tests are only available at specialized university centers, but such equipment will become more widely available in the next few years.

Assessment of poor performance is a complex and often time-consuming activity. In some cases, after extensive investigations including treadmill exercise testing, a precise diagnosis cannot be made. However, the steps delineated above are very useful in most cases for establishing a diagnosis and planning rational therapy.

Recumbency or Inability To Rise

S.L. Green

One of the most distressing problems encountered by a horse owner is an animal's apparent inability to rise. Other parts of this book discuss specific questions to ask, immediate recommendations for the client, and suggestions about emergency veterinary care of the horse that has experienced repeated episodes of collapse or one that has lost consciousness. This section focuses on the recumbent horse or foal that remains unable to rise but does not necessarily suffer an alteration in consciousness.

Several important questions should be asked under these circumstances: When did the animal become recumbent and unable to rise? Are there any known traumatic incidents, previous illnesses in the affected animal or herdmates, exposure to potential toxins, intramuscular or intravascular injections or contributing factors, such as protracted exercise or a substantial increase in the environmental temperature and humidity? Such information enables the veterinarian to relay appropriate instructions over the telephone and to provide immediate care on arrival at the scene. Some early considerations and instructions are as follows:

- A recumbent horse can be dangerous, is often anxious, is sometimes in pain and may be struggling uncontrollably. Clients, especially children and novice horse owners, should be advised to keep clear of the horse. If, however, the animal is fairly quiet and is otherwise safe to approach, clients can be instructed to offer the horse small amounts of hay and water that may help calm the animal; this is provided that colic does not appear to be an associated problem.

- Clients should be instructed not to make any attempt to force the animal to move unless absolutely necessary. The goal is to keep the animal quiet until the veterinarian arrives. Deep bedding and strategically placed hay bales may prevent the animal from injuring itself and may provide support for an animal that is more comfortable in sternal recumbency.

- Clients should be advised to remove any tack from the recumbent horse. If it is necessary to control the animal's head so that rolling can be discouraged, this should be accomplished with a soft halter.

- Small foals that are thrashing can be restrained gently to prevent self-trauma. Recumbent neonatal foals, which may be hypothermic and are prone to hypoglycemia, should be kept warm and be bottle fed if a suckle reflex is present.

- If heat exhaustion is a consideration, perhaps contributed to by anhidrosis or exercise, shade should be provided and the animal sponged down with cool water.
- If the animal appears to be hypersensitive or is experiencing tetanic spasms, plugging its ears with cotton and eliminating loud noises may allow the animal to relax.

Upon arrival at the scene of the recumbent horse, attention should first be given to any emergency veterinary care required (see recommendations for Acute Collapse earlier in this chapter). Once the animal is stabilized, a thorough physical examination should be performed. Care should be taken to look for subtle abnormalities identifying an underlying disease as a complicating factor. A neurologic examination should be performed as indicated. Though sometimes multifactorial in origin, problems causing recumbency generally can be grouped into those producing spinal cord lesions and those producing neuromusculoskeletal lesions.

Trauma to the cervical and thoracolumbar spinal cord, especially injury to the atlantooccipital region, may render the animal recumbent. Cervical vertebral malformation (wobblers) or occipitoatlantoaxial malformation can produce signs of spinal cord disease. Often these signs are subtle and unrecognized by the client before an observed traumatic incident. When exacerbated by observed or supposed (unobserved) trauma, the syndrome renders the animal recumbent and the client ascribes recumbency to trauma rather than the malformation. The degrees of paresis and pain depend on the severity and location of the cervical lesion. Such an animal lying in lateral recumbency may or may not be able to lift its head off the ground or roll into a sternal position. Palpable or audible crepitus or obvious malalignment of the vertebrae is sometimes present. Fracture of the pelvis or an injury to the T3-L6 vertebrae may result in an animal that can "dog-sit" but is unable to stand. Occasionally such injuries are detectable by rectal palpation.

Inflammatory disorders involving the spinal cord, such as protozoal myelitis, vertebral osteomyelitis, bacterial meningitis, aberrant parasite migration and equine herpesvirus-1 myelitis, also may be associated with paralysis. Ingestion of toxic plants, such as sorghum, bracken fern (*Pteridium equalinum*) or horsetail (*Equisetum arvense*), is a rare cause of spinal cord disease that may result in recumbency.

Exertional rhabdomyolysis is one of the more common causes of recumbency that can be grouped in the general class of neuromusculoskeletal lesions. In addition, postanesthetic myoneuropathy, botulism, tetanus or white muscle disease can cause tetraplegia. Metabolic disorders, hypoglycemia and electrolyte derangements (hypocalcemia, hyponatremia, hypokalemia and hyperkalemia) may cause recumbency due to the associated generalized muscle weakness. These electrolyte disturbances usually are manifestations of an underlying problem, such as endotoxemia, sepsis and severe renal or liver disease.

Recumbency also may be associated with pain from colic, laminitis or musculoskeletal injuries. In some cases, debilitation and malnutrition should be considered. Based on the initial examination and a list of differential diagnoses, the diagnostic and therapeutic plan for the recumbent animal can then be approached accordingly.

Respiratory Noises and Difficulties

P.T. Colahan

Excessive or abnormal noise during respiration is caused by turbulent flow of air and/or vibration of fluid or tissue in response to air movement. Respiratory distress is caused by inadequate oxygen delivery to the body, particularly to the brain.

Because obstruction of the airway can be life threatening, a client's concern about a horse's making an abnormal respiratory noise and/or having difficulty breathing must be categorized quickly into emergency or nonemergency situations. To determine if the horse is in severe respiratory distress, appropriate questions should be asked regarding the horse's body position, mental state and respiratory rate, duration of respiratory distress, color of oral mucous membranes, and the presence, amount and nature of any nasal discharge.

Various conditions can cause obstruction of the airway or malfunction of the respiratory system of sufficient severity to be life threatening. In that the cause of the problem dictates the emergency therapy required and thus the drugs and equipment needed to treat the animal, it is important to establish the most likely cause of respiratory obstruction during the telephone conversation. Further, this must be done before the client is given any emergency instructions and before the veterinarian leaves to attend the horse. Life-threatening conditions include pneumothorax, pleuritis, pulmonary edema, obstruction of a main airway with blood, mucus or pus, crushing or collapse of the trachea or nasal passages, foreign body obstruction of the upper airway, and edema of the nose or upper airway. Consequently, appropriate questions should be asked to determine if there is a recent history of injury or snakebite, signs of preexisting or concomitant disease, such as pneumonia, or recent administration of drugs or exposure to toxins.

Once a clear picture of the horse's status and possible causes of the problem is established, instructions can be given to the client. It is advisable to caution clients to be very careful around horses in respiratory distress because the horse's behavior can be erratic, violent and very dangerous. First-aid instructions to the client generally are limited, as the appropriate therapy can only be determined by a veterinarian's physical examination and most effective therapies, such as tracheostomy or epinephrine injection, are only administered by a veterinarian. Usually little can be done by the client other than attempting to calm the horse and prevent it from injuring itself.

The general aims of emergency therapy are to establish a patent airway, reverse pulmonary dysfunctions, and increase the percentage of oxygen in inspired air. The specific procedures accomplishing these goals, such as tracheostomy, oxygen insufflation and drug therapies, are discussed elsewhere in this text.

Respiratory noises or difficulties that are not emergency situations usually involve reduced athletic performance or chronic respiratory diseases. Generally these problems require surgical intervention or prolonged medical therapy. The age and use of the horse determine the most probable cause of the problem. Young athletic horses usually make respiratory noises during exercise and have reduced exercise tolerance due to obstruction of the upper airway. The specific cause of the condition may be obvious on endoscopic examination or may require extensive examination, including observation during and evaluation after exercise. It must be remembered that endoscopic examination provides information about the upper airway under static conditions. Caution must be exercised to avoid immediately attributing the cause of the horse's reduced performance to any abnormality seen during endoscopy. Other methods in addition to endoscopy may be needed for diagnosis. Older horses not in athletic training most commonly develop respiratory distress with minimal noise as a result of chronic obstructive pulmonary disease.

Though the above generalizations tend to hold true, younger horses can certainly develop respiratory distress due to various pulmonary disorders and older horses can develop laryngeal hemiplegia and other obstructive upper respiratory diseases. Under some circumstances, signs of respiratory distress may be due to problems not involving the respiratory system. For instance, an increased respiratory rate may be due to pain or metabolic acidosis. The ultimate determination of any problem causing respiratory distress or noise requires use of all the tools of the diagnostician, including the history, physical examination and ancillary aids.

Excessive Salivation

P.T. Colahan

Clients infrequently seek veterinary assistance because a horse is salivating excessively. Generally they report that the horse is "slobbering" or "drooling." Under most circumstances, excessive salivation is accompanied by signs that help determine if the situation is an emergency. Consequently, careful or persistent questioning during the telephone conversation may be required to elicit these accompanying signs, particularly if they are subtle. For instance, a client may notice that a horse is drooling but not notice a small wound at the angle of the jaw where the horse was kicked and the jaw broken.

Excessive salivation is an emergency situation requiring immediate attention if the saliva is mixed with feed material or stomach contents and most of the saliva exits the nose rather than the mouth. Other emergency situations are if the saliva is accompanied by hemorrhage from the mouth, neurologic signs are also observed, or the horse or, more commonly, the foal is grinding its teeth. Feed in the saliva indicates esophageal obstruction. Gastric dilatation with pending gastric rupture is sometimes accompanied by regurgitation of stomach contents. Hemorrhage from the mouth may indicate trauma to the mouth with open fractures. Severe peripheral or central nervous system disease can interfere with swallowing and cause loss of saliva from the mouth. Grinding of the teeth usually is a sign of gastrointestinal ulceration, especially in foals. Such serious problems have possibly fatal implications for the horse and, in the case of some neurologic problems, such as rabies, serious implications for exposed people as well.

Drooling or loss of saliva from the mouth can occur because excessive saliva is produced in response to irritation or infection of the mucous membranes. Vesicular diseases and ingestion of feed contaminated with caustic agents cause irritation of the mouth and excessive salivation. The pain and edema accompanying such diseases interfere with function of the tongue and with swallowing; this causes the saliva to drool from the mouth.

Mechanical irritation by foreign bodies, such as plant awns, wooden splinters or metal wires, also cause pain and inflammation but of a more localized nature. However, the effect is similar to that of generalized irritation. Loss of saliva from the mouth may be particularly evident if a foreign body is embedded in the tongue, not only because the mouth is irritated and saliva production is increased, but also because function of the tongue may be nearly lost. Though sharp dental points also cause oral irritation, slobbering occurs while the horse is eating because irritation is greatest during mastication. Often the saliva is mixed with food and the client reports that the horse is "quidding." Continual slobbering occurs with minimal oral irritation when a stick or other foreign body becomes wedged between adjacent teeth or between the upper arcades of teeth across the palate.

Dysphagia and excessive salivation may occur when the hyoid bone is fractured or infected, or the temporohyoid articulation is arthritic and saliva cannot be effectively swallowed. Fractures of the jaw also can prevent deglutition. Most horses with maxillary or mandibular fractures have bleeding into the mouth as well as salivation.

When a thorough physical examination reveals neurologic signs, several neurologic disorders that interfere with swallowing and cause drooling must be considered. These include botulism, hepatoencephalopathy, yellow star thistle poisoning, and rabies and other encephalitides. Distinguishing the cause of the problem in these cases requires a careful neurologic examination. When the signs originate because of dysfunction of cranial nerves V, VII and XII, drooling only saliva can be the primary sign. If feed material also is regurgitated and most of the discharge is from the nose rather than the mouth, cranial nerves IX and X more likely are involved.

Some esophageal and gastric disorders cause severe drooling. Typically the drooling is accompanied by grinding of the teeth. The most common disorders causing this are gastric or duodenal ulcers and esophageal erosions due to gastric reflux secondary to a gastric outflow problem. These are uniformly serious problems with guarded prognoses.

Scratching and Rubbing

D.E. Bevier

When a client contacts a veterinarian because a horse is pruritic, it generally is because the horse is making a spectacle of itself by rolling on the ground, scratching itself behind the ear with a hind foot, nibbling its fetlock region, or rubbing against a fence hard enough to bend or break the fence. Alternatively, the client may report that the horse constantly swishes its tail, twitches its skin or rubs against the client. Generally there is a great deal of variability in the client's tolerance of these responses to pruritus. Some clients may find any signs attributable to pruritus unacceptable, whereas other clients, especially those in temperate regions, expect and accept a certain amount of skin disease in their horses. Even so, a severely affected horse may become nervous, anxious and unfit for riding or working. If the condition is ignored, these horses may develop a rattail or rubbed-off mane. Consequently, something must be done to diagnose the cause and develop a rational therapeutic plan.

In most instances, the horse's responses to pruritus are troublesome but seldom constitute a true emergency. Exceptions to this include acute urticaria and toxic epidermal necrolysis. Urticaria is important, as this condition may progress to angioedema and compromise respiratory function. Because toxic epidermal necrolysis, characterized by a fever and exfoliative dermatitis, may be associated with administration of certain drugs, the veterinarian must be aware of any recent or current drug administration.

Use of a standardized history questionnaire is invaluable as a diagnostic aid in horses with dermatologic problems. The most important questions to ask include: Is the problem seasonal? Is more than 1 horse affected? Is the problem localized or does it involve the entire body? Was pruritus the first abnormality noticed? How severe is the pruritus (intermittent or constant)? Have any treatments been given? If so, what was the response?

These questions can be asked by an assistant during the initial telephone contact. Under most circumstances, once it has become apparent that the primary problem involves the animal's skin, it is important to request that the client not bathe or medicate the horse for several days before the veterinarian's visit. If the horse is extremely pruritic, however, it may be necessary for the client to prevent the horse from further self-trauma. This can be accomplished by soaking the affected horse with cool water with or without colloidal oatmeal (Aveeno) or by applying a light blanket. If the horse is pastured and rubs against trees, it may be helpful to move the horse into a stall until the veterinarian can examine the horse and its environment.

Before examining the animal, the veterinarian should review the pertinent history and consider carefully the season of the year. Because some pruritic skin diseases require histologic examination of skin biopsies or skin scrapings for diagnosis, the necessary instruments should be available at the time of the initial examination. Generally the cause for the pruritus is either allergic or parasitic, or a bacterial, fungal or seborrheic dermatosis. In most instances, horses with allergic and parasitic dermatoses are moderately to severely pruritic. The

degree of pruritus is variable for bacterial, fungal and seborrheic dermatoses.

One of the initial aims of the examination should be to determine the pattern of distribution of the lesions and to determine if specific regions of the body are primarily affected. On examination, the most obvious lesions are caused by self-trauma. To determine if primary lesions, such as papules, pustules, bullae or wheals, are present, it often is necessary to clip the hair from an area adjacent to one of the traumatized regions. This area then is examined closely for lesions with a hand lens, if necessary. Though various diagnostic tests and laboratory procedures may be used to assess a dermatologic problem, the diagnostic procedures used most commonly in evaluation of a horse with pruritus are skin scrapings, impression smears, intradermal skin testing, acetate tape preparations, skin biopsy, and bacterial or fungal cultures. The rationale for use of each of these procedures is discussed in the chapter on Diseases of the Skin.

Rarely, neurologic disorders cause pruritus and even self-mutilation. Three such examples are rabies, polyneuritis equi and self-mutilation syndrome. These diseases are discussed in the chapter on Diseases of the Nervous System.

Straining or Tenesmus

A.M. Merritt

Conditions that can cause a horse to "strain" (show tenesmus) most often involve the gastrointestinal, urinary, genital or nervous systems. In general, tenesmus is not a common clinical sign in horses, especially in adults. Consequently, it is important to have the client identify the age and gender of the animal and describe the clinical signs as thoroughly as possible. If a mare is affected, the client should be asked if the mare is in estrus or due to foal. If there is any question about the client's ability to distinguish abnormal from normal behavior, these animals should be seen as emergencies. Because of the particular body systems likely to be involved, it is best not to suggest to the client any potential methods of emergency therapy.

Neonatal foals with meconium impaction or a ruptured bladder sometimes adopt a rather characteristic "sawhorse" stance and strain. An experienced client readily recognizes the problem and can provide the historical information required for diagnosis. Because of the chance of traumatizing the foal's rectum, the client should be instructed not to administer enemas to foals with suspected meconium impaction. In either condition, a complete physical examination is necessary. If a ruptured bladder is suspected, measurement of serum sodium, chloride and potassium concentrations is indicated. If laboratory facilities are available to measure creatinine, the creatinine concentration in the peritoneal fluid of the foal with a ruptured bladder far exceeds that in the serum. Also, it should be remembered that most foals with a ruptured bladder are males 3-6 days of age. Other causes of straining are occasionally seen in foals. Older foals with severe colitis may strain while defecating. Idiopathic self-limiting tenesmus has been observed in 2- to 4-month-old foals.

The most common cause of straining in adult horses is parturition. Fortunately, the incidence of dystocia is <4% of all deliveries. Consequently, it is important for the attending veterinarian to be aware of the characteristics of the 3 stages of parturition, to be able to identify and correct fetal abnormalities causing dystocia, and to identify and respond to premature separation of the chorioallantoic membrane.

Aside from parturition, the most common cause of tenesmus in adult horses is cystic calculi. A careful rectal examination performed immediately after the bladder has been drained should permit identification of the calculus. Endoscopy is the most direct method of confirming the condition. Cystitis due to sorghum grass or blister beetle intoxication causes dysuria and tenesmus. The vagina of nonpregnant mares should be examined for evidence of trauma or diffuse vaginitis. Straining occurs in horses with cauda equina syndrome caused by fractures of the sacral vertebrae or polyneuritis equi. In these cases, the straining is caused by accumulation of feces in the rectum and distal small colon, as well as urinary bladder distention. Loss of tail tone and perineal scalding due to urinary incontinence are strong indications of such problems. A thorough neurologic examination provides the information necessary for diagnosis.

Tetanus and intoxications with strychnine or bracken fern induce signs that resemble severe straining. A complete physical examination, evaluation of a detailed recent history, and examination of the environment permit identification of these causes.

Sudden Death

C.D. Buergelt

A healthy horse found dead in the stall or pasture is an unexpected event that is distressing to the owner and puzzling to the practitioner called to the scene. Though the cause of death may be discovered at necropsy, in some cases a thorough necropsy may yield no immediate explanation. "Sudden death" without premonitory signs should be distinguished from "found dead." The former term is applicable only when death has occurred in a closely observed and apparently healthy animal; the latter applies to an animal with clinical signs of disease before it was found dead. This section addresses management of sudden death cases.

Before beginning the necropsy, consider the circumstances surrounding the death. Initial attention should be given to the history and physical conditions of the horse. This information may indicate and ultimately confirm the immediate cause of death in a few typical situations. For example, an older breeding stallion, after his first services of mares in the spring, may collapse unexpectedly because of a ruptured aorta, with massive hemorrhage into the septal myocardium, pericardium or thoracic cavity, depending on the site of the typical triangular aortic transmural tear (see the chapter on Diseases of the Cardiovascular System).

Sudden death in a pregnant mare at term may be the result of massive hemorrhage from a ruptured middle uterine artery or a tear of the broad uterine ligament (see the chapter on Diseases of the Reproductive System). On the other hand, in each of these situations, the animal might have died from a ruptured alimentary viscus (see the chapter entitled Diseases of the Gastrointestinal System).

A third scenario might involve a young stallion with a history of rearing up when passing by the stable of an older stallion, only to fall over backward and strike its poll on the ground. This animal may die within minutes. At necropsy, one may expect to find basilar skull fractures (see the chapter on Diseases of the Nervous System).

An animal kept on an unfamiliar, slick stable floor may slip and/or rear up to fracture the pelvic bones, with bony fragments lacerating iliac vessels. Such an animal might have bled into the abdominal cavity. Staggering with sudden collapse immediately after an intravascular injection suggests intracarotid injection, resulting in a cerebrovascular accident (see the chapter on Diseases of the Nervous System). Identification of the carotid puncture site (fresh needle mark) may be difficult but should be attempted, in addition to careful dissection of the jugular groove and removal of both jugular veins and carotid arteries for analysis of the drug injected. The so-called anaphylactoid reaction (adverse drug reaction) should also be considered in this situation. Training and racing animals may die acutely of pulmonary hemorrhage (see the chapter on Diseases of the Respiratory System), abdominal hemorrhage, or ventricular fibrillation (see the chapter on Diseases of the Cardiovascular System).

Finally, prolonged serious disputes between management and farmhands may result in sudden loss of one or more horses, usually overnight, with resulting suspicion of intentional gunshot wounds or poisoning for malicious reasons. Outer tissue lacerations and hematomas of internal organs give a clue as to where any projectiles might be located. However, their retrieval may be difficult when they are lodged in bulky organ systems or within gut contents. Radiographs may help localize and retrieve projectiles, and may be indicated if legal action is expected.

The few examples mentioned above have good correlation between typical histories and typical causes of sudden death. Unfortunately, they usually constitute exceptions rather than the rule. More investigative work usually is necessary.

The immediate environment where the horse was found dead should be considered next. Investigation of environmental causes of sudden death should include the search for faulty wiring that could cause electrocution (the horse might have had prior contact with water from exercise pools or sponging down after training). The evaluation also should consider lightning strike in the field or barn after thunderstorms; such toxic plants as Japanese yew (often found in the mouth of dead horses); such animal toxins as blister beetles (cantharidin) or snakebites; organic or chemical toxins from feed, water supplies or containers; toxic fumes; erroneous inclusion of growth promotants in the feed, such as the ionophore monensin to which horses are particularly susceptible; and access to excessive carbohydrate-rich feed (grain overload). The appearance of the stable walls, bedding or pasture around the dead animal should be assessed for signs of blood or agonal thrashing. An undisturbed surrounding suggests instant demise without struggling, as with death from electrocution.

Following collation of historical information and clues from environmental inspection, the next approach should center on spontaneous internal injuries. This necessitates a complete, meticulous and objective necropsy. Regardless of whether the necropsy is done in the field or in a diagnostic laboratory, each body system should be examined carefully and with equal intensity, despite the likelihood that some systems may be involved more consistently than others. In this setting, the systems more frequently involved include the gastrointestinal tract (ruptured viscus), cardiovascular system (massive hemorrhage), respiratory system (hemorrhage, laceration, pneumothorax), and central nervous system (trauma, skull fractures).

Before opening the carcass, an astute prosector may obtain some valuable clues from a careful external examination. External observations should include: extent of rigor mortis; abnormal color of visible mucous membranes; foreign material in the oral cavity; blood and froth exiting the nostrils; swelling of the medial aspect of the thigh or distal extremities; skin abrasions over bony prominences; abdominal distention; singe marks on the skin on the medial aspect of the legs; small hemorrhages in the skin over the head and chest; watery material or blood exiting the oral, rectal or genital orifices; and unusual body odor or unusual odor from body cavities. Obvious internal injuries may be evident when the body cavities are exposed. All too often, however, no gross lesions are evident after careful examination of all organ systems.

Negative findings at necropsy should alter the strategy significantly in that these circumstances demand extensive tissue sampling for histopathologic and toxicologic analyses. Histopathologic examination could reveal indications for toxicoses (chemicals, plants), serum hepatitis (Theiler's disease), metabolic disturbances (lipidemias), viral encephalitides (Eastern encephalomyelitis, equine herpesvirus infection), exercise-induced pulmonary hemorrhage, shock and endotoxins. Negative histopathologic results necessitate toxicologic screening for potential lethal toxins. Modern toxicologic laboratories are well equipped to perform a variety of panels, but toxicologists initially rely on the clinician's and the pathologist's judgment on what toxins to screen for. Often the situation focuses on finding the "needle in the haystack" in that neither the pathologist nor the toxicologist has sufficient clues initially to know in which direction to go, other than to apply routine screening panels.

The situation may become complicated if foul play or malicious intent is suspected. Certain substances known to kill horses without struggling such as insulin, potassium, calcium, acetylcholine, succinylcholine and ricin, are difficult to discover, but toxicologic laboratories using modern techniques can detect many toxic compounds. Other substances, such as endotoxins, are virtually undetectable due to rapid decomposition in the tissues samples. Similarly, asphyxiation from a bag intentionally placed over the nose of a tranquilized horse is extremely difficult to confirm as a cause of death (no diagnostic criteria).

Maliciously used natural substances become "outdated" from time to time and no longer used when it becomes common knowledge that modern techniques can detect them. They may be replaced by other substances unknown (for a while) to the profession. In these circumstances, the toxicologic laboratory should be contacted to obtain updated information and to discuss the availability and costs of analytic methods, as well as the appropriate tissues to sample and how to ship tissue samples.

Despite extensive detective investigation into the cause of sudden death, some cases remain undiagnosed. Such negative findings may be acceptable to insurance companies. However, the reasons for such findings must be explained to all parties involved, especially the owners, so that they are assured that all detectable causes have been ruled out with a reasonable degree of certainty. The honest answer, "I do not know what killed the horse," ultimately may prevail and put the owner's suspicions to rest if everybody involved has been convinced that all possible avenues have been adequately explored.

Sweating Abnormalities

I.G. Mayhew

Production of too much or too little sweat with respect to the ambient environment is not commonly noted by a client in the absence of other problems. The single exception to this is the syndrome of anhidrosis, which occurs frequently in very hot and humid climates. Though excessive sweating is readily detectable by the client, the problem of too little sweating may only be evident because the horse has a rapid respiratory rate, performs poorly or fails to cool down adequately after exercise.

The consequences of excessive sweating can be profound with respect to alterations in blood electrolyte concentrations. This reflects the high salt content of equine sweat. In contrast, though the syndrome of anhidrosis may reflect a water and salt imbalance, the blood electrolyte concentrations are changed surprisingly little in horses with prominent anhidrosis.

Neurohormonal control of sweating in horses is not completely understood. However, for practical purposes, 2 major factors control sweating in horses: peripheral blood flow and concentration of circulating epinephrine. Peripheral blood flow, rather than cutaneous congestion, promotes sweating by exposing the sweat glands to circulating epinephrine. Thus, dilated vessels may indicate increased volume of blood within the cutaneous vasculature but do not necessarily indicate an increased volume of blood bathing the sweat glands per unit of time.

Excessive sweating is characterized by diffuse whole-body sweating, patchy sweating, or clearly demarcated focal sweating. Even with diffuse sweating, sweat production tends to be highest in the areas of skin that contain the greatest concentration of sweat glands. These areas include the skin around the ears and mane, and the skin of the brisket region, saddle region and groin. Excessive sweating is commonly caused by overexertion frequently precipitated and compounded by inadequate conditioning. Hyperhidrosis may occur before the onset of anhidrosis. Many diseases associated with elevated concentrations of circulating epinephrine, including stress and colic, as well as administration of various drugs, cause excessive sweating typically of a diffuse nature.

It is very difficult to determine what should be considered excessive patchy sweating. Often the skin on one side of a horse or of one quarter may produce more sweat than the rest of the body. Usually no explanation is evident. The effects of ambient breezes, air flow from an air conditioner or fan, or blocking of air circulation by a wall are given as possible but unproven causes.

Well-demarcated, focal areas of excessive sweating should immediately suggest either an alteration in local blood flow or, more frequently, a loss of sympathetic innervation (decentralization) of the affected skin. In either situation, the cutaneous vessels are more prominent and there is an increase in the warmth of the affected area. With severe spinal cord lesions, excessive sweating may occur on one or both sides of the body caudal to the lesion. Peripheral nerve lesions affecting nerves containing sympathetic fibers may result in strips or areas of excessive sweating. Horner's syndrome frequently is characterized by excessive sweating on the side of the head and neck down to the level of the second cervical vertebra, or C_2 (postganglionic lesion) or the level of C_2-C_3 (preganglionic lesion).

Too little sweating in a horse living in a cool climate usually occurs in conjunction with heat exhaustion or other systemic problems causing hypovolemia. One notable exception is grass sickness, a disease that occurs in certain areas of Europe. Affected horses with this autonomic neuropathy may be presented with excessive sweating, anhidrosis or patchy sweating. Though these alterations in sweating are quite variable, generally they are associated with signs of gastrointestinal dysfunction.

The syndrome of anhidrosis in a hot humid climate can be somewhat enigmatic in its earlier stages, as the clinical signs are similar to those associated with septic pleuropneumonia and chronic obstructive pulmonary disease. Differentiation of these 3 syndromes, which are usually characterized by an increased respiratory rate, is assisted by comparing the body temperature, pulse and respiratory rates and the degree of respiratory difficulty, as outlined in Table 2.

Specific neurologic diseases associated with excessive sweating, especially those associated with well-demarcated focal sweating, are discussed in the chapter on Diseases of the Nervous System. Anhidrosis is discussed in detail in the chapter on Diseases of the Skin.

Swellings

A.H. Parks

Swellings are encountered commonly in equine practice, as the sole cause for the client's concern or accompanied by other abnormalities. In most cases, swellings alone are seldom life threatening. If the ini-

Table 2. Typical changes occurring early in the course of pleuropneumonia, chronic obstructive pulmonary disease (COPD) and anhidrosis. 0 = no change. + = increased.

Disease	Temperature	Pulse Rate	Respiratory Rate	Respiratory Difficulty
Pleuropneumonia	+	+	+	0
COPD	0	0	+	+
Anhidrosis	+	0	+	0

tial contact with the client is by telephone, the veterinarian should first determine the site of the swelling and overall health of the horse; the presence of accompanying abnormalities determines the urgency of the call. If the client reports that the horse has difficulty breathing, has markedly enlarged limbs or head, or is nonweightbearing on a limb, the animal should be seen immediately. Otherwise the animal can be seen on a routine call. A more detailed history must be obtained and, following a routine physical examination, detailed inspection of the swelling(s) should be performed. This determines if the swellings are single or multiple, diffuse or localized, fluctuant or firm, inflamed, mobile, attached to underlying structures or excoriated. Following physical examination, swellings may be conveniently classified into 4 broad categories.

Usually all 4 limbs are involved in diffuse dependent swelling and there may or may not be involvement of the brisket and ventral abdomen. This pattern of edema results from disturbances of normal microvascular hemodynamics and tissue fluid pressures, namely, hypoproteinemia, increased capillary permeability, increased small vessel hydrostatic pressure and decreased lymphatic drainage.

The specific causes of such generalized edema in each of these categories are extremely diverse. Therefore, treatment, if feasible, is directed toward the primary condition. However, pressure wraps help control distal limb edema.

Swellings restricted to one part of the body (eg, 1 limb) yet diffusely involve that part may be caused by inflammatory or noninflammatory processes. If the cause is inflammation, examination of the area permits evaluation of heat and pain associated with the swelling and other clinical signs, such as lameness and fever.

The main distinction to be made for inflammatory swellings is between trauma and infection because both may have an acute onset accompanied by varying degrees of lameness. If the cause of swelling is trauma, palpation and manipulation of the area often pinpoint a specific source of pain or crepitus. Localized infection, or cellulitis, is more diffuse and may vary from mild to severe, with or without involvement of deeper structures. Pain, warmth and lameness vary from minor to severe. Crepitus may be present if an infection involves a gas-producing microorganism or if skin penetration has occurred. Systemic responses (eg, fever, increased WBC count) are more likely to be present with infection than trauma. The diagnosis of infection usually is based on physical examination findings and elimination of trauma as the cause.

Impairment of venous or lymphatic drainage from an area causes localized noninflammatory edematous swelling. A good example of this is facial edema following bilateral jugular vein thrombosis. Dependent edema also may be present in a distal limb or along the ventral trunk secondary to migration of edema fluid from an inflammatory process located more proximally or dorsally, respectively.

Localized fluctuant swellings generally are hematomas, seromas, abscesses, cysts or distended synovial sacs. Hematomas and seromas commonly are associated with a known history of trauma. Initially the inflammatory response may be intense but decreases fairly rapidly to leave a cool fluctuant swelling. In most instances, aspiration is inadvisable if a hematoma is suspected because of the risk of introducing infection. If the initial diagnosis is uncertain, a period of observation may help distinguish a hematoma or seroma from an abscess.

An abscess often runs a less acute course than a hematoma and the inflammatory response persists unless the abscess ruptures. Cysts are usually slowly enlarging, noninflammatory masses that are fluctuant and turgid.

Pathologic distention of a horse's joint, tendon sheath or bursa with synovial fluid may cause the client some concern, especially if the structure is not normally palpable. Aspiration of synovial fluid should be performed if sepsis is suspected. Hygroma, an accumulation of subcutaneous fluid generally caused by repeated trauma, also should be considered. Hygromas are most commonly seen on the dorsal aspect of the carpus and over the most prominent aspects of the calcaneus and olecranon.

All firm swellings require careful inspection to permit identification of defects in the integument and old scars. These swellings should be palpated for size, mobility in relation to underlying tissue, and evidence of inflammation. Generally these firm swellings are tumors, exuberant granulation tissue, fibrous tissue or osseous tissue.

Tumors may be localized or invasive, and attached or unattached to deeper structures. The skin may or may not be ulcerated and seldom is inflamed.

The distal aspects of the limbs of horses are particularly susceptible to formation of exuberant granulation tissue. A biopsy may be needed to distinguish this from habronemiasis, phycomycosis and sarcoids.

Dense fibrous tissue formed after trauma may be recognized by scar tissue on the surface of the integument. These firm swellings are seldom removed unless they interfere with adjacent soft tissues, such as tendons or ligaments. Swelling associated with chronic tendon strains and ligament sprains can be identified by palpation.

New bone formation may result in a firm osseous swelling, as in metacarpal/tarsal periostitis ("splint") or callus formation about a fracture site. Alternatively, a swelling may occur secondary to displacement or remodelling of bone, as occurs, for instance, with a maxillary sinus cyst or an enlarged dental alveolus.

The clinical relevance of most swellings can be ascertained from a good physical examination; however, definitive diagnosis often requires ancillary diagnostic aids, including radiography, ultrasonography, needle aspiration and biopsy.

Radiography of firm swellings associated with skeletal structures is advisable before more invasive procedures are considered. Such situations include swelling over a splint, sudden onset of severe synovial effusion in a joint, or mandibular swelling. Positive-contrast radiography medium injected into fluctuant swellings can help identify the structure if it is not otherwise apparent.

Ultrasonography can be used to identify normal soft tissue structures and the size, shape and composition of structures such as abscesses, hematomas and cysts. Ultrasonography also may be used to delineate sinus tracts.

Needle aspiration is a simple and inexpensive technique with few contraindications, as long as strict aseptic technique is observed. The diagnostic advantage of needle aspiration over a biopsy is that, by "fanning" the needle during aspiration, a larger volume of tissue can be sampled. Needle aspiration is most useful in identifying specific cell types (*eg*, mast cells or neoplastically transformed cells). Though false-negative results may be obtained, false positives in diagnosis of neoplasia are rare. Further, aspiration of fluctuant swellings may help differentiate hematomas, abscesses and cysts.

Several biopsy techniques are available. These include incisional wedge, excisional, punch and needle biopsies. The advantage of a biopsy is that the structural integrity of the tissue remains intact. Biopsies should include the full range of tissue, from normal to abnormal, at the site of the swelling. If this is not done, necrotic tissue or normal tissue may be sampled, resulting in either no diagnosis or an incorrect diagnosis.

Abnormalities of Urine and Urination

B.D. Brewer

Though abnormal urination is reported to equine practitioners quite often, these complaints frequently come from an inexperienced client who observes cloudy urine or the normal posturing of horses during urination, estrus or masturbation. The complaint also may relate to organ systems other than the urinary system. For example, a colicky horse may stretch repeatedly as if straining to urinate or may appear to look at its kidneys. Consequently, abnormal urination and production of abnormal urine should be considered as 2 separate issues.

Specific historical points are crucial to determine which diagnostic procedures and differential diagnoses are pertinent to each particular case. It is important to determine if previous disease could have resulted in renal failure or if environmental exposure to toxic plants (young, fast-growing sorghum or Sudan grass), blister beetle-contaminated alfalfa hay, or heavy metals has occurred. Similarly, it is important to determine if there is a history of previous administration of drugs or fluids, a history of trauma, or the presence of respiratory disease or abortion on the farm. Finally, one should learn if any attempts to perform an alcohol tail block have been made. The client should be questioned about other clinical signs accompanying the abnormal urination, as well as about any history of chronic colic. The type and quality of feed and water available to the animal should be noted.

A complete physical examination should be performed, with particular attention paid to rectal palpation of the bladder (for fullness and for calculi after voiding or catheterization), the ureters (which should not be palpable normally), and the pelvis and sacrum for abnormalities suggestive of traumatic injury. Patency of the urethra should be assessed via catheterization or endoscopy. In mares, vaginal examination should be performed to check for pneumovagina, urine pooling and perineal urine scalding. The prepuce and penis of male horses should be examined completely for external obstructions by smegma, neoplasia or habronemiasis. The horse may require sedation with xylazine or detomidine.

If no obstruction can be identified, a complete neurologic examination is indicated, emphasizing evaluation of function of the cranial nerves and first 3 sacral nerves. Cranial-nerve abnormalities often occur in conjunction with urination problems in horses with neuritis of the cauda equina. Hypotonia, hypalgesia, analgesia, hyperesthesia or hyporeflexia of the tail, anus or perineal region indicate sacrococcygeal neural involvement. Rectal dilatation and failure to pass feces also may be noted.

If abnormal urination takes the form of stranguria or dysuria, several processes deserve primary consideration, including colic, obstruction of the urinary tract, reproductive disorders, normal estrual behavior, cystitis (rarely primary in origin), blister beetle toxicosis and neurologic disease. If the major complaint is polyuria and polydipsia, differential diagnoses should include acute and chronic renal failure, endocrinopathies including pituitary adenomas, and psychogenic water drinking or salt eating. If incontinence is the major problem, neurologic diseases, alcohol epidural neural block and congenital malformations should be considered. If oliguria or anuria is present, particularly in foals, one should consider rupture of the bladder, urethra or urachus, urinary obstruction, renal failure, or shock and dehydration secondary to other serious diseases.

Common causes for production of abnormal urine include administration of drugs (phenothiazines and DMSO) or other substances (copper), access to toxic plants (red maple, wild onion or bracken fern), previous blood transfusion, equine infectious anemia, and strenuous exercise associated with rhabdomyolysis.

The client should be questioned concerning when, during the course of urination, the abnormal coloration appears. If hematuria is noted only at the beginning of urination, the problem is likely to be the lower urinary or reproductive tracts. If, however, the urine is uniformly bloody, the kidneys may be the source. If hematuria is evident only at the end of voiding, the bladder is the most likely source. If the urine was noticed to be discolored only after it was collected or seen (*eg,* in the snow), remember that equine urine commonly becomes red or brown in the presence of oxidizing agents.

Hematuria must be distinguished from myoglobinuria and hemoglobinuria. If hematuria is present, red blood cells are seen on microscopic examination and the supernatant should be clear after the urine has been centrifuged. It should be noted, however, that some red blood cells may lyse and release their hemoglobin. If hemoglobinuria or myoglobinuria is present, the urine does not clear when centrifuged. If the discoloration is due to hemoglobin, the animal's serum is likely to be discolored and the serum creatinine phosphokinase activity is within normal limits. When myoglobinuria is present, the serum is not discolored but the serum creatinine phosphokinase activity is markedly elevated. When the type of the pigmenturia is identified, a plan for further diagnostic workup can be formulated.

Progressive Weight Loss

A.M. Merritt

One of the more interesting diagnostic challenges in equine medicine is the horse that has progressive weight loss, especially if the animal does not have diarrhea. Age is an extremely important factor, as it has implications regarding parasites, neoplasia and various bacterial infections. Consequently, when the client first contacts the veterinarian's office with this complaint, the receptionist should obtain information about the animal's presenting clinical signs.

It might also be prudent to ask a few specific questions: What is being fed? How much? Has there been a change in the source or type of feed? Has the animal's appetite been the same, increased or decreased? Has the weight loss been rapid or slow? Is only 1 animal involved?

Once the veterinarian arrives on the farm, additional special historical questions *must* be asked regarding a horse with chronic weight loss. These questions can be posed while the affected animal is being examined: What is the deworming program? When were the horse's teeth examined last? Has there ever been any diarrhea or colic just before or after the weight loss was noticed? Has there been a noticeable increase in water intake or urine volume? Has there been any evidence of ventral edema?

A horse with progressive weight loss provides a perfect example of the critical importance of a systematic routine for clinical examination. If the same routine is not followed for every case, the diagnosis may be missed. Implicitly, therefore, the first step is a complete physical examination.

A complete, unhurried rectal examination is an absolute must in evaluating a horse with chronic weight loss. Animals that will not relax their rectum sufficiently may require treatment with 30-45 mg of propantheline bromide IV or 15 ml of 2% lidocaine in 45 ml of water instilled into the rectum. As with the rest of the physical examination, an established routine for performing the rectal examination is necessary to make sure all areas are examined.

With development of longer and more sophisticated endoscopic equipment, examination of the upper airway, esophagus and stomach is a diagnostic alternative available to many clinicians.

Often, however, careful evaluation does not reveal the cause of the problem and use of the clinical pathology laboratory is necessary. Rather than performing an exhaustive number of tests on every horse, the initial battery of laboratory tests should serve as a general guide to more involved diagnostic procedures. Initial assays should include: complete blood count, full serum chemistry panel, routine urinalysis, peritoneal fluid analysis, rectal examination for parasite eggs and blood, and fecal culture for *Salmonella, Yersinia* and *Campylobacter* spp.

Because these procedures are readily available to most practitioners, they should be performed initially in every horse with chronic weight loss unless they present an undue financial burden on the owner. An additional pertinent test that should be included in this initial survey is a carbohydrate absorption study. Either glucose or xylose may be used, with each carbohydrate having its own unique problems with regard to sensitivity. If the results of the physical examination and the initial serum chemistry panel suggest hepatic disease, measurement of serum bile acids, conjugated bilirubin and sorbitol dehydrogenase concentrations is indicated. If migrating strongyle larvae are suspected, serum protein electrophoresis is indicated.

Ultrasonographic examination of the thorax should be used to corroborate abnormal findings encountered on auscultation and percussion of the chest. Transabdominal and transrectal ultrasonography of the abdomen also is becoming accepted practice. For the latter, some degree of resolution must be sacrificed for the required depth of penetration, but intraabdominal abscesses and tumors can be imaged with diagnostic clarity.

If the history and physical examination findings suggest thoracic disease, thoracic radiography is indicated. Because of the bulk of the horse's abdomen, abdominal radiography generally is restricted to foals and young horses. Even with this restriction, techniques using plain films and special contrast procedures can yield important diagnostic information.

Percutaneous biopsy of the liver and kidney always should be considered for further diagnostic clarifications when the findings of other diagnostic tests warrant this approach. Though not a totally innocuous procedure, percutaneous biopsy is safe in experienced hands.

Finally, it must be remembered that some causes of chronic weight loss defy diagnosis after application of all of the previously discussed procedures. The client must be made aware of this possibility at the onset of the examination. In such situations and if the client's desire and finances permit, exploratory laparotomy may be indicated. Though a flank approach under local anesthesia on a standing animal is arguably less expensive for the client, it is far more restrictive with regard to palpation, visual inspection and biopsy. The alternative is a ventral midline celiotomy with the horse under general anesthesia.

In order of decreasing probability of involvement, systems to eliminate as the source of the chronic weight loss are: gastrointestinal, hepatic, cardiac, pulmonary, urogenital, nervous and reproductive.

Wounds

A.H. Parks

Managing wounds is an inevitable aspect of equine practice. Wounds elicit various responses from different clients, especially if the wound is accompanied by much hemorrhage; a little blood goes a long way. Large lacerations may appear much more daunting than small puncture wounds, yet they may be accompanied by less underlying damage. Thus, the initial telephone contact with the client should help determine the nature of the wound, indicate the urgency of the call, and suggest first-aid measures that the client should undertake immediately. Questions should be posed to determine the duration and site of the injury, extent of any hemorrhage, and any functional incapacity. It is also important to determine if the animal is sufficiently distressed or fractious to be dangerous. If so, the client should be advised first to ensure that handlers are not harmed.

If the wound involves the distal limbs, pressure wraps should be applied to control bleeding. One must emphasize the necessity for adequate padding to distribute the pressure. Hemorrhage elsewhere on the body may be controlled by direct pressure with a clean towel. Tourniquets are to be discouraged because they seldom are necessary and often are more deleterious than beneficial when used by inexperienced personnel. Bandaging or supporting skin flaps on fresh wounds helps preserve tissue viability by keeping the tissue warm and moist and minimizing further contamination. If the horse can be walked without further trauma, it should be moved to a well-lit stall if it is not already there.

All recent wounds benefit from rapid treatment, while old wounds causing little or no functional incapacity seldom warrant immediate attention. It is helpful to classify wounds into 3 broad categories to help formulate a diagnostic and therapeutic plan.

Incised Wounds: An example is a cut made by glass or sharp metal. Incised wounds often are not that painful initially, though hemorrhage may be profuse and important underlying structures often are transected.

Lacerations: A good example is a degloving injury of the metatarsal region. There is often loss of tissue, hemorrhage usually is only moderate, and underlying structures may or may not be damaged. Contamination often is substantial.

Puncture Wounds: The most common example is by a nail. Puncture wounds often are painful, hemorrhage usually is minimal, and the small entry wound often masks the extent of trauma to underlying structures. Contamination may be substantial.

Upon arriving at the farm, the veterinarian must take charge of the situation and the often-frantic client. A calm but assertive manner with the client and horse usually allows the severity of the wound to be assessed and an appropriate plan of therapy instituted with minimal delay. If necessary, a fractious or excited horse can be sedated. Xylazine, acepromazine or butorphanol is suitable alone or in combination for this purpose. Caution should be used if hypovolemia is suspected from severe hemorrhage, as tranquilizers may cause or potentiate hypotension. Ligation of major bleeding vessels is desirable, if possible. If there is unilateral involvement of a jugular vein or digital artery, the vessel usually may be ligated without permanent untoward effects. Regional anesthesia of the distal limb may be useful to reduce the pain of exploring the wound while locating the source of hemorrhage. If the vessel cannot be ligated, hemorrhage must be controlled by direct pressure.

After any immediately life-threatening crises are controlled, the veterinarian should perform a physical examination to determine the systemic status of the patient and examine the wound more thoroughly. It may be beneficial to sedate the animal at this stage. The margins of the wound should be clipped or shaved after a water-soluble gel (*eg,* K-Y Jelly) has been applied to the wound surface to prevent adherence of hair to the wound. Gross contamination should then be removed by lavage, preferably with a sterile dilute antimicrobial solution. Finally, the wound should be prepared aseptically before examination to determine the extent of injury and involvement of deeper structures. Exploration without adequate preparation of the skin wound may further contaminate the deeper portions of the wound. Flexible metal probes are useful to identify the depth and direction of small chronic sinuses but are best avoided or used with extreme caution in acute puncture wounds because they may readily disseminate local contamination.

Expression of a viscous amber fluid from the wound may indicate the involvement of a synovial structure; this may be confirmed by sterile irrigation of the synovial structure through a needle placed at a distant site. Radiography should be considered when the location of the wound or altered limb function suggests a fracture or sequestrum. Exploration of deep puncture wounds may require general anesthesia.

Finally, the veterinarian should devise a therapeutic plan with the aim to save the life of the patient, prevent infection, close the wound and correct functional deficits. Treatment of life-threatening complications, such as hemorrhage, are discussed in more detail under Bleeding earlier in this chapter. Tetanus prophylaxis should be provided in all cases unless there is a history of recent vaccination. Immediate use of antibacterials is prudent in all acute cases except minor abrasions. For clean wounds, procaine penicillin G usually is adequate, while broad-spectrum antibacterials are desirable when more serious contamination has occurred. The duration of antibacterial treatment should be determined by the response to treatment but should be maintained for a minimum of 3 days. Horses with acute wounds benefit from nonsteroidal antiinflammatory drugs that minimize the inflammatory response to the injury.

Particulate debris may be removed by lavage using sterile saline, 1% povidone-iodine in saline or 0.05% chlorhexidine in sterile water. Devitalized tissue, recognized by its abnormal color, absence of hemorrhage or evidence of desiccation, should be excised by sharp dissection. If doubt exists as to tissue viability, it is preferable to err on the side of caution by debriding less. Further debridement can be performed at a later date, if necessary.

A difficult decision regarding many wounds is whether to attempt primary closure. The following guidelines are useful indications for primary closure: tissue apposition is possible without excessive tension; the wound is <6-8 hours old; the wound is minimally contaminated and can be adequately debrided; and traumatized tissue can be removed *in toto* by wide excision.

Incised wounds that comply with all of the above criteria are good candidates for closure, as are lacerations with minimal tissue defects. Alternatively, lacerations with tissue deficits may be partially closed. Though puncture wounds usually have minimal tissue defects, contamination may be considerable. Therefore, closure of puncture wounds usually is contraindicated because lack of drainage potentiates the likelihood of cellulitis.

Closure should appose the tissue planes with the least quantity of buried suture material needed to reduce deadspace; drains are seldom required on the distal limbs. Preferably an absorbable monofilament material should be used. The skin may be sutured with simple-interrupted sutures, preferably of a monofilament nonabsorbable material, except where excessive tension exists. Vertical or horizontal mattress sutures or quill sutures are advisable in these instances. Wounds not sutured immediately may be treated by delayed closure or allowed to heal by secondary intention. These wounds should be protected with a nonadhesive dressing.

Referral to a hospital facility is necessary when restoration to normal function requires reconstructive surgery under general anesthesia (eg, severed flexor tendons) prolonged intensive care or casting (eg, laceration of a joint capsule or disruption of collateral ligaments) or with wounds that require extensive exploration and debridement (eg, deep puncture wounds, especially those to the thorax and abdomen. A wound causing instability of a limb requires immobilization by splinting or casting before transporting the patient so as to prevent further trauma. Clients should be advised that injuries of this nature may involve considerable expense.

This page is intentionally left blank.

2 Principles of Patient Evaluation and Diagnosis

R.J. Rose and J.D. Wright

One of the most commonly neglected procedures in veterinary medicine is the physical examination. The curricula at all colleges of veterinary medicine emphasize the importance of conducting a complete examination; however, the combination of time constraints and client pressure often leads to an incomplete physical examination being conducted by the veterinarian in practice. The old adage "when all else fails, do a clinical examination" certainly is a lesson that we all learn. Despite this, it is surprising how often aspects of the complete physical examination are forgotten or ignored. The important thing about the physical examination is that it should be complete. It often is tempting to stop the examination when a major problem tying in with the presenting history is discovered. However, the importance of always conducting a logical and sequential examination cannot be overemphasized. First, a data base of the range of normality for various body systems must be established. Second, a set of examination techniques must be adopted to avoid the possibility of overlooking an important problem.

The important steps in establishing an initial diagnosis are: recording the presenting complaint and establishing the history relating to the problem; undertaking a complete physical examination to localize the problem(s); establishing, in order of likelihood, a series of differential diagnoses; and undertaking any diagnostic tests, such as hematologic examination and plasma biochemical assays, that add further information to the clinical data base. Only after these basic diagnostic steps are taken should any therapy be commenced. Of course, specific emergencies, such as severe hemorrhage, shock and colic, warrant immediate intervention. However, even in these acute problems, the general principles of examination still should be followed through, once the initial therapy has been undertaken.

This chapter provides an overview of general patient evaluation, including the physical examination, and provides some general principles of diagnosis and therapy referable to the acute clinical problem. Additionally, mortality and insurance examination, physical restraint, anesthesia, and some principles of nutrition are covered. It is written with the general equine/mixed practitioner in mind. It is not assumed that specialized facilities and equipment, such as may be found at university teaching hospitals, are available.

HANDLING THE EMERGENCY CALL

A veterinary revision of Murphy's law states that if an emergency is going to happen, it is sure to occur after hours and particularly when the veterinarian is asleep. When such situations arise, it is important to give the client instructions that could help prevent further injury to the animal or that could be lifesaving. If a veterinarian is unavailable at the hospital, it is wise to have some specific information for a receptionist to give to clients.

51

This section is not meant to encompass all the possible emergencies that are likely to occur but rather to give a guide to providing instructions to the client who is waiting for the veterinarian to arrive.

Trauma

In many practices, the most common emergency calls relate to trauma. The first thing to establish by telephone is whether there is serious bleeding or not. Clients frequently are confused about the amount of blood lost and tend to overestimate the seriousness of blood loss. Rather than trying to get a client to estimate the amount of blood loss, it probably is better to find out the type of blood (bright red arterial blood or darker venous blood) and whether the blood is dripping or coming in a steady stream. Unless major arteries are cut, most horses will not bleed to death from common laceration sites. However, if it is clear that an artery has been cut, then it is important to have the client apply a clean pressure bandage over the area. If the wound is in a region that cannot be bandaged, directions can be given to apply digital pressure over the site using a clean towel. Tranquilizers must not be administered, as the phenothiazine derivatives (*eg*, acepromazine) all cause peripheral vasodilation, which will result in a serious decrease in blood pressure, particularly in a horse that has suffered serious blood loss and may be in shock. Further, make sure that instructions are given *not* to apply disinfectants to the wound, as they may irritate the tissues and compromise wound healing.

If the trauma may have caused a fracture and the horse cannot bear weight on the affected limb, the main consideration should be to prevent a simple fracture from becoming compound, with the bone protruding through the skin. This is most likely to happen with mid-shaft fractures of the third metacarpal bone, radius and tibia. Instructions should be given for the client to keep the horse still and protect the affected region of the limb by effective bandaging. This is done most easily using several cotton rolls to pad the limb and bandaging with an elastic bandage. Because splints may be applied improperly and may worsen the fracture in many cases, it is important that no attempt be made to move the horse until the veterinarian arrives and can immobilize the fracture more effectively.

Colic

Most horse owners are reasonably experienced at dealing with horses that show signs of colic. Advice usually can be given to keep the horse walking and to prevent it from rolling. Any attempt to drench the horse or to give such remedies as "Dr. Bell's Veterinary Wonder" should be discouraged. While waiting for the veterinarian to arrive, the client should note such signs as how frequently the attacks of pain occur and the duration of any abdominal distension.

PRESENTING CLINICAL SIGNS

Many factors may predispose a horse to disease. Diagnosis may be assisted by considering the horse's age, breed and sex, and purpose for which the horse is used. These factors may help eliminate specific diseases as differential diagnoses or at least reduce their likelihood as probable causes of the presenting clinical signs. The presenting clinical signs should alert the veterinarian to the most likely differential diagnoses. Before an unusual condition is diagnosed, remember that "common diseases occur commonly."

Age is of particular importance when evaluating a horse for skeletal disease. Certain conditions, such as septic arthritis involving multiple joints, osteochondrosis and angular limb deformities, are most common in young horses, whereas the incidence of degenerative joint disease increases with both age and degree of use. Age also is important in determining the extent and severity of various respiratory diseases. Infectious respiratory disease tends to be more severe in the neonatal and adolescent periods. This, when separated from specific immunologic factors and prior antigenic exposure, is thought to be related to reduced immunocompetence. In contrast, a condition such as chronic obstructive pulmonary disease is found principally in middle-aged horses that have had repeated exposure to specific allergens.

Though congestive heart failure is found most commonly in older horses, congenital heart disease may not manifest itself until the horse is worked. Thus, even with such conditions as interventricular septal defects, the problem may remain undetected until the horse is 2 years of age.

Age also has a significant impact on the incidence and type of gastrointestinal abnormalities. Gastric ulceration, pyloric stenosis and ascarid impaction must be considered carefully in foals with colic. Similarly, volvulus and intussusception of the small intestine occur more commonly in horses less than 3 years of age. Conversely, pedunculated lipomas and incarceration of intestine through the epiploic foramen are common causes of small intestinal obstruction in horses over 9 years of age. Gastric neoplasia, though uncommon, does occur in young horses.

Breed predilections exist for some conditions causing lameness. Bucked shins are common in young Thoroughbreds and Quarter Horses in training. Chip fractures of carpal bones also are diagnosed more frequently in Thoroughbreds and Quarter Horses than in Standardbreds. On the other hand, Standardbreds have a much higher incidence of hind limb lameness and fractures of the distal phalanx (pedal bone) than do Thoroughbreds or Quarter Horses. Quarter Horses appear to have a very high incidence of navicular disease, while Arabians tend to be less affected. In ponies, laminitis and upward fixation of the patella are more common than in other breeds. Breed also plays an important role in neurologic disease, with Thoroughbreds having a high incidence of cervical vertebral malformation (wobbler syndrome). Arabians have an assortment of familial and congenital problems, including cervical malformations and cerebellar degeneration.

Though few respiratory diseases are breed specific, combined immunodeficiency is found primarily in Arabian foals. Many of these foals are presented with signs of adenovirus pneumonia. Laryngeal hemiplegia is more common in Thoroughbreds than in other breeds and generally is noticed first between 2 and 3 years of age.

Sex of the horse is slightly less important in predisposing to disease. However, some conditions, such as inguinal hernias, obviously occur only in colts or stallions. In contrast, the hormonal changes associated with pregnancy and lactation may play a role in the onset of some diseases in mares.

The *use* of the horse is of major importance in determining the likelihood of various types of abnormalities. Clearly, this interacts with the horse's breed.

Finally, *management, husbandry and geography* play important roles in determining the types and incidence of disease. For example, postnatal respiratory infections are more common on stud farms where there is overcrowding. *Rhodococcus (Corynebacterium) equi* infections occur more commonly in certain geographic areas. This may be related to soil type, as infections are more common in foals kept on sandy soils.

THE HISTORY

Before any examination, a thorough and accurate history should be obtained. History taking is an important skill that must be developed. The ability to ask the right questions sometimes can be of great importance in guiding you to the ultimate diagnosis. It requires some practice and expertise to avoid asking leading questions to which the client may be tempted to give a positive (but incorrect) response. Misleading histories are very common, as many clients already have made a decision about their horse's problem before its presentation to the veterinarian.

History taking can be divided into 2 major components: past and recent. Both may be of equal importance in correct diagnosis and appropriate therapy. The *recent history* begins with a discussion of the presenting clinical signs and an assessment as to whether the problem is static, regressing or progressing. The detail and extent of the history collected depend upon the duration of the problem and need for any immediate therapy. For example, many details of the history have little relevance to the immediate treatment of a horse with severe colic and signs of shock.

Past history should commence with the history immediately before the onset of the problem and should include selective details from months to years previously, depending on the nature of the problem. Pertinent facts about the horse's appetite and history of weight gain or loss are important aspects relating to many different body systems.

While it is not possible to illustrate specific questions that should be asked with diseases of each system, we will typify history collection by discussing 3 common problems: gastrointestinal disease, lameness and respiratory disease.

Gastrointestinal Disease

Specific questions should determine the rapidity of onset and duration of the problem.

Special attention must be paid to descriptions of prior episodes of abdominal discomfort. Horses with verminous arteritis, enteroliths, intraabdominal adhesions or mesenteric abscesses often have recurrent episodes of abdominal pain. Information should be gained concerning the horse's appetite and fecal production and consistency, and if these functions are influenced by external factors, such as changes in exercise routine, housing or bedding.

In horses with gastrointestinal problems, an accurate history relating to internal parasite control is of major importance. The types and frequency of anthelmintic use should be documented carefully, together with any information on the efficacy of such treatment. Management and husbandry practices may lead to parasite-related disease. For example, overcrowding due to high stocking rates is often associated with parasite-related disease, especially if pasture conditions are poor.

Knowledge of the quality and type of pasture may aid diagnosis. Horses on coarse roughage, especially if the soil is sandy, may be prone to large-bowel impactions. Other questions relating to feed type should be asked, together with inquiries about changes in the amount of feed offered and tooth care.

Lameness

In musculoskeletal problems, an accurate history is of great assistance in eliminating some diagnostic possibilities. The history may help determine if the problem was associated with a single traumatic incident, specific activity (jumping, racing), or breeding. Questions should include: How recently was the horse shod? Were there any changes in the type of shoe? Has the horse received any medication and, if so, was there any improvement? Was the onset of the problem related to a particular period of exercise? Is lameness more obvious before, during or after exercise? Is lameness static or progressive? Is there any past history of lameness?

Respiratory Disease

In horses with respiratory disease, an accurate history may help differentiate upper respiratory from lower respiratory problems. Additionally, in functional upper respiratory diseases, history of the type, onset and progress of respiratory noise can be almost diagnostic. Of interest in history taking are: duration of signs; presence of nasal discharge; exercise tolerance; presence or absence and character of any cough; presence or absence of respiratory noise and its relationship to exercise intensity; and details of any vaccination program.

Environmental influences may exert a considerable effect on both the onset and course of respiratory disease. In particular, horses with chronic allergic respiratory disease show exacerbations and remissions, depending on their housing and/or the particular season. Other environmental considerations include exposure to other horses with respiratory disease (including strangles) and the possibility of the horse's grazing in company with donkeys, which may lead to lungworm infection.

The character of a cough, whether dry, moist, productive or nonproductive, can indicate the likelihood of pneumonia. If there is nasal discharge, the odor and character of the discharge, and whether it is unilateral or bilateral are important in establishing a diagnosis. Any recent history of transportation may be significant, as pneumonia and pleuritis occur more commonly after the stress of transportation.

Despite careful and detailed history collection, the information obtained should be viewed with healthy skepticism. It is common for conflicting details to be given when a second veterinarian questions the same client. It is also important to avoid using any veterinary jargon. A client may respond negatively when asked if the horse has received any medication but admit that it has "had bute and penicillin." Often it is worthwhile to confirm a particularly important piece of history later in the examination procedure by again asking the same question in a slightly different manner.

REFERRALS AND SECOND OPINIONS

One area that provides great potential for conflict between veterinarians is referral of cases or requests by the client for a second opinion. No criticism of a colleague should ever be made to a client. For referrals to work effectively, it is essential that good communication be established between the referring and consulting veterinarians.

Clients often take their horse to another veterinarian without consulting the first clinician. This can cause many problems because the clients usually are unaware of the full details of treatment and frequently provide a distorted view of the care their horse has received. In such circumstances, the second veterinarian should not be trapped into making statements that are detrimental to a colleague. Rather, as a matter of professional courtesy, the primary veterinarian should be telephoned and details of previous care sought. Clients obviously have the right to request a second opinion, and the first veterinarian should not be offended if a client seeks another opinion. The only reason to fear a client's seeking a second opinion is if the initial treatment was substandard.

The Referral Process

Whether the client requests the examination or the referral is initiated by the primary veterinarian, a series of steps should be followed. Initially, a colleague or an expert in the horse's particular problem at the referral clinic should be suggested to the client. A full written history should be supplied in the referral letter, as well as a clear description of the matters on which a second opinion or request for treatment are being sought. In acute emergency cases, a written report may not be possible, and a telephone call may suffice. However, the referring veterinarian must inform his colleague fully on important clinical findings and any treatment initiated.

The referring veterinarian is entitled to a written report and appropriate telephone discussions about the progress and/or outcome of a case. The findings should be transmitted directly to the referring veterinarian and not by way of the client. Referring veterinarians should realize, however, that once a case is referred, the consulting veterinarian is solely responsible for the type of treatment selected.

As specialization becomes a more common part of equine practice, the ready availability of specialists makes it necessary for practitioners to consider specialists' opinions to improve case management. Seeking such expert opinions for diagnosis or treatment enhances the reputation of the referring veterinarian with the client.

PHYSICAL RESTRAINT

The need for physical restraint of horses becomes obvious when anything other than minor procedures must be performed. In the past, the lack of reliable short-acting tranquilizers, as well as problems associated with general anesthesia, resulted in many procedures being done without general anesthesia. Many forms of physical restraint still are appropriate today, despite the array of sedatives and general anesthetics available.

The importance of a confident approach when dealing with horses cannot be overemphasized. Many horses are nervous, suspicious creatures and quickly detect a lack of confidence on the part of the handler. While veterinarians are not expected to be horse breakers, they should know techniques to control horses. In addition, assurance in handling the horse engenders the client's confidence in the veterinarian. Clients may not be able to assess diagnostic and therapeutic skills, but they are in a position to judge competence in handling their horse.

Holding the Head

In equine practice, it is common to have a client holding the horse's head while such procedures as stomach tubing and teeth floating are performed. The client must be given clear instructions about where to stand so that all involved are protected. The person controlling the head of the horse always should stand on the same side as the operator; then, if the horse starts to misbehave, its head can be pulled toward the handler, and the horse's body will move away from the operator.

Lifting the Limbs

Lifting the limbs can be a very useful form of restraint to carry out minor techniques, such as nerve blocks, removing sutures and bandaging. If a forelimb is to be worked on, the opposite forelimb is lifted. If a hind limb requires attention, a forelimb on the same side is lifted.

Forelimbs: To lift a forelimb, the examiner stands beside the forelimb to be picked up, facing toward the rear of the horse (Fig 1). Starting at the shoulder, the hand closer to the horse is used to run down the lateral side of the limb until the pastern is reached (Fig 2). At that stage, the examiner can lean a shoulder against the horse, encouraging it to transfer weight to the opposite forelimb. This allows the limb to be lifted easily (Fig 3). At that stage, if examination of the foot is required, the distal forelimb may be held between the examiner's knees (Fig 4).

If an additional person is not available to hold the foot, a knee strap can be used (Fig 5). This is applied around the pastern, near the midforearm, and buckled on the lateral aspect of the limb. Alternatively, a leg rope may be used by the handler at the head of the horse to hold up the forelimb (Fig 6).

Hind Limbs: To lift up a hind limb, one starts by moving from the shoulder region to the level of the tuber coxae. Standing close to the horse and facing toward the rear, the hand nearer the horse is placed on the tuber coxae (Fig 7). With this hand so placed, the horse can be pushed away if necessary and weight transferred to the other hind limb. The other hand is run down the outside of the limb until the plantar aspect of the pastern is grasped in the palm of the hand (Fig 8). The

Figure 1. To lift a forelimb, begin by placing the hand closer to the horse at the top of the shoulder.

Figure 3. Leaning against the horse's shoulder, the examiner can transfer weight to the opposite forelimb. The limb can then be lifted.

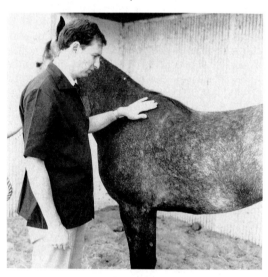

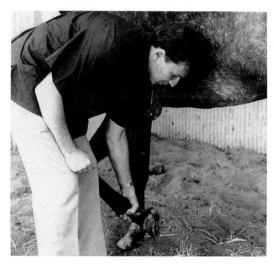

Figure 2. After running the hand down the outside of the limb, the pastern region is held in the palm of the hand closer to the horse.

Figure 4. The examiner holds the horse's foot between his knees to examine the foot.

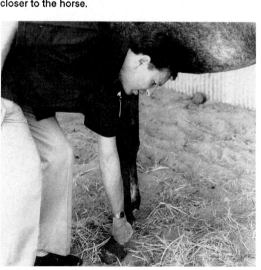

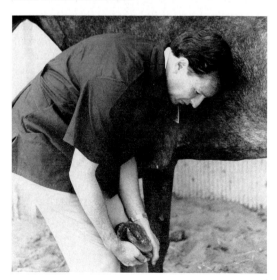

Figure 5. Restraint of the left forelimb using a knee strap.

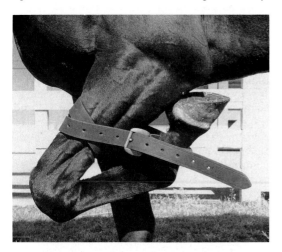

Figure 7. To lift the left hind limb, begin by placing the left hand on the tuber coxae, leaving the right hand free to move distally.

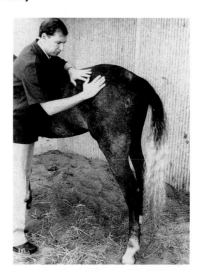

Figure 6. Restraint of the left forelimb using a leg rope secured at the pastern and applied around the withers.

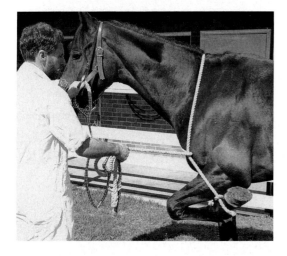

Figure 8. The right hand is moved distally to the plantar aspect of the pastern.

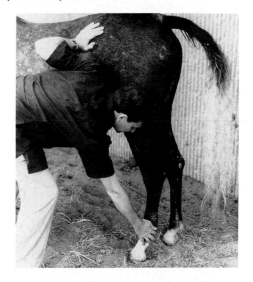

limb then is lifted and brought forward, so that the operator is standing with the horse's hind limb in the flexed position (Fig 9). In this position, the horse may balance itself and usually gives an indication as to whether it is likely to kick. If the limb is lifted for restraint, this is the best position in which to hold it. However, if the distal part of the limb requires examination, the operator can step forward quickly so that the leg closer to the horse moves to the inside of the elevated hind limb (Fig 10).

Applying the Twitch

Various forms of twitches have been used to restrain horses. Though the exact mechanism of action is unknown, it has been shown recently that endorphins are released during twitch application. The twitch is very effective restraint during such procedures as stomach tubing, injection of local anesthetic, and various minor procedures that may cause transitory pain. The simplest twitches can be constructed using an axe handle and cotton rope. A selection of various twitches is shown in Figures 11 and 12. Chain twitches are very popular and less likely to slip off the lip (Fig 13). Regardless of which type of twitch is used, it should allow the person holding the twitch to stand at the level of the horse's shoulder. In such a position, the horse holder has maximum control and is unlikely to be injured if the horse should strike.

The twitch should be applied while standing to the side of the horse. One hand should be on the twitch handle as all the fingers except the index finger are passed through the loop (Fig 14). Leaving the index finger outside the loop prevents the loop from slip-

ping down over the wrist. The twitch handle must be held at all times; otherwise, if the horse suddenly throws its head up, the twitch handle can swing around and injure either the person applying the twitch or the person holding the lead rope. Once applied, the twitch and lead rope are held together (Fig 15) and a series of half hitches may be formed around the twitch handle. Some horses tend to strike when a twitch is applied. For this reason, it is important to stand at the side rather than in front of the horse as the twitch is applied. For such horses, another method of restraint might be tried.

Figure 9. Pushing the left hand against the tuber coxae causes the horse to transfer weight to the opposite hind limb. The left limb can then be picked up and brought forward.

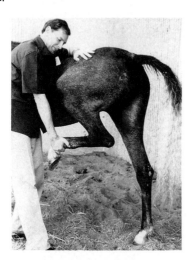

Figure 10. Position of the hind limb for examination of the foot.

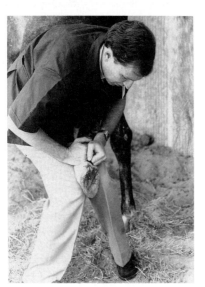

Figure 11. A ring twitch applied to the upper lip.

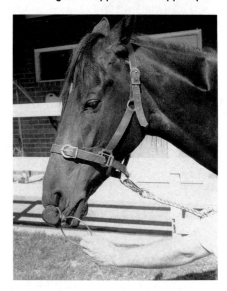

Figure 12. A clamp twitch fixed to the halter.

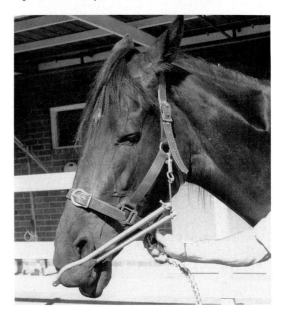

Figure 13. A chain twitch being applied to the upper lip.

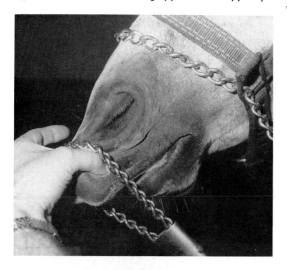

Figure 15. Chain twitch applied, showing position in which the handler should stand.

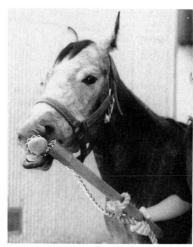

Figure 14. Position of the fingers for twitch application.

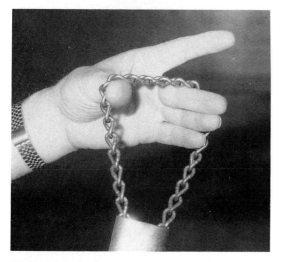

Figure 16. Twisting an ear for restraint.

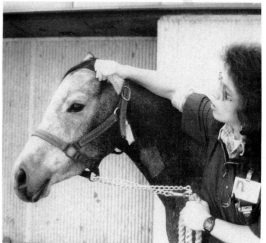

Twisting an Ear

In foals, one of the most effective means of restraint is to back the animal into the corner of a stall and gently twist both its ears simultaneously. This technique permits blood sample collection and stomach tubing with little or no movement by the foal. In adult horses, when a twitch does not provide sufficient restraint, additional restraint may be achieved by twisting the animal's ear. To use this technique, the handler faces the front of the horse and gradually runs the hand up toward the ear on the same side. The horse's ear is twisted at the base whenever additional restraint is required (Fig 16).

Grasping a Fold of Skin

An alternative to twisting an ear for temporary restraint is grasping a fold of skin on the neck (Fig 17). This technique is useful only for very short-term restraint but is sometimes worthwhile in horses that respond adversely to needles.

Restraint of Stallions

A lead rope with a chain at the end may be used to restrain stallions and horses that are difficult to handle. The chain is attached to the halter and then passed over the dorsal aspect of the nose (Fig 18). Pressure should not be applied to the chain until the horse requires restraint, when a sharp tug can be given to the lead rope. A variation of this technique is to pass the chain from the lead rope under the upper lip (Fig 19). The latter procedure is particularly useful in stallions that are difficult to restrain. An alternative to lead rope chains is a rearing bit, applied in combination with a halter and lead rope (Fig 20). The principle is similar to that of a nose chain in that a single, sharp tug is applied to the bit when restraint is needed, rather than using continuous pressure.

Yankee War Bridle

The Yankee war bridle is used infrequently but can be very effective in horses that resist the twitch and are head shy. A 1/4-inch nylon rope with a loop in one end is passed around the back of the ears and through the mouth (Fig 21). When restraint is needed, the free end of the rope is pulled down firmly so that pressure is applied to the commissures of the lips. This technique is worthwhile in horses that tend to strike when a twitch is applied.

Figure 17. Grasping a fold of skin for restraint.

Figure 19. Restraint using the chain of the lead rope, passed under the upper lip.

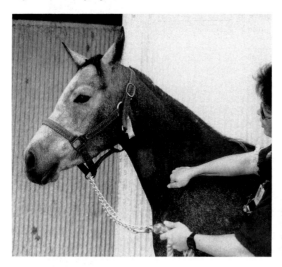

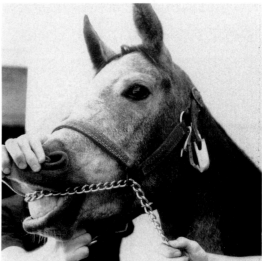

Figure 18. Restraint using a chain passed over the dorsal aspect of the nose.

Figure 20. Restraint using a rearing bit.

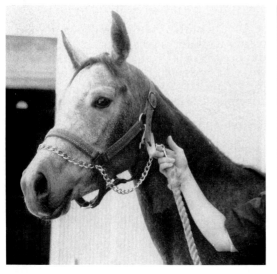

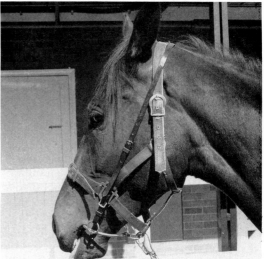

Figure 21. Yankee war bridle applied for restraint.

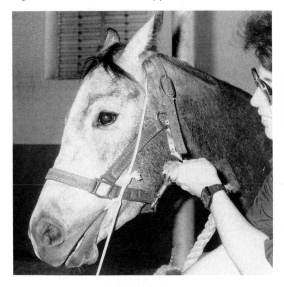

Figure 23. Sideline applied for restraint. A bandage has been used around the distal hind limb to prevent possible skin abrasion from the rope.

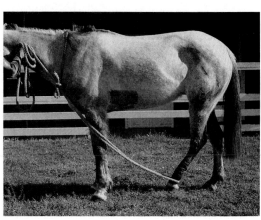

Figure 22. Bowline nonslip knot used for a single sideline.

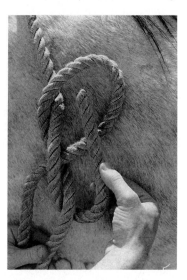

Figure 24. Figure-eight knot used for double sidelines.

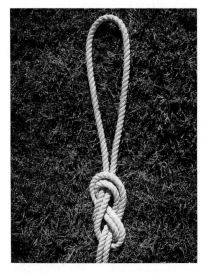

Single and Double Sidelines

When stocks are not available, sidelines are often used for restraint. A single sideline is useful for standing castration and may be applied with a 20-ft-long cotton rope. Initially, a bowline knot is tied around the horse's neck, after which the free end of the rope is taken between the horse's hind limbs and back up through the loop around the neck (Fig 22). The rope is loosened gradually so that it slips down the hind limb to rest around the pastern. Some tension is applied to the rope, bringing the restrained hind limb for-ward 6-8 inches in front of the unrestrained hind limb (Fig 23).

Double sidelines can be used as a form of "breeding hobbles" and may be useful for rectal examinations in fractious horses. A figure-eight knot is tied in the middle of a 40-ft-long cotton rope (Fig 24). The 2 free ends of the rope are taken around the inside of the respective hind limbs, above the hocks. The ropes are passed distal to the hock so that movement of the hock is effectively restricted (Fig 25), then back up through the neck loop and tied or held by the person at the head.

61

Figure 25. Double sidelines applied as a form of breeding hobbles.

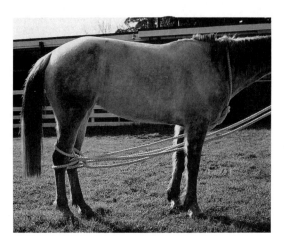

Tail Restraint

Lifting the horse's tail up over its back is useful when performing rectal or reproductive examinations (Fig 26). The tail can be held up by a third person or by a tail rope. The tail rope also is useful during induction of anesthesia when a horse is to be placed against a vertical operating table.

Restraint of Foals

The simplest technique to restrain young foals (up to 2 months of age) for minor procedures is to have the handler twist both of

Figure 26. Tail restraint with the tail held up over the back.

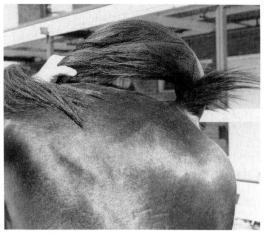

the foal's ears (see above) while the foal's rear end is positioned in the corner of a stall. Alternatively, if only restriction of movement is required, one arm placed around the chest of the foal and the other holding the tail up over its back can be quite effective.

Handling Unbroken Horses

Situations may arise when an unhandled or unbroken horse may require veterinary treatment. In many cases, lacerations or injuries may dictate use of a general anesthetic, but the horse may be difficult to approach. In these cases, the Jeffery method of horse handling is invaluable.[1] This method requires a catching rope 20-25 ft long. With the horse in a restricted area, a large loop is formed in the catching rope and the rope is placed over the horse's head, using a long stick (Fig 27). Throwing the rope at the horse should be avoided, as this frightens the animal. Once the horse is accustomed to the rope around its neck, the handler can exert the first "control pull." This pull must be short, sharp and applied when the horse's long axis is at right angles to the rope (Fig 28). This "control pull" causes the horse to face the handler, whereupon any tension in the rope should be released. The handler then moves to a different spot and applies another "control pull." After 4-5 of these pulls, the horse tends to face up to the handler when the handler moves.

At this stage, the process of advance and retreat can begin. With the horse facing you,

Figure 27. Use of a catching rope placed over a stick to catch an unbroken horse.

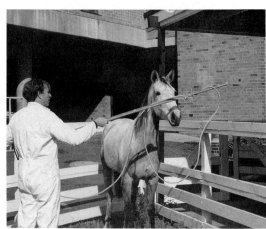

Figure 28. Use of the catching rope to produce a "control pull," as in the Jeffery method of horse handling.

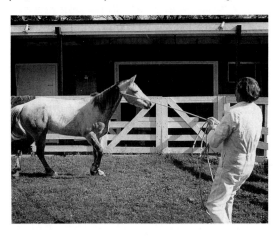

the idea is to advance toward it a little at a time but to retreat before the horse moves. The process is repeated so that the handler gets increasingly closer to the horse, until the horse extends its nose to smell the advanced hand (Fig 29). The handler can then move to the side and begin to stroke the animal gently all over its body. The time required for this varies but with most unbroken horses is 15-20 minutes. If the horse moves at any stage, a few "control pulls" are given to regain control of the horse. At this point, it is a simple matter to give preanesthetic tranquilizers or any other necessary treatment.

Figure 29. Final step in the advance and retreat technique of the Jeffery method of horse handling. Once contact is made, the horse is rubbed all over its body.

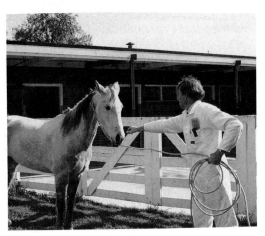

The Jeffery method of horse handling also is useful in horses that have been broken but have some handling difficulties, such as not letting a handler pick up a limb. A few "control pulls" with the catching rope soon have the horse responding to the handler, at which stage the general principle of advance and retreat can be applied to picking up the limb or handling the body part about which the horse is shy.

Use of Stocks

Stocks or "crushes" provide good restraint for such procedures as rectal examination, abdominocentesis, ultrasound examination, intravenous fluid administration, and minor surgical procedures. An ideal set of stocks provides maximum restraint and protects the operator while providing access to most areas of the horse's body. Stocks are most commonly used in equine hospitals and on stud farms. A typical set of stocks is shown in Figure 30. These stocks have been designed to fit most large-breed horses and have adjustable bars at the side that can be raised or lowered. Bottles or bags of fluid can be suspended from the bars above the stocks.

Clinicians accustomed to working with horses in stocks to do stomach tubing and teeth floating should exercise caution when carrying out these techniques where less restraint is available. One becomes used to standing in front of the horse rather than to the side and, without stocks, there is a greatly increased risk of being struck by the horse.

Figure 30. Well-designed set of stocks constructed to fit most sizes of horses.

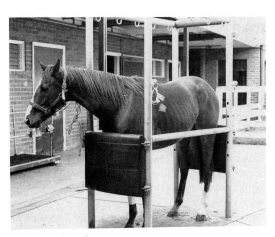

RECORD KEEPING AND THE PROBLEM-ORIENTED MEDICAL RECORD

Accurate medical records are fundamentally important to a veterinary practitioner. Apart from the legal implications of maintaining accurate records, record keeping provides an ongoing history of each animal and enables busy practitioners to keep track of services rendered so they may be fully compensated. The ideal record system must be simple and not require excessive paperwork. Information from records should be easily retrievable, and the problem(s), clinical findings and therapeutic plan should be clear to a third party unassociated with the case. Unfortunately, these ideals seldom are achieved.

Practitioners frequently examine a number of animals at a farm or stable. As such, it may be impractical to have an individual medical record for each horse. A duplicate record system of all service calls is recommended. At termination of each call, the veterinarian should update the record and, on completion, provide a copy to the client and keep the original. The date, owner's name, and name and description of each horse are recorded. Also provided is a brief description of the service or complaint, together with diagnosis, therapy and treatment plan. The same form can be used to record charges. However, charges are more likely to be accurately recorded and billed when record and billing systems are maintained separately.

Problem-oriented medicine is a broadly defined, organized approach to a veterinary practice. The problem-oriented medical record defines a set of rules and directions for methodical writing and organization of medical records. The system usually has 4 components based on 4 phases of medical action: data base, problem list, plans and progress notes.

The *data base* includes the presenting complaint, history, patient profile, physical findings for each body system, laboratory data and a review of previous information that may be relevant to the current problem. The *problem list* is a table of factors that can be considered a threat to the patient's health and, therefore, require management or further evaluation. Associated with each problem, a *plan* of action is designed, generally divided into diagnostic, therapeutic and client information sections. *Progress notes* are divided into 4 categories: subjective data, objective data, assessment of the problem, and a treatment plan. Notes should be dated and numbered, and the specific problem defined.

Such a system goes a long way toward achieving some of the goals of record keeping. The problem-oriented medical record allows specific problems to be identified clearly and the progress followed. Further, the therapeutic plan and response should be evident to an independent observer.

PHYSICAL EXAMINATION

When a horse is first presented to the veterinarian, the main consideration is to determine which systems are or are not affected by disease. Discussions of detailed examination of the various body systems are presented in other chapters of this book.

A number of different approaches may be used for the initial examination. A systemic approach can be taken, with each body system examined sequentially, or a more general approach can be implemented, starting at the front of the horse and working toward the rear. Regardless of which technique is used, examination should be logical and sequential. We find it easier to work from the front to the rear of the horse, without consideration to specific body systems. The time spent examining a particular area, to a large extent, is dictated by the history and presenting complaint. Nonetheless, many problems involve multiple body systems. For example, in a horse presented for poor performance, it is quite common to find several contributing problems involving different systems. Thus, even with the most obvious problem, it is important to perform a thorough physical examination.

The initial part of the examination should involve an overview of the horse. Is the horse alert, depressed or showing signs of pain? Note any asymmetry, swellings or other irregularities before beginning the more detailed examination. The horse should be examined from a distance of 6-8 ft and viewed from the front, both sides and rear. After noting any obvious abnormalities, the horse should be closely examined.

Examination of the Head and Neck

The nares should be checked for symmetry and air flow. Additionally, the examiner should smell air exiting the horse's nares to detect any abnormal odors that could indicate infection of the conchae. The mouth is examined and, initially, light digital pressure is applied to the mucous membranes dorsal to the upper corner incisor teeth for 1-2 seconds to determine capillary refill time. Normal refill time is 1-2 seconds. The teeth then can be examined using a 1-hand technique (Figs 31, 32), with the back of the hand pushing ventrally between the mandibles such that the horse's tongue is forced between the teeth on the opposite side of the mouth. Any abnormalities of wear or any sharp edges on the labial side of the upper cheek teeth and

Figures 31 and 32. One-handed technique for examination of the mouth. The back of the hand is introduced into the interdental space so that the tongue is pushed over to the opposite side of the mouth.

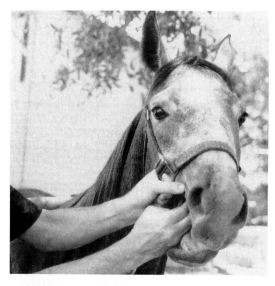

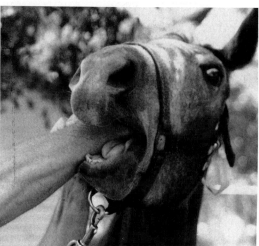

lingual side of the lower cheek teeth should be noted. At this time, the age of the horse also can be determined.

Percussion over the maxillary and frontal sinuses may elicit evidence of pain or a dull sound that could indicate sinusitis (Fig 33). During this part of the examination, the fingers of the other hand are inserted in the interdental space, causing the horse's mouth to open, resulting in better resonance. The eyes should be examined for corneal scars, conjunctivitis, iridocyclitis or cataracts. A menace response should be elicited and consensual pupillary light response determined. The third eyelid should be examined by applying digital pressure to the eyeball via the upper eyelid (Fig 34).

The pulse should be felt in the facial artery as it passes ventral to the horizontal ramus of the mandible. The important things to note are pulse character, strength and regularity. The area between the rami of the mandibles and in the region of Viborg's triangle should be palpated to determine if the mandibular and pharyngeal lymph nodes are enlarged. The larynx also should be palpated to detect atrophy of the dorsal cricoarytenoid muscle (Fig 35). With atrophy of this muscle, as in laryngeal hemiplegia, the muscular process of the affected arytenoid cartilage is more prominent than on the unaffected side. Any scarring or thickening of skin could suggest previous laryngoplasty or laryngotomy and should be noted.

Figure 33. Percussion of the maxillary sinus.

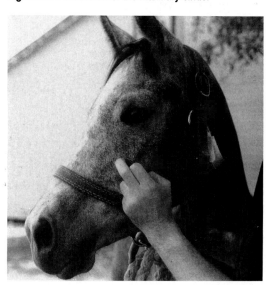

Figure 34. Examination of the third eyelid by application of digital pressure against the upper eyelid.

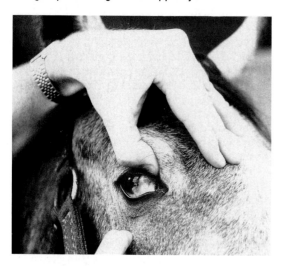

The lateral processes of the cervical vertebrae are palpated and the range of lateral movement and degree of neck flexion noted, along with any indications of pain. The trachea also can be palpated in the cervical region, and signs of narrowing observed. Both jugular veins should be checked for patency and any evidence of an increased jugular pulse, which could indicate congestive heart failure.

Examination of the Forelimbs

The forelimbs should be inspected for swellings, particularly from the carpus dis-

tally. The radiocarpal and intercarpal joints, second metacarpal bone, flexor tendons, interosseous (suspensory) ligament and fetlock joint, including the palmar pouch, are inspected and palpated. It is important to compare findings with those in the opposite forelimb.

Examination should commence at the foot. After assessing the digital pulse and checking for signs of increased heat around the hoof wall and coronary band, hoof testers should be applied around the foot and across the frog to determine if pain can be elicited (Fig 36). With the limb held up, the lateral cartilages should be palpated to check for ossification. The pastern should be flexed and rotated to see if pain can be evoked. The fetlock joint is flexed to examine the range of movement and detect pain (Fig 37). The flexor tendons and interosseous ligament are palpated for heat, swelling and pain (Fig 38). Note that firm pressure on the interosseous ligament near its point of bifurcation produces a painful reaction in normal horses. The second and fourth metacarpal bones are palpated to detect swellings ("splints"), and the dorsal aspect of the third metacarpal bone is palpated to detect pain from "bucked shins." The area of the inferior check ligament, just distal to the carpus at the palmar aspect of the proximal third metacarpal bone, also should be palpated.

Next, the carpus is examined closely. Any distension of the joint capsule over the dorsal aspect of the radiocarpal and intercarpal

Figure 35. Deep palpation with the index finger in the dorsal laryngeal region permits palpation of muscular process of the arytenoid cartilages.

Figure 36. Examination of the foot using hoof testers. The testers are being applied across the middle third of the frog to test for pain in the navicular region.

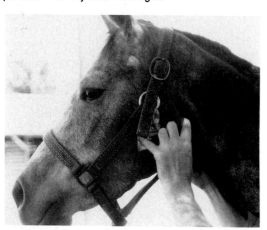

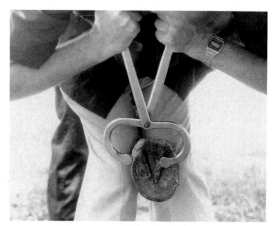

Figure 37. Flexion of the fetlock joint to determine range of movement and to check for pain.

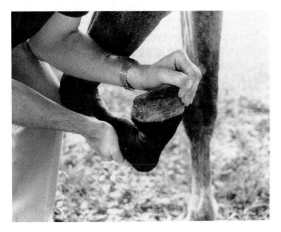

Figure 39. Palpation of the dorsal aspect of the radiocarpal joint to detect swelling and pain in the joint capsule.

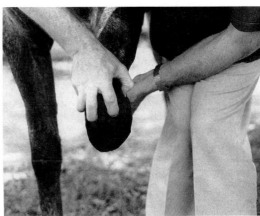

Figure 38. Palpation of the flexor tendons and interosseous ligament. This examination should be performed with weight off the limb.

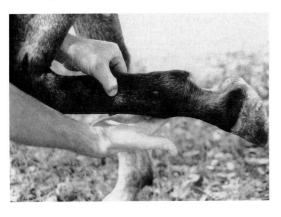

Figure 40. Extreme carpal flexion to detect pain and/or restricted movement in the carpus.

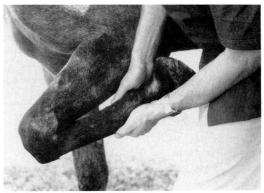

joints should be noted; the joints should be palpated carefully (Fig 39). In some acute injuries, pain can be elicited by firm digital pressure over the affected carpal bone. The horse's carpus is flexed so that the foot is taken up proximally, past the point of the elbow. In many chronic carpal injuries, pain is not evident until the last few degrees of carpal flexion. A normal horse does not show any response to even extreme carpal flexion (Fig 40). The area above the carpus is difficult to examine as far as finding localizing signs. Flexion, extension and abduction of the proximal forelimb can be performed to check for pain (Fig 41).

Examination of the Thorax

When examining the thorax, the most important part of initial assessment is to note the character and frequency of respiration. In the absence of lower respiratory disease, a horse at rest has a respiratory rate of 8-16 breaths per minute, with very little thoracic wall movement. Any prolonged inspiration or expiration should be observed. Initially, the heart should be auscultated with the stethoscope diaphragm placed deep to the triceps muscles (Fig 42). Both sides of the thorax should be auscultated. The heart should be auscultated for at least 1 minute over at least

67

Figure 41. Extension of the proximal limb to detect pain.

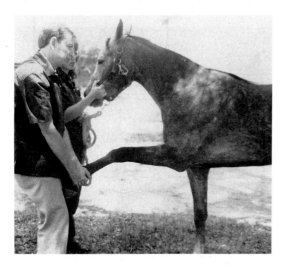

3 sites, noting particularly any disturbances of rhythm or the presence of murmurs. The normal resting heart rate ranges from 28 to 36 beats per minute in the adult horse.

Next, the trachea and both lung fields are auscultated. In most normal horses breathing quietly at rest, few sounds are heard except over the hilar area and during auscultation over the trachea. If there is any suspicion of abnormal sounds (crackles or wheezes), a plastic bag can be placed over the horse's nose to stimulate respiration due to rebreathing of carbon dioxide. This technique increases both the frequency and depth of respiration and permits abnormal lung sounds to be heard more easily. Additionally,

the nares can be occluded for a short time, causing the horse to take several deep breaths when the nares are released.

If there is any suspicion of a respiratory abnormality, the thorax should be percussed using a dessert spoon or a similar utensil for a pleximeter, plus a rubber hammer (Fig 43). With the spoon placed over the dorsal aspect of a rib, the hammer is used to tap the spoon as it is moved ventrally. A dull sound may indicate fluid in the thorax. Alternatively, one may use the tips of the first 2 fingers of one hand as the plexor to strike a middle finger of the other hand, which is pressed firmly between adjacent ribs. If the results of the examination suggest severe intrathoracic disease, one should observe the breathing movements from above the back of the animal to assess the symmetry of thoracic expansion.

Examination of the Abdomen

Examination of the abdomen is very difficult. If an abdominal problem is suspected, various specialized procedures are necessary. However, at the initial examination, note should be taken of the abdominal outline so that any distention can be detected. The abdomen should be auscultated on the left and right sides, over both the paralumbar fossae, and over the ventral flank regions. Over the right paralumbar fossa, ileocecal valve sounds may be heard every 30-60 seconds. In general, it is important to determine whether gut sounds are normal, increased, decreased

Figure 42. Auscultation of the heart using a stethoscope.

Figure 43. Percussion of the chest using a rubber hammer and dessert spoon as a pleximeter.

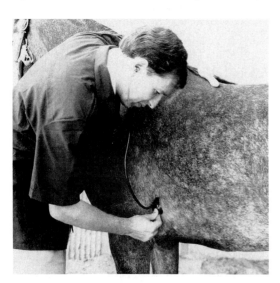

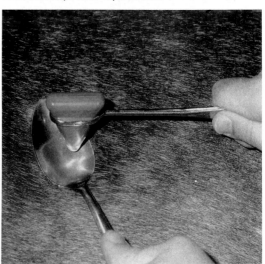

or absent. If abdominal distention is present, percussion over the area of distention can help determine if there is a gas-filled viscus.

The rectal temperature should be measured at this stage. The normal range is 98-102 F (36.5-39 C) for adult horses. The rectal temperature of foals tends to be at the high end of the normal temperature range for adults.

Examination of the Back

The back should be checked for scoliosis, lordosis or kyphosis. These structural abnormalities can be viewed best by standing behind the horse while it is bearing weight evenly on its hind limbs. It is useful to stand on something so the back of the animal can be viewed from above.

The dorsal spinous processes should be palpated over the thoracic and lumbar regions and firm pressure applied over the tuber sacrale. In horses with hind limb weakness or sacroiliac pain, mild pressure at this site causes the horse to crouch away from the examiner. Stroking the horse's thoracolumbar area with the blunt end of a ballpoint pen (or a similar object) causes extension of the thoracolumbar vertebral column. Stroking the caudal sacral region causes the horse to flex its thoracolumbar vertebrae. An abnormal response is found when the horse holds its back rigid, sinks very low as if weak, grunts, or demonstrates some other painful response.

Examination of Genitalia

Unless the history indicates the possibility of a urogenital problem, detailed examination of the genitalia is not necessary. In both stallions and geldings, the preputial area should be examined for any evidence of discharge that could indicate an infection, squamous-cell carcinoma or habronemiasis. In stallions, the testicles should be palpated to make sure the horse is not a cryptorchid. In fillies and mares, the conformation of the perineum should be noted to determine the likelihood of ascending infection or pneumovagina. The presence of current or previous Caslick operations also should be investigated. If there is any discharge from the vulva or "scalding" around the hind limbs, a more detailed reproductive examination with a speculum and a rectal examination are indicated.

Examination of the Hind Limbs

The distal hind limbs, below the hocks, are examined in the same manner as the forelimbs. The hock is the most common site of chronic hind limb lameness and thus should be inspected carefully for any swelling. Areas to be checked include the medial aspect of the tarsometatarsal and distal intertarsal joints, as well as the tibiotarsal joint. The stifle should be examined by careful palpation among the 3 patellar ligaments. The medial femoropatellar pouch is situated between the medial and middle patellar ligaments, while the lateral femoropatellar pouch is found between the middle and lateral patellar ligaments (Fig 44). In stifle joint disease, the most common finding is distension of one or both of these femoropatellar pouches. Finally, the symmetry of the hind limbs should be checked as in many chronic hind limb lamenesses, the gluteal muscles will be atrophied.

Assessing the Gait

After completing the general examination, the horse's gait should be assessed. Of course, the extent of this evaluation depends on whether or not there is a history of a musculoskeletal or neuromuscular problem. A basic minimum examination should include walking the horse toward and away from the investigator to determine if there are any signs of incoordination, and trotting the horse on a firm surface to detect lame-

Figure 44. Palpation of the femoropatellar pouches showing fingers placed between the middle and medial, and middle and lateral patellar ligaments.

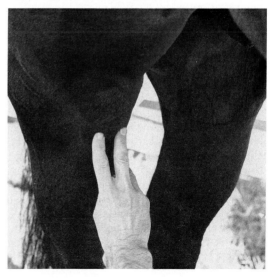

ness. It is also useful to lunge the horse if a musculoskeletal problem is suspected. Many hind limb lamenesses become more evident when the horse is lunged with the affected limb on the inside of the circle.

Rectal Examination

Rectal examination is not part of the routine examination procedure but should be performed when there is a history of weight loss or when a gastrointestinal, reproductive or urinary system problem or a sacral, pelvic or lymphatic disorder is suspected. The horse must be adequately restrained and, if necessary, tranquilized. Propantheline, given IV at 0.1-0.2 mg/kg, or an enema of 15-20 ml of 2% lidocaine in 30 ml of water may be worthwhile if relaxation of the animal's rectum is required. Restraint is most safely achieved in stocks, though use of tail restraint with or without a sideline is quite effective.

Because disposable shoulder-length gloves vary in quality, it is important to make sure that the joined edges (seams) are not sharp. If this is the case, the gloves should be turned inside out. The examiner's fingernails must be short to minimize the chances of rectal mucosal laceration. Liberal amounts of lubricant must be applied to the glove, and the fingers should be shaped into a cone as the hand is introduced through the anus. Any feces in the rectum should be removed with the palm of the hand facing dorsally. Following application of more lubricant, with the fingers forming a cone shape, the arm is introduced slowly into the rectum to the brim of the pelvis. If the horse strains, the hand should not be pushed cranially, as this is the most likely time the rectum will rupture.

The left lateral abdominal wall then can be palpated. With further cranial exploration, the caudal pole of the spleen and, dorsally, the caudal border of the left kidney can be felt. Though variable, the pelvic flexure of the large colon usually is palpable on the left side of the ventral caudal abdomen. On the right side of the abdomen, the small colon can be discerned by the presence of fecal balls and the fact that it is quite mobile. Depending on the degree of distension of the cecum, different portions can be palpated. If severely distended with gas or impacted food, the base can be felt toward the dorsal abdominal wall. However, in most conditions, the only reliable finding is the ventral taenia.[2] Palpation

of the cranial mesenteric artery is quite difficult in most large horses and impossible if there is abdominal pain. In stallions, it is always wise to check the integrity of the internal inguinal rings, which can be felt on the lateral part of the ventral abdominal wall just cranial to the femoral canal. After completing a rectal examination, it is very important to inspect the glove for blood, which could indicate a rectal tear or rupture.

PREPURCHASE EXAMINATION

In the past, examination of a horse before purchase has been called a "soundness examination." Because the term "soundness" implies freedom from any fault whatsoever, the term has been replaced by "prepurchase examination" or, in some cases, "examination for serviceability." The sale of a horse often depends on the veterinarian's findings; therefore, a complete examination should be performed in a methodical manner. Considerable care must be taken not only with the examination but also with recording the findings. Complaints and litigation are more likely in this area of equine practice than in most others.

The technique of prepurchase examination described here accentuates physical examination without sophisticated diagnostic aids. Use of such diagnostic aids as radiography, endoscopy, ultrasonography and electrocardiography always should be discussed with the client and the advantages of such tests explained. Depending on the value of the horse and the particular use for which it is intended, some or all of these tests may be indicated. However, such specialized procedures should not be regarded as part of the routine prepurchase examination.

Legally, the veterinarian is required to demonstrate that reasonable care has been taken to ensure that the examination was as thorough as the circumstances allowed. There may be variations in examining conditions but such variability should be noted on the certificate. The law recognizes differences in skill among members of a profession but requires each veterinarian to perform the examination to the level considered to be standard practice.

A prepurchase examination should be carried out only on the behalf of a potential buyer. Any attempt by a seller to obtain an examination for an unknown purchaser should be resisted. By questioning the client (buyer) carefully, the veterinarian can discern the purposes for which the horse is to be used. Information gathered from a prepurchase examination must be supplied only to the person or agent who employed the veterinarian. Such information is confidential and should be passed to other parties only after permission has been obtained from the buyer.

Horse Identification

As with a routine physical examination, the prepurchase examination should be performed carefully and methodically. Of great importance is adequate identification of the horse.

Height: The height of a horse is taken at the withers. If a measuring stick is not available, an estimate of the height should be given in hands. (Note that 1 hand equals 4 inches or 10 cm.)

Coat Color: The following descriptions of coat color may be used:

Bay. Though variations in coat color may range from dull red to a color approaching chestnut, generally the mane, tail, tips of the ears and distal limbs are black.

Black. There is uniform distribution of black hair color on the body, limbs, mane and tail.

Brown. The distal limbs, mane and tail usually are black, but the trunk is uniformly brown.

Chestnut. The coat may vary from a light, washy yellow through various reddish shades to a dark liver color. However, the pigment is distributed evenly. The mane and tail are chestnut but may be either lighter or darker than the trunk.

Gray. The body color is an uneven admixture of colored and white hairs. Young foals have one of the basic coat colors (brown, bay, black or chestnut) but white hair gradually predominates with increasing age. The basic coat color is reflected in the color of the mane, tail and points. Transitional stages between the basic coat color and white should be designated as gray-black, gray-brown, gray-bay or gray-chestnut.

Roan. The trunk is a fairly even mix of colored and white hairs. A roan horse should be described on the basis of its primary color, either roan-black or black-brown ("blue roan"), roan-brown, bay-brown or bay ("red roan") or roan-chestnut ("strawberry roan"). This is the basic color that is permanent and does not change with increasing age.

Pied, Paint or Pinto. The trunk has areas without pigment, alternating with areas showing one of the basic colors. Thus, horses should be described as pied-black (piebald), pied-brown (skewbald), etc.

Dun. The trunk is essentially yellow, in one of many shades. Such a color is produced by dilution of one of the basic colors, generally with a dorsal stripe of basic color. Occasionally, some evidence of this coat color may also be seen on the carpi and hocks.

Cream. A dilution of brown or bay produces a cream animal with black points. Palomino is a cream horse with silver mane and tail, and represents dilution of chestnut. In such horses, the iris may be deficient in or devoid of pigment, with a resultant pinkish or bluish eye hue.

White. Foals may be born white or predominantly white but with evidence of base pigmentation of the poll, ears and tail. In some cases, the iris is blue.

Albino. In contrast to white animals, albino horses are snow white or cream, with pink skin and light blue, dark blue, brown or hazel eyes. There is no pigment in the skin. This color occurs randomly among many breeds, but some animals breed true to color and their offspring consistently are albino.

Appaloosa. This color is characterized by a spotted coat, the pattern of which varies from horse to horse. There are 8 basic patterns: spotted blanket, white blanket, marble, leopard, near-leopard, few spot, snow flake and frosted tip.

Sex

Description of color is generally followed by notation of sex. A colt is an uncastrated male up to and including the age of 3 years, whereas a stallion is an intact male animal 4 years of age or older. A filly is a female up to and including 3 years of age. On turning 4 years, the filly becomes a mare.

Age

The examining veterinarian should check the age supplied by the owner, brand or tattoo against the age estimated by inspection of the teeth. An excellent description of horses' teeth and the variations that occur with age is provided elsewhere.[3]

A foal is an animal less than 1 year of age but, if weaned, may be described as a weanling. Horses officially 1 year of age are referred to as yearlings.

Natural Markings and Congenital Peculiarities

An accurate description of markings enables rapid identification of the animal and is of great importance for subsequent verification that a particular animal was examined. All markings and their extent and location should be defined accurately. If the markings contain varying amounts of hair of the general body color, they should be described as "mixed," while, if circumscribed by a border of mixed hairs, as "bordered." Relationships to any whorl or whorls should be noted. Markings on the head are described as follow:

Star: This is a solid marking on the forehead that should be denoted by position, size, shape and intensity. Patches of white hairs should be described separately, if only limited in number.

Stripe: Stripes may be continuous (conjoined) with or separated from (interrupted) a star. A stripe is a solid white marking no wider than the flat surface of the nasal bones running down the dorsal aspect of the face. Such a description should not include patches of mixed hairs or a few white hairs on the site where a stripe would be located. When no star is present, the point of origin of the stripe should be indicated. The point of termination and any variation in width or direction should be described, together with the presence of any colored markings in the white.

Blaze: This is a solid white marking covering the major portion of the forehead between the eyes, extending down the front of the face, usually to the muzzle, and involving the width of the nasal bones. Description of a blaze is similar to that for a stripe.

Snip: A snip is an isolated white marking, independent of those previously mentioned. It is situated between or in the region of the nostrils.

Note also that any white markings of the lip and muzzle must be described accurately and drawn on an appropriate diagram (Fig 45).

The description of markings on the head is followed by a similar record of those on the limbs. The extent and location of white markings should be described, with special reference to variation in the height of the marking on various aspects of the limb. Any colored markings within the white should also be noted. Numerous other markings are observed commonly and require careful description. *Flesh marks* are patches where the pigment of skin is absent, whereas *whorls* are permanent irregular settings of coat hairs found on the forehead, nose, throat, neck, shoulder, chest, stifle and/or buttocks. Whorls may be described as simple (clockwise or counterclockwise) or feathered, and may occur singly or in groups of 2-3. The description of these markings involves notation of location, type and relationship to other structures and markings, such a description being of special importance in whole-colored animals.

Ticking is the presence of isolated white hairs distributed throughout the coat. Small collections of white hairs distributed irregularly on any part of the body are referred to as *flecking*. *Spots* are small and more or less circular collections of hair, differing from the general body color. The presence of odd-colored hairs in the mane and tail must be recorded.

Congenital abnormalities and peculiarities should also be noted at the time of examination. Examples of such conditions include: wall-eye, Roman nose, partly colored hoof, undershot or overshot jaw and muscle indentations.

Brands

Before they are allowed to race, Thoroughbred horses in the United States and Canada are tattooed inside the upper lip with a letter representing the year of their birth ("A" represents the years 1945 and 1971) and their American Jockey Club registration number. Thoroughbred horses bred in Europe, the United Kingdom or Ireland are unlikely to carry brands or tattoos unless raced in the United States or Canada.[4] In Australia and New Zealand, Thoroughbreds usually are branded on their right and left shoulders.

Standardbreds also are tattooed inside the upper lip with a letter (representing year of birth) and 4 numbers: eg, "A" following the numbers represents 1961, and "A" preceding the numbers represents 1982. In Australia,

Figure 45. Certificate of suitability for prepurchase examination, recommended by the Australian Equine Veterinary Association.

CERTIFICATE OF SUITABILITY

Owner and Address (if known) _____

Animal Presented as: _____ Breed: _____

If Animal Unnamed: Sire: _____ Dam: _____

Color: _____ Age: _____ Sex: _____

Person Requesting Examination: _____

Place of Examination:_____

Draw Brands and/or Markings: Mark whorls as O, scars as X

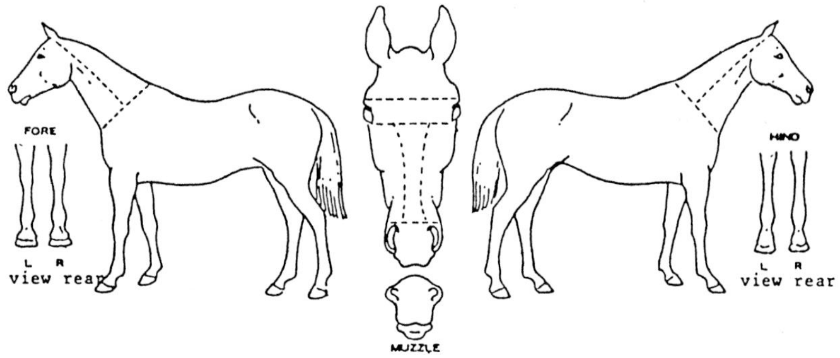

FORE

HIND

L R
view rear

L R
view rear

MUZZLE

CLINICAL EXAMINATION

Purpose of Examination_____

_____

Abnormalities (describe) _____

_____

_____

_____

Remarks: _____

_____

_____

_____

_____

Note: No radiologic or other specialized techniques were included.

Address _____

_____

_____

I find the horse to be suitable/unsuitable for the purpose for which it has been examined.

Signature _____

VETERINARY SURGEON

New Zealand and recently Canada, Standardbreds are identified by alpha-angle freeze branding on the right side of the neck.[5] In the United States, Arabian horses are identified by a freeze brand on the neck. To identify such brands accurately, it often is necessary to clip the hair over the brand. All brands and other permanent acquired markings require careful description and should be noted on the sketch of markings.

Sketch of Markings

A sketch of a horse featuring all markings should be part of the certification process. An outline of the horse from several different angles should be shown, as demonstrated in Figure 45. The position of whorls may be indicated by a circle, with an arrow showing direction of hairs. A few white hairs can be indicated by several lines, and flecking and ticking by small, light lines scattered over the area. Bordering should be noted by drawing a double outline, whereas colored spots or markings on the body are best indicated by drawing the outline. White markings on the face and limbs should be further highlighted by light shading. Flesh marks are best shown by drawing the outline with heavy shading. A small cross (x) can denote position of a scar.

Examination Procedure

If possible, a statement should be obtained from the vendor (or agent) regarding the history of the horse, including a schedule of medication (Fig 46). If an animal is to be examined for athletic serviceability, it is important to note the level of previous exercise training in the months before inspection. Many lamenesses are less obvious following a period without work, especially if the horse has been restricted to a stall.

A number of stages are necessary for a complete prepurchase examination:

Initial Examination

The examination is best conducted in the horse's own environment, preferably in a stall. The horse should have been rested for at least an hour before the examination. The horse's demeanor, general appearance and condition are noted. At this time, evidence of such vices as crib-biting, windsucking and weaving may be observed.

During these preliminary stages of the examination, an accurate description and estimated age (from the teeth) are recorded. Note should also be made of the horse's temperament.

Clinical Examination

The clinical examination is the next stage of the procedure. A careful and thorough examination must be performed, as detailed in the above section on Physical Examination. A check list, such as that recommended by the American Association of Equine Practitioners, helps ensure that no part of the examination is excluded (Fig 46). It is also important to note any conformational abnormalities.

Observing the Gait

The gait is assessed by observing the horse at the walk and trot, and while turning and backing. A firm, even surface is required for this assessment, which should include observation of gait with the horse being led away from as well as toward the examiner. It is most important to look for ataxia, which generally can be accentuated by walking and turning the horse on an incline, particularly with its head elevated.

Flexion tests should be part of the examination, with particular joints being held in flexion for 1-2 minutes, after which the horse is trotted off. If lameness results, the affected area can be examined further and radiographs made, if necessary. Such problems as early navicular disease and various joint problems can be detected in this way.

Inspection With Exercise

Inspection during and after exercise is the final stage of the examination. This final part of the examination often is not performed because of difficulties in exercising the horse in a suitable site. If the horse cannot be exercised at the intensity required for the athletic event for which the horse is intended, the horse should be lunged for at least 10 minutes. The level of exercise undertaken should be noted on the certificate. In hot climates, the horse's ability to sweat after exercise also should be recorded.

Exercise, of sufficient intensity for the intended use of the horse, is required to elevate heart and respiratory rates so that abnormalities can be detected more easily. If examining a horse at the track, the veterinarian should take up a position so that the horse passes close by on each circuit. Immediately after exercise, the horse's thorax should be auscultated to detect abnormal respiratory sounds, cardiac arrhythmias or heart murmurs. Low-grade systolic ejection murmurs often are found in performance horses and are of no consequence. These murmurs usually occur during early systole and do not involve either the first or second heart sounds.

After the immediate postexercise examination, the horse is returned to its stall, where it is allowed to rest for about 30 min-

Principles of Patient Evaluation and Diagnosis

Figure 46. Form recommended by the American Association of Equine Practitioners for prepurchase examination.

Name of Horse   **Breed**   **Tattoo**   **Sex**   **Color**   **Age**   **Markings**

_____

Seller's Statement Before Examination:

_____

Seller's Name   **Address**   **Phone Number**

_____

Do you have knowledge of present or past_____Diseases_____Lameness_____

How long have you been acquainted with this animal?_____

Treatments _____Vices (stable or being ridden)_____

Disabilities_____Medications _____

Eccentricities_____

Do you have knowledge of past performances of this animal for the proposed use?

_____

Do you have a personal estimate of the suitability of this animal for this purpose?

Unique _____ Exceptional _____ Adequate _____ No opinion _____

Signature of Seller _____ Date _____

Address _____

Buyer's Statement:_____

Buyer's Name   **Address**   **Phone Number**

_____

To what use do you intend to put this horse? (degree of work, hours to be used) _____

_____

What is the age, size, ability and experience of the intended rider? _____

_____

How long have you been acquainted with this animal?_____

_____

How long have you tried this animal?_____

How many of the proposed uses have you tried? _____

Of what relative importance are the following to you?

Appearance of the horse including (and any) blemishes _____

Performance _____ Temperament _____

How do you rate the suitability of this horse for the intended purpose?

Unique _____ Exceptional _____ Adequate _____

What type of care (stabling) is anticipated for this horse?

Intensive (continual care and supervision) _____ Average (stabled daily for feeding, etc.) _____

Casual (on pasture most of the time) _____

Signature of Buyer _____ Date _____

Address _____

Physical Examination

Place _____ Date _____ Time _____

Weather _____

General Health and Appearance

Approximate Height _____ Approximate Weight _____

Certificate of Height (Pony) _____ Temperature (Rectal) _____

N — Normal   AB — Abnormal   NE — Not Examined

Bilateral Symmetry

Head and Neck ____
Body ____
Legs ____
Feet ____

Eyes

Symmetry ____
Reflexes ____
Lids ____
Mucous membranes ____
Cornea ____
Ophthalmoscopic exam ____

Mouth

Lips ____
Tongue ____

Teeth ____
Gums ____
Mucous membranes ____
Odor ____
Bite ____

Nasal & Paranasal

Symmetry ____
Air flow ____
Odor ____
Mucous membranes ____
Percussion ____
Exudate ____

Pharynx, Larynx, Trachea

Palpation ____
Cough induction (reflex) ____

Auscultation at rest ____
after exercise ____
after recovery ____

Cardiovascular

Palpation (heart, pulse) ____
Auscultation (at rest) ____
after exercise ____
after recovery ____
Pulse rate & quality ____

Pulmonary

Percussion ____
Auscultation ____
exercise ____
recovery ____
Respiratory (rate rest) ____

Digestive

Percussion ____
Auscultation ____
Inspection of feces ____

Genital — Urinary

External ____
Inspection & palpation ____
Breeding soundness — Mares
  barren ____
  maiden ____
  foaling ____
Rectal exam ____
Speculum exam ____
Culture ____
Breeding soundness —Stallion
Rectal exam ____
Test breeding ____
Culture ____
Semen exam ____
Inspection & palpation ____

Integument

Note especially "used" marks
(interference with the saddle,
girth sores, firing or other
treatment, dermatoses, etc).
Insignificant scars need not be
enumerated.

Musculoskeletal

Vertebral column
  Symmetry ____
  Palpation ____
  Manipulation ____
Limbs
  Symmetry ____
  Palpation ____
  Manipulation ____
Gaits
  Symmetry ____

Freedom of movement
  on hard surface ____

on soft surface ____
on a straightaway ____
turning both ways ____

Vices

Cribbing
Weaving ____
Digging ____
Savaging ____
Other ____
Stable manners ____
Field manners ____

Nervous System

Inspection ____
Has horse been nerved ____
If so, where ____

Conditions other than normal found in the animal (list by title) _____

_____

_____

_____

_____

_____

ECG_____

Endoscopy _____

Radiographs_____

Rectal exam _____

Nerve blocks _____

Laboratory studies _____

Other_____

_____

_____

_____

In my opinion, at this time, this horse is:

_____ reasonably healthy for the use intended

_____ unhealthy for the use intended

_____ unhealthy temporarily for the use intended

_____ purchased at the Buyer's discretion understanding the abnormalities described in section

_____

My opinion does not consider the horse's aptitude, ability or temperament. These are at the Buyer's discretion.

Signature _____

Address _____

Date _____

utes. The final phase of the examination involves further observation of the horse while it is walked, trotted, turned and backed. Of particular interest is whether the exercise caused any stiffness or lameness.

Records and Certificates

In addition to details of the actual examination, summaries of telephone and other communications with the client should be kept as a permanent record. However, the certificate itself should contain only details of the examination findings. Many problems arise when veterinarians prepare certificates in haste and do not check all the details carefully. The certificate of examination generally reflects the care and detail with which the examination itself has been performed.

Each certificate must be dated and written or typed on letterhead stationery, showing the name of the practice and certifying veterinarian. The name and address of the person requesting the certificate and the date and place of examination should be provided. Unless ownership of the horse is clearly defined, care is required in assigning ownership status. Identification of the animal to which the certificate relates requires a full description involving breed, color, height, sex, distinguishing marks, and brands or tattoos. Such a description also may include a diagram showing the horse's markings (Fig 45). The horse is not described by name unless proof of identity is present. Abnormalities detected on examination must be detailed carefully and precisely. Though discretion should be used in expressing an opinion as to the potential loss of function associated with observed abnormalities, the client should be provided with some interpretation of the significance of the findings.

The certificate must be signed and the examining veterinarian's registered qualifications added. Use of the term "in my opinion" as a qualifying statement has no legal value as a disclaimer. The phrase is an admission by the veterinarian that there may be other interpretations of the facts but does not reduce the responsibility of careful observation and application of professional expertise. *A certificate that is false, misleading, inaccurate or inadequate places the veterinarian at risk of litigation and charges of professional misconduct.*

INSURANCE EXAMINATION

When an insurance examination is requested by the client, the veterinarian is not required to attest to the insurability of the horse but only to report the medical facts to the insurance company. The insurance underwriter then has the option, upon review of the application and veterinary certificate, to accept or reject the application.

One of the difficulties facing the veterinarian conducting an insurance examination is, though the horse owner is paying for the examination and is thus the client, the information belongs to the insurance company. This can create a conflict of interest, especially where information about past treatment of the horse is required and may affect the animal's insurability. If such a situation exists, the client should be asked to consult an independent veterinarian.

The intended use of the animal should be considered when interpreting the significance of any abnormalities. For example, a horse may have conditions that would be acceptable in a breeding animal but not in a racing animal. Evidence of firing, blistering, neurectomy or other surgery should be noted and their significance pointed out to the insurance company. Interpretation depends on whether insurance is sought for mortality or for loss of use. A copy of all the findings should be kept as part of the case record.

The examination involves positive identification and a thorough and systematic inspection, similar to that for prepurchase examination. Foals should be similarly examined except that the foal cannot be exercised. Instead, it can be observed running with its dam in a large yard or paddock. Confirming passive transfer of maternal immunoglobulins at 24 hours of age is strongly recommended before passing a foal as suitable for insurance.

Anesthesia and elective surgery should not be performed without permission from the insurer. However, it is the owner's responsibility to advise the insurer of a diagnosis or intended treatment.

DIAGNOSTIC AIDS

Though diagnostic aids can be useful, improperly applied diagnostic aids, such as inappropriate bacteriologic samples, may result in use of costly and potentially harmful therapy. In a busy practice, it is tempting in a puzzling case to simply take blood for a hemogram and plasma/serum biochemical profile so that a diagnosis may be made. However, this is no substitute for an adequate clinical examination. Once the examination is complete, the abnormalities in one or more

body systems identified, and a list of differential diagnoses established, diagnostic aids may be required to confirm a diagnosis.

The various diagnostic aids are discussed in the chapters on the individual body systems. Figure 47 on the following page presents a flow chart of the different diagnostic aids that could be used to diagnose disorders of the various body systems. This list is not comprehensive but is designed as a guide to the tests that may be used.

References

1. Wright M: *The Jeffery Method of Horse Handling.* Breakthrough Publishing, Briarcliff, NY, 1975.

2. Kopf N, in Robinson NE: *Current Therapy in Equine Medicine.* 2nd ed. Saunders, Philadelphia, 1986. pp 23-27.

3. Dyce KM *et al: Textbook of Veterinary Anatomy.* Saunders, Philadelphia, 1988.

4. Thoroughbred Racetrack Protective Bureau: Personal communication, 1988.

5. United States Trotting Assn: Personal communication, 1988.

Additional Reading

Restraint

Federation Equestre Internationale: *Identification of Horses.* 1st ed. FEI Headquarters, Bollingenstrasse 54, CH 3000, Berne 32, Switzerland, 1981. pp 1-48.

Leahy JR and Barrow P: *Restraint of Animals.* 2nd ed. Cornell Campus Store, Ithaca, NY, 1953.

Miller WC and Robertson EDS: *Practical Animal Husbandry.* 7th ed. Oliver and Boyd, Edinburgh, 1959.

Medical Records

Huffman EK: *Medical Record Management.* 6th ed. Physicians Record Co, Berwyn, IL, 1972.

Priester WA: A summary of diagnosis in the ox, horse, dog and cat from twelve veterinary school clinics in the U.S. and Canada. *Vet Record* 86:654-657, 1970.

Weed LL: Medical records that guide and teach. *N Engl J Med* 278:593-600, 1968.

Weed LL: *Medical Records, Medical Education and Patient Care.* Yearbook Medical Publishers, Chicago, 1971.

Physical Examination

Cazalet E: Recent developments in the law relating to veterinary certificates of soundness. *Equine Vet J* 3:125-128, 1971.

Craven JR: Significance of lesions of the cornea and lens in the examination for soundness. *Equine Vet J* 3:141-143, 1971.

Evans LH: The soundness examination and soundness examination form. *Proc 13th Ann Mtg AAEP,* 1968. pp 57-80.

Figure 47. Diagnostic aids that can be considered in disorders of different body systems.

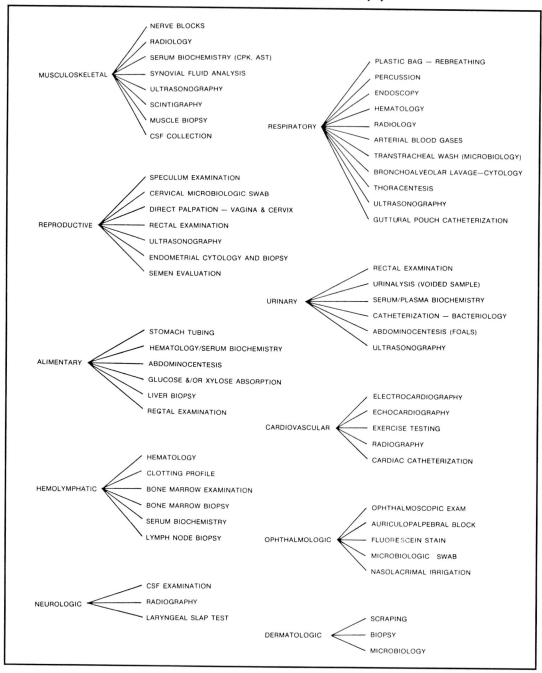

Flynn DV: The issuance of a soundness certificate - ethical and medicolegal considerations - scope, wording and distribution. *Proc 15th Ann Mtg AAEP*, 1969. pp 175-191.

Flynn DV: The purchase examination: historical background. *Proc 24th Ann Mtg AAEP*, 1978. p 569.

Fregin GF: The purchase examination: the cardiovascular system. *Proc 24th Ann Mtg AAEP*, 1978. pp 583-590.

Glendinning ESA: Significance of clinical abnormalities of the heart in soundness. *Equine Vet J* 4:21-30, 1972.

Koch SA: The purchase examination: the eye. *Proc 24th Ann Mtg AAEP,* 1978. pp 571-581.

Mayhew IG: The purchase examination: the nervous system. *Proc 24th Ann Mtg AAEP,* 1978. pp 619-632.

Porter ARW: Some aspects of the law relating to equine practice. *Equine Vet J* 1:223-230, 1969.

Porter ARW: When is an opinion a representation? *Equine Vet J* 2:125-127, 1970.

Proctor DL: The purchase examination: the musculoskeletal system of the standardbred. *Proc 24th Ann Mtg AAEP,* 1978. pp 615-618.

Raker CW: The purchase examination: the respiratory system. *Proc 24th Ann Mtg AAEP,* 1978. pp 591-611.

Reid CF: A field form for soundness examination. *Proc 15th Ann Mtg AAEP,* 1969. pp 169-174.

Reid CF: Radiography and the purchase examination in the horse. *Vet Clin No Am* (Large Anim Pract) 2:151-202, 1980.

Teigland MB: The purchase examination: the musculoskeletal system. *Proc 24th Ann Mtg AAEP* 1978. p 613.

The Veterinary Role in Equine Insurance. AAEP, Rt 5, 22363 Hillcrest Circle, Golden, CO 80401, 1985.

Constitution, By-Laws, Ethics and Professional Guidelines. AAEP, Rt 5, 22363 Hillcrest Circle, Golden, CO 80401, 1982.

Guide to Professional Conduct. Royal Coll Vet Surgeons, 32 Belgrave Sq, London SW1X 8QP, UK, 1987.

A Guide to Examination of Horses. Australian Equine Vet Assn, 134-136 Hampden Rd, Artarmon, NSW 2064, Australia.

ANESTHESIA AND CHEMICAL RESTRAINT

M.A. Brownlow and D.R. Hutchins

Indications for Chemical Restraint and General Anesthesia

In equine practice, the need frequently arises for chemical restraint or general anesthesia to control an uncooperative patient during diagnostic procedures, such as radiography, ultrasonography, arthrocentesis or endoscopy, to provide analgesia during examination of a horse with colic, or to immobilize a horse for minor surgical procedures. Consequently, drugs are used to produce tranquilization, sedation, hypnosis and analgesia.

In other instances, general anesthesia may be required for diagnosis (eg, cervical or pelvic radiography) or in surgical treatment of specific conditions. Because the duration of anesthesia required for specific procedures varies from a few minutes to several hours, numerous anesthetic techniques have been devised.

The following questions should be considered in selection of standing chemical restraint or short term general anesthesia to control horses:

- *Is the horse's temperament such that deep sedation will be required?*
- *Can the procedure be completed with the horse standing?*
- *How much time is required to complete the procedure?*
- *Does the surgical site place the surgeon in a dangerous position?*
- *Is general anesthesia safer?*

The answers to these questions dictate the choice of drugs and their dosages.

Agents for Standing Chemical Restraint

The objective of chemical restraint is to provide sedation, standing immobilization and some analgesia so that clinical examinations or minor surgical procedures can be performed. Generally, the drugs chosen for chemical restraint are selected from the tranquilizer, hypnotic-sedative, and narcotic or narcotic-like analgesic groups. These drugs can be used alone (Table 1) or in combination (Table 2) to produce the desired response. If used alone, however, pharmacologically excessive doses may be necessary. At such levels, adverse effects become more pronounced and, in some horses, the desired effect is not achieved. To provide better standing chemical restraint, 2 or more drugs frequently are administered in combination. Though many drug combinations have been recommended, no technique is accepted universally. The choice of combination and dose is determined by evaluating the temperament of the patient and the procedure to be performed.

Xylazine

Xylazine is a potent sedative with analgesic and muscle relaxant properties. Xylazine induces sedation and analgesia by direct stimulation of central alpha2-adrenergic receptors, which probably decreases neurotransmitter release.[1,2] Nociceptive transmission in the spinal cord is inhibited by a descending alpha-2-noradrenergic analgesic mechanism.[3] Because drugs of this type stim-

Table 1. Characteristics of drugs used in combination or alone for standing chemical restraint.

Drug Group	Drug	Analgesic Activity	IV Dosage	Onset of Action	Peak Effect	Duration of Action
Narcotic analgesics with agonist activity	morphine Morphine (Lilly)	1	0.05-0.12 mg/kg	20 min	15-30 min	3-4 hr
	meperidine Demerol (Winthrop)	0.1	0.1-1.0 mg/kg	10-15 min	15-30 min	2-3 hr
	oxymorphone Numorphan (DuPont)	10	0.015-0.03 mg/kg	5-10 min	15-30 min	3-4 hr
	methadone Dolophine (Lilly)	1-3	0.05-0.12 mg/kg	10-15 min	15-30 min	2-3 hr
Narcotic-like analgesics with agonist-antagonist activity	pentazocine Talwin-V (Winthrop)	0.25	0.4-0.9 mg/kg	2-3 min	5-10 min	3 hr
	butorphanol Torbugesic (Bristol)	5	0.01-0.1 mg/kg	3 min	15-30 min	3-4 hr
	buprenorphine Buprenex (Norwich Easton)	30	0.004-0.006 mg/kg	15 min	30-45 min	up to 8 hr
Tranquilizers	acepromazine	0	0.04-0.08 mg/kg	5-15 min	15-20 min	up to 8 hr
Sedatives	xylazine	NA	0.2-1.1 mg/kg	5-10 min	10-30 min	45-60 min
	detomidine[130] Domosedan (Farmos)	NA	0.004-0.04 mg/kg	3-5 min	15 min	30-120 min
	chloral hydrate	0	15-30 mg/kg			dose dependent

NA = not available

ulate specific receptor sites, their pharmacologic actions can be reversed by specific antagonists acting upon these same receptors. The most well-known antagonist to xylazine is yohimbine.

Xylazine is an extremely useful drug because it has sedative and analgesic effects at the full dosage (1.1 mg/kg IV). At this dosage, xylazine produces sedation in 95% of horses. It also produces a characteristic "stupor," with lowered head, relaxed facial muscles, dropped lower lip and, in males, penile protrusion from the prepuce. Though skeletal muscle relaxation is pronounced and mild incoordination occurs, recumbency is uncommon. However, stimulation of an apparently sedated horse may produce a sudden return of awareness with well-directed kicks and avoidance responses.[4]

At the full recommended dosage, xylazine has profound effects on the cardiovascular system. Time- and dose-dependent selective activation and inhibition of parasympathetic and sympathetic divisions of the autonomic nervous system occur. This reduces the heart rate, ventricular contractility and cardiac output, and increases central venous pressure and peripheral vascular resistance.[5,6] Mean arterial pressure increases for 15-20 minutes and then decreases for a longer period.[5,6]

The dysrhythmogenic effects of xylazine (sinus bradycardia and atrioventricular block) are ascribed to drug-induced increases in vagal tone and can be abolished by atropine. Xylazine's central stimulatory effects are believed to be responsible for the increases in peripheral vascular resistance and

Table 2. Narcotic, narcotic-like analgesic, tranquilizer and sedative combinations for standing chemical restraint in horses.

Drug Combination	IV Dosage (mg/kg)
Morphine	0.1-0.5
Xylazine	0.5-1.0
Meperidine	0.5-0.6
Acepromazine	0.04-0.05
Oxymorphone	0.02
Acepromazine	0.04
Methadone	0.1
Xylazine	0.06
Meperidine	1.1
Xylazine	0.66
Butorphanol	0.01-0.1
Xylazine	1.1
Morphine	0.66
Xylazine	0.66
Chloral hydrate	22
Buprenorphine	0.004
Acepromazine	0.02
Buprenorphine	0.006
Xylazine	0.07
Meperidine	0.3
Xylazine	0.2
Acepromazine	0.04
Buprenorphine	0.006
Xylazine	0.2
Acepromazine	0.04
Xylazine	0.6
Acepromazine	0.02
Chloral hydrate	12-30
Acepromazine	0.04-0.06
Xylazine	0.5-1.0
Chloral hydrate	15

arterial pressure. The dramatic 30% decrease in cardiac output is presumed to be directly related to the decreased heart rate. It also may be partially attributed to increases in arterial pressure.[6] These effects must be taken into account when considering use of xylazine in high-risk or heavily-muscled patients before prolonged or extensive surgical procedures. Xylazine should be used with caution in old or debilitated horses; horses in shock may be compromised if inadequate supportive treatment is given.

Intramuscular administration of xylazine results in less profound disturbances of cardiovascular function. Though there is no initial increase in arterial pressure, hypotension occurs 15 minutes after administration. More important, significant increases in peripheral vascular resistance also occur at this time.[4] The sedation resulting from IM injection of xylazine is less profound than after IV administration and probably less than that achieved by IV administration of acepromazine.[6]

At recommended dosages, xylazine reduces respiratory rate and tidal volume sufficiently to alter arterial blood gas concentrations.[6,7] In addition, respiratory stridor due to upper airway obstruction has been reported. Xylazine also relaxes the larynx and suppresses the cough reflex.[6]

Xylazine induces a dose-related diuresis, with decreased urine osmolality. Hyperglycemia and hypoinsulinemia also occur, but glucosuria is absent.[8] Because yohimbine prevents these effects, presumably they are the result of alpha2-adrenoreceptor stimulation. Further, xylazine decreases serum antidiuretic hormone concentration coincidentally with diuresis.[9]

Xylazine has an oxytocic effect on the uterus and may induce early parturition in cattle if administered in the last trimester of pregnancy. Though this does not appear to be a problem in mares, xylazine should not be used indiscriminately in mares near term.[9]

In cattle and horses, administration of xylazine at recommended dosages produces ileus lasting 30-45 minutes.[5] Further, xylazine may compromise small intestinal vascular function by simultaneously increasing splanchnic peripheral vascular resistance, intestinal motility and oxygen consumption. These effects appear to be dose dependent.[10] These effects on the splanchnic circulation may be important in horses with intestinal hypoperfusion associated with colic.

Administration of xylazine may be followed by profuse sweating. This effect has been attributed to the diffuse autonomic actions of xylazine. Sudden death, respiratory distress characterized by hyperventilation and wheezing, and cardiac arrhythmias also have been reported in horses after IV administration of xylazine.[5,11] Respiratory complications could be the result of bronchoconstriction caused by intense drug-induced cholinergic stimulation.[5] Though bradyarrhythmias are common after IV administration of xylazine, treatment usually is unnecessary.

Xylazine is extensively metabolized by the liver and excreted in the urine. The plasma half-life is about 75 minutes in horses.[5]

Dosage: The recommended IV dosage for standing restraint is 1.1 mg/kg. Clinically, the peak effect occurs within 3 minutes of IV administration. Normal behavior resumes within 30 minutes at a dosage of 0.5 mg/kg and within 60 minutes at 1.1 mg/kg.

An IM dosage of 2-3 mg/kg produces less profound sedation that develops over 10-15 minutes.[12] Higher dosages increase the duration rather than the depth of sedation and prolong recovery time. Recovery usually is complete within 2 hours, even after the use of the higher dosage.

Precautions: Because the undesirable effects of xylazine are dose dependent, it is advisable to use the smallest dose possible to achieve the degree of sedation required. Generally, dosages of 0.22-0.33 mg/kg or 100-150 mg/450 kg are sufficient for anesthetic premedication.

Acepromazine

The phenothiazine derivative tranquilizer, acepromazine, is used extensively in equine practice for both standing chemical restraint and anesthetic premedication. Acepromazine is one of the safest central nervous system depressants and induces behavioral changes that render the animal quiet, calm and relatively indifferent to its surroundings. Acepromazine does not provide analgesia.

Phenothiazine tranquilizers exert a wide variety of effects on the central nervous system. The predominant sites of action appear to be extrapyramidal and involve the basal ganglia, hypothalamus, limbic system and brainstem.[5] The mechanism of action is by interference with or blockage of dopamine receptors.

After administration of acepromazine, horses become less reactive to external stimuli, but there are minimal effects on consciousness, motor ability and coordination. There is a substantial decrease in alertness and responsiveness, making most animals easier to handle.[13] Some horses, however, may become excited or violent in response to painful stimulation.[14] In our experience, acepromazine produces predictable and consistent responses in 75% of horses.

Clinical signs of tranquilization include lowering of the head and extension of the neck, relaxation and drooping of the lower lip, and slight prolapse of the third eyelid. In males, the penis drops from the prepuce, with full extension occurring in about 30 minutes and correlating directly with peak tranquilizer effect and dose rate. The penis may remain extended for up to 2 hours and gradually retracts as the effect of the drug wanes.[13] It should be emphasized that the clinical signs of tranquilization are dose related up to a total dose of about 30 mg.

Generally, a change in the animal's demeanor is observed within 5 minutes after IV administration of acepromazine. The peak effect, however, may require 30 minutes or longer. A horse may appear somnolent if left undisturbed but is readily aroused and moves freely with minimal ataxia.[9] In general, the actions of the phenothiazines are dose dependent and tend to be of relatively long duration, from 4-8 hours.

Acepromazine has peripheral anticholinergic, antiadrenergic and antiganglionic activities. These actions lead to generalized central nervous system depression, interference with temperature regulation and a wide variety of clinically important cardiovascular effects.[5]

Phenothiazine tranquilizers act centrally and peripherally to induce a dose-related decrease in arterial blood pressure that tends to be more evident in horses with increased sympathetic tone. Specifically, hypothalamic depression, peripheral antiadrenergic activity, alpha-adrenergic blockade and a direct vasodilatory effect upon blood vessels act in concert to reduce blood pressure.[15] The reduction in pressure is substantial; blood pressure is reduced by 30% after injection at 0.06 mg/kg (30 mg/450-kg horse). The maximum effect occurs 15 minutes after IV administration of the drug.[16] The accompanying changes in heart rate and cardiac output are not significant.[6]

Phenothiazines have antiarrhythmic activity but the mechanism is poorly understood. This effect may be mediated by myocardial depression, a quinidine-like action, myocardial local anesthetic effect or indirectly by alpha-adrenergic blockade.[17]

Acepromazine produces a decrease in respiratory rate in horses. This usually is compensated for by increases in tidal volume. Minute volume, and thus arterial oxygen and carbon dioxide levels and arterial pH, is maintained near normal values.[5]

84

The effects of phenothiazine tranquilizers on the gastrointestinal tract are negligible.

Acepromazine is extensively metabolized in the liver, and metabolites are identifiable in the urine for 3-4 days after a single dose.[18]

Dosage: The recommended IV dosages of acepromazine vary from 0.02 to 0.1 mg/kg. In our experience, a dosage of 0.035 mg/kg is satisfactory for routine use and provides adequate anesthetic premedication for most horses. Though the IM route may be used, it is not as popular due to the long wait before the full effects are evident.

Precautions: After acepromazine has been given, the horse should be left undisturbed in quiet surroundings. Once the desired effect has occurred, the horse still should be handled gently to prevent excitement. A low dosage (0.035 mg/kg) is recommended, as it provides adequate tranquilization for anesthetic induction in most horses without causing severe hypotension. Because of its propensity to cause hypotension, acepromazine should not be given to old, debilitated, frightened, excited or hypovolemic horses. In such situations, alpha-adrenergic blockade may result in a precipitous fall in arterial blood pressure.

By far, the most noted and potentially most devastating effect of phenothiazine tranquilizers is their ability to produce penile paralysis.[19] This side effect is believed to occur due to central antiadrenergic activity, cholinergic predominance and blockade of dopamine receptors.[20] Though propionylpromazine and propiopromazine are noted for these effects, administration of acepromazine in association with other drugs has been reported to produce penile paralysis.[21] However, the incidence of penile paralysis is too low for acepromazine to be contraindicated for use in stallions and geldings.[22]

Detomidine

Detomidine is a relatively new drug that is satisfactory for standing chemical restraint. Like xylazine, it is nonnarcotic, with sedative and analgesic properties. It produces clinical effects resembling those of xylazine but of longer duration. Detomidine is a potent alpha-adrenoreceptor agonist causing sympathomimetic effects.[23,24] The cardiopulmonary effects of detomidine at dosages of 20, 80 and 160 μg/kg have been investigated. Bradycardia occurs at all dosages, with heart rates as low as 10-12 bpm.[25] Bradycardia is associated with degrees of atrioventricular blockade and arterial hypertension.

Following administration of detomidine, the respiratory pattern changes dramatically, as 30-second periods of apnea are followed by 3-8 closely spaced breaths. There is a decline in P_aO_2 coinciding with the greatest degree of clinical sedation and analgesia.[25] Like xylazine, detomidine induces hyperglycemia and diuresis.[9]

Clinically, detomidine induces dose-dependent depression of the central nervous system, providing more profound and longer sedation and analgesia than xylazine.[26] For standing chemical restraint, a higher dosage can be used to prolong the effect but the dosage should not exceed 80 μg/mg.[25] In clinical trials, xylazine provided reliable analgesia to the forelimbs of two-thirds of horses and to the rear limbs and perineal area in only half the horses.[24] Detomidine provides better sedation and more reliable analgesia of the entire horse than xylazine, and the intensity and duration of these effects can be more easily controlled by varying the dosage.[24]

Combinations of Agents

Narcotics and narcotic-like analgesics serve as the nucleus for many of the combinations that provide standing chemical restraint. If used alone in healthy pain-free horses, these drugs have unpredictable effects and may cause excitation, with mydriasis, sweating, restlessness, violent behavior and even convulsions.[5] These effects may become apparent within 3-10 minutes of drug administration and gradually diminish over the next 15 minutes. However, in some horses, excitation persists for several hours, with muscle tremors, pacing, pawing or sweating. The central nervous system effects of this group of drugs cause a variety of behavioral and analgesic responses primarily dependent on the individual's temperament and the presence or absence of pain. In horses experiencing pain, the response to these agents is usually sedation and analgesia.[5,9]

To provide more reliable effects, narcotics and narcotic-like analgesics usually are combined with acepromazine, xylazine, chloral hydrate or combinations of these. In combination, these agents have synergistic sedative-hypnotic-analgesic effects and blunt the excitatory effects of the narcotic.[5,9] It has been recommended that acepromazine always be added to any narcotic or narcotic-like analgesic combination.[22] This is because the motor activity induced by narcotics and narcotic-like drugs appears to be caused by activation of central dopaminergic receptors, which are effectively blocked by acepromazine.[27] The 8-hour duration of action of acepromazine also is beneficial when narcotics with a relatively long duration of action are chosen. Conversely, if xylazine, which has a relatively short duration of action, is used in combination with narcotic or narcotic-like analgesics, excitation may occur in some horses 60 minutes after receiving the drug combination. If this occurs, supplemental doses of xylazine or a narcotic antagonist, such as naloxone, should be administered. The various drugs and their individual characteristics are presented in Table 1. Table 2 is a summary of combinations used for standing chemical restraint and recommended dosages. In general, the actions of most combinations are more predictable than those of the individual drugs used alone.[5,6,9,22]

When a drug combination is being selected, the respective onset of action of each drug in the combination should be considered. Because the excitatory effects of narcotics occur rapidly following IV administration, narcotics should not be given until the full effect of the tranquilizer or sedative-hypnotic has occurred. This requires 15-20 minutes for acepromazine and 5-10 minutes for xylazine.[5,9]

Though these combinations induce excellent sedation and analgesia, they also may cause incoordination. It is advisable to place the horse in stocks so that support can be provided when necessary.

These combinations have many desirable qualities but they should be used with consideration of their net effects. The cardiovascular effects of narcotic agonists in healthy, pain-free horses is dose related. An exception is pentazocine, which causes a significantly increased heart rate and cardiac output for 15 minutes, followed by a gradual decline to baseline values.[4] For all combinations, mean arterial pressure and peripheral vascular resistance tend to increase and remain above normal for at least 60 minutes after drug administration.[9] Similarly, there is a significant increase in respiratory rate but little alteration in arterial blood gas tensions. These cardiopulmonary effects contrast with those reported for people and dogs, in which depression is more common.[4,5,9] These spe-

cies differences have been attributed to the stimulatory action of these drugs on the cardiorespiratory and vasomotor centers in horses.[6]

The physiologic effects xylazine-morphine and xylazine-acepromazine combinations have been examined in depth. Generally, these combinations provide cardiopulmonary stability despite causing a significant reduction in cardiac output.[6] Further, the sedative and analgesic effects of these combinations are superior to those effects of either drug given individually.[6] Other drug combinations have yet to be investigated thoroughly.

In general, narcotics and narcotic-like analgesics increase gastrointestinal muscle and sphincter tone, enhance nonpropulsive contractions of the intestine, and decrease propulsive contractions. The overall result is delayed transit of ingesta and increased water absorption from the feces.[4,5,9]

Considerations in General Anesthesia

The objectives of general anesthesia are to:
- Provide sufficient hypnosis, analgesia and muscle relaxation for the surgical or diagnostic procedure to be performed.
- Interfere minimally with cardiovascular and respiratory functions.
- Allow recovery without untoward effects after termination of anesthesia.

Special problems confronting the equine anesthetist include the temperament, size and weight of horses. These 3 factors dictate an approach to anesthesia that is quite different from that used for small animals. To be safe and to maintain physiologic normality, induction agents must be reliable and predictable. Excitement and struggling under light planes of anesthesia can have disastrous consequences for both the horse and personnel. Similarly, during recovery from anesthesia, the horse must lie quietly until sufficient coordination is regained to rise without injury. Because prolonged recumbency is not well tolerated by horses, premedication, positioning of the horse, intraoperative monitoring and anesthetic recovery must be planned carefully. Thus, a thorough knowledge of equine anesthesia-associated pathophysiology is mandatory.

Common equine anesthetic problems include hypoventilation, hypoxemia, hypotension and postoperative neuromuscular damage.[21,27-29] Thus, special attention must be paid to inherent cardiopulmonary depressant effects of anesthetics and to maintenance or enhancement of peripheral perfusion.

Though systemic arterial pressure often is monitored in horses under general anesthesia, undue reliance should not be placed upon the values obtained. While arterial pressure may provide a rough index of the vigor of cardiac contraction, it fails to indicate the adequacy of flow through peripheral tissues.[30] Pressure and resistance determine tissue blood flow and perfusion. This relationship between flow, pressure and resistance is expressed in the following equation:

Change in pressure = flow x resistance = cardiac output x total peripheral resistance

The adequacy of the circulation is judged by the capacity of flow to meet tissue cellular demands. The relationship of blood pressure to vascular resistance, therefore, is more important than a simple measurement of pressure alone.[31] Just as a high blood pressure is no guarantee of adequacy of perfusion, neither is a low pressure necessarily associated with hypoperfusion. Thus, the vital factor in the relationship is vascular resistance. If tissue perfusion becomes inadequate, cellular hypoxia, lactic acidosis and, ultimately, cell death result. Consequently, the veterinarian must keep the relationship of blood pressure to resistance in perspective when selecting drugs to be used in the anesthetic regimen.

Pathophysiology of Anesthesia

Respiratory depression and impaired oxygenation occur to some degree in all animals under general anesthesia. In horses, arterial carbon dioxide levels (P_aCO_2) may be elevated substantially and arterial oxygen levels (P_aO_2) can fall far below predicted levels. This has certain implications for anesthetic management during surgery and into the recovery period. The following discussion highlights the clinically relevant aspects of the physiologic responses of horses to general anesthesia and recumbency.

Alveolar Hypoventilation

Alveolar hypoventilation accompanies inhalation anesthesia in horses and causes elevated P_aCO_2 with an associated reduction in

pH.[32] Hypercarbia generally occurs because the chemoreceptor normally stimulated by hypoxemia to cause an increase in alveolar ventilation while breathing air is blunted when horses breathe oxygen-rich mixtures. Thus, reduction of this hypoxemic drive causes reduced alveolar ventilation and retention of CO_2. Retention of CO_2 is evident during recumbency, regardless of the horse's body position. The magnitude of CO_2 retention is much greater in horses than in people and dogs.[33] P_aCO_2 levels commonly exceed 50 mm Hg and may reach 100 mm Hg during deep levels of anesthesia in horses. Generally, P_aCO_2 values above 65 mm Hg are of concern.[34]

The causes of hypoventilation may be identified when one considers the factors in the following equation:

Minute alveolar ventilation (V_A) = (tidal volume (V_T) - dead space (V_D) x respiratory rate (R_f)

When a horse is under general anesthesia, all of the factors governing minute ventilation may be altered. For instance, *drug-induced respiratory depression* may occur, reducing the tidal volume and respiratory rate. Many authors have emphasized the particular sensitivity of horses to the respiratory depressant effects of general anesthetics.[21,28,32] Due to the depressant effects of most anesthetic agents on the central nervous system, there are decreases in both respiratory rate and tidal volume, and a diminished ventilatory response to accumulation of CO_2.[35] The degree of hypercarbia is related to the dose of the anesthetic; the P_aCO_2 tends to increase in direct proportion to the depth of anesthesia. After an initial increase in P_aCO_2, horses maintained at constant alveolar concentrations of halothane have little change in P_aCO_2 for up to 2-3 hours and a gradual increase thereafter.[21,36]

Increased physiologic dead space (V_D/V_T) occurs commonly in anesthetized horses. This means that a greater proportion of the tidal volume does not contribute to gas exchange. V_D/V_T values are high in anesthetized horses, with up to 60% of the V_T being dead space.[37] Further, exhaled CO_2 may be rebreathed if the dead space of the anesthetic apparatus is excessive. This happens when a low gas flow is used with a "to-and-fro" anesthetic system or if there is defective absorption of CO_2 in a circle system.[38]

A *reduction in functional residual capacity* may occur for several reasons during general anesthesia. Regardless of the cause, this effectively reduces the volume of gas available for gaseous exchange. General anesthesia alters chest wall expansion and movements of the diaphragm, resulting in a 50% reduction functional residual capacity in horses, in comparison to 16% and 27% in other species.[35,39] Consequently, this reduction of functional residual capacity leads to airway closure, with trapping of gas in alveoli, alveolar collapse, and an increase in right-to-left intrapulmonary shunt.[40]

Resistance to respiration increases 3-4 fold as a direct result of the anesthetic delivery system and results in a corresponding fall in ventilation. The diameter of the endotracheal tube, size of the inspiratory and expiratory limbs of the anesthetic circuit, pattern of gas flow along the flexible tubing, and design of valves and the soda lime canister all influence resistance.[38]

The consequences of moderate to severe hypercarbia (P_aCO_2 of 65 = 100 mm Hg) are associated with the ubiquitous nature of CO_2 and its diverse effects and sites of action. At P_aCO_2 values up to 150 mm Hg, cerebral blood flow and cerebrospinal fluid pressure increase and there is progressive depression of central nervous system activity. At higher tensions, excitation and convulsions culminate in progressive depression and unconsciousness.[31,41-43]

Hypercarbia causes an increase in sympathetic adrenergic activity. The effect on the circulation is mixed, as hypercarbia within the central nervous system causes vasoconstriction and hypertension. Peripherally, however, increases in P_aCO_2 cause vasodilation.[42] There usually is a close correlation between cardiac output and P_aCO_2 levels; cardiac output increases as the P_aCO_2 rises. This relationship is particularly marked in response to acute changes, as may occur during general anesthesia.[31,41-43]

The effects of hypercarbia on skin and skeletal muscle balance between direct vasodilator effects of CO_2 and vasoconstrictor effects secondary to sympathetic adrenergic activity. During anesthesia, however, the response is predominantly vasodilation in skin and vasoconstriction in muscle.[42,43]

Some factors can be manipulated by the anesthesiologist to minimize hypercarbia. Premedicant and induction drugs having pronounced respiratory depressant effects can be avoided and a minimum concentration of inhalation agent for maintenance of anesthesia used. Further, anesthetic apparatus with minimal dead space and resistance to respiration should be used. Though inherent increases in V_D/V_T and reductions in functional residual capacity may be beyond manipulation, it is useful to be aware of their possible contributions to hypoventilation.

In the clinical setting, hypoventilation and hypercarbia can be ascertained by measurement of tidal volume, arterial blood gas tensions or end-tidal CO_2 concentration. Clinically, with moderate to severe hypercarbia, the horse may sweat profusely and have a progressive rise in arterial pressure and jerky respiratory movements.[34] Generally, horses that develop the greatest degree of hypercarbia are athletically fit and have a pronounced degree of cardiopulmonary depression with halothane anesthesia. Though the plane of anesthesia in these animals appears quite light and they have brisk palpebral reflexes and nystagmus, they often "hold their breath" for prolonged periods. If allowed to breathe spontaneously, these horses may have respiratory rates as low as 1-2 breaths/minute without surgical stimulation. Surgical stimulation may increase the respiratory rate to 4-6 breaths/minute.

Methods of increasing the patient's respiratory frequency, other than with positive-pressure ventilation, include twisting its ear firmly, changing the pressures in the circle system using the "pop-off" valve, and gently striking the horse's flank. Of these, twisting the patient's ear is particularly effective.[34]

Not all horses develop severe hypercarbia under general anesthesia. Pony breeds, most foals and many adult horses not in athletic condition routinely have P_aCO_2 values below 65 mm Hg. Use of controlled or assisted ventilation is controversial because positive-pressure ventilation decreases cardiovascular function and this may outweigh the advantages of normocarbia. Consequently, P_aCO_2 values up to 65 mm Hg should not be considered deleterious. With a well-designed anesthetic apparatus and by using minimal concentrations of inhalation agents, spontaneous ventilation can result in P_aCO_2 levels <65 mm Hg.

Impairment of Oxygenation

General anesthesia and recumbency markedly decrease the efficiency of respiratory gas exchange in horses. This impairment of oxygenation is characterized by an arterial oxygen tension (P_aO_2) well below the alveolar partial pressure of oxygen (PAO_2).[27,28,32, 37,44,45] Theoretically, horses breathing high inspired concentrations of oxygen (90%) during inhalation anesthesia should have P_aO_2 tensions of 500-600 mm Hg (Fig 48). Under clinical conditions, however, many horses have P_aO_2 values much lower, even in the range of 150 mm Hg. This disparity between calculated P_aO_2 and measured P_aO_2 is called the alveolar-to-arterial oxygen tension difference or $P(A-a)O_2$. During inhalation anesthesia, this difference may range from 100 to 450 mm Hg.[34,45,46] This $P(A-a)O_2$ difference develops within the first 30-60 minutes of anesthesia and increases no further thereafter.[36,46,47] Horses in dorsal recumbency may have lower P_aO_2 tensions than horses in a lateral position.[27] The $P(A-a)O_2$ differences

that occur during anesthesia have been attributed to hypoventilation, ventilation-perfusion inequalities, right-to-left vascular shunts, reductions in cardiac output or all of these. While the $P(A-a)O_2$ differences may result in hypoxemia, other factors governing tissue oxygenation also must be considered.

Oxygen Flux: The factors governing tissue "oxygen flux" are blood flow and blood oxygen content.[43] Blood flow is dependent on cardiac output, while oxygen content is determined by the concentration of hemoglobin and its saturation with oxygen (Fig 49). Therefore, the saturation of hemoglobin with oxygen, as determined by the P_aO_2, is only 1 of 3 important factors in tissue oxygenation.

In conscious horses, a 50% decrease in hemoglobin or saturation of hemoglobin with oxygen usually can be tolerated because a compensatory increase in cardiac output generally maintains tissue oxygenation. If all 3 components (hemoglobin concentration, hemoglobin saturation, cardiac output) decrease simultaneously, as may occur in an

Figure 48. The oxygen cascade in an anesthetized horse.

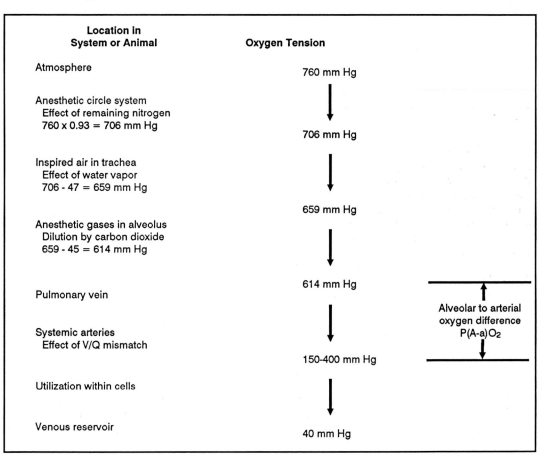

Figure 49. The determinants of oxygen flux.

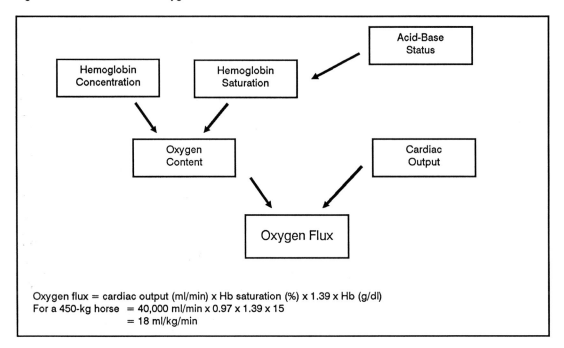

Oxygen flux = cardiac output (ml/min) x Hb saturation (%) x 1.39 x Hb (g/dl)
For a 450-kg horse = 40,000 ml/min x 0.97 x 1.39 x 15
                    = 18 ml/kg/min

acutely ill patient, reductions of as little as 30% may prove fatal unless rapidly corrected.[48]

Thus, a reduction in P_aO_2 alone can be compensated if cardiac output is not decreased substantially and hemoglobin is normal. During general anesthesia in horses, cardiac output commonly decreases by 30-40%. This decreases oxygen flux substantially.

Significance of Hypoxemia: Because horses breathe high oxygen concentrations during inhalation anesthesia, lower-than-predicted P_aO_2 tensions seldom are a problem. This is because, while breathing 90% oxygen, most horses have P_aO_2 tensions above 150 mm Hg and oxyhemoglobin saturation of 98% or more. Because increased P_aCO_2 and body temperature and decreased pH tend to shift the oxyhemoglobin dissociation curve to the right and thereby reduce hemoglobin saturation, the anesthetist should aim to maintain P_aO_2 values >150 mm Hg during general anesthesia.

Hypoxemia is most likely to occur during induction of anesthesia with IV agents, during recovery from inhalation anesthesia, and when the horse is allowed to breathe room air. For recovery, if horses are moved to the recovery stall in a light plane of anesthesia,

with brisk palpebral reflexes, rapid nystagmus and an ear reflex, cardiac output should increase substantially and reduce hypoxemia. In this situation, routine use of oxygen during the recovery period may be unnecessary. The obvious exception is when very low P_aO_2 values are very low. Further, unless relatively high oxygen flow rates are used, the actual elevation in P_aO_2 is minimal. This has been shown in a study in which oxygen insufflation at a flow rate of 10 L/min did not improve P_aO_2 values.[10] Results with demand valves capable of delivering a mixture of air and oxygen at flow rates of 50 L/min and 280 L/min are much better but the technique requires intubation.[49,50]

Recommendations to Optimize Oxygenation: Following are recommendations to optimize oxygenation:

- *Establish and maintain a patent airway.*
- *Maintain a minimum depth and duration of anesthesia,* especially if the horse is breathing gas mixtures not supplemented with oxygen. Avoid techniques that substantially decrease cardiac output. Thus, administration of xylazine during recovery should be minimized or avoided.
- *Ensure a rapid recovery.* Most horses, regardless of ventilation (spontaneous, assisted or controlled) and operative body

position, are hypoxemic immediately post-operatively. Improvement in cardiac output generally compensates for any decrease in P_aO_2. Horses most at risk are those with a depressed cardiac output, metabolic acidosis and low hemoglobin concentration.

- *Maintain oxygen flow through the anesthetic circuit at a rate exceeding oxygen metabolism by the horse.* Flow rates of oxygen of 10 ml/kg/min are well above these metabolic demands. Therefore, provide 4-5 L/min to a 450-kg horse.

- *Provide adequate denitrogenation in the initial stages of inhalation anesthesia.* Because oxygen is displaced substantially by nitrogen within the anesthetic apparatus, high oxygen flow rates should be used and frequent flushing of the rebreathing bag performed during the first 10 minutes of anesthesia. The importance of denitrogenation in quickly elevating the inspired oxygen concentration is well documented.[47,51] Conversely, the low oxygen flow rates commonly used during maintenance of anesthesia tend to have the opposite effect.

- If possible, *select a lateral position over dorsal recumbency.*

- *Consider the horse's condition when selecting an anesthetic.* The normal healthy horse should be able to tolerate general anesthesia breathing air for periods of up to 1 hour. "Topping up" with an additional IV dose of a drug to increase the duration of anesthesia further decreases cardiac output. Consequently, a horse anesthetized by this route may benefit from supplemental oxygen via a nasal catheter at flow rates exceeding 15 L/min. On the other hand, an acidotic horse with an elevated temperature benefits most from inhalation anesthesia because high inspired oxygen tensions can be provided and blood circulation is supported by fluid administration.

- *Use controlled ventilation carefully.* Controlled ventilation does not increase P_aO_2, as it has no effect on the $P(A-a)O_2$ difference. Rather, it decreases P_aCO_2. Because of the substantial reduction in cardiac output caused by controlled ventilation, it may act to decrease oxygen flux.

- *Minimize oxygen demand during recovery.* Factors increasing demand for oxygen during recovery include hypothermia and postoperative pain. Hypothermia is a common complication of general anesthesia, particularly when body cavities are exposed for prolonged periods. While this may cause few problems during anesthesia, the severe shivering that occurs to correct the temperature deficit once consciousness is regained substantially increases tissue oxygen demand. Thus, minimizing intraoperative hypothermia is an important challenge for the equine anesthetist and surgical team. Postoperative pain, from the surgery or such complications as myopathy or neuropathy, may cause violent recoveries and dramatic increases in oxygen demand.

Arterial Hypotension

Arterial hypotension is a common complication during equine anesthesia.[34,52-54] In general, reductions in arterial pressure are proportional to the depth of anesthesia. Consequently, if horses are kept in the lightest plane of anesthesia compatible with the surgical procedure, arterial pressure should be satisfactory. Occasionally, however, even though a light plane of anesthesia is achieved, some healthy surgical patients become hypotensive, with mean arterial pressures as low as 50-60 mm Hg. Athletically fit horses are particularly prone to intraoperative hypotension.

Hypotension probably develops from the additive effects of anesthetic agents and adjuncts, as these drugs, with the exception of ketamine, cause hypotension. Drugs with the most pronounced hypotensive effects are acepromazine, xylazine, thiobarbiturates and, particularly, halothane. Because these hypotensive effects are dose related, using smaller doses of the drugs reduces the likelihood of hypotension.

Hypotension generally is most pronounced immediately after induction. This is especially true with induction techniques that include thiobarbiturates. Care should also be taken to avoid excessively high levels of halothane for maintenance of anesthesia.

Hypotension has many effects. A mean blood pressure of at least 60 mm Hg is required to ensure adequate blood flow to the kidneys and gastrointestinal tract.[53,54] At lower pressures, there is loss of autoregulation to vascular beds, altering cerebral, coronary and renal blood flow.[55] Arterial hypotension also has been implicated in the postoperative myopathy syndrome.[56,57]

Because of the relationship between pressure, blood flow and vascular resistance, it must be emphasized that on some occasions lower pressure with good peripheral perfusion is more advantageous to the patient than a higher pressure with poorer perfusion solely due to increased resistance. Thus, maintenance of blood pressure without considering the adequacy of peripheral perfusion may be detrimental to the patient and increase the likelihood of postoperative complications.

Preanesthetic Considerations

Evaluation of Temperament and Health

The temperament and health of the patient influence the choice and dose of the premedicants and anesthetic agents to be used. Classifying the physical status of the patient helps prepare the surgical team for problems that may arise during surgery. Following is a classification system used to describe the preoperative status of equine patients.

Grade 1: Good health and minor elective surgery.

Grade 2: Minor impairment, *ie,* horses with slight to moderate systemic disturbances that may be associated with the surgical complaint. For example, a simple fracture.

Grade 3: Moderate impairment, *ie,* horses with slight to moderate systemic disturbances that may be associated with the surgical complaint but that may interfere with normal activities. For example, meconium retention.

Grade 4: Major impairment, *ie,* horses with systemic disturbances (may or may not be related to the surgical complaint) that interfere seriously with the patient's normal activities and threaten the animal's life. For example, ruptured bladder and intestinal obstruction.

Grade 5: Moribund.

For each grade, the anesthetist may adopt a different approach and require additional support. Horses classified in grades 4 and 5 require thorough monitoring, vigorous fluid therapy and ancillary medication. By classifying each patient preoperatively, the necessary staff, ancillary equipment and drugs can be assembled so that any complications can be handled efficiently.

Patient Preparation

Preoperative Preparation of Surgical Site: To decrease total anesthetic time, the surgical site should be prepared as thoroughly as is possible before surgery. In most cases, the surgical site can be clipped and scrubbed. This practice can reduce total anesthetic time by 20-30 minutes.

Preanesthetic Restriction of Food Intake: Various conflicting recommendations have been made regarding withdrawal of food from horses scheduled for elective surgery. These range from complete withdrawal of all food but not water for 12 hours preoperatively, to much less stringent and flexible recommendations.[58-60]

The reasons for withholding food in small animals and ruminants are quite clear, namely, vomiting and regurgitation. However, these are not problems in horses. Gastrointestinal distention has been observed in horses but occurs mainly in fit horses in full training that receive a large concentrate ration before anesthesia.[58,59] The pathogenesis of this intestinal distention and the influence of anesthetic drugs and anesthetic regimens may be critical. Consequently, large quantities of grain should be withheld from all horses before general anesthesia. Postoperative cecal rupture has been reported but it is not known whether this is related to specific food restriction practices or lack thereof, intraoperative cecal distention, postoperative cecal impaction or concurrent administration of antiinflammatory drugs. All horses should be monitored carefully postoperatively for normal patterns of defecation.

Alveolar hypoventilation is enhanced by decreases in functional residual capacity. Withholding feed for 18 hours increases functional residual capacity by as much as 30%.[61] Though it is well recognized that many factors may alter functional residual capacity, these findings support the practice of fasting horses for elective surgery of long duration.

Though it is the practice in North America and the United Kingdom to restrict food intake before anesthesia, we believe the indications for and period of starvation required remain unclear. Our aim in not fasting horses is to reduce, as much as possible, any stress associated with general anesthesia. In our clinic, the incidence of intraoperative and postoperative gastrointestinal dysfunction is negligible. This includes the incidence of postoperative salmonellosis, despite carrier incidence of 2.8% in hospital populations.[34]

Preanesthetic Medications

The major aim of preanesthetic medication is to calm the horse and make it tractable despite unfamiliar handlers, complex manipulative procedures and strange environments. Though effective preanesthetic medication makes the induction procedure safer for both the horse and personnel, a large dose of premedicant is not a substitute for good handling techniques. A quiet approach, an experienced person at the horse's head, and a knowledgeable team of people generally allow safe anesthetic inductions with minimal premedication. The general aims of premedication are:

- To select a drug that reliably and predictably calms the patient.
- To minimally depress the cardiopulmonary system.
- To minimally depress the gastrointestinal system.
- To minimize undesirable reflex autonomic activity under general anesthesia.
- To potentiate the effects of other anesthetic agents thereby reducing the doses required.
- To control emotional disturbances effectively and thereby minimize the release of catecholamines. This smooths the whole course of anesthesia, and reduces excitement and struggling during the recovery period.

No chemical agent meets all of these criteria. Some drugs or drug combinations have some of these properties. Because each premedicant may affect many body systems, we must select agents whose benefits outweigh any detrimental effects in a particular patient.

The choice of premedicant always should be tailored to the individual horse's requirements. Some patients may not require premedication. In aged, critically ill and neonatal animals, premedication generally is not used because the adverse effects become more significant.

Quiet horses of draft breeds, donkeys or pony breeds are unusually sensitive to routine premedicant doses based on body weight. These animals tend to become "stupefied" and have prolonged recoveries. Also, for pain-free procedures in ponies, the premedicant dose often must be greatly reduced or a premedicant not used at all. Usually there are no apparent difficulties encountered with induction or recovery; the latter is rapid and excitement free.

Acepromazine

Acepromazine is used extensively in equine practice for anesthetic premedication. It induces behavioral changes that render the animal quiet, calm and relatively indifferent to its surroundings. Generally, a change in the animal's demeanor is observed within 5 minutes after IV administration of acepromazine. The peak effect, however, may require 30 minutes or longer.

Dosage: The recommended IV dosages of acepromazine vary from 0.02 to 0.1 mg/kg. In our experience, a dosage of 0.035 mg/kg is satisfactory for routine use, providing adequate tranquilization, smooth intraoperative course, and quiet recovery for most horses.

Though IM administration has been used before anesthesia, it is not popular. A dosage of 0.04 mg/kg given 1 hour before induction has been recommended.[22] This time requirement restricts the IM route to hospital use.

Precautions: Acepromazine produces consistent results in most horses. Some unruly horses, however, may not respond as expected and require alternative premedication (Table 1).

After acepromazine has been given, the horse should be left undisturbed in quiet surroundings. Once the desired effect has occurred, the horse still should be handled gently to prevent excitement. A low dosage of acepromazine (0.035 mg/kg) is recommended, as it provides adequate tranquilization without causing severe hypotension. Though some decrease in blood pressure accompanies tranquilization, this usually is manageable with IV administration of fluid given intraoperatively. Generally, the benefits of enhanced peripheral perfusion outweigh the detrimental aspects associated with this minor reduction in blood pressure.

Advantages as a Premedicant: Acepromazine has numerous advantages. It is effective and reliable in 75% of horses. Extension of the penis in stallions and geldings is a good indication of onset of action. It potentiates other general anesthetic agents, allowing use of reduced doses.

Evidence of tranquilization is apparent within 10-15 minutes after IV administration and lasts about 2 hours. Anesthesia is safely maintained, in terms of anesthetic depth. Peripheral perfusion and cardiac output are maintained. Finally, acepromazine facilitates a smooth recovery from anesthesia.

Disadvantages as a Premedicant: Acepromazine is not reliable in highly excitable or unruly horses. If this drug must be used in aged or debilitated horses, it should be given cautiously at greatly reduced dosages.

Arterial pressure must be monitored and IV fluids given intraoperatively because of the drug's hypotensive effect. If acepromazine premedication is combined with excessive doses of drugs for induction and maintenance of anesthesia, hypotension could be severe. Though acepromazine smooths recovery from anesthesia, the recovery period tends to be prolonged.

Xylazine

Xylazine is a potent sedative with analgesic and muscle relaxant properties. Consequently, xylazine is used widely as a premedicant (Table 3).

Dosage: The recommended IV dosage for preanesthetic use is 0.25-0.5 mg/kg.[12] Clinically, the peak effect occurs within 3 minutes of IV administration.

An IM dosage of 2-3 mg/kg produces less profound sedation that develops over 10-15 minutes.[12] Higher dosages increase the duration rather than the depth of sedation and prolong recovery time. Recovery is usually complete within 2 hours, even after use of higher dosages.

Precautions: Because the undesirable effects of xylazine are dose dependent, it is advisable to use the smallest dose possible to achieve the degree of sedation required. Generally, dosages of 0.22-0.33 mg/kg or 100-150 mg/450 kg are sufficient. When xylazine is used as a premedicant, induction techniques should be adjusted to avoid unnecessary cardiopulmonary depression.

Advantages as a Premedicant: After IV administration, xylazine produces dose-dependent sedation and muscle relaxation with varying degrees of analgesia. The rapid onset of action in 2-3 minutes allows rapid induction of anesthesia.

The drug has consistent effects in most horses. Though sedated animals can be aroused by sufficiently strong stimuli, they tend not to panic, and become calm again when the stimulation ceases. Because the duration of action is about 40 minutes, if xylazine is used as a premedicant in procedures of less than 60 minutes' duration, recoveries are fast and smooth.

Disadvantages as a Premedicant: Xylazine's effects on the cardiovascular system are profound but dose related. The most important of these effects are reduction in cardiac output and increased peripheral resistance. Dose-dependent increases in small intestinal vascular resistance, motility and oxygen consumption also are of concern.

The respiratory rate is depressed. If xylazine is used as a premedicant for inhalation anesthesia, the animal may wake up as the effect begins to wane (about 40 minutes).

Atropine

Such parasympatholytic drugs as atropine are not routinely used as premedicants because horses do not salivate excessively, are not subject to laryngospasm and seldom develop bradycardia during anesthesia.[5] Further, atropine decreases gastrointestinal motility, causing intestinal distention and ileus. Therefore, there is no justification for routine use of atropine as a preanesthetic medication in equine anesthesia.

Chloral Hydrate

Chloral hydrate is a sedative-hypnotic that produces generalized depression of almost all cellular functions. The effects on the central nervous systems range from mild depression and muscle relaxation to total unconsciousness and coma (Table 3).[5]

Chloral hydrate produces dose-dependent depression of all aspects of autonomic regulation, both centrally and peripherally. Central sympathetic and parasympathetic ganglia, peripheral autonomic neuroeffector functions and adrenergic functions are all depressed.

When administered IV at sedative doses, there appears to be little effect on the gastro-intestinal tract. In larger doses, there is a decrease in glomerular filtration rate and an increase in the force and frequency of uterine contractions. In addition, chloral hydrate can cross the placental barrier easily, but the above effects are negligible on the foal when the drug is given in sedative doses.[5]

Chloral hydrate is metabolized in the liver to trichlorethanol, which then undergoes hepatic metabolism to trichloralic acid and is excreted in the urine.[62]

Sedative doses of chloral hydrate produce bradycardia (due to increased parasympathetic tone), do not alter cardiac output, and tend to be hypotensive. The latter is due to central depression, decrease in cardiac contractility and vascular smooth muscle relaxation.[5,63]

Chloral hydrate remains one of the safest, least expensive and most useful drugs in equine practice. At sedative doses, it induces minimal cardiopulmonary depression and is compatible with many anesthetic agents. One of its major advantages is its predictable effects. In addition, it can be used to calm excited or fractious horses when other drugs have failed.[9] Its augmentation of the muscle relaxation produced by inhalation anesthetics and its prolonged duration of action, lasting through the postsurgical recovery period, make it a satisfactory choice for use as an anesthetic premedicant. When used for sedation, chloral hydrate decreases the respiratory rate, with minimal alteration in arterial blood gases.[5]

Dosage: The recommended IV dosage for restraint is 40 mg/kg. The premedication IV dosage is 15-30 mg/kg.[5,27] Dosages as high as 44 mg/kg (20 g/450 kg) produce excellent sedation with little ataxia.[64] Because there is a delay of several minutes before the full effects become apparent, it has been suggested that two-thirds of the estimated dose be given and then the infusion stopped to assess the effect. To determine the effect of the dose already given, the horse may be pushed. If the animal is easily moved and buckles at the carpus, the dose given is sufficient. The horse should not be given enough chloral hydrate to produce recumbency.[63]

A combination of a tranquilizer, such as acepromazine (0.03-0.04 mg/kg), and chloral hydrate (15-30 mg/kg IV) has been recommended for unruly animals.[27]

Precautions: Chloral hydrate has lost popularity due to the large volume that must be administered, the severe irritation that occurs if the drug is administered perivascularly, its long duration of action, and the degree of ataxia that accompanies sedation.[9]

Chloral hydrate is extremely irritating to tissues. If injected perivascularly, it causes phlebitis and tissue necrosis. Great care should be taken to ensure intravascular injection; 7-12% solutions should be used.[9]

Advantages as a Premedicant: Chloral hydrate provides a predictable response to unit dosage by body weight. It does not cause excitement, and has a wide safety margin and can be given to effect. The drug has minimal cardiovascular and respiratory effects, is compatible with most other anesthetic agents, and is inexpensive.

Disadvantages as a Premedicant: The peak effect of chloral hydrate occurs 2-3 min-

Table 3. Pharmacologic characteristics of premedicant drugs used intravenously in horses.

Drug	Dosage	Onset of Action	Duration
Acepromazine	0.033 mg/kg	10-20 min	2-6 hours
Xylazine	0.25-0.35 mg/kg	2-5 min	40 min
Acepromazine, xylazine	0.02 mg/kg 0.22 mg/kg	2-5 min	90-120 min
Chloral hydrate	15-30 mg/kg	5-15 min	2-4 hours
Detomidine	0.02 mg/kg	2-5 min	60 min

utes after IV administration; therefore, over-dosage can occur rapidly. It is extremely irritating if given perivascularly. Infusion of large volumes requires more time than a single bolus injection and is less convenient.

Detomidine

Because detomidine exerts its effects through alpha2-adrenoceptors, it is often used in the same manner as xylazine (Table 3). When given 3-5 minutes before ketamine, the quality of anesthesia produced was similar to that of xylazine-ketamine except that the time to recumbency was longer and some horses made several attempts before standing.[65] In another study, use of detomidine as a premedicant reduced the dosage of guaifenesin and thiobarbiturate needed to induce anesthesia, and lower halothane vaporizer settings were required to maintain anesthesia.[25] Because of its excellent analgesic properties, detomidine has been used to control pain in horses with colic.[66,67] Many of these horses subsequently were anesthetized with various agents for abdominal surgery, without any apparent ill effects from preoperative use of detomidine.

Dosage: Though information about the clinical use of detomidine is sparse, dosages of 20 μg/kg (0.02 mg/kg) or less should be adequate for premedication before anesthesia is induced with ketamine, or guaifenesin and a thiobarbiturate.

Xylazine with Acepromazine

The aim of using this combination of drugs for premedication is to combine the desirable qualities of acepromazine with the more reliable sedative effects of xylazine. Reducing the dose of xylazine minimizes its dose-related cardiovascular effects. For premedication, this combination is satisfactory in highly excitable, unruly horses.[34] This combination of drugs provides greater intraoperative stability, a quieter but perhaps longer recovery and, most important, better peripheral perfusion than that seen with xylazine alone (Table 3). The behavioral changes produced after IV administration of xylazine and acepromazine are similar to those associated with xylazine.[6]

The combination of xylazine IV at 0.55 mg/kg and acepromazine IV at 0.05 mg/kg initially decreases heart rate and cardiac output. These values return to baseline by 15 and 30 minutes, respectively.[6] The initial increase in arterial pressure observed with xylazine alone is abolished and a stable arterial pressure below baseline values is maintained.[6] Central venous pressure first increases and then falls below baseline values.[6] The initial increase in pressure is attributed to a xylazine-evoked decrease in heart rate and cardiac output. The subsequent decrease in pressure reflects peripheral vasodilation due to the alpha blockade effects of acepromazine.[6] Thus, this drug combination does not decrease cardiac output as much as xylazine alone, does not decrease arterial pressure as much as acepromazine alone, and does not increase total peripheral resistance as much as xylazine alone.

The respiratory effects of the combination of xylazine and acepromazine are similar to those of each drug individually. Though respiratory rate decreases, adequate compensatory increases in minute alveolar ventilation occur.[6]

Dosage: The recommended IV dosage for premedication is acepromazine at 0.02 mg/kg (9 mg/450 kg) and xylazine at 0.22 mg/kg (100 mg/450 kg). These agents can be mixed in the same syringe. This combination tends to produce a reliable calming effect in most excitable horses. The IV dosage of xylazine may need to be increased to 0.5 mg/kg (225 mg/450 kg) for extremely fractious horses. It has been suggested that the dosage of acepromazine should not be increased.[34] The onset of tranquilization is apparent within 3-5 minutes, and the maximum effect is evident by 10 minutes.[34]

Advantages as a Premedicant: The profound dose-related cardiovascular alterations produced by xylazine are minimized by reducing its dose while utilizing its reliable sedative effect. The combination is more effective in highly excitable or fractious horses than is either agent alone. Blood pressure and cardiac output remain closer to baseline values than after administration of either drug alone. Peripheral perfusion is better than with xylazine alone.

Disadvantages as a Premedicant: This combination decreases blood pressure and cardiac output.

Xylazine with Butorphanol

A combination of xylazine and butorphanol was developed to combine the excellent analgesic properties of both drugs, minimize the undesirable side effects characteristic of either drug when used alone, and render the patient more amenable to induction of general anesthesia (Table 3). Butorphanol tartrate is a synthetic opiate with agonist and antagonist properties. Butorphanol is more potent than morphine, meperidine and pentazocine, and causes little depression of cardiovascular or respiratory systems.[8]

The combination of xylazine and butorphanol provides excellent analgesia while reducing depressant effects of xylazine on cardiopulmonary function and marked behavioral effects of butorphanol alone.[69] It appears to produce consistently adequate restraint and sedation for minor standing surgeries, diagnostic procedures, minor dental work, ocular examinations and joint lavage, and can be used as premedication before general anesthesia.[70] When used as an adjunct to xylazine-ketamine anesthesia for castration of stallions, the combination enhanced analgesia and muscle relaxation.

Dosage: Though there is considerable variation in the dosages of the 2 drugs used in clinical situations, generally xylazine is given IV at about 0.55 mg/kg and butorphanol at 0.03 mg/kg. Many equine practitioners administer both drugs simultaneously in the same syringe, while others give butorphanol 3-5 minutes after xylazine.[70] In one clinical study, side effects were more frequent when both drugs were given simultaneously.[70] In the initial experimental trials, the dosages of xylazine (1.1 mg/kg) and butorphanol (0.1 mg/kg) were considerably higher than those now used. Even at these higher dosages, the combination produced minimal and transient hemodynamic effects, with no evidence of respiratory depression.

Advantages as a Premedicant: This combination produces a consistent degree of sedation and has minimal effect on cardiopulmonary function. The dose of xylazine can also be reduced

Disadvantages as a Premedicant: Some horses given this combination have become recumbent.

Agents for Induction of Anesthesia

Several important factors must be considered when selecting agents for induction of anesthesia. These include ease of administration, duration of induction, quality and duration of anesthesia produced, character of recovery, and cost (Table 4). The choice of induction agent also depends on the procedure to be performed (short surgical procedure versus a prolonged procedure requiring use of inhalation agents). The facilities available also influence the induction technique.

Short anesthetic regimens generally require:

- Administration of small quantities of an induction agent.
- Adequate quality and duration of anesthesia to allow completion of minor surgical procedures.
- Minimal cardiovascular and respiratory depression.
- A rapid, excitement-free recovery.
- Predictable results.
- Safety for both patient and personnel.

For induction before inhalation anesthesia, the requirements are less exacting:

- Sufficient duration to permit endotracheal intubation, connecting the patient to the inhalation apparatus and sufficient immobilization to permit the inhalation agents to take effect.
- Minimal cardiovascular and respiratory depression to add to the effect of the inhalation agents.
- Safety, especially in high-risk patients.
- Predictable results.

The method of administration, general effects, cardiovascular and respiratory effects, advantages and disadvantages of each induction technique are discussed below.

Ultrashort-Acting Thiobarbiturates

Thiamylal sodium and thiopental sodium are similar in their chemistry, dosage and response, though generally thiamylal is considered more potent than thiopental. Barbiturates depress impulse conduction in the central nervous system, principally through inhibition of synaptic transmission. The precise molecular mechanisms involved remain speculative.[71]

Distribution of thiobarbiturates is rapid, depending on the circulatory patterns of the patient. Depression of the central nervous system lasts until the anesthetic agent is redistributed to other parts of the body, when consciousness returns.[72]

Table 4. Pharmacologic characteristics of induction agents used in horses.

Drug	Dosage	Induction Time	Duration of Anesthesia
Thiobarbiturates, thiamylal, thiopental	7.5 mg/kg	25-35 sec	5-10 min
Guaifenesin-thiobarbiturate mixture	Guaifenesin up to 110 mg/kg Thiobarbiturate 4-6 mg/kg	1.5-2 min	10-15 min (depends on amount given)
Guaifenesin to effect with thiobarbiturate bolus	Thiobarbiturates 4-6 mg/kg	1.5-2 min	10-15 min (depends on amount given)
Xylazine-ketamine	Xylazine 1.1 mg/kg Ketamine 2.2 mg/kg up to 2.75 mg/kg excitable horses	1-2 min after ketamine	8-20 min
Xylazine and guaifenesin to effect	Xylazine 0.5-1.1 mg/kg IV or xylazine 2.2 mg/kg IM, then guaifenesin 55 mg/kg IV followed by ketamine 1.7 mg/kg	1.5-2 min	10-20 min

Protein binding of thiobarbiturates is decreased by acidosis, uremia and hypoalbuminemia. This increases drug availability, enhances central nervous system depression and prolongs recovery.[73]

Untoward effects include respiratory arrest and cardiovascular collapse due to relative or absolute overdosage. In addition, tissue irritation and necrosis result when thiobarbiturates are injected perivascularly. Stormy recoveries sometimes follow thiobarbiturate inductions.

Thiobarbiturates are potent cardiovascular and respiratory depressants, depending on the dose, rate of injection and physical condition of the patient. All barbiturates directly depress the myocardium and, hence, decrease contractility, cardiac output and mean arterial pressure. These depressant effects are cumulative with repeated doses. Heart rate generally increases, particularly in horses with low resting heart rates.[22,72-75]

Thiobarbiturate anesthesia depresses the response to arterial carbon dioxide, thereby decreasing respiratory rate and tidal volume. Severity of this depression is proportional to the dose and rate of administration.[73]

In healthy mature horses, thiobarbiturates have no direct effect upon gastrointestinal, renal or hepatic function.[22]

Dosage: Anesthetic premedication is mandatory to avoid excitement during induction and recovery. Recommended IV dosage of ultrashort-acting barbiturates is 6-8 mg/kg.[73] A dosage of 7.3 mg/kg is satisfactory. Thus, a total dose of 3.5 g for mature Thoroughbreds generally is used, though athletic horses may require an additional 0.5 g to ensure excitement-free induction.[34] This dose produces surgical anesthesia for 5-10 minutes, with recovery in 30-45 minutes. Anesthesia can be prolonged by repeated incremental doses of 0.1-1.0 g for adult horses; this also prolongs the recovery period substantially.

Administration: Using the so-called "crash" induction technique, the calculated dose, based on body weight and condition of the patient, is given as rapidly as possible as an IV bolus of a 5-10% solution. The animal falls to the ground in about 30 seconds.

Induction Characteristics: Administration of a subanesthetic dose of thiobarbiturate results in excitement. Overdosage results in central nervous system depression requiring cardiopulmonary resuscitation.[29]

"Crash" inductions of horses with thiamylal or thiopental can be divided into 3 groups. About 80% of the horses sink to the ground quickly, with adequate cardiovascular and respiratory function. About 15% of the horses experience excitement on induction, have vigorous involuntary limb movements and require additional barbiturate and/or high initial concentrations of an inhalant agent. The remaining 5% of the horses attain a very deep level of anesthesia, often are apneic when connected to oxygen, and have cardiovascular depression.[27]

Though thiobarbiturate induction is convenient and easily administered, the complicated inductions in 20% of patients are not desirable. This is particularly true for inductions performed onto a vertical tilting table. These difficulties are not as critical for induction of anesthesia in an open area, as an experienced handler at the head of the horse usually can prevent injuries.[34]

Recoveries are generally smooth, but paddling and premature attempts to rise are common. Consequently, sensory stimulation during recovery must be minimized.

Precautions: Careful evaluation of dose and condition of the patient are important because overdosage may be fatal. The irritant nature of alkaline thiobarbiturate solutions necessitates use of catheters rather than needles and requires careful catheter placement to avoid perivascular drug deposition. Because about 15% of horses are not deeply anesthetized just after induction, it is advisable to have other drugs available immediately to control excitement and struggling.

If thiobarbiturate anesthesia is performed in the field, it is the responsibility of the veterinarian to supervise recovery and assist the horse during the occasionally stormy recovery.

Advantages: A bolus of thiobarbiturate is convenient to administer, requiring small quantities of drug and few personnel. The length of anesthesia is suitable for minor surgical procedures. Repeated doses can be used to prolong anesthesia, but this may prolong recovery.

Disadvantages: "Crash" induction using bolus administration of thiobarbiturates can result in overdosage. Therefore, great care is necessary with high-risk patients. Thiobarbiturates cause tissue necrosis when injected perivascularly.

Thiobarbiturate anesthesia is not entirely predictable as about 20% of patients do not have a smooth induction, or are too deeply or insufficiently anesthetized initially. Cardiovascular and respiratory depression are directly proportional to the dose and rate of administration.

Guaifenesin

Guaifenesin (glycerol guaiacolate) is a decongestive and antitussive agent used as a muscle relaxant in equine anesthesia. It has little primary anesthetic or analgesic activity.

This centrally acting muscle relaxant acts by selective depression of nerve impulses at the internuncial neurons of the spinal cord, brainstem and subcortical regions of the brain.[76] Additionally, a degree of sedation and slight potentiation of anesthetic agents result from its action on the reticular formation of the brainstem.[77] Some analgesia is produced.[78,79]

Guaifenesin has some sedative effects and potentiates the effects of other preanesthetic and induction agents. Guaifenesin crosses the placental barrier to some extent. Thus, minimal and transient fetal depression can be expected.[80] Guaifenesin apparently increases gastrointestinal motility but has no evident effect on liver and renal function. It is excreted in the urine after conjugation in the liver to glucuronide. Guaifenesin has a shorter half-life and recovery time in female ponies than in males.[81,82]

Minor untoward effects include hemolysis caused by IV injection of concentrated solutions and thrombophlebitis after perivascular injection.

When given IV alone, guaifenesin (50-100 mg/kg) causes recumbency, insignificant depression of cardiac output and arterial blood pressure, and minimal increases in heart rate.[80] However, when used in a clinical setting, it is always combined with preanesthetics and induction agents, and often with inhalation agents, all of which depress cardiovascular function. Though the hypotensive effect of the guaifenesin-thiobarbiturate combination is not as profound as that of the thiobarbiturate alone, it is prolonged.[72,83] In one study, use of guaifenesin following xylazine (1.1 mg/kg IV) premedication accentuated cardiopulmonary depression.[80] The respiratory effects of guaifenesin are minimal.

Dosage: Guaifenesin alone or in combination with other induction agents usually is administered IV to effect. It is a white, crystalline powder that is poorly soluble in water, tending to precipitate when stored in solution.[77] The major disadvantage of this drug is that the large-volume infusions required are inconvenient, increase induction time and require more personnel to administer. Though attempts have been made to increase the concentration of guaifenesin solutions, concentrations above 16% cause hemolysis.[84] The mechanism of hemolysis is unknown; it appears unrelated to total dose but rather to the concentration of the solution.[76]

Guaifenesin solutions used most frequently in Australia are chemically stabilized. These solutions are made either as a 10% solution in a propylene glycol/ethyl alcohol base or a 15% solution in a lactimide base. In the United States and Canada, the most popular diluents are 5% dextrose and sterile distilled water.[85]

The average IV dosage of guaifenesin required to cast a horse is 110 mg/kg (range, 73-139 mg/kg); the duration of action is 15-30 minutes.[77,78,81] Horses given the drug at 182 mg/kg had violent extensor spasms; death may occur at dosages of 460 mg/kg.[2,77] Because the rate of administration affects the dose required for induction, rapid infusion under pressure reduces by 30-50% the total volume required for induction.[72]

Guaifenesin Infusion and Thiobarbiturate Bolus

Guaifenesin is infused IV by gravity flow or under pressure until the horse becomes ataxic and relaxed. Then, anesthesia is induced with a bolus of thiamylal or thiopental (4-6 mg/kg). Anesthesia is induced within 60 seconds of administration of the thiobarbiturate. It is relatively easy to predict, and the fall of the patient can be controlled. The danger of hypoventilation, apnea and hypotension is increased when the thiobarbiturate is given as an IV bolus.[75]

Infusion of Guaifenesin and Thiobarbiturate Mixture: A mixture of guaifenesin with the thiobarbiturate (4-6 mg/kg) is infused IV rapidly until the horse becomes ataxic. The rest of the mixture is given to effect. This method of administration allows the dose to be titrated to effect, using the minimal amount of drug to produce anesthesia. The disadvantage of this technique is that the infusion apparatus must stay attached to the patient as the animal collapses or must be detached before recumbency. For field inductions, the apparatus is best detached once the patient has had sufficient drug for a smooth induction.

This technique is ideally suited for tilting-table inductions and for patients that can be steadied against a wall and allowed to slide down quietly with the infusion apparatus still attached. This method also permits gradual introduction to inhalation agents, thereby avoiding high initial concentrations of the inhalant anesthetic gas. The safety of this technique, especially by gravity infusion, makes it reliable for induction of anesthesia in high-risk patients.[34]

Recovery from guaifenesin-thiobarbiturate anesthesia is less traumatic than from anesthesia produced solely with thiobarbiturates. One of the major advantages of this combination is fewer complications during the recovery period.[86]

Xylazine Premedication, Guaifenesin Infusion and Ketamine Bolus: After sedation with xylazine, given IV at 0.5-1.1 mg/kg or IM at 2.2 mg/kg, guaifenesin is infused IV until ataxia develops or the legs buckle slightly. Ketamine is then given as an IV bolus at 1.8-2.2 mg/kg. There is a short lag period before the horse becomes recumbent. Infusion of guaifenesin may be continued until the desired effect is achieved.[76] Alternatively, the ketamine can be mixed with the guaifenesin and the solution infused to effect. This technique results in short recovery periods even after prolonged inhalation anesthesia.

Infusion of Guaifenesin, Ketamine and Xylazine Mixture: Anesthesia can be induced by rapid IV infusion of a mixture of guaifenesin, ketamine (2.2 mg/kg) and xylazine (1.1 mg/kg). The mixture is infused at 1 ml/kg. Anesthesia is maintained by continuous infusion at 2 ml/kg/hour.[9,73] Addition of guaifenesin to the xylazine-ketamine combination reduces excitability and increases muscle relaxation.

Precautions: In combination with a thiobarbiturate given by bolus injection or in the mixture, guaifenesin produces safer, smoother induction and recovery than thiobarbiturates alone. The mixture of guaifenesin and a thiobarbiturate is recommended because it can be infused to effect. The key to good induction with this combination is to administer half of the total volume as rapidly as possible, so as to minimize the ataxic phase. The remainder is then given at a slower rate until the desired anesthetic depth is achieved. For high-risk patients, the thiobarbiturate dose is reduced and the solution is given by gravity infusion. Though induction time is prolonged using this technique, titrating the dose to the patient's requirements is relatively easy. Apnea and cardiovascular collapse seldom are encountered using this technique in healthy or sick patients.[34]

Care must be used during catheter placement because guaifenesin causes thrombophlebitis and tissue necrosis if injected perivascularly. Additionally, administration of the solution under pressure carries the risk of air embolism. This is unlikely with experienced operators but must be considered.

Advantages of Guaifenesin as an Induction Adjunct: Guaifenesin is reliable and safe in all horses, sick and healthy. The toxic dose is 3-4 times the therapeutic dose. Because guaifenesin can be administered to effect, the dose can be tailored to the horse's requirements.

The drug produces excellent and consistent skeletal muscle relaxation. During induction, the sedative effect reduces reactions to unexpected stimuli. After a brief period of unsteadiness, the horse sinks to the ground without excitement; similarly, recoveries are smooth and uneventful.

Guaifenesin by itself causes minimal cardiovascular or respiratory depression. When used as an adjunctive induction agent before inhalation anesthesia, guaifenesin allows low initial concentrations of inhalant anesthetics, thereby minimizing further cardiovascular and respiratory depression.

The xylazine-guaifenesin-ketamine combination smooths induction, provides muscle relaxation and avoids the excitation occasionally observed with xylazine-ketamine induction.

Disadvantages of Guaifenesin as an Induction Adjunct: Guaifenesin can cause hemolysis when used as a highly concentrated solution. Large-volume infusion necessitates use of a large-gauge catheter or wide-bore infusion set, or administration under pressure. Inductions require more equipment and are less convenient than other techniques. Induction time is prolonged. Most horses be-

come unsteady as they relax but are unwilling to fall. This is more apparent with slow infusions. Three people are required to induce anesthesia.

Xylazine with Ketamine

Ketamine depresses the thalamoneocortical system and activates the limbic system. Consequently, ketamine anesthesia frequently is characterized by dysphoria, hallucinations, delirium or excitement. Anesthesia is induced by functional disruption of the central nervous system, producing a "cataleptoid state." However, the ketamine-induced clonic muscle activity, tremors and convulsions preclude use of ketamine as the sole anesthetic in horses.[9] The sedative effects of xylazine, given before ketamine, mask these undesirable effects such that a combination of xylazine and ketamine results in an exceptionally smooth induction, an anesthetic time of about 20 minutes and a smooth recovery.[22]

Administration and Induction Characteristics: Xylazine is given IV at 1.1 mg/kg 4-5 minutes before IV injection of ketamine at 2.2 mg/kg. The delay between the 2 injections allows development of the full sedative effects of xylazine. The horse gradually becomes laterally recumbent in about 90 seconds.[22,87] In high-strung horses, the dosage of ketamine should be increased to 2.75 mg/kg.[9]

Horses anesthetized with this combination become recumbent gradually. This is quite different from the progression to recumbency produced by other induction techniques. The horse may sit back on its haunches or kneel down and then slowly sink to its sternum before rolling over into lateral recumbency. There may be extensor rigidity and 1-2 vigorous limb movements before the horse finally lies still. However, once recumbent, the horse becomes unconscious.[22,34]

During the anesthetic period, the horse appears to be in a light plane of anesthesia, with palpebral, corneal and swallowing reflexes maintained. In spite of this, endotracheal intubation is not difficult. The eyeball is rotated ventrally and often there is rapid nystagmus. Muscle relaxation is generally poor and the patient is responsive to sound.

Termination of a surgical plane of anesthesia may be very abrupt. The horse first lifts its head, then rolls up on its sternum and stands, usually on the first attempt. Recovery is remarkably free from excitement. Once the horse is standing, there is little evidence of ataxia.

Problems with this technique may include excitement during induction, insufficient duration of anesthesia, muscular rigidity and incoordination during recovery. To avoid these problems, some authors have recommended that either diazepam or guaifenesin be incorporated into the technique.[9,88,89] Adequate sedation with xylazine before ketamine administration is the key to a satisfactory induction, adequate duration of anesthesia, and a safe recovery with this regimen.[87]

If required, up to 1 hour of additional anesthetic time may be achieved by several methods:

- Give one-third to one-half the original dose of both xylazine and ketamine IV at 20-minute intervals.[9,72]
- Give guaifenesin and thiobarbiturate (2 g) as a mixture IV to effect.[9,34]
- Give a 5% guaifenesin solution containing xylazine at 0.25 mg/ml and ketamine at 1 mg/ml to effect.[89]

Generally, analgesia is sufficient with this combination but muscle relaxation is poor. Recumbency usually lasts 12-18 minutes and may last for up to 20-25 minutes without surgical stimulation.

Redistribution of ketamine to muscle tissue is the major determinant of its duration of action. About 60% of the ketamine dose is metabolized by the liver, while 40% is eliminated unchanged in the urine.[9]

Ketamine produces changes in almost all measurable hemodynamic indices. Heart rate, systemic and pulmonary blood pressures, peripheral vascular resistance, cardiac output, cardiac contractility and myocardial oxygen consumption all increase after administration of ketamine.[90] Xylazine causes bradycardia, hypotension, depression of cardiac output, and increased peripheral vascular resistance. Consequently, combining the 2 drugs increases mean arterial pressure by increasing total peripheral resistance; cardiac output decreases.[34,87]

Though ketamine has minimal effect upon hypoxic and hypercarbic ventilatory responses, it induces an apneustic pattern of respiration accompanied by mild hypoventilation and hypercapnia when the horse breathes air. This respiratory insult is compounded by prolonged recumbency.[9] Thus, hypoventilation with respiratory acidosis develops during the anesthetic period.[87]

Precautions: Xylazine must produce obvious signs of sedation before ketamine is given. An alternative induction method should be selected if xylazine produces no sedation. The combination should not be administered to an excited horse.

The dosage of ketamine is critical. Underdosage results in inadequate anesthesia, while overdosage results in marked depression and prolonged recumbency. Thus, accurate evaluation of body weight is important. The horse should be left in a quiet environment and not be disturbed until fully recovered from anesthesia.

Though xylazine and ketamine can be mixed in the same syringe, the mixture has a shorter duration of action and produces less profound anesthesia. When the 2 drugs are administered simultaneously, anesthesia is characterized by muscle rigidity and tetany.

A guaifenesin-thiobarbiturate mixture should be used to prolong xylazine-ketamine anesthesia because evaluation of anesthetic depth is easier.

Advantages in Xylazine and Ketamine: Xylazine and ketamine produce rapid and quiet induction in an adequately sedated animal. The combination provides a short recumbent period with good analgesia. It is convenient to use because small quantities are required, little equipment is needed, and one person can induce anesthesia and provide restraint during induction and recovery periods. The drugs are not excessively irritating if injected perivascularly. Both xylazine and ketamine are compatible with guaifenesin and the thiobarbiturates.

Arterial blood pressure is maintained. Recovery is rapid. Once the horse is standing, it is alert and steady on its feet.

Disadvantages in Induction: The adverse cardiovascular effects of the full dose of xylazine are not completely reversed by ketamine. Though arterial pressure is maintained, cardiac output is reduced by 23%. Both drugs increase peripheral resistance. Thus, blood pressure is maintained but at the expense of peripheral perfusion and flow.

The procedure for prolonging anesthesia is more complex than with other techniques; therefore, other drugs must be available. Severe side effects may occur. These are minimized by adequate sedation with xylazine.

Care must be taken not to overdose with ketamine on a body weight basis. Correct estimation of body weight with this technique is critical.

In <0.1% of horses, anesthesia cannot be induced. The response in mules and donkeys is apparently unpredictable. Injection of 3 times the horse dose results in stimulation or no response.[72]

Depth of anesthesia tends to be more difficult to control because the classic signs of anesthesia are not recognizable. There is always a ventral eyeball position and brisk palpebral responses, and often nystagmus. If inhalation anesthesia follows xylazine-ketamine induction, the transition phase tends to be abrupt, is often difficult to anticipate, and may result in movement. Subsequent inhalation anesthesia appears to be more unstable than when other induction drugs are used and tends to require higher concentrations of inhaled gases to maintain unconsciousness.

Propofol

A new intravenous anesthetic agent, propofol, has been used successfully in ponies and horses. Propofol is a nonbarbiturate, nonsteroidal, nonopioid drug licensed for use in cats and dogs in Great Britain (Rapinovet: Coopers). Intravenous administration of propofol, by bolus injection or rapid infusion of the induction dose diluted in isotonic saline, rapidly produces recumbency. Premedication with xylazine (0.5 mg/kg) or detomidine (20 μg/kg), followed by administration of propofol IV at 2.0 mg/kg, produces smooth, excitement-free induction of anesthesia.[91,92] A quiet recovery from anesthesia can be expected in 20-30 minutes. If needed, anesthesia can be maintained with IV infusion of propofol at 0.2 mg/kg/min. There is a considerable amount of interest in propofol because anesthesia time can be prolonged by administration of incremental doses of the drug without altering the time to recovery and because propofol is not irritating if injected perivascularly.[91]

Tiletamine-Zolazepam

A combination of a cyclohexamine anesthetic agent, tiletamine, and a benzodiazepine tranquilizer, zolazepam, is available for use in veterinary practice (Telazol: Robins). Because this combination includes an agent with properties similar to those of ketamine and because the combination of xylazine-ketamine has proven well suited to equine species, the combination of tiletamine-zolazepam has been studied in horses. When horses were premedicated with xylazine (1.1 mg/kg) and then given an IV bolus of tiletamine-zolazepam at 2.2 mg/kg, they rapidly became recumbent and remained unresponsive to stimuli for 20 minutes.[93] Using this combination, anesthesia lasted longer and muscle relaxation was greater than with xylazine-ketamine.

Etorphine-Acepromazine

A combination of the opiate etorphine and the phenothiazine tranquilizer acepromazine has been formulated for use in Great Britain. This combination induces neuroleptanalgesia and causes stiffness, strong muscle tremors, and recumbency within 1 minute. Heart rate and arterial blood pressure are increased after administration of this combination. The packed cell volume increases substantially, further indicating the effects on the sympathetic nervous system.

The effect of the opiate is reversed with diprenorphine; horses generally stand within 2 minutes after IV administration of the antagonist. Excitement and compulsive walking may occur several hours later due to enterohepatic recycling of the etorphine. Because very small doses of etorphine can be fatal to people, extreme care must be used when handling this combination and in discarding contaminated needles.[94]

Design of Anesthetic Apparatus

The need for specially developed large animal breathing systems has been apparent for many years.[95-98] In view of the size of horses, the inspiratory and expiratory flow rates generated, the comparatively large tidal volumes and the physical dimensions of equine airways, it is clear that anesthetic circle systems designed for people and small animals are inadequate.[99]

Three major considerations are fundamental to the design of any anesthetic apparatus: minimize resistance to respiration; minimize apparatus dead space; and provide adequate capacity for carbon dioxide absorption. Increased resistance is manifested in the anesthetized patient by labored respiration and sweating. This is particularly notable after prolonged anesthesia. The effects of increased dead space and inadequate carbon dioxide absorption are more subtle and are accurately determined only by the measurement of P_aCO_2.

The design of an ideal anesthetic apparatus is based on certain theoretical considerations. The primary objective is to minimize the resistance to respiration. This is accomplished by reducing turbulent air flow.[100] Components of the anesthetic apparatus that cause turbulent rather than laminar air flow are: internally corrugated tubes; abrupt changes in the direction of air flow (the more gently the direction of flow changes, the quicker the flow becomes laminar); tubing of insufficient diameter; and restricted air flow caused by changes in cross-sectional area. Thus, it has been proposed that anesthetic apparatus should have a larger diameter than the trachea of the patient.

Because resistance is inversely proportional to the radius of the tubes raised to the fourth power, the larger the diameter, the lower the resistance.[101] Doubling the radius decreases resistance by 16 times.[100-102] Because the tracheal diameter of adult Thoroughbreds ranges from 4 to 7 cm, 6.2 cm should be an adequate endotracheal tubing diameter for most horses.[38] Resistance also is directly proportional to the length of the tubing. Thus, the length of the limbs of the circle system should be kept as short as possible but must be long enough to conveniently connect the patient to the apparatus.

Resistance at the inspiratory and expiratory valves may be significant. To minimize turbulent flow, the cross-sectional areas should be the same in the airway and the valve casing. Though the soda lime canister provides only 10-15% of the total resistance of the system, locating the canister on the expiratory side of the circuit places the work of overcoming this resistance on the passive exhalatory phase of respiration.[38] This reduces the energy required to move the gas across the soda lime.

The ideal design of a circuit should consider the positions of the exhale relief ("pop-off") valve, the oxygen inflow tube, and the unidirectional valves. The "pop-off" valve should be placed on the expiratory limb so that exhaled gas is vented before carbon dioxide is absorbed; thus, soda lime use is more economical. This "pop-off" valve should be of sufficient diameter to facilitate rapid and complete evacuation of the rebreathing bag. The oxygen inflow tube should be positioned to add fresh gas to the circuit on the inspiratory limb, so that fresh gas flows to the Y-piece during expiration. Though this may slightly reduce the humidity, it prevents diffusion of carbon dioxide from the expiratory limb to the inspiratory limb of the circuit during the long expiratory pause seen in horses.[38] The inspiratory and expiratory valves should be placed between the patient and the reservoir bag to prevent rebreathing of expired gases.

Certain concepts concerning adequate absorption of carbon dioxide must be appreciated. A canister correctly packed with soda lime has an intergranular and intragranular air space totalling 40-60% of the canister's volume.[100] Therefore, to accommodate the exhaled air, the soda lime canister must be approximately twice as large as the tidal volume of the patient. However, it is not necessary to accommodate gas that contains no carbon dioxide. Thus, the required size of the canister is $(V_T - V_D) \times 2$, where V_T is tidal volume and V_D is dead space. A canister of this size provides adequate carbon dioxide absorption initially. As the carbon dioxide absorption capacity of the soda lime is exhausted, however, carbon dioxide is not fully eliminated. Consequently, it has been proposed that a dual charge of soda lime be used to provide complete carbon dioxide elimination. This also results in considerable economy over a single canister or a "to-and-fro" system.

To construct such a system for horses, it was hypothesized that 50 L of soda lime would be required; this would be impractical. The design of the canister was then modified to suit the average horse with a tidal volume of 10 L. Using the above equation, $(V_T - V_T) \times 2 = (10 - 3.5) \times 2 = 13$ L. Thus, a dual charge of soda lime is 26 L or about 20 kg. When a larger-than-average horse is anesthetized, the apparatus no longer provides a true dual charge but is adequate nevertheless. If the gas passes through the canister from top to bottom, the efficiency of carbon dioxide absorption is improved because water, released by the soda lime as carbon dioxide is absorbed, flows downward and activates unused soda lime. This also eliminates aggregation of granules at the bottom of the canister if gas flows from bottom to top.

All modern circle absorbers have transparent canisters. This enables the anesthetist to observe the color change of the soda lime as it becomes exhausted. It is debatable whether color changes are reliable. Probably the only true indication of carbon dioxide absorption is the exothermic reaction. This is more readily detected in a metal canister because heat conduction is more efficient through metal. Metal also tends to be more durable than plastics, which become less transparent and more fragile with use.

Inhalation anesthesia in horses imposes complex physiologic alterations, causing hypoventilation and a concomitant increase in P_aCO_2. Drug-induced respiratory depression, surgical stimulation, anesthetic apparatus design and anesthetic depth interrelate in the pathophysiology of hypercarbia. All of the above factors, with the exception of machine design, are highly variable. Because of this, good machine design is the "cornerstone" of equine anesthetic practice.

Inhalation Anesthesia

General anesthesia may be maintained by IV supplementation with the original agents, as previously described, or with inhalation agents (Fig 50). While IV methods are simple, cheap and quite satisfactory for short-term procedures, inhalation anesthesia offers distinct advantages for those of long duration. Inhalation agents offer greater control of dosage and thus depth of anesthesia. Also, they offer greater versatility because varied surgical procedures can be performed with rapid recoveries, even after prolonged anesthesia.

Respiratory depression and impairment of oxygenation usually occur with general anesthesia to some extent in all animals. In horses, however, the partial pressure of arterial carbon dioxide (P_aCO_2) increases and the partial pressure of arterial oxygen (P_aO_2) usually decreases. The significance of the reduced P_aO_2 is dependent in part upon the inspired oxygen tension. Thus, the potential for hypoxemia is greater if the inspired oxygen tension is low, as when the horse is breathing air (21% O_2). On the other hand, horses connected to an inhalation apparatus are breathing greater than 90% O_2 in the inspired gaseous mixture after adequate denitrogenation. Hence, the potential hazards of hypoxemia are reduced in horses con-

Figure 50. Methods of maintaining anesthesia in horses.

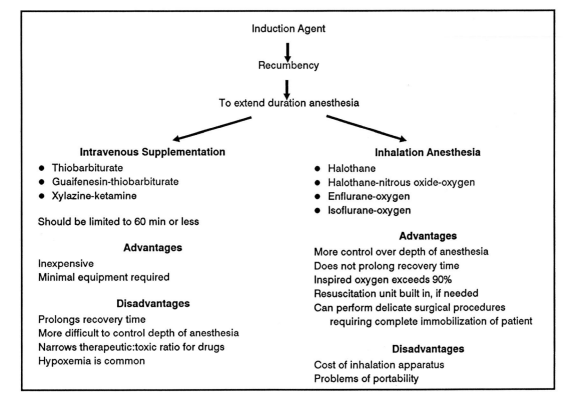

Induction Agent

↓

Recumbency

↓

To extend duration anesthesia

Intravenous Supplementation
- Thiobarbiturate
- Guaifenesin-thiobarbiturate
- Xylazine-ketamine

Should be limited to 60 min or less

Advantages
Inexpensive
Minimal equipment required

Disadvantages
Prolongs recovery time
More difficult to control depth of anesthesia
Narrows therapeutic:toxic ratio for drugs
Hypoxemia is common

Inhalation Anesthesia
- Halothane
- Halothane-nitrous oxide-oxygen
- Enflurane-oxygen
- Isoflurane-oxygen

Advantages
More control over depth of anesthesia
Does not prolong recovery time
Inspired oxygen exceeds 90%
Resuscitation unit built in, if needed
Can perform delicate surgical procedures
        requiring complete immobilization of patient

Disadvantages
Cost of inhalation apparatus
Problems of portability

nected to an anesthetic machine. The major deterrent to inhalation anesthesia is the initial cost of equipment and its lack of portability.

Studies of the effects of halothane, enflurane and isoflurane in horses have provided much useful clinical information.[14,21,27,103-105,107,108] Halothane remains the most widely used inhalation anesthetic agent. Enflurane, while offering rapid induction and recovery, has cardiovascular and respiratory depressant effects similar to those of halothane. Isoflurane has been extensively studied and appears promising.

Regardless of the inhalant agent used, excess or "waste" gases must be removed from the anesthetic system. To protect personnel working in the surgical suite, these waste gases should be removed with a capture device or eliminated using a vacuum line or passive air-flow line. In most instances, the waste gases are vented to the outside through tubing that passes from the anesthetic system to the disposal site.

Halothane

This inhalation agent is used widely in equine practice. Its high volatility, intermediate solubility in blood and moderate potency allow close control of the depth of anesthesia (Table 5). Eye position, presence or absence of nystagmus, palpebral reflexes and tear production are reliable indicators of anesthetic depth (Fig 51). Additionally, halothane-induced arterial hypotension is dose related, and measurement of arterial blood pressure provides a reasonable clinical assessment of anesthetic depth.[104] However, there is little change in heart rate with changes in halothane concentration. Consequently, within the confines of clinical levels of anesthesia, there is little correlation between heart rate and depth of anesthesia.[21] Recoveries are generally quiet and fairly short (20-30 minutes).

Halothane causes cardiovascular depression proportional to the concentration administered. It reduces myocardial contractility, stroke volume and cardiac output, and causes peripheral vasodilation. These effects are additive, causing arterial hypotension.[21]

Halothane substantially reduces cardiac output. Reductions of 40% in the first 15 minutes and 30% at 1 hour have been observed in spontaneously breathing horses. If ventilation is controlled, reductions in cardiac output are more pronounced, with decreases of 56% and 60% at light to moderate planes of anesthesia, respectively.[21,108] These changes greatly exceed halothane-induced decreases in cardiac output in people and dogs.[21] In halothane-anesthetized, spontaneously breathing horses, there is a time-related circulatory adaptation, improving both arterial pressure and cardiac output over a 5-hour period.[109] It is not known if this adaptation occurs to the same extent with use of cardiodepressant premedications and induction agents.

Halothane causes dose-related depression of both respiratory rate and tidal volume, with a resulting increase in arterial carbon dioxide tension. This alveolar hypoventilation is one of the most common problems in

Table 5. Physical and pharmacologic characteristics of inhalation agents used in horses.

| Agent | MAC[1] (%) | Solubility[2] Blood/Gas | Effects of 1.0 MAC | | |
			Systolic Arterial Pressure (mm Hg)	Respiratory Rate (breaths/min)	P_aCO_2 (mm Hg)
Halothane	0.88	2.3	139 ± 4.0	13 ± 1	62 ± 3
Enflurane	2.12	1.9	111 ± 12	6 ± 1	67 ± 2
Isoflurane	1.31	1.4	137 ± 4	9 ± 1	60 ± 4

1 – MAC = Minimum alveolar concentration that prevents gross purposeful movements in response to a painful stimulus. Figures are estimated for young, healthy, unsedated, spontaneously breathing horses.[106]

2 – Solubility = The solubility coefficient (blood/gas) defines in part the speed of anesthetic induction and recovery. The similar low figures for enflurane and isoflurane indicate that induction and recovery for these agents should occur more rapidly than with halothane.

spontaneously breathing horses maintained with halothane.

The motility, tone and peristaltic activity of the gastrointestinal tract are decreased by halothane anesthesia. There are slight decreases in renal, pancreatic and small intestinal blood flow as the concentration of halothane is increased.[110] Halothane readily passes the placental barrier and reduces uterine tone. Halothane may retard uterine involution postpartum.

Though halothane is readily absorbed and excreted through the lungs, up to 12% of inspired halothane is metabolized by liver microsomes, producing trifluoroacetic acid and bromide and chloride radicals. These are excreted in the urine for many days. Metabolites persist in the liver for some time.

Malignant hyperthermia, a potentially life-threatening pharmacogenetic myopathy, has been reported in horses subjected to halothane anesthesia. The syndrome is characterized by a rapid rise in body temperature, muscle rigidity, hypercapnia, hypoxemia, tachypnea, ventricular dysrhythmias, metabolic acidosis and hyperkalemia.[32]

For a smooth transition from anesthesia induced by injectable agents to inhalation anesthesia, halothane concentrations up to 5%, delivered by a precision vaporizer, usually are required. Concentrations of 1.5-2.0% generally are adequate for maintenance of anesthesia. Because halothane is a moderate

Figure 51. Guidelines in assessing anesthetic depth during halothane-oxygen anesthesia after induction with guaifenesin and thiamylal.

Anesthetic Depth	Eye Reflexes	Eye Position Medial Lateral	Other Signs	Heart and Respiratory Rates	Blood Pressure
Too light	Palpebral reflex +++ Nystagmus +++ Tear production ++ Eye position ventromedial		Limb movement ± Ear movement ±	Heart rate 45-50/min Resp rate 5-10/min	Systolic 100-120 mm Hg
	Palpebral reflex ++ Nystagmus ± Tear production + Eye position medial to ventral		Suitable depth for radiography, casting legs, minor wounds	Heart rate 40/min Resp rate 4-6/min	Systolic 95 mm Hg
	Palpebral reflex + Nystagmus – Tear production – Eye position ventral		Depth required for painful procedures, fracture reduction, laparotomy	Heart rate 40/min Resp rate 4-6/min	
	Palpebral reflex ± Nystagmus – Tear production – Eye position lateral		Indicates deepening level of anesthesia	Heart rate 40/min Resp rate 4-6/min	Systolic 50 mm Hg
Too deep	Palpebral reflex – Corneal reflex persists Tear production – Eye position central Dilated pupil Dry pitted cornea		Dangerously profound depth of anesthesia	Depressed resp rate and tidal volume; heart rate unchanged	Decreased pulse pressure

– = absent
± = may or may not be present
+ = minimal
++ = moderate
+++ = maximal

to poor analgesic, increased concentrations may be required for painful procedures.

Advantages as an Inhalation Agent: Halothane is safe, potent and nonirritating to the respiratory tract. It is nontoxic and relatively inexpensive. Halothane has good induction and recovery characteristics. It is easy to determine the depth of halothane anesthesia, as eye signs are reliable and arterial blood pressure correlates with depth (Fig 51).

Disadvantages as an Inhalation Agent: Halothane produces dose-related cardiovascular and respiratory depression. Gastrointestinal motility is decreased. Malignant hyperthermia has occurred in some horses.

Enflurane

This inhalation agent does not appear to have any substantial advantages over halothane in terms of cardiopulmonary depression or margin of safety (Table 5).[104] Cardiovascular depression with enflurane is equal to or greater than that produced by halothane; some investigators have reported profound respiratory depression with this agent.[14,103,104,107]

A pattern of central nervous system depression, followed by excitation leading to electroencephalographic abnormalities, overt seizures and then depression, is unique to increasing alveolar concentrations of enflurane. Fortunately, the incidence of enflurane-induced seizures is minimized or abolished by premedication or induction of anesthesia with a thiobarbiturate.[111]

Enflurane does have a few advantages over halothane, as it is a fair to moderate analgesic, has better muscle relaxant properties, and induction and emergence from anesthesia are usually more rapid. Some authors have commented that though the recoveries are very rapid with enflurane, they may be associated with more excitement ("emergence delirium"), shivering and incoordination than seen after halothane anesthesia.[22]

A surgical plane of anesthesia is produced with concentrations of 4-6%, delivered by precision vaporizer. Anesthesia is maintained with a concentration of 1-3%. Enflurane is substantially more expensive than halothane, and anesthetic depth is more difficult to ascertain clinically, as the horse's eyes tend to remain central.

Isoflurane

This volatile anesthetic agent is the "fastest gas" in the group (Table 5). Its high volatility, low solubility and medium potency combine to give extremely responsive control of anesthetic depth.[22]

Isoflurane produces dose-dependent depression of cardiopulmonary function. Respiratory depression produced by isoflurane tends to be more profound than that produced by halothane and similar to that of enflurane.[104,106,111] Though cardiovascular depression is less than that observed with halothane or enflurane, there still is a decrease in mean arterial pressure and peripheral vascular resistance with increasing depth of anesthesia.[103]

Though a respiratory depressant, isoflurane is inert, nontoxic and an excellent skeletal muscle relaxant. It produces cardiovascular stability even with controlled ventilation. The real advantage of isoflurane is the exceptionally rapid recovery it provides.

Induction concentrations of isoflurane usually are 3.5-4.5% from a precision vaporizer; maintenance levels are 1-3%. Isoflurane is particularly expensive.

Nitrous Oxide

In people and small animals, nitrous oxide is used extensively in conjunction with halothane and oxygen because it provides some analgesia and allows reduced halothane concentrations. However, one cannot safely extrapolate these facts to horses. More important, addition of nitrous oxide to the inhalant gas mixture decreases the inspired oxygen tension (which in part determines arterial oxygen tension) in proportion to the concentration of nitrous oxide in the gas mixture.[105] In horses, an alveolar nitrous oxide concentration of 50% reduces the anesthetic requirements of halothane by about 25% but results in an average P_aO_2 of only 113 mm Hg. This suggests that an inspired concentration of 50% is the upper limit for spontaneously ventilating horses. This may be extended to 60% for controlled ventilation.[105] Because one must not exceed these concentrations in horses, the potency and usefulness of nitrous oxide is limited severely.

The tendency toward increased intestinal gas volume with continued inspiration of nitrous oxide could be deleterious in long procedures. Expense also must be considered, as nitrous oxide is more costly than oxygen.

Intraoperative Anesthetic Considerations

Before Induction of Anesthesia

Because the anesthetic apparatus has a large internal volume, it is advisable to fill the system with halothane and oxygen so that it is ready when the patient is connected. Generally, the rebreathing bag is filled with 3.5% halothane or isoflurane in oxygen.

After Induction of Anesthesia

Immediately after induction of anesthesia, the patient is intubated and connected to the circle system. High initial oxygen flow rates are recommended (>12 L/min). This "washes in" halothane and denitrogenates the patient. This high-flow/open system is used for the first 8-10 minutes of anesthesia. Thereafter, the oxygen flow rate may be reduced to 10 ml/kg (4-5 L/450 kg/min) for maintenance of anesthesia.

It is good practice to ensure an adequate depth of anesthesia at this time because surgical stimulation always arouses the patient. Generally, the anesthetist should aim for ventrolateral eyeball position, absence of nystagmus and a slight palpebral reflex (Fig 51). If arousal occurs at the onset of surgery, it is more difficult to stabilize the patient in the face of surgical stimulation.

Measurement of intracompartmental muscle pressures of anesthetized horses has revealed values exceeding the critical closing pressure for capillary perfusion in dependent limbs. This causes relative ischemia of those muscles, with the potential for muscle degeneration. Certain methods of positioning and padding help reduce these intracompartmental pressures in dependent muscles.[112-114] Positioning of anesthetized horses is critical in prevention of myopathy and peripheral neuropathy (Fig 52). This is an essential part of the anesthetic routine and should not be taken lightly.

When the horse is in lateral recumbency, the head should be well cushioned to avoid trauma to the dependent eye or pressure-induced ischemia of the facial nerve. Halters always should be removed once recumbency is achieved. The dependent forelimb should be pulled as far cranially as possible, as this reduces pressure on the triceps muscles. The upper (nondependent) limb is elevated until parallel with the table and is pulled slightly caudal to the dependent limb. This maneuver also relieves pressure on the dependent limb.[112-116] Such positioning reduces intracompartmental muscle pressures to acceptable levels and facilitates venous return from the distal limbs.[115,116] The upper (nondependent) hind limb should be elevated so that it is parallel with the dependent hind limb.

Care should be taken to ensure that the horse is not leaning to one side when in dorsal recumbency. Improper positioning results in excessive pressure on various muscles, particularly the gluteal and longissimus dorsi muscles. If necessary, the forelimbs may be crossed and each tied to the opposite side to steady the horse. Positioning of the hind limbs is controversial. Some anesthetists recommend extending the hind limbs and tying them to poles. The effect of this position on the blood supply to the distal limb is unknown. Others prefer to leave the hind limbs in a relaxed, flexed position. If the latter technique is used, the limbs must never be tied laterally or excessive pressure inadver-

Figure 52. Horse with postanesthetic localized myopathy and signs of a radial nerve paralysis. The horse was anesthetized in lateral recumbency. The muscles affected reflect the contact points of the supporting surface. The triceps and muscles over the rib cage are swollen, hard and painful on palpation.

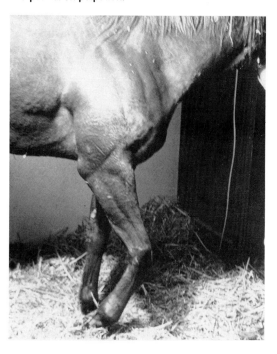

tently applied by surgeons or assistants leaning on the limbs.

Attention should be paid to the surface on which the patient is placed. Water-filled mattresses create an excellent conforming contact surface that cushions the horse. The results of studies comparing the effects of 4 surfaces (concrete, foam rubber, air dunnage bag, water-filled mattress) on forelimb intracompartmental muscle pressure indicated that the water mattress caused the least elevation of intracompartmental pressure, while foam rubber caused the most.[113] However, other authors report that foam padding is better than no padding at all.[114]

Intraoperative Arousal

Horses occasionally wake up during surgery due to misjudgment of the depth of anesthesia. Though these periods of arousal obviously should be avoided if possible in healthy surgical patients, periods of arousal may be unavoidable in lightly anesthetized sick horses. The potential for injury to personnel and the adverse effects of sympathetic stimulation on the animal should be considered in maintaining the depth of anesthesia. Because of the large internal volume (30-70 L) of the equine anesthetic apparatus, there is a considerable lag period before inspired concentrations of halothane can be increased.[34,117] For this reason, an IV injection of an anesthetic agent or a combination of agents, such as a mixture of guaifenesin and thiamylal, given to effect, allows control of the situation. Though hypotension can result from this technique, it is dose dependent. Consequently, care must be exercised if IV drugs are administered during arousal.[118] Alternatively, ketamine, in increments of 200-500 mg, may be used and is less likely to cause hypotension. A disadvantage of ketamine is that it makes evaluation of the depth of anesthesia far more difficult and arousal may occur again when its effect wanes.

**Fluid Therapy and
Cardiovascular Support**

Hypotension is treated by IV infusion of fluids and judicious use of vasoactive drugs. If the mean arterial pressure is 50-70 mm Hg but there is adequate peripheral perfusion (as evidenced by warm extremities, especially the ears, good mucous membrane color, rapid capillary refill time and palpable digital pulses), generally only IV fluid therapy is required. It may be necessary to use 2 IV fluid lines to deliver the adequate fluid volume rapidly enough to improve the blood pressure. If possible, the patient's depth of anesthesia should be reduced. In spite of being hypotensive, horses that have good pulse pressures and that are not hypothermic have few postoperative complications or intraoperative crises.

If, however, the mean arterial pressure is 50-70 mm Hg, pulse pressure is poor and peripheral perfusion is inadequate (as characterized by cool extremities and prolonged capillary refill times), the anesthetist must act promptly. The anesthetic concentration should be reduced or gas flow discontinued, and the circle system evacuated and flushed with fresh oxygen. Vigorous fluid volume support is mandatory, using at least 2 gravity-flow IV fluid lines or an infusion pump to deliver the fluids.

The choice of fluid generally is at the anesthetist's discretion. In normal horses, where minimal blood loss is anticipated, an isotonic maintenance solution can be used. If some blood or plasma loss is likely, a fluid with an electrolyte content approximating that of plasma is recommended. Care should be used in administration of alkalinizing solutions (4.2% $NaHCO_3$) to horses under general anesthesia because of their tendency to predispose to hypoventilation.

The rate of fluid infusion is arbitrary, but 10 mg/kg/hour generally is satisfactory. The saphenous and cephalic veins are ideal for fluid administration and save the jugular veins for postoperative therapy, if necessary.

Vasoactive drugs, such as dopamine, dobutamine and isoproterenol, are indicated with imminent cardiovascular collapse. Because time is crucial, it is better to act prematurely when a downward trend in arterial pressure is detected than to wait until definite signs of acute hypotension become evident.

Dobutamine and dopamine are effective drugs that may be given during anesthesia to increase blood pressure. Either of these can be given by IV infusion, with the dose titrated to produce the desired response. In most instances, IV dosages of 2-5 μg/kg/min are safe and effective. Generally, the effects occur within 30 seconds and dissipate 3-5 minutes after the infusion is discontinued. Both dopamine and dobutamine increase skeletal muscle, splanchnic and renal blood flow, and increase cardiac output.[55] For additional information, the reader is referred to 2 excellent reviews of cardiopulmonary resuscitation in horses.[53,54]

Horses occasionally become hypotensive during surgery while not appearing to be profoundly anesthetized. The dilemma in this situation is how to maintain the animal in a surgical plane of anesthesia and prevent movement while simultaneously alleviating hypotension. Infusion of IV fluids and vasoactive drugs generally are indicated under these circumstances.

Monitoring During General Anesthesia

Extensive reviews of monitoring techniques have been published.[52,119] For clinical practice, the following monitoring techniques should be considered.

Monitoring the depth of anesthesia is critical to patient safety. Accurate assessment of anesthetic depth develops with experience. Depth is not determined by the setting on the anesthetic vaporizer, as this is only a crude guideline. To monitor the depth of anesthesia, the following indicators are used:

Eye Signs: The position and responses of the eyes are particularly reliable with halothane anesthesia (Fig 51). The eyeball may assume various positions within the orbit (medial, ventral, lateral or central strabismus), and there may be varying degrees of sensitivity of the palpebral reflex, tear production and the presence or absence of nystagmus.

Eye position is medial immediately after induction (Fig 53). As the depth of anesthesia gradually increases, the eye moves ventrally (Fig 54), then ventrolaterally (Fig 55). When the horse is deeply anesthetized, the eye is positioned centrally (Fig 56) and widely open with a dilated pupil and a glazed, pitted cornea. Generally, surgical planes of anesthesia exist when the eye is in the ventral to ventrolateral positions. If the eye is medial, the horse may become aroused with sufficient surgical stimulation. A central eyeball position indicates an excessive depth of anesthesia that is unnecessary for any surgical procedure.

The palpebral reflex also is quite reliable during inhalation anesthesia. To correctly elicit the palpebral reflex, the conjunctival border of the eyelashes should be stimulated gently. Frequent stimulation fatigues the re-

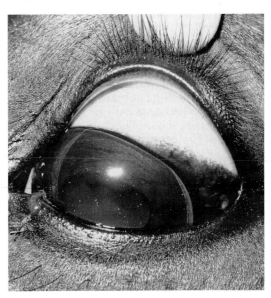

Figure 53. At a light plane of anesthesia, the globe is rotated medially and a large amount of sclera is visible. The palpebral reflex usually is maximal at this stage.

flex, so the response should be checked only once every 5 minutes. At light planes of anesthesia, the palpebral reflex is brisk. It gradually diminishes with increasing depth of anesthesia until it disappears altogether. A centrally positioned eye with no palpebral reflex usually indicates deep anesthesia.

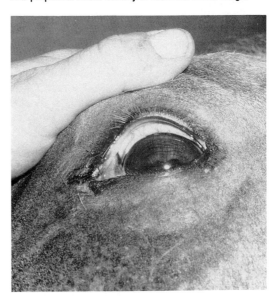

Figure 54. At a moderate plane of anesthesia, the globe is rotated ventrally and a large amount of sclera is visible. The palpebral reflex usually is reduced at this stage.

The corneal reflex is always present at clinical levels of anesthesia in horses. In fact, this reflex persists until death and therefore is not tested routinely.

The presence or absence of nystagmus can be confusing because 2 types of nystagmus are observed under general anesthesia in horses. Rapid nystagmus always is seen under very light planes of anesthesia in association with brisk palpebral reflexes, medial to ventral eyeball positions, lacrimation and ear movement. These findings generally indicate that the horse is about to move. Slow nystagmus may occur at any stage of anesthesia and generally occurs when the eyeball changes positions with increasing or decreasing depth of anesthesia. This does not necessarily dictate altering the level of halothane but indicates that the depth of anesthesia is changing.

Ear Movement: Often the first sign of sudden intraoperative arousal is ear movement. When ear movement is present, the eye is usually widely opened, with a medial to ventral eyeball position and brisk palpebral reflex. Nystagmus may or may not be present. This combination always implies the horse may move. In recovery, ear movement indicates that anesthesia is light enough for the horse to have a swallowing reflex and that the endotracheal tube can be removed. With IV anesthesia, ear movement indicates need for additional anesthetic to prolong anesthesia.

Figure 55. At deeper planes of anesthesia, the globe is rotated ventrally and somewhat toward the lateral canthus, with only a little sclera visible. The palpebral reflex is minimal at this depth.

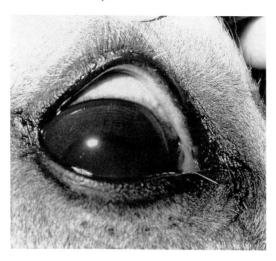

Figure 56. At a dangerously profound plane of anesthesia, the globe is centrally positioned, with a widely dilated pupil, sclera visible only at the medial margin, and almost no palpebral reflex. This plane of anesthesia usually is not necessary for any surgical procedure.

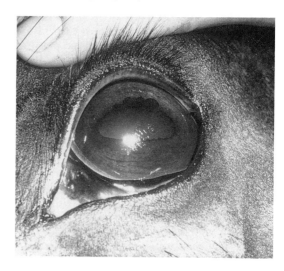

Limb Movement: Limb movement is a very crude determinant of anesthetic depth. It always dictates that additional anesthetic agents are needed to control the horse if recovery is not desired.

Anal Sphincter Tone: The tone of the anal sphincter is detected by touching the anus and observing sphincter contraction. At lighter planes of anesthesia, this response is quite brisk and the sphincter may contract several times from a single stimulation. This response is gradually reduced and is of less value with increased depth of anesthesia. At deep levels of anesthesia, the response is negligible and the anus is flaccid. Under surgical planes of anesthesia, the anal reflex always should be present, but assessment of tone is extremely subjective. There is individual variability between patients in the response, and variation between anesthetists in the intensity of the stimulation. Consequently, anal tone is only a very crude aid in assessing anesthetic depth.

Response to Surgical Stimulation: The response to surgical stimulation is extremely important in evaluating the depth of anesthesia. Surgical stimulation should always produce a response, but the patient should not move. Generally, upon initiation of surgery, the horse immediately takes a breath, eyeball position changes, the horse blinks involuntarily and slow nystagmus may begin. If the patient fails to react at all to surgical stimulation, the concentration of the anesthetic inhalant should be decreased.

Heart Rate: In horses, the heart rate is relatively useless as an indicator of depth of anesthesia. Heart rates are elevated (45-65 beats/min) at induction. As anesthesia stabilizes, the rate decreases to 40-50 beats/min. Generally, heart rate may change only at very deep levels of anesthesia or upon arousal. Consequently, these changes tend to occur too late to help assess the depth of anesthesia.

Respiratory Rate: Usually the respiratory rate is a more reliable indicator than heart rate and tends to increase at lighter planes of anesthesia. The character of respiration is quite important. At light planes of anesthesia, there is a normal thoracic-abdominal respiratory effort. This pattern is replaced by a more pronounced abdominal component at deeper levels of anesthesia.

Pulse or Arterial Pressure: The intraoperative arterial pressure provides a reliable indicator of depth of anesthesia because arterial pressure varies directly with the inspired concentration of inhalant anesthetics, particularly halothane. It should be emphasized, however, that hypercapnia and surgical stimulation increase arterial pressure.

Arterial blood pressure changes are of such importance that measurement of arterial pressure probably is mandatory for equine anesthesia. Numerous measuring devices are available. These include indirect Doppler or oscillometric devices, and direct fluid-filled catheters and transducers. Whichever technique is used, its advantages and disadvantages should be appreciated.

All of the aforementioned signs are important in providing an overall appraisal of anesthetic depth. No single criterion, including blood pressure, should be relied upon. Making the observations is critical; the more careful the scrutiny, the greater are the accuracy and objectivity. In any case, an anesthetic record must be used to help detect trends during long procedures. A chronologic recording of vital signs and physiologic values also permits retrospective analysis.

The cardiovascular system can be monitored quite simply and adequately by sight and palpation. By palpating the pulse, the pulse rate and more important, pulse pressure, can be determined. Much useful information can be obtained by direct digital palpation of a peripheral artery. The major criticism of simple palpation is that mean arterial pressure may fall without a reduction in pulse pressure.[52] Fortunately, this is not often the case, as the first sign of deterioration in cardiovascular status is narrowing of the pulse pressure, followed by a fall in mean pressure. Some experience and consistent attention by the same anesthetist throughout the anesthetic period are required for accuracy. It is a technique that should not be supplanted by sophisticated monitoring equipment but rather should be used in conjunction with these instruments.

Adequacy of peripheral perfusion is assessed by feeling the temperature of the skin, noting the color of mucous membranes and determining capillary refill time. However, these evaluations are subjective and vary between observers. It is often difficult to discern subtle trends by simple palpation and observation.

The cardiovascular system also can be monitored by more sophisticated and expensive techniques that require technical expertise. These techniques provide both quantitative and qualitative information and allow trends to be observed more readily. If problems do arise, these techniques allow more accurate assessment of the problem and evaluation of specific treatments. The major disadvantage of monitoring equipment is that the anesthetist tends to look at the equipment and not at the patient.

The electrocardiogram (ECG) detects precise rate and rhythm of the heart but gives no information about the vigor of cardiac contraction. Thus, the usefulness of the ECG is limited.

Measurement of arterial pressure gives information about the force of cardiac contraction but not about perfusion. There are many techniques to measure pressure, including direct cannulation of the artery with fluid-filled catheters connected to mechanical or electrical sensing devices and indirect, Doppler or oscillometric devices.[52,119] Indirect devices offer the advantage of being noninvasive. Though their precision has been questioned, they accurately detect trends in blood pressure changes. Direct measurement of arterial pressure is performed easily in horses. It is more accurate and dependable, and provides systolic, diastolic and mean pressure readings and visual display of the pressure wave. The last can provide information about cardiac performance.

Pulse pressure, the difference between systolic and diastolic pressure, is determined by the ratio of stroke volume (cardiac contraction) to the compliance of the arterial tree. Any condition affecting either cardiac output or peripheral resistance also affects the pulse pressure.

Assessment of peripheral perfusion provides information about blood flow. Indicators of peripheral perfusion in the anesthetized patient are warmth of the skin and distal extremities (especially hooves and ears), mucous membrane color and capillary refill time. Bleeding at the surgical site also is a good indication of flow. Hypotension reduces bleeding; dark blood in the surgical wound indicates circulatory collapse.

The adequacy of ventilation and oxygenation is difficult to assess without facilities for arterial blood gas analysis. Blood gas and acid-base measurements give quantitative information about PaO_2, $PaCO_2$ and pH, but the necessary equipment is complex and expensive.

Minute ventilatory volume, the product of respiratory rate and tidal volume, determines the efficacy of CO_2 elimination. Therefore, measurement of respiratory rate and subjective assessment of tidal volume from thoracic excursion and movement of the reservoir bag give some indication of the adequacy of ventilation.

Oxygenation is more difficult to assess clinically. Mucous membrane color is an indicator of oxygenation. Cyanotic mucous membranes indicate an excessive amount of reduced hemoglobin (at least 5 g reduced hemoglobin/dl) in the blood. The color of the blood in the surgical wound may also be another indicator of oxygenation, but it is not reliable.

Controlled Ventilation

C.M. Trim

Controlled ventilation (intermittent positive-pressure ventilation, artificial ventilation) often is required in general anesthetic management of equine patients. Under certain circumstances, controlled ventilation may be preferable to spontaneous ventilation. Principally, controlled ventilation is used to treat hypoventilation when respiratory acidosis is contributing to decreased cardiovascular function.

Hypoventilation commonly occurs in horses anesthetized with halothane or isoflurane. Severe hypoventilation is more prevalent in horses that have not had food withheld before anesthesia.[51] Hypoventilation may be more pronounced and arterial oxygenation lower in horses positioned in dorsal recumbency.[27] Use of controlled ventilation allows maintenance of a normal $PaCO_2$ and usually increases the PaO_2.[21] Controlled ventilation also may be used to reverse or prevent collapse of the lung, or decrease the patient's work of breathing. The latter need for controlled ventilation may arise if the horse is very old or depressed, or has significant pulmonary disease.

Controlled ventilation is not without some inherent adverse effects. Generally, the adverse effects of controlled ventilation on the function of the cardiovascular system are more pronounced in large animals than in small animals. Cardiac output is decreased because venous return to the heart is impeded by the positive pressure needed to inflate the lungs.[21] The negative pressure in the thorax that normally occurs during inspiration and promotes blood flow to the heart is completely abolished. Further, improperly applied positive-pressure ventilation can cause emphysema, bullae, pneumothorax or pneumomediastinum. Thus, controlled ventilation should be used when needed and used with care to avoid delivery of excessive volume or pressure to the lungs.

Types of Ventilators: The basic design of a ventilator consists of a reservoir bag within a canister and a source of compressed air. The compressed air enters the canister, generates positive pressure within the anesthetic circuit, and forces the contents of the reservoir into the animal's lungs (Fig 57). A common classification of ventilators separates them according to the mechanism responsible for terminating inspiration: volume, pressure or time.

Volume-cycled ventilators force the gas into the circuit until a preselected tidal volume has been delivered. The Ohio Metomatic ventilator is a volume-cycled ventilator, with a secondary pressure-limiting adjustment, that can be used to ventilate foals.

Pressure-cycled ventilators deliver gas into the circuit until a preselected airway pressure is achieved. Once this pressure is attained, a valve opens and the inspiratory portion of the respiratory cycle ceases. The Bird ventilators (J.D. Medical Distributing, Phoenix, AZ) are examples of pressure-cycled ventilators used to ventilate anesthetized horses.

Time-cycled ventilators operate by terminating inspiration at a preselected time. The North American Drager (Telford, PA) large animal ventilator is a time-cycled ventilator with a secondary ability to limit tidal volume. The newest version of this ventilator allows the anesthetist to adjust the inspiratory:expiratory time ratio (Fig 58). The time ratio is set at 1:2 in older models. When the anesthetist alters the respiratory rate, the ventilator adjusts the initiation and termination of inspiration.

To ensure that oxygen and anesthetic gas are delivered to the patient during inspiration, the circuit "pop-off" valve must be closed. A separate, specially designed valve attached to the ventilator bellows is employed to prevent pressure buildup (Fig 57). This valve is closed during inspiration by pressure derived from the ventilator canister. The pressure decreases to zero during expiration, the valve is no longer shut, and excess gases can then leave the circuit. It should be noted that waste gases must be collected into the scavenging system from 2 sites on the anesthesia machine to prevent room pollution.

Figure 57. Basic design of a mechanical ventilator.

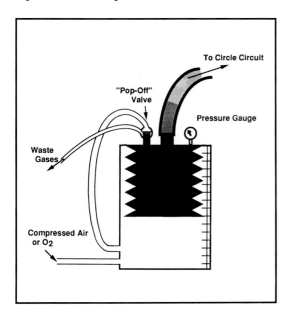

Figure 58. The Narkovet E Large Animal Control Center (North American Drager, Telford, PA) incorporates an anesthesia machine and a mechanical ventilator. The hose leading to the reservoir bag (a) used for spontaneous breathing is disconnected and reattached to the bellows (b) of the ventilator. The "pop-off" valve (c) is closed and the controls (d) used to adjust frequency of ventilation, duration of inspiration and tidal volume.

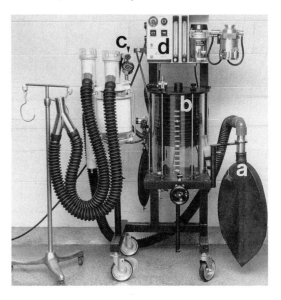

Technique of Controlled Ventilation: When a respiratory rate of 10-12 breaths/minute is used in adult horses, the tidal volume should be 10-12 ml/kg to maintain normal P_aCO_2. A larger tidal volume should be delivered when a slower respiratory rate is used. A tidal volume of 11 ml/kg usually is achieved with a peak inspiratory pressure of 20-25 cm H_2O. A higher pressure (up to 40 cm H_2O) may be necessary to provide adequate ventilation in obese horses or horses with abdominal distention. Foals should be ventilated at 12 breaths/minute and a tidal volume of 15 ml/kg.

Inspiratory time always should be shorter than expiratory time to minimize the depressant effects on cardiac output. An inspiratory time of 1.5-2 seconds is ideal for normal horses. If intermittent positive-pressure ventilation is being instituted because of hypoventilation (increased P_aCO_2), the vaporizer setting should be reduced to avoid substantially increasing the depth of anesthesia. If the animal has been breathing spontaneously and is to be switched to controlled ventilation, it is good practice to lower the patient's P_aCO_2 first by manually squeezing the reservoir bag several times. This reduces the patient's ventilatory drive and helps avoid the animal's "bucking" the ventilator.

Finally, it is good practice to make sure that the animal's chest moves in concert with the inspiratory portion of the ventilator's cycle. Some ventilators continue to cycle normally even when the endotracheal tube is disconnected or the "pop-off" valve is open. Under such conditions, the animal is receiving neither oxygen nor the inhalant anesthetic gas.

Toward the end of surgery, the anesthetist must "wean" the patient from controlled to spontaneous ventilation. If controlled ventilation was initiated because of hypoventilation, it is good practice to wait until surgery is nearly complete so that the depth of anesthesia can be decreased before the animal is allowed to breathe spontaneously. Abruptly discontinuing controlled ventilation results in apnea, with the potential for hypoxemia to develop before the P_aCO_2 accumulates sufficiently to stimulate breathing.

Ideally, the vaporizer setting should be decreased substantially and the respiratory rate decreased to 4-6 breaths/minute. The tidal volume should be unchanged to minimize collapse of the lungs. Finally, the anesthetist should make sure that the animal is in a position that will not impair breathing. If the horse has been positioned on its back during surgery, it should be rolled into lateral recumbency first. Eventually the ventilator is turned off and the reservoir bag filled with 100% O_2. The horse should be observed until it has begun to breathe spontaneously and deeply. The horse then can be moved to the recovery stall.

High-Frequency Ventilation: High-frequency positive-pressure ventilation, high-frequency jet ventilation, and high-frequency oscillatory ventilation are modes of ventilation that use tidal volumes equal to or less than the dead space at low inspiratory pressures and at frequencies several times greater than the normal respiratory rate. The intention is to provide adequate alveolar gas exchange without adversely affecting cardiovascular function. These techniques have been employed successfully in intensive care of neonatal foals but there is limited experience in ventilation of adult horses.[120,121]

Demand Valve for Ventilatory Support: A demand valve (Matrix Medical, Orchard Pk, NY; Hudson Oxygen Therapy Co, Wadsworth, OH) can be attached directly to the endotracheal tube and, when connected to an oxygen source at 50-80 psi, used to assist ventilation during recovery from anesthesia or during emergency resuscitation.[50,122,123] Ventilation can be achieved on demand by allowing the horse to breathe spontaneously, or ventilation can be controlled by manual triggering of the valve at a constant number of breaths per minute. The latter technique is recommended.[122,123]

Termination of Anesthesia

M.A. Brownlow and D.R. Hutchins

Anesthesia should be managed such that concentration of the inhalant gas administered is progressively decreased near the end of surgery. The anesthetic rebreathing bag then should be evacuated completely and filled with fresh oxygen several times. The anesthetist aims to move the horse into the recovery area on the verge of movement but with a medial eyeball position, brisk palpebral reflexes and rapid nystagmus.

Once ear movement occurs and the swallowing reflex is present, the endotracheal tube can be removed. In our experience, about 10% develop some degree of upper respiratory tract obstruction. These horses must have an endotracheal tube replaced. The cause of this obstruction is presumed to be due to soft palate displacement, pharyngeal collapse and/or edema of the turbinates.[34]

Recovery from Anesthesia

C.M. Trim

As the horse is moved into the recovery area at the end of surgery, another critical part of the anesthetic period begins. Because of their nature, some horses may panic during the emergence from anesthesia and try to stand up prematurely. Consequently, the anesthetist should ensure that the recovery room is dark and quiet to minimize extraneous stimuli.

The recovery room should be large enough to permit 1-2 people to stay with the horse, if necessary, and yet small enough to prevent the horse from injuring itself if it has difficulty standing on the first attempt. A reasonable size for a recovery room is 14 x 14 ft. At least one escape door for personnel should be present. The walls of the recovery room and escape door should be smooth and well padded. If possible, low-wattage ceiling lights should be available to allow the people in the recovery room to see. The floor of the recovery room should provide the horse with sufficient traction to allow the horse to stand and should not be slippery when wet.

We have found that recovering horses on a 10-inch-thick foam pad has helped reduce injuries associated with recovery. The horse is moved from the surgery room and is placed on a large pad that supports the horse's head and body. The horse's legs rest on 2 smaller pads and the 3 pads are covered by a single fitted vinyl sheet. Once the anesthetist decides that sufficient time has elapsed to allow the horse to regain its coordination (usually 40 minutes), the horse's head is restrained while the 2 small pads are removed from the room and the vinyl sheet tucked under the edge of the large pad. The horse is then free to roll into sternal recumbency and stand. The quiet, darkened surroundings and soft foam pad prolong the time before the horse tries to stand and thus increases its chance of standing on the first attempt.

Once the horse has stood successfully, the anesthetist can enter the recovery room and put a halter on the horse. With the horse under control, assistants can then lean the large foam pad against one of the walls to prevent the horse from tripping on it. Alternatively, the horse may be allowed to stand on the mats, or only the single large mat may be used.

As the horse stands up, greater control can be achieved with ropes. With one system, only the horse's head is controlled. A halter is applied early in recovery and a rope attached to the halter is passed through an opening in the recovery room wall. When the horse attempts to stand, tension is applied on the rope by someone outside recovery, preventing the horse from moving around. Greater control of the horse's movements can be achieved with individual ropes attached to the tail and halter. These ropes are threaded through metal rings high on the recovery room wall; traction on the ropes provides some extra lift when the horse attempts to stand. As long as the ropes are tied securely and tension on the ropes is maintained, this procedure should not increase the chance of injuring the horse or personnel in the room.

It is standard practice in our clinic to provide oxygen to the horse during the recovery period. Initially, oxygen is supplied (15 L/min/450-kg horse) through a soft rubber tube placed within the endotracheal tube. When the horse regains the swallowing reflex, the endotracheal tube is removed and the rubber tube inserted into the ventral nasal meatus.

Because ventilation may be depressed early in the recovery period, assisted ventilation using a demand valve attached to the endotracheal tube may be beneficial. When increased airway resistance due to nasal edema is evident after extubation, either the endotracheal tube should be reinserted or a smaller endotracheal tube inserted through the nasal meatus and into the trachea. These tubes may be left in place until the horse stands up, if necessary.

Complications Associated with General Anesthesia

M.A. Brownlow and D.R. Hutchins

Postanesthetic Myopathy

Myopathy is a possible sequel to general anesthesia in horses, especially if the procedure exceeds 2 hours. The reported incidence of postanesthetic myopathy is 1-3.4%, ranging from slight stiffness noted after the animal is standing to inability or unwillingness to attempt to stand.[57,124,125] Though the affected muscles generally are those that were in contact with the surgery table, muscle groups in the nondependent limbs occasionally are affected severely.

Affected muscles are firm and swollen, and the horse shows pain when bearing weight on that limb. Clinical signs of postanesthetic myopathy may be apparent during recovery or may be delayed for 60 minutes or more, depending on the severity of the condition. Horses with moderate to severe myopathy may exhibit violent behavior during recovery. Increased serum activity of creatine phosphokinase and myoglobinuria commonly accompany myopathy.

If the horse has been anesthetized in lateral recumbency, the triceps or masseter muscles and muscles over the ribs, flank and proximal portion of the pelvic limb may be affected, singly or in combination. Gluteal and longissimus dorsi muscles are most commonly involved in horses developing myopathy after anesthesia in dorsal recumbency.

Fortunately, most affected horses recover if given sufficient time and appropriate therapy. In some instances, however, the animal's violent response to its inability to bear weight may necessitate euthanasia. In severely affected horses, the muscles may subsequently undergo atrophy, fibrosis and contracture. Consequently, the effects of postanesthetic myopathy may range from temporary discomfort during recovery, to partial loss of function, to death.[124,126]

Simple physical factors, such as prolonged compression of the muscle, may diminish local blood flow and cause myonecrosis. This is particularly true in dependent areas of the body that bear most of the weight when the animal is in lateral or dorsal recumbency. Decreases in systemic arterial pressure from both positional and drug-related reductions in cardiac output also may diminish local blood flow. These alterations in local perfusion likely are time related. Consequently, relatively short periods of ischemia may not cause clinical signs, whereas more prolonged periods result in myopathy. The relative importance of tissue compression, systemic hypotension and local hemodynamic factors has yet to be determined.[57,126]

It has been hypothesized that postanesthetic myopathy in horses may be a manifestation of the "compartmental syndrome," which is defined as local muscular ischemia due to edema and increased pressure within an osteofascial compartment.[115,127] In people, this syndrome occurs after trauma, exercise or ischemia and commonly in comatose patients. Apparently, the muscle pressures measured in the dependent limbs of horses during anesthesia are sufficient to induce this syndrome.

A syndrome of generalized or extensive myopathy affecting forelimb and/or hind limb muscle groups bilaterally has been identified. Though this syndrome has not been associated with the patient's position during anesthesia, affected horses shared a common history. Generally, these animals were athletically fit, of average body size and weight, and anesthetized relatively soon after a race.[57,128,129] They had an unexpected period of arousal, with movement, shaking or rigidity, and evidence of pronounced cardiovascular depression during the anesthetic period.[57] In certain cases, body temperature increased substantially. Signs exhibited by these horses upon recovery from anesthesia included generalized weakness, muscle rigidity, violent behavior and pain that became more pronounced with exertion.[57]

The cause of this generalized form of postanesthetic myopathy is likely to be complex. It has been postulated that individual horses may have a genetic metabolic defect rendering them uniquely susceptible to the syndrome. This proposed susceptibility has been likened to the predisposition of certain people and porcine breeds to malignant hyperthermia and porcine stress syndrome.[124,128] It has also been hypothesized that diffuse rhabdomyolysis may be initiated either directly by the anesthetic agent or by the spreading of a localized myopathy within a dependent muscle group.[115,128]

Prevention: Because postanesthetic myopathy may be a serious, life-threatening complication, the anesthetist should take precautions to prevent it. Therefore, consideration should be given to the following points:

Because there is a direct correlation between duration of recumbency and development of myopathy, the anesthetist should *keep the surgical team aware of the duration of the procedure.* In a study of 50 clinical cases, the duration of recumbency in affected horses was 2.92 hours, vs 2.06 hours in horses that did not develop the syndrome.[57]

Proper positioning of the horse is essential and should not be overlooked. Everything possible should be done to minimize development of excessive intracompartmental muscle pressures.

Because horses fed high levels of concentrate feeds before anesthesia appear to be at increased risk for developing the syndrome, *preoperative grain intake should be restricted.*

Care must be taken to *avoid intraoperative hypotension.* Consequently, the patient should be maintained in the lightest plane of anesthesia that is compatible with the surgical procedure. It is also advisable to administer fluids intraoperatively to minimize the effects of hypovolemia and dehydration.

Treatment: Once muscle damage has occurred, management of postanesthetic myopathy is largely symptomatic. If muscle damage is mild, rest is usually sufficient to allow return of function. Nonsteroidal anti-inflammatory drugs are indicated to reduce inflammation in the muscle and decrease pain. Local application of heat and massage of the affected muscles also may help restore function.[115]

In more severely affected horses, symptomatic support must be extended to maintain the animal's hydration and nutritional status, prevent continuing muscle damage, and prevent renal tubular damage caused by myoglobin release from the affected tissue.[115] It may be necessary to administer narcotics, nonsteroidal antiinflammatories and acepromazine to provide analgesia and reduce stress associated with the condition. Care should be taken with use of nonsteroidal antiinflammatories as hypovolemic horses are particularly prone to develop renal complications caused by these drugs.[115]

Muscle relaxants may be helpful in relieving pain and improving muscle perfusion. Though methocarbamol and guaifenesin, 2 centrally acting muscle relaxants, may help minimize muscle spasms, they must be used carefully, as they can cause ataxia. Dantrolene sodium, a hydantoin derivative, causes muscle relaxation by reducing release of calcium from the sarcoplasmic reticulum, reducing segmental contractions. Dantrolene is likely to be most effective when administered IV at 10 mg/kg before anesthesia.[115]

Dexamethasone given IV at 1-2 mg/kg, though controversial and of unproven value, has been used frequently in treatment of horses with severe muscle necrosis. The purpose of this form of treatment is to reduce inflammation and maintain membrane integrity. Other drugs used for this purpose include vitamin E, selenium and topical or systemic DMSO. Because the last drug has been incriminated as a cause of acute renal failure in people, it should not be used indiscriminately.[115]

Any existing fluid or electrolyte imbalances should be addressed and IV fluid therapy instituted to maintain circulating blood volume, soft tissue perfusion and renal function. Though administration of bicarbonate-rich solutions is indicated with metabolic acidosis, generally this has not been necessary in this syndrome.[115]

One of the most important aspects of therapy is good nursing care. Recumbent horses unable to stand should not be forced to move. These horses should be made comfortable, offered food and water, and encouraged to attain sternal recumbency intermittently to permit muscle perfusion. Horses may remain recumbent for as long as 48 hours before they can stand.[115]

Peroneal Nerve Paralysis

Excessive pressure on the dependent rear limb or caudal traction on the hind limbs during the anesthetic period may cause peroneal nerve paralysis. On recovery from anesthesia, the horse can stand but cannot extend its rear leg or flex the hock. This complication of anesthesia can be prevented by padding the dependent limb and elevating the upper (nondependent) hind limb.

Facial Nerve Paralysis

The superficial course of the facial nerve along the masseter muscle renders this nerve particularly prone to injury if the horse's head is laid on hard, flat surfaces during anesthesia. Halters always should be removed and the horse's head adequately cushioned during anesthesia.

Skin Reactions

Skin reactions, such as edematous plaques, "hair ruffling," necrosis and burns, occasionally become apparent after general anesthesia in certain horses. These reactions may be evident immediately upon recovery, as is generally the case with edematous plaques, or may develop within 24 hours, as occurs with "hair ruffling," skin necrosis and burns. These lesions classically occur over contact points, are transient and heal uneventfully. The hair over the contact points appears matted and "ruffled," and resists attempts to make it lie flat.

Some horses develop a lesion similar to a burn with full-thickness loss of skin. Often these lesions require skin grafts for healing to take place.[34] It has been suggested that body temperature over contact points increases markedly when anesthetized horses are placed on an insulated vinyl surface or pulled across a rubber floor, and that these local changes in the coefficient of friction cause shearing forces that burn the skin.[58] Consequently, attention should be paid to contact points.

Edematous plaques usually are large, raised areas that develop over the contact points. These plaques generally disappear within 24 hours. These lesions have been associated with prolonged anesthetic periods and likely reflect insufficient padding. It has been hypothesized that these lesions develop from localized areas of hyperthermia, vasodilation and edema.[130]

Postanesthetic Myasthenic Syndrome

Postanesthetic myasthenic syndrome is rare in horses. Affected animals have generalized muscle weakness and recover slowly from anesthesia. The muscles of the face, tongue, pharynx and body generally are affected. Often, a combination of aminoglycoside antibiotics, halothane and succinylcholine has been used in these animals; hypocalcemia and prolonged or complicated surgeries are consistent features in the history. Calcium-dependent inhibition of acetylcholine release at the neuromuscular junction, combined with a decrease in the sensitivity of the postsynaptic membrane to acetylcholine, has been implicated in the paralysis. Though treatment with calcium gluconate and neostigmine may be indicated, good nursing care is the most important aspect of therapy.

Colic

In our experience, most horses with postoperative colic have cecal or large colon impaction. This is not surprising when one considers that most preanesthetic and anesthetic drugs substantially reduce gastrointestinal motility. Perforation of the cecum has been reported in horses after routine anesthetic periods for elective surgeries. The proposed mechanism for this condition is alteration in cecal outflow, leading to cecal impaction and eventual perforation.[131] The effects of nonsteroidal antiinflammatory drugs in the pathogenesis of this condition cannot be ruled out; consequently, these drugs should be used judiciously and horses monitored closely postoperatively for feed intake and defecation.

Salmonellosis

Colitis caused by *Salmonella* is a serious infectious disease in horses. The most common clinical syndrome is acute colitis with severe diarrhea. Horses of all ages may be affected; mortality is high. Stress appears to play a major role in initiating the disease. Possible predisposing factors include transportation, general anesthesia, surgery, concurrent illness, and antibiotic use.

The possibility that horses may contract salmonellosis during treatment in veterinary hospitals cannot be ignored. Horses should be monitored postoperatively for fever, appetite, depression, leukopenia and fecal character. Stress should be minimized as much as possible.

References

1. Ruskoaho H and Karppouen H: Xylazine-induced sedation in chicks is inhibited by opioid receptor antagonists. *Eur J Pharmacol* 100:91-96, 1984.

2. Tranquilli WJ and Thurmon JC: Alpha-adrenoreceptor pharmacology. *JAVMA* 184:1400-1402, 1984.

3. Stenberg B: The role of alpha adrenoreceptors in the regulation of vigilance and pain. *Acta Vet Scand* 82:29-30, 1986.

4. Muir WW *et al:* Narcotic agonists, partial agonists and sedatives in horses. *Proc 24th Ann Mtg AAEP*, 1978. pp 173-182.

5. Muir WW: Standing chemical restraint in horses. *Vet Clin No Am* (Large Anim Pract) 3:17-44, 1981.

6. Muir WW *et al:* Hemodynamic and respiratory effects of a xylazine-acetylpromazine drug combination in horses. *Am J Vet Res* 40:1518-1522, 1979.

7. Garner HE *et al:* Effects of Bay Va 1470 on cardiovascular parameters in ponies. *VM/SAC* 66:1016-1021, 1971.

8. Thurmon JC *et al:* Xylazine causes transient dose-related hyperglycemia and increased urine volume in mares. *Am J Vet Res* 45:224-227, 1984.

9. Thurmon JC and Benson GJ: Injectable anesthetics and anesthetic adjuncts. *Vet Clin No Am* (Large Anim Pract) 3:15-36, 1987.

10. Stick JA and Chou CC: Effects of xylazine on equine intestinal vascular resistance, motility and oxygen consumption. *Proc 2nd Symp Equine Colic Res*, 1987. pp 105-111.

11. Fuentes VO: Sudden death in a stallion after xylazine medication. *Vet Record* 102:106, 1978.

12. Clarke KW and Hall LW: Xylazine-A new sedative for horses and cattle. *Am J Vet Res* 85:512-517, 1969.

13. Tobin T: Pharmacology Review: The phenothiazine tranquilizers. *J Equine Med Surg* 3:460-466, 1979.

14. Heath RB: Clinical pharmacology of tranquilizers. *Proc 24th Ann Mtg AAEP*, 1978. pp 189-191.

15. Klein L and Sharman J: Effects of preanesthetic medication, anesthesia and position of recumbency on central venous pressure in horses. *JAVMA* 170:216-219, 1977.

16. Kerr DD *et al:* Comparison of the effects of xylazine and acetylpromazine maleate in the horse. *Am J Vet Res* 33:777-784, 1972.

17. Muir WW *et al:* Effects of xylazine and acetylpromazine upon induced ventricular fibrillation in dogs anesthetized with thiamylal and halothane. *Am J Vet Res* 36:1299-1303, 1975.

18. Maylin GA: Metabolism of phenothiazine tranquillizers. *Proc 24th Mtg AAEP*, 1978. pp 193-203.

19. Pearson H and Weaver BMQ: Priapism after sedation, neuroleptanalgesia and anaesthesia in the horse. *Equine Vet J* 10:85-90, 1978.

20. Bolz W: The prophylaxis and therapy of prolapse and paralysis of the penis occurring in the horse after administration of neuroleptics. *Vet Med Rev Leverkusen* 4:255-263, 1970.

21. Steffey EP and Howland D: Cardiovascular effects of halothane in the horse. *Am J Vet Res* 39:611-615, 1978.

22. Hall LW and Clarke KW: *Veterinary Anaesthesia.* 8th ed. Balliere Tindall, London, 1983.

23. Jochle W: Domosedan: A new sedative and analgesic drug for horses with dose-dependent duration of effects. *Proc 30th Ann Mtg AAEP*, 1984. pp 221-224.

24. Hamm D and Jochle W: Sedation and analgesia in horses treated with various doses of Domosedan: Blind studies on efficacy and the duration of effects. *Proc 30th Ann Mtg AAEP*, 1984. pp 235-242.

25. Short CE *et al*: Cardiovascular and pulmonary function studies of a new sedative/analgesia (Detomidine/Domosedan) for use alone in horses or as a preanesthetic. *Acta Vet Scand* 82:139-155, 1986.

26. Savola JM: Cardiovascular actions of detomidine. *Acta Vet Scand* 82:47-57, 1986.

27. Steffey EP *et al*: Body position and mode of ventilation influence arterial pH, oxygen and carbon dioxide tensions in halothane-anesthetized horses. *Am J Vet Res* 38:379-382, 1977.

28. Hall LW: Disturbances of cardiopulmonary function in anaesthetized horses. *Equine Vet J* 3:95-98, 1971.

29. Klein L: A review of 50 cases of post-operative myopathy in the horse-intrinsic and management factors affecting risk. *Proc 24th Ann Mtg AAEP*, 1978. pp 89-93.

30. Kellman GR: *Applied Cardiovascular Physiology.* 2nd ed. Butterworths, London, 1977. pp 178-207.

31. Scurr C and Feldman S: *Scientific Foundations of Anaesthesia.* 2nd ed. William Heinemann Medical Books, London, 1974. pp 165-188.

32. Gillespie JR *et al*: Cardiovascular dysfunction in anesthetized, laterally recumbent horses. *Am J Vet Res* 30:61-72, 1969.

33. Steffey EP *et al*: Adequacy of ventilation in equine anesthesia. *Proc 21st Ann Mtg AAEP,* 1975. pp 157-160.

34. Brownlow MA and Hutchins DR: Unpublished observations, 1987.

35. Soma LR: Equine anesthesia: Causes of reduced oxygen and increased carbon dioxide tensions. *Compend Cont Ed Pract Vet* 2:557-564, 1980.

36. Steffey EP *et al*: Time-related responses of spontaneously breathing, laterally recumbent horses to prolonged anesthesia with halothane. *Am J Vet Res* 48:952-957, 1987.

37. Hall LW *et al*: Alveolar-arterial oxygen tension differences in anesthetized horses. *Brit J Anaesth* 40:560-568, 1968.

38. Brownlow MA *et al*: The "Turner" circle absorber: An anesthetic breathing system for the horse. *Equine Vet J* 17:225-227, 1985.

39. McDonell WN and Hall LW: Functional residual capacity in conscious and anesthetized horses. *Brit J Anaesth* 46:802-803, 1976.

40. Hall LW: General anesthesia. Fundamental considerations. *Vet Clin No Am (Large Anim Pract)* 3:3-15, 1981.

41. Prys-Roberts C, in Gray TC and Nunn JF: *General Anaesthesia.* 3rd ed. Butterworths, London, 1971. p 164.

42. Cullen DJ *et al*: The cardiovascular effects of carbon dioxide in man, conscious and during cyclopropane anesthesia. *Anaesthesiol* 31:407, 1969.

43. Nunn JF: *Applied Respiratory Physiology with Special Reference to Anaesthesia.* Butterworths, London, 1972. pp 288-325.

44. Mitchell B and Littlejohn A: The effect of anaesthesia and posture on the exchange of respiratory gases and on the heart rate. *Equine Vet J* 6:177-178, 1974.

45. Weaver BMQ: Equine anaesthesia. *Equine Vet J* 1:39-42, 1968.

46. Hodgson DS *et al*: Effects of spontaneous, assisted and controlled ventilatory modes in halothane-anesthetized geldings. *Am J Vet Res* 47:992-996, 1986.

47. Grandy JL *et al*: Arterial blood PO2 and PCO2 in horses during early halothane-oxygen anesthesia. *Equine Vet J* 19:314-318, 1987.

48. Freeman J and Nunn JF: Ventilation-perfusion relationships after hemorrhage. *Clin Sci* 24:135-147, 1963.

49. Mason DE *et al*: Arterial blood gas tensions in the horse during recovery from anesthesia. *JAVMA* 8:989-994, 1987.

50. Riebold TW *et al*: Evaluation of the demand valve for resuscitation of horses. *JAVMA* 176:623-626, 1980.

51. McDonell WN *et al*: Radiographic evidence of impaired pulmonary function in laterally recumbent anaesthetised horses. *Equine Vet J* 11:24-32, 1979.

52. Klein L, in Mansmann RA and McAllister ES: *Equine Medicine and Surgery.* 3rd ed. American Veterinary Publications, Goleta, CA, 1982. pp 282-300.

53. Muir WW and Bednarski RM: Equine cardiopulmonary resuscitation - Part I. *Compend Cont Ed Pract Vet* 5:228-234, 1983.

54. Muir WW and Bednarski RM: Equine cardiopulmonary resuscitation - Part II. *Compend Cont Ed Pract Vet* 5:287-295, 1983.

55. Hubbell JAE *et al*: Perianesthetic considerations in the horse. *Compend Cont Ed Pract Vet* 6:401-414, 1984.

56. Grandy JL *et al*: Arterial hypotension and the development of postanesthetic myopathy in halothane-anesthetized horses. *Am J Vet Res* 48:192-197, 1987.

57. Klein L: A review of 50 cases of postoperative myopathy in the horse-intrinsic and management factors affecting risk. *Proc 25th Ann Mtg AAEP*, 1979. pp 89-94.

58. Heath RB: Complications associated with general anesthesia in the horse. *Vet Clin No Am (Large Anim Pract)* 3:45-47, 1981.

59. LaMont RL and Prasad B: Experience with dome-shaped osteotomy of upper tibia for multiplane correction. *Clin Ortho Rel Res* 91:152-157, 1973.

60. Gabel AA and Jones EW, in Catcott EJ and Smithcors JF: *Equine Medicine and Surgery.* 2nd ed. American Veterinary Publications, Goleta, CA, 1972. pp 659-660.

61. McDonell WN: *The effect of anesthesia on pulmonary gas exchange and arterial oxygenation in the horse.* PhD thesis, University of Cambridge, 1974.

62. Lumb WV and Jones EV: *Veterinary Anesthesia.* 2nd ed. Lea & Febiger, Philadelphia, 1984. pp 307-331.

63. Gabel AA *et al:* Effects of promazine and chloral hydrate on the cardiovascular system of the horse. *Am J Vet Res* 25:1151-1158, 1964.

64. Hall LW: *Wright's Veterinary Anaesthesia and Analgesia.* 5th ed. Balliere Tindall, London, 1964.

65. Clarke KW and Taylor PM: Detomidine: A new sedative for horses. *Equine Vet J* 18:366-370, 1986.

66. Trim CM *et al:* A retrospective study of anaesthesia in horses with colic. *Equine Vet J* 7:84-90, 1989.

67. Jochle W *et al:* Comparison of detomidine, butorphanol, flunixin meglumine, and xylazine in clinical cases of equine colic. *Equine Vet J* 7:111-116, 1989.

68. Jeffcott LB and Whitwell KE: Twinning as a cause of foetal and neonatal loss in the thoroughbred mare. *J Comp Pathol* 83:91-105, 1973.

69. Robertson JT and Muir WW: A new analgesic drug combination in the horse. *Am J Vet Res* 44:1667-1669, 1983.

70. Geiser DR and Henton JE: Xylazine and butorphanol: Survey of field use in the horse. *Equine Pract* 10(1):7-11, 1988.

71. Saidman LJ, in Eger EI: *Anesthetic Uptake and Action.* Williams & Wilkins, Baltimore, 1974. pp 264-284.

72. Short CE: Intravenous anesthesia: Drugs and techniques. *Vet Clin No Am* (Large Anim Pract) 3:195-208, 1981.

73. Thurmon JC *et al:* Injectable anesthesia for horses. *MVP* 65:745-750, 1985.

74. Dundee JW and Wyant GM: *Intravenous Anesthesia.* Churchill Livingstone, New York, 1974. pp 64-128.

75. Muir WW *et al:* Evaluation of thiamylal, guaifenesin, and ketamine hydrochloride combinations administered prior to halothane anesthesia in horses. *J Equine Med Surg* 3:178-184, 1979.

76. Westhues M and Fritsch R: *Animal Anaesthesia.* Oliver and Boyd, Edinburgh, 1961. p 186.

77. Funk KA: Glyceryl guaiacolate: A centrally acting muscle relaxant. *Equine Vet J* 2:173-178, 1970.

78. Roberts D: The role of glyceryl guaiacolate in a balanced equine anesthetic. *VM/SAC* 63:157-162, 1968.

79. Gertsen KE and Tillotson PJ: Clinical use of glyceryl guaiacolate in the horse. *VM/SAC* 63:1062-1066, 1968.

80. Hubbell JA *et al:* Guaifenesin: Cardiopulmonary effects and plasma concentrations in horses. *Am J Vet Res* 41:1751-1755, 1980.

81. Davis LE and Wolff WA: Pharmocokinetics and metabolism of glyceryl guaiacolate in ponies. *Am J Vet Res* 31:469-473, 1970.

82. Funk KA: Glyceryl guaiacolate: Some effects and indications in horses. *Equine Vet J* 5:15-19, 1973.

83. Muir WW *et al:* Evaluation of xylazine, guaifenesin and ketamine hydrochloride for restraint in horses. *Am J Vet Res* 39:1274-1278, 1978.

84. Schatzmann U *et al:* An investigation of the haemolytic effect of glyceryl guaiacolate in the horse. *Equine Vet J* 10:224-228, 1978.

85. Grandy JL and McDonell WN: Evaluation of concentrated solutions of guaifenesin for equine anesthesia. *JAVMA* 176:619-622, 1980.

86. Geiser DR: Practical equine injectable anesthesia. *JAVMA* 182:574-577, 1983.

87. Muir WW *et al:* Evaluation of xylazine and ketamine hydrochloride for anesthesia in horses. *Am J Vet Res* 38:195-201, 1977.

88. Butera TS *et al:* Diazepam/xylazine/ketamine combination for short-term anesthesia in the horse. *VM/SAC* 73:490-499, 1978.

89. Green SA *et al:* Cardiopulmonary effects of continuous intravenous infusion of guaifenesin, ketamine, and xylazine in ponies. *Am J Vet Res* 47:2364-2367, 1986.

90. Muir WW: Cyclohexanone drug mixtures. The pharmacology of ketamine and ketamine drug combinations. *Proc 2nd Intl Cong Vet Anes,* 1985. pp 5-11.

91. Nolan AM and Hall LW: Total intravenous anaesthesia in the horse with propofol. *Equine Vet J* 17:394-398, 1985.

92. Nolan AM and Chambers JP: The use of propofol as an induction agent after detomidine premedication in ponies. *J Assn Vet Anaesth* 16:30-32, 1989.

93. Hubbell JAE *et al:* Xylazine and tiletamine-zolazepam anesthesia in horses. *Am J Vet Res* 50:737-742, 1989.

94. Crispin S: Methods of equine general anesthesia in clinical practice. *Equine Vet J* 13:19-26, 1981.

95. Schebitz H: Zur Narkose beim Pferd unter besonderer Benicksichtigung der Narkose im geschlossenen System. *Mh Veterinaermed* 10:503-508, 1955.

96. Fisher EW and Jennings S: A closed circuit anesthetic apparatus for adult cattle and for horses. *Vet Record* 69:769-773, 1957.

97. Weaver BMQ: An apparatus for inhalation anesthesia in large animals. *Vet Record* 72:1121-1125, 1960.

98. Fowler ME *et al:* An inhalation anesthetic apparatus for large animals. *JAVMA* 143:272-276, 1963.

99. Purchase IFH: The measurement of compliance and other respiratory parameters in horses. *Vet Record* 78:613-615, 1966.

100. Adriani J: *The Chemistry and Physics of Anesthesia.* 2nd ed. Charles C Thomas, Springfield, IL, 1963.

101. Thurmon JC and Benson GJ: Inhalation anesthetic delivery equipment and its maintenance. *Vet Clin No Am* (Large Anim Pract) 3:73-96, 1981.

102. Orkin LR *et al:* Resistance to breathing by apparatus used in anesthesia. *Curr Res Anaes Analgesia* 33:217-222, 1954.

103. Steffey EP *et al:* Enflurane, halothane and isoflurane potency in horses. *Am J Vet Res* 38:1037-1039, 1977.

104. Steffey EP: Enflurane and isoflurane anesthesia. A summary of laboratory and clinical investigations in the horse. *JAVMA* 172:367-373, 1978.

105. Steffey EP and Howland D: Potency of halothane-N20 in the horse. *Am J Vet Res* 39:1141-1146, 1978.

106. Steffey EP and Howland D: Comparison of circulatory and respiratory effects of isoflurane and halothane anesthesia in horses. *Am J Vet Res* 41:821-825, 1980.

107. Orsini JA and Taylor JI: Enflurane anesthesia in the pony. A comparative study between enflurane and halothane. *Cornell Vet* 70:50-66, 1980.

108. Hillidge CJ and Lees P: Cardiac output in the conscious and anaesthetised horse. *Equine Vet J* 7:16-21, 1975.

109. Steffey EP *et al:* Time-related responses of spontaneously breathing, laterally recumbent horses to prolonged anesthesia with halothane. *Am J Vet Res* 48:952-957, 1987.

110. Goetz TE and Manohar M: Renal, adrenal, intestinal, and pancreatic blood flow in controls and during 1.0-1.5, and 2.0 minimum alveolar concentration halothane-O2 anesthesia. *Proc 2nd Symp Equine Colic Res,* 1987. pp 258-263.

111. Kelly AB and Steffey EP: Inhalation anesthesia. Drugs and techniques. *Vet Clin No Am* (Large Anim Pract) 3:59-71, 1981.

112. Lindsay W *et al:* Equine postanesthetic forelimb lameness: Intra-compartmental muscle pressure changes and biochemical patterns. *Am J Vet Res* 41:1919-1924, 1980.

113. Lindsay WA *et al:* Effect of protective padding on forelimb intracompartmental muscle pressures in anesthetized horses. *Am J Vet Res* 46:688-691, 1985.

114. White NA and Suarez M: Change in triceps muscle intracompartmental pressure with repositioning and padding of the lowermost thoracic limb of the horse. *Am J Vet Res* 47:2257-2259, 1986.

115. White NA II: Postanesthetic recumbency myopathy in horses. *Compend Cont Ed Pract Vet* 4:544-550, 1982.

116. Heath RB *et al:* Protecting and positioning the equine surgical patient. *VM/SAC* 67:1241-1245, 1972.

117. Steffey EP and Howland D: Rate of change of halothane concentration in a large animal circle anesthetic system. *Am J Vet Res* 38:1993-1996, 1977.

118. Pascoe PJ *et al:* Hypotensive potential of supplemental guaifenesin doses during halothane anesthesia in the horse. *Proc 2nd Intl Cong Vet Anes,* 1985. p 61.

119. Manley SV: Monitoring the anesthetized horse. *Vet Clin No Am* (Large Anim Pract) 3:111-133, 1981.

120. Wilson DV *et al:* Effects of frequency and airway pressure on gas exchange during interrupted high-frequency, positive-pressure ventilation in ponies. *Am J Vet Res* 49:1263-1269, 1988.

121. Dodman NH *et al:* Gas conductance during high-frequency oscillatory ventilation in large animals. *Am J Vet Res* 50:1210-1214, 1989.

122. Waterman AE *et al:* Use of a demand valve for post-operative administration of oxygen to horses. *Equine Vet J* 14:290-292, 1982.

123. Watney GCG *et al:* Effects of a demand valve on pulmonary ventilation in spontaneously breathing, anaesthetised horses. *Vet Record* 117:358-362, 1985.

124. Johnson BD *et al:* Serum chemistry changes in horses during anesthesia: a pilot study investigating the possible causes of postanesthetic myositis in horses. *J Equine Med Surg* 2:109-123, 1978.

125. White KK and Short CE: Anesthetic/surgical stress-induced myopathy (myositis). Part II: A post anesthetic myopathy trial. *Proc 24th Ann Mtg AAEP,* 1978. pp 107-114.

126. Short CE and White KK: Anesthetic/surgical stress-induced myopathy (myositis). Part I: Clinical occurrences. *Proc 24th Ann Mtg AAEP,* 1978. pp 101-106.

127. Mubarak S and Owen CA: Compartmental syndrome and its relation to the crush syndrome: A spectrum of disease. *Clin Ortho* 113:81-89, 1975.

128. Waldron-Mease E: Correlation of post-operative and exercise-induced equine myopathy with the defect malignant hyperthermia. *Proc 24th Ann Mtg AAEP,* 1978. pp 95-99.

129. Lindsay W *et al:* Intra-compartmental muscle pressure in the anesthetized horse. *Proc 24th Ann Mtg AAEP,* 1978. pp 115-126.

130. Riebold TW *et al: Large Animal Anesthesia. Principles and Techniques.* Iowa State Univ Press, Ames, 1982. pp 99-104.

131. Ross MW *et al:* Cecal perforation in the horse. *JAVMA* 187:249-253, 1985.

NECROPSY

C.D. Buergelt

Every necropsy should be viewed as the beginning, not the end, of understanding a disease. It should confirm a clinical diagnosis, pinpoint an equivocal one, or provide new insights into the cause of disease or death. The necropsy may alter the major clinical diagnosis in some instances. Consequently, it should be considered a major tool for quality assessment in clinical medicine. A necropsy should always be thorough and complete. A partial necropsy gives only partial answers. Gross examination alone often provides an incomplete diagnosis. Additional histopathologic, toxicologic, parasitologic, microbiologic and virologic examinations are need to confirm the final diagnosis.

The equine necropsy can be divided into 3 types: the disease-oriented necropsy, the insurance necropsy and the medico-legal necropsy. A medico-legal necropsy must be conducted under the premise that the case may end up in court. The events of the necropsy should be substantiated through meticulous compilation of recorded physical findings, photographs, radiographs, preserved specimens and laboratory results. The same procedure should be followed for insurance necropsies and in cases where no clear answer can be obtained by performing a gross examination.[1] Authentication requires adequate records, specimen labelling, signatures of participants and witnesses, and the exact date and time of the necropsy.

General Considerations

Before necropsy, a complete clinical abstract concerning the history of the case should be studied. Failure to do this may result in overlooking an important detail essential to the necropsy in question. The clinical abstract should include the animal's breed, sex, age, color, markings, tattoo and use, clinical signs and precise medication history. Though background information is important, one should not overinterpret or be biased by the clinical history. The most detailed clinical history is not a substitute for an objective, complete necropsy. An orderly necropsy requires adequate exposure of the organs under optimal environmental conditions. Under field conditions, one should select even, solid ground, with access to plenty of water and good lighting. This is particularly important for necropsies performed at night. Needless to say, the proper protective attire and the right set of necropsy instruments are important prerequisites.

Ideally, the necropsy should be performed by an impartial party, *eg*, a prosecutor not involved with clinical treatment of the horse. In all cases, written or telephone-witnessed permission should be obtained from the owner or a legitimate representative and the insurance company before starting the necropsy. The dates and times that these contracts are made and the names of persons contacted for such permission are to be recorded. The name and address of the insurance company or agent should be secured as well. Careful attention should be paid to details of the history, special instructions, and special requirements given for the examination. If the necropsy is performed in the field, a second veterinarian may assist or witness the necropsy.

An important goal is to conduct the necropsy within a reasonable period after death, preferably immediately after death, to avoid tissue decomposition. If the animal is to be euthanized just before the start of the necropsy, the carcass should be bled out before the postmortem examination is begun. The reader is referred to other sources for discussion of methods of euthanasia.[2] I generally prefer intravenous euthanasia. Regardless of the necropsy technique used, the approach should always be the same so that no tissues and organs are overlooked. The procedure described here is taught at the University of Florida. Other methods have been described elsewhere.[3-5]

Positioning, Examining and Opening the Carcass

After obtaining or estimating the body weight, the animal should be positioned in left lateral recumbency. All body orifices, ocular sclerae, hooves (including coronary bands), and the condition of the haircoat are examined. The tattoo or brand, if obtainable, is transcribed, and the general color of the visible mucous membranes is recorded. Valuable information can be obtained from the very start by carefully looking at all visible mucous membranes for signs of possible internal disease and organ involvement. Thus, yellow mucosae suggest blood dyscrasia or liver failure; white mucosae suggest blood loss or deficient bone marrow function; blue mucosae suggest insufficient oxygen supply or inadequate circulation; pinpoint red foci suggest septicemia, toxemia, thrombocytopenia or vascular permeability disturbance. Likewise, dermal abrasions over bony structures (ocular arch, ileal wings, extremities) suggest antemortem pain or neurologic disturbances, with struggling before death. Careful examination of the jugular grooves and the rest of the neck, as well as the skin over the gluteal musculature, may reveal injection sites. The injection sites should be saved for eventual toxicologic analyses if malicious intent or faulty injections are suspected.

The necropsy proceeds with a ventral midline incision made through the abdominal skin. The incision is extended caudally toward the right coxofemoral joint, which is opened by incising the joint capsule and the ligament of the head of the femur. The right rear limb is reflected. The animal is skinned over the abdomen and thorax, with the knife blade resting on the inside of the cutis to avoid dulling the blade against the skin. In male horses, a cut is made around the penis and sheath, reflecting both caudally over the ischial arch. The testes are removed from the scrotum, together with each epididymis and ductus deferens. In the female, the entire mammary gland is removed with the skin attached. Immediately, several sections are cut through the mammary gland parenchyma and teats. The right front leg is reflected by cutting into the periscapular subcutis and muscles. The midline incision is extended along the neck toward the head. The exposed subcutaneous and muscular tissues are examined for nutritional and hydration status. The exposed superficial lymph nodes and, in young horses, the umbilicus are examined.

The abdominal cavity is opened by a small incision through the peritoneum; the incision must be large enough to inspect the entire cavity. The incision is extended dorsolaterally and parallel to the last rib (costal arch). Puncturing the abdominal viscera is avoided by placing the back of the hand over viscera and slicing the peritoneum between fingers via the palmar side of the hand. The incision is extended through the abdominal midline and parallel to the transverse processes of the lumbar vertebrae.

The amount and character of the peritoneal fluid are assessed. Clear, straw-colored peritoneal fluid (100-200 ml) is to be expected. If excessive fluid or exudate is discovered in the abdomen, a specimen should be obtained aseptically for culture and sediment examination of cells or bacteria. Fluid should be described in terms of viscosity, turbidity, color and approximate volume. The abdominal viscera, in particular the intestinal tract, are checked for relative normal positions. Portions of the large intestines (colon, cecum) are partially removed from the abdominal cavity to investigate other abdominal viscera, in particular those located in the left side of the abdomen. The

sternal, diaphragmatic and pelvic flexures are examined at this point.

The diaphragm is punctured; an in-rush of air indicates normal negative thoracic pressure. With rib cutters or pruning shears, the entire right thoracic wall is opened in one piece. This is done by cutting each rib close to the attachment to the thoracic vertebrae and through the costochondral junctions. A small intercostal window for the lifting hand helps when grasping the rib wall, which is to be pulled from the body. The exposed thoracic cavity now is examined for the amount and nature of pleural fluid. Approximately 100 ml of straw-colored pleural fluid may be expected. The anatomic relations of the organs of the thoracic cavity are examined. Samples for culture and smears are obtained if necessary, as well as *in-situ* photographs of both the thoracic and abdominal cavities for documentation purposes.

Evisceration and Examination of Abdominal and Pelvic Organs

The right adrenal gland is located medial and parallel to the right kidney. It is removed gently with scissors, avoiding excessive finger pressure on the medulla. Two general methods are used to check the cranial mesenteric arterial root for patency and smoothness of its intima. In one procedure, the branches of the ileocecocolic artery are lifted with one hand and cut transversely with a knife. Immediately, the dorsal portion of the tributary is opened with scissors by cutting toward the aorta. The distal end of the cecocolic artery is examined at a later time. Alternatively, the radicle is lifted and stretched with one hand. After dissection of perivascular tissue, the vascular branch is opened with scissors by cutting in dorsal and ventral directions (Fig 59). To obtain a clear view of the arterial intima, one must avoid cutting into the caudal vena cava or portal veins. Employing the second procedure, the abdominal aorta is opened and followed caudally toward the cranial mesenteric artery, which is opened from its origin by directing the scissors ventrally (Fig 60).

After examining the cranial mesenteric root, the entire gastrointestinal tract is removed from the abdominal cavity by dissecting through its mesenteric attachment

Figure 59. Opening the cecocolic artery to expose the cranial mesenteric artery. Lift the branches with one hand, remove perivascular soft tissue and open the vessels with scissors, directing them dorsally toward the aorta. P = pancreas, L = liver, J = jejunum.

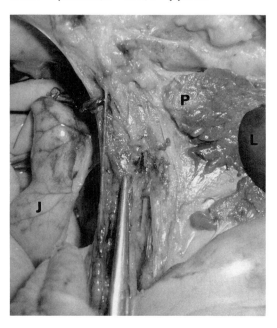

adjacent to the serosa. The small colon is ligated or cut near the pelvic inlet, and the distal esophagus is cut at the cardiac zone adjacent to the diaphragmatic hiatus. The nephrosplenic ligament is severed, and the spleen is removed, attached to and together with the stomach. The liver is removed by cutting it from the diaphragmatic crura. The left adrenal gland and both kidneys are removed with the ureters attached. The ureters are cut close to the entry site into the urinary bladder. The mesenteric root and lymph nodes are severed from their dorsal attachment.

In cases where it is unnecessary to perform a detailed examination of the organs of the pelvic cavity, the urinary bladder is opened *in situ* and the mucosal surfaces are examined. The approximate volume of urine in the bladder is recorded, along with color and turbidity. The uterus and ovaries are removed by pulling the female tract cranially and cutting caudally to the cervix. Should it become necessary to examine the organs of the pelvic cavity more carefully (*eg*, with a rectal tear), the bones of the pelvic cavity are cut with a handsaw. Two saw cuts are made parallel to the symphysis of the pubic bones and continued through each obturator foramen and the ischial ramus. The segment of pelvis is removed from the cadaver, and the urogenital tract and rectum are removed *in toto* (including anal orifice and female external genitalia) by severing them from the soft tissue dorsally and ventrally.

Individual organs of the abdominal cavity (and other cavities) are examined by recording their shape, dimensions, color, edges, consistency, nature of their cut surfaces and, where appropriate, degree of symmetry, weight and precise measurements (length, width, height).

One should judge which organ should be given immediate attention, according to the case history and disease, to avoid accelerated tissue decomposition. For example, if the case history and internal gross examination suggest gastrointestinal disease, one

Figure 60. Opening the cranial mesenteric artery, starting from the abdominal aorta. The scissors are placed in the origin of the cranial mesenteric artery. C = celiac artery.

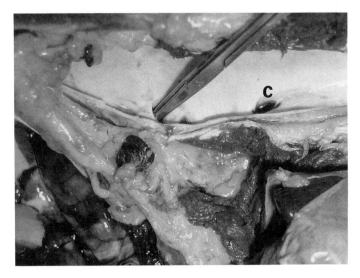

should immediately proceed with a complete, thorough investigation of this system. If this is not the case, dissection of the gastrointestinal tract should be performed after other, more decomposition-susceptible organs are examined, preferably at the end of the necropsy.

If circumstances require immediate examination of the gastrointestinal tract, the length of this organ system requires cutting it into 4 segments: small and transverse colon; large colon and cecum; small intestinal loops; and stomach with spleen attached. The spleen is detached from the stomach, and the stomach is opened along the greater curvature. The nature of the gastric contents and condition of the mucosa are recorded. One may rinse the gastric mucosa gently with water or fixative, but excessive water pressure should be avoided so as not to disturb the mucosal integrity. A similar practice is recommended for examination of intestinal mucosa. The small intestinal tract is opened opposite to its mesenteric attachment, and the nature of the intestinal contents is recorded. The pancreas is removed from the base of the cecum, and its approximate dimensions, color, consistency and degree of lobulation are noted.

Before the large colon and cecum are opened, one should examine the colonic lymph nodes, veins and arteries, if necessary. The cecum, ventral and dorsal colon segments and, last, the transverse and descending small colon are opened. The mesenteric lymph nodes are examined within the root of the mesentery. Multiple slices, 1-2 cm apart, are made through the liver and spleen. The cut surfaces are examined for evidence of structural abnormalities. The amount of blood exuding from the cut surfaces should be judged and recorded. The splenic lymph nodes are sliced and examined.

The kidneys are weighed and measured before being sectioned. Each kidney is cut sagittally with a single knife stroke from the outer cortex toward its pelvis. Delineation and color of the cortex and medulla should be recorded. The shape of the renal pelvis, the extent to which it is dilated, and the appearance of its contents and mucosa are described. It is of the utmost importance to strip the renal capsule to assess adhesions as well as the appearance of the

outer cortex. Often, important minute changes are best revealed on the renal cortical surface. Both adrenal glands are sliced sagittally, and care is taken to avoid crushing the glands with excessive finger pressure. The width and appearance of the cortex and medulla are recorded.

The dimensions, consistency and degree of bilateral symmetry of the ovaries and testes should be described. Both ovaries are sliced and the structure noted on cut section is recorded. The uterus and uterine horns are opened, and the endometrial surface described. If present, any fetus and fetal membranes are removed from the uterus and examined.

For gross examination of the testes, the spermatic cord and epididymis should be dissected from the gonad after these structures have been examined for gross lesions. Then the testes are weighed and measured. A midsagittal incision is made into the testes so that the mediastinum testis is exposed. The cut surface of a mature testis should bulge considerably above the surface. After the midsagittal cut, each half should be cut transversely into slices 0.5-1 cm wide, so that small lesions in the testis, including early tumor formation, are not overlooked. The appearance of the male accessory organs, penis and prepuce should be noted as well.

Removal and Examination of the Thoracic, Cervical and Oral Cavity Organs

The entire pluck is removed *en bloc*, starting by loosening the tongue from the oral cavity. Using a sharp knife, the tongue is removed caudoventrally by cutting vigorously through the periglossal tissue parallel to the medial aspect of the mandibular ramus. Visibility of the mandibular space is improved if the neck is extended forcibly. The glossal frenulum is severed. The stylohyoid apparatus is disarticulated by localizing the greater cornua at the base of the tongue via finger palpation. The knife is inserted into the joint, and the cartilaginous portion is disarticulated by jiggling the knife over the joint. The larynx, trachea and esophagus are freed to the thoracic inlet. The cut is continued dorsal to the aorta, toward the diaphragm. The pericardial sac is dissected from its sternal attachment, and

127

the entire pluck is lifted out of the thoracic cavity.

The parietal pleura between and over the ribs is examined for moisture and transparency. If a thymus can be identified, its dimension and lobulation are recorded. The volume of any fluid in the pleural space is estimated. If necessary, samples of pleural fluid are collected for culture, and smears made on slides for cytologic examination.

Several cuts are made transversely through the tip of the tongue. The esophagus is opened along its entire length and removed from the trachea. Both thyroid glands are identified and examined, and a midsagittal cut is made through the thyroid glands to permit assessment of their degree of activity and to look for small tumors. Because the parathyroid glands of horses are dispersed, they are difficult to distinguish from small cervical lymph nodes. A set of cranial parathyroid glands is located cranial and medial to the thyroid glands. A set of caudal parathyroid glands usually is associated with the bicarotid trunk ventral to the trachea, cranial to the thoracic inlet, and close to the first rib. Sampling of the various pea-sized, tannish, round structures along the cervical trachea is recommended if it appears that microscopic examination of parathyroid tissue will be important. The tonsils, pharynx, larynx, epiglottis and dimensions of the retropharyngeal lymph nodes (draining the head) should be routinely described.

The pericardial sac is opened through a small incision to assess volume and nature of pericardial fluid. A sample of the fluid is obtained for culture, if necessary. The heart is removed from its vascular suspensions. This facilitates detailed examination of the interior of the heart after residual blood is rinsed off. The trachea is opened through its entire length, and the incision is extended into the bronchial tree. The tracheobronchial lymph nodes are assessed. The lungs should be palpated, sectioned and palpated.[3] Palpation for changes in texture differentiates normal from diseased tissue. The color, degree of collapse and presence of fluid exuding from cut surfaces are recorded. Multiple transverse incisions are made through the lung parenchyma to search for small internal lesions. The branches of the pulmonary arteries can be opened with scissors on the ventral side of the lungs if it is necessary to search for thromboemboli.

There are several methods of thorough dissection of the heart. Care should be taken not to destroy major cardiac structures, regardless of which method is chosen. The left and right sides of the heart should be identified before the chambers are opened. In horses, the pointed cardiac apex clearly identifies the left ventricle. The appearance of the epicardium and coronary grooves is recorded. The pulmonary arterial outflow tract is identified and incised. This incision is extended caudally into the right ventricle. The knife or scissors are turned at a 180-degree angle, and the incision is continued along the interventricular septum toward the right atrium. The left ventricle is opened by a continuous knife cut starting laterally and slightly above the apex. The cut is directed toward the left atrium, with the tip of the knife passing underneath the septal mitral valve leaflet toward the aortic ostium. The mitral valve leaflet is severed, and the ascending aorta is opened. The interior of the heart is rinsed with water, and the appearance of all internal structures (endocardium, valves, chordae tendineae, papillary muscles) is recorded. The circumference of each valve ring can be measured, as can the ventricular wall thickness at the midpoint of its longitudinal axis (distance from anulus fibrosus to apex). The degree of myocardial contraction and its integrity can be determined by slicing tangentially into the myocardial muscle mass.

Examination of the Locomotor System and Bone Marrow

Even if a detailed examination of joints, tendons or muscles is not necessary, one should routinely open 5 joints. The scapulohumeral, coxofemoral, femorotibial, tibiotarsal and atlantooccipital joints usually are selected as references for routine examination. Knowledge of joint anatomy guarantees a direct, safe approach to any joint.[6]

The skin of the entire limb should be reflected before opening a joint. This guarantees better visibility and sterility should it be necessary to culture joint fluid. All major limb joints are opened from the medial side and, in the case of the atlanto-occipital joint, from the ventral side. A medial patellectomy is performed before exposure of the stifle joint. Normally, a slight amount of viscous, straw-colored joint fluid oozes from the opened joint. Healthy articular cartilage has a smooth, light bluish-white surface. Care should be taken to differentiate pathologic alterations of the joint surface from normal synovial fossae between trochlear and condylar structures. The synovial fossae vary in size and are particularly prominent in the olecranon of the ulna and in the atlas.[7]

In cases of laminitis, the hooves can be sawed proximal to the coronary band, and the os pedis can be exposed by splitting the hooves into halves with a handsaw. Cut surfaces are cleaned with a hand brush or towel to determine the structural relationships between the os pedis and hoof wall and between the horny and sensitive laminae.

Additional joints are examined when the clinical history identifies their involvement in lameness. Similarly, tendons and muscles are examined when deemed necessary. A general statement should be made regarding the color and consistency of skeletal muscles. The cortical strength of the bones is judged from their resistance to the rib cutter or by breaking a rib against its convex surface in young animals. The bone marrow is exposed by scoring the cortices sagittally with a saw, after which the marrow can be easily "cracked out" with rongeurs. The bone marrow is best fixed in small, perforated plastic cassettes.

Examination of the Head and Brain

Decapitation is performed at the atlantooccipital joint. Then the guttural pouches just dorsal to the occipital condyles are inspected. The severed head is placed tightly into a vise or against a rigid object, such as a wall or raised table corner. The skin, soft tissues and temporal muscles are removed from the skull cap. A handsaw is used to open the dorsal calvaria for removal of the brain. A standard technique for making saw cuts includes a transverse cut through the frontal bones just caudal to the zygomatic arches (supraorbital processes) and 2 laterally angled then sagittal lines on the right and left sides of the calvaria connecting the frontal bone transverse marking with the inner (medial) angle of both occipital bone condyles (Fig 61). The skull cap is loosened with a chisel and pried off. Care must be taken to separate the skull cap from the meninges. The surface of the meninges is examined, and a sterile swab is placed on the meningeal surface to collect a sample for culture.

The head is tilted and the brain is removed from the cerebral cavity by severing the vascular, meningeal and cranial nerve attachments. More rewarding places for swabbing are the basal surface of the meninges and the area of the brainstem. The ventral surface of the brain is examined. After the brain has been removed, the pituitary is lifted with forceps and severed from the basal fossa (sella turcica). The optic chiasm is examined for symmetry. The brain is

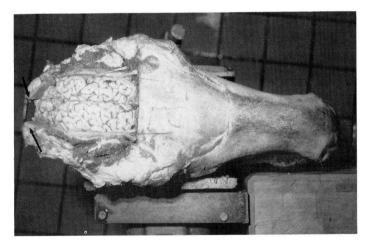

Figure 61. Saw marks to open the dorsal calvaria. Arrows denote the medial angle of the occipital condyles. The entire head is fixed tightly, preferably in a vise. Skin and muscle have been trimmed from the skull cap.

Figure 62. Processing the brain. Three transverse cuts can be made through the removed brain, as indicated, before it is fixed *en bloc* in a large volume of 10% buffered, neutral formalin.

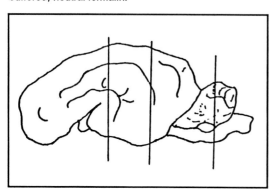

Figure 65. Brain halves after removal of the dura mater. Both sections are ready for gross examination and fixation.

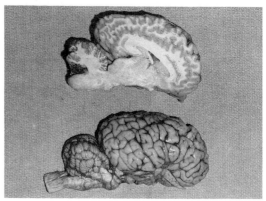

Figure 63. Saw marks for midline sectioning of the calvaria for removal of the brain. The mandible has been removed from the head (Figure 69), which then is placed flat on a firm surface. Trimming of skin is not necessary, and handsaw cuts are made where indicated with white tape. Molar and incisor teeth should be avoided.

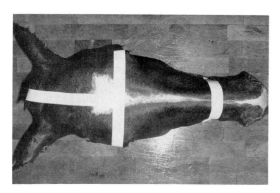

Figure 64. *In-situ* illustration of a midline saw cut through the calvaria and brain. Both cerebral hemispheres and cerebellar halves are exposed. The ethmoid plate (E) has been halved, and a frontal sinus is exposed (F).

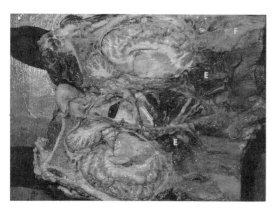

cut in transverse sections (Fig 62) and fixed *in toto,* unless fresh tissue is needed for microbiologic, virologic or toxicologic analyses. A brain fixed for 1 week is best suited for detailed morphologic examination of its interior structures.

Alternative methods for brain removal are: making a longitudinal handsaw cut through the median plane of the head, with subsequent removal of the 2 halves of brain from the cranial cavity by cutting through the vascular, meningeal and cranial nerve attachments (Figs 63-65); and making a transverse craniotomy through the middle of the head caudal to the last visible molar tooth toward the palatine bone and oral cavity, thus splitting the head into rostral and caudal parts (Figs 66-68).[8] Both of these alternatives are easier to perform after the mandible has been removed from the head. Care must be taken to avoid cutting the teeth when making saw cuts.

The mandible can be removed from the maxilla and the rest of the head by cutting, with a knife, through the soft tissues of the cheeks and across the pterygomandibular folds toward the temporomandibular joints (Fig 69). The mandibular coronoid process, which is loosely embedded in the masseter muscles, is exposed. When disarticulating the mandible, it should be kept static while the head is pulled away in an upward (dorsal) direction. This technique allows inspection of the entire oral cavity. The dorsal part of the head now can be sawed longitudinally, and the nasal cavities, sinuses, ethmoids and guttural pouches investigated. The cerebral hemispheres, cerebellum and brainstem also can be removed by this method. The ocular globe is removed by grasping the skin around the eye with forceps, using minimal traction, and cutting deeply around the orbit, close to the bone, using scissors. The eye is removed from its orbit by transecting the optic nerve and is cleansed of its surrounding soft tissue for fixation *in toto*.

Examination of the Spinal Cord and Peripheral Nerves

One of the more challenging tasks at necropsy is removal of the spinal cord. Institutional laboratories usually have an electric bandsaw, which facilitates access to the spinal cord without damaging it. The usual approach is through a dorsal laminectomy

Figure 66. Transverse craniotomy. White tape delineates the saw mark.

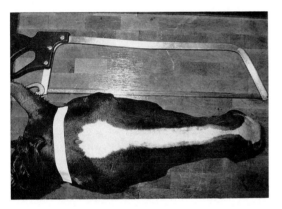

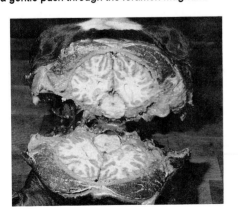

Figure 67. Completion of transverse craniotomy. With the cranium open, both rostral and caudal portions of the cerebrum are exposed and easily removed. The tentorium between the cerebrum and cerebellum then is cut at its osseous attachments. The cerebellum and brainstem then are slid out of the cranial vault, assisted by a gentle push through the foramen magnum.

Figure 68. The brain samples are relatively untraumatized. C = caudal cerebrum, R = rostral cerebrum, Cl = cerebellum, P = pituitary.

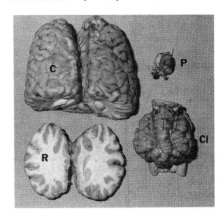

Figure 69. Removal of the mandible. Knife cuts are made (as indicated by white tape) for disarticulation of the mandible. The mandible is freed by pulling on the head.

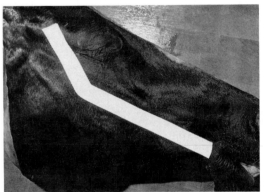

after removal of limbs, ribs and surrounding muscle bulk from the vertebral column.

The spinal cord can also be safely removed under field conditions in various ways. One procedure is to split the vertebral column sagittally just lateral to the spinal cord, using a meat cleaver.[2] The technique has the disadvantage that the intense manipulation of the bony structures may so damage the spinal cord as to prevent adequate histologic examination. An alternative and preferable method is to divide the vertebral column into 3-4 major sections (cervical, thoracic, lumbar) with a handsaw. Depending on the location of the lesion (see Neurologic Examination), one or all of these sections are cut transversely with a handsaw through the arches and bodies of adja-

131

cent vertebrae, leaving the intervertebral articulations intact (Figs 70, 71). The vertebral canal is identified and the dura lifted from one end with a pair of forceps. The spinal cord segments are then removed by cutting with scissors through the vertebral nerves in the epidural fat (Fig 72). This method can be repeated on as many vertebrae as necessary. Each section of spinal cord then is labelled separately, and the dura is opened dorsally and longitudinally to facilitate rapid penetration of the fixative. The spinal cord is cut transversely into sections (Fig 73).

A third method is to saw the defleshed vertebral column into sections 6-12 inches long, bag the segments in formalin, and mail them expeditiously to a laboratory equipped with a bandsaw for removal of the spinal cord for histologic examination.

In the case of "wobblers," the cervical vertebrae can be disarticulated. Cervical radiographs made before or after death can assist greatly in identifying the likely site(s) of spinal cord compression associated with cervical vertebral malformations, fractures and vertebral osteomyelitis lesions. Disarticulation can be performed after the vertebrae are sectioned (Figs 70-72) or can be performed with each vertebra intact. With the latter technique, each spinal cord segment is removed during disarticulation. A scalpel and sharp surgical blades are used in the procedure. The dorsal articular capsules are cut first and the articular surfaces examined for symmetry and shape (Fig 74). The exposed dorsal intervertebral space

Figure 70. Preparation of the cervical vertebral column for removal of the spinal cord. After trimming the soft tissue from the vertebral section, the handsaw is used to make cuts through the center of adjacent vertebrae.

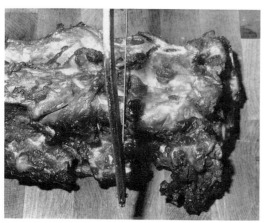

Figure 71. Dorsal view of sawed slices through adjacent vertebrae.

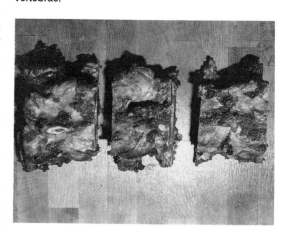

Figure 72. Removal of spinal cord segments from the vertebral canal. Forceps are used to grasp the dura mater, and scissors are used to cut through the spinal nerves within the epidural space.

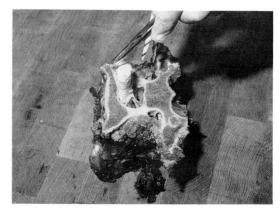

Figure 73. Preparation of the spinal cord for gross examination and fixation. The dura mater is opened with scissors dorsally, leaving the spinal nerve roots (N) attached to the dura.

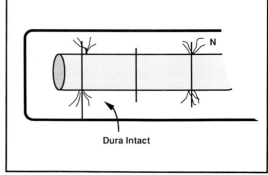

Dura Intact

Figure 74. Disarticulation of cervical vertebrae. The dorsal articular surfaces are exposed by cutting the joint capsules with a scalpel.

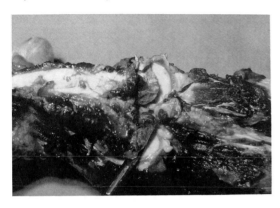

then is examined for the presence of epidural fat, which indicates that compression of the spinal cord is less likely to have occurred at that site.

The spinal cord is severed with a sharp cut, with the scalpel inserted through the intervertebral space before disarticulation of the tight fibrous intervertebral disk (Fig 17). The fibrous disk often is resistant to the scalpel blade and requires loosening by flexing and rotating the adjacent vertebra. The diameter of the vertebral canal is examined for narrowing at both ends of the disarticulated vertebra. The atlantoaxial joint is disarticulated by cutting the strong ligaments of the dens using a ventral approach. Each removed vertebra and spinal

Figure 75. Disarticulation of cervical vertebrae. The spinal cord is severed with a scalpel, the intervertebral disk (D) is loosened by flexion, and the fibrous disk cut with a scalpel or sharp knife.

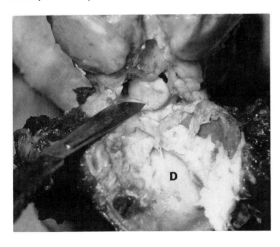

cord segment is labelled separately for precise localization of the disease process.

The peripheral nerves usually examined are the sciatic, just caudal to the femur, and those of the brachial plexus, lying on the medial surface of the scapula.

Ancillary Examinations and Tissue Collection

The nature and number of tissues collected and the type of ancillary special examination required depend upon how much the completed necropsy reveals regarding the cause of death and whether an etiologic diagnosis must be substantiated (Table 6). Special examinations include bacteriologic, virologic, serologic, parasitologic, toxicologic, radiographic, histologic and photographic assessments.

Bacteriologic and virologic samples must be collected and handled in an aseptic manner, using an alcohol flame and sterile containers or swabs. To help ensure asepsis, the surfaces of organs to be cultured should be seared with a red-hot spatula. The seared surface then is incised with a sterile scalpel blade and the specimen for culture is obtained with sterile scissors, swab or needle (fluid aspiration). Ideally, samples should be processed immediately by an appropriate laboratory.

If immediate delivery is not feasible, the sample should be shipped in Whirlpaks, Ziploc bags or heat-sealed plastic bags surrounded by abundant quantities of dry ice or freezer packs, using the fastest available transportation. Serum should be refrigerated or frozen when sent for serologic analyses. Whole blood should never be frozen. Samples for virus isolation attempts should be preserved at -70 C before processing. The samples should be sealed in airtight bags to decrease exposure to CO_2 and should be shipped cold, preferably on dry ice.

Direct fecal flotation and Baermann's methods are recommended as checks for gastrointestinal endoparasitic ova and lungworm larvae, respectively. For helminth identification, parasites from different organs should be placed into different, labelled containers that have been filled with physiologic saline (0.85% NaCl). The containers are placed in a refrigerator for several hours to allow the parasites to relax.

Table 6. Toxic compounds, necropsy findings and samples useful for diagnosis of some toxicoses of horses.[9]   (Courtesy of Veterinary Learning Systems and Dr. C.M. Brown)

Toxic Compounds	Necropsy Findings	Samples
Chemicals		
Arsenic and arsenicals	Intense hyperemia of gastrointestinal tract, fluid hemorrhagic feces	Liver, kidney
Chlorinated hydrocarbons	Nonspecific, random petechiae	Blood, liver, fat, brain, stomach contents
Fluoracetate	None	Stomach contents, liver, kidney
Nicotine	Nonspecific	Blood, liver, kidney, gut contents
Organophosphates and carbamates	Nonspecific, excessive fluid in lungs and gastrointestinal tract	Blood for cholinesterase, urine, brain, gut contents
Warfarin and other anticoagulants	Massive hemorrhage into a space or viscus	Liver, kidney, whole blood
Strychnine	Rapid onset of rigor mortis	Stomach contents, liver, kidney
Animal Toxins		
Cantharidin (blister beetle)	Severe gastroenteritis with sloughing of mucosa, fluid gut contents, pale kidney, inflamed renal pelvis, bladder inflammation, myocardial degeneration	Foodstuffs (alfalfa hay), gut contents, urine
Snakebite and insect bite	Nonspecific; possible local swelling or evidence of acute anaphylaxis	None
Plant Toxins		
Black nightshade (*Solanum nigrum*)	Nonspecific	Plants, gut contents to examine for poisonous plant
Blue-green algae	Nonspecific	Water sample
Castor bean (*Ricinus communis*)	Nonspecific; fluid gastrointestinal contents	Plants, gut contents to examine for poisonous plant
Chokecherry and other cyanogenic plants (*Prunus* spp)	Bright red mucous membranes	Plants, gut contents to examine for poisonous plant
Oleander (*Nerium oleander*)	Nonspecific	Plants, gut contents to examine for poisonous plant
Red maple leaves (*Acer rubrum*)	Icterus, splenomegaly, swollen black kidneys, brown urine, tubular nephrosis with hemoglobin casts	Plants
Poison hemlock (*Conium maculatum*)	Nonspecific	Plants, gut contents to examine for poisonous plant
Water hemlock, cowbane (*Cicuta* spp)	Nonspecific	Plants, gut contents to examine for poisonous plant
Yew	None; food often in mouth	Plants, gut contents to examine for poisonous plant
Pigweed (*Amaranthus retroflexus*) and other plants containing nitrate	Dark brownish blood and mucous membranes	Plants, gut contents to examine for poisonous plants

Trematodes and cestodes then should be fixed in AFA solution (85 ml of 85% ethanol, 10 ml commercial formalin, 5 ml glacial acetic acid). Specimens in this solution may be mailed to a parasitologist. Nematodes should be dipped in hot 70% ethanol and then transferred into glycerine-alcohol (90 ml of 10% ethanol, 10 ml glycerine). They may be stored in this solution indefinitely. If blood parasites are suspected, smears of blood and spleen should be prepared.

Tissue collection for toxicologic analyses should be generous and encompass a variety of organs and body fluids. It is recommended highly that duplicate samples be collected; one set is kept in the event that repeat tests become necessary or other laboratories become involved. All material must be placed in clean, sealed glass containers. These must be identified properly, labelled and shipped frozen or on ice packs. Samples should be stored in a freezer that can be locked or otherwise properly secured. Records should accurately document the animal, case number, nature of specimens, collector and name of laboratory involved.

The following samples and quantities are recommended for submission to a toxicology laboratory:[9]

Urine: all available or 50 ml	Liver: 0.5-1.0 kg
Serum: (clot removed): 10 ml	Kidney: 0.5-1.0 kg
Heart blood: 25-50 ml	Spleen: 0.5-1.0 kg
Body fat: 100 g	Heart: 0.5-1.0 kg
Stomach contents: 500 g	Intact eye with
Intestinal contents: 500 g	aqueous humor
Brain: 1/2 in formalin and 1/2 frozen	Lung: 0.5-1.0 kg

Nonanimal samples that should be considered include:[9]

Feed: 5 lb

Water: 1 qt

Bedding: 5 lb

The toxicology laboratory should be contacted concerning costs and types of analyses to be performed. Toxicologic analyses are expensive and the fee should be discussed with the client for approval before authorization of the tests.

For histopathologic examination, care should be taken to choose the right tissues, appropriate sample size (blocks of 1 x 1 x 0.5 cm), appropriate fixative *eg,* 10% buffered formalin or Bouin's fixative (Table 7), and a spacious container with a wide mouth. There should be at least 10 times as much fixative as tissue. Tissues should be allowed to fix for 24-48 hours, and the formalin should be changed once during that time. As a rule, altered organs should be examined histopathologically if the gross lesion requires microscopic identification. In the absence of gross lesions, any organ that may be associated with the clinical signs noted before death also should be examined histopathologically. Fixed tissues should be shipped in sealed plastic bags with cotton soaked in formalin. Tissues being submitted for histopathologic examination must not be frozen.

Postmortem radiographs are helpful in localizing bullets from gunshot wounds and lesions in the skeletal system, especially those of the distal limbs and the vertebral column (*eg*, wobblers). Radiographs and projectiles should be retained in a safe place.

Photographic documentation of pathologic changes is helpful in insurance or medico-legal necropsy cases. A simple Polaroid camera delivers immediate, good-quality color pictures of pathologic changes. The pictures can be retaken immediately if the first set is not satisfactory. They can be stored along with the necropsy record for future reference.

Recording the Findings

When the necropsy has been completed, all observations should be written down or tape-recorded immediately, preferably before disposal of the carcass and organs. All normal organs should be identified precisely. All gross findings should be documented in a necropsy record as objectively as possible because the record becomes a legal document. Gross necropsy findings should be descriptive in nature, thus allowing the reviewer to form a mental image of what the prosector saw. The description should be accurate, complete, organized, systematic and logical. It should incorporate all abnormal findings and include the nature of the cut surfaces, dimensions, shape, color and consistency of the tissues.

Terms understandable to the layman should be used, and medical terms added in parentheses. Descriptions should be made in the present tense. Statements concerning the meaning of the findings should be

Table 7. Formulae of commonly used fixatives.

10% Neutral Buffered Formalin:

37-40% formaldehyde solution*	100 ml
Distilled water	900 ml
Sodium phosphate, monobasic (NaH$_2$PO$_4$)	4 g
Sodium phosphate, dibasic anhydrous (Na$_2$HPO$_4$)	6.5 g

This is the fixative of choice for routine histologic studies

*37% formaldehyde = 100% formalin

Bouin's Fixative:

Picric acid, saturated aqueous solution	750 ml
37-40% formaldehyde solution*	250 ml
Glacial acetic acid	25 ml

* 37% formaldehyde = 100% formalin

Bouin's fixative hardens tissue and is preferred for soft tissues, such as reproductive tract tissues and bone marrow. The acetic acid removes some of the calcium, such as that in bone spicules within the bone marrow cavity. The tissues are placed in Bouin's solution for 24-48 hours, then transferred to 10% formalin for storage.

Fixed tissues can be shipped most easily by placing the fixed material in small cloth bags (colorless), which are labelled properly. Only enough fixative is needed in the bags to keep the tissue moist. The bags can be placed in plastic bags, tied or sealed, and inserted in waxed cardboard freezer boxes. The boxes should be placed in a larger box so they are protected against compression during shipment. Samples intended for histologic examination should never be submitted frozen or on ice, as freezing disrupts the cellular architecture by ice crystal formation.

---

avoided and reserved for the comment section of the report. All pathologic anatomic findings associated with individual organs should be summarized in a gross diagnosis or diagnoses. The diagnosis for each organ should include duration, type or quality, severity, distribution and a possible etiology. The primary diagnoses should be listed in order of their importance, with all subordinate diagnoses arranged in descending order of their importance.

The comment section contains a narrative and is the interpretation of all necropsy findings. It is the interpretive conclusion and discussion of both the case and the significance of the gross lesions. Its objective is to identify the probable cause of death and nature of the disease. It should correlate morphologic with clinical findings and explain any incongruities. All incidental findings and/or background pathologic lesions should be listed and their potential contribution to the disease process discussed.[10] Likewise, postmortem changes should be listed.

Insurance and Medico-Legal Necropsy

These types of necropsy deserve special attention, require complete dissection and necessitate meticulous recordkeeping.[1] To be protected from the very outset, 4 major considerations should be observed: the necropsy should be performed within 6-8 hours after death or euthanasia of a horse (the earlier, the better); the prosector should be qualified and, preferably, should be a veterinary pathologist; the events of the necropsy should be fully documented with written observations that include all normal findings; and the written report should be authenticated with the valid signature of the prosector as well as the date the necropsy was performed, the time it was started, the time it was concluded, and the names of witnesses to the necropsy, if any.

As a neutral investigator, the prosector should complete a meticulous, full-length report of what was seen, including normal findings and weights and measurements of organs. Normal findings help in recalling the case should it surface years later in litigation. Care should be taken to correctly identify organ anatomy and the right and left dual organs. Whole-body photographs and photographs of the animal's identifying marks (lip or neck tattoo, earmarks, natural markings) should be obtained before starting the necropsy. Photographic documentation of major pathologic lesions should be procured in addition to written descriptions. Photographs of the immediate area where the animal was found dead also may be necessary.

A systematic dissection is imperative and all organ systems should be examined with careful attention to detail. A thorough histologic tissue examination should be performed in the absence of gross lesions.[11] Selected tissue samples and body fluids should be frozen at necropsy for potential toxicologic or microbiologic analyses. Samples should be properly labelled.

The signed, final necropsy report should list all aspects of the final diagnosis or diagnoses and contain, as comment, a scientific interpretation of all findings, including a reasonable conclusion as to the cause of death or nature of disease. The report also should list the results of all ancillary testing (histopathologic, toxicologic, parasitologic, microbiologic, virologic), specimen photographs taken, and the nature of specimens retained. Specimens should be frozen and stored in a safe environment for up to a year.

Finally, insurance companies and other third parties (*eg,* attorneys) may be eager to obtain information and a copy of the final report from the prosector soon after completion of the necropsy. To avoid legal improprieties, information relative to the case should not be released without the owner's signed permission. The form granting this permission should be signed before the start of the necropsy, if possible.

If conducted correctly, the insurance or medico-legal necropsy can produce results edifying to both owner and interested third party, and ultimately contributes to professional pride. The report constitutes a valid legal document useful for depositions or expert witness testimonies in court.

References

1. Edwards WC and Johnson BJ: Equine insurance examination. *Equine Pract* 8:19-22, 1986.

2. Andrews JJ: Necropsy techniques. *Vet Clin No Am (Food Anim Pract)* 2:27-29, 1986.

3. Rooney JR: The equine necropsy. *Vet Scope* 8:2-11, 1963.

4. Rooney JR: *Autopsy of the Horse.* Krieger, Huntington, NY, 1976.

5. King JM *et al:* Necropsy of the horse. *MVP* 59:897-899, 1978; 60:29-32, 1979; 60:109-112, 1979.

6. Rooney JR *et al: Guide to the Dissection of the Horse.* Veterinary Textbooks, Ithaca, NY, 1977.

7. McIlwraith CW, in Stashak TS: *Adams' Lameness in Horses.* 4th ed. Lea & Febiger, Philadelphia, 1987. pp 339-485.

8. Anderson BC and Christensen KW: A simple method to remove the brain for necropsy. *Vet Med* 79:1404-1407, 1984.

9. Brown CM and Taylor FR: Sudden and unexpected death in adult horses. *Compend Cont Ed Pract Vet* 9:78-85, 1987.

10. Roth L and King JM: Nonlesions and lesions of no significance. *Compend Cont Ed Pract Vet* 4:451-456, 1982.

11. Tobin T: Sudden death in racing horses: the "Swale Syndrome." *J Equine Vet Sci* 7:184-185, 1987.

This page is intentionally left blank.

$\underset{\text{3}}{\text{3}}$ Principles of Therapy

R.J. Rose and J.D. Wright

FLUID AND ELECTROLYTE THERAPY

Many situations arise in practice in which fluid and electrolyte therapy is required immediately. In cases of trauma involving blood loss, shock associated with colic, or exercise-related exhaustion, appropriate fluid therapy can be life saving. This section provides an overview of fluid and electrolyte therapy. Specific indications in different diseases are covered in the individual chapters on the body systems.

Intravenous Catheterization

An appropriate vein must be catheterized very carefully, paying attention to sterile technique. Such complications as phlebitis and septicemia can arise from inadequate catheterization techniques. The most common vein used for administration of intravenous fluids is the jugular vein. Other veins that can be used for long-term fluid administration include the cephalic and lateral thoracic veins (Figs 1, 2).[1]

The hair over the vein should be clipped and/or shaved, after which the skin is given a 2-minute scrub with povidone-iodine. Our method of surgical preparation includes application of 70% alcohol, followed by dilute tincture of iodine. Local anesthetic (0.5-1.0 ml of mepivacaine or 2% lidocaine) then is injected intradermally and the skin disinfected again with alcohol and dilute tincture

Figure 1. Catheter in position in the left cephalic vein.

Figure 2. Catheter placed in the left lateral thoracic vein.

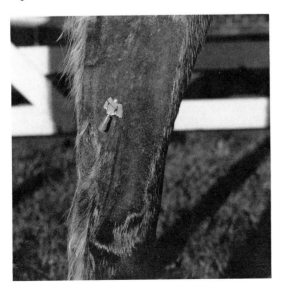

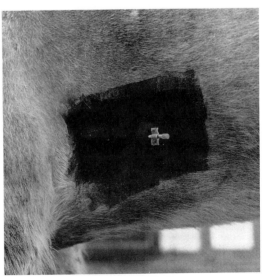

of iodine. The operator then uses sterile gloves to insert a 12- to 14-ga, 3- to 12-inch catheter. The longer catheter is used if long-term fluid therapy is planned, and the larger gauge is selected if large volumes are to be infused or rapid fluid infusion is desired. Extension tubing is connected to the catheter. Sterile gauze swabs, to which a povidone-iodine ointment has been applied, may be placed over the area and the region bandaged. However, leaving the site uncovered has proven to be efficient, effective and economical. The extension tubing is connected to an extensible plastic or rubber tubing. This extensible tubing allows the fluid containers to be set up at some distance from the horse, so the horse can move around the stall freely.

Fluid and Electrolyte Balance

Total body water, which constitutes about two-thirds of the body weight, usually is thought of as being in 2 main compartments: the intracellular fluid (ICF) and extracellular fluid (ECF).

Though these 2 compartments greatly differ in electrolyte composition, water moves freely between the compartments. The ECF has a high sodium concentration with very low concentrations of potassium, while the reverse is true for the ICF. Interpreting plasma or serum electrolyte values often is difficult; therefore, we will discuss briefly the function of the major electrolytes.

Sodium: The average 450- to 500-kg horse has a total body sodium content of about 28,000 mEq, half of which probably is not available due to its localization in such areas as bone. Virtually all of the exchangeable sodium (14,000 mEq) is in the ECF. Plasma or serum sodium values give no reliable guide to sodium deficits or excesses but probably are more reflective of water movement. In people, this relationship exists:[2]

$$\frac{serum\ Na}{(mEq/L\ H_2O)} = \frac{exchangeable\ Na + exchangeable\ K}{total\ body\ water}$$

The same relationship appears to exist in horses.[3] Thus, the serum sodium level is affected by both sodium and potassium status, as well as the total body water. This equation is important because the total body potassium deficit can be estimated if the serum

sodium level is known and the extent of dehydration can be estimated.

Potassium: Plasma or serum potassium values do not reflect the total body potassium status, as the ECF contains less than 2% of total body potassium. Changes in potassium concentration in the ECF have clinical relevance, as they affect neuromuscular conductivity. While hyperkalemia is rare in horses, hypokalemia is more common, particularly in horses with diarrhea. Total body deficits of potassium can be estimated using the equation above.[2] Following is an example of how this could be used and illustrates the potential for large potassium deficits without obvious clinicopathologic changes.

A 500-kg horse is 5% dehydrated (barely detectable clinically) due to anorexia. The plasma sodium level is 140 mEq/L and plasma potassium level is 3.8 mEq/L. Assume the same plasma sodium value before dehydration. In the calculations below, the symbol "I" refers to initial values and "D" to dehydrated values.

$$
\begin{aligned}
\text{Water deficit} &= \text{weight loss x 0.9} \\
&= (500\ \text{kg x 5\%}) \text{ x 0.9} \\
&= 25\ \text{kg x 0.9} \\
&= 22.5\ \text{L}
\end{aligned}
$$

Total body water $(TBW)_I$ = 300 L (60% of body weight)
TBW_D (after dehydration) = 278 L

Using the above equation, plasma sodium concentration x $(TBW)_I$ = exchangeable Na (Na_e) + exchangeable K (K_e). Thus

$$
\begin{aligned}
140\ \text{x}\ 300 &= Na_e + K_e\ (I) = 42,000\ \text{mEq} \\
140\ \text{x}\ 278 &= Na_e + K_e\ (D) = 38,900\ \text{mEq} \\
\text{total deficit of Na + K} &= 3100\ \text{mEq}
\end{aligned}
$$

How can this deficit be apportioned between Na and K? As a general rule, in diarrhea, about 60% of Na + K loss is sodium. In exercise-induced dehydration, about 70% of the loss is sodium, whereas in food and/or water deprivation, about 30% of the loss is sodium. Thus, in this example, the 3100 mEq Na + K deficit can be apportioned as follows:

$$
\begin{aligned}
\text{Na deficit} &= 1000\ \text{mEq} \\
\text{K deficit} &= 2100\ \text{mEq}
\end{aligned}
$$

Because virtually all the exchangeable sodium is in the ECF and all the exchangeable potassium is in the ICF, the following calculations can be made concerning compartmental fluid distributions:

$$Na\ content_D = 14,000\ mEq$$
$$(140 \times 100\ L\ ECF) - 1000\ mEq$$
$$= 13,000\ mEq$$

$$ECF_I = 100\ L\quad ICF_I = 200\ L$$
$$ECF_D = \frac{Na\ content_D}{Na\ mEq/L_D}$$
$$= \frac{13,000}{140} = 93\ L$$
$$ICF_D = TBW_D - ECF_D$$
$$= 278\ L - 93\ L = 185\ L$$

Overall Deficits

TBW deficit = 22.5 L

ECF deficit = 7 L

ICF deficit = 15 L

Na deficit = 1000 mEq

K deficit = 2100 mEq

Thus, a substantial total body potassium deficit can exist in the face of normal serum potassium values. This and the fact that the equine kidney normally excretes a large amount of potassium should alert the clinician that large total body potassium deficits may occur. Such potassium deficits may be a problem when the horse is not eating or does not have access to green feed. In these circumstances, oral administration of 40-50 g potassium chloride for several days can restore potassium balance.

Use of the above equation can give very valuable insights into fluid and electrolyte disturbances.[2] For accurate calculations, the horse must be accurately weighed. Response to therapy also can be assessed by monitoring the weight of the horse so that the amount of fluid retained is known.

Chloride and Bicarbonate: Chloride and bicarbonate are the principal anions of the ECF. Though chloride tends to play a passive role, extensive chloride losses may occur in such conditions as diarrhea and exercise-associated dehydration. In general, chloride and bicarbonate are inversely related: in metabolic acidosis, bicarbonate levels are decreased and chloride elevated, while the reverse is true in metabolic alkalosis.

Bicarbonate values usually are assessed from total CO_2 measurements in plasma. In most situations, the plasma bicarbonate level is about 95% of the total CO_2 level. In the unanesthetized horse, measurements of total CO_2 provide an accurate guide to changes in acid-base status. Because primary respiratory acid-base disturbances are very uncommon in the unanesthetized horse, an increase in the total CO_2 level indicates metabolic alkalosis, while a decrease signifies metabolic acidosis.

Oral vs Intravenous Fluids

Once it has been determined that fluid therapy is necessary, the route of administration must be decided. If rapid blood volume expansion is not needed and if the gastrointestinal tract is functioning normally, oral fluids should be considered. Isotonic glucose-glycine-electrolyte mixtures are very effective for oral administration. These mixtures were formulated for calf diarrhea but are useful for fluid and electrolyte therapy in horses, as the mixture is available in powder form and only has to be mixed with an appropriate volume of water to make an isotonic solution. The glucose and glycine in the mixture enhance uptake of fluid and electrolytes from the small intestine. Most horses will not drink these mixtures, but 8-10 L can be given at one time by stomach tube. Such fluid and electrolyte mixtures are absorbed rapidly in horses with experimentally induced fluid and electrolyte deficits.[4]

Type and Volume of Fluid

A wide range of fluids is available but 2 main fluid types should be considered. *Replacement fluids* are polyionic, with an electrolyte composition similar to that of plasma. Such fluids should be used in situations of acute fluid loss or shock. *Maintenance fluids* have a much lower sodium but higher potassium concentration than replacement fluids. If maintenance with intravenous fluids is required over several days, a high sodium concentration in the fluid is contraindicated. Use of a replacement fluid in these situations may not correct dehydration because the excessive sodium is excreted together with water.[5]

Normal (0.9%) saline should not be used for routine intravenous fluid administration unless no other fluid is available. Saline infusion may cause dilutional acidosis due to dilution of the body's base reserves.

Volume and type of fluid to be administered vary with the particular condition. Some guidelines are presented in Table 1.

Use of Bicarbonate: Sodium bicarbonate is frequently overused because of concern about rapid treatment of metabolic acidosis. The main indication for use of sodium bicarbonate is in conditions causing bicarbonate loss, such as diarrhea. In shock or ischemic colic, bicarbonate may not be indicated because metabolic acidosis is the result of reduced tissue perfusion, leading to increased lactate production. In these cases, expansion of the ECF is required to improve microcirculation. If bicarbonate is administered, it should be used sparingly. Remember that an equal number of milliequivalents of sodium also will be given (as sodium bicarbonate), which could be detrimental.

To calculate the amount of bicarbonate to give, the following equation generally is used:

$$\text{Bicarbonate required} = 0.3 \times \text{body wt(kg)} \times \text{base deficit}$$
$$\text{(mEq)} \qquad\qquad\qquad\qquad \text{(mEq/L)}$$

The base deficit is calculated by subtracting the plasma or serum bicarbonate level from 22 mEq/L (lower end of the normal range). In severe acidosis, the plasma bicarbonate concentration may fall to 10 mEq/L. Thus, the calculated bicarbonate requirement in a 500-kg horse would be:

$$0.3 \times 500 \times (22\text{-}10) = 1800 \text{ mEq}$$

It is usual practice to replace half the calculated deficit so that acidosis is not overcorrected. Thus, 900 mEq (1.5 L of a 5% solution) of sodium bicarbonate are given, and the laboratory evaluations repeated to assess the combined effects of volume expansion and bicarbonate replacement.

ANTIBACTERIAL THERAPY

Of all the drugs used in equine practice, antibacterials probably are the most widely abused group of drugs. Inappropriate antibacterial use has resulted in increased bacterial resistance and such problems as superinfection, which is the appearance of a second bacterial infection during the course of therapy for an unrelated infection. Organisms involved in superinfections usually are part of the normal flora and are resistant to the antibacterials used to treat the initial problem. Such organisms then multiply unchecked by either the antibacterial or by competition from other bacteria.

A much more careful approach to antibacterial use is required in practice. Rather than the "shotgun" approach to therapy, using a large number of different antibacterials, a particular antibacterial should be selected on the basis of the cause of infection. Thus, collection of bacteriologic samples for culture and sensitivity testing should be done early in the course of disease rather than as a last resort after days or weeks of ineffective antibacterial treatment. While such culture techniques may not always be possible or practical in the field, too frequently they are undertaken too late or not tried at all.

Approach to Therapy

The most important consideration in initiating antibacterial therapy is to determine if the horse has a bacterial infection. Antibacterial therapy often is initiated in a horse with nonspecific clinical signs and an elevated temperature. In our clinic, we have noted frequently that if such horses are left untreated, the fever abates and clinical signs resolve spontaneously. This is particularly true in horses during the first 4-5 days after surgery. Steps to consider before starting antibacterial therapy follow.

Establish a Diagnosis

Various diagnostic techniques should be considered to establish a bacteriologic cause of the disease. Such techniques as blood culture, transtracheal aspiration, thoracentesis, abscess aspiration and joint fluid collection may be useful, depending on the particular problem. Samples taken for bacteriologic evaluation often are inappropriate and may confuse the therapeutic plan. When collecting samples for bacteriologic examination, discharging purulent exudates *never* should be sampled. Such samples invariably grow a mixed bacterial flora and give no indication of the causative organism. Thus, with suspected osteomyelitis, the sequestrum of bone should be submitted for culture at the time of surgery rather than any of the discharge from the wound.

It also is important that the sample is not contaminated during collection. The most

Table 1. Likely fluid and electrolyte deficits, alterations in clinicopathologic values and fluid requirements associated with common disturbances of fluid and electrolyte balance (Rose, 1981).

Clinical Condition	Estimated Deficits			Likely Alterations in Hematologic and Plasma Electrolyte Values						Suggested Type and Amount of Fluid Required
	H_2O (L)	Na (mEq)	K (mEq)	PCV	TPP	Na	K	Cl	HCO_3	
Diarrhea – mild	20-30	1500	800	↑	N	N	↓	N	N	10-12 L of polyionic[b] fluid IV, followed by oral fluids containing 60 g KCl.
– severe	50-60	5000	2000	↑↑	↓	↓↓	↓	N	↓↓	20 L of polyionic fluid, 10 L half-strength saline with added KCl (15-20 mmol/L), 3-5 L 5% $NaHCO_3$ and 5-10 L of plasma or plasma volume expanders IV.
Food and water deprivation – 1 day	5-20[a]	200-1000[a]	300-800[a]	N	N	N	N	N	N	5-10 L of oral fluids containing 5-25 g NaCl and 10-30 g KCl BID.
– 3 days	15-50[a]	800-3000[a]	600-2000[a]	N	↑	↑	N	↑	↓	5-10 L of polyionic fluids, 5-10 L of 5% dextrose IV and remainder of deficit with 25-30 L of oral fluids containing 60-180 g KCl and 60-90 g NaCl.
Colic – impaction of LI for 3-5 days	5-20	200-1000	300-800	N	N	N	N	N	N	5-10 L of polyionic fluids IV plus 3-9 L of oral fluids containing 20-60 g KCl.
Shock – impairment of intestinal vascular supply	15-30	Fluid accumulation in transcellular compartment results in functional "loss" of fluid and electrolytes		↑↑	↑↑	N	N	N	↓↓	15-25 L of polyionic fluid, 5 L plasma or plasma volume expanders IV and 3-4 L 5% $NaCO_3$ IV if plasma HCO_3 <10 mmol/L.
Shock – torsion of intestine	20-50			↑↑	↑↑	N	N	N	↓↓	20-40 L polyionic fluids, 5 L plasma or plasma volume extenders and 2-4 L 5% $NaHCO_3$ IV if plasma HCO_3 <10 mmol/L.
Post-exercise dehydration – after 3-10 km (fast exercise)	2-10[a]	200-1000[a]	100-500[a]	↑	↑	↑	↑	N	↓	2-10 L of oral fluids containing 10-14 g KCl if diet is deficient in herbage.
– after 80-160 km (endurance exercise)	20-50	2000-5000[a]	1000-2500[a]	↑	↑	N↓	↓	↓↓	N	10-20 L of polyionic solution IV if severely dehydrated, otherwise 20-50 L oral fluids containing 130-300 g NaCl and 80-200 g KCl.

a — Higher figures represent losses during high environmental temperatures.
b — Polyionic fluids include Ringer's lactate, Harmann's solution, Normosol R, Multisol R and Dilusol R.

Oral fluids are those consumed voluntarily or administered via stomach tube.
LI — Large intestine.
N — Normal values.

↑ Increased values

↑↑ Greatly increased values

↓ Decreased values

↓↓ Greatly decreased values

143

common sources of contamination are from the hair of the horse or from the person taking the sample. Contamination can be avoided by careful attention to surgical preparation of the area to be sampled and appropriate sterile techniques, such as the operator's wearing sterile gloves, cap and mask. Remember that a bacteriologic swab frequently is not the best sample to submit. If possible, a sterile syringe containing the fluid or exudate is more useful. When the sample is collected, a Gram stain can help guide initial antibacterial selection.

Many sites, such as the respiratory and reproductive tracts, have a normal bacterial flora, so merely finding bacteria on culture does not necessarily indicate infection. Note should be made of the cytologic findings and the degree of bacterial growth.

Once an organism has been established as the cause of infection, antibacterial sensitivity testing usually is required. However, some equine pathogens have known sensitivities. Such organisms include *Streptococcus* spp, *Clostridium* spp, *Actinomyces* spp, *Fusobacterium* spp and *Eubacterium* spp, almost all of which are sensitive to benzylpenicillin.[6]

Bactericidal vs Bacteriostatic Drugs

In most situations, it is wise to select a bactericidal over a bacteriostatic drug. When there is compromised host phagocytic activity (septic arthritis, pleuritis) or possible immunologic impairment (foal diseases), bacteriostatic drugs may be ineffective. Commonly used bacteriostatic drugs include chloramphenicol, erythromycin, tetracyclines and sulfonamides. Bactericidal drugs include benzylpenicillin, semisynthetic penicillins (amoxicillin, ampicillin), isoxazolyl penicillins (cloxacillin, flucloxacillin) and aminoglycosides (streptomycin, neomycin, amikacin, kanamycin, gentamicin).

Broad-Spectrum vs Narrow-Spectrum Antibacterials

Though use of broad-spectrum antibacterials is widely advocated, this is an unwise and potentially dangerous practice. Broad-spectrum antibacterials, which include amoxicillin, ampicillin, erythromycin and tetracyclines, may kill off the normal bacterial flora and can result in superinfection.

Additionally, they encourage emergence of resistant bacterial strains. If the cause of the infection is not known, a narrow-spectrum antibacterial always should be chosen in preference to one with broad-spectrum antibacterial activity. In most situations, the best and least expensive first-choice antibacterial is penicillin.

Effective Antibacterial Levels

Treatment of bacterial infection requires effective drug levels. Because it is difficult to determine drug concentrations at the affected tissue site, efficacy is usually based on maintaining effective blood concentrations of the drug during the treatment period. It is generally accepted that the blood concentration that should be maintained is 2-4 times the minimum inhibitory concentration (MIC) of antibacterial for the particular bacteria. With most antibacterials, this requires treatment 2-4 times daily. The so-called "long-acting antibacterials" do not maintain adequate blood concentrations.

Efficacy Against Equine Pathogens

Once the bacteria have been identified, Kirby-Bauer disc sensitivity testing or determination of MICs is necessary for accurate antibacterial selection. However, some general principles apply in selection:

Amoxicillin and Ampicillin: Most Gram-negative equine pathogens are resistant to these antibiotics due to their production of beta-lactamase. Thus, the semisynthetic penicillins have an effective spectrum of activity similar to that of benzylpenicillin, but are less potent and much more expensive.

Chloramphenicol: Whether given intravenously, intramuscularly or orally, chloramphenicol has such a short half-life that it provides effective antibacterial levels only for less than one hour after administration. Therefore, it is not a very useful antibiotic for treating horses.

Streptomycin: Streptomycin is still widely used in combination with penicillin. However, most Gram-negative pathogens are resistant to it; therefore, unless sensitivity tests indicate otherwise, this drug should not be used in horses.

Oral Antibacterials: With the exception of trimethoprim-sulfadiazine, oral antibacterials generally should not be used in adult horses. Variable absorption and the likelihood of inducing diarrhea usually dictate against their use. However, combinations of trimethoprim and a sulfonamide are useful. In foals up to 2 months of age, amoxicillin trihydrate syrup is useful and convenient. Where penicillin is indicated or if sensitivity tests show that amoxicillin may be used, amoxicillin syrup is well tolerated and absorbed by foals.[7] Erythromycin and rifampin given orally can be used to achieve adequate serum concentrations in foals and even in adult horses. Oral metronidazole is effective for certain anaerobic bacteria.

Duration of Therapy

The traditional practice of giving a 5-day course of antibacterials has no therapeutic justification. The duration of therapy should be tailored to the specific problem being treated. As a general guide:

Postsurgical prophylaxis: 12-24 hours
Acute infection: 5-7 days
Septic arthritis: 10-21 days
Urinary tract infection: 14-28 days
Chronic pneumonia: 1-3 months
(*eg, Rhodococcus equi* in foals)

Antibacterial Prophylaxis

Prophylactic use of antibacterials is difficult to justify. Unless a specific problem has been identified, such as a particular neonatal foal infection on a stud farm, prophylactic antibacterial use cannot be condoned. Routine antibacterial prophylaxis, such as after surgery, is without justification. Each surgical case should be considered by taking into account site, operating time, degree of tissue trauma, and likelihood of contamination. For example, when no antibacterial prophylaxis was used in a series of prolonged castrations performed by veterinary students, there was a 60% postoperative infection rate, with *Streptococcus zooepidemicus* most commonly isolated. We then instituted procaine penicillin prophylaxis, giving a dose before and 12 hours after surgery. Additionally, greater care was taken in presurgical skin preparation and disinfection. These changes eliminated the wound infection problem.

One of the great controversies in antibacterial use is whether prophylaxis should be considered when a horse has viral respiratory disease. At this time, there have not been any clinical trials in horses to support or refute use of antibacterials in this situation. However, in principle, it is difficult to advocate prophylactic use of antibacterials in viral respiratory disease.

Antibacterial Dosages

The dosages of various commonly used antibacterials, together with some specific considerations in their use, are presented in Table 2.

ANTIINFLAMMATORY AND ANTIPYRETIC THERAPY

Drugs that suppress or reduce the inflammatory response are used frequently in equine practice. The compounds can be broadly classified into 3 groups: nonsteroidal antiinflammatory drugs (NSAIDs); corticosteroids; and a miscellaneous group that includes sodium hyaluronate, orgotein and polysulfated glycosaminoglycans. The last group of drugs will be discussed in the chapter on the Musculoskeletal System, as their major use is in treatment of joint disease.

Nonsteroidal Antiinflammatory Drugs

The major NSAIDs can be chemically classified into 2 major groups: enolic acids (phenylbutazone) and carboxylic acids (flunixin, meclofenamic acid, naproxen).[8] Aspirin and other salicylates also are regarded as NSAIDs.

All NSAIDs have analogous modes of action, accounting for their similar therapeutic and toxic effects. These drugs block some part of the cyclooxygenase pathway and thereby suppress synthesis of several chemical mediators of inflammation, such as thromboxane, prostacyclin and prostaglandins. The NSAIDs markedly reduce prostaglandin-dependent heat, swelling, edema, erythema and pain in inflamed tissues. Because of their antiinflammatory, antipyretic and analgesic effects, NSAIDs are used widely for treatment of soft-tissue injuries and for reducing body temperature.[8-10]

Specific Uses

While the NSAIDs have similar modes of action, some appear to be more effective in treatment of specific conditions than others. *Meclofenamic acid* is reportedly effective in

Table 2. Antibacterial dosages for horses.

Drug	Dosage	Treatment Interval	Route	Specific Instructions
Na or K benzyl penicillin	20,000 IU/kg	QID	IM, IV	Blood levels maintained better after IM than IV. Muscle soreness can develop with IM therapy.
Procaine penicillin	15,000 IU/kg	BID	IM only	Best "first-choice" drug for Gram-positive pathogens.
Long-acting penicillin (benzathine or benethamine penicillin)	DO NOT USE — ADEQUATE LEVELS NOT MAINTAINED			
Na amoxicillin or ampicillin	15-40 mg/kg	TID	IM, IV	Both drugs have same spectrum of activity. Not as potent as penicillin against Gram-positive organisms.
Amoxicillin trihydrate syrup	20-30 mg/kg	TID	PO	Good absorption, easily given by clients. Use in foals only.
Na cloxacillin or oxacillin	30 mg/kg	TID	IM, IV	Used to treat beta-lactamase-producing *Staph* infections.
Cephalothin or cephapirin	10-20 mg/kg	TID	IM, IV	Useful for penicillinase-producing staphylococci.
Kanamycin	5 mg/kg	TID	IM, IV	Useful for some Gram-negative pathogens.
Gentamicin	2-3 mg/kg	TID	IM, IV	Useful for *Pseudomonas*, some *E coli* and some *Klebsiella* infections.
Amikacin	7 mg/kg	BID to TID	IM, IV	Use only if sensitivity tests show no other aminoglycoside is useful.
Chloramphenicol	DO NOT USE — EFFECTIVE BLOOD LEVELS CANNOT BE ACHIEVED			
Rifampin	5-10 mg/kg	BID - adults SID - foals	PO	Use only in combination with erythromycin for treating *R equi* infections.
Erythromycin gluceptate	5 mg/kg	QID	IV	Use in foals in combination with rifampin for *R equi* infections.
Erythromycin estolate	25 mg/kg	QID	PO	Use in foals only, as for erythromycin gluceptate.
Oxytetracycline hydrochloride	5 mg/kg	BID	IV	Use only if sensitivity tests show no other choice. May cause diarrhea.
Trimethoprim-sulfa	15-20 mg/kg of combined drugs	BID	PO, IV	Wide spectrum of activity. Bactericidal at high dosages. May cause diarrhea if administered orally.
Metronidazole	15 mg/kg loading dosage 7.5 mg/kg maintenance	QID	PO	Use for anaerobic infections, particularly pleuritis. Use in combination with penicillin.

treatment of acute and chronic laminitis, as well as other musculoskeletal problems.[9,11] *Naproxen* is more effective than phenylbutazone against experimentally induced myositis and clinical cases of "tying up."[12] *Flunixin* is recommended specifically as an analgesic for treatment of colic and in management of endotoxic shock.[13-15] *Aspirin* has not been used extensively in horses because of its short half-life. A single dose of aspirin at 20 mg/kg prolongs bleeding time and decreases platelet aggregation.[16] *Phenylbutazone* is by far the most commonly used NSAID and is probably the first choice of most practitioners. This is based partly on cost but predominantly on years of clinical experience that indicate its efficacy and dependability in a variety of conditions.

Because NSAIDs do not suppress the cellular inflammatory response, they have been used to reduce postoperative inflammation. They appear to have no detrimental effect on wound healing. Because of their antipyretic effect, NSAIDs have been used extensively for reducing elevated body temperatures. While this improves the horse's demeanor and appetite, care should be exercised when they are used this way. If an infection is being treated with antimicrobial therapy, NSAID suppression of the body temperature precludes using a temperature drop as an indicator of positive response to therapy. Also, fever is a defense mechanism of the body and should not necessarily be suppressed.

Toxicity

The toxicity of phenylbutazone has been investigated thoroughly in recent years, following the initial report of toxicity in ponies.[17] Though less is known about the toxic side effects of other NSAIDs, it would be wise to assume that similar potential for toxicity exists with prolonged use or high dosages. A decrease in plasma protein levels has been observed in ponies receiving meclofenamic acid.[18,19] Hypoproteinemia also has been reported in a pony mare treated with flunixin.[20] However, at flunixin dosages of up to 5 times those recommended, no clinical or biochemical abnormalities were found in horses.[21]

Though phenylbutazone had been thought to be a very safe drug, recent studies in both horses and ponies have demonstrated that the drug has a narrow therapeutic index.[22]

Breed differences may be observed in the susceptibility to toxicity; pony breeds could be more vulnerable.[23,24] However, in the pony studies, dosages as high as 14.6 mg/kg were used, so the severe effects noted may be the result of the very high dosages. Toxicity is particularly likely if large doses are given for more than a few days.[10,17,23]

Signs of phenylbutazone toxicity include anorexia, lethargy, weight loss, melena, diarrhea, gastrointestinal ulceration, protein-losing enteropathy and, terminally, death from shock. Other toxic effects include toxic neutropenia, hepatotoxicity and nephrotoxicity.[17,18,23,25-31] In foals 3-10 months of age, phenylbutazone administered orally at 10 mg/kg caused gastrointestinal ulceration.[32] Concurrent administration of NSAIDs and aminoglycoside antibiotics may potentiate the risk of nephrotoxicity.[8]

Though signs of toxicity can persist for several weeks after withdrawal of phenylbutazone, the prognosis for recovery is good, provided severe gastrointestinal ulceration has not occurred. A good indicator of toxicity is the total plasma or serum protein level, as the earliest clinicopathologic change in phenylbutazone toxicity is a decrease in total protein concentration.[18]

The recommended dosage for phenylbutazone is a loading dosage of 4.4 mg/kg on the first day, followed by 2.2 mg/kg BID for 4 days, then 2.2 mg/kg SID for 7 days. No significant toxic changes were found at these dosages.[18] In some specific situations, as in treatment of laminitis, potential toxicity must be weighed against the dosage required to alleviate clinical signs. Some of the newer NSAIDs appear to have a greater safety margin than phenylbutazone, but conclusive toxicity studies have yet to be performed.

Interaction With Other Drugs

All NSAIDs are highly bound to plasma protein.[33] This is highly relevant clinically, as it is the free or unbound drug that has biologic activity. Prior exposure or concurrent administration of other drugs that are highly protein bound (eg, some antibacterials, warfarin) may lead to higher unbound concentrations of one or both drugs. For example, use of warfarin in combination with phenylbutazone can cause fatal hemorrhage.

Route of Administration

With phenylbutazone, blood levels are similar after oral and intravenous administration.[34] Because intravenous forms of NSAIDs have low pK$_a$ values, inadvertent perivascular administration causes severe phlebitis. Thus, oral administration is recommended in most clinical circumstances. However, in such situations as treatment of colic and shock, NSAIDs should be given IV.

Absorption from the gastrointestinal tract is influenced by the dose and the relationship of dosing to feeding.[35] Paste preparations may produce more reliable blood levels than powders or tablets, as one can be sure that the horse receives the full dose. Additionally, the preparation can be given on an empty stomach for more rapid absorption.[36] When phenylbutazone is given at the time of feeding, there is also much more variability in the peak plasma levels. This could be a potential source of therapeutic failure with all NSAIDs.

Dosages

From suggested NSAID dosages for horses, NSAIDS are ranked in order of potency as follows: flunixin > meclofenamic acid > phenylbutazone > naproxen > aspirin.[8] Recommended dosages are given in Table 3. The dosage for an individual drug may vary considerably, depending on the particular condition being treated. For example, the dosage of flunixin for treating endotoxemia is less than that needed to alleviate the pain associated with colic. Readers should consult the chapters on individual body systems for specific recommendations.

Dimethylsulfoxide

The physiologic and pharmacologic properties of dimethylsulfoxide (DMSO) are not fully understood, and experimental models have not conclusively demonstrated its antiinflammatory activity.[37,38] There are, however, many reports on the clinical usefulness of DMSO in treatment of acute musculoskeletal injuries, acute traumatic and inflammatory disorders of the central nervous system, postoperative pain and swelling, and certain septic conditions.[39-44] Less consistent responses have been observed in chronic inflammation.[38]

The antiinflammatory effect of DMSO apparently is due to its ability to scavenge free radicals, together with inhibitory properties on the influx of polymorphonuclear and mononuclear cells into the sites of inflammation.[45] DMSO-mediated effects on immune responses also may contribute to its antiinflammatory effects.[43] Its systemic toxicity and teratogenicity are considered low. How-

Table 3. Nonsteroidal antiinflammatory drug dosages for horses.

Drug	Formulation and Route	Recommended Dosage and Clinical Use
Phenylbutazone	Powder, tablets, paste. Oral use.	Loading dosage Day 1, 4.4 mg/kg BID, followed by 2.2 mg/kg BID for 4 days, then 2.2 mg/kg daily thereafter.
	Injectable. IV only.	2.2-4.4 mg/kg for not more than 5 successive days. Note: causes necrosis if administered perivascularly.
Flunixin meglumine	Powder, injectable. IV or IM.	1.1 mg/kg daily for up to 5 days. 0.25-1.1 mg/kg, depending on condition.
Meclofenamic acid	Powder. Oral only.	2.2 mg/kg daily for 5-7 days, then 2.2 mg/kg every other day.
Naproxen	Powder. Oral only.	10 mg/kg daily for up to 14 days.
Phenylbutazone and isopyrin	Injectable. IV only.	4.2 mg phenylbutazone component/kg once daily for 1-4 days. Combination with isopyrin increases plasma half-life of both drugs. Should be administered very slowly IV (30 seconds), as can cause excitement.
Aspirin	Powder, tablets. Oral only.	5-50 mg/kg daily.

ever, rapid intravenous administration can induce seizures. Also, intravenous use of concentrated solutions or large doses may cause hemolysis.[46] Topical DMSO often causes transient skin irritation, erythema and vasodilation, associated with histamine release from mast cells.[43]

Because of DMSO's proven effectiveness as a penetrant carrier, great care should be taken when using DMSO in combination with other agents. DMSO enhances penetration of nonionized molecules of low molecular weight, such as corticosteroids and some antibiotics, across the skin and blood-brain barrier.[43] The effects of some hepatotoxic agents and carcinogens are potentiated by DMSO. Addition of corticosteroids to topical DMSO produces systemic levels consistent with parenteral corticosteroid therapy.[38] In horses, a 10% solution of DMSO in normal saline was safe as a rapid intravenous infusion of 1.0 g/kg.[46] Based on its half-life, DMSO should be given at 12-hour intervals for treatment of increased intracranial pressure and cerebral edema.[44]

The following are recommendations for use of DMSO:[38]

- Only veterinary preparations of DMSO should be used, as industrial preparations may contain impurities.
- Because DMSO is rapidly hydrolyzed, it should be kept in an air-tight container.
- DMSO should be applied only to clean, dry, unmedicated skin surfaces. On damp skin, DMSO may produce excessive heat and discomfort.
- DMSO should be applied with sterile or clean cotton to minimize contamination with potentially dangerous substances.
- Rubber gloves should be worn to apply DMSO. Note that some compounds in solution with DMSO penetrate rubber gloves.

In horses, acute swelling due to trauma is the only condition for which DMSO is recommended and approved by the Food and Drug Administration (FDA). Topical application is the only recommended and FDA-approved route of administration.

Corticosteroids

Two classes of synthetic corticosteroids are available for parenteral administration. Water-soluble succinate and phosphate esters are used in treatment of conditions where rapid attainment of high serum and tissue levels is essential, as in shock, anaphylaxis and allergic reactions. Insoluble esters, such as acetate, are absorbed, metabolized and excreted more slowly.[47,48]

Mode of Action

The antiinflammatory effect of corticosteroids is thought to occur at the cellular level, where they stabilize and maintain the integrity of cellular, lysosomal and mitochondrial membranes. Corticosteroids inhibit the enzyme phospholipase A_2, which is involved in release of arachidonic acid from cell membranes.[9,49] Other effects include maintenance of microcirculation, stabilization of capillary permeability, and modification of the response to histamine release.[55]

Clinical Use

If corticosteroids are used primarily for their antiinflammatory effects, it must be realized that they act nonspecifically and may cause undesirable side effects. One of the contentious areas of corticosteroid use is in treatment of shock. Decreased peripheral resistance, increased venous return, and increased cardiac output have been reported in experimental studies of shock. Corticosteroid use for treatment of endotoxic shock in horses has detractors and supporters.[51,52]

One of the major clinical applications for corticosteroids is in treatment of some dermatologic conditions. In addition, intraarticular use of corticosteroids may be considered for acute synovitis. Other conditions in which corticosteroids can be considered are rhabdomyolysis, some ocular conditions, some chronic pulmonary diseases, and nervous system trauma. Chapters on the individual body systems should be consulted for specific recommendations.

Undesirable Side Effects

If corticosteroids are used for their antiinflammatory actions, one must also be aware of their undesirable side effects. These include:[53]

- Inhibition of fibroblast proliferation and an increase in collagen breakdown. These combined effects adversely affect wound healing and wound strength.
- Inhibition of bone growth, matrix formation and calcification.

- Reduction in calcium absorption and increased renal secretion of calcium.
- Reduction in the number of circulating lymphocytes and eosinophils.
- Suppression of the hypothalamic-pituitary-adrenal system. Soluble forms of corticosteroids cause adrenal suppression for 1-5 days. In contrast, insoluble esters (*ie*, long-acting corticosteroids) can depress adrenal activity for as long as one month.
- Electrolyte imbalances, most notably sodium retention and increased potassium excretion.

References

1. Spurlock GH and Spurlock SL: A technique of catheterization of the lateral thoracic vein in the horse. *Equine Pract* 9(6):33-35, 1987.

2. Edelman IS *et al*: Interrelations between serum sodium concentrations, serum osmolality and total exchangeable sodium, total exchangeable potassium and total body water. *J Clin Invest* 37:1236-1256, 1958.

3. Carlson GP: Personal communication, 1983.

4. Rose RJ *et al*: The use of an oral glucose-glycine-electrolyte solution for experimentally-induced dehydration in the horse. *Vet Record* 119:522-525, 1986.

5. Carlson GP and Rumbaugh GE: Response to saline solution of normally fed horses and horses dehydrated by fasting. *Am J Vet Res* 44:964-968, 1983.

6. Love DN *et al*: Serum concentrations of penicillin in the horse after administration of a variety of penicillin preparations. *Equine Vet J* 15:43-48, 1983.

7. Love DN *et al*: Serum levels of amoxycillin following its oral administration to thoroughbred foals. *Equine Vet J* 13:53-55, 1981.

8. Lees P and Higgins AJ: Clinical pharmacology and therapeutic uses of non-steroidal anti-inflammatory drugs in the horse. *Equine Vet J* 17:83-96, 1985.

9. Snow DH: Non-steroidal antiinflammatory agents in the horse. *In Practice* 3:24-31, 1981.

10. Tobin T *et al*: Phenylbutazone in the horse: a review. *J Vet Pharmacol Therap* 9:1-25, 1986.

11. Conner GH *et al*: Arquel (CI-1583): A new non-steroidal antiinflammatory drug for horses. *Proc 19th Ann Mtg AAEP*, 1973. pp 81-90.

12. Killian JG *et al*: The efficacy of Equiproxen (naproxen) in a unique equine myositis model. *Proc 20th Ann Mtg AAEP*, 1974. pp 210-215.

13. Vernimb GD and Hennessy PW: Clinical studies on flunixin meglumine in the treatment of equine colic. *J Eq Med Surg* 1:111-116, 1977.

14. Bottoms GD *et al*: Endotoxin-induced hemodynamic changes in ponies: effects of flunixin meglumine. *Am J Vet Res* 42:1514-1518, 1981.

15. Fessler JF *et al*: Endotoxin-induced changes in hemograms, plasma enzymes, and blood chemistry values in anesthetized ponies: Effects of flunixin meglumine. *Am J Vet Res* 43:140-144, 1982.

16. Judson DG and Barton M: Effect of aspirin on haemostasis in the horse. *Res Vet Sci* 30:241-242, 1981.

17. Snow DH *et al*: Phenylbutazone toxicity in ponies. *Vet Record* 105:26-30, 1979.

18. Lees P *et al*: Biochemical and haematological effects of phenylbutazone in horses. *Equine Vet J* 15:158-167, 1983.

19. Snow DH and Douglas TA: Studies on a new paste preparation of phenylbutazone. *Vet Record* 112:602-607, 1983.

20. Webbon PM and Wolliscraft GJ: Cautious use of flunixin advocated. *Vet Record* 115:45, 1984.

21. Houdeshell JW and Hennessey PW: A new non-steroidal anti-inflammatory analgesic for horses. *J Eq Med Surg* 1:57-63, 1977.

22. Jeffcott LB and Colles CM: Phenylbutazone and the horse - a review. *Equine Vet J* 9:105-110, 1977.

23. Snow DH *et al*: Phenylbutazone toxicosis in Equidae: a biochemical and pathophysiologic study. *Am J Vet Res* 42:1754-1759, 1981.

24. Sullivan M and Snow DH: Factors affecting absorption of non-steroidal anti-inflammatory agents in the horse. *Vet Record* 110:554-558, 1982.

25. Gabriel KL and Martin JE: Phenylbutazone: short-term versus long-term administration to thoroughbred and standardbred horses. *JAVMA* 140:337-341, 1962.

26. Gabel AA *et al*: Phenylbutazone in horses: a review. *J Eq Med Surg* 1:221-225, 1977.

27. Wanner F *et al*: A preliminary report: demethylation, hydroxylation and acetylation in the horse. Side-effects of repeated phenylbutazone medication. *Proc Third Int Symp Equine Med Control*, Lexington, KY, 1979.

28. Gerring EL *et al*: Pharmacokinetics of phenylbutazone and its metabolites in the horse. *Equine Vet J* 13:152-157, 1981.

29. MacKay RJ *et al*: Effects of large doses of phenylbutazone administration to horses. *Am J Vet Res* 44:774-780, 1983.

30. Collins LG and Tyler DE: Phenylbutazone toxicosis in the horse: a clinical study. *JAVMA* 184: 699-703, 1984.

31. Gerber H: Ethical problems for veterinary surgeons at equestrian events. *Equine Vet J* 16:25-27, 1984.

32. Traub JL *et al*: Phenylbutazone toxicosis in the foal. *Am J Vet Res* 44:1410-1418, 1983.

33. Lambert MBT and Kelly PP: The binding of phenylbutazone to bovine and horse serum albumin. *Irish J Med Sci* 147:192-196, 1978.

34. Chay S *et al*: The pharmacology of non-steroidal anti-inflammatory drugs in the horse: flunixin meglumine (Banamine). *Equine Pract* 4(2):16-23, 1982.

35. Lees P *et al*: Pharmacokinetics of phenylbutazone in Welsh Mountain ponies. *Equine Vet J* 17:83-96, 1985.

36. Rose RJ *et al*: Bioavailability of phenylbutazone preparations in the horse. *Equine Vet J* 14:234-237, 1982.

37. Alsup EM and DeBowes RM: Dimethylsulfoxide. *JAVMA* 185:1011-1014, 1984.

38. Brayton CF: Dimethylsulfoxide (DMSO): a review. *Cornell Vet* 76:61-90, 1986.

39. Teigland MB and Saurino VR: Clinical evaluation of dimethylsulfoxide in equine applications. *Ann NY Acad Sci* 141:471-477, 1967.

40. Koller LD: Clinical application of DMSO by veterinarians in Oregon and Washington. *VM/SAC* 71:591-597, 1976.

41. Mayhew IG and MacKay RJ, in Mansmann RA and McAllister ES: *Equine Medicine & Surgery*. 3rd ed. American Veterinary Publications, Goleta, CA, 1982.

42. Faddock JA and Mullowney PC: Dermatologic diseases of horses. Part I. Parasitic dermatoses of the horse. *Compend Cont Ed Pract Vet* 5:S615-S621, 1983.

43. Hillidge CJ: The case for dimethylsulfoxide (DMSO) in equine practice. *Equine Vet J* 17:259-261, 1985.

44. Blythe LL *et al*: Intravenous use of dimethylsulfoxide (DMSO) in horses: clinical and physiologic effects. *Proc 32nd Ann Mtg AAEP*, 1987. pp 441-446.

45. Wong LK and Reinertson EL: Clinical considerations of dimethylsulfoxide. *Iowa State Vet* 46:89-95, 1984.

46. Blythe LL *et al*: Pharmacokinetic disposition of dimethylsulfoxide administered intravenously to horses. *Am J Vet Res* 47:1739-1743, 1986.

47. Mason RL: The use of anti-inflammatory drugs in horses. *Proceedings 39*, Post-Grad Comm Vet Sci, Univ Sydney, 1978. pp 635-643.

48. Toutain PL *et al*: Dexamethasone and prednisolone in the horse: pharmacokinetics and action on the adrenal gland. *Am J Vet Res* 45:1750-1756, 1984.

49. Mazue G *et al,* in Ruckebusch Y *et al*: *Veterinary Pharmacology and Toxicology*. MTP Press, Boston, 1983. pp 321-331.

50. Jones EW and Hamm D: Steroidal and non-steroidal anti-inflammatory drugs for wounds and traumatic inflammation. *N Zeal Vet J* 25:317-319, 1977.

51. White NA: Management of postoperative complications in equine colic. *MVP* 64:743-746, 1983.

52. Burrows GE: Endotoxaemia in the horse. *Vet Record* 100:262-264, 1981.

53. Sloane DE *et al*: Sodium retention and cortisol (hydrocortisone) suppression caused by dexamethasone and triamcinolone in equids. *Am J Vet Res* 44:280-283, 1983.

Additional Reading

Fluid and Electrolyte Therapy

Brownlow MA and Hutchins DR: The concept of osmolality: its use in the evaluation of "dehydration" in the horse. *Equine Vet J* 14:106-110, 1982.

Carlson GP: Fluid therapy in horses with acute diarrhea. *Vet Clin No Am* (Large Anim Pract) 1:313-329, 1979.

Carlson GP, in Snow DH *et al*: *Equine Exercise Physiology*. Granta, Cambridge, 1983. pp 291-309.

Carlson GP *et al*: Clinicopathologic alterations in the horse produced by food and water deprivation during periods of high environmental temperatures. *Am J Vet Res* 40:982-985, 1979.

Mitchell AR: Understanding fluid therapy. *Irish Vet J* 37:94-103, 1983.

Rose RJ: A physiological approach to fluid and electrolyte therapy in the horse. *Equine Vet J* 13:7-14, 1981.

Rumbaugh GE *et al*: Urinary production in the healthy horse and in horses deprived of feed and water. *Am J Vet Res* 43:735-737, 1982.

Antibacterial Therapy

Adamson PJ *et al*: Susceptibility of equine bacterial isolates to antimicrobial agents. *Am J Vet Res* 46:447-450, 1985.

Baggot JD *et al*: Selection of an aminoglycoside antibiotic for administration to horses. *Equine Vet J* 17:30-34, 1985.

Baggot JD and Prescott JF: Antimicrobial selection and dosage in the treatment of equine bacterial infections. *Equine Vet J* 19:92-96, 1987.

Bertone AL *et al*: Comparison of various treatments for experimentally induced infectious arthritis. *Am J Vet Res* 48:392-402, 1987.

Brown MP *et al*: Kanamycin sulfate in the horse: serum, synovial fluid, peritoneal fluid, and urine concentrations after single-dose intramuscular administration. *Am J Vet Res* 42:1823-1825, 1981.

Brown MP *et al*: Oxytetracycline hydrochloride in the horse: serum, synovial, peritoneal and urine concentrations after single dose intravenous administration. *J Vet Pharmacol Therap* 4:7-10, 1981.

Brown MP *et al*: Gentamicin sulfate in the horse: serum, synovial, peritoneal and urine concentrations after single-dose intramuscular administration. *J Vet Pharmacol Therap* 5:119-122, 1982.

Brown MP *et al*: Trimethoprim-sulfadiazine in the horse: serum, synovial, peritoneal, and urine concentrations after single-dose intravenous administration. *Am J Vet Res* 44:540-543, 1983.

Brown MP *et al*: Chloramphenicol sodium succinate in the horse: serum, synovial, peritoneal, and urine concentrations after single-dose intravenous administration. *Am J Vet Res* 45:578-580, 1984.

Brown MP *et al*: Amikacin sulfate in mares: pharmacokinetics and body fluid and endometrial concentrations after repeated intramuscular administration. *Am J Vet Res* 45:1610-1613, 1984.

Brown MP *et al*: Pharmacokinetics of amikacin in pony foals after a single intramuscular injection. *Am J Vet Res* 47:453-454, 1986.

Gronwall R *et al*: Body fluid concentrations and pharmacokinetics of chloramphenicol given to mares intravenously or by repeated gavage. *Am J Vet Res* 47:2591-2595, 1986.

Editorial: The antibiotic jungle. *Equine Vet J* 12:98-99, 1980.

English PB and Roberts MC: Adverse reactions to antimicrobial agents in the horse. *Vet Res Commun* 7:207-210, 1983.

Hillidge CJ: Review of *Corynebacterium* (*Rhodococcus*) *equi* lung abscesses in foals: pathogenesis, diagnosis and treatment. *Vet Record* 119:261-264, 1986.

Koterba AM *et al*: Clinical and clinicopathological characteristics of the septicaemic neonatal foal: review of 38 cases. *Equine Vet J* 16:376-382, 1984.

Koterba AM *et al*: Nosocomial infections and bacterial antibiotic resistance in a university equine hospital. *JAVMA* 189:185-191, 1986.

Ricketts SW and Hopes R: Selection of antibiotics for use in equine practice. *Vet Record* 114:544-546, 1984.

Rose RJ: *Horses*. Vade Mecum 1. Univ Sydney Post-Graduate Foundation Vet Sci, Sydney, 1983.

Rose RJ and Love DN: Staphylococcal septic arthritis in three horses. *Equine Vet J* 11:85-89, 1979.

Stover SM *et al*: Aqueous procaine penicillin G in the horse: serum, synovial, peritoneal, and urine concentrations after single-dose intramuscular administration. *Am J Vet Res* 42:629-631, 1981.

Sweeney RW *et al*: Pharmacokinetics of metronidazole given to horses by intravenous and oral routes. *Am J Vet Res* 47:1726-1729, 1986.

Antiinflammatory and Antipyretic Therapy

Meschter CL *et al*: Vascular pathology in phenylbutazone-intoxicated horses. *Cornell Vet* 74:282-297, 1984.

Sandford J: DMSO: an alternative perspective. *Equine Vet J* 17:262, 1985.

Sweeney RW *et al*: Pharmacokinetics of metronidazole given to horses by intravenous and oral routes. *Am J Vet Res* 47:1726-1729, 1986.

Vaala WE: Aspects of pharmacology in the neonatal foal. *Vet Clin No Am* (Equine Pract) 1:51-75, 1985.

PRINCIPLES OF NUTRITION

D.T. Galligan

Nutrition is an important factor in determining the health and performance status of equine patients. A selection of nutritionally related disorders is listed in Table 4. Most of these diseases can be prevented by sound nutritional management. Feeding for performance is more complicated and requires constant monitoring of the feeding program by the farm managers and veterinarian. This chapter describes a protocol to evaluate the nutritional management of horses. The main components of this protocol are:

Farm visit, including evaluation of the feeding program and management, the physiologic condition and use of the horses, necessary medical examinations, and sampling of feedstuffs.

Ration evaluation.

Ration formulation, with recommendations to the manager on diet for each class of horse.

Farm Visit

A farm visit is crucial to define the feeding management program.[1] An intensive inspection of the feeds and feeding management, along with examinations of the horses on a farm, is essential for identifying likely causes of a problem and available options for improvement.

Evaluation of Feeding Management

The farm manager and other personnel must be interviewed to gather background data and make an initial appraisal of the feeding program. The uses of the horses must be clearly defined, and historical information on diseases and performance problems documented. General feeding management practices, such as the time and frequency of feeding, should be recorded. Most horses are fed once or twice daily, though those with heavy grain intake should be fed 3-4 times a day. Farm policies regarding the administration of rations should be elucidated for each class of horse. Careful questioning regarding when ration changes are made, and on what age, weight, height, reproductive status, and use criteria these decisions are made help construct this policy.

From this interview, one can assess the overall understanding of the manager's problem. However, attention should not be confined to problems perceived by the farm manager. Other problem areas in nutrient delivery or ration imbalance may become apparent as specific areas are examined. A tour of the facilities confirms information gleaned during the interview and better defines any problem areas.

Table 4. Nutritionally related disorders.

Disorder	Associated Factors
Laminitis	Excessive intake of highly fermentable feeds.
Colic	Sudden changes in feeding programs. Also, poor-quality hay, rich diets, consumption of sand.
Azoturia	Full rations during period of inactivity.
Agalactia and thickened uterus	Fescue pasture for last 90 days of gestation.
Chronic obstructive pulmonary disease	Dusty, moldy hay; subtropical pastures.
Secondary hyperparathyroidism	Excessive phosphorus intake.
Night blindness	Vitamin A deficiency.
Developmental bone diseases	Excessive energy and/or protein; Ca:P imbalances; Cu and Zn deficiency.
Rhabdomyolysis and steatitis	Vitamin E and/or selenium deficiency.
Equine degenerative myeloencephalopathy	Low vitamin E status.

Evaluation of feeding management also involves inspection of the feeds (cereal grains, supplements, hays, pastures), storage facilities, and the feed-delivery system. This entails sampling and weighing feeds, and calibrating scoops and flakes. A spring scale, hay bore, drill, polyethylene bags, marker pens and a bucket are basic tools necessary for a complete evaluation.

Feed Evaluation

Cereal feeds are examined for physical attributes, such as color, odor, kernel integrity, molds and foreign material. There should be minimal evidence of rodent, insect and bird activity, and cats should not be allowed access to grain bins. Processed feeds should be examined for fineness of grind and dustiness. Examination of the feeding tubs shows if "settling" of fine grains is occurring. If settling of mineral components is occurring, molasses should be increased to a minimum of 5% of the grain mix. Minimal dust should be observed when grains are poured. Subsamples of each grain are taken from several bags or bins and thoroughly mixed. A composite sample for each grain then is submitted to a forage laboratory for proximate analysis for dry matter, crude protein, total digestible nutrients, Ca and P content. If the samples must be retained for several days before submission, they must be refrigerated. Previous nutrient analyses of feed and nutrient specification slips from commercial mixes should be obtained when available.

Grains should be stored in a dry environment. Those with high molasses content must be used on a first-in/first-out basis and have a maximum turnover time of 2 weeks. Plastic and metal storage cans are good if they are emptied completely, frequently and between fillings. The capacity and flexibility of the storage facilities should be noted in case additional grains are necessary.

Commercial supplements often are part of the ration and deliver certain micronutrients and vitamins.[2] Use of these products in the feeding program should be identified and labels of the supplements reviewed for information regarding their nutrient content. These products have highly concentrated nutrients and so are potentially toxic if administered or mixed inappropriately. Their administration should be supervised carefully by the feeding manager.

Hay inspection involves opening several bales and examining them for leafiness, blossoms, mildew, odor, weeds and dust. Hay quality correlates closely with palatability and digestibility; hay maturity correlates closely with quality. Stems should be pliable, not woody, as in overmatured hays. When inspecting bales, one should look for buds (small, white, fuzzy structures near the stem tips) as a sign of proper harvest timing. A predominance of flowers indicates a poorer-quality hay (too mature when harvested). The external surface of bales may be bleached from sunlight, but the internal color should be green. Vitamins A and E are lost when hays are bleached excessively.

There should be no evidence of insects or foreign bodies (dead rodents) in the bales. Blister beetles are attracted to flowers and may be found in mature alfalfa hays. The toxin cantharidin is found in blister beetles, alive or dead, and is very stable.[3]

Heating within bales occurs if there is excessive moisture at harvest (>13% moisture). This causes loss in dry matter and encourages moldiness. Moldy hays are unpalatable and a frequent cause of chronic coughing.

For an accurate assessment of hay quality, a sample for proximate analysis is obtained by core drilling about 5% of the bales. Flakes and clippings of hays are not representative samples and should not be used for proximate analysis. Because energy and fiber density are inversely related, hays containing high crude fiber (>39%) are poor quality and do not even provide maintenance energy requirements of adult horses.

Pastures are evaluated for their potential as a source of nutrients. In general, if there is less then 1 acre of pasture available for each horse, primary use of the pasture is considered to be for exercise. They vary greatly in productivity by the kind of pasture and season. Table 5 is a general guide to the carrying capacity of various pastures through the seasons.[4] Grazing management practices, such as stocking density (number of animals per acre) and grazing times for each season, are recorded. Continuous use of a single large area is not recommended and results in overgrazing (grazing too close to the roots). Pasture acreage should be divided into smaller paddocks so that horses can graze in one area for 10-14 days and then moved to a new area. Mowing and dragging

153

practices are noted. In general, if pastures are grazed rotationally, mowing after grazing maintains uniformity and improves quality for subsequent grazing.[4]

Seed mixtures (proportions) used in seeding the pasture are noted if available. This information, along with nutrient composition tables from the National Research Council (NRC), is useful to determine nutrient content of the pasture as well as its potential palatability.[5,6] Further, certain pasture types are associated with specific problems. For instance, agalactia and thickened placentas were observed in broodmares grazing fescue pastures throughout gestation.[7]

Feed Delivery

After feedstuffs are evaluated, the feed-delivery management is analyzed by checking feed allocation and weighing procedures. Major goals of evaluating feed delivery are to accurately determine intake (pounds) of the various feeds used in the current ration for each class of horse and to evaluate the potential for management to carry out any feeding recommendations that may be necessary.

Most horses are fed by volume measurements, such as coffee can scoops of grain and flakes of hay. All feeds commonly used for horses vary greatly in density; thus, actual dry matter delivered to the animals varies. Volumetric measurements of grain and hay commonly result in inappropriate nutrient delivery. Feed-measuring devices used in feed delivery should be calibrated for each feed. A scoop of mare's grain ration may differ in weight from a scoop of the creep feed grain ration, because of different cereal feeds used. For example, many mare grain mixes contain bran, which weighs 0.5-0.6 lb/qt, as compared to corn and soybean meal, which weigh 1.5-1.9 lb/qt.

Hay is commonly fed by the flake, which can vary in weight from day to day. The bales themselves vary in weight (25-80 lb), depending on the type of hay, harvest maturity and packing pressure; therefore, an average bale weight is calculated from the weights of several bales. The approximate "flake weight" can be calculated by knowing the number of flakes in a bale.

If group feeding is practiced, the horses should be adequately separated to avoid overfeeding of aggressive individuals and underfeeding of timid animals. Bag feeding requires more management but ensures each horse the opportunity to consume its grain allotment.

Feed mangers and water bowls should be evaluated for their safety, availability and ease of cleaning. Feed mangers at approximately shoulder height of the horse allow easy access, yet are safe. Ideally, hay should be fed from manger racks. Ground feeding of hay is discouraged to avoid parasite contamination and to reduce sand and soil intake. Furthermore, the greatest losses of hay occur when it is fed on the ground.

Salt and water should be available on a free-choice basis, giving the horses opportunity to regulate their Na and Cl intake. Management factors in feed delivery, such as routine feeding times, individual animal evaluation, and proper attention to weighing of feeds, determine whether your feeding recommendations will result in the horses' having access to a properly balanced ration.

Individual Horse Evaluation

Individual horses are evaluated nutritionally for feed intake, use and current body condition. Body condition is an indicator of relative balance between nutrient intake and

Table 5. Carrying capacity of pastures.[4]

Type of Pasture	Yield (tons*/acre/season)	Acres per Horse**				
		May	June	July	Aug	Sept
Bluegrass - white clover (unimproved)	1.0	0.8	1.0	2.0	3.5	3.0
Timothy (with added nitrogen fertilizer)	2.0	0.4	0.4	1.0	3.0	1.5
White clover - timothy	1.5	0.5	0.6	2.0	3.0	2.0
Empire birdsfoot trefoil - timothy	2.0	0.6	0.5	0.5	0.8	1.7

* 15% moisture content.

** 1000-lb horse with intake of 20 lb of hay equivalent/day.

requirements. Body condition scoring is based on examination of body regions reflecting changes in body fat. A system used for horses is presented in Table 6.[8] In conjunction with body condition, body weight is estimated by tape girth measurements (Table 7). Managers should be encouraged to

tape-weigh all horses on a monthly basis. These measurements can be used to see if progress is being made in terms of weight loss or gain for animals placed on special diets. Photographs also can be taken for future reference.

Laminitis or stress rings on the hooves are an indication of stress from diets, diets containing highly fermentable nutrients, or disease. Hoof quality and coat condition also are observed. Manure is examined closely and, if necessary, broken up to look for fiber and undigested grain, which indicate poor feed processing. Large stems and uncracked grain cereals are found in the manure of horses with dental disease. Excessively firm manure is an indication of low salt and/or water intake.

Blood samples rarely are taken on routine nutritional consultations. Though the concentration of certain nutrients in plasma may suggest a deficiency or excess of the nutrient in the ration, it is of little value in assessing nutritional status for a horse or the adequacy of the ration for most nutrients.[3]

Table 6. Body condition scoring of horses.[8]

Score	General Condition	Appearance
1	Emaciated	Dorsal and transverse vertebral processes, ribs, tailhead, hooks and pins prominent. Bone structure of withers, shoulder and neck easily noticeable. No fatty tissue palpable.
2	Very thin	Dorsal and transverse vertebral processes, ribs, tailhead, hooks and pins prominent. Slight fat covering bases of spinous processes. Bone structure of withers, shoulder and neck discernible.
3	Thin	Transverse vertebral processes cannot be felt nor can individual vertebrae be identified. Pin bones not distinguishable.
4	Moderately thin	Ribs only faintly discernible. Hook bone not discernible.
5	Moderate	Ribs not distinguishable but easily palpated. Shoulders and neck blend smoothly into body.
6	Moderate to fleshy	May have a slight crease down fleshy back. Fat deposition behind the shoulder and along sides of the withers and neck.
7	Fleshy	May have a crease down back. Individual ribs can be felt, but noticeable filling between ribs with fat.
8	Fat	Crease down back. Difficult to feel ribs. Fat deposited along inner buttocks. Area behind shoulder filled in flush. Thick dorsal neck.
9	Extremely fat	Obvious crease down back. Patchy fat over ribs. Flank filled in flush. Fat along inner buttock may rub. Bulging crest of fat on dorsal neck.

Nutritional Evaluation of the Ration

When evaluating the feeding system, one should inquire about daily intake of all feeds for all classes of horses on the farm. The major classes of horses, on a nutritional basis, are:[9]

- Mature horses at maintenance
- Mares in the last 3 months of gestation
- Lactating mares, first 3 months
- Lactating mares, last 3 months

Table 7. Girth tape measurements related to the weight of Thoroughbred horses.[3]

Girth (inches)	Weight (lb)
30.0	100
40.0	200
45.5	300
50.5	400
55.0	500
58.5	600
61.5	700
64.5	800
67.5	900
70.5	1000
73.0	1100
75.5	1200
77.5	1300

- Nursing foals
- Weanlings
- Yearlings
- Long yearlings
- 2-year-olds
- Horses in work

The most accurate and reliable means of determining the nutritional status for an individual or the adequacy of the ration for one horse or a class of horses is to compare the level of nutrients in the ration being fed to the level required.[3]

For each class of horse on the farm, the total nutrient intake (lb of dry matter, lb of crude protein, lb TDN, lb of Ca, lb of P), the nutrient density, and the percent of NRC requirements met by the ration all are calcu-

lated.[9] These calculations are based on the weighed intakes and nutrient analysis of each feed.

An example of these calculations is presented in Figure 1 for evaluation of a weanling ration. The ration consists of 6.5 lb of a 14.6% crude protein grain mix and 6 lb of mixed hay. The feed analysis of the samples established by proximate analysis is listed on an as-fed basis. Nutrient contributions of each feed ingredient are calculated by multiplying the intake (as-fed lb) by the nutrient density (as-fed basis). The resulting nutrient contributions are added across all feed ingredients to calculate total nutrient intake. Total nutrient intakes are expressed as a percent of the total dry matter intake and then compared to the nutrient densities re-

Figure 1. Evaluation of a weanling ration.

Daily Ration: 6.5 lb (as fed) of grain and 6 lb (as fed) of mixed hay					
Nutrient Requirements[1]					
	Dry Matter	TDN	Crude Protein	Calcium	Phosphorus
Density (%)		70	16.0	0.70	0.50
Nutrients (lb)[2]	11	7.7	1.76	0.077	0.055
Feed Analysis (% as fed)[3]					
Grain (%)	88	70	14.6	0.35	0.38
Hay (%)	89	46	14.2	1.34	0.22
Contributions[4]					
Grain (lb)	5.7	4.55	0.95	0.023	0.025
Hay (lb)	5.3	2.76	0.85	0.081	0.013
Total (lb)	11	7.31	1.8	0.104	0.038
% Requirement	100	95	102	135	69
Nutrient Density (%)[5]	100	66	16.4	0.945	0.345

1 — NRC nutrient requirements for weanling with adult weight of 1100 lb.
2 — Nutrient (lb) = dry-matter intake (lb) x nutrient density (%).
3 — As-fed basis from proximate analysis.
4 — Calculation: lb of feed (as-fed basis) x nutrient density (as-fed = amount of nutrient).
5 — Calculation: total amount of nutrient/total lb of dry-matter intake.

quired (Table 8).[9] In general, the NRC nutrient requirements are viewed as minimal, rather than optimal for performance animals.

High-protein diets, excessive caloric intake, and imbalances of major and trace minerals in the diets may cause abnormal bone formation.[10-12] Nutrient imbalances have been found on farms improperly using commercial supplements.[2] Supplements often are added to rations without evaluation of their total nutrient contribution to the ration. Part of the problem is market pressure for sale of "growthy" yearlings. Rapid growth rates, along with nutrient imbalances, may reveal genetic predisposition to certain growth abnormalities, such as epiphysitis and splints.[1]

Calcium to phosphorus ratios varying from 1:1 to 6:1 Ca:P do not appear detrimental to mature horses if P intake is at the requirement level (NRC). Young stock (ponies) have been fed Ca:P ratios up to 3:1 without problems.[13]

It is difficult to evaluate the nutrient contribution to the ration of feeding systems for which feed intakes are unknown or when horses are fed in groups, not individually.

One can estimate the intake of feeds to approximate the predicted dry matter intake and then review the level of all nutrients.[9] Underconditioned horses often are found when energy intake is low relative to requirements or when a horse is parasitized. Overconditioning primarily results from excessive energy intake and lack of exercise.

Ration Formulation

New rations are formulated on the basis of the initial ration evaluation, feed analysis, and the feeding system on the farm.

The nutritional requirements listed in NRC publications serve as a guide in formulation.[9] Nutritional requirements for maintenance and activity (reproduction, growth, work) must be satisfied for horses to maintain a constant body weight and composition. Lack of adequate nutrients, as well as nutrient imbalances, affects performance.

Energy requirements of working horses as listed by the NRC are considered to be low by 30-50%.[8,14] The vitamin A levels for growing horses also appear low in the NRC guide; horses should be fed 18-60 μg retinol/kg body

Table 8. Nutrient concentrations recommended by the National Research Council, 1978 (100% dry-matter basis).

	TDN* (%)	Crude Protein (%)	Calcium (%)	Phosphorus (%)	Dry Matter Intake (lb/day) Adult Weight (lb)			
					440	880	1100	1320
Mature animals at maintenance	50	8.5	0.30	0.20	8.2	13.9	16.4	18.8
Mares, last 90 days of gestation	55	11.0	0.50	0.35	8.1	13.7	16.2	18.5
Lactating mares, first 3 months	65	14.0	0.50	0.35	11.5	18.4	22.2	26.0
Lactating mares, last 3 months	60	12.0	0.45	0.30	11.0	17.1	20.6	23.9
Nursing foals, creep feed	80	18.0	0.85	0.60	5.0	7.8	9.2	10.2
Weanlings	70	16.0	0.70	0.50	6.3	9.2	11.0	12.0
Yearlings	65	13.5	0.55	0.40	6.4	10.9	13.2	14.8
Long yearlings	60	11.0	0.45	0.35	6.8	12.2	14.3	16.2
Two-year-olds	65	10.0	0.45	0.35	6.8	11.8	14.5	16.3
Horses in work								
Light	55	8.5	0.30	0.20				
Moderate	65	8.5	0.30	0.20				
Intense	70	8.5	0.30	0.20				

* 1 Mcal of digestible energy = 0.5 lb of TDN

weight.[2] Low levels of the amino acid lysine decrease weight gains in growing animals.[15,16] Thus, lysine is considered to be a requirement (0.7% of dry matter). Fortunately, most feeds used in horse rations are relatively high in lysine.

Grain mixes are formulated to balance the nutrients from forages. Commercial mixes can be used if they are appropriate for the forage type and intake. If supplements are used to supply specific nutrients, their total nutrient contribution must be considered.[2]

Individual feeding should be considered. Managers should be instructed about the need for constant reevaluation of peculiarities of each individual horse. Recommendations are a guide, and the feed manager must be instructed to adjust the feeding program as needed. One should try to reformulate the diet with the fewest possible changes in the feed staples and delivery system. Generally, only the relative proportions of roughage to concentrate require change.[1] Any changes in the rations should be made over a 7- to 10-day period.

Grains should be fed by weight and nutrient content, rather than by volume. Changes in amounts of grain fed per day should not exceed increases or decreases >0.5 lb. Furthermore, if the total amount of concentrate fed exceeds 8 lb at a feeding, increased feeding frequency should be encouraged. A minimum roughage allowance of 1% body weight should be maintained for all classes.

References

1. Kronfeld DS: Feeding on horse breeding farms. *Proc Ann Mtg AAEP*, 1978. pp 461-464.

2. Donoghue S and Kronfeld DS: Vitamin-mineral supplements for horses with emphasis on vitamin A. *Compend Cont Ed Pract Vet* 8:S121-S126, 1980.

3. Lewis L: *Feeding and Care of the Horse*. Lea & Febiger, Philadelphia, 1982.

4. Seaney RR and Reid WS: *Pasture Improvement and Management for Horses*. Information Bulletin 171, College Agri and Life Sci, Cornell Univ, Ithaca, NY.

5. Archer M: Preliminary studies on the palatability of grasses, legumes and herbs to horses. *Vet Record* 89:236-240, 1971.

6. Archer M: Studies on producing and maintaining balanced pastures for studs. *Equine Vet J* 10:54-59, 1978.

7. Heitman ED *et al:* Selenium and reproductive abnormalities in pregnant pony mares grazing fescue pasture. *Proc 7th Equine Nutrit Physiol Symp*, 1981. pp 62-67.

8. Henneke DR *et al:* A condition score relationship to body fat content of mares during gestation and lactation. *Proc 7th Eq Nutrit Physiol Symp*, 1981. pp 105-116.

9. *Nutrient Requirements of Horses*. National Academy of Sciences, Washington, DC, 1978.

10. Auer JA and Martens RJ: Angular limb deformities in young foals. *Proc Ann Mtg AAEP*, 1980. pp 81-84.

11. Wagner PC *et al:* Contracted tendons (flexural deformities) in the young horse. *Compend Cont Ed Pract Vet* 4:S101-S104, 1982.

12. Mayhew IG *et al:* Nutrition, bones and bone pathology. *Cornell Vet* 68:71-102, 1978.

13. Jordan RM *et al:* Effect of calcium and phosphorus levels on growth, reproduction, and bone development of ponies. *J Anim Sci* 40:78, 1975.

14. Winter LD and Hintz HF: A survey of feeding practices at two thoroughbred racetracks. *Proc 7th Eq Nutrit Physiol Symp*, 1981. pp 136-140.

15. Hintz HF *et al:* Comparison of a blend of milk products and linseed meal as protein supplements for young growing horses. *J Anim Sci* 33:1274-1277, 1971.

16. Breuer LH and Golden DL: Lysine requirement of the immature equine. *J Anim Sci* 33:227, 1971.

4 Systemic Diseases Involving Multiple Body Systems

R.J. Rose and J.D. Wright

SEPTICEMIA

Septicemia is a systemic disease caused by multiplication of pathogenic bacteria and their toxins in circulating blood. Septicemia caused by pyogenic organisms is known as pyemia and may result in multiple abscesses.

Septicemia in Foals

Septicemia primarily is a disease of neonatal foals. In foals the infection is acquired *in utero* or shortly after birth.[1-5] Mortality associated with neonatal septicemia has been estimated at 75%, with most infections due to Gram-negative bacteria, principally *Escherichia coli* in the United States.[5,6] In Britain, most cases of septicemia are due to *Actinobacillus equuli* and *Streptococcus* spp.[1] Various other organisms also have been identified in foal septicemia, including *Klebsiella* spp, *Pseudomonas aeruginosa*, *Salmo nella* spp, *Rhodococcus* (*Corynebacterium*) *equi*, *Staphylococcus aureus* and *Pasteurella hemolytica*.

Most neonatal infections are opportunistic, stemming from failure of transfer of passive immunity. The principal portals of entry of infection are the umbilical cord, alimentary canal and respiratory tract.[7] However, failure of passive transfer appears to be less important in the pathogenesis of infections by *Rhodococcus equi* and *Salmonella typhi murium*, which tend to affect older foals.[7,8]

Septicemia in Adult Horses

Septicemia occurs far less commonly in adult horses than in neonates. *Salmonella* infections are one of the most common causes of septicemia. Diarrhea usually is preceded by fever, mild abdominal discomfort and anorexia. Together with an elevated pulse rate, there may be signs of septic shock due to absorption of endotoxins from the damaged bowel or release from circulating bacteria. The most dramatic clinicopathologic finding is marked neutropenia, which often precedes diarrhea.[9]

Septicemia secondary to release of Gram-negative bacteria and their endotoxins is the major cause of death in strangulating intestinal obstruction in horses.[10,11] Other isolated cases of septicemia associated with a number of different organisms have been reported. Of more recent note are the rickettsial organisms, *Ehrlichia* (Potomac horse fever), which produce enterocolitis in horses of all ages.[12]

Diagnosis

Diagnosis of neonatal septicemia is very difficult because there is no single criterion that specifically and consistently identifies a septicemic foal. Early signs, such as decreased appetite and slight lethargy, often are missed, particularly when other problems also are present.[5] *E coli* and *S typhimurium* often invade joints and/or physes, causing swollen joints and lameness. Signifi-

159

cant indicators of infection include failure to suck, abdominal pain, diarrhea, uveitis and seizures. In foals, however, the presenting clinical signs are nonspecific, and fever is not always present.

The hemogram generally shows neutropenia, with <4000 segmented neutrophils/μl. Most septicemic foals have an increased number of band neutrophils (>200/μl) and toxic changes in neutrophils, such as Doehle bodies, basophilic cytoplasm, and cytoplasmic vacuolization.[5] However, these changes are not specific for septicemia and are observed frequently in other diseases. A WBC count within the normal range (6000-12,000/μl) is common in foals with positive blood cultures. Persistent, severe pneumonia and septic arthritis may be responsible for prolonged leukocytosis.[5]

One characteristic finding in foals with septicemia is hypoglycemia. The clinician should be aware of this and use reagent dip sticks for early detection of low blood glucose levels.

Septicemia is definitively diagnosed by blood culture. To undertake this procedure, an area over the animal's jugular vein should be clipped and shaved. After full presurgical skin disinfection, blood is collected using a 19-ga needle and a new, sterile 20-ml syringe. It is absolutely essential that this procedure be carried out using full sterile technique; otherwise, bacterial skin contaminants will confuse culture results. A blood smear should be made from residual blood for Gram staining after the blood is deposited into aerobic and anaerobic enrichment media. Such broths are available commercially as blood culture bottles. Subcultures are performed at 24-hour intervals for up to one week, as some bacteria take a long time to grow. Multiple blood cultures, particularly if samples are taken while the body temperature is rising or during persistent fever, increase the likelihood of positive results.

Treatment

Septicemia in neonatal foals has very high mortality. This is due partially to involvement of Gram-negative organisms, which may be resistant to commonly used antibacterials. This problem may be exacerbated further by inadequate penetration of antibacterials into the cerebrospinal fluid if meningitis is part of the clinical picture.[13]

When infection is suspected and culture results are pending, a bactericidal drug should be given. As Gram-negative infections are common causes of septicemia, aminoglycosides usually are the drugs of choice. The duration of antibacterial therapy should depend on the response to therapy and negative blood cultures. With certain infections, such as pneumonia with abscessation, osteomyelitis, septic arthritis or meningitis, long-term antibacterial therapy for up to one month may be required. Even then, the prognosis for full recovery is poor.[8,13,14]

In foals with partial or total failure of transfer of passive immunity, oral colostrum (if the foal is <12 hours old) or intravenous plasma should be given. If plasma cannot be used from the dam because of concern about neonatal isoerythrolysis, a universal donor (usually an unrelated gelding) is best. The ideal donor is an adult horse that has been blood typed and has no major RBC antigens or antibodies to the major equine blood types. Commercial frozen plasma also is available.

At least 2 L of plasma should be infused IV at a rate of 10-20 ml/kg/hour. This is 600-1200 ml/hour in an average-sized foal a few days old. If frozen plasma is available, partially thawed plasma provides immunoglobulins while reducing the overall volume to be administered.[15] About 90% of the immunoglobulins are found in the initial 50% of the thawed plasma. Plasma should be given at room temperature and care taken to prevent volume overload. Anaphylaxis is very uncommon. Generally, the only noticeable side effects are an increased respiratory rate and shivering, both of which disappear if the flow rate is reduced.[5]

In most cases of septicemia in foals, intravenous fluid administration is required to maintain serum electrolyte and glucose levels, acid-base balance, and urinary output. The composition of the electrolyte solutions used depends on any serum electrolyte and acid-base derangements in the foal.

Treatment of septicemia in adult horses consists of specific antibacterial therapy, dictated by the particular organism involved, and appropriate supportive therapy. Because septicemic salmonellosis in adults is accompanied by severe diarrhea, treatment is primarily oriented toward continuous intravenous fluid therapy. In these cases, it is important to monitor the changes in serum protein and electrolyte levels and acid-base balance. Small doses of flunixin may also be considered for its antiendotoxemic effects. The value of antibacterials in salmonellosis is controversial. Such drugs appear to have little effect on resolution of diarrhea or the course of the enteric infection but may prevent bacterial seeding of other tissues. Antibacterial therapy is only useful early in the course of septicemia.

SHOCK

For clinical purposes, shock can be considered as failure to maintain cardiac output.[16] While there is usual coincident arterial hypotension, the most important consideration in therapy is to restore cardiac output and prevent tissue hypoperfusion. Vasopressor agents may restore arterial pressure at the expense of cardiac output but they cannot be recommended for shock because tissue perfusion may be worsened.

Two main types of shock are encountered in equine practice: hypovolemic shock and endotoxic shock.

Hypovolemic Shock

The most common cause of hypovolemic shock in horses is blood loss resulting from external trauma, such as wire cuts involving major vessels. In newborn foals, hypovolemia may occur due to severance of the umbilical cord during delivery.[17] Horses can sustain a loss of about 20% of their blood volume (about 12-14 L in a 1000-lb horse) without undue physiologic disturbances.

In acute hypovolemia, RBC are released from the spleen under the influence of increased circulating catecholamines. Thus, despite extensive blood loss, no decrease in RBC values may be found on initial examination. However, this effect is short lived and, within 24 hours, the hematocrit decreases significantly. Physiologic responses to hypovolemia include increased heart rate, reduced pulse amplitude, and movement of fluid from the interstitial spaces and intracellular fluid into the circulation. In the early phases of hypovolemic shock, arterial pressure may be maintained due to vasoconstriction in target organs, such as the kidneys, gastrointestinal tract and muscles. However, peripheral perfusion, as assessed from capillary refill time, often is decreased considerably. Other signs include hypothermia, increased respiration, and pallor of the mucous membranes.

The priority in therapy for hemorrhagic shock is reestablishment of circulating blood volume. This takes precedence over transfusion of RBC, because horses can tolerate decreased oxygen-carrying capacity associated with blood loss better than the irreversible changes associated with hypovolemia. Therefore, initial therapy should consist of rapid intravenous infusion of polyionic fluids at 30-50 ml/kg, depending on the severity of shock. If available, plasma should be given intravenously at 10-20 ml/kg in addition to isotonic electrolyte solutions. Plasma provides longer-term benefits, since the expansion of blood volume is more prolonged. Plasma infusion should not exceed 15 ml/kg/hour. Electrolyte solutions can be infused at up to 50 ml/kg/hour without overloading the circulation. To achieve such fluid flow rates, 12-ga catheters must be placed in at least 2 large veins.

Note that if severe hemorrhagic shock has been present for more than 6 hours, severe and irreversible changes associated with tissue hypoxia may have occurred. This may be evident as circulatory overload at high intravenous infusion flow rates, due to a component of cardiogenic shock.

After therapy has been given to combat hypovolemia, whole-blood transfusion can be considered after blood collection from a suitable donor. Donor and recipient blood should be cross-matched and a donor selected that does not cause agglutination, though alloantibodies on equine erythrocytes behave more as hemolysins than agglutinins.[18] Detection of hemolysins is not feasible in the practice laboratory; however, if agglutination does not occur, most single blood transfusions do not cause adverse reactions. About 10 L of blood can be collected from an adult donor horse without causing adverse effects. Blood should be infused into the recipient at a rate not exceeding 10-15 ml/kg/hour.

Endotoxic or Septic Shock

In severe septicemia, hypotension can be followed by a vicious cycle of circulatory events leading to shock. Endotoxic shock may occur in severe septicemia and with various gastrointestinal disorders in which endotoxins are released from Gram-negative bacteria. In such instances, the clinical findings are similar to those of hypovolemic shock previously discussed. Because septicemia occurs more frequently in foals than in adults, endotoxic shock is more common in foals. Endotoxic or septic shock may be present in septicemic animals with an elevated heart rate, increased respiratory rate, decreased pulse pressure, and prolonged capillary refill time.

Tissue perfusion is best restored by giving intravenous polyionic electrolyte solutions at 40-60 ml/kg/hour. Fluid volumes of 50-100 ml/kg often are necessary to restore peripheral perfusion. The main difficulty with such volumes is that the plasma protein level is lowered and edema may develop due to reduction in plasma oncotic pressure. The total plasma protein concentration must be monitored during large-volume electrolyte infusion. If the plasma protein level falls below 4.5 g/dl, the flow rate must be slowed or consideration given to intravenous infusion of plasma. Intravenous dextrose may be necessary to combat the attendant hypoglycemia of endotoxemia, especially in foals.

Because it inhibits generation of vasoactive metabolites of arachidonic acid, intravenous flunixin should be considered early in endotoxic or septic shock. The role of corticosteroids in treatment of endotoxic shock is more controversial. Though corticosteroids have a protective effect against experimental endotoxic shock in dogs, sheep and rats,, recent studies in people have not supported use of corticosteroids. In a controlled study of methylprednisolone, no differences were found in prevention or reversal of shock, or overall mortality.[19] In people with increased serum creatinine levels (>2 mg/dl), those treated with methylprednisolone were more likely to die. In general, more deaths were due to secondary infections than in the placebo-treated group. Though no such clinical trials have been undertaken in horses, use of corticosteroids for treatment of endotoxic shock cannot be recommended.

DISSEMINATED INTRAVASCULAR COAGULATION

Disseminated intravascular coagulation (DIC) can involve many body systems. After formation of excessive thrombin, the various coagulant factors are depleted. Fibrin formation in small blood vessels results in obstruction of the microvasculature and, in extreme cases, lack of clotting ability. A wide range of diseases may produce DIC, though gastrointestinal disorders and laminitis are the most common predisposing conditions.[20-26] Other conditions in which DIC should be considered include endotoxemia, neoplasia, septicemia and severe acid-base disturbances. A hypercoagulable state may exist in periparturient mares, as it does in women; therefore, DIC should be considered as a potential complication of diseases in mares just before and after foaling.[26]

Clinical Signs

Few clinical signs suggesting DIC are found early to midway through the course of the disease. Rather, signs of the primary problem, such laminitis or colic, predominate. Later, when the coagulation system fails, hemorrhage and large-vein thrombosis may indicate the end stage of DIC. Because of this, reliance must be placed on laboratory investigations when DIC is a suspected complication of a primary disease.

Clinicopathologic Changes

As a screening measurement, platelet numbers give a good guide to the presence or absence of DIC. Normal platelet numbers are >100,000/μl. If low values are found, DIC should be suspected. Plasma fibrinogen levels, which usually are decreased in people with DIC, may be elevated during the early phase of DIC in horses. If platelet numbers are lower than normal, a full clotting profile should be performed. Usually this would include prothrombin time (PT), partial thromboplastin time (PTT) and, if possible, fibrin/fibrinogen degradation products (FDP). In DIC, the PT and PTT are increased, with a variable increase in the concentration of FDP.

Therapy

The main aim of therapy is to treat the underlying condition contributing to DIC. Fluid therapy is very important to correct any hypovolemia and reduced tissue perfusion, and dilute thrombin and FDP. Isotonic polyionic fluids should be given initially at 40 ml/kg. Potent inhibitors of arachidonic acid metabolism, such as flunixin, meclofenamic acid or phenylbutazone, may be indicated to reduce platelet aggregation. Additionally, nonsteroidal antiinflammatory drugs, particularly flunixin, have beneficial effects in combating endotoxemia. Because plasma antithrombin III (ATIII) concentrations are reduced, administration of fresh plasma (4-20 ml/kg) may be indicated to replenish ATIII. Low dosages of heparin (5-10 units/ kg) given IV also should be considered, though the benefits of this therapy have not been proven in horses. Theoretically, heparin potentiates the action of plasma ATIII, which inactivates thrombin and other clotting factors.[27]

For successful treatment of DIC, early diagnosis and therapy are necessary.[28] Once DIC has progressed to the stage of severe hemorrhage, death is almost certain despite treatment. Therefore, it may be appropriate in high-risk cases to initiate therapy as though DIC were present. This is particularly so when access to laboratory facilities is limited.

References

1. Platt H: Septicaemia in the foal. A review of 61 cases. *Brit Vet J* 129:221-229, 1973.

2. Platt H: Joint-ill and other bacterial infections on thoroughbred studs. *Equine Vet J* 9:141-145, 1977.

3. Wenkoff MS: *Salmonella typhimurium* septicemia in foals. *Can Vet J* 14:284-286, 1973.

4. Baker JR and Ellis CE: A survey of postmortem findings in 480 horses 1958-1980: causes of death. *Equine Vet J* 13:43-46, 1981.

5. Koterba AM *et al*: Prevention and control of infection. *Vet Clin No Am* (Equine Pract) 1:41-50, 1985.

6. Koterba A *et al*: Clinical and clinicopathological characteristics of the septicaemic neonatal foal. Review of 38 cases. *Equine Vet J* 16:376-392, 1984.

7. Platt H: Acute infections in young foals. *In Practice* 5:41-49, 1983.

8. Prescott JF and Sweeney CR: Treatment of *Corynebacterium equi* pneumonia of foals: A review. *JAVMA* 187:725-728, 1985.

9. Smith BP: Equine salmonellosis: a contemporary view. *Equine Vet J* 13:147-151, 1981.

10. Sembrat R *et al*: Acute pulmonary failure in the conscious pony with *Escherichia coli* septicaemia. *Am J Vet Res* 39:1147-1154, 1978.

11. Templeton CB *et al*: Effects of repeated endotoxin injections on prostanoids, hemodynamics, endothelial cells and survival in ponies. *Circ Shock* 16: 253-264, 1985.

12. Palmer JE: Update on equine diarrheal diseases: salmonellosis and Potomac fever. *Proc 12th Ann Mtg Am Coll Vet Intern Med, 1984.* pp 126-132.

13. Morris DD *et al*: Therapy in two cases of neonatal foal septicaemia and meningitis with cefotaxime sodium. *Equine Vet J* 19:151-154, 1987.

14. Leitch M: Musculoskeletal disorders in neonatal foals. *Vet Clin No Am* (Large Anim Pract) 1:180-209, 1985.

15. Thomas KW and Pemberton DH: A freeze-thaw method for concentrating plasma and serum for treatment of hypogammaglobulinaemia. *Aust J Exp Biol Med Sci* 58:133-142, 1980.

16. Kelman GR: *Applied Cardiovascular Physiology*. 2nd ed. Butterworth, London, 1977.

17. Rose RJ and Leadon DP: Severe metabolic acidosis manifested as failure to adapt in a newborn thoroughbred foal. *Equine Vet J* 15:177-179, 1983.

18. Becht JL and Gordon BJ, in Robinson NE: *Current Therapy in Equine Practice*. 2nd ed. Saunders, Philadelphia, 1986.

19. Bone RC *et al*: A controlled clinical trial of high-dose methylprednisolone in the treatment of severe sepsis and septic shock. *N Eng J Med* 317:653-658, 1987.

20. McClure JR *et al*: Disseminated intravascular coagulation in ponies with surgically induced strangulation obstruction of the small intestine. *Vet Surgery* 8:78-83, 1982.

21. Meyers K *et al*: Circulating endotoxin-like substance(s) and altered hemostasis in horses with gastrointestinal disorders: an interim report. *Am J Vet Res* 43:2233-2238, 1982.

22. Morris DD and Beech J: Disseminated intravascular coagulation in six horses. *JAVMA* 183:1067-1072, 1983.

23. Pablo LS *et al*: Disseminated intravascular coagulation in experimental intestinal strangulation obstruction in ponies. *Am J Vet Res* 44:2115-2122, 1983.

24. Johnstone IB and Blackwell TE: Disseminated intravascular coagulation in a horse with postpartum ulcerative colitis and laminitis. *Can Vet J* 25:195-198, 1984.

25. Johnstone IB and Crane S: Hemostatic abnormalities in equine colic. *Am J Vet Res* 47:356-358, 1986.

26. Johnstone IB *et al*: Early detection and successful reversal of disseminated intravascular coagulation in a Thoroughbred mare presented with a history of diarrhoea and colic. *Equine Vet J* 18:337-340, 1986.

27. Ruehl W *et al*: Rational therapy in disseminated intravascular coagulation. *JAVMA* 181:76-78, 1982.

28. Sullivan M and Snow DH: Factors affecting absorption of non-steroidal anti-inflammatory agents in the horse. *Vet Record* 110:554-558, 1982.

Additional Reading

Septicemia

Becht JL and Semrad SD: Hematology, blood typing and immunology of the neonatal foal. *Vet Clin No Am* (Large Anim Pract) 1:91-116, 1985.

Carlson GP: Fluid therapy in horses with acute diarrhea. *Vet Clin No Am* (Large Anim Pract) 1:313-329, 1979.

Carter PL *et al*: A haemolytic variant of *Actinobacillus equuli* causing an acute septicaemia in a foal. *N Zeal Vet J* 19:264-265, 1971.

Dickie CW and Regnier JO: Equine myositis and septicaemia caused by *Acinetobacter calcoaceticus* infection. *JAVMA* 172:357-359, 1978.

Harris MC and Polin RA: Neonatal septicaemia. *Pediat Clin No Am* 30:243-258, 1983.

Koterba A: Prevention and control of infection. *Vet Clin No Am (Large Animal Pract)* 1:41-50, 1985.

Koterba A: Neonatal infection. *Proc 9th Bain-Fallon Memorial Lectures,* Australian Equine Vet Assn, 1987. pp 164-170.

Koterba A: Immunity in the neonatal foal and failure of passive transfer. *Proc 9th Bain-Fallon Memorial Lectures,* Australian Equine Vet Assn, 1987. pp 171-175.

Liu IKM: Management and treatment of selected conditions in newborn foals. *JAVMA* 176:1247-1249, 1980.

McClure JJ *et al*: Immunodeficieny manifested by oral candidiasis and bacterial septicemia in foals. *JAVMA* 186:1195-1197, 1985.

Pemberton DH and Thomas KW: Hypogamma-globulinaemia in foals: prevalence on Victorian studs and simple methods for detection and correction in the field. *Aust Vet J* 56:469-473, 1980.

Rooney JR: Joint-ill. *JAVMA* 141:1259-1268, 1962.

Van Pelt RW and Riley WF: Clinicopathologic findings and therapy in septic arthritis in foals. *JAVMA* 155:1467-1480, 1969.

Yelle MT: Clinical aspects of *Streptococcus equi* infection. *Equine Vet J* 19:158-162, 1987.

Shock

Bottoms GD *et al*: Endotoxic-induced hemodynamic changes in ponies: effects of flunixin meglumine. *Am J Vet Res* 42:1514-1518, 1981.

Brigham KL *et al*: Methylprednisolone prevention of increased lung vascular permeability following endotoxemia in sheep. *J Clin Invest* 67:1103-1110, 1981.

Dunkle NJ *et al*: Effects of flunixin meglumine on blood pressure and fluid compartment volume changes in ponies given endotoxin. *Am J Vet Res* 46:1540-1544, 1985.

Hunt JM *et al*: Incidence, diagnosis and treatment of postoperative complications in colic cases. *Equine Vet J* 18:264-270, 1986.

Meagher DM: Clinical evaluation and management of shock in the equine patient. *Vet Clin No Am* 6:245-255, 1976.

Moore JN and White NA: Acute abdominal disease: pathophysiology and perioperative management. *Vet Clin No Am* (Large Anim Pract) 4:61-78, 1982.

Morris DD *et al*: Endotoxemia in horses: protection provided by antiserum to core lipopolysaccharide. *Am J Vet Res* 47:544-550, 1986.

Rooney JR *et al*: Exhaustion shock in the horse. *Cornell Vet* 56:220-235, 1966.

Schoeb TR and Panciera RJ: Blister beetle poisoning in horses. *JAVMA* 173:75-77, 1978.

Smith BP: Understanding the role of endotoxins in Gram-negative septicemia. *Vet Med* 81:1148-1161, 1986.

Todd TR *et al*: Pulmonary capillary permeability during hemorrhagic shock. *J Appl Physiol* 45:298-306, 1978.

Veterans Administration Systemic Septis Cooperative Study Group: Effect of high-dose glucocorticoid therapy on mortality in patients with clinical signs of systemic sepsis. *N Eng J Med* 317:659-665, 1987.

Weld JM *et al*: The effects of naloxone on endotoxic and hemorrhagic shock in horses. *Res Commun Chem Pathol Pharmacol* 44:227-238, 1984.

Whitlock RH: Colitis: differential diagnosis and treatment. *Equine Vet J* 18:278-283, 1986.

5 Diseases of the Cardiovascular System

P.W. Physick-Sheard

DETAILED EXAMINATION OF THE CARDIOVASCULAR SYSTEM

P.W. Physick-Sheard

There is a tendency to look upon the heart as the center of activity when considering the cardiovascular system, with the blood vessels a secondary set of conduits. However, the heart is simply a pump, though an extremely important and complex one. In a vessel-centered view of cardiovascular function, blood vessels are seen as primary determinants of system behavior.[1] For the clinician, the important consideration is that system evaluation cannot proceed without a thorough evaluation of both components. Too often, a cardiovascular examination is limited to auscultation of the heart, and many important clinical signs are missed. In this chapter, both parts of the system are emphasized.

Much of the material upon which interpretation of cardiovascular signs in the horse is based tends to be subjective, representing opinion rather than scientific fact. Some of this opinion is accurate, while other observations may be open to question. Some of the original studies on the relationship between cardiovascular function in the horse and clinical manifestations must be repeated using new methods of monitoring physiologic values. Excellent original work has been contributed by various investigators. However, much of what is presented below represents opinion based upon limited studies. Reference occasionally is made to the human literature to amplify observations and to provide access to some of the work upon which many of our current veterinary interpretations depend.

When reviewing cardiovascular problems in the horse, 3 fundamental considerations must be kept in mind. First, cardiovascular disease can be primary or secondary; problems can originate in the cardiovascular system or may be secondary to systemic disease or disease in other body systems. All disorders with systemic components and all disorders of the respiratory system and blood impose an increased load on the heart by increasing functional demands and directly compromising cardiovascular function. Thus, the heart must work at an increased level under adverse circumstances. Sometimes the consequence is permanent damage, especially if a horse is worked while subclinically diseased.

Second, the horse is first and foremost an athlete, and insults to the cardiovascular system in general, and the heart in particular, have the potential to reduce functional capacity. It is the functional and dimensional capacity of the cardiovascular system that makes the greatest contribution to the superlative capacity for work in the horse.[2,3] Thus, in clinical examination, all deviations from normal can be clinically significant. The implications of any abnormality, in part, depend upon the use to which the animal is put.

Third, because the horse has exceptional cardiovascular reserve, disease usually must be severe before clinical signs become evident at rest. Mild damage is not always functionally evident unless the animal is asked for a measured maximal effort. The clinician may be lulled into a false sense of security when considering the implications of cardiovascular disorders.

Primary cardiovascular disease, such as congenital heart diseases, acquired valvular disease or aorto-iliac thrombosis, is characteristically difficult to treat and, especially in the case of the heart itself, often represents a permanent disability. The major contribution made by the clinician in such cases is early definition of the problem and prognosticating to allow rational career and financial management. While secondary cardiovascular disease, such as toxic myocardial degeneration, can represent a major diagnostic and therapeutic challenge, in this type of abnormality the clinician can make the greatest therapeutic contribution by minimizing damage and optimizing the chances that the horse will have the opportunity to express its true genetic potential.

Whether primary or secondary, the major difficulty facing the clinician is determination of the clinical significance of an observation. The size and rate of contraction of the equine heart and other physical factors, such as the relationship between blood viscosity and vessel diameter, together with a propensity toward apparently benign variations in rate and rhythm, present the clinician with a bewildering array of signs. Current definitions of normality are inadequate. The problem is compounded by great variation in the physical effort required of different types and breeds of horse and by the multiplicity of factors influencing the outcome of performance events, even within a defined performance category. Interpretation and the proffering of advice are further complicated by a lack of information on the natural history of most cardiovascular diseases in the horse.

The increasing use of treadmills in measurement of functional capacity and advancement in the application of diagnostic ultrasound provide very promising options that probably will not be available to most general practitioners for some time. Accumulation of large volumes of clinical data contributes little in the absence of benchmark standards for definition and diagnosis of clinical entities. However, experimental studies quantifying the effects of standard-ized insults, together with increased use of noninvasive methods for routine monitoring and definition of natural history in spontaneously occurring disease supplement the clinician's judgment with objective data. In the interim, the equine clinician can use a wide range of techniques, starting with careful and detailed clinical examination, to detect abnormality and evaluate the potential for compromised function.

Reasons for Examination

Reasons for performing a detailed examination of the cardiovascular system include a history or clinical signs suggestive of cardiovascular insufficiency (see below) or detection on general physical examination of a discrete cardiovascular abnormality, such as a murmur or pulse deficit. Examination also may be indicated during the course of severe systemic illness, such as colitis with its associated fluid, acid-base and electrolyte disorders. Thorough evaluation of cardiovascular function is indicated in cases of syncope, unsteadiness during exercise, suboptimal performance, limited exercise tolerance, abnormally low or fast heart rate or any abnormal cardiovascular finding detected on routine physical examination. If routine physical examination does not pay sufficient attention to the cardiovascular system, many problems will be missed. Careful palpation of pulses and auscultation of the heart on both sides of the thorax are essential.

Cardiovascular Anatomy and Physiology

A thorough knowledge and understanding of normal anatomy and physiology and an awareness of gross and histologic pathology are fundamental to objective examination and appropriate interpretation of findings in any body system. Specific pathologic findings will be reviewed during discussion of relevant conditions. General observations on cardiovascular pathology will be made during discussion of clinical examination. While the reader is referred to anatomy and physiology texts for detailed discussion, some features of equine cardiovascular form and function must be examined here if accurate description and correct interpretation of cardiovascular abnormality are to be achieved. Further discussion of anatomy is found below under Auscultation.

The heart of the horse constitutes 0.7-1.1% of body weight and is absolutely larger in the racehorse than in other breeds.[4,5] Because of the heart's size, large stroke volume and low rate of contraction and because of the shape of the thorax, cardiac activity is easily detected by inspection, palpation and auscultation. This accessibility is compromised only by the close apposition of the forelimb to the thorax (see below).

The relationship of the heart to the chest wall, diaphragm and lungs is shown diagrammatically in Figures 1 and 2. Diagrammatic representations of the heart and its internal structure are presented in Figures 3 and 4 (also see Figures 50 and 51, presented with the discussion of Congenital Heart Disease). Though the 2 sides of the heart are functionally described as right and left, they might be described more accurately topographically as cranial and caudal, in that the right ventricle lies cranial to the left. The ventricular septum thus runs obliquely from the left side of the thorax to the right (Figs 2, 4).

The heart also lies slightly to the left of midline; the area contacting the left thoracic wall is much greater than that contacting the right. On the left, both ventricular

Figure 2. Frontal section of the equine thorax at a level just ventral to the shoulder joint and viewed from above (dorsal to ventral). Note the large area of contact between the heart and chest wall on the left as compared with the right. Note also the large area of cardiac auscultation covered by the muscles of the forelimb. (See horizontal line in Figure 1 for level of section).

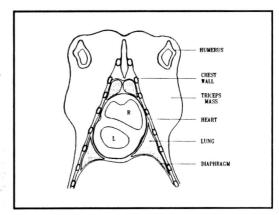

chambers contact the thoracic wall. The area of contact is from the third rib to the fifth intercostal space/sixth rib. On the right, only the right ventricle touches the wall; the contact area is from the third to the fourth intercostal space. Contact with the chest wall extends approximately 10-12 cm or one-quarter to one-third the way up the thoracic cavity on the left and one-quarter to one third of the way up on the right.

Figure 1. Relationship between the ribs, heart, diaphragm and lungs viewed from the right and left sides. The jugular vein is also included to indicate its relationship to the base of the heart. The horizontal line shows the level taken for the section shown in Figure 2.

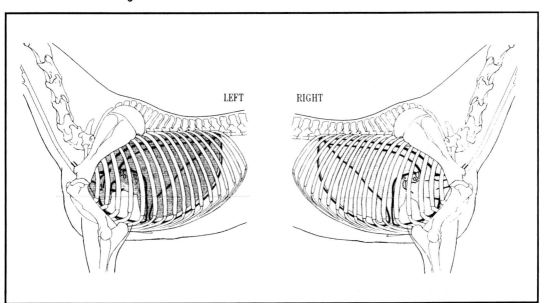

The heart may be said to radiographically span 5 ribs and 4 intercostal spaces, which is the perspective gained if the cardiac silhouette is projected to the body surface (see further discussion under Auscultation).

Dorsoventrally, the apex of the heart lies close to the sternum, just dorsal to the level of the point of the elbow. The heart occupies about one-half of the dorsoventral dimension of the thoracic cavity though, when the great vessels are considered, this proportion seems more like two-thirds (Fig 1). These features of anatomy, plus the fact that the cardiac notch in the left lung is much larger than on the right, mean that, for palpation and auscultation, most information can be derived on the left side. The function of all 4 valves can be monitored from the left, including the right atrioventricular valve. It should be noted that the pulmonic valve is closer to the left chest wall than is the aortic valve (Fig 4).

While of importance in the evaluation of all clinical conditions, these features of anatomy take on particular importance in the evaluation of congenital cardiac disease. To fully appreciate thoracic topography and the structure of the heart, the clinician is strongly encouraged to take every opportunity to examine these anatomic features closely during routine postmortem examination.

The basic features of the equine cardiac cycle are shown in Figure 5. The critical importance of fully understanding the events represented in this diagram cannot be overemphasized. Most misconceptions in clinical interpretation stem either from an incomplete understanding of topographic anatomy or from a failure to fully understand the events of the cardiac cycle. Particularly close attention should be paid to the relationship between pressure changes and heart sounds, the contour of the pulse wave as represented by pressure changes in the aorta, and the differences between systole and diastole. These terms refer to the *mechanical* or pressure events of the cardiac cycle, as opposed to the *electrical* events. Ventricular systole starts with the first heart sound, S_1, and terminates with the onset of the second sound, S_2 (Fig 5). These sounds roughly coincide with closure of the atrioventricular valves (S_1) and the semilunar valves (S_2, see discussion of Heart Sounds below).

An understanding of pressure changes in the right atrium and cranial vena cava also is essential if pulsation in the jugular veins is to be interpreted correctly. Reference should be made to this diagram during discussion of clinical examination and evaluation of abnormalities of cardiac rhythm and valve function.

Figure 3. Views of the heart from the right (R) and the left (L). The profiles are those presented to the chest wall *in situ*. The lines B-B, C-C and D-D indicate the planes for the sections shown in Figures 4b, 4c and 4d, respectively.

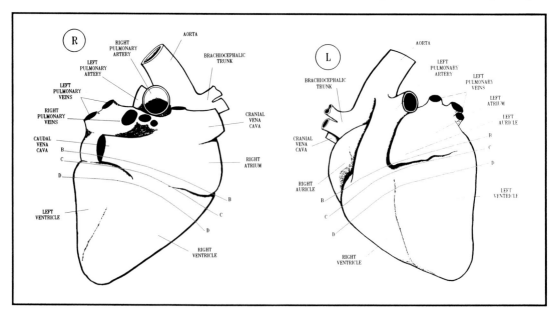

Figure 4. A view of the base of the heart (a) and 3 views as successive layers are dissected away (b, c, d). All views survey the heart from above (cranial to caudal) with the planes of the sections about parallel to the heart base. The top of each view is thus cranial, with the left to the left. In (a) only the pericardium and excess fat have been removed. The orientation of the great vessels and atria is clear. In (b) the aorta and pulmonary artery have been trimmed to a level just cranial to the valves, and the atria have been removed just cranial to their base, as per the line B-B in Figure 3. The central position of the aortic valve and the proximity of the pulmonic valve to the left side are clear. Note that the valves do not all lie in the same plane. In (c) a curved section has been taken through the base of the ventricular chambers (C-C in Figure 3) so as to remove the valves but preserve the ridge of muscle, the crista supraventricularis, which divides the inflow and outflow tracts of the right ventricle. The interventricular septum is relatively thin to the right immediately beneath the aortic valve. Section (d) (D-D in Figure 3) is taken about 2 cm below (c) and shows the ventricular chambers and the orientation of the interventricular septum, which runs obliquely across the thorax.

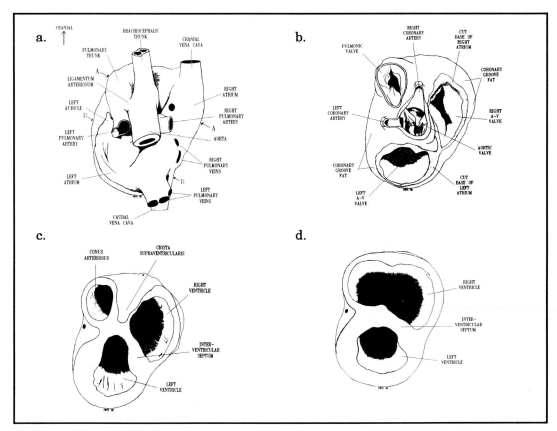

Cardiovascular Examination

In examination of the cardiovascular system, the clinician is tempted or pressured to reach for diagnostic aids to arrive at a clinical interpretation and course of action. However, the most valuable aids to clinical diagnosis are the results of a thorough clinical examination interpreted in the light of knowledge and experience. While such aids as laboratory studies, electrocardiography, echocardiography and an exercise test can be very informative and often essential parts of an in-depth cardiovascular examination, they should be applied only after the clinical examination and interpreted in the light of clinical findings and history.

A detailed examination of the cardiovascular system starts with a review of the history. Inspection, palpation and auscultation are then carried out, followed by examination of the respiratory system, application of special techniques (*eg*, electrocardiography, echocardiography) and laboratory estimations and, in appropriate cases, an exercise test. This approach has the advantage of ensuring completeness and consistency and of avoiding the grave error of rushing for the stethoscope at the beginning. Dogmatic adherence to this sequence is not nec-

Figure 5. Basic features of the cardiac cycle. Special attention should be paid to the temporal relationship of electrical, pressure and sound events. The vertical lines mark the beginning and end of ventricular systole. A = aorta. LA = left atrium. LV = left ventricle. PA = pulmonary artery. RV = right ventricle. RA = right atrium. P = phonocardiogram. ACS = atrial contraction sound.

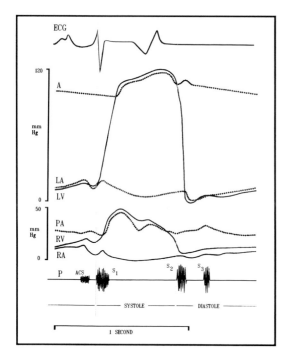

after a period of rest. Current performance should be assessed and plateaus or evidence of deterioration in performance defined. Congenital abnormalities overlooked in the neonatal period may be associated with consistently suboptimal performance; their detection in a racing animal may not necessarily provide an etiologic reason for recent deterioration.

With racehorses, race records can be of tremendous help in interpreting the significance of clinical findings, especially for horses that perform frequently, such as the Standardbred. The clinician may detect a pattern that puts the clinical problem into context and helps explain its contribution to suboptimal performance. Of particular importance is the patient's success in relation to peers of equivalent talent, allowing performance to be examined in relation to season. In animals with chronic and not necessarily progressive cardiac disease, deterioration in performance may in fact be only relative. The cardiac problem may have "capped" the animal's ability to respond to the progressive training effect of competition.

The current training or exercise program and the horse's response to this work should be discussed with the owner/trainer. Questions are aimed at obtaining an overview of the animal, the standards of training applied, and whether the training program has been appropriate for the work expected. Exercise history, and thus level of athletic condition, can affect cardiovascular function, such as strength and quality of cardiac impulse and resting heart rate. Correct application of an exercise test depends upon knowledge of the animal's level of fitness.

Periods of rest should be viewed especially critically because, as mentioned above, clinical signs sometimes are manifested on return to training, while periods of rest may modify clinical signs. Owners and trainers must be encouraged to present animals for examination as soon as a problem is recognized, while the horse is still in condition, rather than after a period of letdown.

Clinical History: Previous disease may have a bearing upon current problems, especially if the episode had severe systemic consequences and/or led to a period of rest. Similarly, previous problems the trainer or owner believes are no longer pertinent may

essary, however, and some overlap is desirable to avoid returning to the same anatomic region repeatedly. Aspects of inspection and palpation are thus combined below.

History

A review of the history must include analysis of exercise/training regimes, consideration of previous clinical problems and general management, and consideration of the history of the presenting clinical problem and other current clinical problems.

Exercise History: Suboptimal performance is a common reason for cardiovascular examination. It is therefore useful to know at what age the animal started training and how long it has been in consistent work since then. In the case of a performance horse, it is helpful to know the animal's best performance time, when and under what circumstances this was achieved, and when and for how long it was last off work. For instance, clinical signs of aorto-iliac thrombosis often become obvious

have considerable bearing on current signs of cardiovascular disease. As an example, recurrent episodes of tying-up as a 2-year-old could be associated with myocardial fibrosis, reduced performance and an increased incidence of arrhythmias.

General Management: Review of general management other than training can be helpful, especially if the onset of clinical signs was coincident with management change, such as putting an animal with marginal reserve into a pasture with a new group of dominant horses. Nutritional history can be invaluable, particularly in the investigation of myocardial degeneration possibly associated with intoxication or nutritional deficiency. A change of environment, trainer or use may have a bearing on the clinical picture.

History of Presenting Problem: The history of the presenting complaint should include a discussion of all clinical signs and circumstances of occurrence. The clinician should cautiously cross-examine clients to determine the accuracy with which they use terminology. In the minds of many horse owners and trainers, any episode of unsteadiness, stumbling or collapse automatically is associated with the heart, yet cardiac problems are an infrequently documented cause of such events. In cases of suboptimal performance, it is necessary to determine whether a problem really exists or whether the real issue is one of unreasonable expectation.

Where a discrete (as opposed to a chronic, progressive) problem has occurred in an animal during maximal exercise, such as a racehorse, review should include details of the clinical episode and of the event during which it occurred. The speed of a race, point at which signs were seen, track conditions, environmental temperature and humidity, and the animal's apparent mental status may help define the problem. A review of environmental circumstances is useful in animals showing signs of possible cardiovascular dysfunction at rest. For example, in an animal experiencing tachyarrhythmia or bradyarrhythmia, syncope often occurs during the excitement just before feeding time. Any medication the horse has been receiving should be noted, as this may relate to the onset of clinical signs or may modify the signs observed.

Inspection and Palpation

Age, Attitude, Condition: Age, breed, sex, apparent degree of fitness, muscling and muscle tone should be noted. Age provides guidance in evaluation of congenital as opposed to acquired conditions, especially in interpreting valvular dysfunction. Breed may be of relevance in congenital cardiac diseases, while there is a sex predisposition in some diseases. Attention is paid to body cover as this relates to both stage of training and the prominence of some signs of cardiovascular function. For example, heavy body cover reduces the intensity of heart sounds. Degree of alertness must be assessed, as arousal and possibly adrenaline release may have far-reaching effects on cardiovascular function. The extent to which there is agreement between the animal's appearance and the history provided by the owner determines the quality of the history and allows the clinical findings to be interpreted more accurately.

Thoracic Conformation: Thoracic conformation and the "set" or position of the forelimb on the chest can affect findings during examination. For example, Thoroughbreds tend to have a deep but relatively narrow thorax but have a large heart in relation to body weight. These factors, together with temperament and usual level of fitness, make cardiac activity very obvious during auscultation and palpation. Because heavy horses have a very wide thorax and a relatively small cardiac weight, heart sounds are generally quiet and the cardiac impulse may not be easily detected.

In some breeds, especially Standardbreds, the forelimbs are positioned well forward on the thorax, changing the relationship between the point of the elbow and the ribs. Because this relationship is used frequently in cardiovascular assessment (such as area of cardiac dullness, location of apex beat), this conformational feature must be noted.

Respiratory Function: Respiratory rate and pattern should be observed, especially for evidence of increased inspiratory or expiratory effort, reduced depth of respiration or asymmetry. Abnormal observations should prompt a detailed examination, as respiratory problems can have a marked effect upon cardiovascular signs and function (see also Pulmonary Edema below).

Edema: Edema may be caused by increased capillary hydrostatic pressure, capillary damage, lymphatic obstruction or decreased colloid osmotic pressure. Edema often is described as pitting or nonpitting. Essentially, all edema "pits"; that is, firm digital pressure leaves an indentation that may take several minutes to disappear. Edema fails to pit only if it has been present for considerable time and the tissues have undergone induration and fibrous organization, at which stage it is questionable whether edema is even the correct term to use. Edema may be passive, as in cardiovascular disease, in which it is cool and nonpainful, or inflammatory, in which it is hot and painful. Passive edema almost invariably is dependent because of the contribution of gravity to local hydrostatic pressure and because of the tendency for free tissue fluid to gravitate through tissue spaces. It must be remembered that clinical examination usually reveals only the involvement of subcutaneous tissues.

Increased capillary hydrostatic pressure is an unusual cause of edema in horses but it does occur in right heart failure and venous obstruction. The latter sometimes is seen, but congestive heart failure is relatively uncommon (see below). Edema is unlikely to be seen with primary atrioventricular valvular insufficiency unless generalized myocardial failure follows, as may occur when insufficiency is sudden and severe.

Edema due to capillary damage is more common, occurring along with damage to larger vessels in the course of systemic viral disease, such as equine viral arteritis, or in some autoimmune problems. It is stretching the point, however, to suggest that local edema due to inflammation is cardiovascular in origin, as the primary insult lies outside the cardiovascular system. During systemic states, such as endotoxemia, in which a generalized increase in capillary permeability may be anticipated, gross clinical edema does not occur often, though this factor probably does contribute to the edema seen with hypoproteinemia in, for example, severe colitis.

Inspection for edema should be supplemented by palpation. A thin plaque on the ventrum can be missed easily. If severe generalized edema is observed, the primary differential diagnosis should be hypoproteinemia rather than heart failure. Symmetric edema of the limbs, especially the hind limbs, should suggest inactivity, possible overfeeding or chronic trauma. This distribution of edema is an infrequent primary sign in congestive heart failure.

Attention should be paid to regional distribution. In cases of venous obstruction, edema occurs in the drainage area of the obstructed vessel. A common observation is ventral edema in the heavily pregnant mare. Tension on the abdominal wall presumably interferes with local venous drainage, promoting fluid accumulation. Mammary development and increased local blood flow are probable contributing factors. An equally common example of venous obstruction, sometimes resulting in edema of the head, is bilateral iatrogenic jugular thrombosis.

Heart-base and mediastinal masses can selectively obstruct the cranial or caudal vena cava, with resultant cranial or caudal distribution of edema. In contrast to the infrequent case of congestive heart failure, in which limb involvement is uncommon, horses with thoracic masses frequently show swelling of the forelimbs. Distribution of edema thus can be of great diagnostic significance. Immediate signs of obstruction of regional veins may later become obscured by the swelling. Severity of swelling and clinical consequences reflect both the speed of onset and the extent of the obstruction. Severe swelling of 1 limb is most likely to reflect inflammatory disease of the lymphatics, especially if of sudden onset and associated with lameness, heat and pain. This is the most massive and rapidly developing form of edema that is encountered commonly.

Pulmonary Edema: A special case of edema and of special relevance to cardiovascular function is pulmonary edema. This accumulation of fluid in the interstitium of the lung can occur as a result of primary left heart failure (an infrequent occurrence in the horse) or left atrioventricular insufficiency. Pulmonary edema rarely is seen in the latter condition, however, unless the valve dysfunction is severe or sudden in onset, as pulmonary lymphatic drainage can accommodate considerable increases in tissue fluid production resulting from increased capillary hydrostatic pressure.[1] Severe arrhythmias also may be a cause of pulmonary edema. Without very obvious cardiac disease, an extracardiac cause of the edema should be sought.

Jugular Veins and Thoracic Inlet: Confusion with regard to interpretation of events occurring visibly at the thoracic inlet and in the jugular veins stems partly from inadequate understanding of anatomy and physiology and partly from inaccurate terminology. It may be best to describe precisely what is seen rather than attempt to apply such terms as "true jugular pulse," the precise meaning of which may not be fully agreed upon. Clinically significant abnormalities of this aspect of cardiovascular function are common, as are misinterpretations of resulting signs. Manifestations of cardiac function in this region in particular, and in the venous system in general, are among the most useful to the clinician in detecting and interpreting cardiovascular dysfunction. It is thus worthwhile to take a few moments to study the factors that influence jugular vein function.

Anatomically, the right atrium is level with the ventral half of the thoracic inlet, approximately level with the point of the shoulder. Thus, most of the jugular vein lies above the level of the right atrium. Pressure in the equine right atrium ranges from -4 to +12 mm Hg during each cardiac cycle, being lowest during ventricular ejection and early diastole and highest during atrial contraction (Fig 6).[6,7] Mean right atrial pressure is 0-4 mm Hg. Bearing in mind the density of blood, peak atrial pressure would be sufficient to support a column of blood about 15 cm high. This can be regarded as the maximum, normal, transient degree of filling one might reasonably expect to see reflected in the jugular veins. Through most of the cardiac cycle, however, pressure is much lower, and filling of the vein is not evident. Above the level of the heart base, gravity collapses the veins. Conversely, pressure in veins below the level of the heart base always is positive.

If the head is lowered below the level of the thoracic inlet, gravity acts against venous return. The veins fill distally until the filling reaches the level of the right atrium, when return from the head to the right heart is reestablished. This occurs within 1 or 2 beats in the normal animal.

Venous return is achieved only to a very limited degree by hydrostatic pressure in the venous system.[1] Most of the energy for venous return comes from the pumping action of skeletal muscles contracting around the veins, which are equipped with a one-way valve system, from the pumping action of the thorax during ventilatory excursion, and from the pumping action of the heart, in which pressure in the right ventricle often falls transiently below zero during ventricular systole. The overall effect of this activity is to both push and pull blood back to the right heart. With normal cardiac function, blood is removed from the great veins at the right atrium as fast as it is presented and the jugular veins appear to be empty most of the time.

The thoracic inlet and proximal jugular veins are not totally devoid of activity. While there are valves in some parts of the jugular veins, there are none between the cranial vena cava, into which the veins drain, and the right atrium. It should be anticipated, therefore, that some of the activity in the right heart will be visible at the thoracic inlet. In fact, in the normal horse with the head erect, cardiac activity often is detectable in the jugular veins by a slow filling during late diastole that passes a maximum of 8-10 cm up the jugular furrow. Sometimes only pulsation at the thoracic inlet is visible, depending on thoracic conformation.

For obvious waves or pulses to be seen in the jugular groove, the veins must be distended to some degree. It is important to remember that *distention* is the primary abnormality when pulsation is seen in the jugular groove, not the pulsation itself. Pulsation is a secondary consequence of filling and could be due to activity of the underlying carotid artery, changes in pressure in the thorax with ventilation, or abnormal cardiac activity. If the jugular veins are collapsed, there is no medium in the jugular groove through which carotid activity or intrathoracic pressure changes can be referred, and no pulsation. Conversely, if the veins are relatively full, even normal cardiac activity results in obvious pulsation in the column of blood they contain.

The following description of movement at the base of the neck is based upon personal observation and upon measurement of jugular and atrial pressure profiles.[6-8] Three waveforms can be seen at the thoracic inlet/lower jugular vein, and only 1 is usually obvious (Fig 6). More complex descriptions found in the literature relate to pressure profiles in the right atrium and describe waveforms *not* visibly transmitted to the jugular veins.

The most obvious wave at the thoracic inlet in the normal horse is a long, slow, filling wave (Fig 6) that may pass 5-8 cm up the jugular veins. This occurs at the end of rapid ventricular filling, the first event in diastole. The wave results when the sudden and rapid flow of blood into the ventricles is checked as the chambers become full and recoil, causing blood to back up into the cranial vena cava and the jugular veins. This is followed by a slight, superimposed, positive wave in the veins at the time of atrial contraction (Fig 6). Shortly afterward, ventricular systole occurs. An early slight positive wave *may* be seen at this point as the right atrioventricular valve bulges transiently into the atrium, but the major effect of ventricular systole is a negative wave or emptying of the jugular veins as the base of the heart moves ventrally, transiently increasing the volume of the right atrium. As this is followed immediately by rapid ventricular filling, the vein empties completely, with the next waveform being the aforementioned slow jugular filling wave at the end of rapid ventricular filling of the next cycle.

The jugular veins should be examined with the horse's head in a normal, erect position. The veins first should be inspected for extent and symmetry of any fluid movement. Thrombosis may be visible but digital palpation of both veins is recommended to detect and quantify any scarring or obstruction. Lack of symmetry may be the first indication of abnormality. Each vein should be obstructed individually at the base of the neck and filling observed. The time taken for filling may provide some indication of rate of venous return, relative blood volume and blood supply to the tissues drained by the jugular veins. Filling normally takes 6-10 seconds with compression of only 1 vein. When compression is removed, the vein collapses immediately as blood returns to the right heart, usually within 1 cardiac cycle in the normal animal.

If the veins are abnormally full, they should each in turn be obstructed halfway up the neck and the blood in the caudal portion milked with the hand toward the heart to empty the vein. Significance may be attached to any tendency of the vein to refill

Figure 6. ECG and simultaneous pressure profiles from the jugular vein just cranial to the thoracic inlet, from the right atrium, right ventricle and proximal pulmonary artery. Note that in the jugular vein, the atrial and ventricular contraction waves, which are very clear in the right atrial and ventricular pressure signals, have become greatly attenuated. The pressure changes visible reflect mainly slow diastolic filling of the jugular vein (1), with atrial contraction (2) terminating this phase, followed by rapid emptying (3). This last phase reflects, in sequence, subsidence of atrial contraction, increased volume of the atria as the base of the heart moves ventrally during ventricular systole and rapid ventricular filling in early diastole. Note that the lowest pressures in the right atrium and jugular vein occur during the second half of right ventricular systole and during early diastole.

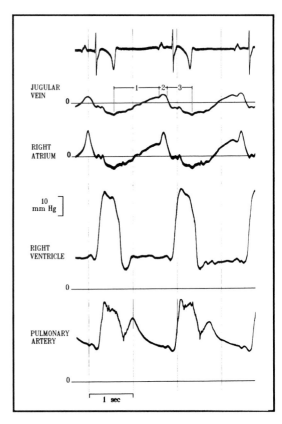

and to the manner in which it does so (see below). Any abnormality detected in jugular vein function should be correlated with the condition of other veins in the body, comparing especially the front and rear end of the animal. Interpretation may be aided by simultaneous observation of the thoracic inlet and auscultation of the heart.

Jugular filling may be persistent or intermittent. Causes of persistent filling are many, but all result from obstruction to venous return (*eg*, intrathoracic mass, severe right atrioventricular endocarditis causing stenosis and insufficiency, pericardial effusion) or elevation of central venous pressure, as with right heart failure or iatrogenic volume overload.

Specific causes of persistent jugular filling cannot be determined by examination of the jugular veins alone; accompanying signs must be taken into account in interpreting findings. For example, intrathoracic obstruction of the cranial vena cava may cause the veins to fill to the point that they do not pulsate. This affects cranial rather than caudal venous drainage. In cases of severely distended, nonpulsatile jugular veins, an intrathoracic mass and pericardial effusion should be the primary differential diagnoses. Elevation of heart rate may be anticipated. Similar venous engorgement and severe tachycardia (>100 bpm at rest) may be seen in advanced congestive heart failure but this problem is uncommon in horses (see below). Significant jugular filling with a normal heart rate and sinus rhythm can occur in association with masses in the thoracic inlet, such as lymphoma, as opposed to those at the heart base. Some respiratory difficulty and possibly dysphagia may be expected in such cases.

In some cases of right atrioventricular insufficiency, an abnormality traditionally described as a "true" jugular pulse may be seen. This terminology is mentioned for the sake of completeness, but it is of questionable value. In right atrioventricular insufficiency, ventricular systole results in regurgitant flow of blood into the right atrium. When and only when this flow is large, pressure may rise sufficiently in the jugular veins to cause filling, with an obvious wave during ventricular systole. If the vein is held off midway up the neck, and the blood in the caudal vein is milked out toward the heart, the vein refills in a *pulsatile* fashion. This "true" jugular pulse confirms (presumably in the presence of a murmur) right atrioventricular insufficiency or regurgitation.

The clinician should be cautious, however, in making this interpretation. First, mild or even moderate insufficiency may not give this result, and in my experience, the sign is uncommon. Where pulsatile refill does occur, it usually reflects either insufficiency accompanying right heart failure, in which case central venous pressure already

is very high, or combined insufficiency and stenosis of the right atrioventricular valve, as may occur in valvular endocarditis. In such cases, venous return is obstructed. Second, the vein also may refill after emptying when central venous pressure is very high but valve function is normal (eg, intrathoracic mass, right heart failure, pericardial effusion). This is especially likely if venous distention has been severe and chronic, and the valves within the jugular veins have become incompetent.

In some cases, the jugular veins manifest intermittent filling or filling that varies from beat to beat. This usually is an indication of arrhythmia, though the sign may be seen in respiratory disease. Differentiation is easily achieved by noting the relationship between the filling wave and respiration. In the simplest and most common example, second-degree atrioventricular block, atrial contraction is not followed by ventricular systole (see below under Arrhythmia). The missed ventricular contraction leads to accumulation of blood in the great veins, as the right ventricle is full. This filling disappears spontaneously as the heart fills after the next cardiac cycle. Similarly, any period of severe bradyarrhythmia or tachyarrhythmia may be associated with temporary filling of the jugular veins as a consequence of reduced cardiac output.

A similar but much more clinically significant observation is made in atrioventricular dissociation, in which the atria and ventricles beat independently. Occasionally the atria contract while the ventricles are in systole and the atrioventricular valves are closed. On the right side of the circulation, this results in reflux of blood into the great veins, seen in the jugular veins as sudden filling referred to as a "cannon A-wave." Careful observation of the behavior of the jugular veins assisted by auscultation of the heart thus can allow the approximate definition of arrhythmias.

Other Peripheral Veins: An observation of fullness of the jugular veins should be correlated with observation of all other superficial veins. In a normal performance horse, as well as in a very fit and possibly excited animal, some distention of the cutaneous veins may be seen as a component of thermoregulation, especially during or after exercise. This is largely a consequence of increased skin blood flow. Thoroughbreds also tend to have finer skin and these veins are more obvious. These factors apart, obvious superficial veins other than the dependent veins on the medial aspect of the limbs (*eg,* cephalic and saphenous veins) should be noted as a possible abnormality and subjected to further examination. Regional distention of cutaneous veins may be seen in an area of arteriovenous anastomosis. Such areas may show pulsation on palpation, but fremitus may only be detectable if moderately large arteries and veins are anastomosed.

A common but infrequently referenced cause of venous distention is the physiologic enlargement of a vein draining an area receiving increased arterial blood supply. This should be considered in cases of asymmetric venous distention and may be seen, for instance, in the digital vein in many cases of hoof abscessation or laminitis. Conversely, venous distention may result from prolonged stall rest, with physical inactivity reducing the efficiency of drainage even in the face of normal arterial supply. In such cases, incompetence of the valves in superficial veins contributes to the clinical signs.

At rest, collapse of veins that should normally be distended, such as the cephalic and saphenous veins, is occasionally seen as a result of local vascular injury to the arterial tree and poor blood supply to the limb. This is more likely to be seen in the forelimb, where there is a less extensive collateral circulation. In severe aortic-iliac thrombosis, however, the saphenous veins may be collapsed after light walking exercise.

Palpation of Arterial Pulses: During routine general physical examination, the pulse is evaluated, usually at the facial artery as it crosses the ventral border of the mandible, ventral to the masseter muscle or on the rostral border of the masseter. The transverse facial artery caudoventral to the eye can be a useful site in horses that refuse to stand still. By putting the hand against the horse's cheek and 2 or 3 fingers along the course of the artery, the pulse can be palpated with ease despite movement of the horse's head. The artery runs in a groove at this site and is relatively immobile.

During detailed examination of the cardiovascular system, pulse palpation is repeated and all available superficial arterial sites are palpated. The objective is to clearly define the rate, rhythm and character of the pulse, and evaluate pulse strength and contour. These findings reflect the integrity of the peripheral circulation.

Because of the slow heart rate of most horses and the long, slow, surging pulse, palpation initially can be difficult, especially for those used to achieving more immediate results as with small animals and small ruminants. This problem is compounded by the tendency for horses to occasionally drop beats. Best results are achieved by first locating the artery, then positioning the fingers over it with gentle pressure and waiting for the pulse to arrive. With experience, the clinician can differentiate a weak, arrhythmic pulse from one that seems to periodically disappear but is in fact normal.

After starting at the head, the pulse should be palpated in the carotid and median arteries, the medial palmar arteries (behind the carpus), the medial and lateral digital arteries in all 4 feet, and the median caudal (coccygeal) and saphenous arteries (the saphenous artery lies beneath the leading edge of the saphenous vein on the medial aspect of the hind limb). The dorsal metatarsal artery also can be palpated on the lateral aspect of the hind limb, where it runs obliquely over the proximal end of the cannon bone just distal to the hock.

While palpating the peripheral pulses, perfusion can be assessed by noting the surrounding skin temperature. A palpable pulse in an extremity is not in itself a reliable indication of adequate tissue perfusion, however.

The clinician should be wary of such statements as "the horse has a digital pulse." Careful palpation nearly always reveals a pulse in the digital arteries. The exceptions are immediately after exercise and when the extremities are very cold, as in cold weather. These comments should not cause the clinician to disregard a digital pulse that seems unusually prominent, however. In inflammatory conditions of the foot, such as laminitis, the abnormality of the digital pulse lies in its character, which is very full and strong. It is often described as "bounding" and is thus relatively easy to detect. Increased arterial supply to an extremity usually is associated with some degree of local venous distention and increased heat when inflammation is involved. Asymmetry also can be some guide to abnormality.

Pulse Rate: The pulse rate should be counted for 15 seconds in all animals and for 30-60 seconds if the rate is very low or the heart beat irregular. The normal resting heart rate of the grade and untrained animal ranges from 28 to 40 beats per minute (bpm). Rates as low as 20 bpm may be seen in older, fit performance horses, though this is unusual. In ponies, the resting pulse rate may be as high as 45 bpm; in any adult domestic horse, a resting pulse rate above this should be viewed with suspicion.

It is especially important to critically evaluate situations in which the pulse rate is inconsistent with the overall clinical picture because it may indicate a serious arrhythmia as opposed to a normal sinus rhythm. Not all arrhythmias are manifested as an irregular cardiac rhythm. For example, a normal or low pulse rate may be detected in a dehydrated, weak foal. In this situation, the relative/absolute bradycardia may be precipitated by hyperkalemia or hypoglycemia, and may reflect the severity of the foal's condition.

In horses recovering from colitis, profound tachycardia is occasionally observed despite the fact that the animal has maintained its own hydration and diarrhea is reduced. While sometimes an indication of myocardial disease, this usually is a reflection of electrolyte disturbance, including a severe total body potassium deficit; the associated arrhythmia is a ventricular tachyarrhythmia (Figs 47-49).

Fetal and Maternal Pulse Rate: Most studies have evaluated fetal heart rate from midgestation only. Fetal heart rate progressively falls with advancing gestation.[9-11] However, if discrete observations are taken on numerous different subjects at different times, no correlation with gestational age is determined.[12] This finding reflects the tendency toward transient episodes of tachycardia in the fetus. These episodes, which do not necessarily have any clinical significance and which may reflect movement of the fetus or a response to transient maternal influences, become more frequent as gestation progresses.[13] Fetal heart rates range from 100-150 bpm at 150-160 days of gestation, to 75-105 bpm near term.[10,11]

Though the lowest fetal heart rates are normally recorded immediately before parturition and can be as low as 60-70 bpm, the absolute bradycardia at this stage in other species has not been recorded in horses.[13-15] A heart rate of 68.8 $\pm$ 2.0 bpm has been observed in the first 5 minutes after birth.[15] In that study of Thoroughbred foals, the heart rate rose to 129.8 $\pm$ 6.2 bpm (range 60-200) over the ensuing hour as foals attempted to rise, but decreased to a mean of 95.8 $\pm$ 1.5 bpm over the next 43 hours. There has been surprisingly little research into the rate at which neonatal heart rates fall to adult levels, but clinical experience suggests that normal adult rates are achieved by 4-5 months.

Maternal heart rate increases as pregnancy advances, but the pattern of rise in maternal rate is unclear.[9,10,13] Significant elevation does not occur until the last third of gestation; the increase is greatest in the last month. A maternal heart rate of 60-80 bpm in the last month of pregnancy should be regarded as normal. A rate persistently above this should be cause for concern, as it may indicate circulatory insufficiency or homeostatic disorders related to systemic disease that could have serious implications for normal parturition and viability of the foal.

Pulse Rhythm: Abnormalities of cardiac rhythm can be detected during palpation of the pulse, though this is not always easy. In many systemic conditions and arrhythmias, the pulse can be very weak or of variable strength. Detection of an arrhythmia during tachycardia also can be difficult. At the same time, the patient may be uncooperative. Under these conditions, selection of a different pulse site and/or combining palpation of the pulse with auscultation of the heart should help. Attempts should be made to confirm a pulse deficit (see below) because of the functional consequences.

Pulse Deficit: The term "pulse deficit" is used rather loosely. Strictly speaking, it refers to a situation in which cardiac (ventricular) contraction is not accompanied by a palpable pulse wave. This situation occurs in arrhythmias when the diastolic interval is too short to allow adequate cardiac filling and stroke volume is very low or nonexistent. The weak pulse found in hypovolemia, shock or a failing heart with a poor ejection fraction is a weak pulse, not a pulse deficit. In common usage, however, the term often is used for any situation in which the pulse appears to be very weak or in which "holes" appear in the regular sequence of pulse waves. It may thus be used erroneously to describe the lack of pulse during the dropped beat of second-degree atrioventricular block. The finding of a *true* pulse deficit is of significance not only in that it indicates possibly serious cardiovascular disease, but also because the myocardium is performing work without the benefit of a normal blood supply. Flow within the coronary arteries depends upon adequate cardiac output to maintain blood pressure and adequate duration of diastole.

If the pulse rhythm is abnormal, the pulse should be palpated simultaneously with auscultation of the heart. There may or may not be a pulse deficit, but this is easily determined, as the first heart sound has a tendency to be loud in cardiac cycles in which the ventricles are relatively empty (see Arrhythmias and Fig 46). This sign may not be obvious during very rapid runs of beats. The most convenient site for palpation of the pulse during auscultation is the median artery, though most clinicians have trouble finding this. Difficulties arise when the examiner expects to palpate the artery itself. The site lies one-third to one-half of the way from the cranial to the caudal aspect of the forearm, on the medial side and at the most proximal area of the limb. At this site, the artery proper cannot be palpated and the pulse is felt *through* the overlying superficial pectoral muscle.

If the median artery pulse cannot be detected, the medial palmar artery may be palpated immediately caudal and slightly deep to the medial palmar vein over the carpal canal on the caudomedial aspect of the carpus. The technique of simultaneous auscultation of the heart and palpation of the pulse also can be very useful in defining murmurs during tachycardia, when differentiation between systole and diastole otherwise may be difficult.

Pulse Character: Pulse "character" consists of 2 components: width and contour. Both can be of value in clinical evaluation. Character depends upon the size of the vessel palpated and its distance from the heart. Moving progressively farther from the heart, there is some enhancement of the height of the pulse pressure wave which facilitates detection, though the duration of the wave falls.[1] As an example, because of its full, surging nature, the pulse in the carotid artery may not be as obvious as the pulse in the digital artery of the hind limb.

The pulse is a pressure wave representing the difference between systolic and diastolic pressures (pulse width or pulse pressure). In palpating the pulse, the pressure wave that precedes blood flow is detected. Flow may be pulsatile but is continuous. Though the tone of the artery may give some idea of mean arterial pressure, the determination of pressure by palpation alone is not possible. It is a fundamental precept of pulse evaluation that *the ease with which a pulse is palpated provides no index of normality.* A wide pulse pressure, as may be seen in a case of aortic insufficiency, may result in a very easily palpable but abnormal pulse. Conversely, the absence of a pulse wave almost always indicates abnormality, though the problem may be local rather than systemic.

The contour of a pulse describes the manner in which the pressure changes with time. The easiest pulse to palpate is one with good strength and rapid change in pressure. The pulse in a normal, physically fit horse is best described as long, surging and full. The pulse contour consists of an initial, rapid, strong rise to a peak. A fall in pressure in the aorta accompanies the fall in ventricular pressure at the end of ventricular systole. This fall is halted because prior closure of the aortic valve closes the arterial compartment and resists flow of blood back into the ventricle. Elastic recoil of vessel walls then causes a second pulse wave, after which pressure falls slowly (Fig 7). The dip in the pressure waveform, referred to as the dicrotic notch, is palpable in most normal horses.

Characterization of the pulse contour can provide information with regard to the functional integrity of the cardiovascular system; however, with the exception of the weak pulse felt in shock, easily detectable pulse abnormalities are not as common as the literature would have us believe. This probably is because statements concerning clinical findings in relation to specific lesions rarely account for variation in the severity of the lesion. For example, an animal with aortic insufficiency sometimes has an exaggerated pulse wave at ventricular ejection. This reflects an increased stroke volume because of elevated end-diastolic volume and a tendency for the pulse to fall away unusually rapidly as blood leaks back into the left ventricle (Fig 7).[17] Unfortunately, while aortic insufficiency can be associated with quite musical, distinct murmurs, the quantity of blood lost into the ventricle may be low, so there may be minimal effect on the pulse wave.

The character of the pulse under circumstances of circulatory failure is a feature of great value in alerting the clinician to the problem. In the animal in shock, the heart rate is high, cardiac output and stroke volume are low, and the force of ventricular contraction is reduced. Systemic blood pressure, both mean and diastolic, is low and the pulse wave is weak, rising relatively slowly, then falling rapidly due to lack of energy to stretch the elastic arteries (Fig 7). The dicrotic notch usually is not palpable. This gives rise to the short, tapping pulse of hypovolemia that, because of the rapid fall in pulse pressure, is not always as difficult to palpate as may be anticipated.

Pulse contour can be of value in the definition of regional abnormalities in arterial supply. Absence of the pulse implies arterial obstruction, which may occur through thrombosis/thromboembolism and some-

Figure 7. Diagrammatic representation of a normal pulse contour (A), an exaggerated pulse as may be found in aortic insufficiency (B), a hypokinetic pulse as encountered in shock and hypovolemia (C), and the flat, prolonged pulse encountered in collateral circulation (D).

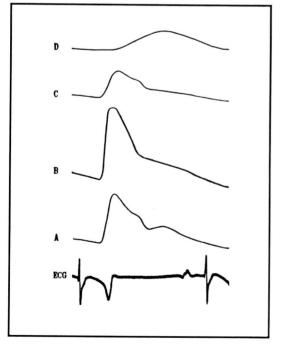

times is associated with fractures in which the displaced bone lacerates an artery or intermittently compresses it. Severe local tissue swelling also can cause arterial obstruction.

Collateral Pulse: In arterial occlusive diseases, such as aorto-iliac thrombosis, development of arterial obstruction often is slowly progressive and collateral circulation develops. The pulse proximal to the obstruction is unusually strong. Total absence of pulse distal to the obstruction does not occur, though it may be very difficult to palpate because it becomes flattened and indistinct, having both a slow rate of rise and fall (Fig 7). This results from the fact that blood arrives at this peripheral site via numerous collateral vessels of varying length and dimension, and often through a very tortuous course. This damps the pressure wave. Detection of such a pulse strongly suggests chronic arterial obstruction.

Examination of Mucous Membranes: Capillary refill time is a crude test of peripheral perfusion and is measured by gently pressing a mucous membrane, usually of the gum, and noting how rapidly the color returns to the blanched area. Accurate timing is impossible and estimation of normalcy is based upon experience. Pressing too hard or repeating the test at the same site too often influences the result. An approximate normal capillary refill time is less than 2 seconds.

The normal color of a mucous membrane is pink but the hue varies with the membrane examined. Those of the mouth are typically pale pink to very marginally bluish and show quite wide regional variation. The membranes of the nasal septum usually are a much brighter and more homogeneous pink than those of the mouth, while the conjunctiva tends to show quite marked variation from horse to horse, generally being a brighter pink than the oral mucosa but not so bright as the nasal septal mucosa. Vaginal mucosae tend to show similar color and variation as the mouth. Regional differences in membrane color suggest regional changes as opposed to generalized cardiovascular disease.

Evaluation of membrane condition as an index of cardiovascular function has some limitations, principally because of 2 factors: red cell volume and condition of the microcirculation. In severely anemic animals, the membranes are pale and measurement of capillary refill time can be difficult. If poor cardiac output is contributing to pallor, a cold periphery and elevated heart rate also are present. However, cardiac workload is increased in anemia because of the reduced oxygen-carrying capacity of the blood. Peripheral temperature and pulse strength thus are more consistently reliable indicators of cardiovascular insufficiency.

With hemorrhagic shock, mucosal pallor may reflect shutdown of peripheral circulation. At this stage, the packed cell volume most likely would be within normal limits. Later, as the animal accommodates to red cell loss, mucosal pallor would be more nearly a reflection of the anemia.

Injected or cyanotic mucous membranes are far more likely to reflect the local effect of a systemic disorder upon the microcirculation than to indicate a primary abnormality of the cardiovascular system. Such membrane discoloration typically occurs during endotoxemia, with dilatation of arterioles, closure of postcapillary sphincters and pooling of blood in the dilated peripheral circulation. Capillary refill time should be interpreted with caution under these circumstances because it reflects the time taken for blood to move back into the dilated capillaries that have been compressed and not true peripheral perfusion. Uncomplicated cardiovascular insufficiency causes pale rather than blue membranes. The only exception to this is cyanosis associated with congenital cardiac disease involving right-to-left shunts.

Cardiac Impulse (Apex Beat): The cardiac impulse represents the point of maximum intensity of the lowest-frequency components of the heart sounds, as detected at the chest wall. The event often can be seen on the left side and should be palpable at this location. Its strength and location can be of diagnostic value, though the degree of abnormality probably must be great before it can be detected easily. Usually the impulse reflects the first heart sound (S_1), though occasionally a particularly strong second sound (S_2) may be palpated also. This finding is not necessarily abnormal.

For examination, the horse should stand squarely on all 4 feet. On the left side in an average horse, the cardiac impulse lies 5-10 cm directly dorsal to the point of the left elbow or slightly caudal to a line drawn vertically through the point of the elbow at the fifth intercostal space. In an animal with a heavy triceps mass, such as in a Quarter Horse stallion, the impulse may be partially or totally obscured (Figs 1, 2). In a fit performance horse, the impulse is located at the fifth or sixth intercostal space about 8-10 cm dorsal to the point of the left elbow and 5-8 cm caudal to a line drawn vertically through the point of the elbow, where it is easily visible and strong on palpation.

On the right side, the impulse usually cannot be seen unless the animal, even if fit, also is very lean or possibly excited. If visible under such circumstances, it lies a little more ventrally than on the left, and well into the triceps muscle. In the normal animal, the impulse on the right always is weaker on palpation than that on the left, and one must invade the axilla with the palm of the hand to palpate it at the fourth intercostal space.

Abnormal location of the impulse on the left or right almost invariably involves caudal cardiac displacement, as the heart cannot move cranially in the thoracic cavity. Causative factors include cranial thoracic masses (lymphoma, pulmonary abscess) and cardiac enlargement. A mass ventral to the heart may displace it dorsally, but this would most likely reduce the impulse because of the widening dimension of the thorax and reduced contact of the heart with the chest wall.

Easily finding the apex beat on the right is significant, as this indicates possible right ventricular hypertrophy or displacement of the heart caudally or to the right. If the impulse is stronger on the right than on the left, this may indicate displacement of the heart to the right and/or some process reducing the intensity of the impulse on the left. In the case of unilateral left pleural effusion or pulmonary abscessation, cardiac displacement and reduced intensity of the impulse on the left may be found together. In my experience, pulmonary abscesses of sufficient size to cause cardiac displacement most often occur in the right cranial lung field, displacing the heart to the left and caudally. Loss of cardiac impulse also may occur with severe increase in lung size due to chronic airway disease and with pleural effusion/pleuritis and pericardial effusion.

Clinically significant causes of increased strength of cardiac impulse other than cardiac displacement include ventricular hypertrophy and any cause of circulatory hyperkinesia. This denotes a pathologic state of increased resting activity, such as may occur during fever, anemia, hypertension or hypovolemia. This is in contrast to increased activity in excitement, which causes the most profound increase in cardiac impulse.

Change in quality of the cardiac impulse is a less distinct but occasionally useful characteristic in some cases. In older horses, especially those of Thoroughbred breeding with several seasons of aerobic training, the cardiac impulse takes on a very "slow" and forceful character, whereby the hand is lifted from the chest wall at each contraction during palpation as opposed to being gently "thumped" by the underlying cardiac activity. This presumably reflects an increased chamber size and stroke volume in response to training. In shock, the impulse lacks strength but can be very obvious and is best described as a hollow "tap" as opposed to a thump. A similar observation is made in heart failure.

Apparent location and strength of the cardiac impulse can be influenced by several factors, limiting the diagnostic value of the observation. In a completely untrained animal or one that is systemically weak and has poor muscle tone, the entire thorax may sink in the pectoral girdle so that the scapulae become prominent dorsally at the withers and the point of the elbow moves dorsally in relation to the sternum. This and the earlier-mentioned differences in set of the forelimb on the thorax must be taken into account when examining the location of the cardiac impulse. Ideally, location should be related to rib space.

As an animal progresses through training, there is a tendency for the cardiac impulse to become more clearly visible and well emphasized. The extent to which aerobic training provides a stimulus for physiologic cardiomegaly (increase in chamber size) is not clearly defined. In our present context, some of the response may be due to loss of superficial fat and increased myocardial contractility. However, in the short term, this response is unlikely to produce the degree of displacement of cardiac impulse that may be related to pathologic cardiomegaly, gross displacement of the heart or a physiologically large heart. Rather,

training has a more significant effect on the intensity and strength of the cardiac impulse.

Other factors influencing strength of cardiac impulse include excitement, which causes the impulse to become strong and radiate widely, and age/body condition. The impulse is strong in young animals and those with a thin chest wall. Arrhythmias cause wide variation in strength (see below). Respiratory disease can confuse the picture; overinflation of the lungs reduces strength of the impulse and hydrothorax obliterates it.

Palpable Thrills: Various grading systems for murmurs are found in the literature. For consistency with discussions of cardiovascular examination in previous editions of this text, the 5-point grading system will be used here.[18] Using this system, a murmur of grade III/V or greater is accompanied by a palpable thrill that usually is most obvious over the point of maximum intensity of the murmur. This may not necessarily coincide with the location of the cardiac impulse and, in fact, usually does not. A reduced intensity of the cardiac impulse may accompany the hemodynamic disturbances associated with the murmur. In some texts the term "precordial," meaning over the heart, is used in describing the thrill.

Palpation in Congenital Cardiac Disease: Palpation of the cardiac impulse on both sides of the thorax simultaneously, a procedure easily achieved in the neonate and not impossible in the adult, often is of value in detection of congenital cardiac disease and should be a routine clinical procedure in foals. In the case of ventricular shunts, shunt flow often can be perceived moving from one side of the thorax to the other and frequently is associated with a palpable thrill.

Area of Cardiac Dullness: The area of cardiac dullness is that area caudal to the left elbow that is dull upon percussion by virtue of the heart's lying directly beneath the chest wall. Percussion may be achieved using a plexor and pleximeter or by flicking the chest wall firmly with a finger. Normally the area does not extend beyond the sixth intercostal space, even in a fit performance horse. Dorsally it extends to a line running horizontally 8-10 cm ventral to the point of the shoulder. A technique for detecting the normal dorsal limit of the area of cardiac dullness by reference to anatomic landmarks has been described.[19,20] The procedure is performed with the animal's left forelimb raised, the point of reference being the junction of the ventral border of the serratus ventralis muscle and the third intercostal space.

The area of cardiac dullness is enlarged with cardiomegaly, caudal displacement of the heart, and pulmonary consolidation or abscessation caudal to the heart. The area is essentially lost with pleural effusion. On the right, there should be no area of cardiac dullness; the presence of one indicates pathologic changes. On either side, cardiac enlargement must be severe before the area is clearly enlarged; displacement of the heart is a more frequent cardiac cause of enlargement.

Hydration Status: Dehydration usually results in reduced blood volume and increased cardiac workload. Usually there also are concomitant electrolyte disturbances and other factors affecting cardiovascular function, such as pain or toxemia. Thus, volume depletion is only one component of a generalized homeostatic disturbance. However, in the context of a detailed cardiovascular examination, dehydration must be considered because of its direct effects upon all aspects of cardiovascular function. Hydration status should be assessed by testing skin turgor at the upper eyelid and the side of the neck. With clinical evidence of dehydration, total serum solids and packed cell volume should be measured.

Auscultation

General Considerations and Approach: To adequately access the area of cardiac auscultation in a horse, it is necessary to protract the limb manually; even then the area is not fully exposed. In many cases, the assistance of a second person is required to adequately auscultate the heart. Failure to do this can cause significant cardiac abnormalities to be missed. *It is of critical importance to fully auscultate both sides of the thorax.* Many cardiac abnormalities may only be evident on one side. For example, some cases of right atrioventricular insufficiency and simple ventricular septal defects are detected only on the right side.

The sequence of evaluation in cardiac auscultation should be: 1) measurement of heart rate, 2) evaluation of intensity and character of sounds and of area of auscultation, 3) evaluation of individual heart sounds by topographic reference to valve areas on each side of the thorax, and 4) evaluation of murmurs. Heart rate should be determined regardless of the previous measurement of pulse rate because heart rate and pulse rate are not necessarily the same. Any significant difference should be explained.

The area over which heart sounds can clearly be heard, the area of auscultation, should be evaluated and compared with the location of the cardiac impulse and area of cardiac dullness. The stethoscope should be slid over the skin rather than lifted from site to site so as to better detect regional differences. An apparent increase in area of auscultation is seen with cardiac enlargement, caudal cardiac displacement, lung consolidation, excitement and circulatory hyperkinesia. Differentiation between these various causes must be made on the basis of other cardiovascular findings and findings in other body systems.

Heart Sound Amplitude vs Frequency: Heart sounds are of low frequency (<500 Hz) and as such are not detected easily by the human ear, which is better attuned to higher frequencies. Thus, the clinician must differentiate between frequency and amplitude. Relatively high-frequency sounds, especially those with a musical or metallic quality, are easily heard but quite often are of little clinical significance. In contrast, very low-frequency sounds may be barely audible yet often are of great clinical significance. Low-frequency sounds must be relatively intense to be detected readily and consequently are easily missed.

Heart Sound Intensity and Character: The intensity and character of heart sounds must be interpreted in light of the type of animal and environmental circumstance. Excitement, exercise, a high level of fitness, hyperkinesia (as in anemia and shock), or lack of body cover cause heart sounds to be more prominent. Lack of athletic condition, excessive body cover, breed (see above under Thoracic Conformation), pericardial or pleural effusion, and myocardial weakness may be associated with a reduced intensity of heart sounds. The cardiac and extracardiac factors that influence cardiac impulse have the same effect upon the intensity of heart sounds.

The character of the sounds may be thudding, as in a nervous horse, or muffled, as in an excessively fat horse or one with pericardial or extensive pleural effusion. Care must be taken to differentiate between muffled and quiet sounds. Muffled sounds have a remote, soft quality that is lacking in sounds that are merely quiet. Muffling implies cardiac displacement or the presence of some intervening medium, such as fluid or air. In shock and heart failure, the sounds often take on a hollow, complex character. Assessment of strength and character should not be finalized until the entire cardiac area has been auscultated. Variation in the intensity and character of sounds from region to region should be noted. The right side of the chest should be auscultated in the same manner and compared with the left. Any murmur detected should be temporarily disregarded, as overconcern with murmurs may cause other abnomalities to be overlooked.

Terms Describing Auscultatory Findings: Certain conventions are used when describing findings upon cardiac auscultation. Sounds that are most easily heard in the dorsal area of auscultation, in the region of the semilunar valves, are described as being prominent at the heart base. Other sounds may be described as being prominent toward the apex. Because both ventricles are auscultated at the left chest wall (Figs 1, 2), sounds may be described as best heard over the right or left ventricle on the *left* side. Murmurs sometimes are described as radiating into the left or right ventricle on the left (a feature that can be of diagnostic value) or toward the right or left apex. The point of maximum intensity describes the location at which an abnormal sound, usually a murmur, is most easily detected. With very intense murmurs, this usually coincides with the location of a thrill. Finally, sounds may be described as radiating cranially toward the thoracic inlet or dorsally along the outflow tracts or as widespread, meaning that they are heard over a large area.

The term "apex" refers to the most ventral "pointed end" of the heart, which lies close to the sternum. Some authors use the term "sternal border" to describe this location, though apex is more descriptive and is used here. If the term "apex" is used, then reference can be made to the apex of both the right and left ventricles, both of which lie at the sternal border.

When describing sounds heard on the right side of the thorax, similar descriptions are used. However, little comment can be made from this side concerning the status of left chamber function. To avoid confusion, descriptions should emphasize the side of the thorax as well as the particular chamber described. For example, a sound may be described as prominent over the right ventricular apex on the left side of the thorax.

Heart Sounds and Valve Areas: Numerous structures are involved in the genesis of heart sounds, which can be heard over wide areas. However, an approach to examination of sounds based upon cardiac topography usually is taken because of the obvious relationship between form and function, and because regional variation in strength and quality of sounds can be of diagnostic significance. Cardiac structures provide points of reference. In describing findings, it is important to mention the relationship to approximate valve location, the cardiac apex or ventricular chambers. Transmission of sound from deep structures to the body surface involves some modification or distortion because of varying density of overlying structures but approximate valve locations still provide a valuable guide.

In working by valve area, it is important to consider the events that give rise to the heart sounds. These are discussed for each sound below. For now, it is sufficient to emphasize the observation that heart valves close "with gentle reverence."[21] Heart sounds are not the result of valves "slapping" together but are generated by cardiac events approximately coincident with the time of valve closure/opening. Thus, though auscultation is *by reference* to valve locations, it is not the activity of the valves *per se* that is being evaluated. A useful view is to consider the sounds as caused by sudden acceleration or deceleration of columns of blood and the resonance of that blood and its containing chamber.[22-24]

At or just after the approximate time of left atrioventricular valve closure in early systole, blood in the left ventricle decelerates as pressure rises and as the closed a-v valve and walls of the chamber suddenly limit the blood's movement (isovolumic contraction). This is followed immediately by acceleration as the aortic valve opens and blood is ejected into the aorta (Fig 5). In that these events give rise to the first heart sound (S_1), the components of S_1 generated in the left heart should be particularly distinct ventral to the left atrioventricular valve over the left free ventricular wall (Fig 8). In that the second heart sound (S_2) is generated by sudden deceleration of columns of blood in the outflow tracts, as elastic recoil of these arteries drives the column of blood against the already closed semilunar valves, then S_2 should be most easily detected dorsal to the semilunar valves over the outflow tracts themselves, as these are the structures whose resonance is primarily responsible for the sound.

For these reasons, the areas of auscultation represented diagrammatically in Figure 8 (open circles) are each located ventral or dorsal to the actual valve by which they are named (filled ellipses). The areas of auscultation reflect the major focus of sound at closure of the associated valve in the *normal* cardiac cycle and overlie rapidly decelerating blood columns. In the diseased

heart, the distribution of sound does not necessarily follow these columns, and direct reference to valve location is necessary. However, consideration of blood columns continues to be of great value, as murmurs tend to radiate into these areas and follow the direction of blood flow. These considerations are discussed below under Abnormalities of Sound.

Auscultation and location of specific cardiac structures are aided by consideration of thoracic topography and the actual location of the heart in the chest and by reference to ribs (Fig 8). Moving dorsally from the skin of the sternum, about 6-7 cm of solid tissue are encountered ventral to the thoracic cavity; the heart extends almost to the most ventral aspect of this cavity. The heart lies with its cranioventral border (free wall of the right ventricle) parallel with and just dorsal to the sternum, while the caudal border (free wall of the left ventricle) is inclined almost vertically at the sixth rib or sixth intercostal space. Caudally, the diaphragm courses cranially to the sixth intercostal space/seventh rib, about 6-7 cm caudal to the point of the elbow, and the heart is usually 1-2 cm cranial to the diaphragm on the midline. Cranially, the heart extends to the second intercostal space or second

Figure 8. Position of the heart valves (filled ellipses) and areas of auscultation (open circles) in relation to the cardiac silhouette and rib spaces. The areas of auscultation reflect the major locus of sound energy at the time of closure of the associated valve in the normal cardiac cycle, and overlie rapidly accelerating/decelerating blood columns. In the diseased heart the distribution of (abnormal) sound does not necessarily follow these columns, and direct reference to anatomic valve location is necessary. A = aortic. P = pulmonic. R = right AV valves. L = left AV valves. See also Figures 4, 50 and 51.

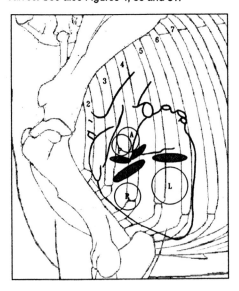
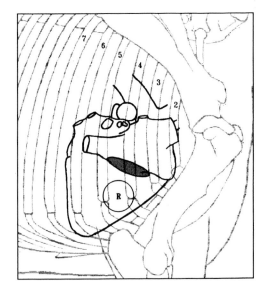

rib. Because the most cranial aspect of the shoulder in the average horse lies at or slightly cranial to the first rib, the cranial border of the heart lies approximately 8-10 cm caudal to the point of the shoulder.

The curve of the vertebral column defines the dorsal limit of the thoracic cavity, with the aortic arch lying in close proximity after the eighth rib. The base of the heart, excluding the great vessels, lies level with the ventral one-third of the thoracic inlet, occupying approximately half of the dorsoventral dimension of the thoracic cavity at this level. Projection of this cardiac silhouette onto the body wall (Fig 8) and consideration of the size of the cardiac notch in the lung (Fig 1) guides auscultation of the heart. Reference to rib spaces and height in relation to the shoulder and point of the elbow may be used to describe findings.

Normal Heart Sounds: The precise origin of heart sounds and the events they denote are controversial. The character of heart sounds may vary from moment to moment and horse to horse. Part of this diversity arises from the slow resting heart rate in horses, and part from the volatility of heart rate and temperament. The following description, based upon clinical experience and limited published studies, should be regarded as a composite picture and open to discussion.[23,25-34]

Consideration of Figure 8 suggests that all 4 valve auscultation areas are accessible on the left, and that both left and right ventricular chambers can be accessed there also. With the exception of the right atrioventricular valve, the valves are located toward the left side of the thorax (Fig 4). Auscultation on the right is principally of value in evaluating right heart events associated with activity of the right atrioventricular valve, though activity associated with this valve also can be detected well cranially and ventrally on the left. Most cardiac sound on either side of the thorax is contributed by the left heart.[33,34] Right heart contributions probably only are prominent during hyperkinetic function of the right ventricle.

Each valve area should be auscultated and the manner in which individual heart sounds change from location to location noted. At least 4 heart sounds may be encountered in the normal horse: the atrial contraction sound, S_1, S_2 and S_3. The prominence of each sound varies according to lo-

cation. In the normal horse, at least 2 and often 4 or more sounds may be heard (see below under Complex Sounds).

The fourth heart sound, S_4, really is the first sound of the cardiac cycle and its name is misleading. In this text, it is described as the *atrial contraction sound*. It may have up to 4 components, though only 1 is likely to be heard upon auscultation. This component occurs just after atrial contraction and is thought to reflect recoil of the ventricular walls after influx of blood from the atria. It is a short, quiet, low-frequency sound best heard over the ventricles (Fig 5).

It is probable that the late components of the atrial contraction sound are, in fact, the early components of S_1. Where the PR interval of the ECG is long, that is, where atrioventricular conduction is slow, the sound can be clearly differentiated from S_1 as a soft "lu." As the PR interval shortens, the atrial contraction sound merges with S_1, extending that sound. This is quite obvious in some cases in which the PR interval varies from beat to beat. When the sound is very close to S_1 yet still distinguishable, it may be mistaken for a split first heart sound. The sound can be very obvious in second degree atrioventricular block in which atrial contraction is not followed by ventricular systole. An atrial contraction sound frequently is present on either side of the thorax and is a normal finding.

The *first heart sound,* S_1, starts shortly after the beginning of ventricular contraction. It is thought mainly to reflect deceleration of blood in the ventricles during the isovolumic phase of ventricular contraction and occurs after closure of the atrioventricular valves. The sound extends at least up to opening of the semilunar (aortic and pulmonic) valves. Some workers have suggested that early ventricular ejection also contributes to the sound. It is of relatively long duration and low frequency and, over the left atrioventricular valve region, is the most intense heart sound. Its lowest-frequency components are palpated as the cardiac impulse.

The *second heart sound,* S_2, occurs after the end of ventricular ejection and occurs after closure of the semilunar valves. It is associated with deceleration of the columns of blood in the great vessels as they recoil against the closed valves. It is a short, intense sound, especially at the heart base, where it may be heard either dorsal or ventral to the semilunar valves. Though its relatively high frequency and short duration make it easy to detect, it is not as strong as S_1. Both S_1 and S_2 are reflections of mechanical (as opposed to electrical) ventricular systole, essentially marking the beginning and end of that event, and occur even in the absence of atrial contraction.

The *third heart sound*, S_3, also known as the ventricular filling sound, occurs at the end of rapid ventricular filling early in diastole. Thus, it is more closely linked to S_2 than to the length of diastole, and is associated with recoil of the walls of the ventricular chambers and deceleration of blood at the end of rapid filling during early ventricular diastole.

Some researchers believe a mitral valve opening sound, is the prominent sound after S_2.[35,36] Others consider this sound to be part of the late components of S_2, and consider S_3 to be a distinct sound. The distinct interval usually noted in most horses between the second sound and the first clearly detectable diastolic sound suggests strongly that this diastolic sound is best interpreted as the ventricular filling sound, S_3.

Little clinical significance is attached to variation in the atrial contraction sound, though, theoretically, atrial hypertrophy might promote a prominent sound. However, with atrioventricular stenosis, the clinical abnormality most likely to cause this problem, atrial systole is likely to be prolonged. This would preclude vigorous recoil of the ventricular walls. The atrial contraction sound may be accentuated in early atrioventricular insufficiency, increased filling of the atria leading to hypertrophy, and more forceful atrial contraction.

S_1 and S_2 both occur as a result of ventricular systole so that they are heard each time the ventricles contract, regardless of whether the atria contract or not. If the atria are not functioning normally, S_1 and S_2 may be modified in intensity and quality. Where the diastolic interval is long and cardiac filling greater than normal (*eg*, after a dropped beat), there is a tendency for S_1 to be quiet and for S_2 to be loud. Conversely, in a short diastolic interval, as with a premature contraction or junctional escape beat, the ventricle is relatively empty, S_1 tends to be very loud and S_2 is sometimes inaudible (Fig 46). The same effect operates

when ventricular contraction is not preceded by atrial contraction even if the diastolic interval is of normal length (see Abnormalities of Rhythm).

A prominent S_3 may be heard during cardiac acceleration and particularly during deceleration. Under these circumstances, it is of no significance. Prominence of S_3 during rest and in the absence of obvious excitement, especially in an untrained animal with a relatively normal heart rate, may indicate reduced compliance as is seen in cardiac hypertrophy or failure. A prominent S_3 may, however, be normal and associated with a very well-toned heart in an athletic horse. In general, the S_3 of pathologic cardiomegaly is more obvious and persistent than that of physiologic response to training. A loud S_3 in cardiac dilatation usually is accompanied by other signs of abnormality, such as tachycardia, jugular filling or valvular insufficiency. An S_3 is as likely to be heard on the right as on the left in the normal animal.

Splitting of Heart Sounds: Apparent splitting of heart sounds may be detected. Splitting of S_2 is often incorrectly diagnosed. S_3 may be detected as a second sound after S_2, following it closely, but careful auscultation usually reveals that it is distinctly separated. S_2-S_3 may be phonetically described as "dup-dup," while a split S_2 is best described as "dudup." A split S_2 also is likely to be most obvious at the heart base, while S_2-S_3 should be most obvious over the ventricles. A split S_2 can be heard in many normal horses by careful auscultation well cranially over the heart base on the left side of the thorax. The splitting varies according to the stage of the respiratory cycle.

Though some studies have suggested that the aortic valve closes before the pulmonic in horses, others have found no difference. This likely reflects individual variation, technique and condition of the respiratory system. As with many cardiac observations, the finding is abnormal only in degree. Thus, easily detected splitting may indicate ventricular asynchrony as may occur when one chamber is working against an increased afterload (arterial pressure).

Splitting of S_1 is unusual. When observed, it usually is an atrial contraction sound followed closely by S_1. Were true splitting noted, it would indicate chamber asynchrony that may reflect changes in preload or afterload. While intraventricular conduction abnormalities are rarely seen in horses, this also is a possible cause of splitting of S_1.

Complex Sounds: Unusually complex sounds are heard in some horses. With splitting of S_1 and S_2, the usual 4 sounds result in 6. The atrial sound also can be double; systolic clicks sometimes can be heard. Interpretation can be especially difficult if there also is tachycardia. However, these do not necessarily indicate an abnormality. If other features of cardiovascular function or the history suggest clinical disease, phonocardiography should be employed for identification. No specific clinical significance can be attached to such complex sounds unless they accompany other signs of cardiovascular disease.

Special Examination of the Respiratory System

The reader is referred to the chapter on Diseases of the Respiratory System for detailed discussion of this system. For the purposes of cardiovascular examination, it is important to detect any acute or chronic respiratory diseases. Chronic small airway disease may be associated with a decreased area of auscultation and cardiac dullness, and with increased load on the right heart. Consequences include splitting of S_2, increased activity in the right heart and perhaps prominence of heart sounds on the right. Pulmonary abscessation may cause cardiac displacement. Pulmonary consolidation increases the area of cardiac dullness and regions over which heart sounds are transmitted. Animals experiencing obvious ventilatory problems are often difficult to auscultate, especially if lung sounds are increased. Caution should be exercised in occluding the nares for auscultation, as the patient may not be able to tolerate interruption to oxygen delivery.

Severely hypoxemic patients may exhibit cardiac arrhythmias, especially if they also are toxic. In the face of severe hypoxemia or moderate hypoxemia of recent onset, tachycardia is a consistent finding unless cardiac arrhythmia is depressing the heart rate (see below under Bradycardia and Arrhythmia). *The combination of tachycardia and hypoxemia should be regarded as a medical emergency.* The primary objective should be to improve oxygenation and reduce the load on the myocardium. In animals with mild to moderate hypoxemia over a prolonged period, resting heart rate usually is normal. The chronicity of the problem is reflected in a depressed venous oxygen level, which appears to be an adaptive response. In the absence of fever, toxemia or any primary cardiac problem, resting heart rate usually does not become elevated until arterial oxygen tension falls below 50-60 mm Hg.

ANCILLARY DIAGNOSTIC AIDS

Electrocardiography

Electrocardiography involves recording the electrical activity of the heart, usually at the body surface, during myocardial depolarization and repolarization. The principal applications of the technique are diagnosing and interpreting arrhythmias, monitoring cardiac activity and detecting changes in myocardial mass, chamber size or workload by evaluation of waveform conformation in multiple standardized ECG leads. Analysis of these multiple scalar ECGs by determination of planar (2-dimensional, 2-D) or spatial (3-dimensional, 3-D) vectors is referred to as vectorcardiography. An understanding of the conduction system of the heart is a prerequisite to application of these techniques.

Depolarization and the ECG

The proximal elements of the conduction system consist of the sinoatrial (SA) node, which is the normal pacemaker, the atrioventricular (AV) node, the atrioventricular bundle (common bundle or bundle of His), the left and right bundle branches, and the Purkinje network (Fig 9). The SA node or pacemaker is located in the right auricle, just ventral to the junction of that structure and the cranial vena cava, in tissue adjacent to the crista terminalis.[37,38] In comparison to that in other species, the SA node of horses is a relatively large structure with a horseshoe shape that curves around the opening of the cranial vena cava.[37] Activity spreads radially from the SA node through the right atrium, generating the first component of the generally bifid P wave in the

ECG.[39,40] Depolarization of the left atrium appears to occur spontaneously, having numerous wavefronts which cancel each other out, so that they do not contribute to the P wave in the body-surface ECG. Instead, the second component of the bifid P wave is thought to reflect depolarization of the interatrial septum.[39] The various conformations of P wave recorded using a base-apex (Y) lead and their relative frequencies of occurrence are shown in Figure 10.[41] These indicate activity of normal SA node origin. Conformation may change if the atrial impulse arises in an abnormal focus.

The pathway for conduction of activity from the SA node to the AV node remains unconfirmed. The existence of specialized conducting (Purkinje) tissue has been demonstrated in the right but not the left atrial subendocardium, which conflicts with observed patterns of depolarization.[39,42] Also, these conducting tissues are not continuous with the SA or AV nodes but blend into the normal atrial myocardium.[37] Their function is thus unconfirmed and conduction of activity between the 2 nodes presumably occurs by both transmission across myocardial cells and by specialized conducting tissue.

The AV node is a very complex structure both anatomically and functionally. It is located in the right side of the interatrial septum, cranioventral to the coronary sinus.[37,42] While conducting tissue in general has the potential for pacemaker activity, this appears only to be true of the distal one-third of the AV node. Delayed conduction though the AV node is responsible for the PR interval of the ECG. Variation in vagal tone is primarily responsible for variation in conduction velocity.[1] The AV and SA nodes have a rich vascular and autonomic nerve supply, both sympathetic and parasympathetic.[37,43] The predominant parasympathetic supply of the SA node comes from the right vagus and that of the AV node from the left vagus.[43]

The AV node is continuous with the atrioventricular bundle or bundle of His, the combined structures representing the only normal pathway through the fibrous septum dividing the atria from the ventricles. The atrioventricular bundle divides into left and right bundles that supply the left and right ventricles, respectively. All of these are enclosed in a sheath of fibrous tis-

Figure 9. Right base (top) and right lateral view (middle) of the heart, showing location of the proximal conduction system.[42] The sinoatrial node (SAN) is horseshoe shaped and located at the junction of the cranial vena cava (C) with the right atrium (RA). A window has been cut into the right atrium and right ventricle (RV) to reveal the atrioventricular conduction system. Bottom: Location of the atrioventricular node (AVN), the common bundle (CB), left bundle branch (LBB) and right bundle branch (RBB).[42] The AVN lies in the base of the atrium, while the common bundle descends into the interventricular septum and represents the only electrical continuity between the atria and ventricles. A = aorta.

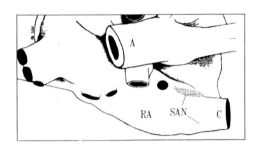

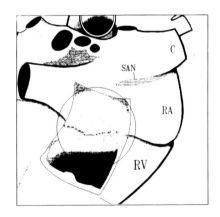

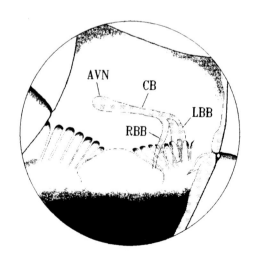

sue that isolates them from the surrounding myocardium and also carries a rich plexus of nerve fibers.[37] These nerve fibers generally are assumed to be sympathetic, with no parasympathetic innervation of the ventricles. However, recent studies suggest that the ventricles are directly influenced by vagal innervation, a view supported by anatomic observations.[43-45]

Slight delay in conduction in the beginning of the atrioventricular bundle may contribute to the PR interval but conduction in the remaining bundle is fast and activity passes quickly to the ventricular myocardium via the terminal Purkinje network. One of the characteristics of the intraventricular conduction system in horses is the very extensive arborization and distribution of this terminal network throughout the myocardium from endocardium to epicardium, in contrast to that of other species.[37] The ramifications of this network and its connections with the branches of the main conduction system have been studied extensively.[37]

After division of the atrioventricular bundle, the right branch passes through the septum to the right free wall and apex without making any contribution to the Purkinje network of the septum. The left branch divides into 3 sub-branches, 1 of which is continuous with the septal Purkinje network. The remaining 2 pass toward the base of the papillary muscles of the left ventricle and then join the terminal Purkinje network within the free walls. With the exception of the limited contribution of the right branch to the septum, the networks of the left and right ventricle probably are continuous.[37] The implications of these observations for electrocardiography in horses are significant.

Ventricular depolarization gives rise to the QRS complex, while ventricular repolarization is reflected in the T wave. Figure 10 shows typical waveform configurations for the base-apex lead for a semiorthogonal lead system.[46-48] The conformation of the waveforms is determined by normal conduction through the conduction system. Origin of the impulse in an aberrant pacemaker or obstruction of part of the conduction system results in abnormal spread of the wave of excitation through the myocardium (see the discussion of Arrhythmias later in this chapter). However, cardiac

Figure 10. Range of waveform conformations encountered in a base-apex (Y) lead. Relative frequencies of occurrence for the P wave and QRS complex are indicated. Frequencies for the P wave are from a population of 50 2-year-old Thoroughbreds.[39] Figures for the QRS complex are from unpublished observations of a population of 286 horses of mixed breeding, mainly Standardbred, aged 3 months to 18 years. T waves are very labile, tending to swing continuously through the forms shown.

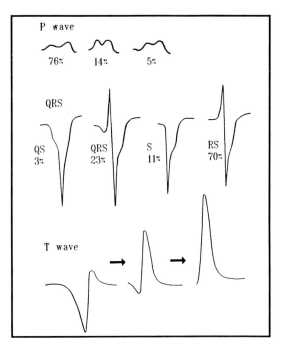

electrical activity is not necessarily evident in the ECG. Myocardial contraction is preceded by myocardial depolarization that involves a change in charge in and around each myocardial cell. A fraction of this change in potential finds its way to the body surface and may be detected by the ECG machine, which measures potential difference (voltage).

For activity to have sufficient strength to reach the body surface, depolarization must proceed across the myocardium as a coordinated wave. The larger the wavefront, the greater the ECG deflection. The longer the wavefront lasts, the greater the duration of deflection. Small wavefronts are not detected at the body surface because they lack the electrical energy to overcome the insulating effect of overlying tissue. In addition, where areas of myocardium depolarize by numerous small wavefronts, the charge is cancelled as the current from one area of tissue meets opposing current from adjacent tissue. Such activity may not be detected even if an exploring electrode is placed directly on the myocardium.

In people and dogs, much of the ventricular depolarization proceeds according to distinct wavefronts that cause recognizable deflections in the body surface ECG, allowing changes in pattern to be related to changes in the myocardium. Not all of the myocardium depolarizes in this manner, however, and the extent to which specific myocardial lesions are accurately reflected in the body surface ECG, that is, the sensitivity and specificity of accepted patterns, is likely to vary greatly. However, in these species, recognition of ECG patterns and diagnosis have been aided by a wealth of experience. Thus, some feeling for strength of associations has been developed.

Because of the nature of the intraventricular conduction system in horses, depolarization of most of the ventricular myocardium is achieved in one explosive event, with numerous local areas of activity cancelling each other out, so that no significant wavefronts of depolarization are generated and there is no body surface signal. That is, so far as the body-surface ECG is concerned, depolarization of the ventricular free walls and apex is electrically silent.[46] Because of the pattern of the main conduction system, any ventricular activity reflected in the body-surface ECG might be expected to originate mainly in the ventricular septum. Studies in which ventricular depolarization has been correlated with the body surface ECG strongly suggest that this is the case.[49] Septal depolarization is felt to give rise to the Q and R waves (apical third of the septum), and S wave (basilar third) of the QRS complex of the base-apex ECG (Fig 10). In addition, some small contribution probably is made by basal regions of the free walls and the region of the conus arteriosus (right heart outflow tract), probably giving rise to hesitation in the ascending limb of the S wave (Fig 10).[50]

Rhythm Analysis and Monitoring

Choice of ECG Lead: Most ECG machines are equipped to take Einthoven's limb leads; this is the system which has generally been used in horses. An ECG lead is a standardized combination of cables, named according to the location on the skin at which electrodes are attached (and not necessarily according to what the lead selection dial on the ECG machine says).

A lead may be described as bipolar or unipolar.[51] A bipolar lead (*eg*, limb leads I, II, III) consists of 2 *cables* with an electrode attached to the end of each, 1 positive and 1 negative. A unipolar lead is theoretically collected when all the limb cables are connected together to the negative pole of the ECG and the remaining (chest) cable becomes the positive "exploring" electrode. Most clinical ECGs are made using simple bipolar leads. When monitoring cardiac rhythm, only 1 lead is required and the operator may attach the electrodes just about anywhere, though if sequential ECGs or samples from different animals are to be compared, standard electrode positions should be used for consistency. The electrodes most often are alligator clips.

Traditionally the limb lead system devised by Einthoven has been used in recording the equine ECG.[18,52] Lead II is most often chosen for rhythm monitoring, as in other species. This is adequate, though movement of the limbs may make other leads more practical. Leads that lie along the principal cardiac electrical axis (about base-apex) tend to give a large, easily read deflection that is less subject to movement artifact. Thus, the Y lead of Holmes' semi-orthogonal system (positive electrode on the xiphoid, negative on the manubrium; Figs 11, 12), is useful for rhythm monitoring.[46] Note that the Y-electrode should be on the *tip* of the manubrium, not between the pectoral muscles. Typical waveform conformations for this lead and their relative frequency of occurrence are shown in Figure 10. When recording the ECG during exercise tests (as opposed to monitoring heart rate), the base-apex lead used most often involves attaching the negative electrode over the horse's forehead and the positive over the croup.

ECG machines commonly used in North America are configured for Einthoven's leads (I, II, III, AVR, AVL, AVF) and the cables are color coded. By selecting the position of the lead-selector dial so that the amplifier is connected to the particular pair of cables you wish to use, it is possible to take any lead. For example, Figure 13 shows the hexaxial system and polarity of the bipolar and unipolar limb leads. If the lead selection switch is set to lead I, the black (left arm, positive) cable and the white (right arm, negative) cable are selected. As shown in Figure 12, for the Y lead, the black would be on the xiphoid, the white on the manubrium. In addition, the green or ground cable should always be attached (the right leg cable on most machines). When using the Y lead, the shoulder area is a useful point for attachment of this cable.

In some cases of cardiac arrhythmia, one or more waveforms may be difficult to identify. A useful technique in such cases is to choose a lead axis with a different orientation to the heart. This may expose the waveform in some cases and should always be taken where one part of the ECG, particularly the P wave, appears to be missing.

Technique: For collection of a resting ECG, the horse should stand quietly, preferably on an insulating rubber mat to avoid any adverse consequences from an improperly serviced machine and to reduce 60-cycle interference. The ground or earth electrode always should be attached. A mains-powered ECG never should be used if the ground circuits in the building are not in good condition. Quite aside from the risk to the users and the horse if the machine malfunctions, severe electrical (60-cycle) in-

Figure 11. Theoretical relationship of the X, Y and Z axes of a semi-orthogonal system to the heart and thorax.[46] The axes are viewed from the left, dorsally and caudally.[54]

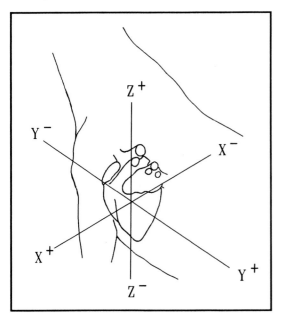

Figure 12. Electrode placement for a semi-orthogonal lead system.[46] The X leads are large plates or saline-soaked sponges laid over the triceps muscle and adjacent thorax, and are used instead of smaller electrodes to defeat proximity effects. The Y lead runs from the xiphoid (+ve) to the manubrium (-ve), the Z lead from the lateral side of the left forelimb (-ve) to the left side of the withers directly dorsal to the limb (+ve), and the X lead from the left forelimb (+ve) to the right forelimb (-ve). The horse should stand square during collection of the ECG.[54]

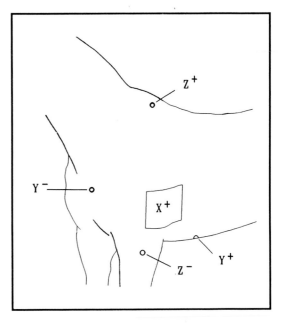

terference will be encountered. Though some of these precautions are not safety requirements for battery-operated machines, they reduce interference. If limb leads are used, the horse must be made to stand squarely on all 4 feet.

The ECG should be recorded at standardized speed and sensitivity (*eg,* 25 mm/sec and 1 mv/cm) to allow comparison of tracings. Because of the low heart rate of horses, recording should be continued for several minutes to detect arrhythmias (see discussion of 24-hour rhythm monitoring below). A calibration signal should be placed on the actual tracing periodically. The completed tracing should be identified and preferably mounted on the medical record immediately. Few things are as useless as an unlabelled ECG several days after the fact.

Vectorcardiography

Electrocardiographic detection of changes in chamber size generally involves the use of multiple leads. The objective is to detect cardiac abnormalities by pattern recognition in the scalar tracings or by deviation of derived planar (*eg*, mean modal vector) or spatial (*eg*, vector loop) values from normal values. The latter approach generally requires computer methods for greatest accuracy. Problems that are theoretically detectable include increase in myocardial mass, chamber enlargement and cardiac displacement. All multiple-lead systems attempt to describe the spatial or 3-D pattern of electrical activity generated around the heart during depolarization/repolarization.

Because most methods of analysis involve resolution of cardiac electrical activity along axes or planes, the term *vectorcardiography* is used to describe the technique. The resultant diagrammatic representation of the ECG is a vectorcardiogram (VCG). The approach taken to VCG analysis is described below. Though used to evaluate all waveforms, the technique finds its greatest application in people and small animals in evaluation of the QRS complex.

The following discussion relates primarily to ventricular depolarization. Vectorcardiography probably is of limited value in horses and is likely to be largely eclipsed by echocardiography. However, because the technique may help support clinical diagnoses, a basic understanding is desirable.

VCG Lead Systems: The body-surface ECG is only a poor reflection of events in the myocardium. This might be expected to limit the diagnostic value of the technique and, in fact, this appears to be the case. It is important to remember that, because the heart is a 3-dimensional (3-D) object, electrical activity generated during depolarization/repolarization also has a 3-D or spatial pattern. Additionally, the pattern changes constantly with time. The objective of vectorcardiography is to record this pattern as accurately as possible. This is subject to several limiting factors.

Overlying tissue has a distorting effect upon both the magnitude and time course of electrical signals that reach the body surface. This problem is compounded by the fact that not all electrode positions are equidistant from the heart. This can exaggerate relatively minor electrical activity that happens to be comparatively close to an electrode (proximity effect). For these reasons, the body-surface ECG can provide, at the

very best, only a very limited approximation to the true distribution of electrical activity.

It thus becomes important to position electrodes so as to provide as accurate a picture of body-surface potentials as possible. To do this, hundreds of electrodes distributed evenly over the entire body surface would be required;[46,47,53] this is an impracticable approach for other than research purposes. Multiple-lead systems are thus a compromise and represent an attempt to collect, as accurately as possible, the greatest possible amount of information with a few leads. All multiple-lead systems are based upon certain fundamental concepts and conventions.

At any instant, the signal registered through an electrode depends upon the polarity of the electrode and its position in relation to the wave of depolarization. If a wavefront passes toward the positive or searching electrode, a positive deflection is recorded. If the wavefront passes away from it, a negative deflection is recorded. Electrical activity passing at right angles to a line joining the electrode pair is not seen. The approximate magnitude and direction of wavefronts of myocardial depolarization can be deduced from knowledge of the location and polarity of electrodes and vectorial analysis. Vectorcardiographic lead systems thus employ multiple spatially distributed electrodes to build a 3-D approximation of cardiac electrical activity.

The main differences in the various lead systems used in horses reflect the extent to which they were designed for use in this species and the extent to which they accurately record the equine body-surface ECG.[48,53,55–62] Early studies in horses used Einthoven's system of limb leads or systems derived therefrom. Adaptations often involved addition of electrodes on the dorsal midline or either side of the thorax to add a third dimension to the essentially 2-dimensional (horizontal) plane of the limb leads. Though used extensively, Einthoven's system was not designed for horses and its ability to adequately detect the equine cardiac electric field has been questioned.[46]

A lead system for use in horses, based upon detailed study of the body-surface ECG, was developed by Holmes.[46-48] In recognition of the fact that true electrical orthogonality cannot be achieved because of the anatomy of the thorax, the system was referred to as semi-orthogonal. The design was based upon the concept that, to determine the shape of a 3-D object, a minimum of 3 different viewpoints or axes at mutual right angles (orthogonal) must be used. The relationship of the 3 orthogonal axes to the heart is shown in Figure 11, while the actual points of attachment of the 3 bipolar leads are shown in Figure 12.

Simple orthogonal axes are adequate only if the object to be viewed has a fairly simple shape. If the shape is complex, additional views are required. The theory on which this technique is based assumes that the heart is equivalent to a single dipole generator (magnet) rotating on a fixed point. This is only approximately true. A better approximation is that the point is not fixed but moves several centimeters or that there are several dipoles.

More recent studies have shown that the semi-orthogonal system of Holmes misses some available information.[53,60] My experience is with the semi-orthogonal system of Holmes, and all examples presented in this chapter were collected using that system. While acknowledging variation among lead systems in terms of the amount of electrocardiographic information gathered, the basic conformation of the loops derived (with other than Einthoven's system) does not appear to differ greatly.

Approach to VCG Analysis: Scalar measurement of waveform amplitude in multiple-lead ECGs represents an attempt to describe in 1-dimensional terms a process that is 3-dimensional and that changes continuously with time. This results in complex tables of values and represents one of the serious limitations of multiple-lead systems. Reduction of each waveform to a mean modal vector is achieved in a 2-dimensional plane by taking any 2 leads and applying the algebraic sum of the waveform in each lead (positive and negative area beneath the curve, though usually only the height of the waveforms is taken) to create a single resultant vector (Fig 13). This is a simpler graphic concept but greatly reduces the value of the ECGs by ignoring the change in the pattern of activation with time.

The vectorcardiogram (VCG) is ideally viewed in the form of 2-D, horizontal and sagittal loops. The loop is referred to as a vector loop because it can be conceived of as an infinite number of instantaneous component vectors, each representing the vector resultant of the dimension of 2 scalar ECG leads at a particular instant during the QRS complex. The loop is formed by joining the tips of all instantaneous vectors. If 3 "orthogonal" ECGs are used, the result is a spatial (3-D) loop. Figure 14 shows the 3 semi-orthogonal leads, X, Y and Z, from a normal horse. In Figure 15, the QRS complexes have been resolved into horizontal and sagittal plane vector loops. Each planar loop is produced by combining a pair of scalar ECG leads.[63] A third, transverse loop could be drawn but is not necessary to visualize the spatial loop.

Because the loop is derived from the scalar ECG, its conformation reflects the principal waveforms of the ECG. The loop can thus be divided into phases that represent the major fronts of activation.[64] These phases are referred to as the Q, R and S phases and approximate but are not entirely

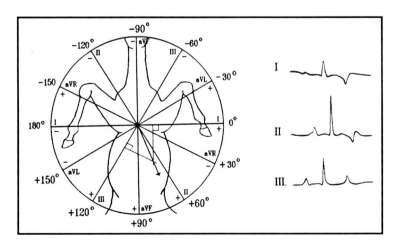

Figure 13. Hexaxial system for the derivation of mean modal vector together with Einthoven's leads I, II and III from a normal horse. The algebraic sums (in this case positive) of leads I and III have been projected onto the positive limbs of the lead-I and lead-III axes, and the direction of the resultant mean modal vector (arrow at 70 degrees) derived.

synonymous with the Q, R and S waves of the ECG. The point of onset of each of these phases is indicated in typical loops in Figure 16.

Because the anatomic location and polarity of the electrodes are known, the phases of the loop also can be spoken of in anatomic terms in relation to the heart. Thus, the usual orientation of these components is: ventral, to the right and cranial (Q phase); ventral or dorsal, to the left, and caudal (R phase); and dorsal, to the left or right, and cranial (the dominant, S phase). These phases can be described and analyzed by reference to their duration, magnitude (both relative and absolute), timing and orientation. They also can be analyzed by reference to their scalar equivalents. For example, the spatial R phase is equivalent to X_r and Y_r, and in the Z lead may occur during Z_q or the early part of Z_r. This approach increases the diagnostic information extracted from the VCG but is not practical for routine use and usually is achieved with computer assistance.

Clinical Correlations: The limited diagnostic value of the equine VCG should be anticipated on the basis of the numerous factors discussed above. Though reference to horses exhibiting ECG vector changes consistent with a specific cardiac abnormality are found in the literature, there is no information that allows the diagnostic value of particular ECG patterns to be deter-

Figure 14. Simultaneously recorded semi-orthogonal leads from a 4-year-old Standardbred mare with normal clinical findings.

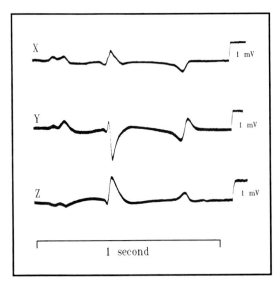

Figure 15. Horizontal and sagittal plane loops for the QRS complex for the ECG shown in Figure 14. The scalar QRS for each lead is shown adjacent to the relevant loop and in the orientation used in constructing the loop. Note that X has been inverted and Y rotated clockwise through 90 degrees to present both loops in the same diagram.

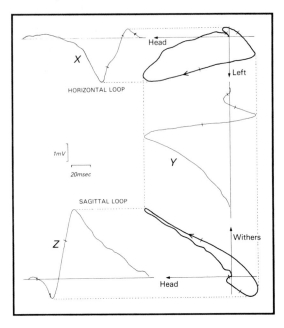

Figure 16. Horizontal (top) and sagittal plane vector loops showing Q, R and S phases.[48] The horizontal loop moves clockwise, the sagittal loop counterclockwise. Orientation of loops is as in Figure 15. F and B indicate the greatest cranial and caudal displacement of vectors, respectively.

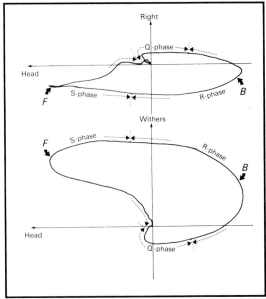

mined with any confidence. It has been suggested that the extent of backward R phase forces may relate to the relative size of the left and right ventricles and to left ventricular hypertrophy, and that some aspects of the distribution of forward S phase forces may relate to right ventricular size/activity.[48,64] In my studies, a group of 52 horses with clinical findings suggesting left ventricular hypertrophy showed a higher incidence of extensive backward vectors than the rest of the population (n = 276, predominantly Standardbred) (Fig 17). For example, evaluation of the upper and lower 20 percentiles for VCG variables in 21 cases of simple ventricular septal defect (mean age 2.97 years, range 0.5-13) revealed significant concentration of cases in the upper range for all values associated with the extent of the R phase. R-phase vectors tended to be distributed extensively to the left, caudally and ventrally. There was a tendency toward reduced absolute and relative S-phase activity and reduced dorsal distribution of vectors. In scalar terms, this is equivalent to large Z_q and Y_r, large Y_r/Y_s ratio, and prolonged duration of Y_r.

Figure 17. Scalar QRS for semi-orthogonal leads and horizontal and sagittal plane vector loops showing extensive backward and leftward distribution of vectors. Though this vector pattern is thought to indicate cardiac enlargement, particularly enlargement of the left ventricle, these tracings came from a clinically normal 3-year-old Thoroughbred stallion with an average performance record, indicating the need for caution in interpretation.

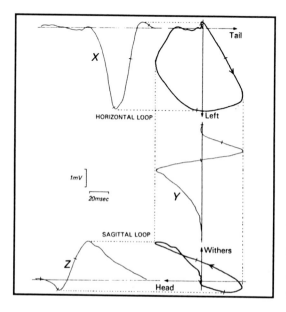

Postmortem examination supported these broad conclusions. However, absolute heart mass had a confounding effect upon all associations. Specifically, total cardiac mass was positively correlated with both the relative and absolute extent of the R-phase loop. The pattern for increasing mass of the left ventricle plus septum (used here as the structural analogue of the left ventricle as a functional unit) differed little from that observed for total heart weight, except that relationships generally were stronger than those found for combined ventricular weights. The dominant influence of the R phase upon the entire equine vector loop and the fact that this appears to be the most expressive component of the equine ECG has been commented upon previously.[64,65] The VCG pattern for right ventricular change was less easily defined and could not be separated from the effects of overall cardiac mass.

In a study of normal horses and horses with confirmed cardiac disease, similar observations were made but only for horses with aortic insufficiency.[66] In other cases of confirmed cardiac disease, no difference in the VCGs between normal and diseased horses could be demonstrated. In my studies, the sensitivity and specificity of R-phase changes appear suspect. Some horses do not have an R wave (Fig 10), a variation that appears dependent upon pattern of terminal arborization of the Purkinje system and that presumably is congenital, while others with no evidence of cardiac disease have a very large R phase.[37,49] It also has been suggested that the same diagnostic information can be derived by use of a single, simple base-apex lead (Y axis) as can be determined from use of all 3 orthogonal leads and that vectorcardiography does not contribute any additional information.[66]

There is general agreement that the Q and R phases make the greatest contribution to variability in the equine QRS complex and are likely to be the most useful source of information. While diagnostic value could be increased were a previous ECG tracing available, that is a rare luxury. A large R wave in the Y lead, especially in relation to the S wave, may be grounds for suspicion of cardiac enlargement. However, because neither the specificity nor the sensitivity of the sign is known, the clinician should proceed with caution at this time.

Studies of foals over the first year of life have demonstrated a progressive swing to the left of the mean modal vector in the horizontal plane. This has been attributed to a shift from the dominance of the right heart *in utero* to the left heart in the adult.[67-69] Despite the distinct nature of the change over time for the mean for the population as a whole (48.5 degrees in 1 study[68]), there appears to have been considerable variation within each age group, illustrating the difficulty in establishing normal values for age. These measurements were determined using limb leads. Because a progressive change was being measured, the appropriateness of the lead system used was not an issue, though the system used allowed changes to be observed in the horizontal plane only and may have contributed to the intragroup variation. The effect of age must be taken into account when following foals with congenital cardiac disease.

Vector changes in response to training have been investigated, though results are confusing because of the use of different lead systems and protocols.[70-74] Also, some studies have not controlled for age effects as opposed to training. The results suggest a shift of the mean modal vector in the horizontal plane toward the left and possibly a reduction in magnitude of the vector, interpreted as indicating a training-induced change in muscle mass distribution in the heart.[73] Studies in horses in their second year of training revealed no further change over that noted after 1 year of training.[74]

Ventricular Ectopic Foci: Multiple-lead systems may be used in investigation of ventricular ectopic foci. The normal transmission of the action potential through the Purkinje network of the ventricle results in rapid depolarization of most of the myocardium and limited fronts of activation, as noted above. If the action potential arises in an unusual location, however, the pattern of depolarization may be abnormal and is characterized by bizarre QRS conformation and prolonged QRS duration as the signal passes through the myocardium by the relatively slow process of propagation from cell to cell (Figs 45, 46).

In general, an ectopic focus originating in the left free ventricular wall generates a deep S wave in the Y lead as it passes forward, while a focus in the right ventricle causes a positive Y lead (large R wave). The

pattern may be complicated by partial Purkinje transmission, block of a major branch of the Purkinje network or ectopic foci arising in the septum. Detection of multiple QRS patterns implies multiple foci of ectopic activity.

Scalar Values

Measurement of intervals on the ECG (*eg,* PR interval, QRS duration) help detect some arrhythmias, especially if there are published and agreed-upon criteria (see discussion of Arrhythmias). Normal interval values for Einthoven's system of limb leads have been published in the literature.[18,75,76] Use has been made of the ratio of the TQ interval (electrical diastole) to the QT interval (electrical systole), the diastolic-systolic quotient, in evaluation of functional capacity of the heart.[77,78] Increase in heart rate shortens diastole to a greater extent than the shortening of systole. A relationship with performance is assumed because well-trained individuals appear able to shorten systole sooner, thus reaching a higher heart rate before the ratio reaches unity. Reduced performance has been associated with widening of the QT interval.[78]

Because depolarization is a spatial event, measurement of waveform amplitude is simply a shorthand way of assessing spatial vectors, while electrode placement obviously can affect the size of waveforms. Height of waveforms cannot, therefore, be expected to have any more value than vectors (see discussion of Vectorcardiography above). A number of factors, including increased chamber size (Brody effect), pericardial and pleural effusion and increased body cover, can reduce waveform magnitude, while amplitude is increased in tachycardia and with sympathetic stimulation.[79] Because many of these factors can operate acutely, standardization of conditions under which the ECG is recorded obviously is essential. The diagnostic criteria used in people and small animals cannot be extrapolated to horses.

T-Wave Changes

T-wave changes in horses should not be overinterpreted, as this waveform is extremely labile.[80,81] Changes occur spontaneously in the resting animal, sometimes in response to environmental stimuli and sometimes for no apparent reason. Because the conformation of any ECG waveform depends upon the particular lead used, this must be specified. In this discussion, reference is to the Y or base-apex lead. Normal values for Einthoven's lead system are available in the literature.[76] The normal T wave in the Y lead in a resting, relaxed horse is biphasic (negative then positive, Fig 10), with the negative component of the wave sometimes greater in amplitude than the S wave of the QRS complex. In such horses, the ST segment most often is elevated above the isoelectric line. The T wave rarely is totally negative. In vector terms, the T loop extends to the right, forward and slightly down.

In conditions of excitement, electrolyte disturbance and increased myocardial workload, and during many arrhythmias, general anesthesia and probably other presently undefined conditions, the negative component of the T wave tends to become progressively smaller and the positive component larger, sometimes to the point where the T wave becomes entirely positive (Fig 10). These changes may occur on a beat-to-beat basis in many arrhythmias. Under such circumstances, a relatively normal, biphasic and predominantly negative T wave would be unusual except during cardiac deceleration after exercise (see below).[81] In vector terms, the effect of these forms of myocardial "stress" is a swing of the vector loop through a horizontal plane, from forward and slightly to the right, to backward and to the left.

Persistent changes in T waveform and polarity sometimes may be found in animals not obviously exhibiting myocardial stress or excitement. It has been suggested that abnormalities occur with high frequency in horses performing poorly.[80,82-84] Criteria for diagnosis of ventricular myocardial disease based upon such changes have been described.[80,85] However, at the present time, a persistently abnormal T wave cannot be associated consistently with a specific clinical entity, though changes in relation to the overall clinical picture might emphasize the need for further investigation. It must be emphasized that, because ventricular repolarization is a spatial event, more than 1 ECG lead must be used to confirm the presence of T-wave changes.[80]

None of the above changes is necessarily associated with changes in heart rate. However, significant change in the T wave does occur as heart rate increases and, in scalar terms, consists of increasing positivity to a tall, spiked form, with a reduced elevation of the ST segment that blends into the S and T waves, and may become depressed (Fig 10). The change is equivalent to a smooth shift in the vector loop from a largely right and forward orientation, to a left and backward position. Any attempt to interpret T waves must be considerate of this rate-related effect.

During postexercise deceleration, T-wave changes vary. An overshoot has been described in which the T-wave becomes more negative than at rest, slowly returning to normal as heart rate approaches resting values.[81] The magnitude of this overshoot is less in a horse recovering from steady-state exercise as opposed to that in an animal just warmed up and showing a degree of tachycardia as much related to excitement as to effort. Exercise-related changes in T-wave polarity subside within 4 minutes in most horses, though return to normal amplitude is unlikely until heart rate approaches normal. The relationship between exercise and T-wave changes requires further investigation, as does the diagnostic value of this waveform and the definition of what constitutes an abnormality.

P-Wave Changes

The P wave also may be examined in vectorial or scalar terms. In scalar terms, the wave is most often bifid (showing 2 peaks) and positive in the Y lead (Y_p). In many normal animals, an early negative component to Y_p also is observed (Fig 10). The 2 positive peaks of Y_p, usually referred to as P_1 and P_2, can be loosely related to the pattern of atrial depolarization though, notwithstanding the discussion of genesis of the ECG above, there is not full agreement as to the areas of the atrial myocardium that contribute to the various components of the P wave in horses.[39,40] The vector loop equivalent of the scalar waveforms is a double loop, both limbs lying roughly parallel to each other and inclining downward, to the left and back.[41]

Horses frequently exhibit a rhythm variation referred to as wandering pacemaker, in which spontaneous changes in P-wave conformation are assumed to reflect change in location of the pacemaker (Fig 35). This phenomenon, along with the fact that areas of both atria depolarize simultaneously and cancel each other's effect on the body-surface ECG, plus an inadequate understanding of the contribution different areas of the atrial myocardium make to the P wave, makes interpretation of P-wave changes difficult. Difficulties sometimes arise when the timing of a cycle suggests a supraventricular premature contraction, as the P wave in such cases may not differ from those seen in wandering pacemaker (see below under Abnormalities of Rhythm and Fig 43).

Changes in P wave that show some correlation to clinical and/or postmortem diagnosis have been described.[86] However, cardiac pathology has not been associated consistently with P-wave changes in horses; at this time, the appropriate interpretation of changes in the waveform is undetermined. Limited contribution of the left atrium probably limits expression of abnormalities of this structure. Increased magnitude of P_2 may occur in left atrial enlargement due to mitral and aortic insufficiency. In right atrioventricular insufficiency, increased duration of the P wave may be seen. It is probable that the diagnostic value of P-wave changes could be increased by consideration of vectorial rather than scalar or mean modal changes.

Fetal Electrocardiography

Recording of the fetal ECG has been recommended as a means of determining fetal viability, detecting twin pregnancies, assessing fetal distress and monitoring the fetus during induced parturition.[9,10,87] Several techniques have been described, most using a bipolar lead with the positive (left-arm) electrode on the back over the mid-lumbar region and the negative (right-arm) electrode on the ventral midline about 6 inches cranial to the mammary gland, and the ECG machine set to lead I.[9]

The fetal ECG complex is small when compared with the maternal ECG. When high gains are used on the ECG machine to amplify the fetal signal, "noise" (movement of the mare, muscle twitching, mains interference) also is amplified. Filtering reduces the amplitude of waveforms and is not a useful strategy. The same precautions should be applied when recording a fetal ECG as described for rhythm monitoring (see above).

Complications in fetal electrocardiography include variation, both in absolute terms and from hour to hour, in the amplitude and conformation of the fetal QRS complex, possibly due to movement of the fetus. It may be necessary in some cases to try several lead positions to obtain a readable fetal signal.[10,12] Changes in fetal heart rate from moment to moment plus the above concerns, suggest that the technique should be repeated on several occasions, minutes to days apart, depending upon the circumstances (see below), before any conclusions are drawn.

Twins can be detected by careful examination of the fetal ECG if the QRS complexes for both fetuses are sufficiently large.[10,88] If difficulty is encountered, using several leads or simultaneous collection of a standard ECG lead from the dam may help in analysis of the tracing. In most cases, the 2 fetal heart rates or the QRS configurations differ, allowing the fetal rhythms to be distinguished.

Use of the ECG to detect fetal distress probably is of limited value unless serial recordings are made; even then, interpretation is equivocal. Tachycardia followed by bradycardia has been reported in a late-gestation fetus that subsequently was aborted.[10] Relative tachycardia was assumed to be an indication of fetal immaturity in a growth-retarded twin foal.[88] Persistent tachycardia in late gestation may indicate imminent fetal death, though the opportunity to take advantage of this information is limited in veterinary medicine. This is in contrast to the situation in human medicine, where fetal ECG monitoring is used more widely. Tachycardia has been associated with rapid or difficult foaling and appears to be transient, while fetal arrhythmias do not seem to occur with any frequency.[10] Fetal heart rate has been discussed above in the section on Heart Rate.

Exercise Testing and Exercise Tolerance

Though the term "cardiovascular" is used in this chapter in recognition of the systemic implications of marginal or reduced cardiac pumping capacity, this section concentrates on evaluation of cardiac function at exercise. Evaluation of vascular function is discussed separately below. The cardiovascular response to exercise has been the subject of several exhaustive reviews.[3,89,743] It is not the intention here to paraphrase these authors, but rather to make some practical observations concerning clinical evaluation of the cardiovascular system under exercise conditions. The reader is directed to the reviews for a discussion of the physiologic response to exercise and training.

Exercise testing should be undertaken only in animals that appear likely to tolerate the stress. The clinician should not feel obliged to use this procedure in an animal exhibiting signs of systemic disease. Horses exhibiting signs of marginal cardiovascular function at rest do not need an exercise test. No matter how sophisticated the test, the animal's response should be observed closely and the test halted if the patient shows signs of distress (*eg,* respiratory difficulty or an inappropriately high heart rate), unsteadiness or difficulty in complying with the instructions of the rider or driver. However, the horse has superlative cardiovascular reserve capacity and, with the exception of patients that are untrained and difficult to manage or those with significant arrhythmias (see below), there usually is no reason to avoid applying an exercise test.

Reasons for Exercise Testing

In the context of cardiovascular examination, exercise testing may be carried out under 4 circumstances:

- To further evaluate murmurs and arrhythmias noted at rest.
- During prepurchase examination.
- During evaluation of animals exhibiting reduced performance.
- To measure functional capacity during standardized exercise tests.

The last of these represents a specialized evaluation under closely controlled conditions. For the first 3, the clinician generally is looking for discrete signs of disease, such as a murmur, arrhythmia and excessive elevation in heart rate, or limited exercise tolerance. The basic issues to be resolved are: is there any evidence of abnormal cardiac function at exercise, and does any observation have any significance in the context of the animal's intended use? Because it cannot be assumed that a cardiac abnormality will necessarily have a clinically detectable effect, findings must be interpreted with adequate appreciation of the nature of the physiologic response to exercise.

Exercise Testing to Detect Reduced Cardiac Functional Capacity

Cardiac Disease vs Functional Capacity: The following discussion assumes that the horse being examined does not exhibit any abnormalities of rhythm other than those commonly encountered in a resting horse (see discussion of Arrhythmias), as these impose a load on the heart that may be neither predictable nor linear. Exercise testing for abnormalities of rhythm is discussed separately below.

A diseased heart functions inefficiently. For cardiac disorders in which rhythm is normal, this inefficiency can be regarded as having the following implications for exercise:

- If the level at which a horse with *acquired* cardiac disease is asked to perform is *well within its aerobic capacity,* ie, requires a rate of oxygen consumption well below its current maximum rate of aerobic working, then there will be no apparent effect upon performance, even though maximum capacity may have been reduced and the heart rate induced by the effort is now higher than before disease onset. If the horse is asked to perform at a rate close to its maximum rate of aerobic working, it will tire, as would any normal horse under the same circumstances, but earlier than expected from previous performance.
- Even assuming no prior objective evaluation of performance capacity, if an acquired cardiac disorder is progressive, reduced exercise tolerance eventually will be noted at a level of effort that subjective examination suggests was previously well tolerated.
- A horse with *congenital* heart disease has a lower maximum rate of aerobic working than with no such anomaly. As long as it is asked to work within this lower aerobic limit, its performance does not appear abnormal.

The relationship between work effort, measured as treadmill speed, load pulled or carried, and heart rate, is linear between about 120-210 bpm (Fig 18).[91] The gradient of this line decreases with training, such that any particular level of submaximal physical effort can be performed at a lower heart rate than before training. Conversely, in the diseased animal, the gradient increases and a higher heart rate is required to perform any particular level of submaximal effort than before the disease occurred. If the horse's performance was measured using a standardized exercise test before onset of cardiac disease and again after the onset of disease, it should be possible to demonstrate a reduced level of performance. However, if the disease has been present for some time and some compensation/adaptation has occurred, its effects may not be easy to detect.

Implications for Exercise Testing: If the clinical effect of a cardiac disorder is to be *measured accurately* by exercise testing, 2 conditions must be met: the test must be standardized, progressive and submaximal where heart rate is measured at a series of submaximal running speeds; and some objective measurement of work capacity before onset of the disorder must be available. If, on the other hand, the objective is simply to *detect* a clinical disorder, that disorder must manifest itself by some detectable clinical sign, such as an arrhythmia or murmur. Otherwise, an exercise test capable of ruling out other causes of performance limitation must be done to confirm the heart problem by a process of elimination. Because it is rare to have a "before and after" set of tests, the clinician most often is left offering an opinion as to the significance of a disorder without the benefit of objective measurement.

In the absence of access to a treadmill facility, field exercise tests, such as the V_{200} test can be applied (see below).[92] It must be emphasized that a *standardized* test is required. Otherwise, using exercise as a cardiovascular evaluation within the realm of submaximal tests most often applied is of value only in monitoring rhythm and heart sounds.

Similar considerations apply to the question of heart rate recovery. If the effort has been performed within the animal's cardiovascular reserve capacity, an oxygen debt has not been incurred and other body systems are normal, recovery is normal in all but the most severe cases, regardless of the degree of cardiac disease. Abnormalities of rhythm, particularly those that tend to appear at particular heart rate ranges, will complicate this situation (see below).

Tests Used for Measurement of Functional Capacity: Lunging and light exercise under saddle, while very convenient, are rarely appropriate for testing functional capacity in animals conditioned for aerobic work. Where significant limitation of functional capacity is anticipated on the basis of signs at rest, light lunging may be sufficient to demonstrate disproportionate elevation of heart rate and may guide the clinician as to the advisability of heavier work. If an animal cannot be subjected to other than this form of exercise, it is not a candidate for functional capacity determination. In all other cases, a standardized test must be performed.

In the application of a standard exercise test, the whole-body response to exercise is evaluated. Such tests of functional capacity,

Figure 18. Relationship between heart rate (HR) and velocity (V, running speed) for an unfit horse or one with a cardiovascular disorder (left, solid curve), a healthy but untrained horse (middle, solid curve) and an aerobically conditioned horse (right, solid curve).[92] Note the change in gradient with increasing performance capacity. Lack of true linearity, increasing with decreasing condition, results in overestimation of velocity at a heart rate of 200 bpm (V_{200}) when extrapolating from heart rate-velocity points determined at lower exercise intensities (dashed lines, thick bars on x axis). Approximate range for linearity of the relationship between HR and V for a fit, fully conditioned horse is shown by the arrows. (HR in beats per minute, velocity in meters per second).

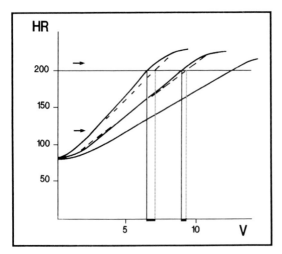

which can be applied noninvasively on a routine basis, use such values as velocity as a measure of work effort and heart rate, and blood chemistry changes as indicators of response. Contributions to the exercise response are made by many organs, including the respiratory tract and blood, as well as by the cardiovascular system. In applying such a test specifically to evaluate cardiac functional capacity, it is assumed that there is no disease in other body systems that could influence the results. It also is assumed that the only component of the oxygen delivery system that has changed between 2 test episodes is the cardiac component.

Though the value used to monitor response to exercise is the heart rate, this does not represent a specific test of cardiac functional capacity. In fact, in submaximal tests (see below), unusual elevation of heart rate is equally likely to reflect disease in other systems, while a slow rate of return to normal is unlikely to be due to cardiovascular disease.[93] Specific response of the cardiovascular system to exercise can be measured but requires invasive methods, such as the use of catheters.

Though there are a number of exercise tests described in the literature, only the V_{200} test is described here as an example.[92,94] The test takes advantage of the linear relationship between heart rate and work effort over the heart rate range of 120-210 bpm.[91] The objective is to obtain 3 or 4 points that allow a regression line to be drawn, relating these 2 variables within this range. Though statisticians may have reservations concerning the accuracy of this approach, it is suitable for practical purposes *provided that no attempt is made to attach great significance to small differences in the results between one test and the next.* Ideally, to allow for experimental error, the test would be repeated several times and the results pooled. Then these results could be compared to those from the same test applied at a later date to evaluate the possibility of progression of a cardiac problem. Under standardized conditions, the speed-heart rate relationship is highly reproducible.[92]

The horse should be worked lightly for several minutes to warm up and settle, then the test should begin. Standardization is achieved most effectively using a high-speed treadmill, though the test can be performed using a measured distance of travel and a stopwatch. Speed can be controlled at each of 3 or 4 selected levels and the horse is free to choose the gait it wishes to use, thus removing one source of error.[95] Speeds should be chosen to give a heart rate response in the range indicated. Below a level of 100 bpm, heart rate response may not fully reflect work effort; above 180-200 bpm, the anaerobic contribution to the work effort cannot be quantified and the relationship loses its linearity.[92] Each speed should be maintained for 2 minutes to allow a steady state to be achieved, with heart rate measured at the end of this time, before moving to the next level. The quantity of work involved may be beyond the exercise capacity of unconditioned horses and it may be necessary to do the test in stages.

In field situations, close synchronization between the rider or driver and the person measuring speed is necessary to ensure that heart rate response and speed can be matched accurately. Establishment of a protocol allows the rider or driver to work the horse in a manner likely to provide the required heart rate response. Standardization of the test extends not only to the test protocol but also to the surface upon which the effort is being performed. Heavy going, as may be encountered in wet weather, may totally invalidate test results.[92,96]

Heart rate can be measured using a Holter apparatus, but currently available heart rate meters provide a preferable alternative for field use. A meter with a memory can record the entire heart rate response to the test; speed and heart rate subsequently can be matched to determine the relationship. Heart rate meters are discussed below. Manual measurement of heart rate is not a viable alternative, as the rate falls very rapidly after exercise ceases. Maximal heart rate can be predicted with reasonable accuracy by measuring it 5 minutes into the resting period.[92] This only is likely to be accurate if the horse has been worked vigorously and would only provide one point for the curve. Radiotelemetry represents an alternative but it is unlikely that such equipment will be available. V_{200} can be predicted from total red cell volume divided by body weight and serum lactate concentration at a speed of 10 meters/second. This can be used in evaluation of the exercise test results.[92]

Interpretation of Results: Results of standardized exercise tests may be evaluated by determining the speed at a chosen heart rate from the heart rate-speed regression line. For V_{200}, this is 200 bpm, a rate believed to reflect both aerobic capacity and maximum rate of working.[92] This point is determined by extrapolation; it is not necessary to work the horse to a heart rate of 200 bpm. A progressive rise in V_{200} would indicate a training effect, whereas a fall would be expected in acquired cardiac disease or with change in any other aspect of the oxygen delivery system. Note that the relationship is not truly linear, even in the stated range (Fig 18). The lower the individual's performance capacity and thus the greater the heart rate response to exercise, the greater the error in estimating V_{200} by extrapolation. This problem can be offset by ensuring that the highest heart rate/velocity point used in drawing the relationship is as high as is reasonably possible.

If a horse manifests any arrhythmia during the test, the results cannot be interpreted because rate does not necessarily reflect physical effort. In cases of myocardial weakness, a degree of tachycardia that is out of proportion to the work effort may be expected, and the animal tires rapidly. With acquired defects, such as valvular dysfunction, the heart rate response does not seem unusual so long as the test limits are within the animals aerobic capacity. Similarly, the rate of cardiac slowing after exercise is normal. In general, horses have superlative cardiovascular reserve; once work is stopped, all of that reserve is available to support recovery.

If the horse has not exceeded its maximum rate of aerobic working and therefore has not incurred a significant oxygen debt, recovery is rapid. Even if a significant debt has been incurred, most patients have sufficient circulatory reserve to fully support normal correction of that debt once exercise stops. If the cardiovascular disorder is severe enough to interfere with recovery, then the test has not been carried out correctly (a heart rate in excess of 180 must have been maintained for a considerable time) or the horse has developed a serious arrhythmia that is limiting cardiac output. If recovery is prolonged, the clinician should investigate other clinical possibilities, such as respiratory disease, or look for some focus of pain or significant metabolic disturbance.

The literature contains little guidance on normal recovery rates, primarily because it is difficult to allow for the condition and temperament of the animal and the environment, even if the test protocol is standardized. As a rule of thumb, a horse warmed up and taken through a standardized exercise test, with the last component as steady state exercise (2 minutes) at a heart rate of about 180 bpm, should have a heart rate in the range of 40-60 within 30-40 minutes after exercise. Recovery rate may be used as an indicator of fitness in horses, whereas the intensity of physical effort correlates with biochemical values.[97,98] As mentioned previously, a prolonged heart rate recovery most likely indicates problems in some system other than the cardiovascular system.

Exercise Testing to Evaluate Abnormal Heart Sound

Subject to the above constraints, testing to evaluate abnormal heart sounds only requires that the heart rate be elevated into mid-ranges; maximal effort is neither necessary nor desirable. The test should be progressive at first, providing light exercise to raise the rate into the 80-120 range. Once the response to light exercise has been evaluated, heavier exercise may be applied. A murmur that cannot be detected at mid-range heart rates is unlikely to be detected after intense exercise, while at very high heart rates the intervals between heart sounds are sufficiently short to make murmur detection a challenge. Conversely, if a sound becomes more intense or changes character with exercise, yet persists, further evaluation at exercise is of value only if functional capacity is to be measured.

Auscultation with Normal Sounds: Auscultation can only be carried out after exercise has ceased. Thus, it is important that the horse be brought to a standstill in a location that facilitates examination. It is very difficult to listen to a murmur with a force-10 gale blowing around your stethoscope. Most horses stand more quietly during auscultation if the duration of the exercise has been sufficient to allow them to settle.

During cardiac deceleration, especially in mid-range heart rates (60-120), a gallop rhythm characteristically is heard. This reflects augmentation of the third and/or fourth sound or summation of the 2, which may produce a sound rivalling the first heart sound in intensity. In most horses, cardiac acceleration is rapid, with the sympathetic drive of excitement or anticipation having more to do with rate than the work. Heart sounds usually are more intense after exercise.

Exercise sometimes is used to evaluate horses exhibiting complex sounds, such as a very intense S_3 or splitting of S_1. Such sounds have their greatest significance at rest and do not change in a diagnostically useful manner with exercise. The presence of extra sounds at exercise, especially at mid-range heart rates, is of questionable significance.

Auscultation with Murmurs: Systolic and diastolic intervals are shortened progressively as heart rate rises, such that even a persistent murmur may not be easy to detect. Variations in cardiac rhythm that can be heard when the patient is not exercised to a steady state may make interpretation of murmurs after exercise difficult, though occasional long diastolic intervals may facilitate detection of sounds that otherwise are difficult to detect. It is important to listen to the heart throughout cardiac deceleration and to thoroughly auscultate both sides of the thorax.

Change in character of a murmur may be as important as its persistence. One that falls in frequency or pitch during postexercise tachycardia when compared with the resting state may be more difficult to detect and of much greater clinical significance than a sound that rises in pitch and becomes more obvious.

Exercise Testing to Evaluate Abnormalities of Rhythm

To the extent that cardiac malfunction is a factor in episodes of collapse or syncope, arrhythmias are the prime cause, not murmurs. Syncope is always a possibility when exercising a horse to evaluate an arrhythmia. If the problem is bradyarrhythmia, such as severe second-degree block, exercise may not carry much risk so long as the arrhythmia disappears as exercise starts.

With ventricular tachyarrhythmias, exercise should not even be attempted. Bearing in mind the possible underlying abnormalities, such as severe myocardial irritation, the consequences could be fatal because exercise tends to increase the frequency of ectopic beats as well as overtax a compromised system.[99,100]

An exercise test typically would be applied to evaluate the significance of *occasional* ectopic beats noted at rest or during excitement-induced tachycardia or to evaluate the significance of dropped beats. The objective usually is to determine whether the arrhythmia becomes worse with exercise or disappears. Evaluation requires a progressive approach, starting with light exercise and working up, stopping the test if obvious increase in cardiac irregularity or any unsteadiness of gait occurs. Such tests ideally involve use of some method of recording heart rhythm, as detection of an arrhythmia is of limited value if an ECG cannot be collected and a definitive diagnosis made. The ideal is to use radiotelemetry, though such equipment can be unreliable and good equipment is expensive. A tape recorder, carried by the rider to store the ECG (Holter monitor), is another option. The ECG is evaluated later after being replayed through a suitable machine. A quick and often quite effective approach is to attach the ECG leads to the horse with alligator clips and start exercise. When the horse comes to a stop, the cable immediately is plugged into the machine. This sometimes is adequate as long as the patient is cooperative. Because appropriate grounding of the horse would be difficult under these circumstances, use of a battery-operated ECG is preferable.

Clinical significance depends upon the particular type of arrhythmia. Arrhythmias rarely persist throughout all heart rates, with atrial fibrillation a notable exception. Expression of an arrhythmia probably depends upon autonomic balance, which changes throughout the cardiac response to exercise and with the circumstances of the test. It is to be expected that some types of arrhythmia will disappear with exercise and that others will be present only in particular ranges of heart rate. Thus, premature contractions, both ventricular and supraventricular, are encountered most often at mid-range heart rates (60-120 bpm).[100,101]

Detection of occasional ectopic beats in this range, however, should not necessarily be taken to indicate a clinically significant abnormality.

The clinician must constantly be aware of the danger of missing an arrhythmia or of misinterpreting a normal finding. An arrhythmia is not necessarily associated with an irregular rhythm. Arrhythmias frequently occur during cardiac deceleration even in normal horses (see discussion of Sinus Arrhythmia later in this chapter), particularly if the exercise applied is submaximal or if the animal is not worked to a steady state.[102] Radiotelemetry or use of a Holter monitor is the only way to evaluate this finding. Further evaluation usually is indicated, and ventricular ectopic activity would be a differential diagnosis. Irregular cardiac deceleration should be interpreted with caution and the animal worked to a steady state and reevaluated.

The extent to which arrhythmias occur at maximal heart rates or are associated with reduced performance has not been fully investigated. However, the occurrence of spontaneous atrial arrhythmias in racing horses suggests that this possibility should be studied more thoroughly.[103] Lack of suitable equipment is the major limiting factor, in that such arrhythmias may be transient and not present during postexercise auscultation.

Heart Rate Meters

Heart rate meters may be used in training, routine monitoring of response to exercise as a means of early detection of problems, or application of exercise tests. They allow the heart rate to be monitored during exercise with varying degrees of accuracy. The output of the meter may be monitored during work as a guide to the horse's response to effort. A meter with a memory may be used to provide a means of reviewing performance after work and as a permanent record of physiologic response by storing the heart rate response curve in a microcomputer.

These meters have been used in a number of research studies and are routinely used by many trainers. They provide a very valuable source of objectivity in the training of horses and are essential if training is to proceed according to scientific principle.

However, all of these applications depend upon the accuracy of the meter, care with which the unit is applied, manner in which the meter is used, and particularly the care and ease with which its output is monitored.

Not all meters are equally accurate;[90,104] yet the average user does not have the opportunity to test their function. In 1 study, under ideal conditions of use, the best case accuracy was ±8 bpm. This variation may be larger than that caused by the training effect a user is attempting to detect. If the trainer simply wishes to achieve a heart rate within a particular range during training, this level of accuracy is quite adequate. However, the accuracy of some meters can be very poor.[104] Dire consequences could result were a horse to be worked solely according to the output from such equipment.

One of the weakest points in application of heart rate meters is the care with which the electrodes are applied. Electrodes with poor skin contact or those that are dirty, poorly maintained or not positioned according to the manufacturer's recommendations can present inaccurate information to the meter. Meters vary greatly in their ability to handle a low-quality signal. Instructions provided by the manufacturers should be followed closely.

Telemetry

Telemetry involves remote monitoring of cardiovascular function, usually heart rate, using a transmitter and receiver. The technique has been used on numerous occasions in veterinary research.[99,101,105-110] Equipment often has been custom designed or adapted, though commercial units also have been used.[111-113] Applications generally have involved monitoring of heart rate and rhythm during exercise or at rest, though rate monitoring at exercise is best achieved with one of the meters referred to above. Perhaps the most useful application of radiotelemetry is monitoring of exercise-associated arrhythmias.[99-101]

Despite the appeal of being able to monitor cardiac rhythm during exercise, some constraints must be anticipated in use of radiotelemetry.[109,112] Range is variously limited by different government regulations; most units typically transmit less than half a mile and some only yards. Use of equipment with sufficient range for a racetrack, for example, may require a special license. Frequency bands assigned to this type of application are narrow and degrees of interference can be expected. Signal-to-noise ratio often is the critical determinant of system performance. Most radiotelemetry systems work best when the distance between transmitter and receiver is minimal and there are no intervening physical obstructions, including the body of the horse or the rider or driver.

The electrode attachment sites and the method of attachment are of great importance in obtaining an artifact-free tracing of diagnostic quality. The same considerations apply as for heart rate meters. However, electrode conditions are more stringent because of the need to obtain an ECG tracing rather than only a semi-computed rate. Most studies have used some form of adhesive to attach cup-like electrodes to the coat. Each electrode has a silver disk at the base and the cup is filled with electrode jelly.[112] One technique involved clipping the hair at the electrode sites and epilation before attaching the electrodes with contact adhesive but this may not be necessary.[111]

Peripheral Vascular Response to Exercise

Studies using labelled microspheres have demonstrated increased blood flow to skeletal muscle, diaphragm and heart, and reduced blood flow to the splanchnic circulation during exercise.[114] In an exercise test, the clinician often is more interested in the manner in which peripheral pulses and venous filling change. These changes have not been critically evaluated.

Most of the peripheral vessels that are accessible to the clinician immediately after exercise supply superficial tissues and/or tissues that experience little or no increase in metabolic rate during work. At maximal effort, therefore, reduced flow through these vessels may be anticipated as blood is redirected to functioning muscle. After intense (race-intensity) exercise, it is usual for the pulses in the digital arteries to be reduced. These pulses return within 30-60 seconds in the normal animal. Failure of the pulse to return may reflect greatly reduced cardiac output or local arterial obstruction. Clinical observation suggests little or no change in peripheral arterial pulse at the end of light to moderate exercise. Palpation of pulses must commence immediately after the horse comes to a halt for results to be meaningful.

Reduced blood flow through the arteries at most peripheral pulse sites leads to reduced filling of veins draining areas supplied by these vessels, while improved function of the muscle and thoracic pumps during exercise contributes to improved venous blood flow. As a result, after intense exercise, the major veins of the limbs are collapsed. In contrast, the cutaneous veins of the trunk and proximal limbs are distended because of shunting of blood from deeper veins and increased skin blood flow to meet the needs of thermoregulation.

The saphenous and cephalic veins should be full immediately after halting from light exercise and should be filled within 10-15 seconds of the end of intense exercise.[115] A regional failure of veins to return to normal within this interval or an asymmetric filling should be regarded as abnormal and suggestive of a local, peripheral circulatory problem, such as failure of regional arterial supply, or of venous obstruction distally. Once again, it is essential that timing of venous filling be started immediately after the horse comes to a halt. To this end, the rider or driver must be encouraged to rapidly stop the horse near the examiner. Determination of venous filling time after exercise is by direct observation of the time it takes the vein to return to a relatively normal degree of distention without any palpation, *not* by milking out the vein and watching refill.

Predicting Cardiovascular Functional Capacity

The dimensional and functional capacity of the oxygen delivery system is a primary limiting factor in aerobic performance; another is the rate at which peripheral tissues can extract and use available oxygen. Though in the elite athlete the capacities of all 3 principal elements of this system (blood, cardiovascular and respiratory systems) probably are closely matched, it can be safely assumed that the horse with a greater than average cardiac pumping capacity (a large heart) has a competitive advantage. Any method, therefore, of predicting performance capacity by predicting heart size has obvious attraction. Heart size theoretically may be predicted by electrocardiography or echocardiography. In considering the concept of performance prediction, it must be remembered that despite the very important contribution of a large heart to functional capacity, heart size is only one factor determining oxygen delivery. The relative contribution of both aerobic and anaerobic mechanisms to any particular type of exercise must be considered. As this has yet to be determined for most equine athletic events, the percentage contribution made by cardiac capacity to different types of equine performance can only be guessed at.

Echocardiography

Little has been published on the relationship between heart size and echocardiographic values. Measurement of wall thickness by echocardiography is intuitively attractive in predicting performance, though in a slaughterhouse study, no correlation between wall thickness measurements and heart weight was observed.[116] This may have reflected technique, however. Similarly, echocardiographic measurement of wall thickness is inaccurate. Measurement of chamber diameter as an approximation to volume is a promising approach and is more likely to correlate with functional capacity.

Heart Score Theory

The heart score theory proposes a relationship between heart mass (and thus pumping capacity) and QRS duration on the basis that cardiac capacity is closely related to aerobic work capacity.[80,117,118] This theory has found application in people, Greyhounds and horses. There is a relationship between the time taken for ventricular depolarization and cardiac mass.[80,117] However, this is confounded by numerous variables, particularly age, breed and sex, and by the influence of pattern of myocardial depolarization (see discussion of the conduction system and generation of the ECG above).[65]

The theory has had many antagonists.[119,120] Recent studies indicate that, while the time from onset of the S phase (approximately the peak of the S wave in

the Y lead or base-apex ECG) to the end of the QRS complex makes the greatest contribution to overall QRS duration, the greatest source of variation in QRS duration comes in the time up to the onset of the S phase.[64,65] Because the R wave dominates the early part of the QRS, R-phase forces probably relate to overall cardiac mass more consistently than S-phase forces. This finding reveals an additional source of error in the heart score theory because not all horses have an R wave, though it also provides a means of increasing the predictive power of the relationship. A horse with no Q or R wave in its base-apex ECG would lack this contribution to its overall QRS duration, which could be expected to be short, whether the horse had a large or small heart. No relationship between pattern of depolarization and cardiac dimension has been demonstrated. In conclusion, the heart score theory should be applied with caution and not used to make decisions concerning an animal's future.

Blood Gas Analysis

Routine procedures in referral centers usually call for collection of a resting venous blood gas sample, primarily for determination of acid-base status, with the venous oxygen tension (PvO_2) being incidental. However, the PvO_2 can be of great diagnostic significance. A level below the normal 40-45 mm Hg indicates increased peripheral extraction. This can only be due to 1 of 3 factors: a significantly increased metabolic rate (which should be evident from heart rate or body temperature), reduced arterial oxygen tension, or insufficient cardiac output to meet resting requirements.

Blood gas analysis is thus of clinical value in evaluation of congenital heart disease and in assessment of animals with cardiac insufficiency. In congenital heart disease, shunts are encountered frequently. If the shunt is from left (systemic arterial) to the right (systemic venous) side of the heart, blood gas tension in peripheral vessels does not change. Where the shunt is right to left, a decrease in both arterial and venous O_2 can be anticipated. The extent of this fall can be of great diagnostic significance in congenital heart diseases and is considered in their discussion later in the chapter. Arteriovenous fistulas cause a rise in the oxygen tension in venous blood downstream from the fistula, but their systemic effect depends most upon the size of the vessels involved and thus the hemodynamic, as opposed to gas tension, effects.

In heart failure, arterial oxygen tension (PaO_2) is normal unless severe pulmonary edema or pulmonary fibrosis secondary to chronic pulmonary edema is present. These are unusual but occasional complications in horses. However, with cardiac insufficiency or congenital heart disease, reduced delivery of oxygenated blood to the periphery or persistent arterial hypoxemia leads to venous hypoxemia as peripheral oxygen extraction increases. Though some fall in PvO_2 occurs rapidly upon a sudden insult, a marked fall over time reflects the chronicity as well as the severity of the primary problem. In acute cases and in chronic cases in which increase in oxygen extraction has been exhausted as a compensatory mechanism, tachycardia is observed. However, in many cases, an increase in the arteriovenous oxygen difference (a-vO_2) meets peripheral requirements without an increase in resting heart rate.

Analysis of the relationship between the a-vO_2 and heart rate thus can provide insight into the severity and chronicity of a clinical disorder. Anticipated basal oxygen requirement can be compared with computed oxygen delivered, though, unless physiologic values can actually be measured, the calculation is only a general approximation. Resting oxygen requirement in a *normal* horse can be assumed to be about 3.5 ml/kg/min.[121] On the basis of a mean resting cardiac output (CO) of 70 ml/kg/min (range 56-85) and a mean resting heart rate of 35 bpm (range 28-40), a stroke index (SI) of 2 ml blood/kg/beat can be derived.[3] PaO_2 and PvO_2 are determined by blood gas analysis with correction for body temperature, and percent oxygen saturation determined from oxyhemoglobin dissociation curves for horses.[122] Arteriovenous oxygen difference then can be determined. Hemoglobin should be measured by hemoglobinometer as blood gas machine estimations of hemoglobin can be very inaccurate. Oxygen content of hemoglobin at 100% saturation can be assumed to be about 1.36 ml/g hemoglobin.[123] These values then can be used in the equations in Table 1.

In performing the calculation, it must be emphasized that it is approximate. There will be variation in cardiac output according to the condition of the myocardium. Jugular venous PO_2 does not necessarily reflect systemic venous PO_2, which usually is likely to be lower, while metabolic rate and thus oxygen requirement vary with age, body size, body temperature and level of resting activity. However, the calculation does provide guidance in clinical management. Thus, a 150-kg foal with congenital heart disease, a resting heart rate of 80, PaO_2 of 45 mm Hg, PvO_2 of 24 mm Hg and a hemoglobin level of 120 g/L has an oxygen consumption of about 1.25 L/min, more than twice the anticipated basal requirement of 0.53 L/min.

The technique of collection of a blood sample for blood gas analysis is critical. The blood must be collected into a heparinized syringe, using care not to allow room air to enter during collection. Any bubble of air that has entered the syringe must be expelled immediately and the syringe tightly

Table 1. Equations for comparison of anticipated basal oxygen requirement with estimated actual oxygen delivery.

$$\text{Basal } O_2 \text{ requirement (L/min)} = \frac{\text{bwt (kg)} \times 3.5}{1000}$$

$$\text{CO (L/min)} = \frac{\text{HR (bpm)} \times \text{SI (ml/kg/beat)} \times \text{bwt (kg)}}{1000}$$

$$\text{Arterial } O_2 \text{ content (L/L)} = \frac{\text{arterial } O_2 \text{ saturation (\%)} \times 1.36 \times \text{Hb (g/L)}}{1000 \times 100}$$

$$\text{Venous } O_2 \text{ content (L/L)} = \frac{\text{venous } O_2 \text{ saturation (\%)} \times 1.36 \times \text{Hb (g/L)}}{1000 \times 100}$$

$$O_2 \text{ delivered (L/min)} = \text{CO (L/min)} \times \text{a-v}O_2 \text{ (L/L)}$$

capped. The syringe then should be rotated for mixing and chilled with cold water or ice until analysis, which should begin within an hour. If delays are anticipated, a heparinized glass syringe, as opposed to plastic, is recommended strongly. Body temperature always must be recorded simultaneously so that oxygen tension can be corrected accordingly.

Arterial samples can be collected from the horse's carotid artery at the base of the neck, the facial artery rostral to the facial crest, the femoral artery in the groin or the dorsal metatarsal artery distal to the hock. The last 2 sites are useful only in foals. For an arterial sample from a site at which the artery itself cannot be clearly seen, a needle large enough to allow free flow of blood should be used as ideally the blood should be allowed to spurt both before and after the collection of the sample to convince the operator that the sample was indeed collected from an artery. A fine needle (23-25 ga) is preferred by some to reduce the arterial spasm that may result from arterial puncture and to reduce hematoma formation. Spasm also can be reduced by prior application of a bleb of local anesthetic over the artery. Both an arterial and a venous sample should be collected to determine the a-vO$_2$ and to reinforce the notion that the arterial sample was truly arterial. Tail veins never should be used for blood gas analysis because of the difficulty in avoiding a mixed sample.

Phonocardiography

Interpretation of auscultatory findings is aided by phonocardiography, which involves recording heart sounds on paper.[30,32] A phonocardiogram (PCG) does not necessarily provide a definitive diagnosis as to the origin of abnormal sound(s) but may aid diagnosis by defining timing in relation to the cardiac cycle. To this end, it is important that a simultaneous ECG be recorded. Normal heart sounds generally are of low (<200 Hz) frequency, though many murmurs have many higher frequency components.[124] One particularly useful application of the PCG, therefore, is emphasis of sounds of very low frequency that sometimes are difficult to interpret by auscultation.

Phonocardiography has not been used routinely, probably because few recorders are commercially available and suitable for practice application. The PCG is of limited value if the ECG cannot be recorded simultaneously as a timing signal. A suitable machine accepts input from a microphone capable of detecting low frequencies and has a frequency response allowing sounds from 10 Hz to 2 kHz to be recorded. The microphone ideally has a profile that allows it to be positioned on the chest wall ventral to the elbow, though this requirement can rarely be met with available equipment, as it was designed for use in people. Therefore, it is necessary to elevate the forelimb for a few moments. A phonocardiogram should also be capable of dividing output into switch-selectable frequency ranges to be recorded simultaneously (Figs 19, 20). This is important because not all heart sounds have the same frequency content. Thus, the atrial contraction sound, S$_1$ and S$_3$ tend to be low-frequency sounds (mainly <200 Hz), whereas S$_2$ and many murmurs tend to be of higher frequency (up to 200-1000 Hz). A machine with a single, fixed, broad-frequency response generates tracings that can be difficult to interpret.

While it has been suggested that recording from the mitral valve area only may be adequate for most purposes, thorough evaluation of murmurs requires that all areas be examined.[32] The horse should stand quietly, with the heart beating at a resting rate, to avoid changes in heart sounds that commonly accompany tachycardia. Clipping of the thorax is not necessary. If possible, the paper speed of the recorder should be 50 mm/sec to allow better separation of sounds, especially important with loud murmurs. Increased amplification should be used with caution, as "noise" is also amplified, which may confuse interpretation.

Notwithstanding the desirability of obtaining a paper record of heart sounds, one should not expect a close correlation between what is heard and what is recorded on the PCG. Sounds may be modified by the recording apparatus, deemphasizing those the operator heard, and recording frequencies not heard through the stethoscope. There is a very wide range in quality of PCGs because of difficulties in standardizing equipment and technique, as well as background noise. It has been suggested that increased diagnostic sensitivity and

Figure 19. Y-lead ECG and 4 phonocardiogram bandwidth channels from a clinically normal 4-year-old gelding during a period of mild tachycardia (HR 60 bpm). The atrial contraction sound (acs), S_1, S_2 and S_3 are all visible. All channels were taken with the same gain. Note that, with the exception of S_1, the sounds tend to be most obvious in the bands accommodating the lower frequencies. Note also the relationship between the heart sounds and waveforms of the ECG. cps = cycles per second.

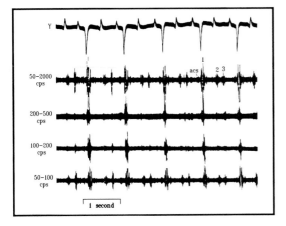

specificity can be obtained by intracardiac phonocardiography, though this is not an option in a practice situation.[33]

The literature contains specific reference to the time intervals encountered in the normal PCG.[27,32,125] Such detailed analysis can be of value in interpreting some murmurs if recordings made from different areas and at several frequencies are compared. However, there is considerable variation, both between horses and with heart rate, and such measurement may be of limited practical value. It is far more useful to examine the general relationship between abnormal and normal sounds. For example, does a murmur interfere with a particular heart sound? These features are discussed in the section on Pathophysiology.

Diagnostic Imaging In Cardiovascular Disease

H. Dobson

The literature on diagnostic imaging of the equine cardiovascular system is sparse in comparison to that of other species. This is largely a direct result of limitations due to size. Despite this, a great deal of useful diagnostic information can be obtained, particularly in the neonate, with the relatively simple equipment available in the practice situation, albeit with some ingenuity and patience on the part of the clinician.

The Heart and Great Vessels

Radiography: Comprehensive radiographic examination of the heart and great vessels, on a practical basis, is limited to the neonatal foal. However, even in the adult, radiography can give a valuable overview of cardiovascular status.

In the foal, diagnostic lateral projections of the cardiac silhouette can be made easily using rare-earth intensifying screens and high-speed film. Radiographic techniques on the order of 70-80 kVp and 10-15 mAs are required and frequently are within the capabilities of the average practice. It is not always appreciated that a neonatal foal may be smaller than an average dog. Where only low-output equipment is available, motion artifact can be reduced by making the exposure at end expiration, as the pause before the next inspiration is longer than that between inspiration and expiration. Recumbent lateral positioning with manual restraint or, if appropriate, chemical sedation or general anesthesia allows both of the patient's forelimbs to be extended, improving the imaging of the cranial cardiac border. Attempts to extend a forelimb in older foals and yearlings in the standing position, with or without chemical restraint, are

Figure 20. Y-lead ECG and 4 phonocardiogram bandwidth channels from a 2-year-old Arab filly with a large VSD and signs of heart failure. Note the delay in onset of S_1 compared with that in Figure 19 (reflecting dilatation and reduced contractility). Systole is occupied by an intense murmur (SM), which extends from S_1 to S_2 and obliterates the latter. Note the variation in murmur intensity in the different frequency bands.

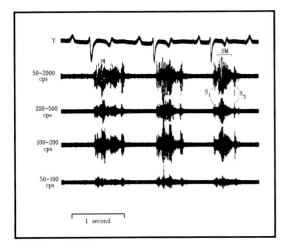

often futile. This can be safely and adequately accomplished only in older horses that have been broken.

Ventrodorsal and dorsoventral projections can be obtained in young foals if sufficiently powerful equipment is available. Frequently the limiting factor is inability to adequately restrain and position all but the smallest foals without use of general anesthesia, which often is contraindicated.

In adult horses, only lateral projections of the heart and great vessels can be obtained. The increasing use by practitioners of mobile rather than portable x-ray generators, particularly of the capacitor discharge type, has led to wider use of these techniques. Use of 28 x 17-inch cassettes (Spectroline Four Square Cassette: Spectronics Corp, Westbury, NY) that hold 2 14 x 17-inch films, produces all of the cardiac silhouette on 1 radiograph. Use of a grid requires a high-mAs radiographic technique, but use of an airgap technique reduces this substantially. A typical technique using a 200-cm film-focal spot distance and a 20-cm air gap is on the order of 120 kV and 20 mAs for a 500-kg horse.

Alteration in the size or shape of the cardiac silhouette may indicate cardiac disease. Unfortunately, only limited objective data are available to aid assessment of cardiac size. In adult horses, usually only the caudal border of the silhouette, which has a slightly convex shape and runs parallel to the long axis of the adjacent ribs, can be evaluated reliably. Using the intersection of lines drawn parallel to the trachea and to the ventral border of the adjacent thoracic vertebrae, the spinotracheal angle can be defined (Fig 21). A 50% decrease in this measurement has been demonstrated in a group of young horses with confirmed congenital heart disease.[126] However, some overlap between the 2 groups did occur and the true value of this measurement as a criterion for diagnosis of cardiomegaly has yet to be determined.

Assessment of the remaining structures of the thorax for abnormalities that may be primary or secondary to cardiovascular disease is essential, particularly the great vessels and the pulmonary parenchyma. An evaluation of pulmonary circulation is extremely subjective and can be strongly influenced by radiographic technique. It is of paramount importance to use a consistent technique and to develop an appreciation for the normal range of appearance, particularly with respect to the size and clarity of the pulmonary vasculature. It has been suggested that changes in the vena cava are the easiest to appreciate.[127]

Pulmonary overcirculation, combined with its associated pulmonary hypolucency and undercirculation with hyperlucency, are recognized in the various manifestations of congenital and acquired cardiac disease. In left heart failure, the progression of pulmonary venous congestion to pulmonary edema is recognized as in other species.

Angiocardiography: Angiocardiography is a valuable diagnostic procedure and is widely used in many species, particularly people, with low complication rates. However, it is not an entirely benign procedure, particularly in an animal with a compromised cardiovascular system. It requires a team approach, with appropriate equipment and careful planning from the outset. When adequately performed in appropriate cases, it can provide valuable information regarding both cardiovascular anatomy and function.

Techniques for positive-contrast angiocardiography, both selective (injection of

Figure 21. Lateral radiograph of the thorax of a normal neonatal foal. The angle A (spinotracheal angle) is formed by the intersection of 2 lines, 1 parallel to the trachea, the other parallel to the ventral border of adjacent thoracic vertebrae.

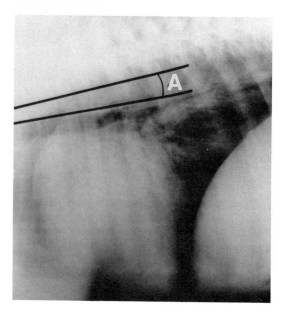

contrast material into a specific vessel or chamber) and nonselective (peripheral injection of contrast) have been described for neonates and adults.[128-130] For neonates, facilities for cardiac catheterization and pressure injection of contrast medium and fluoroscopy, cineradiography or a rapid film changer are required. Though these techniques are likely to be beyond the scope of most private practices, they usually are available at referral institutions. Sophisticated facilities for angiocardiography in standing and anesthetized horses are available only at a small number of institutions.[131] In view of the current development of nuclear angiocardiography and diagnostic ultrasound, it is unlikely that further development of these techniques will be pursued in adult horses.

To avoid dilution of contrast medium in angiocardiography, a bolus injection is rapidly given using a large-bore, short catheter. Reported dosages are about 200 mg of iodine/kg body weight.[128-130] Any of the water-soluble iodine-based contrast agents may be used. However, these preparations are irritating and it is prudent to use the newer, low-osmolality agents in a compromised animal.

Nuclear Medicine Imaging: Nuclear imaging is rapidly becoming a standard diagnostic technique in equine practice. Though new equipment is extremely expensive, rapid technologic developments have placed used equipment within the reach of many institutions and some private practices. The techniques are no more invasive than an intravenous injection and can be performed in the standing animal with minimal, if any, chemical restraint.

In nuclear angiocardiography, the simplest techniques give a subjective analysis of cardiac function; with computer support, quantitative analysis of the dynamic aspects of cardiac function can be performed. This last approach is likely to be used increasingly in investigation of selected cases of cardiac disease in adult horses. First-pass nuclear angiocardiography is the technique used most commonly. More complex techniques, such as gated-equilibrium nuclear angiocardiography, in which temporal separation of data acquisition is triggered by the ECG, are widely used in people and have been used in horses and dogs but are less applicable to routine diagnosis.[126]

First-pass nuclear angiocardiography involves rapid injection of a small-volume bolus of technetium-99m. Passage of the bolus through the heart and great vessels is recorded using a gamma camera, which detects radiation emitted by the technetium. Sequential images, made over periods of 0.5-3 seconds, allow viewing of the bolus as it passes sequentially through the right heart, lung and left heart during a total examination period of about 30 seconds. Details of these techniques have been described.[126,132]

Valvular dysfunction or myocardial failure results in enlargement of one or more chambers or prolonged transit time. Cardiac shunts allow simultaneous visualization of both ventricles or slow the clearance from compartments downstream to the shunt.[126]

Peripheral Vessels

Peripheral angiography, the injection of contrast material into peripheral vessels, is within the scope of most private practices, including those with limited equipment. Under some circumstances, examination may be done in the standing animal but general anesthesia usually is required.

In ideal circumstances, either cineradiography or rapid film changers are required. Fluoroscopy provides a more flexible approach, particularly in nonstandard examinations; with a good image intensifier and high-quality video equipment capable of frame-by-frame replay, the results can be comparable to those of cineradiography. With sheet film, subtraction techniques can be employed to improve the diagnostic sensitivity. Where available, digital subtraction angiography can provide exquisite detail.

With minimal improvisation using a simple cassette tunnel with lead shielding, a series of regular cassettes can be pushed through the tunnel manually and exposures made at 1-second intervals.[133] Under these circumstances, it is vital to ensure that each cassette is correctly identified with lead markers. Team work is vital to coordinate movement of the cassettes correctly with the exposure; with forethought, excellent results can be obtained.

Maximum absorption of radiation by iodinated contrast agents occurs at 60-70 kVp.[130] Before injection of contrast material, test exposures should be made to determine a satisfactory technique. Percutaneous arterial injection can be used, but a cut-down approach is recommended to minimize arterial trauma. A compromise must be reached between use of a small-bore catheter to minimize trauma and a large-bore one to allow rapid bolus injection. The catheterization site, particularly in examination of the extremities, should be as close to the heart as practical because vascular abnormalities, especially development of a collateral circulation, may be located more centrally than clinical signs may suggest. Particularly in the hind limb, where difficulty is experienced in locating a vessel, it may be possible to make a retrograde injection in the opposite femoral or saphenous artery, with the contrast material forced into the aorta and from there carried into the affected limb.

Typically, 20-50 ml of contrast material containing 250-300 mg of iodine per ml are injected rapidly as a bolus. If a rapid film changer is used, exposures should commence at the beginning of contrast agent injection and then at 1-second intervals. If only a single radiograph can be made, this is exposed at the end of the injection.

Figure 22. Peripheral angiogram of the left hind limb of a 3-year-old Standardbred gelding with aortoiliac thrombosis. The catheter was placed in the femoral artery via the saphenous artery. The white arrow marks the completely occluded popliteal artery. The black arrow identifies development of a collateral circulation, indicated by the tortuous vessel.

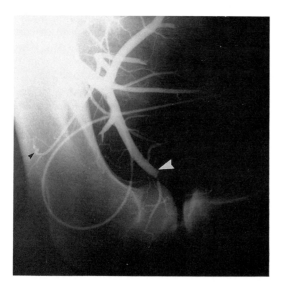

The normal angiographic anatomy of the carotid and cerebral vessels and selective techniques for specific vessels have been described.[134] The principal indications are investigation of guttural pouch mycosis and selected central nervous system diseases. Peripheral angiography is indicated in any vaso-occlusive condition, such as trauma, frostbite or thromboembolism, to determine the site and the degree of vascularization peripheral to the lesion and the development of collateral circulation. Radiographically, a partial obstruction is recognized as an abrupt narrowing of the contrast column, distinct from the gentle tapering toward the periphery seen in the normal vascular tree. A complete obstruction appears as a sudden termination of the contrast column (Fig 22). A developing collateral circulation is identified by tortuous vessels of fine caliber (Fig 22).

Complications due to angiography are uncommon and usually are related to arterial spasm or embolism following trauma at the injection site. Care must be taken not to confuse arterial spasm due to trauma with a true occlusive lesion.

Serum Enzyme and Isozyme Measurements

P.J. O'Brien

Determination of the serum activity of enzymes with unusually high concentration in the heart may aid diagnosis of acute myocardial injury. In people, creatine kinase isozyme 2 (CK-MB) and lactate dehydrogenase isozyme 1 (LDH-H4) are commonly used for this purpose. However, CK-MB is found in much lower concentrations in equine myocardium and therefore has less diagnostic value.[135] Nevertheless, combined isozyme analysis of CK and LDH may identify the tissue causing increased serum activity. In cardiac disease, there is mildly to moderately increased serum LDH-H4 activity, while serum CK-MB activity may be mildly increased. In contrast, muscle disease is characterized by mildly to markedly increased serum LDH isozyme 5 (LDH-M4) and CK isozyme 1 (CK-MM) activities. Hemolysis likely increases serum LDH-H4 activity, as this isozyme occurs in erythrocytes. In digestive disease, there is mildly to moderately increased serum CK-MB (smooth muscle) and LDH-M4 (liver) activity.

Total activity determinations for other tissue-specific enzymes may supplement LDH and CK isozyme data and facilitate diagnosis, especially if there is multiple tissue involvement. Aldolase (ALD) and alanine transaminase (ALT) are found in much higher levels in equine muscle, whereas alpha-hydroxybutyrate dehydrogenase (HBD) is found in higher levels in the heart. Thus, in myocardial injury, the ratio of serum LDH and/or HBD activity to ALT and/or ALD activity is more increased than in skeletal muscle disease. If the serum ratio and myocardial and muscle tissue ratios are known, one may be able to comment on the most likely source of enzyme leakage.

Following injury, the different enzymes are released from myocardium and cleared from the blood at different rates. Serum CK and AST activities peak after 12-24 hours and return to normal within 3-4 days, whereas serum LDH activity peaks after 24-48 hours and returns to normal within 7-10 days. Thus, acute serial samples (obtained every 12 hours for 36 hours after injury) are likely to have greatest diagnostic value.

Reference ranges must be established for serum activities of LDH and CK isozymes and other tissue-specific enzymes in horses before using these determinations in diagnosis of acute myocardial injury. They should be used with caution and only with other diagnostic tests until a larger data base has been accumulated. Application of LDH isoenzyme analysis in investigation of cardiac disorders has been described.[136-138]

Twenty-Four-Hour Rhythm Monitoring

V.B. Reef

Cardiac arrhythmias occur in horses and may be frequent, intermittent or persistent. Persistent cardiac arrhythmias are documented easily using routine electrocardiographic techniques in which a resting ECG is obtained from the horse over a 5- to 10-minute period. Many horses, however, have cardiac arrhythmias that are transient or intermittent, and a routine resting ECG may not detect the abnormality. Longer periods of electrocardiographic monitoring are indicated in these animals to document the arrhythmia.

Twenty-four-hour continuous electrocardiographic (Holter) monitoring is a means of recording the rhythm to detect many of the transient or intermittent cardiac arrhythmias that may not be appreciated during routine electrocardiography. This technique should be considered in horses in which previously auscultated cardiac arrhythmias are not detectable during subsequent examination and in horses with a history of collapse, syncope or poor performance in which no other abnormalities have been found.

A light-weight portable tape recorder (Holter Recorder Model #445A: Del Mar Avionics, Irvine, CA) is used to obtain a continuous ECG tracing over a 24- to 26-hour period. The ECG is recorded on magnetic tape that is then analyzed with the help of a computer. Individually grounded flat bipolar electrodes normally used with heart rate monitors (EQB, Doe Run Rd, Unionville, PA) are adapted to connect to the Holter monitor. The electrodes are held in position under a blanket surcingle and connected to the recorder, and the recorder is strapped to the rings on the surcingle. A base-apex ECG is obtained by placing the negative electrode near the left side of the withers in the saddle area and the positive electrode over the left cardiac apex. Alcohol is used as a conducting agent and the electrodes are sprayed every 4-6 hours or as needed, depending on the weather and the horse's haircoat. Events occurring during monitoring can be marked by pressing an event-marking button on the Holter recorder and noting the event in the time log book, allowing arrhythmias to be related to the daily events (eg, feeding, exercise).

The Holter monitor report on the 24-hour recording is generated by computer analysis through a commercial laboratory (Cardio Data Systems, Box 200, Haddonfield, NJ) and contains an hourly reading of high, low and mean heart rate, the rhythm during that hour, and the number of supraventricular or ventricular premature beats occurring during that time. Paired, single, multiform and R-on-T ventricular premature beats, supraventricular premature beats and ventricular tachycardia can all be differentiated. The laboratory performing the analysis provides sample ECGs of any of these events, as well as any periods of bradycardia or tachycardia or any other arrhythmias, and a random sampling of the normal periods. Heart rate and ventricular arrhythmias also are plotted over time.

Supraventricular and ventricular arrhythmias frequently are detected in horses in which no abnormalities were detected on routine electrocardiography. Thus, continuous 24-hour rhythm monitoring can be a helpful diagnostic aid and also can be used to evaluate therapy.

Echocardiography

V.B. Reef

Echocardiography is a widely used non-invasive technique for evaluation of cardiac size and function in horses.[139-143] The normal appearance of the valves and chambers have been described using M-mode and 2-dimensional real-time techniques, as well as normal flow profiles using pulsed-wave Doppler echocardiography. Echocardiographic examination is performed from the right and left cardiac "windows," which are areas of the thorax where the heart lies directly against the chest wall without any lung intervening.

The left and right sides of the thorax are clipped closely in the fourth to fifth intercostal space between the level of the point of the shoulder and the elbow. An aqueous coupling gel is applied to the skin to provide air-free contact between the skin and transducer for optimal imaging. A 2.5-mHz or lower-frequency transducer is optimal for imaging the heart of an adult horse, while a 3.0- or 3.5-mHz transducer is preferable for foals or yearlings. The highest frequency transducer that will penetrate to the desired depth should be used, as image resolution increases with higher frequencies but penetration of the ultrasound beam decreases. A simultaneous ECG should be obtained with the echocardiogram for timing.

There are 2 modes of echocardiographic imaging (M-mode and 2-dimensional real-time) and 2 types of Doppler echocardiography (pulsed and continuous wave). These can be used alone or in combination. M-mode echocardiography provides a 1-dimensional view of the heart that changes with time and is used to obtain accurate measurements of intracardiac structures.[139-141] Two-dimensional real-time echocardiography is used to obtain a 2-dimensional cross section of the heart in motion. Pulsed-wave Doppler echocardiography usually is combined with imaging to provide information about direction, location and velocity of intracardiac blood flow.[143] High-velocity blood flow cannot be observed using pulsed-wave Doppler echocardiography; in these instances, continuous-wave Doppler is needed to determine peak velocity. Color-flow Doppler echocardiography is a combination of 2-dimensional real-time imaging and Doppler technology that depicts blood within the heart flowing toward and away from the transducer as different colors.

The standards of the American Society of Echocardiography have been adapted to horses for M-mode and 2-dimensional imaging. Standard M-mode views are obtained from the right cardiac window (fourth intercostal space) and include the aortic valve, mitral valve and ventricular position. The aortic root (AR) position includes the right ventricular (RV) free wall, right ventricular outflow tract (RVOT), cranial aortic wall, aortic valve leaflets within the aortic root, caudal aortic wall and left atrium (LA) (Fig 23). The mitral valve (MV) position includes the RV free wall, RV chamber, interventricular septum (IVS), septal (cranial) leaflet of the mitral valve, free wall (caudal) leaflet of the mitral valve, left ventricular (LV) free wall, and pericardium (Fig 24). The left ventricular position includes the RV free wall, RV chamber, interventricular septum, LV chamber, chordae tendineae of the mitral valve, LV free wall above the papillary muscle and the pericardium (Fig 25). Measurements of wall thickness, chamber size, fractional shortening, vessel size and valve motion can be made from these views.

Two-dimensional echocardiography can be used to obtain both long- and short-axis views from both the right and left sides.[139-142] From the right cardiac window, the images most closely resemble those seen in people The transducer is placed in the fourth intercostal space just ventral to the level of the point of the shoulder. The plane of the sector is dorsocranial to ventrocaudal. In most horses, the transducer is tilted cranially about 20-30 degrees from vertical to obtain the long-axis views. The left ventricular outflow tract view (right caudal long axis) is obtained by aiming the transducer directly perpendicular to the long axis of the horse or slightly cranial to this imaginary line.[139,142] In this view, the right atrium (RA), TV, RV, IVS, left ventricular outflow tract (LVOT), LV, aortic root, AV and LA can be imaged (Fig 23). These same structures can be seen in short axis by rotating the transducer 90 degrees cranially and scanning from apex to base.

The 4-chamber view (right caudal long axis) is obtained by angling the transducer slightly caudal to the LVOT position. In this view, the RA, TV, RV, IVS, LV, MV and LA can be imaged (Figs 24, 25).[139] Turning the transducer 90 degrees cranially and scanning from apex to base will result in a short-axis image of these structures at this position. The long-axis view of the right ventricular outflow tract can be obtained by angling the transducer cranially from the LVOT position in the direction of the point of the left shoulder (Fig 26). In some horses, the third intercostal space must be used for

Figure 23. Normal echocardiogram from a 3-year-old Thoroughbred filly, made at the aortic root position. Top: Two-dimensional real-time echocardiogram showing the aortic root (AR), aortic valves (AV), left ventricle (LV) in the area of the left ventricular outflow tract, left atrium (LA), right atrium (RA) and right ventricle (RV). The dotted line represents the location at which the M-mode echocardiogram (bottom) was obtained. Bottom: M-mode echocardiogram at the aortic root position showing the tricuspid valve (TV), aortic valve (AV) and left atrium (LA).

Figure 24. Normal echocardiogram from a 3-year-old Thoroughbred filly, made at the mitral valve position. Top: Two-dimensional real-time echocardiogram showing the 4 cardiac chambers. RA = right atrium. TV = tricuspid valve. RV = right ventricle. LA = left atrium. MV = mitral valve. LV = left ventricle. The dotted line represents the location at which the M-mode echocardiogram (bottom) was obtained. Bottom: M-mode echocardiogram of the mitral valve position showing the tricuspid valve (TV), mitral valve (MV) and left ventricular outflow tract (LVOT).

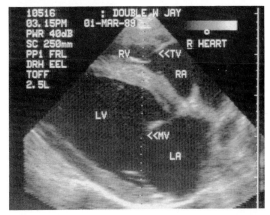

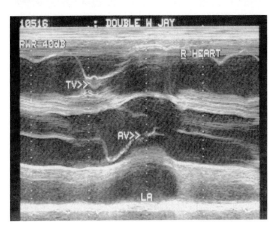

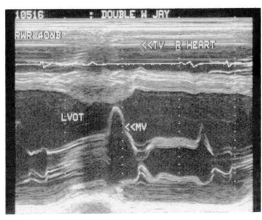

this view in which the RA, TV, RV, pulmonic valve, pulmonary artery and aorta can be imaged. A short-axis view of this area can also be obtained by rotating the transducer cranially 90 degrees.

Long- and short-axis views of the heart also can be obtained from the left cardiac window (third to fifth intercostal space between the level of the point of the shoulder and elbow). A 2-chamber view of the left heart can be obtained from the fourth (or fifth) intercostal space with similar positioning of the transducer as used on the right side (Fig 27). In this 2-chamber view,

the LA, MV and LV can be imaged in long or short axis.[139-142] Moving slightly cranially, a reverse 4-chamber view can be obtained. Angling the transducer cranially obtains a view of the LVOT, AV, aorta, LV and LA (Fig 28). The pulmonic valve and pulmonary artery can also be imaged but the third intercostal space must be used to obtain this view, angling slightly cranially (Fig 29). In this view, the PA, PV, RVOT, RV, TV, RA and aorta are seen.

Pulsed-wave Doppler echocardiography combined with 2-dimensional real-time imaging allows the echocardiographer to eval-

Figure 25. Normal echocardiogram from a 3-year-old Thoroughbred filly, made at the left ventricular position. Top: Two-dimensional real-time echocardiogram showing the 4 cardiac chambers. RA = right atrium. TV = tricuspid valve. RV = right ventricle. LA = left atrium. MV = mitral valve. LV = left ventricle. The dotted line represents the location at which the M-mode echocardiogram (bottom) was obtained. Bottom: M-mode echocardiogram of the left ventricular position showing the right ventricle (RV) and left ventricle (LV).

Figure 26. 3. Normal echocardiogram from a 3-year-old Thoroughbred filly, made at the right ventricular outflow tract and pulmonary artery (long axis) Top: Two-dimensional real-time echocardiogram of the right ventricular outflow tract and pulmonic valve in diastole. RA = right atrium. TV = tricuspid valve. RV = right ventricle. PV = pulmonic valve. PA = pulmonary artery. Bottom: Two-dimensional real-time echocardiogram of the right ventricular outflow tract and pulmonic valve in systole. RA = right atrium. TV = tricuspid valve. RV = right ventricle. PA = pulmonary artery.

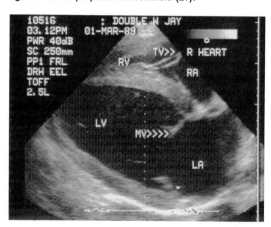

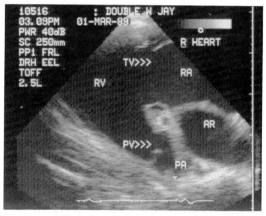

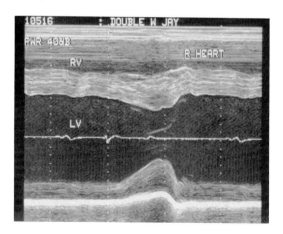

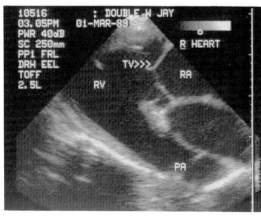

uate the cardiac valves for evidence of valvular insufficiency (most common) or stenosis and the interventricular and interatrial septa for shunts.[143] The scanner head is placed on the atrial side of the atrioventricular valves and on the ventricular side of the semilunar valves to listen for any evidence of valvular insufficiency. The views used are those described above for 2-dimensional imaging. An abnormal signal is a turbulent, harsh, prolonged sound composed of varying frequencies. The abnormal flow is mapped by moving the scanner head

Figure 27. Normal two-dimensional real-time echocardiogram of the left atrium (LA), mitral valve (MV) and left ventricle (LV) in a 3-year-old Thoroughbred filly, made at the left cardiac window.

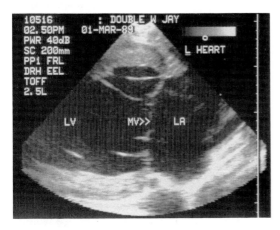

Figure 28. Normal two-dimensional real-time echocardiogram of the aortic valves and left ventricular outflow tract in a 3-year-old Thoroughbred filly, made at the left cardiac window. AR = aortic root. AV = aortic valve. LV = left ventricle. RA = right atrium. RV = right ventricle.

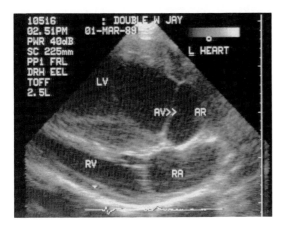

Figure 29. Normal two-dimensional real-time echocardiogram of the right ventricular outflow tract and pulmonary artery in a 3-year-old Thoroughbred filly, made at the left cardiac window. PA = pulmonary artery. PV = pulmonic valve. RA = right atrium. RV = right ventricle. TV = tricuspid valve.

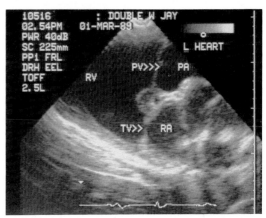

around the associated cardiac chamber to depict the entire area of regurgitant flow. Normal flow profiles within the equine heart have been described using pulsed wave Doppler echocardiography and can be used as a reference for horses with suspected cardiac disease. The scanner head can be placed on the ventricular side of the atrioventricular valves and the aortic or pulmonic side of the semilunar valves for horses with suspected valvular stenosis (rare). Flow mapping of shunts at the atrial or ventricular level also can be performed using the same technique. Color-flow Doppler echocardiography provides a pictorial display of the blood flow abnormalities detected with flow mapping.

High-velocity blood flow cannot be resolved with pulsed-wave Doppler echocardiography because the signal becomes distorted with velocities exceeding about 1.5 m/sec. Though normal blood flow velocities in the equine heart generally are less than this, turbulent flow associated with valvular insufficiency, stenosis or shunts exceeds this velocity.[143] Continuous-wave Doppler echocardiography is needed to observe these high velocities. This technique is a blind technique without 2-dimensional imaging and is best performed after localizing the abnormal flow with pulsed-wave Doppler echocardiography, using that information to guide the ultrasound beam.

Measurement of Blood Pressure

P.J. Pascoe

Blood pressure can be subjectively assessed by digital palpation of superficial arteries. The facial artery, lying between the masseter muscle and ramus of the mandible, is most accessible, but the median and digital arteries also are readily palpable. Pulse strength is related to its pressure, which is the difference between systolic and diastolic pressures. Normally, as mean blood pressure falls, pulse pressure also falls; hence, the pulse feels weaker. In some circumstances, the systolic-diastolic gap may be reduced at high mean pressures and may be widened at lower pressures, giving an incorrect subjective evaluation of the pulse strength. To overcome this problem and to obtain more accurate information, several methods can be applied to measure blood pressure. It may be determined invasively (directly) by arterial puncture and insertion of a catheter connected to a suitable transducer, or noninvasively (indirectly) by use of Doppler ultrasound or oscillometry.

Direct Measurement

Direct pressure measurement is not suitable for practice, as it demands invasion, special skills and highly specialized equipment, though this is the most accurate method of measurement. It can be done with an intraarterial, fluid-filled catheter connected to an external transducer or with a transducer-tipped micromanometer.[144] The latter can enhance frequency response and is less subject to artifact than a fluid-filled system, but the catheter is delicate and relatively expensive.[6] The system has the advantage over fluid-filled systems of not needing correction to any standard reference point because the micromanometer measures pressure at the catheter tip. However, some idea of the approximate location of the transducer in the vascular system obviously is necessary.

Indirect Measurement

Noninvasive indirect measurement of blood pressure relies on use of a cuff to occlude the artery and a detection device to detect the return of flow as pressure in the cuff is reduced. In an unanesthetized animal, the cuff usually is applied to the base of the tail. It is important to use the correct size of cuff for the measurement technique being employed. If the cuff is too small, it produces falsely high values, while an overly wide cuff gives falsely low values. The cuff must be wrapped firmly around the tail; too tight or too loose an application interferes with the measurement. The center of the occlusive bladder should be directly over the vessel; in the tail, this is located ventrally on the midline.

The measurement obtained is the pressure at the head of the tail. This is slightly lower than the central pressure. This is not important if the measurement is being used on an individual horse or if it is being used to compare pressures in a relatively standard group of animals. If it is being used among horses with a wide variation in size, the measurement should be corrected to central pressure by determining the difference in vertical height of the shoulder joint and head of the tail in centimeters and multiplying by 0.77 to convert to mm Hg. This value should be added to the tail measurement obtained.

It also is important that the horse stands with its head in a normal position because blood pressure falls as the head is lowered. In 1 study, measured blood pressure was 11 mm Hg lower when the horse's head was in a grazing position.[145]

Doppler Detection: Resumption of flow into the vessel beneath the cuff is detected with high-frequency ultrasound transmitted and received by a hand-held detection probe. As the vessels are relatively superficial, it is necessary to use frequencies in the 8- to 10-MHz range. After the cuff has been placed around the tail, aqueous ultrasound gel is applied to the face of the probe, which is placed against the skin on the ventral surface of the tail just distal to the edge of the cuff. The probe is moved around until a clear signal is obtained. Then the cuff is inflated until the signal disappears and deflated slowly until a short sound is heard with each pulse. To obtain an accurate reading, the cuff should be deflated at a rate of 2-4 mm Hg per heart beat. Because the heart rate is so slow in horses, it is often useful to use faster deflation to get a rough idea of the systolic pressure and then to reinflate the cuff to a pressure just above this value. The reading on the sphygmomanometer at the first return of a signal is taken as the systolic pressure. The cuff is deflated further until the sound of the pulse returns as a continuous signal; this indicates the diastolic pressure. This latter measurement is very subjective and requires a crystal-clear signal at the start.

The correct cuff bladder width for this technique is 0.34 times the circumference of the tail for systolic pressure and 0.98 for diastolic pressure.[146] A bladder width of 9-10 cm, about 0.48 times tail girth, accommodates most adult horses, with overestimation of diastolic pressure and underestimation of systolic pressure by about 9%.[146]

The cheapest application of the technique is to use a hand-held ultrasonic stethoscope (Ultrasound Stethoscope BF4A: Medasonics, Mountain View, CA). The main disadvantage of this method is that it can be difficult to hold the probe on the vessel while taking the measurement in an unanesthetized animal. A flat probe attached to an ultrasonic detector (Ultrasonic Flow Detector 811: Parks Medical Electronics, Aloha, OR) makes it simpler to hold the probe in place or to attach it to the tail with tape or a Velcro strip. One other device, which is supposed to detect arterial wall motion (Arteriosonde, Kontron Medical, Everett, MA), has the probe incorporated in the cuff. However, the cuff must be inflated to get a signal and this makes it less convenient to use.

Oscillometry: Oscillometry analyzes the pulse-induced variation in pressure within the cuff as it is deflated. In horses, this requires a machine that can cope with the low heart rates normal to this species. Most machines designed for human use do not provide a measurement if the heart rate falls below about 45 bpm. One machine has been specifically adapted for use in horses (Dinamap Research Monitor 1255: Critikon, Tampa, FL). Because it is detecting the pressure changes associated with the flow through the vessels beneath the cuff, any tail movement interferes with the measurement. In studies using this equipment, best results were obtained with the machine set for low heart rate and high sensitivity; however, it did not function if the heart rate was below 25 or if the pulse was arrhythmic. The bladder width recommended for the oscillometric technique is 0.2-0.5 times the tail circumference.[147]

Some variation is found in the literature concerning normal blood pressures recorded using indirect methods and is mainly a result of variation in technique. In particular, accuracy of estimates can be enhanced by correction for cuff width:tail circumference ratio.[148] However, normal *coccygeal* blood pressures determined by ultrasonic (Doppler) methods in the resting adult horse have been reported in ranges of 85/42 to 138/97 mm Hg and 79/49 to 145/106.[148,149] Thoroughbreds tend to have significantly higher pressures than Standardbreds (10 mm Hg), which in turn have slightly higher pressures than grade horses (7 mm Hg).[148] In foals, blood pressure is low at birth (81/35) and rises to 104/40 by 1 week of age. Diastolic pressure continues to rise until about 1 month of age.[150]

Clinical Utility of Blood Pressure Measurement

In people, blood pressure is a component of a routine physical examination, but it has not been used in this fashion in horses. Hypotensive or hypertensive diseases do not appear to be common in horses, and the equipment required to detect them tends to be specialized. In the critically ill animal, however, evaluation of blood pressure is of great benefit in guiding therapy and defining prognosis.

In equine colic, for example, a distinct correlation has been shown between circulatory status and the likelihood of survival. Various indices of circulatory status have been used (capillary refill time, temperature of the extremities, strength of peripheral pulse, blood lactate levels) but one of the most objective, simple and accurate is measurement of blood pressure. This variable is directly correlated with prognosis.[151] In horses with a systolic pressure ≥100 mm Hg, the likelihood of survival was 95% vs 69% at 80 mmHg and 10% at 60 mm Hg. Though no evaluation has been attempted in other circulatory shock states in horses, it is probable that blood pressure monitoring could help guide decisions regarding therapy and prognosis.

PATHOPHYSIOLOGY AND PRINCIPLES OF THERAPY

P.W. Physick-Sheard

Abnormalities of Cardiac Sound

Abnormalities of cardiac sound frequently are encountered during clinical evaluation and represent a significant source of concern when evaluating serviceability during prepurchase examination or determining the cause of poor performance. The principal questions are: is the sound an indication of structural abnormality of the heart as opposed to some benign variation in function; does the sound indicate reduced functional capacity; and will the problem progress? These questions cannot be answered with accuracy, and interpretations remain subjective and imprecise. However, critical and systematic appraisals of sound abnormalities often narrow the range of diagnostic possibilities to manageable proportions and provide insight into clinical interpretation. In the future, evaluation will be aided by echocardiography and Doppler ultrasound; at present, the resources for application and interpretation are limited.

Abnormalities of sound may be divided into variations in normal sounds and murmurs.

Variation in Normal Sounds

Normal heart sounds are often described as "transients" and are of short duration (Fig 19). Particularly wide variation in these sounds is encountered in horses; occasionally 6 or more sounds are heard in each cycle (atrial contraction sound, split S_1, split S_2, S_3). These can overlap, producing a sound resembling a murmur or, alternatively, individual sounds can be relatively prolonged and soft, again sounding "murmur-like." Listeners who have difficulty detecting low frequencies may have trouble differentiating these sounds. In most cases, differentiation is aided by an obvious change in intensity and degree of duplication of such complex "transients" as heart rate and autonomic tone change. Because murmurs are associated with blood flow, they tend to persist longer than complex

sounds and to change much more gradually with variation in heart rate.

Murmurs

Guidelines in Interpretation: There can be many pitfalls in interpretation of murmurs, including application of "rules of thumb," that lead to erroneous conclusions. Errors in interpretation are more likely to lead to a potentially useful animal being discarded than to injury to a rider, yet fear of litigation may cause the examiner to paint a more bleak picture than is warranted clinically. Guidelines that attempt to relate prognosis to such factors as distribution, intensity or quality of a murmur often oversimplify the problem. Also, while a widespread murmur or one that can be heard on both sides of the thorax may be associated with valve damage and possibly multiple valve involvement, neither the murmur nor the associated valve changes necessarily provide any guidance to prognosis.[152] An alternative approach is to encourage critical examination. In this way, each murmur can be evaluated on its merits, with due regard to possible hemodynamic consequences and underlying causes.

Heart sounds are evaluated carefully over the entire cardiac area on both sides of the thorax and described as outlined below, using only standardized terms. Use of standard terminology allows efficient communication of findings. However, if the examiner is unsure of the correct terminology, it is safer to simply describe what is heard, as this avoids confusion. Findings are then related to the events of the cardiac cycle, especially the hemodynamic events, and to cardiac and thoracic topography. Consideration of the history and presenting clinical signs further reduces the list of diagnostic possibilities. Even a definitive diagnosis will not necessarily allow you to provide a client with an accurate prognosis, but it should be possible to provide general guidance for monitoring the animal and career planning. Any statements regarding prognosis must relate to and are presented with the individual conditions discussed later in the chapter.

Sources of Murmurs: A murmur may be defined as an abnormal cardiac sound consisting of a relatively prolonged series of audible vibrations that vary from case to case in intensity, duration, frequency and quality, and in their relationship to normal heart sounds and in the shape of the sound "envelope" (see below). The physical processes underlying the genesis of murmurs are still under debate, but it is generally accepted that they represent some manifestation of nonlaminar blood flow, variously described as disturbed flow in jets, vortex shedding and periodic wave fluctuations. Though turbulence has been offered as an explanation for murmurs, research suggests that inadequate energy is released by turbulent flow to generate the intensity of sound often observed, whereas vortex shedding, in which eddies are formed, and jet impaction can generate sound.[153,154]

As vessel diameter or flow velocity increases, the tendency toward nonlaminar flow increases. Likewise, a decrease in blood viscosity or rise in blood density increases the tendency for murmurs to develop. At constant cardiac output, reduction in vessel diameter enhances the tendency toward flow disturbance, while high cardiac output is associated with increased flow velocity at constant vessel diameter.

In circumstances under which stroke volume is increased (*eg,* aortic regurgitation leading to increased end-diastolic volume), the increase in flow rate may precipitate a systolic murmur that is essentially functional because it has occurred without any lesion or change in the size or shape of the aortic valve. Such sounds are referred to as functional murmurs. Conversely, with a reduction in the size of the opening through which blood is moving, flow velocity must increase if flow volume is to remain constant. These considerations must be kept in mind because horses with quite distinct murmurs may have no identifiable lesion of any valve at postmortem examination.[152]

Local conditions at the blood-tissue interface, such as a minor irregularity in the surface of a valve, may be sufficient to cause a flow disturbance. The amount of sound energy released at the site is enhanced as flow velocity increases, fluid density rises or viscosity falls. A minor abnormality of a valve may give rise to a very distinct murmur in a colicky horse with anemia, for example. However, in interpreting murmurs, it must be remembered that the behavior of blood cannot be divorced from that of the surrounding structures, such as valve margins

or the edges of shunt defects. Because of their tendency to vibrate, these too participate in the character and distribution of the sound generated.

Describing Murmurs: The protocol by which murmurs are described is quite critical because the features of the sound may relate to causative factors. Unusual clinical circumstances are detected more readily if the technique of examination is consistent. There is no hope of interpreting a murmur correctly if the events of the cardiac cycle are not understood (Fig 5).

Murmurs may be described by 8 features: intensity, frequency, character, timing, topographic location, shape, pattern of interference with normal heart sounds, and presence or absence of a palpable thrill.

Several systems have been used to classify the *intensity* of murmurs. The system used here, both in the interests of consistency and because it appears to be the easiest to remember, is a 5-point system based upon that described in a previous edition of this text.[18]

Grade I. The softest audible murmur, heard only after careful auscultation and often limited to a small area of the thorax.

Grade II. A faint murmur, clearly audible after a few seconds of auscultation.

Grade III. A murmur that is audible immediately when auscultation begins and is heard over a fairly wide area. A palpable thrill accompanies the most intense murmurs within this grade. (This is the widest grade and, when used, the clinician should indicate whether the sound is simply very distinct or also loud and whether a thrill was detected).

Grade IV. The loudest murmur that becomes inaudible when the stethoscope is removed from direct contact with the thoracic wall. A thrill is always present.

Grade V. The loudest murmur. It remains audible when the stethoscope is removed from contact with the thoracic wall but is held near it. A pronounced thrill is always present.

The *frequency* or *pitch* of a murmur can be diagnostically useful and should always be reported; however, caution should be employed to avoid confusing frequency with intensity and shape. Because of the limited human auditory range, many murmurs of low frequency may be difficult to detect even though such sounds may be of clinical significance (see below). Conversely, higher-frequency sounds, especially those of musical quality, may be heard easily but often have limited importance. Many murmurs are noisy and by definition have a very mixed-frequency spectrum. The murmur that falls in frequency markedly during its course, for example, may appear to be decrescendo even though its intensity is, in fact, increasing. *A low-frequency sound that is heard easily generally is likely to have greater significance than a high-frequency sound of equivalent intensity because, in general, low-frequency sounds tend to accompany larger disturbances of valve integrity, particularly in the atrioventricular valves.* Unfortunately, the means to objectively measure the intensity of a murmur are not readily available, though phonocardiography eliminates some of the subjectivity.[30] Variation in murmur intensity with frequency is evident from Figure 20.

The *quality* of a murmur is its character, described by such terms as noisy, soft and blowing, harsh, musical or rumbling. Some murmurs tend to have characteristic qualities, such as the harsh, noisy murmur of a ventricular-level shunt or the soft, blowing sound of some atrioventricular insufficiencies.

The following terminology, standardized by the American College of Cardiology, describes the relationship between a murmur and the events of the cardiac cycle, ie, the *timing* of murmurs. Because the markers used for components of the cycle are the normal heart sounds, the timing of murmurs approximates the mechanical (hemodynamic), as opposed to electrical events of the cycle.

Systolic murmur. Begins with or after S_1 and ends before or with S_2.

Early systolic murmur. Begins at the time of S_1 and ends about or before the middle of systole.

Late systolic murmur. Begins about the middle of systole and ends at or just before S_2.

Midsystolic murmur. Begins clearly after S_1 and ends clearly before S_2.

Holosystolic (pansystolic) murmur. Begins with S_1 and ends with S_2, ie, it occupies all of systole.

Diastolic murmur. Begins with or after S_2 and ends with or before S_1 of the next cycle.

Early diastolic murmur. Begins with the aortic or pulmonary component of S_2.

Mid-diastolic murmur. Begins clearly after S_2.

Late diastolic (presystolic) murmur. Confined to the period immediately before S_1.

Additionally, the term "pandiastolic" is found in the veterinary literature and is used to describe those murmurs that last throughout diastole.

There is no consistent and dependable association between the *location* of a murmur and an etiologic diagnosis, as distribution is profoundly influenced by the condition of tissues overlying the heart, position of the heart in the thorax, and other cardiac lesions, such as cardiomegaly. However, the shape of the thorax of most quadrupeds and location of the heart in a rotated position, especially in horses, place the right ventricle cranially and the left ventricle caudally, allowing for some differentiation of murmurs on the basis of the location of the point of maximum intensity (Figs 2, 4, 8). That is, some disorders tend to have a fairly characteristic distribution of sound.

Murmurs generated in the outflow tracts tend to follow the tract dorsally, while their higher-frequency components tend to radiate back toward the apex of the ventricular chamber of origin.[155] This helps differentiate pulmonic from aortic murmurs. Murmurs generated in the atrioventricular valves tend to be heard best immediately dorsal and ventral to the valve of origin, with greatest intensity following direction of the regurgitant stream as in valvular insufficiency. Thus, an intense left atrioventricular regurgitation murmur tends to have its point of maximum intensity on the left side of the thorax at the fifth to seventh intercostal space at about the level of the shoulder. Murmurs of right atrioventricular origin tend to be loudest on the right side of the thorax, though often they also can be detected ventrally and cranially on the left (Fig 8). Murmurs associated with shunts tend to have a wider distribution, but the direction of the shunt often can be inferred from the point of maximum intensity (see discussion under congenital heart disease).

The configuration or *"shape"* of a murmur is a reference to the shape of the intensity envelope (Fig 30). This envelope can be characterized by auscultation and phonocardiography. Thus, a crescendo-decrescendo murmur becomes loud, then quiet. A crescendo murmur progressively increases in intensity. A decrescendo murmur starts out relatively loud and becomes progressively quieter.

Shape traditionally has been used as a major diagnostic feature. A murmur of an outflow tract stenosis, for example, often is referred to as an ejection or crescendo-decrescendo murmur. While such guidelines can be very helpful, they should be used with caution, as there is considerable overlap (see below under Factors Influencing Murmur Characteristics).

When it can be detected, the precise temporal relationship between a murmur and normal heart sounds often is of diagnostic value. Murmurs should be described as to the extent that they *interfere* with normal sounds. The murmur of aortic stenosis, for example, starts very shortly after the first heart sound; the main events that give rise to S_1 have passed before ejection commences. Reversal of pressure gradients across the valve precedes aortic valve closure. Because forward flow would have ceased before this closure, the murmur must end before S_2. In this instance, there is no interference with the normal transients. If there is marked splitting of sounds and especially if one component of the split sound is very soft, some interference may be present. In contrast, the murmur of a ventricular-level shunt persists as long as there is any pressure gradient, starting with S_1 and often overriding S_2, sometimes obliterating both sounds.

The more intense murmurs are associated with *palpable* vibrations referred to as *thrills*. These are detected most easily at the point of maximum intensity of the murmur and represent intense low-frequency components of the sound. They always are of clinical significance. The term "precordial" sometimes is found in the literature and is borrowed from human terminology, referring to the precordium or lower sternothoracic region. It has no true equivalent in horses. The location of a thrill should be described as for the location of a murmur.

Figure 30. Intensity envelope or "shape" of various murmurs.

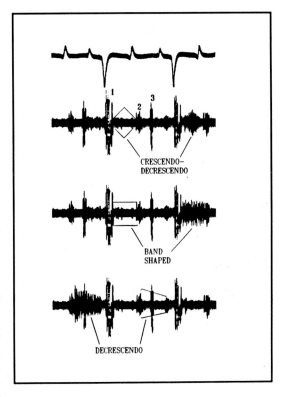

CRESCENDO-DECRESCENDO

BAND SHAPED

DECRESCENDO

Severe flow disturbances are associated with *systemic consequences* as a result of congestion in peripheral tissues. Thus, left atrioventricular insufficiency may result in pulmonary congestion and edema, with increased respiratory rate and effort and an obvious expiratory lift. Right atrioventricular insufficiency occasionally leads to venous hypertension, jugular engorgement and edema. These clinical signs are further discussed in the sections on Heart Failure and under specific valvular abnormalities. If cardiac disease has progressed to this extent in a horse, the precise relationship to any murmur encountered may be extremely difficult to determine because the sound could be primary or secondary to the failure.

Types of Murmurs: Before categorizing murmurs, some general comments must be made. *The presence of a murmur does not necessarily indicate significant cardiac disease in a horse, while the absence of a murmur does not necessarily mean all is well.* Similarly, a murmur can only infrequently provide guidance as to the condition of the myocardium. Horses are prone to benign flow sounds and also to quite intense sounds during stress, such as colic. Murmurs therefore should be interpreted with caution and evaluated critically. Mentioning to an owner that a horse has a murmur can be devastating, yet in my experience, many of the abnormal sounds observed in horses are not associated with any structural change in the valves, while the presence of a murmur does not necessarily mean that there will be any material impact upon the animal's ability to perform. These observations are amplified below.

As mentioned previously, the diagnostic accuracy of auscultation in horses is undetermined. The wide application of ancillary diagnostic methods that aid definitive diagnosis in other species has not yet taken place in equine cardiology, and the opportunity to follow a horse with a murmur throughout life to necropsy is rare. Further, valvular abnormalities detected at postmortem examination cannot always be assumed to have been the cause of sounds heard upon auscultation. Diagnostic interpretations thus are based upon limited objective data.

Holosystolic murmurs. For a murmur to be holosystolic, there must be a pressure differential and continuous flow from S_1 to S_2. Thus, a holosystolic murmur usually indicates restricted flow down a pressure gradient from an area of relatively high to an area of relatively low pressure. Under these circumstances, the duration of the murmur results largely from the steep pressure gradient. The murmur of atrioventricular insufficiency most often is soft, blowing and of low frequency, and does not radiate widely (Fig 31). It tends to be of consistent intensity or band shaped. In contrast, the murmur of a ventricular level shunt (*eg,* VSD) tends to be harsh, widespread and bow-shaped (louder in the middle) with very mixed frequencies (Fig 20). However, exceptions are described later in the chapter. Other examples include the systolic component of persistent ductus arteriosus (the diastolic component of this sound is inaudible in some cases), and the infrequently encountered systolic component of the sound generated when aortic aneurysms dissect into a heart chamber. In these last 3 examples, the duration of the murmur is additionally aided by the fact that the defect across which flow is occurring is patent at all times. Holosystolic murmurs almost always indicate a lesion.

Caution should be exercised because shape, quality and intensity of sound cannot be used as reliable guides to interpretation. The larger the "hole" through which blood is flowing (and hence the greater the pathologic changes), the quieter the murmur may become. Theoretically, complete absence of the interventricular septum would result in no noise at all from a left-to-right shunt. Similarly, complete absence of the left atrioventricular valve would not be associated with a murmur. Conversely, a relatively small defect with normal pressure gradients could be expected to generate an intense, relatively high-frequency murmur; left atrioventricular insufficiency can occasionally have these characteristics. If the defect were at the base of the valve between the main and commissural cusps, as frequently is the case, the murmur may be soft and blowing. If a ruptured chorda tendinae has allowed the free margin of the primary cusp to vibrate freely in the regurgitant flow, the murmur may be quite noisy and coarse, with a "buzzing" component.

Holosystolic murmurs most often are band shaped and of uniform intensity. Yet if the defect in a valve or septum is small and pressure gradients steep, the sound can take on a crescendo-decrescendo contour. In such cases, it is possible to miss the fact that the sound is holosystolic rather than mid-systolic. Also, while these murmurs occupy all of systole, they can obliterate one or both heart sounds and appear to continue beyond S_2. A very intense ventricular shunt may be associated with a quiet, almost undetectable S_1 because movement of blood from the left to the right ventricle modifies the normal rapid deceleration of blood with which the sound is usually associated. Marked splitting of S_2, as a result of delayed completion of systole in the left heart combined with a soft aortic component to S_2, creates the impression that the murmur continues into diastole.

Finally, where the holosystolic sound is part of a continuous murmur, the diagnostic options generally are narrower (see below). However, complications include patent ductus arteriosus, in which pulmonary hypertension has reduced diastolic shunting, and atrioventricular insufficiency, in which increased flow across the atrioventricular valve during ventricular filling may generate a low-frequency functional diastolic murmur.

Early systolic murmurs. Early systolic, crescendo-decrescendo murmurs that do not extend far into systole, typically have a very early peak of intensity and do not exceed grade II in intensity have been referred to as innocent systolic murmurs (Fig 32).[156] They can be heard best at the heart base over the aortic and pulmonic valves and may become slightly exaggerated during excitement or exercise. Their origin is unclear but it has been proposed that they reflect the normally rapid flow through the aortic valve. A similar sound has been detected on the surface of the aorta and also from the aortic root during intracardiac phonocardiography though, in the latter study, spread of the murmur to the chest wall was not demonstrated.[34] A similar murmur has been detected in foals and usually subsides gradually, though it may be detected for 3-4 months and up to 10 months.[36,150,157] This murmur is distinct from that associated with patent ductus arteriosus in the neonatal foal (see below) and is of unknown though likely little clinical significance.

Figure 31. Simultaneous ECG and phonocardiogram from a 3-year-old Standardbred filly presented because of suboptimal performance. The clinical diagnosis was right AV insufficiency. There is a low-frequency, pansystolic murmur of relatively constant intensity (band shaped) and of a soft, blowing quality upon auscultation. The first and second heart sounds are not obvious in this tracing, made at the point of maximum intensity at the right fourth intercostal space.

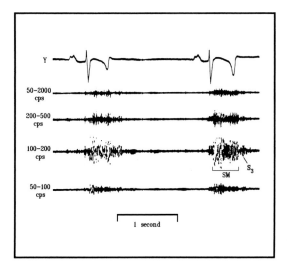

Figure 32. Early systolic, crescendo-decrescendo murmur recorded from a clinically normal, 2-year-old Standardbred colt. The murmur was an incidental finding on routine precastration evaluation. (Heart rate 38 bpm).

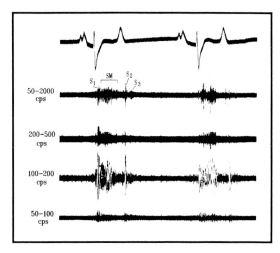

Midsystolic murmurs. These also may be referred to as ejection murmurs, which causes confusion since this term may also be used to refer to the innocent flow sounds that occur in early systole (see above). The term "ejection murmur" refers to the shape of the sound that follows the velocity of ejection of blood from the ventricular chambers and is thus descriptive rather than any indication of clinical significance or etiology. The classic example of a mid-systolic murmur is aortic stenosis, which can produce a harsh, intense, crescendo-decrescendo (diamond-shaped) murmur of relatively high frequency best heard at the heart base on the left side of the thorax. The vibrations radiate back into the chamber of origin and can be followed along the outflow tract, occasionally being detected at the base of the neck over the carotid arteries and at the withers. A similar sound, though of lower intensity and with a more limited area of distribution, is heard with pulmonic stenosis. True aortic or pulmonic stenosis is exceedingly rare in horses.

An outflow tract valve need not be stenotic or even diseased to be the source of a murmur. Even mild irregularity of a valve may cause abnormal flow under conditions in which stroke volume or velocity of ejection are increased. Thus, very soft mid-systolic murmurs may be intensified during hyperkinetic circulatory states as seen during colic. Such murmurs generally are not evident after exercise unless the exercise is associated with excitement. A distinct outflow tract murmur detected immediately after saddling, for example, may no longer be present upon postexercise auscultation.

Early diastolic murmurs. Diastolic murmurs in horses are early diastolic, pandiastolic or biphasic and, in general, not common. When present, however, they are detected with greater ease than in other species because of the low heart rate and long diastolic interval of horses. Such murmurs are likely to vary markedly in intensity and character with changes in heart rate. Early diastolic murmurs may be caused by semilunar valve insufficiency or by atrioventricular stenosis. Murmurs of semilunar insufficiency begin with or immediately after S_2 and extend for varying periods into diastole. Some last until the next cycle (see below under Pandiastolic Murmurs). The sound is characteristically decrescendo and often very musical, of high frequency and widespread, though on occasion it can have very low-frequency and coarse underlying vibrations that can be quite intense. The murmur usually is loudest at and ventral to its valve of origin, radiating into the respective ventricular chamber. An early diastolic, decrescendo musical or high-frequency murmur originating over the heart base and starting with or immediately after S_2 is safely diagnosed as semilunar insufficiency.

Murmurs of atrioventricular stenosis usually are not detected, as they are of very low frequency and intensity. Also, such a valvular abnormality is rare in horses. The murmur is most intense early in diastole during rapid ventricular filling, and always starts after S_2 and again during atrial contraction late in diastole; it is thus biphasic.

Pandiastolic murmurs. The term "pandiastolic" may be superfluous because this is simply an early diastolic, decrescendo sound that extends through much of diastole, often to S_1 (Fig 33). The factor determining this behavior is the persistence of a pressure gradient to drive regurgitant flow. Pandiastolic murmurs most often indicate insufficiency of a semilunar valve. If valve leakage is severe, pressure differences disappear rapidly, quickly curtailing the sound. Persistence of the sound throughout a double interval when the horse drops a beat suggests that the volume of the regurgitant

flow is low and that the duration of the murmur may not accurately reflect its hemodynamic significance. Conversely, failure of a decrescendo early diastolic sound to last well into systole does not necessarily indicate severe insufficiency because the regurgitant flow may be modified by changes in the relationship of the valve cusps.

Other diastolic sounds. An early diastolic "squeak" has been referred to in the literature as the "2-year-old squeak." This sound has never been explained satisfactorily nor has the frequency with which it occurs been fully investigated. In 1 survey, it occurred in 10% of a group of 94 horses.[158] It is heard in early diastole between S_2 and S_3, and is inconstant.

A particularly significant though, thankfully, uncommon diastolic murmur is that due to aneurysms in the aorta when these dissect into a heart chamber (see Aortic Ring Rupture). The sound may or may not be continuous. For example, an aneurysm dissecting into the right ventricle may not be patent during systole as contraction of the ventricular myocardium closes the defect. During diastole, however, blood regurgitates into the right ventricle. In other cases, flow may occur throughout both phases of the cycle and the murmur is continuous. The topographic location of such murmurs varies considerably, depending upon the path of dissection and the chamber(s) involved. The sound, however, is characteristically harsh and noisy.

Continuous murmurs. In addition to the rare dissecting aortic aneurysm, a more common cause of a continuous (or machinery) murmur is persistent ductus arteriosus. Most newborn foals manifest a murmur due to flow across this natural defect but the sound usually disappears by 3-4 days of age, correlating with the time of anatomic closure of the communication.[16,150, 157] The sound usually is not present immediately after birth, but in 1 study it was detected between 1 and 24 hours of age in all 10 foals examined.[16]

The diastolic component may not be obvious and is often of low grade, in which case the murmur will not be continuous. The systolic component can be very intense, with a typical shunt quality (harsh, noisy and band shaped, starting with S_1). The sound often runs through both S_1 and S_2 and can be up to grade IV in intensity. It

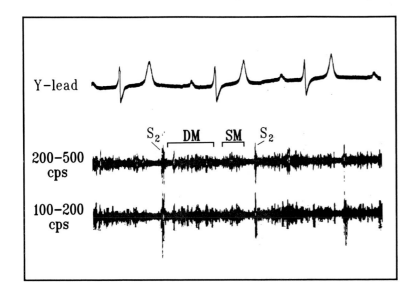

Y-lead

S_2 DM SM S_2

200–500 cps

100–200 cps

Figure 33. Pandiastolic murmur (DM) recorded at the left heart base of a 17-year-old Thoroughbred gelding. The murmur had been present for 2 years and was interpreted clinically and echocardiographically as an aortic insufficiency. The diagnosis was confirmed at necropsy. There is a distinct pause after S_2 before the start of the murmur. Note the absence of an obvious S_1, reflecting greatly increased end-diastolic volume, and the presence of a systolic murmur (SM). The latter reflects increased stroke volume and resultant functional stenosis of the aortic valve. (See Figure 67 for lesions in this horse.)

can be differentiated easily from murmurs originating in the outflow tracts by virtue of this shunt quality. It is loudest at the heart base level with the point of the shoulder and at or just cranial to the line of the triceps.

Methods of Evaluating Murmurs: Murmurs can be evaluated by auscultation and palpation, phonocardiography, exercise tests, Doppler ultrasound and cardiac catheterization. They also can be evaluated by the systemic clinical signs with which they are associated.

The general approach to exercise testing has been discussed elsewhere in this chapter. Interpretation of the changes that a murmur may undergo as a result of exercise represents a challenge. It sometimes is assumed that, if a murmur persists or is louder during immediate postexercise tachycardia, its clinical significance has been confirmed; however, there is no scientific evidence to support this interpretation. Increased cardiac output and rate of flow may be expected to augment the predisposition to flow disturbance so that some increase in murmur intensity ought not to be surprising. Persistence of the murmur can be taken to indicate that the flow disturbance is still present at the rates over which the heart was auscultated and that some unquantifiable hemodynamic consequences may influence both progression of the underlying abnormality and the animal's capacity to perform work. Beyond this, it is not possible to interpret persis-

tence of the murmur objectively after exercise, other than to acknowledge that a marked increase in intensity and a change in quality to a harsh, coarse or noisy character should be regarded as a poor prognostic sign.

Conversely, if the murmur disappears at exercise, this is diagnostically more valuable because a sound that subsides is likely of limited immediate clinical significance in the context of the horse's athletic potential. It is assumed that loss of the murmur reflects alterations in the physical relationship of the valve cusps with changes in myocardial tone and blood pressure. Caution is required, however, because the flow disturbance actually may have become worse, with the combined effects of reduced systolic/diastolic time interval and a fall in sound frequency having led to an *apparent* reduction in murmur intensity. Also, while the disappearance of the sound *may* indicate little or no flow disturbance at work, it tells us little regarding prognosis or the nature of the underlying lesion.

Diagnostic ultrasound is discussed elsewhere in this chapter. In most cases in which a valvular abnormality gives rise to a murmur in a horse, the lesions are very mild and usually not detectable by current echocardiographic techniques. However, Doppler ultrasound, particularly color Doppler, provides a very sensitive tool to evaluate, for example, the extent of regurgitant flow and other functional consequences of flow disturbance. This procedure is in its infancy in veterinary medicine.

The advent of catheter tip-mounted transducers has facilitated intracardiac recording of sound and may allow more critical examination of the source of the vibrations.[6] However, remembering that flow disturbances cause multiple cardiac structures to vibrate, it may not be possible to locate the offending structure precisely by this means. Theoretically, changes in pressure contours in cardiac chambers also are of diagnostic value in interpreting murmurs, though it is probable that a valvular abnormality would have to be fairly advanced to allow definitive diagnosis on this basis. Pressure evaluation appears to be of inconsistent value in diagnosis of murmurs associated with congenital heart disease.[159]

Murmurs also may be evaluated on the basis of systemic consequences. However, most murmurs in horses, even when quite loud, are not associated with any clinically detectable changes in the circulatory system or other organs at rest. As noted above, systemic consequences of exercise can be measured only with sophisticated methodology. By the time a murmur is associated with obvious clinical consequences, the horse is in serious trouble and athletic activity is not an option. Management, if that is an option, is directed at the clinical problem of heart failure rather than the primary valvular disorder.

Principles of Management: Obvious murmurs detected in very young animals almost invariably indicate congenital heart disease and always should be interpreted as of probable clinical significance (see specific discussion of congenital abnormalities elsewhere in this chapter). Murmurs heard in old horses occasionally are congenital abnormalities but most likely indicate acquired valvular disease, with the probability that there is already some compensatory change, especially in the case of aortic or atrioventricular insufficiency.[116,152,160,161] In general, the greater the valvular dysfunction, the more the horse will have to compensate for the problem by chamber enlargement/hypertrophy. The more vigorously the horse is asked to perform, the more rapidly this compensation will progress to an endpoint of decompensation. However, because a tendency to tire or detection of the murmur will likely cause the horse to be moved

down in class or withdrawn from active competition, a state of decompensation may never be reached.

Most outflow tract murmurs do not progress rapidly. Inflow tract insufficiencies carry a good chance of progressing and are also associated with development of atrial arrhythmias, notably atrial fibrillation, as a consequence of atrial distention.[162,163] Murmurs of aortic insufficiency should be regarded with equal concern. Murmurs associated with *complex* congenital heart disease always carry a poor prognosis, with probability of progression because of pressure changes and accompanying hypoxia.

While horses with *simple* congenital defects are likely never to perform at the level they might have achieved in the absence of the defect, in general the problem is not likely to progress rapidly. In less arduous athletic events, these horses can be expected to perform adequately. These horses should be subjected to periodic examination and, ideally, to objective and easily repeated performance evaluations to monitor progress. Attention also should be paid to the level of performance the animal is achieving. The greater the work effort the animal is asked to perform and the more serious the cardiac abnormality, the more frequent the examinations. In all cases, the horse should be reexamined at least every 6 months. If more objective methods of evaluation, such as echocardiography, are available, they should be used.

Adventitial Sounds

Not all "murmur-like" sounds are of cardiac origin. Pericarditis, pleuritis and pneumonia all can cause sounds that may be mistaken for murmurs. Friction rubs sometimes can sound remarkably like ventricular-level shunts. All of these so-called adventitial sounds are variable in their character, duration from cardiac cycle to cycle and precise relationship to normal heart sounds. They also tend to come and go. Careful auscultation usually allows differentiation from true murmurs.

Abnormalities of Heart Rate

Abnormalities of heart rate are encountered frequently in clinical practice; however, in horses, these rarely indicate primary cardiovascular disease, and more frequently reflect excitement or secondary involvement of the cardiovascular system in other disease states. Where the finding is persistent, the following check list should be considered. The significance of the questions will be apparent from the discussion below of tachycardia and bradycardia.

Is there evidence of pain or anxiety?

Is the animal showing profound depression?

Is there evidence of homeostatic disturbance?

Is the rectal temperature normal?

Is there evidence of disease within the respiratory system?

Is heart rate consistent with other clinical signs?

Is the heart beat rhythmic?

Is the cardiac rhythm sinus in origin?

Are there any definitive signs of cardiovascular disease?

Tachycardia

Though precise thresholds have limited meaning because of varying circumstances, elevation of heart rate can be present when the resting rate exceeds 45 bpm. From a physiologist's perspective, there are 3 basic causes of tachycardia: increased body temperature, increased sympathetic/reduced parasympathetic activity in the autonomic nervous system, and toxic conditions of the heart.[1] Though autonomic mechanisms, for example, can be invoked as the immediate cause of elevation in rate under most clinical circumstances, the clinician attempting to determine pathogenesis and arrive at a rational therapeutic approach should view tachycardia from an etiologic rather than a mechanistic perspective. Causes of elevation in resting heart rate may thus indicate increased demand for cardiac output, reduced ability of the heart/myocardium to meet resting demands, or arrhythmia. This classification encompasses physiologic elevations due to exercise, excitement and elevation in body temperature, and also pathologic circumstances.

Pathologic circumstances include situations in which myocardial function is compromised by direct insult, primary cardiomyopathy or valve dysfunction, or by such external factors as an intrathoracic mass or pericardial effusion. Additionally, lesions

may be manifested as arrhythmias associated with tachycardia.

Under most circumstances, the reason for elevation of heart rate will be evident from the results of a clinical examination and review of the history. Where clinical manifestations indicate secondary involvement of the cardiovascular system, the degree of tachycardia usually correlates with the degree of systemic disturbance and thus provides guidance as to the extent and urgency with which therapeutic intervention is necessary. However, elevation of heart rate is not always directly related to extent of homeostatic disturbance or increase in demand on the cardiovascular system and the quality of the disturbance must be taken into account. For example, severe depletion of total body potassium, often compounded by dissociative ventricular tachyarrhythmias, can occur without any ongoing disturbance of fluid balance. *Therefore, it is desirable to record an ECG in all cases of severe elevation of heart rate to confirm that tachycardia is indeed sinus in origin.* Similarly, even where systemic disease appears to be the cause of tachycardia, the actual heart rate may not appear to correlate with the clinical signs. *In all such cases, an ECG should be recorded to detect tachyarrhythmias.* Tachyarrhythmias occurring in association with disturbances of homeostasis, toxemia and septicemia always are serious and potentially life threatening.

Elevation of rate purely as a reflection of cardiovascular insufficiency is as uncommon in horses as is heart failure but always is serious because it indicates decompensation and a poor prognosis. This finding is dealt with in detail under heart failure below. Elevation in sinus rate in association with systemic disease rarely exceeds 120 bpm; a horse maintaining a rate this high is extremely ill. Rates in excess of this level are far more likely to reflect a serious arrhythmia than sympathetic drive in response to pain or myocardial weakness.

Bradycardia

Bradycardia may be relative or absolute. It is an uncommon finding in adults and only occasionally occurs in foals. Absolute bradycardia in adults is associated with third-degree heart block when ventricular rate drops to 12-16 bpm. At this rate, episodes of syncope can be expected (see below). In my experience, very fit older racehorses that have undergone several seasons of aerobic training and those used for endurance work, such as 3-day events, often exhibit a relative bradycardia (heart rates of 24-28/min). A rate of 18/min was observed in a healthy 13-year-old Standardbred just retired from active competition with an excellent race record.

Bradycardia also may be seen in hypoglycemic foals and in association with hyperkalemia, increased intracranial pressure and stimulation of the vagal nerves. The last may be seen after surgical manipulation of the vagosympathetic trunk and occasionally after deep perijugular injection of irritants. In cases of hydrocephalus and cranial trauma, the effect of intracranial pressure upon heart rate can partially mask the homeostatic disturbances often found in comatose patients, thus obscuring the need for supportive care to the casual observer. Once again, an ECG always should be taken to confirm sinus rhythm and probable etiology of the low heart rate.

Abnormalities of Cardiac Rhythm

Most common arrhythmias in horses are benign, and are abnormal only in degree. Abnormalities of cardiac rhythm, however, are second only to abnormalities of sound in causing confusion and anxiety in interpreting findings made during clinical examination. Specific treatment sometimes is necessary, especially in cases of ventricular tachyarrhythmia. In most cases, treatment is directed primarily at the underlying disorder rather than at the arrhythmia itself. In such cases, the objective of specific therapy is stabilization of life-threatening situations while the condition of the myocardium improves. Therefore, an understanding of equine arrhythmias is necessary if case management is to be rational. Numerous reviews concerning their clinical significance and management may be found in the literature.[18,36,52,156,164-176]

Pathophysiologic Basis of Arrhythmias

The pathophysiologic basis of abnormalities of rhythm can be viewed from structural or mechanistic perspectives. The role

played in clinical arrhythmias by many of the cellular mechanisms remains to be demonstrated.[177,178] For routine interpretation of arrhythmias in horses, an understanding of current theories of arrhythmogenesis is not as important as an appreciation of predisposing factors and clinical associations, combined with the ability to recognize the electrocardiographic features of the abnormalities. Thus, the following general observations concerning underlying mechanisms are included only for the sake of completeness. Because most clinicians approach the diagnosis and management of arrhythmias from other than a mechanistic viewpoint, the discussion of specific arrhythmias that follows deals with particular diagnoses, proceeding anatomically with supraventricular and then with ventricular arrhythmias, rather than attempting to classify the abnormalities by underlying pathogenesis. It must be recognized by those interested in a more traditional approach that this is a classification of convenience.

Structural Basis of Arrhythmias: An association between pathologic changes and common abnormalities of rhythm has been proposed.[162,179-184] The frequent occurrence of arrhythmias and myocardial lesions provides some support for the concept of such a structural basis.[116,160,171,172,185-189] The functional basis for participation of such lesions in arrhythmogenesis involves anatomic obstruction of the conduction system or some abnormality of impulse formation associated with areas of scarred/infarcted/inflamed myocardium. The result can be ectopic impulses, abnormal conduction or refractory period and such phenomena as reentry and decremental conduction.[190]

There is little doubt that areas of recently damaged myocardium can serve as a focus for impulse generation. Myocarditis in association with ionophore intoxication or A-equi-2 influenza are examples in horses.[191,192] Such arrhythmias usually are ventricular and can be of great clinical significance (see below). However, despite recent attempts to demonstrate a relationship between myocardial changes and supraventricular arrhythmias, the evidence in support of a role for focal myocardial scarring/fibrosis in the genesis of some of the more chronic, benign, atrial arrhythmias requires further investigation.[184,193-197] Also, myocardial lesions are not always associated with arrhythmias though failure to monitor cardiac rhythm for long enough or during exercise may preclude detection in many cases (see discussion of 24-hour Rhythm Monitoring).[100,188,198] The extent to which such arrhythmias come and go in individual horses must be investigated. However, as stated earlier, it is probable that the slow heart rate and high vagal tone in horses are more potent factors in genesis of these arrhythmias.

Functional Basis of Arrhythmias: In addition to the following, some cases of arrhythmia almost certainly represent a combination of mechanisms. The reader is referred to the discussion of the conducting system and genesis of the ECG earlier in this chapter for background information.

Abnormalities of impulse formation involve enhancement or depression of normal automaticity (unusually rapid or slow depolarization in pacemaker tissue), abnormal automaticity (tissues abnormally acting as pacemaker tissue, referred to as escape beats when associated with marked slowing of the normal pacemaker), or events induced or triggered by activity in adjacent myocardium.[190] Automaticity is enhanced by increased temperature, hypoxia, hypercapnia, stretching of the myocardium and increased sympathetic activity. It is reduced by decreased temperature and, for the atria only, by increased parasympathetic tone. Injury currents, which are regional changes in membrane polarization secondary to damage-induced changes in local extracellular electrolyte concentration and manifested in the ECG as ST segment shifts and T-wave changes, also enhance automaticity and may be important in the genesis of arrhythmias seen in myocarditis.[199]

While the term *"abnormalities of impulse conduction"* sometimes is interpreted as implying abnormal function of the conduction system proper, it can imply abnormal propagation of the action potential in any area of the myocardium. Thus, for example, some theories of the pathogenesis of atrial fibrillation propose abnormal conduction such as reduced velocity and abnormal refractory period in the atrial myocardium, as the mechanism for this arrhythmia without assuming any abnormality of the conducting system. Disturbances of impulse conduction occur in horses and are evidenced by such phenomena as partial heart block, the variation in size/conformation of the ventricular QRS complex that may be associated with some supraventricular arrhythmias and by some ventricular arrhythmias. These may include fixed coupling of ventricular ectopics with normal complexes, an example of reentry (Fig 46). Specific malfunction of the conduction system generally is not seen in horses, with the possible exception of occasional cases of total AV nodal block and preexcitation syndrome. Bundle branch block is very uncommon.

Clinical Consequences of Arrhythmias

The clinical consequences of arrhythmias are primarily hemodynamic, though only limited specific investigation has been done in horses.[6,7,200,201-205] The effects relate to changes in ventricular performance and cardiac output, often with a secondary reduction in myocardial perfusion as a consequence of lowered blood pressure, shortened diastolic interval and inefficient ventricular contraction. These are of particular importance in ventricular tachyarrhythmias, with some contractions following very short diastolic intervals, resulting in minimal stroke volume and pulse deficits. The reduction in efficiency of myocardial perfusion thus conflicts with an increase in myocardial workload. Conversely, many equine atrial arrhythmias not associated with major changes in heart rate have minimal consequences.[204-206] The marked cardiovascular reserve of horses appears to have some protective influence insofar as the myocardium is concerned; reports of heart failure resulting solely from arrhythmias are rare. All the same, a horse experiencing a prolonged bout of tachyarrhythmia is in danger of developing secondary myocardial damage, with subsequent long-term implications for reduced reserve capacity and performance. In many cases, arrhythmia accompanying organic heart disease undoubtedly contributes to the animal's deterioration.

Systemic consequences of arrhythmias are primarily those of syncope. This may occur during bradycardia or runs of tachycardia. The episode also may be brought on in an animal with an otherwise stable arrhythmia because of a sudden increased demand for cardiac output and a fall in pressure. (Syncope is discussed in more detail elsewhere in this chapter.) Thus, while a horse with a heart murmur may present limited danger to the rider, a horse with a predisposition to arrhythmias may represent a considerable risk.

Evaluation of Arrhythmias

Clinical Examination: The ideal approach to accurate diagnosis of arrhythmias is electrocardiography, which also provides a permanent record of the abnormality and an objective means of monitoring progress and response to treatment. The equipment is inexpensive and readily available. Virtually everyone with a telephone has access to transtelephonic ECG analysis services. However, even under circumstances in which such equipment is not available, progress can be made in evaluation of abnormalities of rhythm by careful auscultation and palpation of pulses and by observation, particularly of the thoracic inlet and jugular veins.[172,175,207] These techniques have been discussed earlier in this chapter, while the specific observations in different arrhythmias are identified below.

Electrocardiography: It is of little consequence which particular ECG lead is used in investigation of arrhythmias, but consistency is to be encouraged to allow comparison of tracings within and between animals, particularly so that the conformation of complexes can be compared. A base-apex lead is most useful because it provides a large, easily identified QRS complex. Collection of more than 1 lead is indicated in difficult cases to allow accurate identification of waveforms that may not be obvious in the base-apex lead. Analysis of a rhythm tracing always should proceed in 3 steps: measurement of the heart rate; examination for evidence of abnormal rhythm; and examination of the individual complexes.

Exercise: Only limited research has been performed on the effect of exercise upon arrhythmias, even though most clinicians use this approach to determine their clinical significance.[99,100,202,208-210] The assumption is that if the arrhythmia subsides with exercise, it is likely to be of limited importance. If the immediate objective is to ascertain the absence of arrhythmias at normal work, this approach is rational. Unfortunately, the evidence to support the assumption is scant, and it is risky to assume that any resting arrhythmia that subsides is insignificant. Arrhythmias can be episodic and

bradyarrhythmias in particular may be very sensitive to the effects of increased sympathetic tone. Most examinations only involve jogging or light exercise under saddle; rhythm at submaximal effort rarely is evaluated. The comments made below concerning the exercise response of specific arrhythmias should be interpreted in light of this caution.

Atrial Arrhythmias

In the absence of electrocardiography, the clinician first detects arrhythmias during auscultation of the heart or palpation of the pulse. Cardiovascular signs then are evaluated to provide clues as to the possible nature of the abnormality. A careful approach would dictate that conclusions not be reached prematurely. The characteristics of cardiac activity that are obvious most immediately are the heart rate and the pattern, if any, of the rhythm disturbance.

With this approach in mind, Table 2 has been generated to provide some guidance as to where to look first. Even if an ECG is available, reference to Table 2 may be helpful in deciding what the most appropriate interpretation might be. Note that some arrhythmias appear in more than one category. Only the commonly encountered ones are discussed below. Various combinations and unusual types of arrhythmias may be encountered, and it may be necessary to refer to texts dealing exclusively with abnormalities of rhythm.

Clinical Associations: The horse is subject to a range of atrial arrhythmias, though those of clinical significance are infrequent. With the exception of atrial fibrillation, preexcitation (Wolff-Parkinson-White syndrome), atrial flutter, atrial (supraventricular) tachycardia and third-degree heart block, most convert to a normal rhythm with even the slightest stimulation and elevation in rate. Thus, persistence of an atrial arrhythmia at elevated rates should be regarded with suspicion.[172] Clinical associations are, in the main, nonspecific. Bradyarrhythmia or tachyarrhythmia may be associated with syncopal episodes and often are paroxysmal, while persistent arrhythmias (eg, third-degree heart block, atrial fibrillation) are associated with poor performance in animals asked to perform vigorously. With acute myocardial injury, ventricular rather than atrial arrhythmias are more likely to be observed. The extent to which chronic myocardial disease underlies atrial arrhythmias is undetermined, though several studies have attempted to demonstrate a causative association. It must be recognized, therefore, that while most atrial arrhythmias in horses are regarded as benign and secondary to variations in autonomic and particularly parasympathetic tone, sometimes they may be associated with pathologic changes according to criteria described above.

Sinus Arrhythmia: The term "sinus arrhythmia" is used rather loosely in the veterinary literature and can refer to a fluctuation associated with respiration or exercise, or a variation in RR interval most often associated with second-degree partial atrioventricular block. In the human literature, the term is used most often to describe the vagally mediated fluctuation in heart rate and PR interval that occur in synchrony with respiration.[1] This particular manifestation should properly be described as "respiratory" sinus arrhythmia since fluctuation in RR and PR intervals can also occur independently.[18] Respiratory sinus arrhythmia rarely is obvious in normal horses. It has been suggested that the animal's low resting tidal volume may be insufficient to significantly affect vagal activity.[45]

An exercise-associated arrhythmia, which is quite normal but a frequent reason for referral, also is referred to as sinus arrhythmia by some workers.[102,172,211] Fit horses worked only lightly rather than to a steady state have a tendency to show irregular cardiac deceleration. Typically, the heart rate slows suddenly, then rises again gradually, so that deceleration occurs in steps (Fig 34). The reason for this is unclear, but it possibly reflects a heart rate that is as much a response to excitement as physical work effort, combined with some hesitation within autonomic feedback loops controlling the rate. This observation has been made more often in hunter-jumpers and event horses than in racehorses. It is a normal finding of little or no consequence, and usually can be eliminated by working the horse again, this time to a steady state. If the arrhythmia persists, radiotelemetry or a Holter apparatus can be used to characterize the rhythm. Because this arrhythmia appears to have nothing to do with respiration, use of the term "sinus arrhythmia," which has quite distinct meaning in other species, is confusing. The prefix "exercise-associated" should be used to avoid misunderstanding.

Sinus arrhythmia has been described as commonly accompanying second-degree AV block in horses, though it is unclear whether this finding should be regarded as a simultaneous occurrence of 2 distinct disturbances or whether variation in RR interval should be seen as a primary component of partial AV block.[166,200,212-215] Studies have revealed no obvious relationship between the occurrence of second-degree partial AV block and respiration;[200] variation in RR in-

Table 2. Arrhythmias classified according to rhythm disturbance and commonly found rate changes.

Disturbance of Rhythm	Heart Rate		
	Low	**Normal**	**High**
None	sinus bradycardia total heart block	sinus rhythm preexcitation, wandering pacemaker, bundle branch block	atrial tachycardia, ventricular tachycardia (atrioventricular dissociation)
Regular	second-degree partial atrioventricular block, sinoatrial block	second-degree partial atrioventricular block, sinoatrial block	exercise-associated sinus arrhythmia
Occasional	sinus bradycardia with escape beats, sinoatrial block with escape beats	atrial premature beats, ventricular premature beats, sinoatrial block with escape beats	premature atrial contraction, premature ventricular contraction
Absolute	sinus arrhythmia, atrial fibrillation, multiple/ frequent premature atrial or ventricular beats	sinus arrhythmia, atrial fibrillation, multiple/ frequent premature atrial or ventricular beats	atrial fibrillation

terval apparently accompanying second-degree partial AV block should be regarded as a manifestation of a nonrespiratory sinus arrhythmia.[215,216] The underlying mechanisms in each rhythm disturbance probably are similar (see discussion of Second Degree AV Block below). In the interests of clarity, the dropping of beats is best regarded as a distinct arrhythmia in which there also may be an underlying variation in sinus rate. Where sinus arrhythmia is very obvious, as may occur in horses with severe chronic respiratory disease, the clinician should first look for extracardiac causes before assuming the presence of primary heart disease.

Wandering Pacemaker: This finding is detectable only by electrocardiography, where it is manifested as variation in conformation of the P wave (Fig 35). This is thought to reflect variation in the location of the pacemaker, either within the large sinoatrial node (SAN) or elsewhere in the atrium, leading to a varying pattern of depolarization in the myocardium. The finding is commonly observed in horses, especially in athletically fit animals, and is regarded as a completely benign variation by most authors.[18,80,156,171,172,185] Underlying pathologic changes have been suspected by some authors and attempts have been

made to associate specific pathological changes in the myocardium with wandering pacemaker, though it is difficult to provide adequate controls for such studies.[166,196,217] The consensus is that wandering pacemaker is an entirely benign normal variation and is probably more common in horses because of the large size of their sinoatrial node and right atrium.[37]

Sinoatrial Block and Sinus Arrest: An example of sinoatrial block is presented in Figure 36. The arrhythmia is characterized in the ECG by a normal rhythm with periodic dropped beats in which there is electrical silence with no P wave or QRS-T. During the blocked interval, there is no auscultable sound, in contrast to second-degree partial AV block. Usually only 1 beat is dropped, though occasionally 2 or 3 may be missed. The only change that might be observed in the normally conducted cycles is variation in the PR interval. The waveforms are normal. When a single beat is dropped, the blocked interval is typically twice the normal length of the RR interval, in contrast to sinus arrest, in which the interval is longer. However, occasionally, the blocked interval is less than twice the normal interval, in which case the arrhythmia

Figure 34. ECG collected by radiotelemetry from a 4-year-old Hanoverian filly referred because an arrhythmia had been noted after exercise during a prepurchase examination. Clinical findings at rest were normal. After a 1-mile warmup at a slow canter, irregular cardiac deceleration was observed. Note the sudden slowing (arrows), followed by acceleration. This pattern of "exercise-associated sinus arrhythmia" is normal and frequently observed in fit animals subjected to only light exercise. Compare this tracing with that in Figure 40.

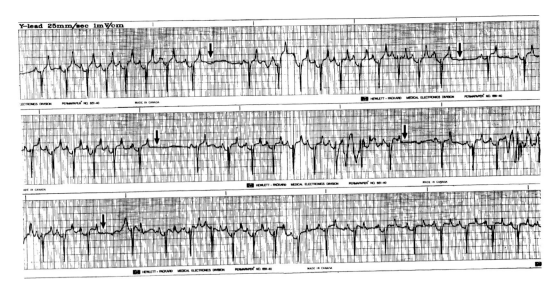

is described as variable sinus node exit block.[172]

Sinoatrial block is difficult to differentiate from sinus arrest, in which variable-length periods of asystole are encountered. If the blocked intervals are infrequent and last for twice the RR interval of the preblock period or less, then sinoatrial block may be presumed. However, where the delay is long and of variable length, differentiation becomes problematic. The issue may appear somewhat academic because such a horse would require full evaluation in either case to explore the possibility of

Figure 35. Wandering pacemaker in a 5-year-old Standardbred mare with a pubic symphysis fracture. There were no cardiac abnormalities and the ECG finding was an incidental observation. Note the change from a bifid to a biphasic P wave in the first strip and its reversal in the third strip. Both P-wave conformations are regarded as normal in horses (see Figure 10).

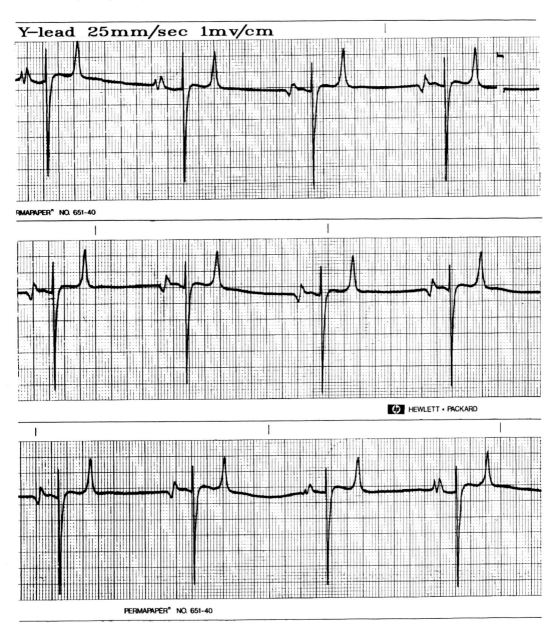

Y–lead 25mm/sec 1mv/cm

RMAPAPER® NO. 651-40

HEWLETT · PACKARD

PERMAPAPER® NO. 651-40

underlying myocardial disease. The implications of the 2 arrhythmias are somewhat different, however, as sinus arrest is more likely to be associated with lesions. Prolonged periods of atrial asystole of variable duration should thus be regarded with great suspicion.

Generally, sinoatrial block is regarded as a benign variation on normal and a reflection of vagal tone.[156] However, in surveys of atrial arrhythmias in horses, sinoatrial block occurs with low frequency, suggesting that it may not represent a typical response to elevated vagal tone.[18,94,166,218] Some authors have suggested a pathologic basis for the arrhythmia.[166,219] If the resting heart rate is normal and the arrhythmia disappears with mild stimulation/light exercise, there should be no cause for concern. Where resting heart rate is very low as a consequence of a severe degree of sino-atrial block/sinus arrest or where blocked intervals are long (>4 seconds, especially where syncope is a clinical problem), the possibility of myocardial lesions or a pathologic degree of vagotonia should be considered and the arrhythmia regarded as pathologic regardless of its response to exercise. Persistence of the arrhythmia at elevated heart rates due to exercise or parasympatholytic agents strongly suggest myocardial disease. Associations with atrial myocardial lesions have been described.[197]

Atrioventricular Block: Atrioventricular block occurs in 3 degrees: first-degree partial atrioventricular block, second-degree partial atrioventricular block, and third-degree (total) heart block. These first 2 disturbances of AV nodal conduction are commonly encountered in horses, with frequencies ranging from 6.4% to 44%.[18,52, 94,156,165,166,185,207,214,218,220] Second-degree partial AV block is more common than first-degree partial AV block. In studies, the criteria for inclusion in the population varied widely and often were not stated. Additionally, a horse generally must be relaxed to manifest these rhythm disturbances, and their true incidence is not known. Third-degree block is encountered infrequently and, in contrast to the first 2, always is of clinical significance.

First-degree partial AV block is characterized by variable PR interval, the interval becoming progressively longer to exceed an arbitrarily determined threshold value of 0.425-0.47 seconds (Fig 37).[207,221] Such threshold values vary according to age and breed.[75,80] The interval then returns to normal. In some cases, the prolonged interval may persist. The effects are minimal but the arrhythmia can be detected upon aus-

Figure 36. Sinoatrial block in a 3-year-old Standardbred stallion presented for elected limb surgery. The arrhythmia was an incidental finding on routine preoperative examination. Resting heart rate was 24 bpm. The animal's performance was regarded as satisfactory by the owner. Note that increased RR intervals are not necessarily simple multiples of the basic sinus (atrial) rate.

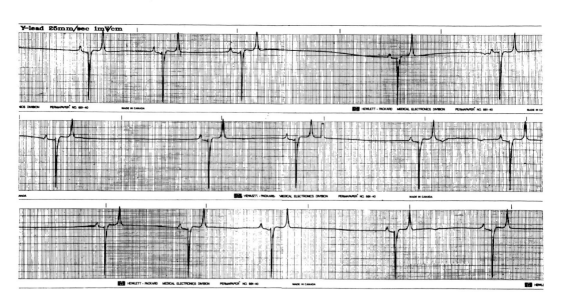

cultation by variation in the interval between the atrial contraction sound and S_1. In cycles associated with a very short PR interval, the atrial sound may not be discernible from S_1; as the interval lengthens, the sound becomes distinct. One may find both first- and second-degree block in the same animal, with first-degree block giving way to second-degree block when the animal is relaxed.

The most consistent feature of *second-degree partial AV block* is dropped beats, in which a P wave is not followed by a QRS-T, *ie,* the wave of depolarization is blocked at the AV node. Upon auscultation, therefore, an atrial contraction sound frequently can be heard as a soft "lu" but is not followed by S_1 and S_2 in the blocked cycle. In addition, there usually is a variation in PR interval and PP interval (sinus rate). This arrhythmia, in particular the inconsistent relationship between the blocked beat and the PR interval of preceding and succeeding cycles, has been the subject of considerable study.[207,215,222] Cases of second-degree partial AV block are divided into 2 types: Type 1 (Wenkebach) and Type 2.

In Type 1 (more common in horses) a progressive lengthening of the PR interval heralds arrival of a blocked beat (Fig 38). Often the PR interval increases until a beat is dropped, then immediately shortens in the first postblock beat. However, commonly, the longest PR-interval in the cycle occurs in the first or second postblock beat, though numerous variations occur.[18,207,214] These variations in relationship between dropped beats and PR interval represent a deviation from the usual presentation of the Wenkebach phenomenon as described in people.[223] The relationship between the longest PR interval and the blocked beat may vary in an individual horse as well as between horses, while the longest interval to be found in a tracing may occur completely independent of any dropped beats. Atrial rate (PP interval) follows the same cycle, being generally slowest at the time a block occurs and fastest afterward; hence the observation that sinus arrhythmia usually accompanies second-degree partial AV block. In contrast to the above, in a Type-2 block, dropped beats occur without any variation in PR interval (Fig 39). Such cases are rare in horses.[18,166,207]

In most cases of second-degree partial AV block, only 1 beat is dropped at a time, but occasionally 2 or more consecutive beats may be dropped. In the latter cases, the relationship of the dropped beats to PR interval and heart rate is the same as for single dropped beats, though immediate shortening of PR interval in the first postblock beat is more likely. Also, horses that show consecutive blocked cycles have been observed to show second-degree partial AV block at a higher atrial rate than those dropping single beats.[214] The atrioventricular conduction ratio (ratio of P waves to QRS-T complexes) ranged from 4:3 to 10:9 in a study of 116 horses with second-degree partial AV block.[214] In a case of severe block, a 3:1 ratio was observed, with a ventricular rate of 17/minute as a consequence.[224]

The mechanism of second-degree partial AV block in horses involves changes in

Figure 37. Prolonged PR interval in a 4-year-old stallion presented for evaluation of low-grade airway disease. The PR interval varied in an inconsistent manner not related to respiration. Criteria for first-degree block are not adequately determined for horses while variation in PR interval with occasionally quite prolonged intervals is common. The longest PR interval exhibited by this horse (0.56 seconds) is at the top of the range reported by one investigator.[75] Pathologic associations with prolonged PR interval are not clearly established in horses.

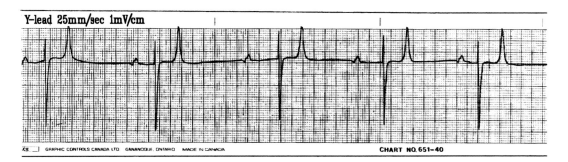

Y-lead 25mm/sec 1mV/cm

GRAPHIC CONTROLS CANADA LTD. GANANOQUE, ONTARIO   MADE IN CANADA   CHART NO. 651–40

vagal tone.[185,214,215,222,225] Elevation in blood pressure over successive cardiac cycles causes reflex increase in vagal tone, leading to decreased activity in the sinoatrial node and progressive decrease in conduction through the AV node. That this autonomic reflex results in AV block before affecting sinus rate may be explained by the assumption that the AV node is more extensively influenced by changes in vagal tone than

Figure 38. A moderately severe degree of type-I, second-degree partial atrioventricular block in a 10-year-old Standardbred gelding. Clinical findings indicated equine rhabdomyolysis syndrome. The horse frequently drops 2 consecutive beats. Resting ventricular rate was 28 bpm, atrial rate 37. This arrhythmia is common in horses but is not usually seen to this degree. Note the variation in PR interval in the first line. Blocked cycles and changes in PR interval are not necessarily related in this arrhythmia.

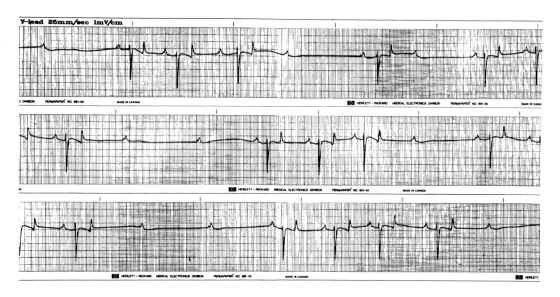

Figure 39. Type-II, second-degree atrioventricular block in a 6-year-old Standardbred gelding with a history of fading during races. There is no change in the PR interval, and blocks are frequent (atrial:ventricular ratio 3:2). Note the varied P-wave conformation. Ventricular rate is 24 bpm. The arrhythmia was not abolished by stimulation (slapping the horse's abdomen), and returned rapidly after light exercise (see also Figure 40).

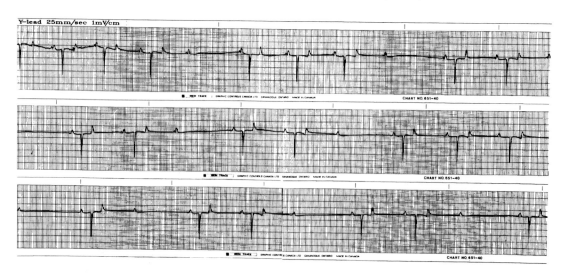

the sinoatrial node.[18] This interpretation is reinforced by the observation that sectioning only the left vagosympathetic trunk, which supplies the AV node with most of its vagal innervation, abolishes the arrhythmia, whereas sectioning the right vagosympathetic trunk, which provides most of the parasympathetic fibers to the sinoatrial node, often induces the arrhythmia.[43,222]

The clinical significance of second-degree partial AV block is the subject of debate. Several investigators have concluded that it is a benign physiologic variant and that a lack of clinical significance can be assumed if the arrhythmia subsides with exercise and does not reappear until heart rates approach normal values.[18,99,207,214,222] Thus, the arrhythmia may be regarded as abnormal only if present in a severe form. However, histopathologic studies have suggested a relationship with myocardial disease, while the arrhythmia has been described as occurring in association with respiratory disease, myocarditis and reduced performance.[80,166,182,188,226,227] It has occasionally occurred to a severe degree and was presumed to be pathologic.[224] Severe Type-2 second-degree partial AV block in a Standardbred gelding is shown in Figure 39. The arrhythmia persisted after exercise (Fig 40). The horse consistently faded in the second half of its races and subsequently was shown to have paroxysmal, exercise-associated atrial fibrillation.

Reports of pathologic association must be interpreted with caution. If the arrhythmia is indeed a common, benign and frequent physiologic variant, it can be expected to occur, by chance, in association with any disease, including myocardial disease, without any cause-effect relationship necessarily being present. Descriptions of histopathologic association must be controlled by thorough investigation of myocardial status in animals manifesting no arrhythmia.[84,188,228] Diseases outside the cardiovascular system associated with a high level of vagal activity or specific damage/irritation of the vagosympathetic trunk or nodal tissue may secondarily induce second-degree partial AV block.

In *third-degree heart block*, the conduction block between the atria and the ventricles is complete. The structures beat independently, the atria at the inherent sinus rate, the ventricles at a low, idioventricular rate. The arrhythmia may be suspected clinically by noting the very low heart rate and by observing the jugular veins. Because the atria and ventricles are beating independently, atrial contraction occasionally occurs during ventricular systole when the atrioventricular valves are closed, resulting in a very prominent regurgitant wave in the jugular veins. The ECG shows P waves with a frequency reflecting the normal sinus rate of 28-40/minute and unassociated rhythmic ventricular complexes with a frequency of 10-20/minute. The conformation of the QRS varies. In cases in which the ventricular pacemaker is located in the conduction system, the complex is normal. Where the pacemaker is outside the conduction system, the QRS complex is widened and may take on a bizarre conformation, reflecting slow conduction through normal myocardium. Ventricular rate is thus very rhythmic in the former cases but can be quite irregular if different foci of ectopic activity initiate systole.

A number of cases of severe heart block associated with syncopal attacks have been described in the literature.[229-244] Total or third-degree heart block is the cause in most instances. The consistent clinical associations are lethargy/weakness, reduced exercise tolerance, syncopal attacks (Stokes-Adams or Morgagni-Stokes-Adams seizures) and bradycardia. Attacks may be recurrent, and may occur over a period of months to years.[237,241,242] They have been presumed to be the cause of death in some cases.[238] Syncope can be anticipated if the period of ventricular inactivity exceeds 12-15 seconds.

The functional and anatomic basis of third-degree AV block has received limited attention in horses, probably because the problem is uncommon. Most interpretations of the pathophysiology are based upon postmortem findings in a limited number of horses. Total heart block has been seen in association with aortic aneurysms, resulting in hemorrhage into the ventricular septum and interruption of the conduction system, with inflammation and degeneration around the AV node and bundle of His, and with pericarditis and myocarditis.[233,238,239] Syncope in a horse with second-degree partial AV block and total block with ventricular tachycardia also has been observed in a horse with lymphosarcoma, though myocardial involvement was not confirmed.[245] In people, complete block is associated with congenital and organic heart disease and surgical sectioning of the bundle of His.[190] Organic lesions appear to be relatively nonspecific and nonselective, involving the intraventricular conducting system by chance and designated as sclerosis of the cardiac skeleton (valve bases and adjacent myocardium). The arrhythmia also is seen with digoxin toxicity; any degree of AV block is a strong indication for extreme caution in use of this drug.

Treatment is not usually attempted because of the limited usefulness of affected animals. However, successful use of cardiac pacemakers in equidae has been described.[242,246,247] Drug therapy is of little value. Despite the generally poor prognosis, the possibility exists that the arrhythmia is a recent result of acute myocardial injury from which the horse could recover.

Figure 40. Radiotelemetry tracing collected after a slow 1-mile race from the horse described in Figure 39. The cardiac rhythm was normal immediately after exercise (maximum rate recorded 180 bpm). When the rate fell to 100 bpm, atrioventricular block became evident. Note the P waves (arrows) in the blocked intervals. Second-degree heart block at elevated heart rates should be viewed with suspicion. This horse subsequently developed paroxysmal atrial fibrillation after intense race miles. Compare this tracing with that in Figure 34. (The inversion of the peak of the T-waves is an artifact caused by overload of the amplifier in the transmitter. Sensitivity was doubled to 1/2 mV/cm halfway through the first strip.)

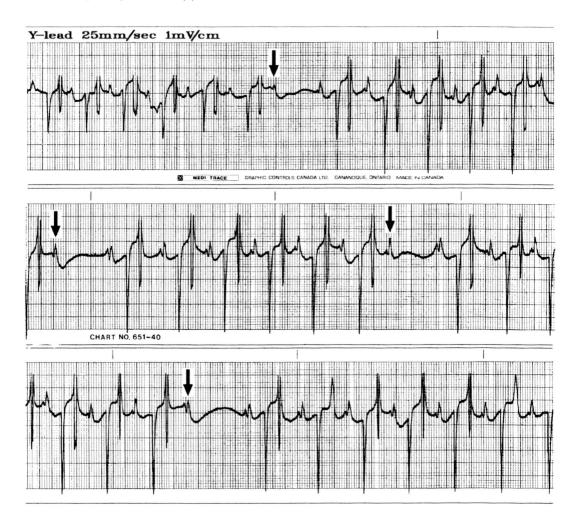

Atrial Fibrillation: Atrial fibrillation is perhaps the most frequently documented arrhythmia in horses (Fig 41).[18,162,163,180, 209,248,249] The estimated incidence in *selected* populations ranges from 0.34% to 2.5%.[162,209,250] The true incidence in the general population is probably much lower than these estimates. Incidences of 5.7-6.2% of horses referred specifically for cardiovascular examination have been reported.[94,162] The numerous reports of the arrhythmia probably reflect its frequent association with organic heart disease and its ease of diagnosis and treatment.

Atrial fibrillation was first recorded in horses in 1911.[251] Subsequent studies have commented upon a predisposition in heavier, larger breeds and types, and the infrequent occurrence in small breeds or ponies.[162,209] A higher incidence in older horses also was observed. These observations support impressions gained from the earlier literature, which could have been biased toward heavier military and commercial carriage/draft horses.

It has been stated that atrial fibrillation rarely develops except in serious heart disease and that it should be considered a grave prognostic sign;[180] associated myocardial lesions are often found.[162] Such observations have been partly based, however, upon limited postmortem studies of horses

and experience in other species. While complicated cases in which there are other signs of cardiac disease do appear to carry a poor prognosis, it is now well established that atrial fibrillation also can occur in an uncomplicated form in apparently healthy horses.[163,172,180,250,252] Many cases have been observed with no other clinically detectable signs of heart disease or myocardial lesions.[162,163,185,202,210,248,250,252,253]

Atrial fibrillation may occur in varied clinical circumstances. The following discussion considers the 2 extremes. Animals with atrioventricular insufficiencies, particularly on the left, may be predisposed and may develop the arrhythmia well before any overt clinical signs of failure develop.[162,163] Attempts to correct the arrhythmia in such animals usually are unsuccessful, and the horse fails to respond or reverts to the arrhythmia shortly after conversion; thus, the prognosis is grave.[163,250,252] In such cases, myocardial disease and dilatation of the atria are assumed to contribute to the onset of the arrhythmia. With the exception of the effect on heart sounds, heart rhythm and pulse characteristics, it is difficult to attribute many of the signs in such cases specifically to the arrhythmia, though the inefficient cardiac filling and subsequently reduced cardiac output undoubtedly contribute to the circulatory insufficiency, espe-

Figure 41. Atrial fibrillation in a 7-year-old Standardbred gelding. The baseline undulations (F waves) characteristic of this arrhythmia are obvious. Note also the clustering of ventricular complexes with long pauses in between. This is a common finding and may cause the arrhythmia to be erroneously diagnosed as second-degree partial AV block upon auscultation, especially if heart rate is low-normal.

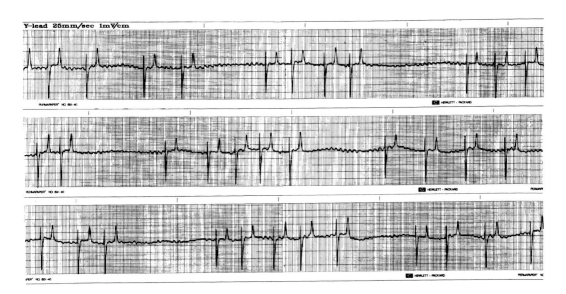

cially at exercise. At the other extreme are fit, younger (<7 years of age) racehorses with spontaneous onset of the arrhythmia and no apparent predisposing factors. Such animals usually respond well to treatment and many show no subsequent detrimental influence upon performance.[163,252,254,255]

Between these 2 extremes are a range of clinical associations. It is generally recognized that the older and larger the horse and the longer it has been fibrillating, the poorer the prognosis for cardioversion. Onset of the arrhythmia in an animal with signs of marginal circulatory function for some time indicates serious deterioration.[162,180,208]

The pathogenesis of atrial fibrillation continues to be the subject of much debate.[190,256] The basic mechanisms proposed involve circus movement and reentry of waves of depolarization, single or multiple foci of spontaneous activity, or combinations thereof. Atrial size is of importance, with a large atrial mass predisposing.[257,258] As with most arrhythmias, autonomic tone plays a role. Vagotonia shortens the refractory period, slowing the sinus rate, which facilitates ectopic activity. Finally, large areas of damaged (ischemic, fibrosed) myocardium may predispose by providing a path for reentry.[259]

Clinical signs depend upon the animal's use and the presence/absence of additional cardiac abnormalities. Horses expected to perform maximally or near maximally, such as racehorses, eventers or field hunters, show obvious exercise intolerance, tiring easily and showing a greatly reduced maximal rate of working.[163,250] Change in exercise tolerance usually is sudden and, in cases of paroxysmal fibrillation, there may be periods of exercise intolerance interspersed with periods of normal performance. Exercise intolerance reflects inability to control heart rate and thus to maintain cardiac output in response to demand.[103] Animals used for lighter exercise, such as hacks and show hunters, may show no obvious signs at work.

Syncopal attacks may occur at rest when the heart rate is very low, or during exercise or excitement, especially if the arrhythmia accompanies another cardiovascular abnormality.[163,209,250] In my experience, there is no reliable way to identify horses prone to syncopal attacks and all horses with atrial fibrillation should be considered potential candidates.

Epistaxis has been described in numerous cases, but it is unclear whether this reflects a cause-effect relationship.[82,163,250, 260,261] Epistaxis is a common problem in racehorses, while those with atrial fibrillation may be expected to find race-intensity exercise particularly stressful. At exercise, particularly if the arrhythmia develops during work, unsteadiness and dyspnea also may be seen.[172,209,250]

Physical examination reveals the characteristic totally irregular rhythm. Heart rate can be low, normal or high, and ranged from 17 to 120 in a study of 106 cases.[250] However, in most uncomplicated cases, the heart rate is normal. Caution is required because most affected horses manifest an underlying waxing and waning of rhythm, with relatively long periods of asystole interspersed with runs of several beats.

Where resting heart rate is normal or low and the examination superficial, the arrhythmia can be mistaken for second-degree partial AV block. However, with atrial fibrillation, there is marked variation in the intensity of heart sounds.[202,208] S_1 is especially loud in some cycles, particularly during a run of fast beats. Pulse strength varies with cardiac output from almost imperceptible to strong. Wide variation in pulse strength may be the initial indication of the arrhythmia. Pulse deficits may be encountered, especially if the heart rate is high or heart failure is present. Observation of the jugular veins reveals filling during variable periods of ventricular inactivity. Because of the tremendous variation in RR interval, interpretation of murmurs in cases of atrial fibrillation can be challenging.

The effects of exercise upon atrial fibrillation have been examined by several authors.[100,172,202,209,210] In all cases, the problem persisted at exercise. Typically, the response to a standardized exercise test shows a much more rapid rate of rise and greater elevation in heart rate than in normal animals; the difference in maximal heart rate response before and after conversion was as much as 30% in 1 study.[209] Most horses reached maximal heart rates at distinctly submaximal efforts, some during only light cantering exercise. Postexercise recovery seems generally unremarkable, as circulatory reserve is still quite sufficient to correct any deficits that may have occurred (see discussion of Exercise Testing). Cardiac rhythm during exercise is still irregular, though less noticeably so, while the high ventricular rate may obscure "f" waves on the ECG.

Some reports comment upon unsteadiness, dyspnea, apparent discomfort during exercise and collapse, and some exercise ECGs reveal ventricular ectopic activity in addition to atrial fibrillation.[202,209,210] The significance of these observations is difficult to determine, though signs of discomfort, in particular, may reflect the primary cardiac disorder (*eg,* myocarditis) rather than atrial fibrillation. In 1 study, ventricular ectopic activity had no influence upon prognosis for response to therapy or freedom from relapse.[163] In a group of young racehorses with atrial fibrillation, I observed no discomfort or collapse, even when affected horses were worked intensively. These animals generally responded well to treatment and returned to previous levels of performance, implying that underlying myocardial disease, if any, was mild.

Diagnosis is confirmed by ECG findings, which are quite characteristic (Fig 41). The baseline shows marked irregularity, with both coarse and fine "f" waves reflecting the random atrial activity and a total absence of P waves. This atrial "ripple" activity may show frequencies of up to 500/minute.[202] Heart rate and RR intervals vary widely. QRS complexes generally are unremarkable, though some variation in amplitude often is encountered. T waves also can vary in amplitude. The tendency of some affected horses to show relatively large, coarse "f" waves when compared with other species has led to use of the expression "flutter-fibrillation," a reference to the fact that the large "f" waves are in some ways reminiscent of atrial flutter. These coarse waves may simply reflect the large size of the equine atria and the relatively long time taken for depolarization to traverse the myocardium, though their presence does imply a wavefront as opposed to multiple simultaneous areas of local depolarization. The atrial complexes in atrial flutter and supraventricular tachycardia in horses are larger and very consistent in size and duration (Fig 42).

Approach to treatment depends upon the presence of other signs of cardiovascular disease. Though the arrhythmia may have only limited hemodynamic consequences at rest, in the absence of other signs of heart disease, horses intended for serious work show greatly reduced exercise tolerance.[206] Thus, treatment is aimed at cardioversion of uncomplicated cases to facilitate their return to useful work. Successful cardioversion in horses with other signs of cardiac disease is questionable because, aside from the limited chances of the horse's converting or staying converted, treatment of the arrhythmia may do little to improve overall prognosis. However, persistence of the arrhythmia could lead to progressive myocardial and possibly valvular deterioration, especially due to poor myocardial perfusion during tachycardia, while the potential for syncopal attacks exists.[162]

Treatment usually is with quinidine sulfate. The myocardial myasthenic effects of quinidine preclude its use in heart failure without prior digitalization; even then, treatment should be approached with caution.[163] The literature contains a number of "recipes." However, the recommended approach involves administration of 10 g PO at 2-hour intervals until cardioversion occurs, until signs of obvious toxicity are encountered, or until a maximum dose of 60-70 g has been given, whichever comes first.[252,262] A test dose of 5 g usually is given the previous day to identify horses that are sensitive to quinidine. An ECG is recorded immediately before each dose and, if possible, every hour, to monitor response to therapy and signs of toxicity. (The toxic effects of quinidine are discussed later in this chapter.) Response to medication is evidenced on the ECG as an elevation in heart rate, typically to 60-70 bpm, and increasing coarseness and reducing frequency of "f" waves. Horses frequently pass through a period of atrial flutter before cardioversion. Heart rate usually falls immediately after cardioversion but does not return to normal for several hours.

Uncomplicated cases in young horses occasionally convert on the test dose. Others, particularly older, heavier animals, may not convert until obvious signs of toxicity are encountered, raising the question of whether or not to proceed. I have seen horses that would not convert after administration of 60-70 g of quinidine, then converting after a much smaller dose several days later. Therefore, if a horse fails to respond, it may be advisable to stop treatment and attempt conversion again a week later rather than risk a fatal outcome. Horses that have relapsed and are retreated may develop obvious signs of toxicity, especially neurologic manifestations, before converting to sinus rhythm.

The reason for this variation in response is not clear. In people, electrolyte disorders, particularly total body potassium deficit, are thought to predispose to the rhythm disturbance. (see discussion of quinidine elsewhere in this chapter).[263,264] I have encountered patients that appeared to have potassium deficits based upon renal fractional excretion ratios and red cell potassium concentrations, and would not convert. Oral administration of 40 g of potassium chloride daily, together with withdrawal from training, led to cardioversion 1-2 weeks later. It must be emphasized that a cause-effect relationship has not been established, however, and such horses might have responded because of a number of factors, including subsidence of myocardial disease and change in autonomic tone or in other aspects of electrolyte status. Because of this difference in response, tremendous individual variation in uptake and the very real potential for toxicity, whenever possible, determination of serum concentrations of quinidine should be accompanied by ECG monitoring. Serum quinidine levels should be kept within the presumed therapeutic range of 2-4 μg/ml (6.16-12.32 μmol/L).[174]

Cardioversion by intravenous administration of quinidine gluconate, dihydroquinidine chlorhydrate or dihydroquinidine gluconate also can be very effective.[265-268] However, if one of these is used, the horse must be kept under supervision and the ECG monitored constantly. Though cardioversion can be achieved much faster by intravenous than by oral therapy and with much less interference with the horse, toxic signs can develop much more rapidly, especially cardiac arrhythmias, serious tachycardia and decrease in blood pressure. Drug administration can be stopped immediately

Figure 42A. Atrial (supraventricular) tachycardia with variable AV conduction in a 12-year-old Arabian mare used for endurance work. The mare had a cardiac arrhythmia after work. Resting heart rate was normal despite the arrhythmia and the horse showed no obvious limitation of exercise tolerance, though the heart rate did not return to resting values as fast as normal after exercise. The arrhythmia might also be interpreted as atrial flutter with variable AV conduction ratio, though the atrial rate of 160-170 is slower than might be anticipated in this arrhythmia. (Courtesy of Drs. H. Staempfli and H. Kloeze).

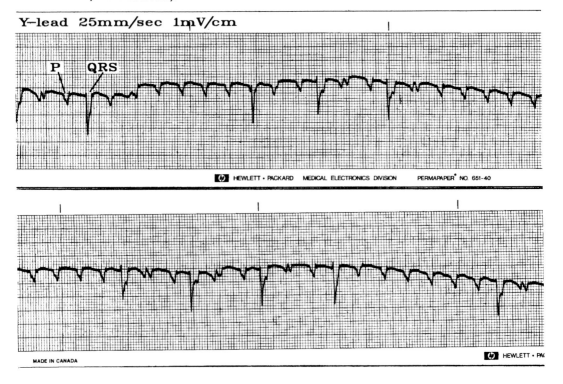

if monitoring detects the onset of serious toxic signs. In view of the potential for deleterious side effects, however, this approach probably should not be used in animals exhibiting signs of circulatory insufficiency. The total dose of dihydroquinidine gluconate administered in 1 study was 3.5-22.0 g, with infusion rates of 0.1-0.68 g/minute leading to cardioversion in 15-120 minutes.[266] Concentration of the solutions used ranged from 0.9% to 2.95%. One author recommends stopping infusion immediately after cardioversion is achieved.[268]

If a horse with a propensity to relapse converts immediately before the next scheduled dose, administration of another half dose may be indicated. Regardless of treatment strategy, however, once cardioversion is achieved, it usually is not necessary to administer further "topping-up" doses. I have used this approach and have not had any relapses in the first few days after treatment when working with a young population of racing animals. Absorption of quinidine sulfate from the gut continues beyond 2 hours

after an oral dose. With a half life of 6.7 hours, plasma levels may rise or stay in the therapeutic range for some time after treatment has stopped.[262] These considerations emphasize the utility of giving the drug every 2 hours as described above.

Recommendations for management after cardioversion vary widely and depend in part upon the presence of other signs of cardiovascular dysfunction. In complicated cases, the extent to which the animal is exercised is determined by underlying abnormalities. For example, a horse with suspected myocarditis requires rest. In uncomplicated cases, a horse can immediately begin 2-3 days of hand walking to ensure that all quinidine has been eliminated, then gradually return to full exercise over 2 weeks. Because arrhythmia often is the only abnormality present, there is little to be gained by withholding exercise.

If there are no other signs of cardiac disease and cardioversion is achieved, the prognosis is difficult to predict. Relapse into fibrillation can happen, sometimes imme-

Figure 42B. The upper tracing was recorded after 20 g of quinidine sulfate were given PO. Atrial rate has decreased to 120 and ventricular rate has increased to 60 (2:1 conduction ratio). Locations of the first 5 P waves are marked by arrows. In the lower tracing, the horse has reverted to sinus rhythm at a heart rate of 48 bpm after 50 g of quinidine PO. Note the change in P-wave conformation. The response to therapy suggests atrial tachycardia with variable AV conduction as the most appropriate interpretation. Quinidine should be given with great caution in this arrhythmia. (Courtesy of Drs. H. Staempfli and H. Kloeze).

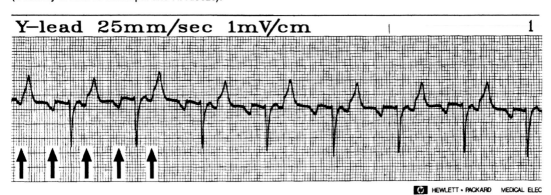

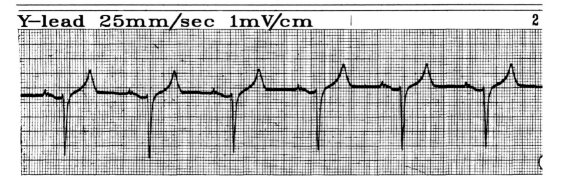

diately after cardioversion or up to months later.[250,252,254,260] The younger the horse when the arrhythmia occurs and the shorter the duration, the better the prognosis for permanent cardioversion.[163,252,254] Conversely, horses with atrial fibrillation for more than 1 month are more likely to show an adverse response to treatment and to relapse. The prognosis for horses with signs of heart failure was poor in all the studies reviewed.

Atrial fibrillation is a stable arrhythmia, and horses with no other cardiovascular abnormalities can continue to work as long as they are not expected to perform intensely. Affected horses have continued to work for prolonged periods without obvious deterioration in performance.[163,166,202,269-271]

Cardiac lesions related to atrial fibrillation have been reported.[162,163,194,202,250,272] A high incidence of atrial fibrillation has been associated with heart failure and atrioventricular insufficiencies, particularly left atrioventricular insufficiency.[162] It also has been associated with a range of primary and secondary cardiac diseases, including valvular abnormalities, myocarditis and endocarditis.[162,180,250,272,273] Histopathologic lesions have included focal and diffuse myocardial fibrosis, thinning and dilatation of the atria, and myocarditis with fatty infiltration.[162,183,269] Detailed examination of the atrial myocardium and cardiac innervation has also revealed alterations in microvasculature, including thickening of the wall and stenosis, and changes in intracardiac and extracardiac nerves.[194,272] These latter changes indicate progressive loss of nerve fibers. The significance of these findings is undetermined, as is their specificity for participation in the pathogenesis of atrial fibrillation. The serious nature of the lesions found in some affected horses should not cause the clinician to offer an overly grave prognosis because, in most affected younger horses, the prognosis for athletic performance after treatment can be excellent.

Paroxysmal Atrial Fibrillation: Some cases of atrial fibrillation appear and disappear spontaneously. When this occurs during exercise, there has been a tendency to use the term "paroxysmal." While "paroxysmal" is more often used to describe brief episodes of arrhythmia of several minutes' du-

ration, most cases described in horses have been present for hours to days. The separate discussion of the paroxysmal form does not imply a different arrhythmia. Rather, the different circumstance of occurrence, *ie,* an exercise-induced arrhythmia that apparently subsides spontaneously, suggests that in such cases the underlying cause may differ significantly from that in nonparoxysmal cases. However, it is possible that any horse that develops atrial fibrillation may persist in the arrhythmia or may convert to sinus rhythm spontaneously. The difference may thus lie in the nature of the processes that promote resolution rather than in the mechanisms causing the arrhythmia.

Paroxysmal atrial fibrillation has been described in numerous reports, including 3 newborn foals, in which the arrhythmia in 2 resolved spontaneously within minutes of birth.[103,166,248,253,274-277] The findings in most of adult patients have been consistent, with horses showing a sudden decrease in performance during work and arrhythmia upon postexercise examination. The arrhythmia persisted for 4-48 hours and all but 1 resolved spontaneously.[103] Most went on to uneventful and often successful performance after spontaneous resolution.

Several published studies make the point that the true incidence of the arrhythmia is unknown, with 1 referring to 37 reported cases out of 75,000 runners over a 19-year period.[103] The clinical associations are assumed to be the same as those previously outlined for the persistent form of atrial fibrillation, though the stress of physical effort and atrial ectopic activity also have been proposed as factors in pathogenesis.[253]

Atrial Flutter, Atrial Tachycardia and Paroxysmal Atrial Tachycardia: Atrial flutter is a supraventricular tachyarrhythmia. In people and dogs, the rate varies from 300-440/minute.[190,278] The atrial complexes, referred to as "f" waves, are regular and consistent in conformation. The resultant baseline undulations on the ECG have a saw-tooth appearance, and are characteristically large and rounded when compared with the normal P wave after conversion. Ventricular rate is lower than the atrial rate, and rhythm is regular or irregular.

There appears to be some uncertainty as to the appropriate diagnostic criteria for atrial flutter in horses.[18,169,183,206,278-280]

Strict adherence to previously published criteria would support the diagnosis in only 1 of the equine reports;[278,281] the remaining cases most closely resemble atrial fibrillation with very coarse "f" waves or atrial tachycardia. The fine line between the "f" waves in atrial flutter and the similar but smaller and less regular "f" waves in atrial fibrillation in horses have led to use of the term "flutter-fibrillation."[278]

The ventricular rate varies from very low to very high, depending upon the degree to which AV conduction allows atrial activity to pass to the ventricles. Conduction ratios (atrial:ventricular) of 2:1 to 6:1 are seen in people. Ventricular rhythm is regular if the AV conduction ratio is constant but irregular if the ratio varies. Clinically, atrial flutter with variable AV conduction may be difficult to differentiate from atrial fibrillation.[156] Most horses undergoing cardioversion for atrial fibrillation go through a transient period of flutter before sinus rhythm is reestablished.

Atrial (supraventricular) tachycardia, on the other hand, is an arrhythmia in which spontaneous onset of rapid (up to 200 beats per minute), firing of an atrial ectopic focus results in a rapid, rhythmic ventricular rate (Fig 42). The term "paroxysmal atrial tachycardia" may be used when the arrhythmia is intermittent. Syncope may occur and the pulse may be weak. Atrial tachycardia must be differentiated from sinus tachycardia in which the origin of the activity is the sinus node. In the latter, the heart rate usually is lower. In atrial tachycardia, P-waves may be difficult to see if they are obscured by the T wave, though in cases with variable AV block there are irregular ventricular complexes, and rapidly recurring P waves are quite obvious between the QRS-T complexes (Fig 42). The P wave is typically of unusual conformation, reflecting the ectopic origin of the impulse, though the natural variation in P-wave conformation in horses may make this difficult to appreciate. Diagnosis sometimes can be very difficult. If there is irregular AV block, the clinical findings may suggest atrial fibrillation. If the AV block is regular or if all atrial activity is conducted, the arrhythmia can be hard to differentiate from atrial flutter with high AV conduction ratio.[278]

The prognosis in these arrhythmias also is difficult to determine because they have been described infrequently.[183] It has been stated that atrial tachycardia usually indicates atrial myocardial disease and the arrhythmia is likely to be encountered in cases of preexcitation, as in people.[156] In people, atrial flutter and atrial fibrillation are viewed as poor prognostic indicators.[190]

Based upon limited experience, atrial tachycardia is treated with digoxin to increase the degree of AV nodal block and reduce ventricular rate. Spontaneous conversion to atrial fibrillation assists clinical management as it allows treatment with quinidine sulfate. Treatment of atrial tachycardia or flutter with quinidine alone must be approached with great caution, as increased AV conduction may cause severe elevation in ventricular rate.

Premature Atrial Contractions: Ectopic activity within the atrial myocardium will

Figure 43. Premature atrial contractions in a 16-year-old Thoroughbred gelding presented for evaluation of a diastolic murmur. The horse remained agitated throughout the examination and showed frequent premature atrial contractions (arrows). Note the spontaneous change in P-wave conformation in the premature cycles. The signals arrive sufficiently early that there is no disturbance of the sinus rhythm.

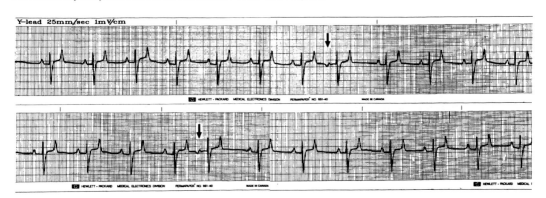

give rise to premature atrial contractions, characterized on the ECG by a short PP interval and an altered P wave (Fig 43). In some cases, however, the P-wave change may be subtle, while the premature signal may arise only slightly earlier than normal. Care must thus be taken in diagnosis, as a combination of wandering pacemaker and sinus arrhythmia may present a similar appearance. The QRS conformation usually is not changed in premature atrial contraction and there is no change in intensity of heart sounds as observed with premature ventricular contraction (see below).

Premature atrial contraction is detected upon auscultation only as a change in rhythm. After a premature atrial contraction, there may be a pause as sinus rhythm is reset or the next sinus signal is blocked. A premature atrial contraction also may be fully intercalated, in which case there is continuation of the regular sinus rhythm. Premature atrial contractions are uncommon in horses. When they do occur, usually they are single events of limited clinical significance. Premature contractions that persist or occur in high frequency after exercise

may reflect atrial myocardial disease, though no specific associations have been established.[168,282,283] An occasional premature atrial contraction does not require treatment.

Pre-Excitation (Wolff-Parkinson-White Syndrome): Though classified here with atrial arrhythmias for the sake of consistency, this abnormality of atrioventricular conduction often is classified with abnormalities of intraventricular conduction. An abnormally short PR interval during sinus rhythm, combined with a prolonged QRS duration with initial slurring (delta wave), are the ECG criteria for the Wolff-Parkinson-White syndrome, also known as accelerated conduction or pre-excitation (Fig 44).[284] Several variations are now recognized.

This conduction abnormality has an anatomic basis, usually consisting of an accessory conduction pathway between the atria and the ventricular myocardium or between the bundle of His and adjacent myocardium. In some cases, there is also a functional basis, characterized as anomalous AV nodal conduction.[256] In people, the arrhyth-

Figure 44. Wolff-Parkinson-White syndrome (ventricular preexcitation) in a 5-year-old Standardbred stallion. The horse had atrial fibrillation and a history of fading. Quinidine therapy revealed ventricular preexcitation. The P wave (arrow) leads directly into the QRS complex without any PR interval. The QRS complex is prolonged (160 msec), as is the T wave. The horse subsequently converted to sinus rhythm but periodically lapsed into preexcitation. In normal sinus rhythm the QRS duration was 80 msec.

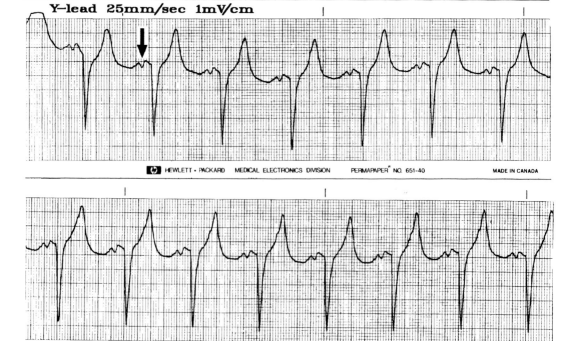

Y-lead 25mm/sec 1mV/cm

HEWLETT · PACKARD   MEDICAL ELECTRONICS DIVISION   PERMAPAPER NO. 651-40   MADE IN CANADA

mia is associated with paroxysmal tachycardia and atrial fibrillation. Though not common, this syndrome has been described in horses on several occasions.[80,166,285-292] In the published cases, it was not always persistent, appearing for several cycles and then subsiding. Significant variation in QRS conformation also was a frequent finding, showing a complete change in direction in some cases.[286,287,291] Patients I have observed have shown minimal or no QRS changes, while 1 horse lapsed into atrial fibrillation repeatedly (Fig 44).

Clinical signs have included unsteadiness during racing and poor performance, though in most affected animals the arrhythmia appears to have been an incidental finding. The arrhythmia persisted in 2 horses that continued to perform successfully.[287,291] The problem is likely of limited clinical significance. By analogy with cases in people, a predisposition to paroxysmal atrial arrhythmias may be anticipated, though this complication has not been described frequently in horses.

Junctional and Ventricular Arrhythmias

Ventricular arrhythmias tend to fluctuate, gradually or suddenly changing from one type into another. It may, therefore, be more important to simply recognize that a ventricular arrhythmia is present because, regardless of electrocardiographic diagnosis, ventricular arrhythmias usually are of clinical significance.

Also there are many considerations in regard to underlying causes and clinical signs that are common to all ventricular arrhythmias. The approach to management often differs only in degree from one arrhythmia to another, with identification and removal of any underlying cause always of primary importance. However, recognition of specific ventricular arrhythmias sometimes is of value in determining the prognosis and the urgency with which therapy must be applied.[18,156,292] Arrhythmias not primarily associated with functional or physical obstruction of the intraventricular conduction system are discussed here as a group.

Clinical Signs: Ventricular arrhythmias are much less common than most atrial arrhythmias.[94,100,218,293] However, they assume greater importance because of their

clinical associations. With the possible exception of occasional premature ventricular contractions, ventricular arrhythmias are best regarded as clinically significant until proven otherwise. Such arrhythmias frequently are encountered in association with myocardial damage, especially where the insult is acute, such as in ionophore toxicity or viral myocarditis.[191-193,198,294] Horses with severe electrolyte disorders, especially disturbances of total body potassium, as in severe cases of diarrhea, are predisposed to ventricular tachyarrhythmias. Arrhythmias sometimes accompany reactions to drugs, particularly agents with a direct effect on membrane function, such as certain anesthetics or digitalis. Hypoxia (severe respiratory disease, severe anemia, acute blood loss) leads to acute myocardial degeneration and arrhythmias, worsening an already serious situation. Endocardial and pericardial inflammation, while capable of causing arrhythmias by virtue of local irritation, are not common in horses. However, where endocarditis involves the left side of the heart, embolic showering via the coronary arteries may be associated with focal myocardial infarction and inflammation, giving rise to an arrhythmia.

Thus, in evaluating horses with ventricular arrhythmias, extracardiac causes should first be ruled out because they are more common than organic heart disease and are often more easily corrected. The presence of significant homeostatic disturbance can worsen the impact of any primary cardiac disorder. Notwithstanding these observations, however, ventricular arrhythmias occasionally are observed in the apparent absence of cardiac or systemic disease and may subside spontaneously without specific treatment.[214,295,296] Horses with ventricular arrhythmias in the absence of other signs of cardiac disease can be expected to perform poorly. If the arrhythmia is intermittent, performance may be equally variable.[80,295]

General ECG Characteristics: For junctional or ventricular arrhythmias, the locus of disturbance is assumed to lie in the AV node or adjacent His bundle (junctional) or below this area, often within the myocardium itself (ventricular). It often is difficult or impossible to determine the precise location of the problem clinically. Because the signal is arising within or below the AV node, the QRS-T complex is not usually accompanied by a P wave. However, retrograde conduction occasionally occurs, especially with junctional activity, and the P wave may occur during or even after the QRS complex.

When the activity of the atria and ventricles is dissociated, both P waves and QRS-T complexes are present, but the 2 bear no consistent relationship to each other. Additionally, some degree of abnormal conduction may exist, such as a partial block or reduced conduction velocity, with the ectopic activity itself often inducing such abnormalities. The degree of abnormal conduction and thus the degree of QRS disturbance may vary from beat to beat.

The conformation of the QRS depends upon the pattern of ventricular depolarization. When this occurs via the normal conduction system, as in most junctional arrhythmias, the conformation is normal. Functional or structural abnormality of part of the Purkinje network may cause a portion of the ventricular myocardium to be depolarized via an abnormal pathway. Where the focus of excitation lies well away from the main conduction system branches, the pattern of spread of the wave of excitation can be completely abnormal, resulting in a very bizarre QRS (Fig 45). An ectopic signal also may be conducted partly by cell-to-cell (myocardial) transmission and partly via the Purkinje system, further complicating the range of possibilities. Additionally, because depolarization of the myocardium is a relatively slow process compared with transmission of the impulse through the Purkinje network, the QRS tends to be prolonged with ectopic signals (Fig 45).

While abnormal duration and conformation of the QRS are frequently observed in ventricular arrhythmias, a relatively normal-looking complex is no guarantee that conduction is normal and *vice versa.* Equally, changes in QRS conformation may result from electrolyte imbalances, drugs or ventricular hypertrophy. However, such changes are rarely as pronounced as those associated with ectopic activity. The more bizarre the QRS complex, the greater the probability an abnormal focus is the origin. An additional guide to clinical significance is the extent to which the QRS varies in conformation, in that 2 or more different patterns usually indicate multiple foci (multiform premature ventricular contractions), which carries a more guarded prognosis.

The other frequently observed characteristic of ventricular arrhythmias, as with many atrial arrhythmias, is abnormal timing or changes in rhythmicity. Aberrant foci of activity may thus fire prematurely before the next anticipated sinus signal, causing a premature ventricular contraction (PVC) (Fig 45). A particularly close temporal relationship between a PVC and the T wave of the preceding cycle (R-on-T) is particularly serious, as this can lead to ventricular tachycardia or fibrillation. A PVC may exhibit a consistent, fixed relationship with the sinus signal or may appear randomly, and can be manifested as sporadic, single complexes or in runs that behave like a pacemaker. Where an abnormal focus has a slow rate of discharge and only occasionally results in an isolated ventricular depolarization during periods of relatively low sinus rate, the term "escape beat" is used. Where the focus displays pacemaker activity, its in-

Figure 45. ECG collected from an 8-year-old Standardbred stallion presented for evaluation of chronic musculoskeletal disease. Occasional premature ventricular contractions were noted as an incidental observation. There were no other cardiovascular findings. The ectopic signal (arrow) has unusual conformation and increased duration. It occurs prematurely, and obscures an underlying P wave just visible in the ST segment. The next sinus signal is delayed, indicating resetting of sinus rhythm.

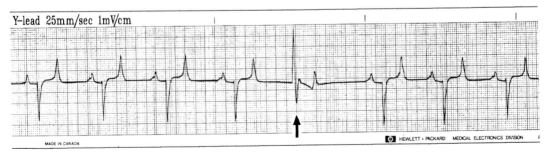

Y-lead 25mm/sec 1mV/cm

MADE IN CANADA

HEWLETT · PACKARD   MEDICAL ELECTRONICS DIVISION

herent rate may be higher or lower than that of the sinus pacemaker, and it may take over heart rhythm, briefly (paroxysmally) or constantly (fixed or permanent ectopic rhythm). Such ectopic pacemaker activity is most characteristic of abnormal foci within the conducting system.

An abnormal focus is only likely to fully capture rhythm if it discharges at a rate much higher than that of the sinus pacemaker or if the sinus pacemaker is very slow or inactive. An ectopic pacemaker with a high inherent rate may still fail to capture ventricular rhythm if its activity is blocked such that only occasional extra signals are seen. Conversely, when heart rhythm has been taken over by an abnormal focus, the sinus pacemaker may still occasionally take over as capture beats.[295] Sinus and ectopic pacemakers also may interfere in other ways. For example, an ectopic signal may enter the conduction system at the same time as a normal sinus signal, both contributing to ventricular myocardial depolarization and resulting in a QRS complex known as a fusion beat.

Premature Ventricular Contractions: Premature ventricular contractions (PVC, ventricular premature beats, ventricular premature systoles), characterized by their premature position in relation to normal

sinus rhythm, absence of an associated P wave and often bizarre QRS conformation, have been described frequently in horses (Fig 45).[94,100,142,164,166,171,218,293,296-298] Resting heart rate usually is normal unless PVCs are associated with systemic illness and/or myocardial disease when rate may be elevated. A PVC typically is accompanied by a loud first heart sound and a soft, often imperceptible, second sound (Fig 46), together with a pulse deficit if the ectopic arrives very shortly after the sinus beat. Where sinus rate is low, the ectopic signal may be fully interpolated, *ie*, there may be no disturbance of sinus rhythm, though usually the next signal is blocked and the ectopic beat is followed by a pause.[172]

Premature ventricular contractions in the absence of detectable signs of cardiac disease have been reported.[164,166,295,297,299,300] A single PVC generally is regarded as of limited clinical significance as long as it is infrequent and does not become more frequent with exercise.[172] It is not known how often such systoles occur in a normal, resting animal but probably not more often than once every 10-15 minutes. Equally, the conformation of the premature QRS complex should be constant. Frequent PVCs, grouping in twos and threes, varying QRS conformation and increased frequency during cardiac deceleration after exercise all have clinical significance and a cause should be sought.[214]

It has been suggested that examination after exercise is a valuable means of exposing ectopic activity in horses with a normal cardiac rhythm at rest.[100,198] Because PVCs occur somewhat unpredictably, the clinician can never be sure that a period of normal auscultation or ECG examination indicates true absence of the arrhythmia (see 24-Hour Rhythm Monitoring). Conformation of the QRS complex in different leads is used in people to help map myocardial damage in such conditions as myocardial infarction.[256] While some investigation of the relationship between QRS conformation and location of ectopic focus has been carried out in horses, currently it is not possible to accurately determine the location of ventricular myocardial lesions.[301]

Ventricular Tachycardia: Ventricular tachycardia, both paroxysmal and permanent, has been described in horses.[80,164,166,193,201,296,302-305] The arrhythmia occurs when

Figure 46. Simultaneous ECG and phonocardiogram from a 12-year-old broodmare with hyperlipemia and hypokalemia. Heart rate is 94 bpm. The ECG showed frequent coupling of ectopic beats (second and fourth complexes in the figure) with normal complexes (first and third complexes). The first heart sound in the ectopic cycles is especially intense, while S₂ is diminished. Note the flattening of the T and P waves in the ECG due to the hypokalemia (1.2 mEq/L).

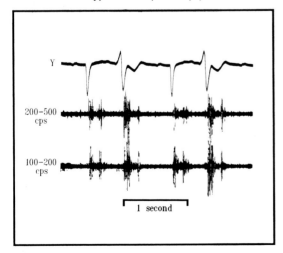

cardiac activity is controlled by an abnormal ventricular focus. QRS complexes are abnormal in conformation unless the ectopic focus is junctional, in which case they may be normal. Regular atrial activity is at a lower rate and independent of ventricular activity; most P waves are obscured by overlying ventricular complexes (Fig 47). The T wave often is quite large and the ST segment short, with the QRS complex blending into the T wave. The heart rate is usually high, often >100 bpm, and the rhythm is regular. Heart sounds are pounding. At high heart rates, the pulse may be weak and cardiac output low. Where the ar-

rhythmia is paroxysmal, the change in heart rate is spontaneous, not gradual. Obvious pulsation may be seen in the jugular groove when the right atrium contracts during ventricular systole. Very high heart rates may be associated with episodes of syncope and respiratory distress; persistence of the problem can lead to myocardial failure.[201] The arrhythmia may be paroxysmal or constant, and may coexist intermittently with AV dissociation and PVC.

Parasystole and AV Dissociation: The existence of 2 pacemakers, sinus and ectopic, creates the circumstances for parasystole and AV dissociation.[18] The nature of the re-

Figure 47. Ventricular tachycardia in a 13-year-old Quarter Horse stallion used for trail riding. The horse had a history of colic, though no signs of abdominal pain were observed during 5 days of hospitalization. The horse repeatedly lapsed into ventricular tachycardia with a ventricular rate of 100 bpm. Capture beats (arrows) are evident, while at the start of the second strip the sinus node recaptured normal rhythm for 2 beats. Serum biochemistry assays revealed marginally low serum potassium levels and significantly elevated muscle enzymes. (Courtesy of Dr. F.D. Horney)

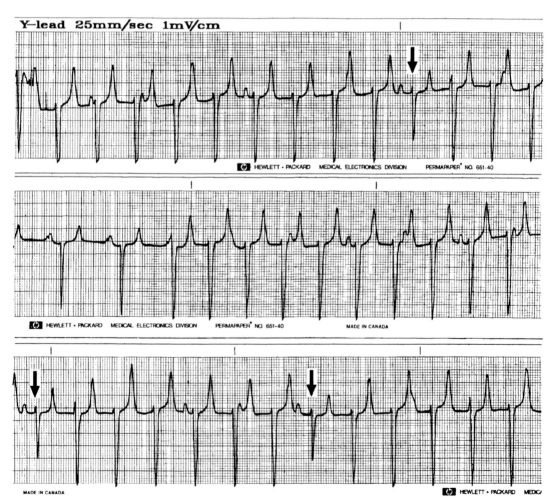

sultant arrhythmia depends upon the relative rates of these pacemakers and interaction between sinus and ectopic signals. In parasystole, the ectopic focus discharges at constant rate and can take over cardiac rhythm. The ectopic focus is protected from the effects of the sinus signal by a phenomenon known as entry block, so that a sinus signal does not influence the inherent rhythmicity or rate of ectopic discharge. During periods of parasystolic rhythm, all cardiac cycles are determined by the ectopic focus and the rhythm is regular. Periodically, the sinus pacemaker regains predominance and a "capture" beat occurs (Fig 48). Under these conditions, activity of the ectopic pacemaker is subjected to exit block but is not reset. It thus subsequently recaptures heart rhythm, with the interval since its last firing being a simple multiple of the inherent rate exhibited by the ectopic before

the sinus capture beats (see second strip, Fig 48).

Criteria for the arrhythmia are a varying coupling interval between sinus and ectopic signals. The constant shortest interval between sequential pairs of ectopics and the interval between any 2 successive pair of ectopics always are a simple multiple of the shortest interval. Additionally, fusion beats are frequent (Fig 48).

AV dissociation is not an electrocardiographic diagnosis and simply describes a circumstance under which the atria and ventricles beat independently (Fig 49). Parasystole, ventricular tachycardia and third-degree block are all dissociative arrhythmias. However, third-degree block is a term reserved for an arrhythmia in which the ventricular rate is lower than the atrial rate, usually very slow. In all other cases, the atrial and ventricular rates are close or

Figure 48. Parasystolic rhythm in a 5-year-old Quarter Horse gelding. The history was vague but suggested unaccustomed exercise 2 days before presentation. The horse showed signs of cardiovascular insufficiency. The serum potassium level was depressed at 1.6 mEq/L. Ventricular tachycardia was diagnosed upon collection of an ECG. This arrhythmia responded to intravenous lidocaine but the horse later developed a persistent parasystolic rhythm. The animal died suddenly and at necropsy had numerous chronic and acute infarcts in the left ventricle. In the top ECG strip, the ectopic focus has captured the rhythm except for a single capture beat (arrow). In the lower strip there are numerous fusion beats (first 2 marked by arrows), in which the ventricles are simultaneously depolarized by both a supraventricular or junctional signal and by firing of the parasystolic focus. The fifth complex in the lower strip (dot in lower margin) is of a different conformation and out of sequence, and may reflect an additional (non-parasystolic?) focus of excitation. All other ectopic signals have a constant frequency of 94/minute. (Courtesy of Dr. T.E. Blackwell)

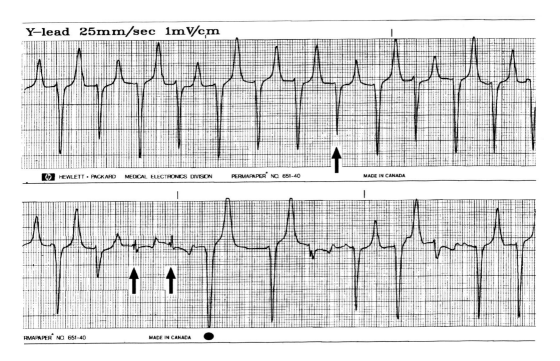

the ventricular rate is faster. The circumstance can be caused by a number of abnormalities of impulse conduction, such as a slow sinus rate together with a focus of ventricular excitation.

An ECG shows complete dissociation if the ectopic pacemaker fully controls ventricular rhythm, and incomplete dissociation if capture beats are present. The terms "ventricular tachycardia" and "parasystole" can be used if the criteria for these arrhythmias are met. Unfortunately, adequate criteria for these rhythm disturbances in horses are somewhat elusive and the reader justifiably may be confused. At present, therefore, it may be advisable to describe the ECG features of ventricular tachyarrhythmias without attempting to put specific labels on them.

Dissociative arrhythmias indicate probable myocardial distress or disease. If untreated, they can lead to ventricular tachycardia and/or fibrillation. However, horses appear to have a remarkable ability to tolerate AV dissociation, which may occur spontaneously and without obvious prodromal signs or evidence of homeostatic disorder in apparently normal animals. Cardiac rhythm often is irregular and rhythm disturbances almost invariably are associated with tachycardia. Heart sounds vary in intensity according to RR interval, with a loud S_1 occurring with short intervals. Syncope is uncommon in contrast to ventricular tachycardia.

Parasystole has been described infrequently in horses.[166,290,298] The clinical impression is that this arrhythmia and dissociative arrhythmias in general occur more frequently in horses than reported. Failure to record the arrhythmia more often may, in part, reflect variation in the application of appropriate ECG criteria.

Ventricular Fibrillation: This arrhythmia may be said to be only of academic interest, as it precedes death by seconds. Its recognition may give the clinician time to take evasive action, however. It is characterized on the ECG by coarse, low-frequency baseline undulations with no recognizable atrial or ventricular complexes. Pulse and cardiac impulse are absent. Little can be done except perhaps when the horse is under anesthesia, when ECG monitoring allows immediate recognition, and venous access and the potential for assisted ventilation may allow immediate management. Electrical defibrillation has been described but is not a practical option under most circumstances.[306]

Figure 49. AV dissociation in a 10-year-old Standardbred mare with acute enteric salmonellosis. Serum sodium, chloride and potassium levels were all depressed. The mare recovered uneventfully. Note the wide, bizarre QRS complexes. Variation in conformation of these waveforms may reflect constant variation in degree of conduction disturbance and/or varying ventricular origin of the focus of excitation. On the second strip there are 2 capture beats, revealing the conformation of the normal QRS (third and fourth ventricular complexes). Locations of atrial complexes are marked by arrows. Atrial rate is 57, ventricular rate (ectopic focus) is 72.

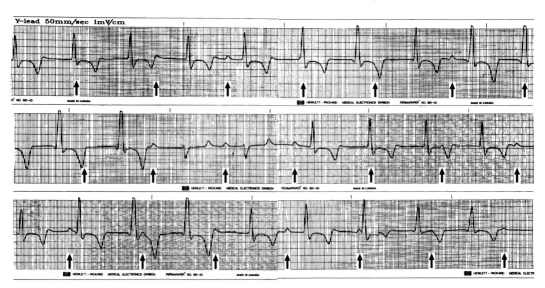

Idioventricular Rhythm: This term applies to any situation in which cardiac rhythm is controlled from within the ventricles, *ie,* by an ectopic pacemaker, and thus is appropriately applied in cases of ventricular tachycardia. However, more common use of the term describes the rhythm of atrial standstill or total AV block. The ventricular rate is low (often 12-16 bpm) and rhythmic; the ectopic pacemaker presumably lies in the intraventricular conducting system. Cases of third-degree block show P waves and unassociated QRS-T complexes of normal or abnormal conformation, whereas in atrial standstill there are no P waves. The rhythm is most commonly seen with third-degree heart block (see above).

Bundle Branch Block: Only 2 rather equivocal reports of the problem in the horse have been published.[18,196,307] The arrhythmia arises when one or more branches of the intraventricular conducting system are interrupted either functionally by, for example, a drug, or structurally by inflammatory or degenerative myocardial disease. As a result, the wave of depolarization is propagated through the myocardium rather than through the conduction system. The obstruction may involve the entire conduction system or only one branch. The general term "bundle branch block" is used to classify the condition, with right bundle branch block and left bundle branch block describing specific obstruction of the right and left bundle branches, respectively.

In most species, this relatively slow myocardial depolarization process and the abnormal pattern by which wavefronts spread result in unusually prolonged and bizarre QRS waveforms.[190,308] Experimental section of the intraventricular conduction system in calves, however, did not lead to obvious changes in QRS conformation, a result attributed to extensive arborization of the Purkinje network in hooved animals.[309,310] On this basis and in view of the normally wide variation in the equine QRS, it has been suggested that bundle branch block may be difficult to diagnose in horses.[18] No experimental studies have been performed in horses to establish ECG criteria for diagnosis of intraventricular block. The true incidence of the arrhythmia is unknown. Were it to occur, ventricular rate and rhythm may be expected to be normal, though asynchrony in contraction in different areas of the ventricular myocardium might be expected to result in some splitting of heart sounds.

Treatment of Arrhythmias

Management of arrhythmias can be addressed from 2 perspectives: general management, including removal of the underlying cause; and specific pharmacologic management.

General Management: Removal of the underlying cause, particularly in the case of ventricular arrhythmias, often is the primary management approach.[171,175] In many cases, this may be all that is required. If the underlying cause is other than organic heart disease (*eg,* electrolyte disorders), the prognosis is excellent. Maintenance of homeostasis is of both general and specific importance as homeostatic disorders and secondary renal dysfunction may be fundamentally involved in genesis of many ventricular arrhythmias and can cause reduced myocardial performance and increased cardiac workload.

Infectious processes may be treated with antimicrobials where appropriate. All cases of inflammation, whether endocardial, myocardial or pericardial, are likely to respond to appropriate antiinflammatory therapy during periods of serious rhythm disturbance. Any arrhythmia that inherently increases myocardial workload should be addressed in part by reducing physical activity, at least until the arrhythmia is under control. This is not only to reduce physical demands on the heart but also to avoid the wide fluctuations in autonomic balance that accompany exercise. As a general rule, active myocardial disease should be allowed at least 60 days for repair *after all signs of active disease have subsided.* Serum enzyme profiles are of limited value in detecting active myocardial damage and inflammation. Recording an ECG is recommended, though the resting tracing may be normal, and light (very light) exercise may be necessary to uncover an arrhythmia.

If the arrhythmia involves bradycardia with associated syncopal attacks, neither exercise nor its avoidance may have any influence upon progress or prognosis. Serious thought should be given to the advisability of retaining such an animal. Installation of a pacemaker may be an option (see above under Third-Degree Heart Block).

Pharmacologic Management: For organic heart disease, drug therapy may be necessary to stabilize cardiac function and reduce myocardial workload, especially in acute cases. The approach taken depends upon factors such as whether the problem is acute or chronic and the nature of the arrhythmia, but the criteria that should be used to define the need for specific drugs are difficult to determine. In general, specific antiarrhythmic therapy should be instituted with ventricular tachyarrhythmia, a resting heart rate above 90-100 bpm, arrhythmia causing significant reduction in cardiac output or syncopal attacks, or a chance for secondary myocardial failure. Myocardial failure is of concern particularly when the heart rate is very high or the rhythm very irregular, with frequent pulse deficits.

Though the most frequently treated arrhythmia in horses is atrial fibrillation, disturbances of ventricular rhythm generally are treated more often by drug therapy than atrial arrhythmias by virtue of frequent association with active myocardial inflammation or degeneration and/or serious electrolyte disorder.[174,175,201,311] However, antiarrhythmic agents in ventricular arrhythmias may be only of temporary value if the underlying cause cannot be removed.

There is a tendency to assume that horses have sufficient cardiovascular reserve to tolerate an episode of tachyarrhythmia; however, acute cases can progress to ventricular fibrillation or result in permanent myocardial damage. At the same time, the expense involved in specific treatment (and constant monitoring) and the potential for an adverse reaction call for caution in using drug therapy. The compromise often adopted is to treat conservatively if the problem is not immediately life threatening. If the arrhythmia is life threatening and permanent myocardial damage is a probable consequence, drug therapy should be instituted.

With the exception of atrial fibrillation, the literature offers only limited guidance in the acute and long-term pharmacologic management of arrhythmias in horses (Table 3).[174,175,176] This may reflect limited experience, the cost of drugs (which often are available only in human dosage units) and also practical limitations. In theory, the full range of therapeutic agents used for pharmacologic management of arrhythmias in people and small animals is available. Some agents, especially when given IV (eg, lidocaine by bolus), can cause systemic reactions or syncope, making their use hazardous in horses. In all cases, drug therapy of cardiac arrhythmias requires use of electrocardiography to confirm the accuracy of the diagnosis and, most important, to monitor response.

The beneficial effects of *digoxin* upon disturbances of cardiac rhythm are direct and indirect. The direct effects involve an increase in parasympathetic tone, causing cardiac slowing in the patient exhibiting tachycardia with heart failure, and antagonism of adrenergic effects at the AV node. Also, it has a direct effect upon the AV node, leading to depressed nodal conduction, with a prolongation of the PR interval in both the normal and diseased heart.[313] The indirect effects are improved myocardial perfusion and reduced workload secondary to cardiac slowing with improved renal function as a result of increased cardiac output. These latter benefits only accrue in the diseased heart.

The main application of digoxin in arrhythmias is to treat supraventricular tachyarrhythmias by reducing AV nodal transmission or atrial activity. Digoxin usually does not have any direct effect upon these arrhythmias and is used primarily to decrease cardiac workload and improve output by reducing rate. The potential for improvement in failure-associated arrhythmias should not be disregarded and prior digitalization often is essential if atrial arrhythmias are to be treated in such cases. Finally, digoxin can cause a range of ventricular tachyarrhythmias, especially ventricular extrasystoles, when large doses are used, and also can cause total AV nodal block. Use of digitalis is discussed in the section on Heart Failure later in this chapter (also see Table 7).

Quinidine is the most widely used antiarrhythmic drug in management of cardiac arrhythmias in horses. It is indicated for treatment of supraventricular and ventricular arrhythmias but is used most often for treatment of atrial fibrillation.[260,262,314]

Quinidine reduces myocardial excitability, conduction velocity and contractility, and it prolongs the myocardial refractory period.[313] These effects are primarily responsible for the agent's antiarrhythmic properties in the case of reentrant arrhythmias and those associated with abnormal automaticity. These direct effects upon the myocardium are accompanied by a vagal blocking action and by some indirect (secondary to fall in blood pressure) elevation in sympathetic activity. The overall circulatory consequences are a fall in blood pressure after oral or intravenous administration and decreased cardiac output after intravenous administration.[174]

Early in therapy, the heart rate may fall slightly but it subsequently rises. Tachycardia is a typical response to the drug and also one of its toxic manifestations (see below). The depressant effect of quinidine upon myocardial contractility and cardiac output may be counteracted by its alpha-adrenergic blocking action, leading to relaxation of vascular smooth muscle and reduction in peripheral resistance.[313]

The pharmacokinetics of quinidine in horses have been investigated.[262] Its biological half-life after intravenous administration is 6.7 hours. An oral dose of 10 g is 50% absorbed by 2 hours, with a peak plasma concentration of about 1.5 μg/ml. An oral

dosage of 20 mg/kg every 2 hours to a total dose of 60 g (or less if toxicity occurs) has been recommended (Table 3).[174] Higher dosages are frequently used in horses with atrial fibrillation to achieve cardioversion. It has been suggested that quinidine is contraindicated in heart failure.[163] In horses, quinidine generally is administered PO as quinidine sulfate, though quinidine gluconate or dihydroquinidine gluconate have been given IV to correct atrial fibrillation.[265,266,268] Intravenous therapy requires close monitoring because of the potential for rapid onset of toxic signs and life-threatening arrhythmias; nonetheless, it sometimes is necessary, as the clinical response to the safer oral dosing is relatively slow.

Toxic effects of quinidine in horses vary widely.[163,174,252] Depression, increased frequency of defecation and a reduction in appetite are typical. Nasal congestion also is quite common and appears to be dose related. Other toxic manifestations are colic, diarrhea, convulsions, laminitis, syncope and sudden death.[18,156,252] Frequent dosing and consequent high plasma levels sometimes are associated with excitement, disorientation and unsteadiness, and occasionally convulsions. In people, these signs are known as cinchonism.[313] Ideally, treatment is stopped well before this point. During treatment, the ECG may be monitored

Table 3. General dosage recommendations for antiarrhythmic agents.

Drug	Route	Dosage	Reference
Propanolol	IV	0.22 mg/kg, bolus[a]	312
	IV	0.1-0.3 mg/kg BID	174
	IV	Days 1&2: 25-mg bolus BID; days 3&4: 50-mg bolus BID; days 5&6: 75-mg bolus BID	176
	PO	Days 1&2: 175-mg bolus TID; days 3&4: 275-mg bolus TID; days 5&6: 350-mg bolus TID	176
Quinidine	IV	0.5-1.0 mg/kg to 2 g total dose[a]	312
	IV	0.5 mg/kg every 10 min to 4-6 mg/kg total dose	174
	PO[b]	20 mg/kg every 2 hours to 60 g total dose	174
	PO	22 mg/kg every 2 hours to 80 g total dose	176
Procainamide	IV	0.25-0.75 mg/kg/min, diluted, as drip[a]	312
	IV	0.5 mg/kg every 10 min to 4-6 mg/kg total dose	174
Lidocaine	IV	1-2 mg/kg as bolus, repeat dose or drip as necessary[a]	312
	IV	0.5 mg/kg at 5-min intervals to 2-4 mg/kg total dose	174
	IV	1.0-1.5 mg/kg as bolus	176

a – Dosage regimens recommended for use in anesthetized horses.
b – See discussion of treatment of atrial fibrillation.

for signs of toxicity, including an increase in QRS duration by more than 25% over resting level, ST segment changes and tachycardia. The true value of these changes in detecting impending toxicity in horses has not been evaluated.

Progressive increase in heart rate is a consistent finding as therapy progresses and may become of concern, especially if there was initial tachycardia, as in heart failure. I set an arbitrary limit of 80 bpm as the ceiling when converting uncomplicated cases of atrial fibrillation. Serum levels can vary greatly from horse to horse with identical dosage regimens. To avoid toxic effects, serum quinidine levels should be monitored if possible to keep them within the therapeutic range of 2-4 μg/ml (6.16-12.32 μmol/L).[174]

Idiosyncratic reactions have occurred in horses, including collapse, urticaria, hyperesthesia, colic and ventricular tachycardia.[163,313] The ever-present potential for this sort of reaction underlies the recommendation that an oral test dose of 5 g be given when possible to evaluate the response before initiating definitive therapy.[18,175,314] However, with the possible exception of urticaria, the range of reactions described as idiosyncratic is essentially the same as that observed with excessively high blood quinidine levels; the difference is that the idiosyncratic reaction occurs very early in treatment, before high blood levels have been achieved. While reactions to a test dose are uncommon, mild side effects, such as nasal congestion, depression and increased frequency of defecation, may be seen early in treatment. If these signs are mild, treatment may be cautiously continued.

In horses exhibiting cardiac arrhythmias with signs of circulatory insufficiency, quinidine should be used with the greatest caution or perhaps not at all, in that its myocardial depressant effects may precipitate overt failure and severe respiratory embarrassment. Prior digitalization may reduce the chances of this complication, though quinidine can raise plasma digoxin concentration and precipitate signs of digitalis toxicity in animals with marginally high plasma digoxin levels. Special caution thus should be employed when using quinidine in digitalized animals, particularly if the arrhythmia being treated could itself be the result of digoxin toxicity (see Atrial Fibrilla-

tion). Acute quinidine toxicity can be treated with IV sodium bicarbonate (0.5-1.0 mEq/kg body weight) to increase plasma binding.[174]

Procainamide is an antiarrhythmic drug with effects very similar to those of quinidine, though it appears to be more effective in ventricular than supraventricular arrhythmias. Suggested dosages for horses are presented in Table 3. Though procainamide occasionally may be of value in initial management of serious arrhythmias, it appears to be of limited practical use in horses. Generally, it is available only in dosage units intended for people. High plasma levels are difficult to achieve in horses.[175] Effective concentrations in tissue preparations are about 10 times as high as equally active concentrations of quinidine.[313] Intravenous administration may be accompanied by a fall in blood pressure though, in people, cardiac contractility and cardiac output are not depressed as much as with quinidine at equivalent therapeutic dosages.

Propanolol is a beta-adrenergic blocking agent with some quinidine-like actions at high dosages. Most of the drug's antiarrhythmic properties are attributed to the first action. Because clinical response depends on the prevailing sympathetic tone at the time of administration and the role played by that tone in the arrhythmia being treated, response to the drug is somewhat unpredictable.[313] Increased refractoriness of the AV node develops regardless of underlying sympathetic tone.[315] The principal use of the agent is in slowing ventricular rate in supraventricular arrhythmia, an effect probably achieved by reduction in sinus rate and by beta1-adrenergic blockade of the AV node.[313] Though use of propanolol to control ventricular extrasystoles and tachyarrhythmias has been suggested, this may not be the agent of choice.[175,176190,313]

Suggested dosages for propanolol in horses are presented in Table 3. Oral bioavailability appears to be low as a consequence of hepatic metabolism. Intravenous administration is the route of choice. The initial intravenous dose should not exceed 0.1 mg/kg and should be administered slowly over 1 minute to reduce the chances of bradycardia, hypotension and muscle weakness in horses with heart disease and high resting sympathetic tone.[174] Pharmacokinetics suggest that therapeutic plasma levels are maintained by TID or QID use, though an adequate antiarrhythmic effect may be achieved with an IV dosage of 0.1-0.3 mg/kg given BID.[174,316]

Toxic effects of propanolol relate principally to excessive beta-adrenergic blockade and reduced cardiac contractility. The negative inotropic effect makes the drug of limited value in heart failure. It should not be given to horses with evidence of heart block, as total block may result. Bradycardia, hypotension, muscle weakness and depression are the most common toxic side effects.[174] Dopamine or dobutamine by slow IV infusion (0.5-3.0 μg/kg/minute) are recommended to treat overdosage. Intravenous atropine (0.45 mg/kg) has been suggested to counteract excessive ventricular slowing or AV block.[176]

Overall, propanolol appears to be of limited value in management of arrhythmias in horses. It might be used diagnostically to evaluate the role played by sympathetic tone in an arrhythmia or to reduce ventricular rate in supraventricular tachycardia if digitalis or quinidine has been unsuccessful.

Lidocaine, primarily a local anesthetic, often is used in people in emergency control of life-threatening ventricular arrhythmias, particularly in cases of myocardial infarction.[190] It is given as an IV bolus during initial management and by slow IV drip in later management. The antiarrhythmic effect of the drug disappears very rapidly after administration is stopped, usually within 10-20 minutes.[313]

Because of limited side effects and a short duration of action that allows the clinical effect to be carefully titrated, lidocaine is regarded as a relatively safe antiarrhythmic agent in people and can be used in a similar manner in the horse, particularly during anesthesia.[176] However, convulsions after IV bolus administration are not uncommon in horses and thus limit usefulness of the drug. If the agent must be used in a life-or-death situation, adequate precautions should be taken to avoid injury to personnel or the horse. Chances of an adverse reaction can be minimized by giving the maximum dosage of 2-4 mg/kg in aliquots of 0.5 mg/kg every 5 minutes.[174] Convulsive episodes are generally of limited duration but are nonetheless dangerous. *Never use the preparation of lidocaine that contains epinephrine.* Because lidocaine has no effect upon supraventricular arrhythmias, its use as a diagnostic agent to differentiate between supraventricular and ventricular arrhythmias in the absence of an ECG has been suggested;[176] a more vigorous search for an ECG may be a safer approach.

Atropine and glycopyrrolate have been suggested for management of bradyarrhythmias in horses, though such parasympatholytic agents may be more useful diagnostically in the evaluation of heart block.[174,176] Vagally induced bradycardias respond to these agents, whereas idioventricular rhythms in third-degree heart block do not. Such drugs may cause gastrointestinal disturbances in horses and therefore are of little or no therapeutic value.

I have used slow IV infusion of *potassium* (as potassium chloride) to control ventricular arrhythmias, often with good results, though the sometimes slow response to this treatment makes it difficult to determine whether the response was due to a direct effect of the ion, an indirect effect on homeostasis and electrolyte levels in general, or a natural progression of the case. Its use is particularly appropriate in ventricular arrhythmias caused by digoxin toxicity.[190] Potassium alters conduction in reentrant arrhythmias or eliminates slow (phase-four) depolarization in ectopic foci.[317]

Administration of potassium should be at a maximum rate of 0.5 mEq/kg/hour. The infusion rate can be adjusted according to electrolyte status, clinical response and seriousness of the arrhythmia. If a total body potassium deficit is contributing to the arrhythmia, an isotonic potassium chloride solution is given with an equal volume of isotonic dextrose to encourage movement of the ion into cells. Simultaneous administration of insulin is not necessary. If the potassium status is normal, potassium chloride may simply be added to the balanced electrolyte solution being administered for hydration. Ideally, dehydration and acid-base disturbances are corrected first and normal renal function established.

Intravenous infusion of potassium involves some risks, including inducing AV block, and atrial, then ventricular, standstill. ECG monitoring can be used to detect toxicity, with obvious prolongation of the QRS and disappearance of the P wave indicating the need to halt therapy immediately. Earlier signs include slight peaking of the T wave, prolongation of the PR interval and depression of the ST segment. The objective in use of potassium to control arrhythmias is to raise serum potassium levels. However, because the ion is potentially toxic, serum levels should be monitored during therapy and care taken to ensure that the patient is not hyperkalemic to begin with.

Syncope and Sudden Death

Syncope is a clinical syndrome in which there is temporary loss of blood supply to the cerebrum, resulting in collapse or fainting. Episodes of collapse are uncommon in horses but, because of the size of the animal, the potential association with work, and the resulting danger to the rider, they tend to attract much attention. The frequency with which the heart is primarily involved in episodes of collapse, *ie,* the frequency with which such events are actually syncopal attacks, is undetermined. Most lay people seem to assume that an affected horse has had some sort of "heart attack," though true heart attacks (massive infarction in people) are very rare because horses do not have significant disease of the major branches of the coronary arteries.[116]

The cause of syncope can be cardiac or extracardiac; arrhythmia is probably the major cardiac cause in horses. It may be associated with bradycardia (*eg,* third-degree heart block) or paroxysmal ventricular tachyarrhythmias, though the latter are an infrequent cause of collapse.[190,232,234,242,243] Other cardiac causes, such as tetralogy of Fallot (see below) or pulmonic stenosis, are very uncommon. Syncope may occur with heart failure and pericarditis.[318]

Extracardiac causes involve the cardiovascular system either indirectly or not at all. Specific obstruction to cerebral blood flow may conceivably result from space-occupying lesions; certain neurologic diseases could lead to marked changes in autonomic tone, causing profound bradycardia. Cerebral dysfunction, either due to primary neurologic disease (*eg,* increased intracranial pressure) or secondary to metabolic disturbances (*eg,* hypoglycemia in the neonate) may also be associated with syncopal attacks. These conditions are discussed elsewhere in this text. Seizures and narcolepsy are some of the other disorders to be considered in acute collapse; acute collapse is covered in the chapters on Common Presenting Complaints and Diseases of the Nervous System.

The relative frequency with which these clinical entities occur in syncope in horses is unknown. In foals with severe respiratory or congenital heart disease, collapse may occur during restraint, exercise or excitement.[319,320] In such cases, hypoxia is probably the primary factor. Even minimal reduction in flow of blood to the cerebrum can be sufficient to induce unconsciousness. In animals exhibiting signs of heart failure, marginal cardiac output is likely the immediate cause. In a 13-year-old Quarter Horse stallion with a moderately large ventricular septal defect, incipient failure and atrial fibrillation, syncopal episodes could be induced by excitement, such as by making the horse wait to go out to pasture. However, in many cases, especially in otherwise healthy working adults, it is not possible to replicate the circumstances that led to a particular episode.

Many so-called syncopal attacks in horses probably are, in fact, stumbling when the animal lands badly after a jump or experiences spasmodic pain from a musculoskeletal problem. The history frequently indicates that the horse began to get up immediately after it had gone down or that it only went down onto its knees. Though subject to some variability, horses experiencing syncopal attacks usually go down completely and are slightly groggy or unsteady for a moment before rising; some may stay down for several minutes.

Nonetheless, every case must be investigated for predisposition to paroxysmal bradyarrhythmia or tachyarrhythmia. The examination ideally should include detailed cardiovascular and neurologic examination, evaluation of cardiac rhythm at exercise and, if available, 24-hour rhythm monitoring. The client should be warned that negative findings do not rule out the possibility of arrhythmia, and also that critical evaluation of the episodes and immediate clinical examination may help determine a cause.

Sudden death might be said to differ from syncope only in that the horse did not get up again, whereas a syncopal attack is, by definition, temporary. Similarly, sudden death may be the result of cardiovascular or noncardiovascular causes. Cardiovascular causes of sudden and unexpected death are numerous, ranging from rupture of coronary vessels to rupture of the heart, through the atria or a ventricle.[18,161,321-331] Rupture of the aorta has been described on numerous occasions, particularly in stallions, as has rupture of the pulmonary artery and vena cava.[332-335] Fatal internal hemorrhage late in gestation or after parturition also has been described, as have myocarditis and coronary occlusion with thrombi secondary to parasitic aortitis.[321,334-338]

The relative and absolute incidence of cardiovascular catastrophes, as opposed to other causes of sudden death, has received limited attention.[321,322,339] In a review of 69 cases that included racehorses, broodmares and foals, 32% had cardiovascular lesions as the cause or contributing to the cause of death.[321] Lesions were internal hemorrhage (10), endocarditis (4), parasite-associated obstruction of the coronary arteries (3), heart valve lesions or myocardial failure (2 each) and polyarteritis (1). Death occurred during or immediately after exercise in 19 of 24 horses in which demise was witnessed, with cardiovascular causes identified in 10. Four cases of internal hemorrhage appeared to be caused by external trauma. In 9, no lesions were found. All of these horses were undergoing exercise or were under some form of physical or emotional stress at the time of death. In all the remaining cases in which death was not observed and in which the horses were presumably at rest, the diagnosis was made at necropsy. The hypothesis that horses in which lesions were absent may have had spontaneous, fatal arrhythmia or abnormalities of the conduction system is unproven.[161,321]

In another study of 25 horses dying suddenly at racetracks, 84% died while racing or training.[322] Lesions thought to cause death were found in only 8, 6 of which were fatal hemorrhage. It was postulated that most of the unexplained deaths were due to exercise-induced acute cardiovascular failure. This interpretation was based in part upon the frequent observation of pulmonary edema, congestion and/or hemorrhage. In many of the cases of hemorrhage in this and the previously cited study, the site could not be identified. In 11 Thoroughbreds that died during racing or training, severe pulmonary hemorrhage occurred in 9 but there was no detectable cardiac involvement.[339] The authors concluded that the cause was exercise-associated pulmonary hemorrhage possibly associated with chronic airway disease. Epistaxis at the time of death was evident in only 4 horses.

Cardiovascular disease can cause sudden death, but the absence of lesions in many cases leaves open the possibility of cardiac arrhythmias or conduction disturbances as the cause. Pulmonary hemorrhage could be of capillary origin or arise from larger pulmonary or bronchial vessels and may reflect primary respiratory disease or acute onset of cardiac insufficiency induced by arrhythmias. The low incidence of chronic cardiac lesions (valvular abnormalities, myocardial fibrosis) implies that these might not be predisposing causes to sudden death in performance horses. However, histopathologic investigations suggest that we have much to learn about the relationship between myocardial lesions and clinical cardiac disease in horses.[228,340] Very thorough postmortem examination of the heart is necessary to eliminate myocardial causes.

Lameness Induced by Vascular Disease

The arterial tree is characterized in many tissues by extensive anastomoses, the degree of which increases as the microcirculation is approached, and in other tissues by the presence of end-arteries that alone supply an area of tissue.[38] Arteries responsible for supplying skeletal muscle generally show significant anastomoses, even of larger branches, though tissue necrosis can still result where obstruction of a large artery occurs rapidly. However, in most clinical cases of lameness associated with arterial disease, obstruction has developed over a period of days to months, and blood supply rarely is totally absent in affected areas because collateral supply has developed in response to demand. Clinical episodes in most cases of lameness secondary to vascular obstruction do not appear to be associated with any tissue breakdown; thus elevation in muscle enzyme activities in serum is not seen (see discussion of Aortic-Iliac Thrombosis).

Only about 25% of the normal flow capacity of an artery supplying muscle is used to meet resting requirements;[341] the remainder is a reserve to meet the demands of intense exercise. In contrast, the flow capacity of collateral vessels in vascular obstruction is only adequate to support resting requirements and a limited amount of exercise, and can rarely fully replace the normal artery. Collateral channels are not new vascular channels but represent greatly augmented flow through existing conduits.[341] Obstruction of small arteries may have little or no clinical effect because extensive local anastomoses may provide several functionally equivalent pathways for blood flow to reach the tissues, while the volume of affected muscle is small.

The larger the vessel that is obstructed, however, the less the chance that an equivalent route will be available, and blood must thus reach the tissue via numerous smaller vessels that typically have a longer and very tortuous course, leading to an attenuated and prolonged pulse wave. Collateral vessels thus have a characteristic coiled or "curly" appearance on an angiogram. The flow is relatively inefficient and only replaces a portion of the lost capacity. Nonetheless, in cases of even total obstruction of the caudal aorta, if obstruction develops slowly, collateral flow may be adequate to support resting function and even moderate exercise.[342] The most commonly described example of lameness associated with vascular disease in horses is aortoiliac thrombosis.[115,342] When demands exceed the flow capacity of collateral vessels, affected muscles must function anaerobically, and accumulation of tissue metabolites leads to rapid fatigue and lameness.

The primary stimulus to development and maintenance of collateral flow is a consistent pressure gradient. Arteries distal to an obstruction remain patent as long as they can still participate in the local anastomotic network. However, they have lost their direct connection to larger arteries and must thus be perfused by adjacent vessels. Blood flows down the steepest pressure gradient, while the vascular bed previously supplied by the obstructed vessel represents an area of relatively low pressure. Flow thus reverses in some components of the vascular network adjacent to the obstructed area and perfusion is achieved. Flow also may reverse in large muscular arteries if an anastomotic branch is available below the area of obstruction. The efficiency of this system depends in part upon the level at which obstruction is present and thus the size of the collateral vessels and, as indicated above, in part upon the length and complexity of the collateral pathway. Flow capacity also is affected by the strength of the stimulus, *ie,* by exercise. Thus, regular exercise (within the horse's limits of tolerance) appears to promote adequate collateral flow, whereas total rest can reduce it. This can occur in a matter of days.

Alterations in Blood Pressure

Alteration in blood pressure is likely to occur in a wide range of systemic disorders, but pressure monitoring is not often done in horses. Measurement is undertaken in the intensive care units of most large equine establishments and has become a routine intraoperative procedure, but this is rarely applied during general clinical or even detailed examination of the cardiovascular system. Routine clinical application of blood pressure measurement may reveal such entities as a tendency toward hypotension in some cases of recurrent syncope. However, syndromes of hypertension or hypotension as seen in people are not recognized in horses, with the notable exception of the hypertension seen in laminitis.

Congenital Heart Disease

The adverse effects of congenital heart disease principally involve 2 consequences. The first involves the hemodynamic results of blood being shunted along abnormal channels, often the result of obstruction to normal flow patterns. The other involves the arterial hypoxemia that results if shunting is from right to left; this occurs most often with complex cardiac disease. Therapeutic options are limited and, in terms of assessing prognosis and providing the client with guidance, the most important diagnostic objectives are to determine whether the defect is likely *simple or complex* and whether there is *arterial hypoxemia*.

Specific congenital abnormalities are discussed later in this chapter. Table 4 summarizes congenital cardiovascular abnormalities seen in horses. The objective here is to provide an overview that may aid the clinician in assigning priority to diagnostic possibilities. There are no firm criteria for interpreting clinical findings, as subtle variations can occur in congenital heart disease, while signs can be modified by growth and intercurrent disease. Thus, the situation can be dynamic.

Identifying a congenital anomaly depends upon age of the animal at examination and signs observed. Simple congenital *abnormalities of the atrioventricular valves* occur with unknown frequency and have the same functional consequences in most cases as other causes of AV insufficiency. Confirming their congenital nature, antemortem may be difficult unless they are detected shortly after birth. *Atrial septal defects* and *persistent foramen ovale* are diagnosed infrequently. When present, they are most often 1 component of a complex defect. As isolated anomalies, they are asymptomatic in neonates unless very large. *Patent ductus arteriosus* can be symptomatic and associated with an obvious, continuous murmur but in fact occurs as a singular lesion infrequently in horses.

Isolated *ventricular septal defect* is the only simple and consequential congenital cardiovascular anomaly diagnosed with any frequency and is in fact the most common congenital anomaly (Table 4, Figs 50, 51). Ventricular septal defect also is frequently one component of complex congenital defects; thus its detection and definition are worth some effort. Understanding of the defect also provides insight into most complex anomalies.

If a simple and relatively small defect in the ventricular septum results in left-to-right shunting, there is mild overcirculation of the lungs and an increased load, primarily on the left ventricle, while direct pressure effects on the right heart may be minimal. Over time, pulmonary hypertension can develop because of the pulmonary overcirculation, leading eventually to a halt and then reversal of the shunt, at which point a horse not worked regularly may first start to show signs. This reversal of flow occurs only infrequently and, even then, only in the presence of large defects. Most horses with simple ventricular septal defect remain asymptomatic and can perform mild to moderate work. Coexisting respiratory disease may predispose to reversal. In performance horses, impact varies, but maximal rate of working is generally limited.

In complex defects, there often is obstruction, functional or structural, to outflow from the right heart. In the case of tetralogy of Fallot with moderate to marked pulmonic stenosis, the right ventricle retains its fetal dominance, pressure in the right heart may equal or exceed systemic arterial pressures, and right-to-left shunting across a ventricular septal defect and cyanosis may be present at birth. Where both ventricular chambers are drained by a single vessel (common outlet heart, persistent truncus arteriosus), the right ventricle must compete against systemic pressures to achieve ejection, with resultant severe right ventricular hypertrophy. Total mixing of arterial and venous blood occurs over the septal defect and in the outflow tract immediately distal to the defect. In total transposition of the great vessels, the effect on the right heart is the same but arterial hypoxia is more severe because blood passes from the ventricles and out of the reversed outflow tracts with incomplete mixing. Most of the systemic venous return thus passes out of the aorta, bypassing the lungs.

All of these defects are associated with loud murmurs and some degree of hypoxemia. The ventricular septal defect, which is almost invariably present, usually represents both the source of much of the flow disturbance causing the murmur and the level at which shunting is occurring. Exercise intolerance is common. Respiratory distress is common and reflected as cyanosis with severe right-to-left shunting and, in some cases, overcirculation of the lungs and congestion. These signs may progress due to inability of the compromised heart to meet the needs of the increasing body mass or the onset of heart failure. Foals with congenital heart disease may appear to grow well initially. Animals surviving into adulthood may show chronically poor condition.

While definitive diagnosis of complex congenital cardiac disease often is only made at necropsy, a simple ventricular septal defect and probable complex cardiac disease can be clinically differentiated in many cases, allowing the client the opportunity to make appropriate management decisions. In most cases of simple ventricular septal defect, the defect is located towards the "right-hand end" of the septum, somewhere beneath the septal cusp of the right AV valve (membranous defect), and occasionally more ventral in the septum, toward the apex (apical defect, Figs 50, 51). The resultant murmur is harsh, noisy, band shaped and loudest on the *right* side of the thorax,

Table 4. Congenital cardiac abnormalities in horses.

Abnormality	Clinical Signs	Reference
Simple Vascular Anomalies		
Associated with a Murmur		
Persistent ductus arteriosus (5 cases)	Continuous murmur (occasionally diastolic or systolic only), loud S_2, congestive heart failure	356, 417-420
Murmur Infrequent or Absent		
Persistent right aortic arch (3 cases)	Esophageal obstruction, regurgitation, inhalation pneumonia; possibly subclinical	411, 421, 423
Aortic coarctation (1 case)	Variable; possibly subclinical or hypertensive, congestive heart failure	432
Interruption of aortic arch (2 cases)	Exercise intolerance, tachycardia, differential cyanosis	364
Complex Vascular Anomalies		
Anomalies of the Origin of the Great Vessels		
Tetralogy of Fallot (high VSD, overriding or dextrorotated aorta, RV hypertrophy, pulmonic stenosis) (4 cases)	Variable; With mild pulmonic stenosis: harsh pansystolic murmur at left heart base, radiating widely, thrill, reduced exercise tolerance, tachycardia With severe pulmonic stenosis: same as above, plus lethargy, dyspnea, cyanosis (especially with exercise), exercise intolerance, poor growth	398, 427, 430, 431
Tetralogy of Fallot with PDA (3 cases)	As for simple tetralogy plus possible diastolic murmur	129, 415, 416
Pulmonary atresia/ pseudotruncus arteriosus (high VSD, dextrorotated aorta, atresia of pulmonic valve and/or artery; RV variable depending upon presence of atrial septal defects) (8 cases)	Harsh, pansystolic or continuous murmur at left heart base, radiating widely, thrill, tachycardia, exercise intolerance with cyanosis, syncopal attacks, dyspnea, poor growth	129, 319, 359, 429, 738
Persistent truncus arteriosus (heart drained by single large vessel, no remnant of other vessel, VSD, biventricular hypertrophy) (8 cases)	Cyanosis, exercise intolerance, dyspnea, harsh widespread machinery murmur, thrill, tachycardia, weakness, poor growth	360, 369, 418, 427, 428, 600
Complex Valvular Anomalies		
Tricuspid atresia (absence of right AV orifice, right ventricular hypoplasia, atrial septal defect, VSD in all cases; right heart outflow obstruction LV and LAV hyperplasia in some cases; PDA in some cases) (13 cases)	Poor growth, lethargy, limited exercise tolerance, cyanosis, harsh,pansystolic murmur at left heart base, occasional diastolic component, tachycardia	129, 320, 362, 368 ,413, 414, 418, 599, 600, 601, 602

Table 4 continued.

Abnormality	Clinical Signs	Reference
Simple Myocardial Anomalies		
With Murmurs		
Ventricular septal defect (39 cases)	Left-to-right shunt Membraneous: pansystolic murmur, point of maximum intensity cranial on right, may radiate ventrally Infundibular: pansystolic murmur loudest cranially on both sides, occasionally distinct point of maximum intensity at left heart base Apical: pansystolic murmurloudest toward apex on right side	18 ,36, 156, 159, 357, 361, 426, 430, 530, 592 , 607, 622, 607, 641,643, 644, 739, 740, 741, 742
	Reduced performance capacity, poor-doing, Eisenmenger's syndrome and congestive heart failure with large defects; small defects asymptomatic	
Without Murmurs		
Atrial septal defect and persistent foramen ovale (Ostium primum defect) (Ostium secundum defect) (Persistent foramen ovale)	Usually asymptomatic: large defect may lead to pulmonary hypertension and secondary right heart failure	603,648
Complex Myocardial Anomalies		
Cor triloculare biatriatum (common ventricle) (Two atria and AV valves; single ventricle; pulmonary outflow chamber) (1 case)	Poor growth, exercise intolerance, hypoxia, pansystolic murmur at left heart base, tachycardia	367
Hypoplastic left heart syndrome (1 case)		365
Hypoplastic right heart syndrome (1 case)	Exercise intolerance, dyspnea, cyanosis, harsh widespread pansystolic murmur, tachycardia	603

often well cranially, deep to the triceps and becoming louder as the stethoscope is advanced. On the left side of the thorax, the murmur is quieter and best heard cranially.

Where the defect is located directly beneath the outflow tract valves (infundibular defect, Figs 50, 51), the murmur tends to be loudest on the *left* at the heart base, in that the defect is at the "left-hand end" of the septum. The sound radiates widely, including to the right side. Such left heart base murmurs often acquire a slightly higher pitch and a crescendo-decrescendo contour.

The observation is important because most complex anomalies of the outflow tracts include a ventricular septal defect in this region. A complex congenital anomaly thus is more often a possibility if a shunt-type murmur is identified at the left heart base; the index of suspicion is increased greatly if arterial hypoxemia is also present.

Arterial O_2 tension is easily measured by blood gas analysis. In the absence of respiratory disease, arterial O_2 tension often reflects the nature of the congenital abnormality and can thus be combined with

Figure 50. View of the right side of the heart.[422] The cranial aspect of the right atrium and the right free ventricular wall have been removed to reveal the interior of the right atrium, right AV valve, right side of the interventricular septum and right heart outflow tract and pulmonic valve. Typical locations for ventricular septal defects are marked. These locations do not encompass all possible sites of septal discontinuity, but cover most circumstances.

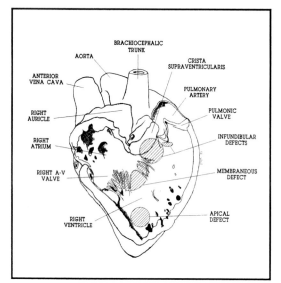

clinical evaluation to narrow the range of diagnostic possibilities. Approximate ranges for arterial oxygen tension in various congenital abnormalities are presented in Table 5. These values should be used for guidance only, in that many factors can influence PaO_2. With respiratory disease, the contribution made by this additional problem to arterial hypoxemia must be assessed and may invalidate the interpretations. Though arterial O_2 tension at normal body temperature is in excess of 100 mm Hg in normal animals, circumstances of collection under hospital conditions often result in values in the range of 85-100 mm Hg. The data presented in Table 5 reflect values obtained from carotid artery samples collected in such a clinical setting.

Blood gas analysis should be employed whenever congenital heart disease is a possibility and not restricted to animals in which a murmur can be detected, as some profound abnormalities (*eg*, total absence of the interventricular septum) may not be detectable upon auscultation. For definitive diagnosis, more involved techniques are necessary, such as echocardiography and cardiac catheterization with angiocardi-

Figure 51. Two views of the left side of the heart. The caudal aspect of the left atrium and left free ventricular wall have been removed. In (A) the septal cusp of the left AV valve is intact. In (B) it and the left atrium have been split to reveal the left ventricular outflow tract and aorta. Typical locations for ventricular septal defects are indicated. Note that, with the exception of the apical defect, most defects open immediately below the aortic valve on the left.

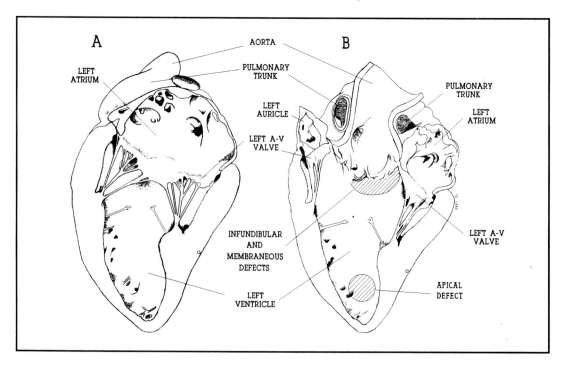

ography, measurement of intracardiac pressures and selective sampling of oxygen tension at different levels in the heart and great vessels.

Rarely is treatment an option in congenital heart disease. Treatment should not be considered until there is clear evidence of the absence of genetic factors. Patient management is optimized by early recognition of the problem, preferably in foalhood, so as to allow appropriate economic decisions to be made by the owner. If complex congenital heart disease is not suggested by initial evaluation, the foal should be given time to mature, as quite bizarre murmurs in neonatal foals can subside.

Cardiovascular Disease and Limitations to Athletic Performance

Horses performing over long distances rely mainly upon aerobic metabolism. A small reduction in their maximum rate of aerobic function has a marked effect on overall performance, especially if their performance for most of the event is close to the so-called anaerobic threshold. In contrast, a sprinter uses predominantly anaerobic metabolism and can tolerate some degree of for example, valvular disease, without obvious deterioration in performance. The average racehorse, which is expected to deliver a maximal or near maximal effort, relies upon both aerobic and anaerobic mechanisms to varying degrees, depending upon the distance of the race. Limitations in aerobic metabolism cause premature use of anaerobic capacity and limit the ability to repay oxygen debt during work. In an endurance or event horse or a field hunter, the complaint is most often described as "tiring," whereas in a racehorse it is described as "lack of finish" or "fading."

Performance implications of cardiac disease also depend upon the class of the animal. The best horses consistently perform much closer to their maximum potential than average animals.[343] A minimal cardiac problem could thus have a significant effect upon racing success in a Standardbred with a record for the mile of 1.54.0 (1 minute, 54 seconds), where the difference between winning and losing may be a matter of a tenth of a second or less. Conversely, mild cardiovascular disease in a horse with average performance may have little or no apparent effect upon race success until the disease has progressed because, at lower levels of athletic competition, the spread of performance standards tends to be relatively wide.

If the horse has had the problem for a long time (*eg*, a damaged valve from a foalhood episode of endocarditis), then it probably always will have performed within its capabilities and a clinical effect will not be seen, despite the fact that the abnormality is limiting maximum cardiac output. If the problem is acquired during the horse's competitive life, performance may deteriorate; however, if the problem is not progressive and the horse is moved down in race class so that it is once again performing within its capabilities, the disorder may become inapparent.

Because of the multiplicity of factors and the difficulty in achieving a definitive diagnosis, the clinician must deal with a great deal of uncertainty when attempting to advise the client. With the exception of some

Table 5. Approximate ranges for arterial PaO2 in congenital heart disease.

Shunt	PaO$_2$	Examples
Mild	55-100 mm Hg	Partial shunting right to left: *eg,* large atrial septal defect, ventricular septal defect or persistent ductus arteriosus with shunt reversal (Eisenmenger's syndrome) secondary to pulmonary hypertension. No cyanosis.
Moderate	34-45 mm Hg	Total mixing or reduced pulmonary artery flow: *eg,* persistent truncus arteriosus, common ventricle, tetralogy of Fallot with mild to moderate pulmonic stenosis +/- PDA, tricuspid atresia. Cyanosis in most cases.
Severe	<30 mm Hg	Reversal of flow or severely reduced pulmonary artery flow: *eg,* total transposition, tetralogy of Fallot with severe pulmonic stenosis, pulmonic atresia. Cyanosis in all cases.

arrhythmias and acute inflammatory myocardial disease, treatment rarely is an option and the case must instead be "managed." In the context of exercise, management usually involves 2 options: campaign the horse so that it can perform within its abilities, recognizing that this will mean competition at a lower level and a limited competitive life, or convert the animal to less demanding use, recognizing the probability that maximal effort could accelerate progression of the problem. In either case, because the problem could eventually lead to syncopal attacks, periodic reexaminations are mandatory.

Heart Failure

Two factors have prevented full appreciation of the significance of heart failure as a syndrome in horses. The first is the fact that a horse in heart failure is of little value except perhaps for its breeding potential if the problem can be stabilized. The second is the infrequency of the syndrome.[116,162,172] This has resulted in a tendency not to recognize the syndrome in its early stages and perhaps to deemphasize the contribution that congenital and acquired diseases can make to cardiovascular dysfunction.[344]

The literature contains many excellent discussions of the mechanisms involved in the systemic syndrome of heart failure.[1,190,256,345,346] Though some of the clinical features differ, the underlying mechanisms appear to be the same for all species studied. This section summarizes the salient features of heart failure in horses.

Definition

Though heart failure is the end result of all progressive cardiac disease, an adequate definition is elusive because there is no clear starting point at which the syndrome is clearly established.[190] In the interests of accurate clinical interpretation and management, a distinction must be made between circulatory failure or insufficiency and heart failure (Table 6). "Circulatory failure" may be defined as a situation in which cardiac output is low in relation to the requirements of the body. While this includes all cases of heart failure, the syndrome need not involve the heart primarily, which may be normal. A horse showing signs as a consequence of a cranial thoracic mass would be a suitable example.

"Heart failure" can then be defined as circulatory failure in which the cause is inadequate pumping by the heart. One major cause is primary *myocardial* failure, such as myocarditis and acute myocardial degeneration.[347,348] The other major cause of heart failure is *mechanical*, as with valvular dysfunction, though the distinction is obscured by the tendency for both factors to be operative, especially in chronic failure.[349,350]

The literature mentions "forward failure," which describes failure of the left heart to maintain adequate peripheral perfusion, and "backward failure," which describes right ventricular dysfunction and systemic congestion/edema.

These terms should be used with caution as failure of either side of the heart has both forward and backward effects. Congestion of the lungs is often a more significant and life-threatening consequence of heart failure than subcutaneous edema. In all cases, both sides are involved to greater or lesser degree. It is, however, useful to speak of left and right heart failure because, in many cases, clinical signs indicate predominant involvement of one chamber of the heart. It

Table 6. Etiologic classification of circulatory failure.[190]

I. Interference with systemic venous return:
  A. Due to factors remote from the heart
    1. Hemorrhage
    2. Peripheral vascular collapse
    3. Shock
  B. Due to factors in the heart region
    1. Pericardial tamponade
    2. Constrictive pericarditis
    3. Tricuspid stenosis

II. Interference with ventricular ejection or filling:
  1. Mitral stenosis
  2. Pulmonic or aortic valve stenosis or insufficiency
  3. Left or right AV valve insufficiency
  4. Pulmonary hypertension
  5. Pulmonary emboli

III. Primary diseases of the myocardium (leading to myocardial failure):
  1. Loss of myocardium (fibrosis, infarction)
  2. Myocarditis
  3. Toxic damage (endotoxemia, ionophore poisoning)
  4. Nonspecific degeneration (cardiomyopathy)

IV. Hyperkinetic states:
  1. Hypervolemia (overzealous IV therapy)
  2. Low peripheral vascular (AV fistula) resistance
  3. Hypoxia, anemia, cor pulmonale
  4. Uncomplicated congenital L-R shunts (PDA, VSD, ASD)

also should be appreciated that "heart failure" is primarily a reference to *ventricular* function.

Cardiac Compensation

Central to an understanding of heart failure is the concept of "compensation," which can be regarded as progressive recruitment of mechanisms that compensate for the effects of functional impairment so as to maintain cardiac output. If the process is successful, the animal achieves *resting* cardiac output, with a normal or even low heart rate. The mechanisms used to compensate for disease are the same as those used to meet the demands of exercise: elevation of heart rate, enhanced contractility, and increased venous return leading to increased filling. Changes in sympathetic nervous activity underlie most of these circulatory adjustments, which include changes in peripheral resistance and redirection of cardiac output.[1] A fourth mechanism, cardiac hypertrophy/hyperplasia, is a delayed response to chronically increased load.[190]

An additional systemic feature of the compensatory response is the retention of salt and water. This expands absolute blood volume. While initially beneficial in terms of promoting increased cardiac output, this contributes significantly to the edema formation that venous hypertension (secondary to increased venomotor tone and reduced myocardial performance) promotes.[1] As an additional compensatory mechanism, the capacity for the heart to recover from an acute insult by tissue repair must not be overlooked, though it is improbable that repair will return the heart to normal functional capacity.

Whether the insult is acute or chronic, successful compensation involves the combined operation of all mechanisms to return the circulatory system to a stable condition. It must be remembered that the system is not normal at this point but is successfully "compensated." As reserve mechanisms are enlisted to meet increased demand, less functional capacity remains available to support increased physical activity; the exercise response may be qualitatively as well as quantitatively compromised. Additionally, a compensated circulatory system does not have the same capacity to respond appropriately to a new insult even if the primary insult has not progressed.

Progression of the primary disorder causes a gradual reduction in reserve, with occasional clinical episodes of failure when the animal is exposed to increased demands through, for example, unaccustomed exercise or stress. The compensatory mechanisms themselves also begin to place an added burden on the heart and to reduce reserve. For example, while fluid retention can, to a limited degree, be beneficial, that benefit is rapidly outstripped by the extra load on the circulatory system that leads to progressive cardiac dilatation, pulmonary congestion, reduced oxygenation and systemic edema.[1] The point is eventually reached at which even the physical demands of daily maintenance become difficult to support. At this point the animal develops overt heart failure or decompensation. One of the clinical features of this stage is an elevated heart rate at rest, which is a very poor prognostic sign.

Because the horse is first and foremost an athlete, a suitable definition of heart failure would be to describe it as the point at which virtually all the reserve functional (pumping) capacity normally used for physical effort above and beyond basal activity has been used, so that the animal walks a narrow path between failure and compensation. A horse thus can have varying degrees of cardiovascular disease and reduced functional capacity. However, such an animal should only be described as being in circulatory failure when it crosses this conceptual "threshold" of exhausted reserve. Such a horse shows obvious limitation of exercise tolerance. On the other hand, an animal that tires because of mild cardiovascular disease is described more accurately as exhibiting signs of *reduced circulatory reserve*.

An investigation of pressures in the pulmonary circulation in horses exhibiting poor performance emphasizes use of hemodynamic and isoenzyme monitoring in cases of suspected cardiac dysfunction.[138] The results from the 21 horses examined showed a pattern of elevation of pressures at rest consistent with a diagnosis of chamber failure, based upon human criteria. These horses had raced poorly within days of the hemodynamic test. Inadequate history and clinical details were provided to determine whether the horses were suffering the effects of recent cardiac insult or how poor their performance was. The concept of failure at rest in an animal still capable of race-intensity exercise, however, emphasizes the difficulties involved in arriving at workable definitions of heart failure.

Whether use of the term "compensation" in cases of reduced circulatory reserve is appropriate is open to question, as a slight reduction in reserve sufficient to reduce maximal rate of working would still leave the animal with a huge reserve, allowing it to perform physical effort at a substantial level. Any "accommodation" such an animal may show to the insult may be brought about by virtue of another component of the oxygen-delivery system taking up the slack, assuming that the horse works frequently at or beyond its maximal rate of aerobic working. For compensatory mechanisms to become active, it is necessary for a circumstance of marginal function to operate for most of the time, which would not be the case for mild problems.

This raises the question of what cardiovascular changes occur in the horse during training. Evidence suggests that increased myocardial mass and chamber size plus increase in blood volume, are appropriate and expected responses to training.[3,743] Such responses mirror closely those of compensation despite evidence of different underlying biochemical mechanisms. The extent to which normal training represents an adequate stimulus for recruitment of compensatory mechanisms in animals with cardiovascular disease requires investigation, in that a compensated system is not normal and may respond inappropriately to excessive workload.

The equine clinician attempting to put functional abnormality of the circulatory system into perspective may be better served by this view of cardiac disease in horses than by the concept of "compensated heart failure" as sometimes used in people.[1] A horse that has progressed far enough with cardiac disease to exhibit obvious exercise intolerance is no longer an athlete. Recognition of a condition of limited exercise tolerance is important because treatment is likely to achieve the best long-term results if started early (see below). It is necessary, therefore, to consider a continuum of clinical signs, from the compromised animal to the patient in overt heart failure or decompensation.

The extent to which a horse might be able to compensate for mild cardiac disease has not been investigated. We have little idea of the actual degree of circulatory impairment associated with different lesions. As noted in the discussion of Exercise Testing earlier in this chapter, the typical absence of objective measurement of reserve before the insult allows only subjective estimates of functional capacity.

Dilatation, Hypertrophy and Hyperplasia

Within limits, increased cardiac filling facilitates a more forceful contraction by increased stretching of myocardial fibers and increased ejection fraction.[1,190] Chronically elevated workload leads to myocardial hypertrophy. The typical response to a pressure overload (outflow tract stenosis, arterial hypertension) is *concentric* hypertrophy, in which the external chamber dimension remains unchanged but myocardial mass increases, leading to some eventual reduction in chamber volume. In a stable situation, cardiac output returns to normal, even in the face of elevated resistance to outflow. Volume overload, as occurs in aortic insufficiency and left AV insufficiency, results in *eccentric* hypertrophy, in which both myocardial mass and chamber volume are increased. In this case, hypertrophy maintains cardiac output at normal levels in the face of an elevated end-diastolic volume. A certain amount of hyperplasia occurs as a pathologic response to chronic cardiac overload.[351,352]

Though these responses are initially beneficial, their progressive development becomes detrimental by virtue of such mechanisms as inadequate coronary blood flow for the increased myocardial mass.[352-354] In the case of severe concentric hypertrophy, reduced filling leads to reduced output. In the decompensated heart, end-systolic and end-diastolic volume progressively increase as the chamber fails, and myocardial stretching exceeds the elastic limit. The chamber thus becomes unable to fully eject all of the blood entering during diastole, and dilatation occurs regardless of the nature of the primary insult.

Acute vs Chronic Failure

Circumstances of acute failure include myocardial failure secondary to hypoxia in severe acute blood loss or respiratory disease, acute myocarditis or toxic myocardial degeneration, cardiac tamponade/pericardial effusion, some cases of severe pleural effusion, and severe acute valve dysfunction, such as rupture of chordae tendineae. In many of these conditions, there either is insufficient time for compensatory mechanisms to offset the extra load or no opportunity for compensation because of the nature or extent of damage.

Acute failure of the left heart is accompanied most often by respiratory signs, including acute pulmonary edema, as the capacitance of the pulmonary venous circulation is inadequate to accommodate the increased volume of blood with which it is presented, especially if right heart function is initially normal. Acute right-sided failure does not lead to rapid onset of subcutaneous edema because of the ability of the systemic venous circulation to accommodate the increased volume as blood shifts to the systemic venous side of the circulation. Subcutaneous edema would only be expected to develop after 3-4 days of circulatory insufficiency in the absence of other factors, such as low serum albumen or loss of capillary integrity. Thus, signs of acute left heart failure are fairly distinct, whereas those of right heart failure may develop more insidiously.

"Chronic" failure refers to a condition in which the primary lesion has been present for weeks to months and numerous episodes of compromised function and compensation have occurred. The term is a misnomer to some degree in that clinical manifestations of decompensation can sometimes be as severe and apparently rapid in onset as in acute cases when ability to compensate is finally exhausted. Evidence of compensation may be apparent clinically.

Finally, the term "exercise-induced acute cardiovascular failure" has been used as a possible explanation for unexplained deaths in horses during training or racing.[322] This interpretation was supported by the frequent observation of pulmonary congestion or edema at necropsy in the absence of other findings. In such a case, the underlying cause may not be apparent, there may be no prodromal signs, and such acute pump failure may have a functional rather than a structural basis, having occurred in an essentially normal heart.

Clinical Associations

Any agent that can damage the heart's ability to function as a pump can be associated with heart failure. Greatly reduced cardiac reserve and overt failure have been associated with congenital heart disease and acquired valvular abnormalities.[129,319, 320,349,350,355-374] Primary myocardial disease has also been associated with signs of failure, as have myocardial disease secondary to bacterial or viral infection, extension of bacterial endocarditis, fungal infection and ionophore intoxication.[328,337,348,375-385] Heart failure also has been associated with dissecting aortic aneurysms and aortic ring rupture.[333,386-388]

Though infrequently reported in the veterinary literature, failure also may occur as a result of severe ventricular tachyarrhythmia.[190] The infrequency of this association in horses may reflect their great circulatory reserve capacity. This should not encourage complacency, however, in that clinical episodes often may not be associated with overt failure but may lead to irreversible myocardial damage and be the immediate cause of death in some presumed cases of acute exercise-associated failure.[321,322] Finally, signs of failure may be associated with chronic respiratory disease in the syndrome known as cor pulmonale.[389,390]

While it has been suggested that diseases of the myocardium are the most frequent causes of heart failure in horses, this cannot be confirmed from literature where congenital cardiac disease and diseases of the left AV valve are described more frequently.[344] However, the possibility that the myocardium is secondarily involved in cases of systemic viral and bacterial disease always should be considered. Critical evaluation in such cases may reveal a greater contribution to the clinical picture by circulatory insufficiency than previously contemplated.

Clinical Signs

In addition to the reports cited under clinical associations above, numerous reports have provided descriptions of heart failure in horses.[320,333,344,362,368,369,378,389-400] Signs may be conveniently divided into left and right failure. Often both are found, but usually one predominates. In both cases, the signs are a consequence of congestion and failure of forward flow.

Failure of the left heart leads to elevated left atrial and pulmonary venous pressure and pulmonary congestion. In early cases, reduced exercise tolerance and a tendency to cough are observed but frank pulmonary edema and signs of right heart failure are improbable. Weight loss or poor condition is observed frequently and can progress to emaciation in chronic cases, the consequence both of poor peripheral circulation and of poor splanchnic blood flow leading to malabsorption (Fig 52). As the condition progresses, weak or imperceptible pulse, cool periphery, pale membranes, anxiety and unsteadiness also are found. Syncopal attacks or episodes of collapse (sometimes incorrectly called "seizures") may occur, particularly upon exertion or where there is an arrhythmia. These are described particularly often in cases of congenital heart disease, especially where cyanosis also is present.[319,320,369,401]

Though advanced cases develop right heart involvement secondary to elevated resistance to flow through the lungs, this complication does not often progress to become clinically evident in horses.[372] The clinician must be aware of the problem, however, especially when managing concurrent respiratory disease or applying fluid therapy.

In acute and in severe cases of chronic left heart failure, pulmonary congestion progresses to pulmonary edema with tachypnea and severe dyspnea. Similar clinical signs have been described in association with arrhythmias, including atrial fibrillation.[250,252] Where edema has been chronically present and uncontrolled, diffuse pulmonary fibrosis causes greatly increased effort on both expiration and inspiration; the clinical picture suggests severe chronic small airway disease. Differentiation may be aided by the fact that horses with chronic left heart failure are unlikely to exhibit expansion of the lung fields. Auscultation may reveal a normal heart rate in early cases but specific signs of heart disease, such as murmurs, arrhythmias and a very prominent cardiac impulse with evidence of cardiomegaly, may be found.

The presence of a gallop rhythm at rest should be taken as strong evidence of cardiac dilatation and/or hypertrophy. Conversely, detection of a prominent third heart sound with a normal rate and no gallop rhythm may be consistent with hypertrophy but also may be normal for the patient. Once the animal has reached decompensation, insufficiency of the AV valves develops and widespread systolic murmurs are detected. The heart may sound like a washing machine. Auscultation at this stage provides little guidance in identifying the underlying cause(s). Paroxysmal coughing, cyanosis and appearance of

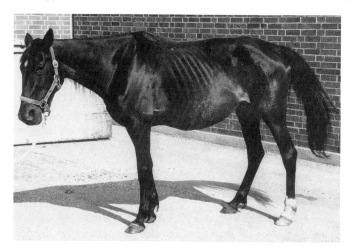

Figure 52. Emaciation (cardiac cachexia) in a 7-year-old Standardbred mare that developed signs of left heart failure secondary to acute onset of left AV insufficiency due to a chordal rupture 2 years before this photograph was taken. The mare died at 8 years of age after successfully foaling twice. At necropsy, 2 old and 1 recent chordal ruptures were found. All involved the right commissural cusps and right papillary muscle.

froth at the nares and mouth are seen in terminal cases. Horses at this stage are in desperate trouble and unlikely to respond to even the most heroic treatment.

Failure of the right ventricle leads to chronic elevation of systemic venous pressure. This is manifested as a tendency to filling of peripheral veins, particularly obvious in the jugular veins. Initially, signs are limited to a tendency for veins and thus pulsation to be particularly obvious at the thoracic inlet, with filling gradually extending up the neck. Except in cases where acute myocardial insult has led to failure, rapid onset of jugular filling to the point the vein is full and nonpulsatile all the way to the angle of the jaw should suggest specific obstruction to venous return, as may occur with intrathoracic masses or rapid development of pericardial effusion, rather than failure of the right ventricle. This degree of jugular filling in right heart failure is uncommon in horses.

Reduced cardiac output in failure (left or right heart) results in reduced renal blood flow and salt and water retention, leading to expansion of total body water. With the added factor of increased systemic venous pressure, decompensation of the right heart is accompanied by congestion manifested as ventral edema, initially in the sternal region and later on the ventral abdomen (Fig 53). Edema of the legs is not a prominent finding in heart failure in horses, while swelling of the hind limbs is a common finding in animals without heart disease. Additionally, heart failure is the least common cause of edema in horses.

The distribution of edema should alert the clinician to the possibility that regional venous hypertension secondary to specific obstruction of venous drainage is the cause, rather than systemic venous hypertension. Ascites, a prominent sign in small animals, is rarely detected clinically in horses because of the naturally high tone of the equine abdominal wall, though increase in fluid in all serous cavities, including the pericardial sac, is present. Hepatomegaly is seen at necropsy but evidence of hepatic dysfunction generally is not detected clinically. Diarrhea occurs in some animals as a result of splanchnic congestion or low blood flow and hypoxic damage.

Circumstances of circulatory failure in which the myocardium is normal and in which failure is due to interference with venous return or cardiac filling may result in some variation in signs. Thus, in cases of pericarditis/pericardial effusion, heart sounds and the cardiac impulse cannot be detected. Pleural effusion also may be sufficiently massive to displace the heart and interfere with filling, causing signs very suggestive of right heart failure. Constrictive pericarditis and endocardial fibroelastosis may be associated with a normal cardiac silhouette on thoracic radiographs and normal auscultatory findings but signs of congestion secondary to inadequate filling. These considerations indicate the need for caution in clinical examination. Finally, signs are modified with biventricular failure. For example, concurrent right heart failure reduces the rate and extent to which left heart failure leads to pulmonary congestion and edema, while a low systemic arterial pressure as a result of left heart failure delays development of systemic edema.

Cor Pulmonale

Cor pulmonale refers to a syndrome of right heart failure as a result of underlying

Figure 53. Resolving ventral edema in a 7-year-old Belgian mare. The animal had colitis but showed minimal edema until it developed acute and initially refractory ventricular tachyarrhythmia, apparently secondary to electrolyte disturbance. Signs of right heart failure included jugular filling and extensive ventral edema. Swelling began to subside after the arrhythmia was controlled. Depressed serum protein levels undoubtedly contributed to the edema in this case. Note the absence of edema in the limbs.

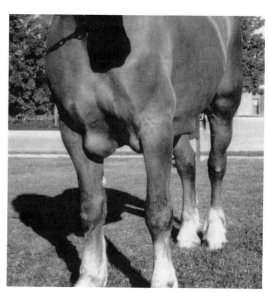

chronic respiratory disease.[391,392,394] The actual cause of the failure is progressive pulmonary hypertension in response to alveolar hypoxia.[402,403] Though the syndrome occurs in cases of uncontrolled small airway disease, more effective management of this problem has resulted in a reduced incidence of cor pulmonale. With the exception of the signs of severe lung disease and a tendency for respiratory excursions to obscure activity in the jugular vein, the signs are typically those of right heart failure. Examination of the respiratory system and review of the history also help differentiate cor pulmonale from the syndrome of acute left heart failure.

Management

General: The following discussion is concerned primarily with heart failure as a cause of circulatory insufficiency. Discussion on other approaches to the correction of circulatory insufficiency are found elsewhere in this text. The literature provides very little guidance on optimal management of heart failure in horses and no reports of long-term maintenance. However, it is feasible to maintain horses in a state of compensation for years. The primary though not the only reasons for such action would be maintenance of breeding animals or pets. Circumstance may dictate the need for modification in practical application while, even in human cardiology, management of the syndrome remains somewhat controversial.[190,256]

Management of heart failure in horses depends somewhat upon the duration of the syndrome. In acute failure, the prognosis may be very good for recovery though guarded for return to previous level of athletic performance, yet the amount of time available to make therapeutic decisions is much less because of rapid progression of the problem. The prognosis in chronic failure usually is poor for significant improvement in cardiac performance but good for achieving stability.

Cases of acute failure are managed initially by removal of the primary insult whenever possible. An essential element in achieving a successful outcome is early recognition of myocardial compromise. Specific treatment depends very much upon the primary cause. Supportive therapy, including oxygen and bed rest, as applied in people

are not options in treating adult horses but affected animals should be confined to a stall. Improvement in respiratory function by use of furosemide to reduce lung fluid and bronchodilators (aminophylline) to assist ventilation support cardiac function. Supplementary salt should be withheld to counteract renal salt and water retention, but a salt-free diet is neither an option nor is it usually necessary. Adequate hydration must be maintained, though renal perfusion is best achieved by improvement in cardiac output because overzealous intravenous fluid therapy in cases of acute failure can have disastrous consequences by overloading an already compromised system and promoting pulmonary edema.

If the clinical circumstance or presence of ventricular ectopic activity indicates myocardial inflammation, antiinflammatory agents, such as flunixin meglumine, are indicated. This therapeutic approach has the added benefits of reducing metabolic rate by lowering temperature in febrile patients and reducing catecholamine levels where pain is a factor. Digitalization (see below) may be necessary to support the remaining myocardium if the primary insult causing cardiovascular compromise cannot be removed rapidly and effectively. However, in horses in acute failure, the clinical circumstances, and frequently the nature of the acute myocardial involvement (*eg,* viral myocarditis), make detection and differentiation of digitalis toxicity difficult.

Digitalization and use of diuretics, together with reduced salt intake and controlled exercise, are the main therapeutic approaches in chronic heart failure. If the problem is detected early before clinical signs of congestion are evident, digitalization and restricted exercise may be all that is required. At this stage, salt restriction is an issue only in animals that habitually consume their salt blocks and in cases of severe left AV insufficiency with respiratory signs. In the latter circumstance, improved cardiac performance in response to digoxin therapy has the potential to promote increased pulmonary venous congestion by increasing regurgitant flow. In some cases, occasional use of diuretics as an adjunct to digoxin during stress or effort-induced pulmonary edema is necessary; in other cases, frequency of such episodes may indicate the necessity for continuous diuretic therapy.

In people, it is thought that edema may develop only when considerable salt and water retention has occurred.[1] The basis of this interpretation is that, in failure, reduced cardiac output leads to reduced systemic arterial pressure and capillary pressure. Increased cardiac output secondary to increased blood volume and improved cardiac filling leads to increased capillary pressure, promoting edema formation in the face of venous hypertension. Because the problem of heart failure often is not identified in horses until signs of congestion have appeared, considerable salt and water retention may already have occurred, necessitating early introduction of diuretic therapy.

Close attention should be paid to respiratory rate and pattern to detect early development of pulmonary edema. Failure to achieve significant improvement in respiratory signs with other therapeutic approaches certainly is an indication to initiate diuretic therapy, as chronic pulmonary edema promotes fibrosis and progressive increase in right heart workload, both accelerating progression of the syndrome and reducing the chances of a satisfactory response to treatment. Review of history and familiarity with the patient should allow differentiation between signs secondary to heart failure and chronic airway disease.

The extent to which systemic hypervolemia, as opposed to pulmonary venous hypertension secondary to poor left ventricular function, contributes to the observed respiratory embarrassment in heart failure in horses has not been investigated. However, the observation that a maximal response to diuretic therapy is not achieved for up to 24 hours after treatment is started may indicate the involvement of systemic/renal factors in addition to local respiratory factors.

Furosemide is the diuretic of choice, administered PO at 0.5-1.0 mg/kg/day in 1-2 doses.[174] Except perhaps at the start of therapy, application of a full dose is rarely necessary and is undesirable, especially in cases in which the horse is depressed and anorectic, as sometimes is the case during digitalization. Water intake should be monitored but need not be limited unless consumption is excessive, when renal function should be evaluated.

Though not classified as a potassium-wasting diuretic, furosemide does increase potassium excretion, which can lead to problems with digoxin toxicity in animals not eating properly. Oral supplementation every other day with 20-30 g KCl appears to be adequate in most cases. Chronic or excessive diuretic therapy also can be associated with hyponatremia, dehydration and alkalosis; thus, regular evaluation of electrolyte and acid-base status is necessary. The clinical signs of these iatrogenic homeostatic disorders can be the same as those of the heart failure, ie, lethargy, weakness and cardiac arrhythmia, necessitating constant vigilance. Potassium status is only reflected in serum potassium levels when severe (as much as one-third) total body depletion has occurred. Red cell potassium concentration may be used as a guide to total body status and can be useful when monitored constantly.[404] However, these values should be interpreted with caution. The ideal but impractical technique is to determine the potassium content of an ashed muscle biopsy sample.

Though seemingly paradoxic, a horse in heart failure can be dehydrated and hyponatremic, especially if circulatory insufficiency is chronic. In such cases, diuretic therapy appears ineffective.[174] Cautious intravenous fluid therapy combined with slow digitalization should be instituted to reestablish normal electrolyte status and renal function.

Affected horses should be stall rested while being stabilized. Once effectively digitalized, they must be protected from sudden changes in amount and type of exercise. Ideally they should have constant access to a very small paddock and a run-in stall. Broodmares in late pregnancy may need some modification of their therapeutic regimen until after foaling. In all cases, changes should be made gradually. If the problem is not detected until signs of overt failure develop, the horse may prove relatively refractory to therapeutic management. Greatest response can be expected if clinical signs have led to critical appraisal and early diagnosis. Early therapeutic intervention can be expected to slow the rate of myocardial deterioration as well as improve functional capacity. Therapy should not be withheld until signs of decompensation have developed but, rather, decompensation should be held at bay by appropriate management.

Digitalization: Cardiac glycosides have 2 main applications in equine cardiology: management of supraventricular tachyarrhythmias and management of congestive heart failure. In the context of heart failure, the primary actions of the drug are its positive inotropic effects and negative chronotropic effects.[313] Digitalization has, for many years, been the most useful pharmacologic approach to management of heart failure. More recently, cardiac glycosides frequently have been used in people in combination with other therapeutic agents, such as afterload reducers, diuretics and angiotensin-converting enzyme inhibitors, especially in refractory cases.[190,256] Newer inotropic agents have been developed but none has eclipsed the cardiac glycosides and none has been tried in horses because of high cost.[174] Cardiac glycosides remain the drugs of choice. The 3 agents used in horses are digitoxin, digoxin and ouabain. Digoxin is most commonly used and the only one for which there is adequate guidance in the literature.

Much of the controversy surrounding use of digoxin relates to 2 factors: the wide variation of effective dosages and the level at which toxic signs are encountered, making patient management sometimes difficult; the drug's narrow therapeutic index causes a wide range of toxic signs, many of which may mimic or worsen the primary cardiac complaint being treated. Detailed accounts of these concerns can be found in the literature.[190,256,313,405]

Dosages for digitalization of horses are presented in Table 7. The wide range in recommendations reflects variation in experimental method in the studies cited and differences in the equations used to calculate dosage regimens from studies of pharmacokinetics. Extrapolation, experimental observations and limited clinical experience suggest that the therapeutic range for digoxin in horses is the same as that for people, or 0.5-2.0 ng/ml plasma.[372,406-408] To be consistent with the data presented in the references cited, most figures in Table 7 are for 24-hour dosing. However, to avoid wide swings in plasma levels and variable response, the drug usually is given in divided doses at 12-hour intervals.[174]

Oral dosing is with a pediatric elixir, which is rather expensive or, more usually, by crushing tablets and administering them in a syrup by dosing syringe. Careful attention is essential to ensure that the horse has received the full dose. Inconsistency in this technique is probably one of the reasons that horses can appear difficult to stabilize orally. Another reason may be varied uptake due to individual variation and differences in bioavailability of the preparation used. The literature suggests that therapeutic plasma levels can be achieved in 3.5-6 days by twice-daily treatment with the oral maintenance dose.[407,408] In most horses in which signs are mild, this approach provides satisfactory results and has been recommended as the approach of choice.[408] Bioavailability of an oral dose varies between 14% and 25% and averages about 20%.[407-409] A double peak in serum concentration after oral dosing probably depends

Table 7. Some recommended dosages for digoxin. All dosages are in mg/100 kg/24 hours unless otherwise stated.

Half Life	Intravenous Loading	Maintenance	Oral Loading	Maintenance	Reference
23 hr	1.0-1.5	0.5-0.76	–	–	406
23.1 hr	1.4	0.7	7.0	3.5	407
28.8 hr	–	0.61	–	1.74	409
16.9 hr	0.425[a] (12-hr dose)	0.165[a] (12-hr dose)	3.86[b] (12-hr dose)	1.5[b] (12-hr dose)	408

a – To provide steady state serum concentration in the range of 0.45-2.33 ng/ml.
b – To provide steady state serum concentration in the range of 0.97-1.67 ng/ml.

upon numerous factors, including those mentioned above.

If severity of clinical signs or acute onset of heart failure dictates the need for rapid digitalization, cautious IV administration of a loading dose may be employed, dividing the dose into 3 parts and administering it slowly, not by bolus, at 1- to 2-hour intervals.[407] Though I routinely employ this technique, it can be hazardous unless facilities for close monitoring are available.[408] Use of loading doses, particularly when given IV, carries the risk of toxicity because of the high initial plasma levels achieved and the prolonged time necessary for levels to return to normal.[410] It has been recommended that loading doses be avoided if possible.[156,407] Intravenous administration may be particularly useful in management of some arrhythmias.

Signs of a clinical response vary according to the patient being treated but include increased pulse strength, improved peripheral perfusion and diuresis. The heart rate decreases in most cases, especially if supraventricular tachyarrhythmias are present, and signs of congestion (cough, dyspnea, peripheral edema) subside gradually. Changes in demeanor are unpredictable because of mild toxic effects. Failure to achieve clinical response is an indication to increase dosage only if there are no signs of toxicity. As noted above, combination therapy, particularly concurrent use of diuretics, can be very effective in severe or refractory cases.

The therapeutic index for cardiac glycosides is narrow and signs of toxicity are common. Limited research has been done on toxic signs specifically in horses and observations are thus based largely upon clinical experience and extrapolation from other species, though signs of presumed digoxin toxicity have been described in one somewhat complex case.[18,156,174,410] Overdosing, widely fluctuating serum levels, low serum protein level (reducing protein binding and increasing active levels of the drug), dehydration, hypokalemia and reduced renal function predispose to toxicity. Early signs include depression, anorexia and mild diarrhea. These can become progressively more severe if treatment at the same level is continued, with the animal exhibiting obvious weakness. Bradycardia due to severe AV block can occur.

Toxicity also can be associated with sinus tachycardia and a predisposition to conduction disturbances and ventricular ectopic activity as a consequence of increased sympathetic tone and interference with the Na-K ATPase-dependent pump.[174] This aspect of the toxicity of cardiac glycosides is of particular concern in management of acute myocarditis and myocardial degeneration because the primary lesion predisposes to the same arrhythmias. Cardiac glycosides should be used with the greatest caution in horses exhibiting ventricular arrhythmias. Ideally, other therapeutic approaches, such as specific antiarrhythmic drugs, antibiotics to treat identified bacterial infection and antiinflammatory agents would be employed first to reduce the ectopic activity, if clinical signs allow this more conservative approach.

As an aid in management, maintaining serum digoxin levels in the therapeutic range of 0.5-2.0 ng/ml is recommended. Many commercial laboratories now are equipped to provide these assays. In the absence of signs of toxicity, collection of a serum sample midway between maintenance doses has been recommended.[408] Instructions with regard to sampling procedure from the reference laboratory should be adhered to closely. Safe use of the drug also may be promoted by use of electrocardiography to establish status at the onset of treatment and to detect signs of toxicity. By analogy with the situation in dogs, increased frequency of second-degree block and ST segment deviation may provide some early indication of toxicity, though the sensitivity and specificity of these signs in horses have not been investigated.[156]

DISEASES OF ARTERIES

P.W. Physick-Sheard

Congenital and Familial Diseases

Congenital Abnormalities of Arteries

Isolated congenital abnormalities of the great vessels (aorta and pulmonary artery) are not common in horses and most often are detected in association with complex congenital heart disease. The following discussion concentrates mainly upon discrete vascular abnormalities. The reader should consult the sections dealing with congenital abnormalities of valves and of myocardium for a more complete view of the participation of the great vessels in congenital cardiac disease. Congenital abnormalities of the cardiovascular system in horses are overviewed in Table 4.

Persistent Ductus Arteriosus

A murmur associated with physiologic patency of the ductus arteriosus is detected clinically in most newborn foals, usually within the first 24 hours.[16,128,150,157] Usually the murmur is absent for the first 15-30 minutes after birth. Anatomic narrowing of the ductus appears to start before birth, with changes in the wall anticipating anatomic closure occurring as early as day 320 of gestation.[4,157] The vessel may remain anatomically patent for several days after birth or may close within 3 days. The variation between foals may reflect the circumstances surrounding birth and the gestational age of the foal at birth.[157] Physiologic closure probably precedes anatomic closure by hours to several days. However, in normal foals physiologic closure is achieved by 3-4 days at latest and the murmur of patent ductus arteriosus (PDA) thus subsides by this time.[16,128,150,157] Logically, therefore, a diagnosis of PDA cannot be safely made in a foal less than 4-5 days of age. If the typical continuous or machinery murmur can be heard after this time, PDA may be suspected. The characteristics of the murmur have been described earlier in this chapter. Both systolic and diastolic components may not always be detected. The diastolic sound may occupy only early diastole, or may be soft and easily missed.

Notwithstanding the frequency with which the murmur is detected in neonates, persistent ductus arteriosus, *ie,* flow patency of the ductus after 4-5 days of age, occurs clinically and as an *isolated* abnormality only very rarely in horses. Of the approximately 28 cases of PDA reported in the literature, most were associated with other cardiac anomalies. These included persistent right aortic arch, interruption of the aortic arch and ventricular septal defect, pseudotruncus arteriosus, tricuspid atresia, and tetralogy of Fallot.[18,129,362,364,411-416] Of these cases, most were diagnosed

in very young foals showing signs of exercise intolerance and cardiovascular insufficiency. In cases of an isolated lesion, ages ranged from 30 days to "aged."[356,417-419] A reported case in a 3-day-old donkey is questionable because of the animal's age.[420]

Because of the wide range of ages and clinical circumstances, a clear clinical picture does not emerge. Where other congenital anomalies are present, the relative contribution of each to the clinical signs is difficult to determine, while the combination of murmurs that can be generated may be complex. In some cases *eg,* tetralogy of Fallot with severe stenosis of the pulmonic ostium, the presence of a large, patent ductus arteriosus is essential for life, allowing blood to reach the lungs. In other circumstances, the vessel may contribute to clinical signs.[421] An inadequate number of cases have been reported to establish clear guidelines, but in uncomplicated cases, signs presumably vary with age and size of the vessel.

Pressure gradients after birth favor a left-to-right shunt throughout systole and diastole, with the murmur fading in late diastole. If the defect is sufficiently large and/or with concurrent primary respiratory disease, pressure in the pulmonary circulation rises and a progressive load is placed on the right heart. Rapid development of pulmonary hypertension causes right heart failure. Slower development eventually leads to Eisenmenger's syndrome, in which pulmonary hypertension due to high pulmonary vascular resistance is associated with reversed or bidirectional shunting across a congenital defect, in this case, the persistent ductus arteriosus.[356,422] Evaluation of the defect can be complicated by changing pressure differentials because the murmur may reduce in intensity or subside as pulmonary artery pressure rises. The diastolic component may disappear or both systolic and diastolic components may become shortened.

The diagnosis is suggested by the murmur and, in mature animals, by a prominent S_2 reflecting pulmonary hypertension. The diagnosis may be confirmed by cardiac catheterization.[356] During catheterization, the pressure differential between the aorta and pulmonary artery (to confirm the direction of the shunt and to detect pulmonary hypertension), and PaO$_2$ levels in the pulmonary artery and the right ventricle (to detect left-to-right shunt) are measured. A technique for angiography in foals has been described.[128] Additionally, echocardiography should have potential for diagnostic application in young foals. Though an attempt at surgical management of persistent right aortic arch has been described in the foal, surgical treatment of PDA has not.[423]

Persistent Right Aortic Arch

In persistent right aortic arch, the right fourth aortic arch persists and gives rise to the arch of the aorta instead of the usual left fourth arch.[424] If the cause of this persistence is situs inversus, in which all viscera are reversed, no vascular ring is formed and the condition is not associated with clinical signs. However, if the left sixth arch (which gives rise to the ductus arteriosus) persists, a vascular ring is formed by the aortic arch and the ductus arteriosus (or ligamentum arteriosum if the duct has closed normally) that encloses the esophagus and trachea.[425] Vascular rings also may be comprised of the right aortic arch and the left subclavian artery when that vessel still arises from a left dorsal (descending) aorta or by a double aorta in which both fourth aortic arches persist.

These anomalies are very rare. The 3 cases in the literature all are examples of right fourth arch and left ductus arteriosus. Two of these occurred in foals and were associated with esophageal obstruction, difficulty swallowing, and regurgitation and inhalation pneumonia.[411,423] In the third case, in a 22-month-old trotter, clinical signs were of exercise intolerance and heart failure believed most likely the consequences of a coexisting ventricular septal defect.[421] In that case, the vascular ring was not tight and caused no clinical signs of obstruction. A persistent ductus arteriosus was observed in 2 of the cases.

Persistent right aortic arch should be considered in cases of nasal regurgitation in foals but would be a relatively unlikely differential diagnosis as compared with such congenital problems as cleft palate.

Abnormalities of the Great Vessels

Abnormality of the great vessels can take several forms and usually comprises one component of a complex defect. Of the numerous possible combinations described in mammals, only 3, tetralogy of Fallot, pulmonic atresia (pseudotruncus arteriosus) and persistent truncus arteriosus, have been described in horses. With the exception of cases of tetralogy in which right heart outflow is minimally obstructed, all have essentially the same consequences and presenting signs and cannot easily be distinguished on clinical grounds.

Persistent Truncus Arteriosus: In embryologic development of the heart, the developing ventricular chambers are drained by a common vessel, the truncus arteriosus. During formation of the definitive outflow tracts, the proximal portion of this vessel is septated by the bulbotruncal septum, while the distal portion is divided by the aorticopulmonary septum. These partitions form in a spiral fashion, forming the definitive aorta and pulmonary artery, which twist around each other.[422] Failure of these septa to develop proximally results in persistence of the common truncus, in which both chambers are drained by a single vessel, forming a persistent truncus arteriosus. Partial failure of the septation process distally results in an aortopulmonary window.

In persistent truncus arteriosus (also called truncus communis, common aorticopulmonary trunk), there is a single semilunar valve, usually functionally competent though with 2-6 cusps, and always an infundibular ventricular septal defect (VSD), discussed below. Failure of truncus division thus is associated with failure of the septum to fully develop. There are several variations in the manner in which the pulmonary arteries arise from the common truncus, with some configurations protecting the pulmonary circulation from excessive pressure and the left heart from volume overload. Such cases are compatible with survival. Excessive pulmonary arterial flow leads to left heart volume overload and failure, while minimal flow results in effective right-to-left shunting and cyanosis with similar consequences.

Too few cases have been described in the equine literature to define prognosis, which must be assessed on a case-by-case basis; generally, it is very poor. Reports on 8 cases have been published. Three are postmortem descriptions, while the remaining 5 describe clinical features of cyanosis, dyspnea and intense machinery (continuous) murmurs.[360,369,418,426-428] In 3 cases, the murmur was loudest at the heart base on the left, in 1 it was generalized and continuous with no obvious point of maximum intensity, and in 1 it was loudest well forward on the right side and pansystolic.[360,369,428] The last case is somewhat unusual, as the source of the murmur in persistent truncus would be most likely to generate a widespread sound loudest at the left heart base.

Possible sources of the murmur in persistent truncus arteriosus include turbulent systolic flow through the VSD located beneath the single outflow tract, flow disturbance due to stenosis of the pulmonary arteries at their point of origin from the common trunk, and diastolic sounds due to diastolic flow between the aorta and pulmonary arteries. Stenosis at the origin of pulmonary vessels is described in 4 cases. Severe limitation of exercise tolerance was evident in most and only one survived beyond 3 weeks. This 2-year-old showed poor development of the hindquarters, which was ascribed to persistent hypoxemia.[428]

Differential diagnoses would include all causes of obstruction to right heart outflow with right-to-left shunt, as all of these conditions may include a PDA. Differentiation from pulmonic atresia, in which the picture is essentially the same but in which there is a ductus arteriosus, indicating development at some point of a pulmonary vessel, may be achieved at necropsy by noting the course of the left recurrent laryngeal nerve and, if present, by noting the atretic pulmonary artery.[319]

Pulmonic Atresia: In atresia of the pulmonary trunk (pseudotruncus arteriosus), the pulmonic valve is vestigial or absent and the pulmonary artery is represented only by a thin cord. It has been described in horses.[129,319,359,429] All cases were accompanied by a VSD and a single large outflow vessel, identified as a dextrorotated aorta in most cases, positioned above the septum and draining both ventricular chambers. Pulmonic atresia may be differentiated from tetralogy of Fallot by the fact that the pulmonary trunk is atretic rather than simply stenotic, and from persistent truncus arteriosus by the presence of the vestige of the pulmonary artery and by the course of the left recurrent laryngeal nerve.[319] A PDA has been present in most cases described.

The embryologic basis of the abnormality is abnormal septation of the truncus.

Clinical signs are typical of congenital heart disease involving right-to-left shunts and abnormality of the outflow tracts, and include lethargy, weakness, poor growth rate, exercise intolerance, cyanosis and a pansystolic murmur with a point of maximum intensity at the heart base on the left. Though survival to 2 years was reported in 1 case, affected animals are symptomatic from birth and generally have a poor prognosis for survival.[359] Diagnosis is achieved as for tricuspid atresia.

Tetralogy of Fallot: Tetralogy of Fallot classically consists of stenosis of the pulmonary outflow tract (subvalvular, supravalvular or valvular), dextrorotation of the aorta, a VSD and right ventricular hypertrophy.[422] Additionally, in the most severe form of tetralogy, pulmonic atresia (complete absence of the pulmonic valve and atretic pulmonary artery) may be present. This causes some confusion in terminology because the literature makes specific reference to pulmonary atresia in horses. To maintain consistency, the term "tetralogy" is used here to describe only cases in which the right ventricular outflow tract and pulmonary artery retain some communication and in which the artery is recognizable and patent. Seven cases have been described in the literature, with consistent signs of a harsh pansystolic murmur loudest at the left heart base and radiating widely.[129,398,415,416,427,430,431] Most affected horses had an associated thrill on palpation. Tachycardia and reduced exercise tolerance were observed in each case.

Cyanosis need not be a constant finding in tetralogy of Fallot. If there is moderate to severe obstruction of the right heart outflow tract, then high right ventricular pressures are associated with severe right-to-left shunting and cyanosis. If pulmonic obstruction is mild, there may be little shunting at birth, with the pulmonary artery still representing a lower resistance outlet for right ventricular blood than the aorta. Right-to-left shunting occurs later as pulmonary hypertension develops secondary to overcirculation of the lungs. The presence of a PDA can also modify signs. The murmur at the left heart base tends to be particularly intense in cases of tetralogy of Fallot as compared with other anomalies of the great vessels, presumably due to the combination of flow disturbance both in the region of the VSD and in the right heart outflow tract. The murmur may take on a crescendo-decrescendo shape in contrast to the coarse, band-shaped sound more typically associated with congenital shunts.

Other Congenital Vascular Anomalies

Though other congenital abnormalities of arteries have been described in horses, they are uncommon. Interruption of the aortic arch, in which the arch fails to form and the descending aorta arises via the ductus arteriosus from the pulmonary artery, has been described in 2 foals.[364] Clinical signs were of limited exercise tolerance and progressive tachycardia. Differential cyanosis (normally arterialized proximal flow via the ascending aorta, cyanosis of tissues supplied by the descending aorta) may be expected in such cases. A ventricular septal defect always is present. Two cases of coarctation (congenital narrowing) of the aorta also are described. An affected 9-year-old pony was asymptomatic and the finding was incidental to physiologic studies.[432] In the other, thrombosis and lameness were assumed to be secondary to congenital narrowing of the aorta discovered at necropsy.[433]

Inflammatory, Infectious and Immune Diseases

Vasculitis

Vasculitis is a general term that refers to inflammation of blood vessels of any size, in any location, regardless of cause.[434] Most vasculitic syndromes in horses have characteristics of hypersensitivity (allergic) vasculitis. They are distinguished by predominant involvement of small vessels, such as venules, capillaries and arterioles. Histologic findings include neutrophilic infiltration of venules in the dermis and subcutaneous tissue, nuclear debris in affected vessels and fibrinoid necrosis.[435] Clinical signs of vasculitis include demarcated areas of dermal and/or subcutaneous edema, skin infarction, necrosis and exudation.[436-438] Edema, hemorrhage and necrosis may occur in muscles, joints, kidney, intestine, lung or the central nervous system. Consequently, clinical

signs exhibited by an affected horse may range from lameness, colic and dyspnea to ataxia.[439] Vasculitis often is complicated by cellulitis, thrombophlebitis and laminitis.

The principal causes of vasculitis in horses include infectious agents, hypersensitivity reactions, immune complexes, drugs and parasites. Purpura hemorrhagica, equine infectious anemia and ehrlichiosis are discussed in detail in the chapter on Diseases of the Hemolymphatic System.

Parasitic Arteritis

Domestic animals are affected by numerous parasitic infections that involve the cardiovascular system directly or indirectly.[455] Several in equidae have been described, including infections by heartworms (*Dirofilaria immitis*), *Trichinella spiralis* (experimental infection), *Sarcocystis* and *Elaeophora bohmi* (forming parasitic nodules in walls of peripheral limb vessels).[455-458] However, with the exception of heartworm infection, which appears to be very uncommon, none of these infections appear to be of practical clinical significance.

Strongylus vulgaris infection, on the other hand, is responsible for a wide range of cardiovascular lesions and clinical problems in horses.[459] The life cycle of the parasite involves migration in the arterial network of the intestine.[460-462] Ingested third-stage larvae exsheath and penetrate the mucosa of the small or large intestine. Within 7 days of infection, they molt to fourth-stage larvae that penetrate submucosal arteries and migrate in or on the intima to the cranial mesenteric artery, arriving by 11-21 days postinfection. Further maturation of the parasite occurs at this site and, after 3-4 months, the larvae molt to the fifth stage and return to the wall of the bowel via the intestinal arteries. Here they undergo a further 6-8 weeks of maturation before returning to the lumen of the bowel as adult parasites. The prepatent period is 6-7 months.

Migration in the arteries is associated with a range of lesions.[455] The most consistent is arteritis of the cranial mesenteric artery. Occasionally there is secondary aneurysm formation as the wall of the artery becomes weakened, and thromboembolism of branches of the artery as thrombi form and detach. Typically, in active cases the wall of the artery is greatly thickened and the lumen narrowed by formation of thrombi. In chronic and resolving cases, the vessel wall becomes hardened, fibrosed and thin, and the lumen increases in diameter. These various effects, plus inflammation of the perivascular tissues with pressure and inflammatory effects on adjacent autonomic ganglia and possibly direct effects of exsheathment fluids on bowel motility, can be associated with bowel dysfunctions, including recurrent mild gassy colic, severe acute colic due to thromboembolism and bowel ischemia, diarrhea, or even fatal peritonitis secondary to rupture of the antimesenteric border of the bowel wall.[459,463,464]

Aberrant parasite migration also occurs and migration tracts may be observed throughout the thoracic and proximal abdominal aorta.[455] The resulting lesions are responsible for many of the clinical consequences of infection. Tracts, endarteritis with thrombosis and fibrous nodules of parasitic origin sometimes are encountered in the bulb of the aorta, usually on its cranial curvature, and in the region of the coronary sinuses.[455,465] These lesions may lead to valvular endocarditis with insufficiency or stenosis (Fig 54), aneurysm and rupture of coronary arteries, coronary obstruction and myocardial infarction and occasionally sudden death.[179,189,321,337,465-467] Involvement of the renal arteries sometimes results in renal infarction, while migration into the brachiocephalic trunk and carotid arteries may lead to parasitic embolism of the brain, with subsequent encephalomalacia and/or encephalomyelitis.[468]

Clinical consequences of infection with *S vulgaris* are likely to be most severe in the young, naive animals exposed to infection for the first time, and when the infecting load of parasites is high. Mild to moderate infections are always associated with vascular lesions but the consistency with which they lead to gastrointestinal disorders and colic is undetermined. Arteritis of the cranial mesenteric artery may be suggested by recurrent low-grade abdominal pain. The index of suspicion may be increased by detection of a hardened, enlarged or painful cranial mesenteric artery on rectal palpation. In cases of endarteritis and embolism, abdominocentesis may demonstrate nonseptic peritonitis.

Though parasite damage to the cranial mesenteric artery can be severe, almost total resolution of the lesion is possible through appropriate use of anthelmintics. Excellent response has been obtained in foals with ivermectin at 0.2 mg/kg.[469] Repeat dosing with benzimidazoles also is effective against fourth-stage larvae.[470-472] Resolution of lesions resulting from thromboembolism and aberrant migration does *not* depend upon use of anthelmintics, however, and a broader approach to parasite control is necessary.

Neoplastic Diseases

Vascular Neoplasia

Vascular neoplasms are uncommon in horses and represent a poorly defined group of lesions.[455,473] The difficulty arises in part

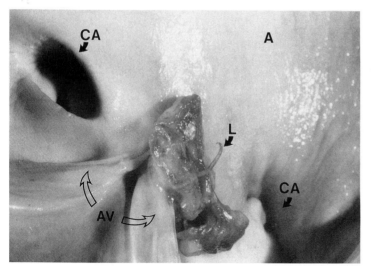

Figure 54. Parasitic endarteritis of the aortic valve. A fourth-stage larva (L) can be seen protruding from a thrombus attached to the cranial (right coronary) cusp of the valve. This animal showed parasitic involvement of the cranial mesenteric artery also. A = aorta. CA = coronary arteries. AV = left caudal and cranial cusps of the aortic valve. (Courtesy of Dr. G. Maxie)

because of the absence of a consistent system of nomenclature and also difficulty in histopathologic differentiation in some cases. Tumorous and tumor-like lesions of the vascular system may be loosely classified into benign angiomas and malignant angiosarcomas.

Angiomas: Many angiomas probably are not neoplastic processes, representing instead hamartomas or developmental malformations of vascular tissue. These may be found in any site and often are present at or shortly after birth.[455,473] They tend to develop with the growth of the animal and, like all other vascular masses, may be pulsatile on palpation. Local infiltration is not a feature of these masses and they may be excised, though their vascularity may present a surgical challenge.

True angiomas or hemangiomas are classified as benign tumors of endothelial cells and may be difficult to differentiate from vascular malformations or granulation tissue.[455] They may occur in any tissue of the body but are most commonly identified in the skin of the legs, head or flank.[473-477] They may be seen at any age, though young animals are usually affected. These tumors appear to be generally slow growing and nonulcerative, and vary from soft, fluctuating, fluid-filled and cystic structures to hard nodules. They are usually discrete, though they vary from sessile or pedunculated localized lesions, to cord-like elongated masses. Such a lesion may be more a blemish than a clinical problem, but rapid growth of a lesion in a young animal may be associated with abnormal development of adjacent structures.[473] Clinical signs are otherwise not necessarily associated with these lesions unless their location leads to trauma and hemorrhage or they are multicentric. It may be difficult to differentiate the lesion from angiosarcoma on biopsy, and local infiltration and/or recurrence after excision may prove problematic.[477] Treatment is an option, though broad-based sessile masses may be difficult to remove.[473,475]

Angiosarcoma: Angiosarcoma (hemangiosarcoma) is classified as a malignant tumor of endothelial cells and is very uncommon in horses. The tumor sometimes is referred to as a malignant hemangioendothelioma. Of 6 affected horses described in the literature, all had metastatic involvement of several organs and tissues, variously including spleen, heart, lungs, brain, liver and bone.[478-482] Seeding of lesions across the peritoneum and/or pleural surfaces and, in 1 case, of the pericardium was observed. Extensive involvement of skeletal muscle also has been described.[479,480] Neoplastic masses were nodular and red, and varied in size up to several centimeters and in consistency from soft to hard. Involvement of skin was not a feature. All cases occurred in mature horses aged 5-22 years.

Clinical signs included weakness, dyspnea, pallor, anorexia and weight loss. The clinical course was short (days to weeks) once signs became evident. Horses with skeletal muscle involvement manifested some degree of external swelling of a fluctuating nature. Affected horses frequently died from the effects of the tumor, with the most frequent cause of death being hemorrhage from neoplastic masses. Pleural effusion and hemorrhage were prominent findings where metastasis to the thoracic organs had occurred.[481,482] Icterus secondary to chronic severe hemorrhage was a prominent finding in some horses.[479-481] In a hemangiosarcoma, local infiltration rather than metastasis was noted.[477] Differentiation between metastasis and multicentric neoplasia usually cannot be achieved.

Multifactorial Diseases

Abnormalities of Coronary Arteries

The pattern of coronary artery distribution and flow, both at rest and exercise, have been investigated extensively.[483-487] Studies have demonstrated the degree of collateralization of the coronary circulation and the existence of significant coronary reserve flow capacity in ponies.[488-490] The results of these investigations, in addition to their comparative interest, help explain why clinical disease associated with the coronary arteries is uncommon in horses.

Most clinically significant abnormalities of the coronary arteries tend to represent sporadic conditions. Congenital abnormality of the coronary arteries has been described.[491-493] Abnormalities usually involve abnormal origin of the arteries, such as a single vessel that subsequently divides to supply both ventricular chambers, and are most often found in association with other complex cardiac abnormalities. Only occasionally do isolated anomalies appear to be responsible for clinical signs and generally these are incidental findings.[418] Coronary artery anomalies can be responsible for death in infancy or adulthood in people.[422] In horses, obstruction of the coronary arteries appears to have been primarily verminous and embolic.[179,321,338,466,467] Sudden death has been the outcome in most cases and the diagnosis is thus made at necropsy. Too few cases are described to confirm predilection for either the left or right coronary artery.

Both primary and secondary acquired degenerative disease of the coronary microvasculature have been reported in horses.[188,494,495] Microembolization and myocardial infarction as a consequence of parasitic thromboendarteritis of the aortic arch have been described.[189] Participation of other factors in coronary arterial degeneration and myocardial fibrosis has been proposed, however, including a role for the autonomic nervous system.[340,496-498] Coronary aneurysm and rupture have been described as a cause of sudden death.[323,499] A role in such cases for medial degeneration of the coronary arteries secondary to malfunction of vasa vasorum has been proposed.[500]

The clinical significance of many of these arterial lesions, which may be age related, remains to be determined.[188] Horses appear prone to focal myocardial fibrosis, which, in turn, also appears to be an aging or age-related change. The predictable consequence of coronary artery disease, namely focal myocardial infarction, may thus provide a link between these pathologic findings. Such clinical signs as serious cardiac arrhythmias or myocardial failure are a very infrequent consequence. The proposal that such lesions are of primary significance in the genesis of common arrhythmias in horses requires further investigation.[182,197,226] These considerations are discussed in more depth under acquired myocardial disease.

Vascular Accidents

Rupture of the Aorta: Rupture of the aorta has been associated with a range of problems, including myocarditis, endocarditis and chronic aortic valvular insufficiency, and necrosis of the arterial media.[325,371,] [375,501-508] With the exception of aortic ring rupture, exercise is an infrequent association. The readiness with which cases are reported should not lead the reader to assume that aortic rupture is a common occurrence, however. Aortic rupture can be conveniently divided into 2 groups: aneurysm/rupture and aortic ring rupture.

Rupture appears to occur most frequently in the root of the aorta just *above* (distal to) the aortic valve.[333,386,508,509] Sudden death can occur as a consequence of cardiac tamponade or hemorrhage into the thoracic cavity. However, this is not necessarily an immediate consequence because the intimal tear and partial destruction of the arterial wall may result in spread of blood between the layers of the wall and formation of a dissecting aneurysm that can extend for variable distances along the wall of the aorta and its major branches.[329,333,386,387] Dissection generally occurs between the media and adventitia.

Infrequently, involvement of the pulmonary artery may lead to necrosis and rupture of that vessel, and formation of an aorticopulmonary fistula.[333,386] This is thought to be a consequence of local pressure necrosis. Affected horses may show evidence of acute thoracic pain and distress at the time the aneurysm first develops and subsequently may develop signs of heart failure.[386,387] The fistula usually is associated with a murmur that typically is continuous and reminiscent of that of patent ductus arteriosus, though it waxes and wanes, and is loudest in diastole.[386]

The cause of the rupture has not been immediately obvious in many of the earlier cases described in the literature, though in a series of 7 cases there was histopathologic evidence of medial necrosis in the region of the rupture.[508] In a review of 4 cases in which the rupture occurred just proximal to the scar of the ductus arteriosus and the aneurysm dissected into the pulmonary artery, medial necrosis was found in both the aorta and pulmonary artery and was thought to be associated with primary thickening and obliteration of vasa vasorum.[333] Though rupture was at a single site, areas of necrosis and change in vasa vasorum were found throughout the entire aorta and pulmonary trunk. The authors concluded that such changes are probably not uncommon in horses but that rupture is an infrequent complication, and that most cases of medial necrosis are subclinical.

In addition to the foregoing, weakening of the arterial wall can occur at any site and may be associated with dilatation and rupture. Aneurysms thus have been encountered in the coronary artery and in the cranial mesenteric artery secondary to parasitic arteritis.

Aortic Ring Rupture: Aortic ring rupture in the stallion, in which there is a separation between the aorta and the fibrous annulus of the heart, as opposed to a rupture of the wall of the aorta itself distal to the valve, appears to be a distinct and separate condition. In a series of 8 cases, all tears were in the right coronary sinus, with dissection into the right ventricle occurring in 2.[388] In the remaining 6, hemorrhage had dissected into the interventricular septum (cardioaortic fistula). It was postulated that, when death was sudden, hemorrhage had interrupted the atrioventricular bundle. In another case in which the problem occurred after swimming exercise, rupture was into the right ventricle with secondary damage to the right AV valve.[375] Detection of an inflammatory reaction in the disturbed tissues led the author to conclude that myocarditis was involved.

If hemorrhage dissects into the right ventricle, the horse may survive for several weeks, and a characteristic pandiastolic murmur loudest on the right side of the thorax may be heard. The heart of a 7-year-old stallion with lethargy, syncopal attacks, ventricular tachyarrhythmia and a pandiastolic murmur is shown in Figure 55. In this horse, the rupture was in the right coronary cusp of the aortic valve. Though medial necrosis was observed in several of the cases described in the literature it appeared to be unrelated to the tear, the etiology of which was unknown.[388] Seven of the cases described occurred shortly after the stallions were used for natural service.[371,388] Arterial hypertension in association with a local anatomic weakness was thought to be a predisposing factor.

Uterine Artery Rupture: Arterial rupture in the pregnant, foaling or recently foaled mare is not rare in the spectrum of arterial ruptures. Affected mares usually are older and multiparous.[321,336] They may manifest varying degrees of discomfort and hemorrhagic shock as blood escapes into the broad ligament, or may be found dead.[321] There may be no association with dystocia, and a mare may appear healthy after a normal foaling, only to collapse later. Postmortem examination reveals extensive hemorrhage and rupture of the uterine branch of the ovarian artery, the middle uterine artery or the external iliac artery.[321,336,509,510] Age-related degenerative changes and, in cases of external iliac artery rupture, repeated episodes of local pressure in multiparous mares have been proposed as predisposing causes.[336] Copper deficiency has been suggested as an additional predisposing factor, though this appears not to be a fully substantiated extrapolation from observations on vascular disease in people and swine.[455]

Pulmonary Hemorrhage and Pulmonary Artery Rupture: A vascular accident involving a large vessel often is assumed to be the cause of death in horses with epistaxis of pulmonary origin at time of death. However, pulmonary hemorrhage rarely causes death, and rupture of the pulmonary artery proper is diagnosed even less frequently. Only a few cases of pulmonary hemorrhage have been investigated, but most seem to

Figure 55. View of the interior of the cranial (right coronary) cusp of the aortic valve of a 7-year-old Standardbred stallion. There is a dissecting aneurysm (open arrow) extending from this site to both left and right ventricles. Clinical signs were of an acute onset of exercise intolerance during a race. The horse had ventricular tachycardia and systolic and diastolic murmurs, loudest on the right side of the thorax. CA = right coronary artery. C = cranial cusp of the aortic valve.

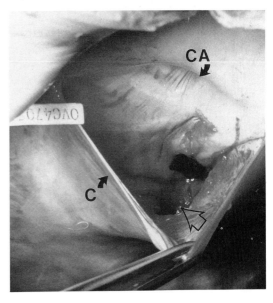

reflect generalized hemorrhage, possibly from microvasculature, rather than the rupture of a single large vessel. In a review of 11 cases of sudden death in racehorses, 9 of which were thought to be the direct result of hemorrhage into the lungs, bleeding occurred throughout much of both lungs and was most severe in the caudal lung.[339] These horses also exhibited evidence of chronic pulmonary disease of a character and degree that seems unusual for horses regularly and successfully undertaking race-intensity exercise. A diagnosis of exercise-induced pulmonary hemorrhage (EIPH) was made.

Previous studies of EIPH have not incriminated the syndrome as a cause of death.[511-514] It would be very difficult to isolate the level at which hemorrhage had occurred in such cases, and the precise cause must remain open. However, a generalized or focally diffuse, rather than a single, discrete, source of hemorrhage must be incriminated. Similar cases of pulmonary hemorrhage of undetermined cause may represent examples of the same pathogenetic mechanisms.[322] The role played by pulmonary artery rupture in cases of sudden death thus remains undetermined.

Only 4 of the horses in the study described above exhibited epistaxis. Epistaxis would not be expected in pulmonary artery rupture because bleeding would be into the pulmonary interstitium or thoracic cavity, not into airways. In 2 studies examining causes of sudden death in groups of 69 and 25 horses, no diagnoses of pulmonary artery rupture were made, though hemorrhage into the thoracic cavity was observed.[321,322] Four documented cases have been found in the literature, 3 of these occurring in very young horses and 1 in association with patent ductus arteriosus in an adult horse.[332,356,515-517] Additionally, secondary pulmonary artery rupture has been described in 5 horses in association with a dissecting aneurysm of the aorta.[356,517] Pulmonary artery rupture thus appears to be very uncommon and usually is associated with other primary cardiovascular lesions. Limited and varying clinical associations would make the condition difficult to diagnose as other than a postmortem finding.

Other Vascular Accidents: Rupture of other arteries generally reflects direct trauma or laceration secondary to fractures,

rather than consistent clinical entities or spontaneous rupture.[321,323,518-523] Rupture of veins also has been reported as a cause of fatal internal hemorrhage.[334,335,524-526]

Other Causes of Arterial Thrombosis and Thromboembolism: In addition to aorto-iliac thrombosis, arterial thrombosis and thromboembolism have been reported in a number of different sites, including the brachial artery and renal artery.[527-531] The causes vary widely, though, with the exception of parasitism and possibly trauma, none is encountered with any frequency. Aberrant parasitism was commonly stated as a cause in many earlier papers. Improved management methods and increased use of anthelmintics have greatly reduced the incidence of such conditions but cases still occur.

Trauma also is a cause of arterial thrombosis. Ischemic necrosis of the distal limb in a horse with arterial occlusion after application of local anesthesia during lameness diagnosis is shown in Figure 56. A thrombus

Figure 56. Ischemic necrosis of the distal forelimb in a Standardbred gelding. The horse had received a sub-carpal block of the check ligament area 3 days before presentation and had subsequently become lame on the limb, with local swelling and coldness distally. At necropsy there was a thrombus in the medial palmar artery just distal to the carpus, with local arteritis.

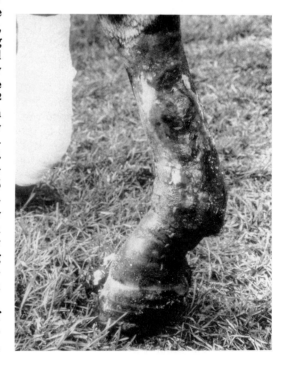

was found in the medial palmar artery at the level of the accessory (carpal) check ligament. Thrombosis of the humeral artery and vein has been described secondary to congenital malformation of the ribs, while thromboembolism of the median artery, presumed to be secondary to atrial thrombosis, has been described as the cause of ischemia and lameness in a foal.[532] Thrombosis also occurs in association with fractures and direct trauma to the vessel wall.

Thrombosis and ischemia have been described as components of the vascular changes that occur in the navicular syndrome in horses.[533,534] Changes in the vascular supply to the foot, including thrombosis and progressive intimal thickening and occlusion, may contribute significantly to degenerative lameness of the distal limb.[535-538] Almost total occlusion of the common brachiocephalic trunk by a well-organized thrombus in a pony was associated with weight loss, swelling of the forelimbs, ventral edema, and aortic sclerosis and calcification.[539]

Pulmonary Thromboembolism: Obstruction of the pulmonary artery by thrombi is most often a consequence of thrombosis elsewhere in the systemic circulation. Embolism, rather than primary thrombosis, may occur more frequently in horses than is clinically appreciated. Thromboembolism is a predictable consequence of iatrogenic thrombophlebitis after venipuncture and jugular vein catheterization, as well as a sequel to local inflammatory processes elsewhere in the circulatory system.[540-543] Postoperative pulmonary microembolism has been described as a consequence of intravascular thrombosis secondary to tissue trauma and local hypoxia and shock.[544]

Consequences of pulmonary embolism depend upon the size of the thrombus, or extent of thrombosis if thrombi are small, the preexisting condition of the pulmonary circulation and the nature of the thrombi. Rapid reduction of the cross-sectional area of the pulmonary arterial tree causes pulmonary hypertension and may lead to cor pulmonale and death.[544] This may be an acute event or may result from progressive obliteration of vessels, as when the lungs are continually showered from a chronically inflamed focus. These outcomes appear to be uncommon in horses, however. Because thrombophlebitis is a common iatrogenic

problem in horses, a higher incidence of circulatory compromise might be expected. Failure to observe such cases may reflect rapid removal of emboli, the size of emboli in relation to the cross-sectional area of the vascular tree, or ability of the right heart to sustain increased effort in the face of obstruction. Pulmonary infarction is not a consequence of pulmonary arterial embolism unless preexisting lung disease has already compromised bronchial artery supply to lung parenchyma.[545]

A more common potential consequence is pulmonary abscessation and pneumonia because emboli frequently are septic.[455,543] The extent to which pulmonary abscessation in adult horses is due to septic thromboembolism has not been investigated. Aneurysm formation and rupture also are a theoretical possibility in thromboembolism of the pulmonary artery.

Clinical signs of pulmonary embolism include persistent or recurrent fever when emboli are septic, though this may be difficult to ascribe to a putative pulmonary complication when the primary focus is still active. However, pulmonary abscessation may develop after the primary infected focus has been brought under control. Sudden showering of the lungs from a septic focus, such as an abscess, can result in toxic shock or sudden death. Extensive obstruction of pulmonary circulation could be expected to cause acute respiratory embarrassment because of circulation-perfusion mismatch, hypoxia and indications of cor pulmonale.

Idiopathic Diseases

Thrombosis

Aortoiliac Thrombosis: Aortoiliac thrombosis is a primary idiopathic thrombotic disease of the terminal aorta and its major branches. The condition is characterized clinically by exercise-associated lameness or stiffness that may appear only at high speeds and disappears with rest.[115] The condition is due to development of a primary thrombus at the aortic quadrifurcation with progressive secondary embolization of the vascular tree of the hind limbs or, alternatively, to development of fibrous intimal plaques with secondary local thrombosis.[342] Despite frequent reports of the problem in the literature, there is virtually no information on the natural history of the condition, which is probably subclinical until obstruction of arteries supplying muscles of the hind limbs occurs, after which clinical progression is seen. The disease usually follows a chronic course, though initial episodes of intimal damage, thrombus formation and embolization may be acute.

Aortoiliac thrombosis has been described in the veterinary literature since the mid-1800s and appears to have been a significant source of wastage.[115,546-558] It has been reported in most breeds and ages of horse. Early literature described the condition in a range of horses from army remounts to draft animals. Most reports in the more recent literature are in young performance animals.[115,342] The condition does not appear to have any geographic predilection. The apparent high frequency among racing breeds suggested by recent reports may be misleading and most likely reflects the probability of clinical signs becoming evident at an early stage in such animals rather than any particular breed predisposition. In many cases, progression of the condition is slow as long as work is maintained; animals never asked for maximal performance may never show clinical signs. Equally, young performance horses are more likely to be closely scrutinized if they develop lameness problems. Lesions have been identified as an incidental finding at necropsy.[342] The condition may go unnoticed in many animals, particularly mares. A clinical impression that faster, more promising colts are predisposed remains unconfirmed, as does the question of sex predilection.

Variation in postmortem findings leaves open the question of pathogenesis.[342,559,560] In some cases, the primary lesion appears to be the formation of a mural thrombus in the terminal aorta, just distal to the origin of the external iliac arteries; at the time that clinical signs secondary to peripheral embolism become evident, the aortic thrombus may or may not be present. The thrombus may be localized or may extend into 1 or more of the 4 iliac arteries, and usually forms on the dorsal wall of the aorta. The size of the thrombus does not necessarily bear any relationship to clinical signs, though severe cases may show total obstruction of the terminal aorta and all branches (Fig 57). Lameness almost invari-

ably is associated with peripheral embolism as pieces of the relatively friable thrombus break off. An embolus lodges most frequently at the bifurcation of the popliteal artery into the cranial and caudal tibial arteries.

In other cases, postmortem findings suggest possible multifocal thrombosis secondary to fibrous intimal plaques.[342] In such cases, the most mature lesions may be in the femoral or internal iliac arteries with limited changes in the aorta. In advanced cases, aortic lesions almost always are present. The severity of clinical signs depends upon the size of peripheral artery obstructed. Clinical experience suggests that sudden unaccustomed exercise or excessive

Figure 57. Diagrammatic representation of the vascular tree of the right hind limb.[342] The gray portions of the vessels show the extent of obstruction in a typical case of aortoiliac thrombosis in a 3-year-old Standardbred stallion. The horse had a 3-month history of exercise-associated hind limb lameness at presentation. A large thrombus at the aortic quadrifurcation (A) occupied 70% of the cross-sectional area of the vessel and extended several centimeters into each of the external iliac arteries (E), which were only partially obstructed. However, both femoral (F) and popliteal arteries were occluded from the origin of the femoral artery to the point of bifurcation of the popliteal into the tibial arteries (T). Obstruction of the internal iliac arteries (I) was total. Major collateral pathways are indicated.

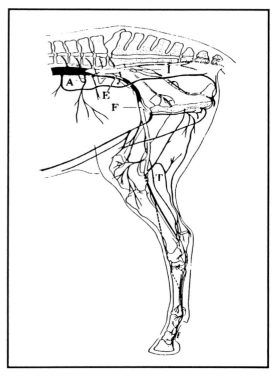

palpation of the aorta during rectal examination of the quadrifurcation may promote detachment of thrombi and sudden worsening of clinical signs.

Though many possible causes of the primary thrombosis have been suggested, including primary degenerative arterial disease, trauma, repeated distortion of the wall of the artery during locomotion, and parasitism, the cause remains undetermined.[342, 556,558-561] Part of the difficulty results from failure to diagnose cases sufficiently early. While irregularity of the aortic wall in the region of the quadrifurcation may be found as an incidental finding in the absence of thrombosis, isolated cases of thrombosis without embolism and suggestive of early development of aortoiliac thrombosis have not been described. This prompts the suggestion that development of a thrombus on the dorsal wall of the terminal aorta leads rapidly to clinical signs of embolism, *ie*, that the subclinical course is short, or that thrombus formation can occur and resolve spontaneously without embolism necessarily being a consequence.

Clinical signs of aortoiliac thrombosis have been described by numerous authors.[115,552,553,558,562] Initially, signs may be very subtle and affected horses commonly have been subjected to a range of diagnostic tests for hind limb/back lameness before attention is focused on the circulation.[115,563,564] If obstruction is confined to a small muscular artery (artery supplying muscle tissue), a slight roughness in the gait at maximal effort may be the only abnormality. As progressively larger areas of muscle become involved, the characteristic signs become evident.

Affected horse typically perform normally up to a "threshold" speed that varies with each case, at which point some stiffness in the affected limb becomes evident.[115,562,565] A tendency to drag the toe and occasionally to knuckle over may be seen. In mild cases, there may be no progression in degree of discomfort even if work is continued. Thoroughbreds may show a tendency to "bunny hop" and Standardbreds to break gait. If a severely affected horse is forced to continue working, it eventually loses the ability to move the limb, knuckles over frequently, stumbles and may go down. If exercise is stopped and the horse is rested, discomfort subsides rapidly and within 15-20 minutes the horse can work again. Other clinical signs include uncharacteristic irritability and a tendency to kick out with the hind limbs after exercise or to stamp a hind foot. The condition may involve one or both hind limbs, though almost invariably signs are asymmetric.

Clinical examination immediately after exercise usually reveals coolness of the hind limb and sometimes a regional absence of sweating. Reduced skin temperature is most evident around the gaskin. Even severely affected horses may appear warm to the touch over the proximal thigh because of warming during light exercise, while the temperature more distal on the leg in the cannon region is not consistent even in normal animals because of the influence of ambient temperature and moisture from the track surface. Failure to sweat is a somewhat undependable sign. It may be detected most easily in animals progressing fairly rapidly from warmup to the threshold speed, while asymmetry also may be of help in a horse showing signs predominantly in 1 hind limb. Though assymetry of muscle mass has been seen, in 21 horses I examined, this was rarely obvious, regardless of duration of the clinical problem.[115]

The only significant variation in this typical clinical picture involves horses that experience a sudden massive episode of thromboembolism, when the degree of arterial obstruction may be too great for adequate collateralization, causing muscle necrosis. Such horses are presented in acute distress, with severe hind limb lameness, firm swelling of muscle tissue, and crepitation upon palpation of the affected area. Such episodes appear to be an infrequent manifestation of the disease.[342]

Palpation of peripheral pulses is an important part of clinical examination and can be very useful in detecting the abnormality even in horses with only early signs.[563,564] The pulse in the hindquarters may be palpated at the coccygeal, saphenous, dorsal metatarsal and digital arteries (Fig 54) and normally is strong and double, with an easily discernible dicrotic notch. With aortoiliac thrombosis, the pulse contour distal to the site of the obstruction is flattened, weak and prolonged. Proximal to the level of obstruction, the pulse may be normal or increased, depending upon the degree and duration of occlusion. Asymmetry of pulses between the hind limbs also can be diagnostically useful.

Pulses should be palpated in the fully rested animal rather than after exercise, as wide fluctuation in pulse strength in response to temperature and exercise is found even in normal horses, while the digital pulse immediately after exercise is reduced in all horses. Because obstruction at the level of the stifle is the most frequent postmortem finding, a collateral pulse in the dorsal metatarsal and digital arteries and a normal or very full pulse in the saphenous artery is typical. However, many variations are found, as embolization can affect any vessel. Thus, for example, the internal iliac arteries may be totally occluded, leading to a loss of normal coccygeal pulse, while flow in the external iliac arteries and their branches may be normal. Also, discrete and localized obstruction of arteries supplying muscle may not alter palpable peripheral pulses.

Rate of filling of the saphenous vein immediately after exercise may reflect arterial obstruction.[115] This filling is measured by bringing the horse to a rapid halt after moderate to intense exercise and timing the rate at which the vein fills. The vein is not manipulated but is simply *observed*. It is collapsed in normal horses after intense exercise but fills within 10 seconds. In diseased horses, the time taken for filling depends upon the extent of arterial obstruction and can exceed 90 seconds. After trotting, the vein usually is full immediately upon coming to a halt but may take several seconds to fill in cases of aortoiliac thrombosis.

Rectal palpation to assess quality and strength of the pulse in major branches of the aorta frequently is valuable. Gentle pressure on vessels frequently reveals their firmness and lack of local pulse even when movement of the aorta transmitted to the branch suggests that a local pulse is present. Badly obstructed vessels may be greatly enlarged and hardened. Care should be taken to follow the major branches throughout their intrapelvic course because obstruction may be peripheral and the proximal pulse actually augmented by the obstruction. In some cases, there may be an aortic thrombus and peripheral thromboembolism but the actual iliac arteries themselves may be normal. Therefore, rectal palpation, while often very helpful, is by no means a definitive diagnostic technique, and rectal findings may require confirmation.

Diagnostic ultrasound, using a routine pregnancy diagnosis probe, can be very rewarding.[141,566,567] The technique is not as simple as one might expect, however, and imaging of normal horses is recommended to increase confidence in interpretation. Arteriography is definitive but requires specialized equipment and facilities (Fig 22). It is especially useful in early cases with minimal or no obstruction of iliac arteries or changes in peripheral pulses. In advanced cases, difficulty is encountered in catheterizing the terminal aorta because of obstruction of all accessible arteries. Advancement of a catheter into the abdominal aorta from the carotid artery precludes rapid injection of contrast medium because of the length of catheter necessary. In cases of partial obstruction, the saphenous artery may provide convenient access.

Clinical laboratory studies of aortoiliac thrombosis are of little diagnostic value. Muscle-derived enzyme activities do not become elevated after episodes of exercise-induced lameness, though these are elevated after acute episodes of thromboembolism-induced muscle necrosis.

Though cures in response to treatment with sodium gluconate have been claimed, the efficacy of the agent has not been confirmed and the diagnosis was not verified.[568-570] Histologic examination of tissue removed from affected horses would suggest that a therapeutic response is highly improbable. By analogy with similar conditions in people, surgical replacement of affected vessels would appear the only option by the time the condition is confirmed; this is not feasible in horses at this time.

Regardless of the possible role of *S vulgaris*, the maturity of lesions found at necropsy suggests that deworming is not likely to help. The only management approach found to be of value is to maintain exercise, as long as this is not causing the animal serious discomfort. Collateral flow is thereby stimulated and maintained. Because of the danger that collateral flow will subside, with resultant worsening of clinical signs, affected horses should *not* be confined to a stall but instead turned out if they are not to be kept in work.

The prognosis and clinical course of aortoiliac thrombosis cases depend greatly upon what the animal is used for, how much exercise it is getting, the rate and circumstances under which pieces of thrombus detach, and the size of vessels obstructed. Mildly affected horses may show very slow clinical deterioration as long as they are kept in steady work. In other cases, deterioration has been rapid, with horses becoming incapable of jogging in a matter of weeks. Acute events associated with episodes of thromboembolism may be superimposed upon an otherwise progressive picture, and the clinical course may thus appear irregular. In any degree, the condition is not compatible with race-intensity exercise. In stallions, infertility may result from obstruction of spermatic arteries or shunting of blood away from these vessels.[571]

Postmortem findings vary according to extent of obstruction and age of lesions.[342,] [559,560] It is as yet undetermined whether there is any proportionality between duration of the clinical syndrome and extent of arterial occlusion. In early and mild cases, the problem may be restricted to a thrombus at the quadrifurcation and thromboembolic obstruction of the popliteal artery at its bifurcation into the tibial arteries, at the level of the stifle. Alternatively, there may be local thrombosis overlying fibrous intimal plaques at various levels in the arterial tree, particularly the femoral artery, with narrowing of the vessel lumen. At least partial obstruction of the branches of one or both internal iliac arteries also is found typically, promoting the idea of embolic cause for peripheral lesions in many cases.

In more advanced cases, there are varying degrees of obstruction of the major branches of all 4 iliac arteries, while in some cases the terminal aorta also is totally occluded (Figs 57, 58). In such cases, the thrombus may extend throughout much of the vascular tree of the hind limb to the level of small muscular arteries (Fig 59). Collateral flow is maintained by anastomoses between the thoracic arteries and caudal superficial and deep epigastrics, the middle artery of the penis and pudendoepigastric trunk, and caudal mesenteric and cranial rectal arteries and the pudendoepigastric trunk. In mares, the ovarian and uterine arteries probably make a very significant contribution to collateral flow. While some mural thrombosis of major arteries may be observed with blood flowing past partial obstructions, occlusion more frequently is centripetal and complete. Postmortem examination has demonstrated no consistent relationship with lesions of parasitic arteritis or aortitis, and parasites have not been observed in thrombi in any of the horses I have examined.

DISEASES OF VEINS

P.W. Physick-Sheard

Diseases With Physical Causes

Rupture of Veins

Rupture of veins is not common because of the low venous pressure and the thin,

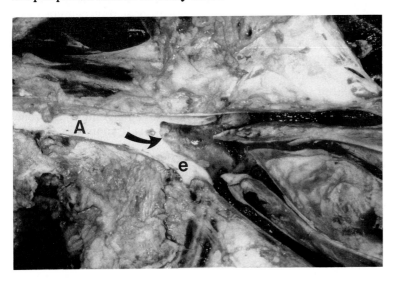

Figure 58. Dissection of the aortic quadrifurcation of a 4-year-old Standardbred gelding. The animal had a history of lameness at fast work for several weeks before presentation. At the time of necropsy the horse had been at pasture for 2 months. The aorta (A) is occluded at its quadrifurcation by a mature thrombus (arrow). The thrombus extends into both external (e) and internal iliac arteries. (Courtesy of Dr. M.G. Maxie)

flexible nature of the wall. The vessel usually yields when subjected to external pressure. However, rupture does occur and may reflect direct trauma, venous hypertension or preexisting disease of the wall of the vein.[321,325,524,526,572,573] Tearing because of tension during hyperextension has been postulated as a cause of rupture of the portal vein in horses.[524] Portal vein rupture also may occur intraoperatively during correction of epiploic foramen entrapment.[574] Spontaneous rupture may occur during exercise and is a possible factor in cases of sudden death.

Because veins are thin-walled and not always easily identified in a body cavity filled with blood, many venous ruptures may be missed and the problem may be the underlying factor in some cases of body cavity hemorrhage of unknown etiology.[322] Rupture of veins is too sporadic for any pattern to be identified, and no consistent etiologic factors emerge from review of published cases.

Multifactorial Diseases

Arteriovenous Anastomosis

Direct communication between an artery and a vein without an interposing capillary network is referred to as arteriovenous anastomosis. The communication may be direct (aneurysmal varix) or via a communicating sac. The lesion may be congenital or acquired.[575-577] The problem is not common in horses but, because it can be acquired secondary to traumatic venipuncture and can lead to heart failure and spontaneous venous rupture, the clinician should be aware of the condition.

Clinical signs vary according to the vessels involved. A fluctuating swelling may be anticipated where aneurysmal dilatation of the vein develops, and palpation may reveal a distinct thrill.[576] The intensity of the vibration may vary with changing body position and may not be constant. Heart failure results if the anastomosis allows a large volume of blood to shunt from the arterial to the venous side of the circulation, causing constant high cardiac output and subsequent high-output failure. In a performance horse, the reduction in cardiac reserve may be significant with even a small shunt as systemic arterial pressure rises with exer-

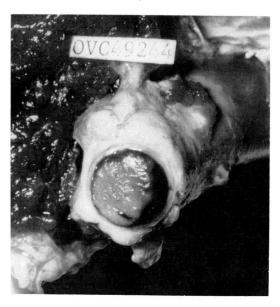

Figure 59. Right femoral artery of a 5-year-old Standardbred gelding. The artery is totally occluded by a thrombus that showed fibrous organization and vascularization adjacent to the vessel wall on microscopic examination. The thrombus was laminated. The smooth muscle of the arterial media showed patchy necrosis. (Courtesy of Dr. M.G. Maxie)

cise. Correction of the problem involves ligation of the communicating structure or of the artery supplying the shunt.

Thrombosis

Phlebothrombosis (thrombosis of veins) occurs all too frequently in horses, most often in the jugular veins, where the problem usually is iatrogenic and frequently associated with inflammation or phlebitis. Venous obstruction can only be directly assessed if the vein is superficial and/or palpable but may be inferred with thrombosis of a large vein by venous engorgement and edema in distal tissues. Phlebothrombosis in the absence of phlebitis is manifested as a firm, filled and relatively obvious vein. Thrombosis may be localized with venous stasis distally or the entire vein may be thrombosed.

Early formation of a thrombus may be detectable by careful palpation. With inflammation, the vein is hot and painful, and frequently there is perivenous reaction as well as inflammation of the vein itself. If the problem is the result of perivenous injection of an irritant solution, as occasionally occurs with jugular venipuncture, extensive cellulitis may obliterate the vessel.

Potential sequelae of venous thrombosis include edematous swelling of distal tissues and thromboembolism of the pulmonary circulation. The former is likely only if a large vein is involved, as smaller veins are subject to extensive anastomosis. When the thrombus is secondary to septic endocarditis, septicemia and pulmonary abscessation are all potential complications.

Iatrogenic thrombophlebitis of the jugular vein is the most common cause of venous thrombosis in horses. Thrombosis of veins is otherwise sporadic. Venous thrombosis may occur in any animal with consumptive coagulopathy, especially in vessels subject to trauma or sluggish flow.[544,578] Venous thrombosis has been described in horses with aortoiliac thrombosis, as has thrombosis of the caudal vena cava secondary to traumatic duodenitis.[115,579]

Spontaneous venous thrombosis, frequently accompanied by inflammation, can be particularly troublesome in some toxic horses. The nature of the disease processes and circumstances associated with this observation (postoperative colic, septic pleurisy and colitis) and clinical signs suggest endotoxemia, though presumably other toxins could be involved. Venous thrombosis follows even the most minor, atraumatic venipuncture, regardless of the size of the vein, while jugular veins can thrombose totally within hours of catheterization. Pregnant or recently foaled mares appear particularly prone to this complication. Though no controlled study of the processes involved has been performed, clinical evaluation at the Ontario Veterinary College has revealed significantly depressed plasma antithrombin III levels and prolonged activated thrombin clotting times in such cases, suggesting coagulopathy. Treatment with plasma appears to be beneficial.

If thrombosis cannot be diagnosed by palpation or diagnostic ultrasound, angiography may be attempted. Treatment of simple thrombosis may be attempted by surgical removal of the thrombus, but this rarely is necessary. Removal of the primary insult, if possible, and symptomatic treatment of edematous swelling usually are adequate. Collateral drainage usually develops over several days, and recanalization, especially of a localized thrombus, occurs frequently.

In severe cases, the result of this process may be multiple communicating channels rather than a single vessel.

Iatrogenic Jugular Thrombophlebitis

G.H. Spurlock

Thrombophlebitis is a relatively common sequela of intravenous catheterization.[401, 541,580,581] The reported incidence in people is 2-35% of catheterized veins, often reflecting differences in definition of thrombophlebitis.[582,583] The incidence in horses has been estimated to be as high as 50%.[584] Given the increasing technology of critical care and resultant increased use of intravenous catheters, it is clear that thrombophlebitis is a significant problem.

Cause: Thrombophlebitis results from mechanical trauma to the vein by the catheter and from chemical irritation of the vein by the infusate.[582] It is promoted by endotoxemia. Bacterial colonization of the catheter undoubtedly plays a role, though it remains unclear whether it is an opportunistic or causative involvement.

Mechanical trauma is related to the catheter composition, length and diameter in relation to the vein.[585,586] The ability of various catheter materials to incite inflammation and thrombosis has been compared and ranked in order of decreasing irritation, as follows: polypropylene, polyethylene, polytetrafluoroethylene, silicone rubber, nylon, polyvinyl chloride, polyurethane.[587] Commercially available polytetrafluoroethylene (Abbo Cath-T: Abbott), polyurethane (L-Cath: Luther Medical Products), and silicone rubber catheters (Centrasil: Baxter) have been studied in horses.[542] The rank order was similar to that previously reported with the exception that the polyurethane catheter incited slightly more inflammation than the silicone rubber catheter.

Softness of the catheter material seems to be paramount in minimizing inflammation and thrombus formation (Fig 60). Endothelial damage occurs wherever the catheter contacts the vein (Fig 61).[585] Stiffer catheter materials contact the vessel wall along most of their length, promoting development of thrombophlebitis, while soft catheters, such as silicone rubber, appear to float freely in the bloodstream, reducing the endothelial trauma.[588] Increasing the catheter length or diameter, particularly of the stiffer catheters, increases the incidence of thrombophlebitis.[586] This effect is offset somewhat by the greater disparity between diameter of the vessel and the catheter in large veins. Rapid dilution of potentially irritating solutions by blood flow in larger veins reduces chemical trauma to the endothelium.

Thrombophlebitis also occurs as a sequel to perivascular injection of irritating medications.[541] This is among the most common reasons for malpractice claims against veterinarians. It can be prevented by proper restraint, good lighting, dampening or clipping of long hair, raising the jugular vein so it can be identified, and placing the needle accurately and directly into the vein. During the injection, the position of the needle can be confirmed by a free flow of blood if the syringe is detached and the vein occluded, or by aspiration with the attached syringe. If a perivascular injection occurs,

Figure 60. A jugular vein catheterized with a soft silicone rubber catheter for 14 days has a short fibrin sleeve (arrow). The endothelium is intact.

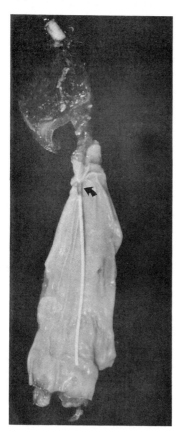

Figure 61. A jugular vein catheterized with a relatively stiff polytetrafluoroethylene catheter for 14 days has endothelial erosions (small arrows) and extensive perivascular inflammation (large arrow).

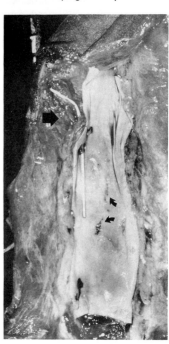

the needle should be left in position and the perivascular medication diluted (6-10 times the amount estimated to have been outside the vein) by infusing saline through the needle.

Rapid or repeated injection of irritating solutions into a vein also can result in thrombophlebitis. Medications most frequently incriminated include phenylbutazone, thiobarbiturates, sulfa solutions, chloral hydrate and tetracycline solutions. Diluting such medications first or injecting them slowly helps minimize this complication. When multiple treatments are anticipated, consideration should be given to alternative routes of administration or use of an intravenous catheter to provide a secure venous access.

Clinical Signs: Clinical signs associated with thrombophlebitis include pain, localized or generalized swelling and a thickened cord-like vein on palpation.[401] Affected horses frequently are febrile and reluctant to move their neck. The degree of vascular compromise varies; total occlusion of the vein results in venous congestion and swelling proximal to the occlusion. Circulation through collateral veins usually resolves this congestion over several days. Purulent material draining from the site of skin penetration is evidence of infection; however, this is not always evident with septic thrombophlebitis. The infection may be limited to the subcutaneous catheter tract or extend into the vein. Expressing the vein toward the catheter insertion may expel purulent exudate from the site of skin penetration, confirming its involvement. Septicemia with periodic fever spikes and general depression usually accompanies septic thrombophlebitis. Bilateral jugular thrombophlebitis is a particularly serious complication. Lack of sufficient collateral venous circulation often results in swelling of the head and respiratory distress.[583]

Treatment: Thrombophlebitis is best managed by prevention. If it occurs, elimination of the inciting cause, usually a catheter, is paramount for successful treatment. Catheters should be removed at the earliest onset of pain, swelling, purulent discharge or palpable thickening of the vein. Delaying removal significantly increases the severity of disease, which may still progress after catheter removal.[589] Dimethyl sulfoxide, applied topically for its antiinflammatory effect and for the exothermic reaction following its application, seems to reduce the pain associated with thrombophlebitis. Oral nonsteroidal antiinflammatory drugs are indicated for relief of pain.

Shedding of bacteria and emboli typically results in periodic fever spikes, with accompanying depression. Aggressive antibiotic therapy is mandatory to prevent the serious consequences of septicemia. Bacterial culture and sensitivity tests should be performed on blood samples, the catheter tip, exudate from the skin penetration site, or a fine-needle aspirate obtained from the vein. Long-term antibiotic administration (4-6 weeks) is indicated for septic thrombophlebitis. Surgical removal of the septic vein has been performed in refractory cases.[541] Aseptic thrombophlebitis usually resolves following 2-4 weeks of symptomatic treatment. Recanalization occurs to some extent in most veins, though months often are required for this to occur.[541]

Preventing catheter-related thrombophlebitis requires recognition of the inciting factors and strict adherence to good management techniques that minimize their impact. Catheter selection is based on the anticipated needs of the patient. Large-volume fluid therapy requires a large-bore catheter; these are available commercially only in the stiffer materials, such as polypropylene and polytetrafluoroethylene. Stiff materials will cause significant trauma to the vein in as little as 48-72 hours. Therefore, it is prudent to remove them at 48-hour intervals and rotate the catheter to an alternate venous site. When volume replacement is not necessary, the less thrombogenic, softer catheters made of silicone rubber or polyurethane should be used. These can be safely used for several weeks if inserted carefully and maintained.[542]

The more experienced the person performing the catheterization, the lower the incidence of complications.[590] Strict adherence to aseptic technique is mandatory for proper placement. This should include an adequate surgical scrub of the patient's skin (5 minutes with a iodophor disinfectant) and wearing of sterile gloves.[589] Once the catheter is inserted, it must be firmly anchored to the skin with sutures. Any motion of the catheter greatly increases trauma to the vein.[591] To-and-fro motion of the catheter also may "seed" the subcutaneous tissue with bacteria, thus increasing the risk of septic thrombophlebitis. The skin penetration site may be dressed with an appropriate topical antiseptic ointment and covered with a nonocclusive dressing in an attempt to reduce this complication. Manipulation of the catheter at its entry point may be reduced by use of venous extension tubing. The injection port should be cleaned with alcohol before puncture.

DISEASES OF THE ENDOCARDIUM AND VALVES

P.W. Physick-Sheard

Diagnostic and Therapeutic Considerations

Acquired Diseases of the Mural Endocardium

There are no common acquired diseases of the mural (nonvalvular) endocardium in horses. In an extensive postmortem study of 1557 horses examined at an abattoir, lesions of the heart were found in 381 or

24.5%.[116,160] Of these, 27 were described as nonvalvular endocardial "jet" lesions, which were intense localized fibrous thickenings seen in areas of turbulence, secondary to valvular disease. The cause of these lesions is assumed to be endothelial damage, with secondary platelet and fibrin adhesion. Examples include fibrous thickening of the septal cusp of the right AV valve in ventricular septal defects shunting blood from left to right, fibrous ridges in the left ventricular outflow tract opposite defective cusps in cases of aortic insufficiency, and fibrous thickening and roughening of the atrial endocardium due to regurgitant jets of blood in AV insufficiency (Fig 62).[350,592-594] The lesions are of limited clinical significance unless they involve valve cusps and lead to progressive scarring and distortion. Thus, regurgitant flow from an aortic insufficiency may damage the septal cusp of the left AV valve, while the shunt flow across a ventricular septal defect may lead to severe distortion of the septal cusp of the right AV valve and secondary insufficiency.

Diffuse fibrosis may be observed subendocardially in chambers subjected to prolonged overload and dilatation. The role that this fibrosis may play in the syndrome of failure is unclear. In examining the heart at necropsy, care should be used in making this interpretation, as the endocardium of the left atrium and ventricle is thicker and paler than that of the right side in normal animals. Calcification of the endocardium may be observed occasionally in horses with extensive mineralization of arteries or subendocardial fibrosis.[455] Extensive endocardial and myocardial calcification were described in 3 horses with suspected exposure to hay containing a vitamin D analogue.[595] Endocardial and valvular calcification also has been associated with splenic lymphosarcoma and pseudohyperparathyroidism.[596]

Endocarditis most often forms initially on the heart valves, from which it may extend to involve adjacent endocardium. Primary mural involvement, which would not necessarily be associated with evidence of valvular dysfunction, also may be seen.

Acquired Diseases of Heart Valves

With the exception of a study published in 1971, the prevalence of valvular abnormalities in horses and the relationship between those lesions and abnormal heart sounds has not been subjected to systematic examination.[116,152,160] Similarly, the natural history of lesions observed and their clinical implications represent essentially unresolved issues.[597] The study referred to above is biased because the population examined comprised horses sent to an abattoir for slaughter, and thus contained a high proportion of mature animals.

Reviewing findings in published clinical cases is unsatisfactory because such a group is highly selected and not necessarily representative of the general population. In these studies, diagnostic methods and criteria vary; so does the terminology used to describe abnormal heart sounds. There also is a wide variation in type and use of the

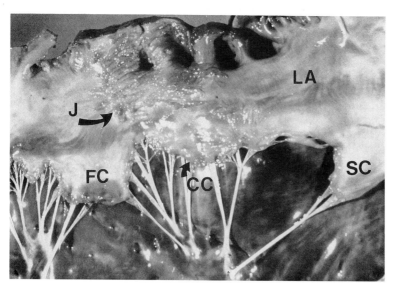

Figure 62. Extensive endocardial thickenings (jet lesions, J) on the endocardium of the left atrium (LA) in a horse with chronic left AV insufficiency. The valvular changes promoting the insufficiency involved primarily the left commissural cusp (CC), which was thickened and shortened. The septal (SC) and free wall (FC) cusps showed minimal changes. The jet lesions extend in a broad band above the commissural cusp.

horses described. Published clinical cases may reflect bias in the interests of the authors, as most reports concentrate on specific valvular abnormalities rather than reviewing all cases observed. However, these sources, combined with clinical experience, represent the only available guidance in interpreting murmurs.

Therefore, it must be remembered that the interpretations herein are based upon limited information and do not necessarily reflect the circumstances in the equine population with which an individual clinician works. The clinical scenarios presented below under discussion of diseases of the individual valves should not be taken to preclude the existence of other clinical circumstances of equal significance.

General Observations: The results of an abattoir study in which the hearts of 1557 horses were examined are shown in Table 8, together with the diagnoses reported in 22 papers published since 1966.[116,152,160] The papers reviewed considered only horses in which clinical signs (in addition to a murmur) caused the animal to be presented for examination. Signs included evidence of heart failure and limited exercise tolerance or a tendency to fade. The diagnosis was confirmed by necropsy and/or echocardiography in all but a small number of animals. Each event recorded in Table 8 represents a valvular lesion rather than a horse. Some horses had involvement of more than 1 valve, and numbers quoted are thus slightly greater than the actual number of horses affected. The series does not include cases in which the primary diagnosis was endocarditis or congenital heart disease. In comparing the 2 data sets, it must be remembered that cases in the general literature were presented with clinical signs, whereas those in the abattoir study usually showed no obvious clinical signs and the history was unavailable.

The frequencies revealed in the 2 approaches are consistent, with the exception that the relative incidence of left AV and aortic valve lesions is reversed. This difference may indicate that lesions of AV valves are more likely to lead to clinical signs of heart failure and/or arrhythmia. Lesions of the aortic valve associated with a systolic as opposed to a diastolic murmur, on the other hand, seem to be infrequently associated with clinical consequences. There appears

to be a very low incidence of pulmonic valve involvement.

The left heart was about 3 (clinically) to 8 times (abattoir survey) more likely to be involved than the right, a difference attributed to the greater valvular trauma likely to occur in the left heart because of higher blood pressure.[116] Increased involvement of the right heart in clinical cases is entirely a result of the frequency of right AV insufficiencies. Changes in the left AV valve occurred about twice as often as changes in the right AV valve. The abattoir study suggested that right AV valve lesions also are much less extensive than those on the left. In a subset of the clinical cases in which horses exhibited atrial fibrillation, the frequency of involvement of AV, as opposed to outflow, valves increased greatly.[162]

For all valves, older horses had a much greater chance of having *lesions*. Though for semilunar valves, even young horses showed a high frequency of involvement (>18% studied).[116] Clinically, however, young horses appeared to be as susceptible as older horses, while some types of valve-related disease, such as syndrome of acute left AV insufficiency, seemed more likely to occur in young horses (see below). Horses often exercised intensely (Thoroughbreds and hunters) had a higher incidence of lesions, though this may reflect bias in the selection of cases, as such animals are more likely to be evaluated thoroughly and asked to perform at a level that would reveal a cardiac abnormality. Also, no accurate and relevant population data on the distribution of breeds are available for comparison.

The prevalence of valvular abnormalities in the general equine population, as opposed to distribution of lesions within affected horses, is not obvious. Of 1557 horses examined in the abattoir survey, 381 (25%) had cardiac lesions, with 93.4% of those having valvular changes detectable grossly. One of the difficulties in evaluating postmortem studies of the incidence of valvular lesions is variation in degree to which valves are inspected and in definition of a lesion. In the abattoir study, many horses were aged. Some pathologists may regard examples of slight thickening of valve margins as a "normal" age-related change in the absence of other signs of valve dysfunction, such as jet lesions or chamber dilatation. Because a murmur is no consistent guide to the presence of a valvular lesion, studies that comment upon the incidence of murmurs can give a false impression of the incidence of endocardial disease.[152,597,598]

In most cases, however, the only indication that a valve defect *may* be present is a murmur. The index of suspicion is increased if other signs of cardiovascular dysfunction are present. All of the horses described in published clinical cases exhibited murmurs with characteristics that generally were consistent with the valvular abnormality revealed by postmortem or echocardiographic examination. However, in the abattoir study, which included horses with murmurs and no lesions and others with lesions and no murmurs, correlation with auscultatory evidence of valve dysfunction was obscured both by the conditions under which auscultation was done (making accurate auscultation difficult) and by the decision of the authors to select cases for inclusion in the discussion of findings made upon auscultation.[152] Horses with valve lesions and no murmurs thus were underrepresented.

Diastolic murmurs tended to be associated with lesions, usually of the aortic valve, and occasionally of the left AV valve. Softer and early systolic murmurs tended to be benign or associated with minimal lesions, whereas loud murmurs and those that were pansystolic or radiated widely were more frequently associated with significant lesions, including distortion of valves by fibrous tissue and involvement of more than 1 valve. Though the point of maximum intensity of most murmurs, together with their timing and character, gave some insight into the possible underlying origin of the sound, the associations were by no means consistent, especially with regard to the pattern of radiation of a murmur. In particular, multiple valve involvement in horses exhibiting both systolic and diastolic murmurs can cause significant diagnostic difficulty.[152] This emphasizes the importance of the history and results of general physical and cardiovascular examination in interpretation, both of cause and of clinical significance. Abnormal sounds cannot be used as a totally reliable guide to structural change. Each case must be evaluated on its merits, as few dependable patterns of association can be used to guide the clinician.

Congenital and Familial Diseases

Endocardial Fibroelastosis

Endocardial fibroelastosis consists of diffuse endocardial thickening of 1 or more

Table 8. Distribution of valve lesions in horses.

Valve Affected/Diagnosis	Clinical Cases[a]		Abattoir Survey[b]
	Number[c]	Percent[d]	Percent[d]
Left AV insufficiency	89	43.4	18.4
Left AV insufficiency	(88)		
Left AV stenosis	(1)		
Right AV valve	38	19.4	8.0
Right AV insufficiency	(35)		
Right AV stenosis	(3)		
Aortic valve	69	35.2	70.7
Aortic insufficiency	(59)		
Aortic stenosis	(10)		
Pulmonic valve	4	2.0	3.0
Pulmonic insufficiency	(1)		
Pulmonic stenosis	(3)		

a – Breakdown of diagnoses made in 22 papers published between 1966 and 1989, in which cases of heart valve disease in horses were described. Diagnosis was confirmed by postmortem and/or echocardiography in most cases. Sources are cited in discussion of the appropriate valve in the text.
b – References 116, 152, 160. See text.
c – Numbers refer to valve affected rather than subjects. Most horses had only one valve involved.
d – Percent of total valves affected.

cardiac chambers by collagenous and elastic tissue. It may occur as an isolated lesion or with other congenital abnormalities.[422] The true nature of this condition is the subject of considerable debate, and its status as a congenital abnormality is open to question in some species.[455] This is because it may be detected only several months or years after birth. Some investigators believe that in many cases the lesion is secondary to a range of congenital or acquired factors, including chamber overload, rather than a primary congenital abnormality.

While endocardial thickening does occur as a consequence of chronic chamber overload, the lesion is primarily fibrous in nature. In endocardial fibroelastosis, extensive elastic tissue is laid down in parallel layers and the thickening becomes particularly marked. The endocardium is dense and milky white, and may have a granular appearance. Trabeculae carneae are emphasized (Fig 63). Chordae tendineae may be thickened, and thickening and incompetence of the AV valve may be present. The lesion may be unilateral or bilateral and of a dilated or contracted type. In people, the dilated type with isolated involvement of the left ventricle is most common.[422] Affected individuals have a poor life expectancy; the cause of death is congestive heart failure. Postmortem findings include marked cardiomegaly, with hypertrophy and marked dilatation of the left ventricle. Left atrial involvement may be present.

Endocardial fibroelastosis has been diagnosed in only 2 horses, in addition to the case presented in Figure 63.[365] Both horses were over 2 years of age and both died suddenly. Both showed predominantly ventricular septal endocardial involvement and no obvious ventricular dilatation or other cardiac lesions. Systemic signs were those of acute heart failure. It was suggested that involvement of Purkinje fibers in the endocardial process was a possible cause of death. In a case observed by the author, signs of weight loss, poor growth rate, lethargy and atrial fibrillation were observed in an 8-month-old Thoroughbred filly. A murmur indicative of left AV insufficiency was detected on the left side, and clinical and radiologic examination revealed severe cardiomegaly. During 3 weeks of observation, signs of congestive heart failure developed and the filly became progressively weaker.

At necropsy, the heart was greatly enlarged and the endocardium of the left ventricle was thickened and pale yellow, and had firm white corrugations running across the surface (Fig 63). The left AV valve was thickened and there was left atrial dilatation and endocardial thickening. Atrial endocardial jet lesions were present. The extensive additional lesions present in this animal reflected left AV insufficiency and subsequent arrhythmia and chronic failure. Critical examination of endocardial changes in hearts of young animals dying with signs of heart failure and in cases of sudden death appears indicated so as to avoid missing this particular abnormality.

Congenital Abnormalities of Heart Valves

The human medical literature describes numerous types of congenital valvular abnormalities.[422] Abnormalities of valves occur both as isolated findings and as components of complex congenital cardiac disease (Table 4). In horses, however, isolated congenital abnormalities of heart valves are uncommon. This section deals only with isolated congenital valvular disease and those complex conditions in which valve changes represent a major component of the anomaly, as found in domestic animals. It should be noted that this is an anatomic arrangement of convenience and does not necessarily follow a pattern considerate of morphogenesis.

Tricuspid Atresia: The complex of tricuspid atresia consists of atresia (absence) of the right AV orifice, right ventricular hypoplasia, and an atrial septal defect.[422] Additionally there is communication between the systemic and pulmonary circulations. Of 13 equine cases reported, this always has taken the form of a ventricular septal defect. Additionally, patent ductus arteriosus was present in 4 cases.[362,413,414,599] The defect in the atrial septum has been described as a patent foramen ovale by some authors.[320,362,368,413,599] However, atrial septal defect is a more appropriate term because the opening in the interatrial septum usually is several centimeters in diameter and occasionally is heavily fenestrated.[129,414,418,600-602] The atrial septal defect represents the only available route for venous blood returning from the systemic circulation. Abnormalities of the right heart outflow tract sometimes also are present.[362,368,414] Various degrees of right atrial and left ventricular hypertrophy and dilatation also exist as secondary consequences of the primary defects.

The functional consequences of the anomaly depend upon the particular combination of defects present. Blood returning from the systemic circulation crosses the atrial septal defect into the left atrium, mixing with oxygenated blood from the lungs and constituting a right-to-left shunt. Blood reaches the lungs by crossing the ventricular septal defect, traversing the hypoplastic right ventricle and exiting via the pulmonary artery. With significant pulmonic stenosis, persistence of the ductus arteriosus is essential to allow blood to reach the lungs if the anomaly is to be compatible with extra-uterine life.[362] Ages of affected animals have ranged from a premature foal to a pony 1 year old at the time of diagnosis, though most have been foals that were symptomatic from birth and were destroyed.[601,602]

Clinical signs include poor growth rate, lethargy, severely limited exercise tolerance and cyanosis. An intense, pansystolic, shunt-type murmur is usually present, with a point of maximum intensity at the left heart base. The precise character and location of the murmur may vary according to the combination of defects present; a diastolic component may be noted. Differential diagnoses include any congenital anomaly with a right-to-left shunt and flow distur-

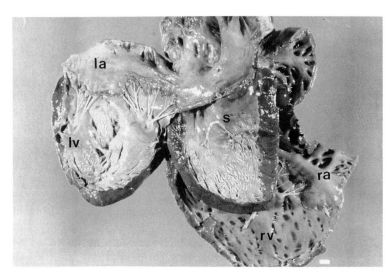

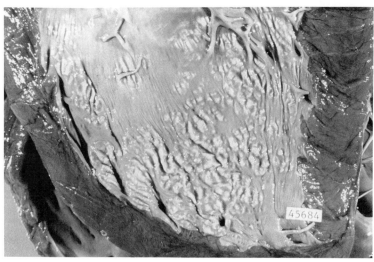

Figure 63. Endocardial fibro-elastosis in an 8-month-old Thoroughbred foal with lethargy, poor growth and signs of heart failure. Atrial fibrillation was detected on clinical examination. Top: Endocardial involvement is only of the left ventricle and is most severe over the interventricular septum, though dilatation of both ventricles was found at necropsy. (la = left atrium. lv = left ventricle. s = septum viewed from left. ra = right atrium. rv = right ventricle.) Bottom: On the left side of the septum the endocardium is thickened and opaque, and shows numerous coarse, white, calcified ridges. Similar endocardial changes may be encountered with chronic chamber overload.

bance beneath the outflow tracts, such as tetralogy of Fallot and persistent truncus arteriosus. The diagnosis cannot be based on clinical signs alone. Blood gas analysis helps confirm hypoxemia but cannot differentiate the different possible causes. Echocardiography and contrast studies can provide a definitive diagnosis, though the results may be confusing to those not entirely familiar with 3-dimensional anatomy of the heart.[320,368] Angiocardiography and catheterization studies also can be applied in an attempt to refine the diagnosis and render a prognosis.[129,362] However, the results may be largely of academic interest, as the prognosis is uniformly poor.

Other Congenital Atrioventricular Valve Abnormalities: With the exception of tricuspid atresia, congenital abnormalities of AV valves appear to be particularly rare in horses. When lesions are found, they are most often part of complex cardiac anomalies, particularly endocardial cushion defects, or are secondary to other congenital lesions. Dysplasia of the right and left AV valves has been observed in a case of atrial septal defect with hypoplastic right heart, in which failure of endocardial cushions to fuse normally was associated with failure of the interatrial ostium primum to close and formation of a cleft in the septal cusp of the left AV valve.[603] Concurrent dysplasia of the right AV valve may have had a separate cause. Congenital stenosis of the left AV valve has been described in a horse with Lutembacher's syndrome (atrial septal defect with left AV stenosis).[604]

Right AV insufficiency in a horse with ventricular septal defect was assumed to be secondary to impingement on the valve of shunt flow through the defect and scarring of the valve.[592] Left AV fibrosis and insufficiency have been associated with congenital absence of aortic origin of the left coronary artery in a yearling.[418] Left AV valve atresia was identified together with aortic atresia as a component of hypoplastic left ventricular syndrome in a 2-day-old foal.[365]

Congenital Aortic Insufficiency: Two cases are described in the literature in which clinical signs and postmortem findings led to a diagnosis of congenital aortic insufficiency. In 1, the diagnosis was made in a yearling Arabian filly with a history of chronic weight loss and debility.[363] Reexamination 1 year later revealed exertio-

nal dyspnea, ventral edema and other signs of cardiac decompensation. A combination of murmurs was detected, including an ejection murmur at the left apex and holosystolic and diastolic murmurs at the left heart base. Postmortem examination led to diagnoses of left and right AV and aortic insufficiencies. In the second case, a holodiastolic murmur in a yearling was ascribed to aortic insufficiency.[605] The diagnosis was confirmed by echocardiography and postmortem examination.

The abnormalities described in these horses did not differ greatly from those observed in an abattoir study, in which bandlike aortic valve lesions were detected even in young horses.[116,160] Fenestrations of the aortic valve observed in the second horse have been seen by others and their significance questioned.[593,597,605,606]

Whether aortic insufficiency occurs as an isolated congenital abnormality in horses remains open to question. Insufficiency sometimes accompanies defects in the bulbar or conal interventricular septum. A lack of support for the base of the valve causes the right coronary cusp to prolapse during diastole.

Other Congenital Abnormalities of Outflow Valves

Though aortic or pulmonic stenosis (subvalvular, valvular and supravalvular) are recognized as congenital abnormalities in other species, these have not been identified as isolated findings in horses.[190,308] Pulmonic stenosis is seen in complex cardiac defects and occurs in tetralogy of Fallot, in tricuspid atresia and hypoplastic right ventricle and atrial septal defect.[129,362,368, 398,414,416,431,603] The anomaly also has been associated with patent ductus arteriosus and right AV stenosis and in a ventricular septal defect in which the valve was also bicuspid.[129,361]

Aortic stenosis (narrowing of the aortic orifice) has not been identified as a congenital lesion in horses. Distortion of the right coronary cusp of the aortic valve was seen with ventricular septal defect in a 7-year-old gelding.[607] The question of whether this was a congenital lesion or secondary to the ventricular septal defect was left open. Aortic atresia (absence of an aortic orifice) has been described once in association with left AV atresia and hypoplastic left ventricle.[365]

Infectious, Inflammatory and Immune Diseases

Endocarditis

Endocarditis is an inflammation of the endocardium. It may be acute or subacute, bacterial or nonbacterial, valvular or mural (nonvalvular). The significance of these terms is explained below. Over 80 equine cases have been described since 1943, though the clinical condition is considered to be sporadic and uncommon in horses.[608] In an abattoir study of 1577 horses, in which some selection for aged and diseased horses may be anticipated, only 2 cases of vegetative endocarditis were encountered out of a total of 447 horses with cardiovascular lesions.[116] The readiness with which endocarditis is reported may reflect the sometimes spectacular nature of postmortem findings and the very definitive nature of the lesion. The extent to which chronic cases of valvular dysfunction reflect previous, healed lesions of endocarditis, however, is undetermined, and mild cases may escape detection.

Endocarditis may be as common in young animals as in adults.[321,608-614] A sex predisposition has been suggested.[608] Of cases in the literature in which sex is given (19 animals), 79% were males. The reason for this predisposition is unclear. Endocarditis does not appear to be consistently associated with any particular clinical entity, is not a frequent complication of thrombophlebitis and may develop with no current or past history of a septic focus.

Cause: Numerous theories have been put forward to account for the development of lesions of endocardial inflammation and infection.[455,615-618] Current concepts favor some form of initial endocardial damage. In this scenario, various agents, including turbulent blood flow, stress and hypersensitivity reactions, cause damage to the endothelium and/or valve substance.[616] Platelet adhesion and fibrin formation follow and may lead to nonbacterial thrombotic endocarditis, in which shallow ulcerations form on the valve margins. Lesions thought to be equivalent to this pathologic entity in people also have been described in horses.[593] These form most frequently on the valve surfaces that come into apposition during ventricular systole. Bacterial colonization of these lesions results in bacterial endocarditis. Factors promoting bacterial adhesion include pathogenicity (serious pathogens with ability for adhesion) and formation of antibody-antigen clumps as a result of chronic exposure of the immune system to bacteria from a primary site.[619] The former mechanism may prevail in acute cases, the latter in subacute cases.

Immune mechanisms may be of particular importance in cases of endocarditis observed in equine serum donors that receive repeated injections of bacterial cultures or by-product.[611,620] In such animals, those showing particularly high serum antibody levels appear predisposed, and a generalized endothelial reaction and spontaneous thrombosis, not of thromboembolic origin, are found.[611,621] The condition may reflect a systemic response of endothelium with secondary colonization rather than a direct effect of inoculum on the endocardium. The role played by coagulopathies in such cases has not been investigated.

Animals with congenital heart disease may be predisposed to endocarditis. While this association is occasionally seen in cattle, it is rare in horses.[622]

Clinical Signs: The clinical signs depend upon the speed of onset, location of the lesion and underlying cause. In people, differentiation between acute and subacute cases is of great clinical importance.[190] This is based upon the observation that subacute cases of insidious onset and progressing slowly usually have some underlying, predisposing heart disease, involve less virulent organisms and have a reasonable prognosis for response to treatment. In contrast, acute cases may have a fatal outcome in a matter of days, can arise spontaneously without underlying cause and often involve more virulent organisms. This dichotomy is not obvious in equine cases. Though examples of acute and subacute endocarditis have been described, most equine cases appear to be subacute.[371,610,612,623,624] The division may help evaluate the clinical course and prognosis.

In subacute bacterial endocarditis, there is variable but persistent fever, weight loss, lethargy and depression.[516,611,612,623] The fever may respond to antibiotics, only to relapse when treatment is withdrawn. These signs are nonspecific and may reflect inflammation in any organ; more specific guidance to a cardiac cause may be provided if a murmur can be detected. However, endocarditis is not always accompanied by a detectable murmur, even if a valve is involved.[611] Some cases involve nonvalvular (mural) endocardium only. If a murmur is detected, the sound may vary from moment to moment throughout the course of the disease.[516] Any valve can be affected; thus the murmur may be systolic, diastolic and sometimes both.[198] Interpretation can be further complicated by concurrent involvement of several valves.[198,374,608,609]

The clinical course in subacute cases may last from weeks to months, with obvious signs of cardiac disease only a terminal event. These signs are those of right or left heart failure, as described earlier in this chapter. Ventral edema early in the course of subacute cases are as likely to reflect such factors as low serum albumin levels and possibly vasculitis, as heart failure. In acute cases, the clinical course can be as short as several days, with severe fever and depression and a reluctance to move that may reflect thoracic discomfort or lameness. Signs of cardiac insufficiency, such as edema and jugular filling, develop rapidly in such cases.

Because of the often friable nature of the vegetative masses forming on the endocardium, embolic episodes are likely, with the pattern of the resulting tissue infarction reflecting the side of the heart involved.[455] Isolated episodes of pulmonary arterial embolism may go unnoticed, to be detected only at necropsy. Embolic showers lead to pulmonary arterial hypertension and ultimately contribute to right heart failure. Coughing and respiratory distress may also be seen. Left-sided lesions may result in embolism of any peripheral tissue, notably the kidneys, myocardium and joints. Signs of renal dysfunction, cardiac arrhythmia and lameness thus may be observed.[198,516,608,612] In acute cases, embolism more often may be associated with abscess formation, reflecting the septic nature of the emboli. In such cases, there are signs of multisystemic disease.

With the exception of parasite damage, clinically significant nonbacterial endocarditis is very uncommon in horses. Parasitic lesions caused by *Strongylus vulgaris* are usually restricted to the endothelium and intima of the bulb of the aorta but may extend to involve the aortic valve and coronary arteries.[189,338] Most parasite-associated changes in the aortic valve are small, sometimes calcified nodules of limited clinical significance. Involvement causing severe valvular dysfunction are uncommon.

The distribution of bacterial valvular lesions in horses contrasts with that in cattle, and has been described as aortic > left AV > right AV > pulmonic.[611,620,625] In 80 cases reported since 1943, 110 valves were involved, with the distribution consistent with previous observations: aortic 55.6%, left AV 27.8%, right AV 9.3% and pulmonic 7.4%. Multiple valve involvement is possible, with both sides of the heart diseased in some cases.[198,374,608,609] Jet lesions may be encountered in chronic cases. Healed lesions are occasionally found at necropsy, while active vegetative lesions sometimes are also an incidental postmortem observation.[607] These findings suggest that endocarditis may occur subclinically or that the diagnosis may be missed, with resolution spontaneously following nonspecific treatment. The frequency with which these events occur is unknown.

Lesions vary with the clinical course. Typically, there are variably sized, vegetative, friable masses attached to the valve margins.[455,608] The masses may be up to several centimeters in diameter and, if small, may be pedunculated, moving to and fro in the blood flow. Larger and acute lesions are sessile, involving the valve broadly and extending toward the valve base. Lesions most often form on the valve margins, on the ventricular surface of the semilunar valves and the atrial surface of the AV valves (Fig 64).

Small lesions may cause minimal valve damage and may not affect valve function. Larger lesions cause variable degrees of valve distortion, depending upon the age of the lesion and amount of secondary fibrosis. In severe cases involving the AV valves, almost the entire valve orifice may be obstructed by the mass (Fig 64). Atrioventricular lesions may extend to involve the chordae tendineae. Any valvular lesion may involve adjacent mural endocardium, but extension to the myocardium is uncommon.

Active lesions consist of masses of fibrin with some platelets superficially combined with granulation tissue and fibrosis in the deeper layers, particularly in chronic cases. Bacterial colonies are evident throughout the mass, especially in acute cases. Heavy infiltrates of mononuclear cells are present. Bacterial culture of the masses frequently is negative and bacteria are best identified by direct smear.[455]

Clinical laboratory findings are nonspecific, reflecting persistent infection, inflammation and antigenic stimulation. Anemia and neutrophilia are common and elevated serum fibrinogen levels are common. Hypoalbuminemia and hypergammaglobulinemia also are present. The extent to which these values deviate from normal provide some indication of the extent to which the lesion is active. Other biochemical abnormalities reflect embolic involvement of other organs.

Diagnosis: The diagnosis is based upon clinical signs. Clinical and laboratory evidence of infection, combined with a heart murmur, are reasonable grounds for suspicion. The diagnosis always should be considered in cases of variable, recurrent fever responsive to antibiotics. A murmur is not always present. When one is encountered, the quality of the sound may vary from beat to beat and day to day. The index of suspicion may be increased by evidence of embolic showering and multiorgan involvement, though in some cases the initial presenting clinical signs may be referable to an organ other than the heart. A typical

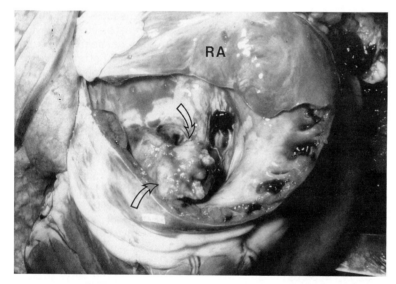

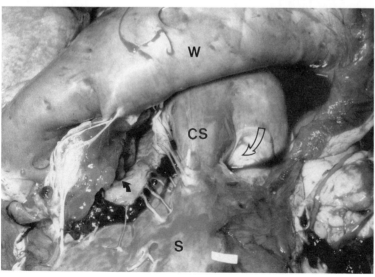

Figure 64. Acute bacterial endocarditis of the right AV valve in a 2-year-old Thoroughbred. Top: View from the right atrium. The vegetative mass (arrows) almost occludes the valve orifice and is located primarily on the atrial surface of the parietal cusp. RA = right atrium. Bottom: View from the right ventricle. There is little or no involvement of the chordae. The dark mass near the septal cusp is a blood clot. Filled arrow = vegetative mass. Open arrow = pulmonic orifice. W = free wall of right venrticle. CS = crista supraventricularis. S = septum viewed from right side.

clinical picture, together with frequent ventricular ectopics or ventricular tachyarrhythmia, should raise the possibility of secondary myocardial involvement via infarction.

Echocardiography is a very simple means of confirming the clinical diagnosis and can provide guidance as to the extent of the lesion. Blood culture always should be attempted, as a positive result aids diagnosis and guides therapy. However, the results frequently are negative. Use of devices to remove antibiotics from blood samples before culture may increase the number of positive cultures though their efficacy remains to be confirmed. Ideally, 3 samples for blood culture, should be collected at 8- to 12-hour intervals, after antibiotics have been withheld for at least 24 hours.

Organisms isolated from cases of endocarditis in horses have been mainly streptococci (usually *Streptococcus zooepidemicus*), staphylococci and *Actinobacillus equuli*.[516, 530,613,626] *Shigella equirulis, Erysipelothrix rhusiopathiae*, fungi, *E coli* and *Pseudomonas* spp also have been isolated sporadically.[608,612,624,627] The full spectrum of bacterial involvement in endocarditis in horses has not been determined because in many cases cultures are negative.

Differential diagnoses include all causes of chronic inflammation, including abscesses and neoplasia. I have observed clinical pictures indistinguishable from endocarditis in 1- to 4-month-old foals with urachal abscesses, parasitic arteritis or severe *Strongyloides westeri* infection. In the last instance, clinical signs may be accompanied by a functional murmur reflecting anemia, fever and circulatory hyperkinesia, further complicating the diagnosis. Additionally, in the case of omphalophlebitis and urachal abscessation, endocarditis may be a secondary complication. Use of diagnostic ultrasound is advised in all cases.

Treatment: Treatment does not carry a good prognosis but may be attempted. On the basis of probable sensitivity of common causative organisms, use of penicillin is appropriate while results of blood culture are awaited. High levels (50,000 IU/kg IV QID) combined initially with gentamicin were successfully used in 1 patient.[516] This regimen should not be expected to be effective against some of the organisms isolated,

however, and treatment ideally should be guided by results of blood culture, though a negative result does not rule out the diagnosis. Failure to observe a fall in temperature within 4-5 days indicates the need to reassess choice or dosage of antibiotic. For any chance of a favorable outcome, treatment must be continued for at least 4 weeks. Echocardiography, hematologic examination and monitoring of temperature may be used to assess response to therapy.

The prognosis remains poor despite any initial response to treatment. Relapse is common, while varying degrees of valve dysfunction, such as chronic valvular incompetence and/or stenosis, can be expected. Cardiac compensation may occur with a stable situation, but progression is more probable with extensive valve distortion. Exercise tolerance is predictably reduced.

Mild lesions that respond to therapy may carry a good prognosis. If the value of the animal warrants the cost of treatment, therapy should be attempted. Treatment should not be attempted in acute cases and in those showing signs of cardiac compromise because of the poor prognosis for satisfactory response, short or long term.

Multifactorial Diseases

Left Atrioventricular Valve Insufficiency

In an abattoir study, diastolic murmurs were encountered more often in horses with aortic valve lesions (63 of 151) than were systolic murmurs in horses found to have left AV valve lesions (44 of 151).[116,152,160] This suggests that, on the basis of auscultable flow disturbance alone, aortic insufficiency was the more common. Similarly, lesions were found on the aortic valve far more frequently than on any other valve. However, as is evident from Table 8, clinical signs (other than a murmur) associated with insufficiency of the left AV valve (left AV insufficiency) have been reported more often than signs from abnormality of any other valve. Review of clinical cases suggests that clinical signs also are generally more severe than with most other valve abnormalities. Thus, left AV valve insufficiancy is frequently associated with signs of heart failure.[349,350,372,373]

Cause: Abnormal function of the left AV valve may involve a range of structural abnormalities. In the abattoir study, lesions of the AV valves were described as fibrous thickening of the valve cusps, with a diffuse, localized or nodular distribution (Fig 65).[116] Thickening of chordae tendineae, either localized or generalized, was observed when valvular disease was advanced. No chordal ruptures were seen. Fenestration, blood cysts and vegetative endocarditis were observed infrequently. Atrial endocardial jet lesions were common findings (Figs 62, 65). Histopathologically, the lesions varied from superficial disruptions of the endothelium to fibrosis extending to various depths into the fibrous skeleton of the valve, causing distortion in severe cases. Few of the lesions exhibited obvious activity. It was concluded that changes represented wear and tear, being both age related and indicative of aging independent of age of the horse.

In a related study in which 45 horses with atrial fibrillation were considered separately, 51.6% had similar lesions of the left AV valve.[162] Comparable lesions have been described in many clinical cases.[188,350,372,623,628] Endocarditis, both acute and chronic, also has been reported as a cause of left AV valve insufficiency.[198,609]

Rupture of chordae tendineae leading to acute valvular insufficiency and respiratory

Figure 65. Septal (S) and right commissural (R) cusps of the left AV valve in a 4-year-old Thoroughbred mare. The horse had signs of bi-ventricular failure and loud pansystolic murmurs on both sides. Generalized thickening of the valve with nodularity of the valve margin is evident (arrows). Endocardial thickening of the atrial surface of the valve is also apparent. LA = left atrium.

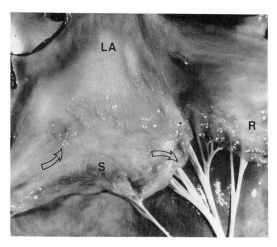

Figure 66. Rupture of a chorda tendineae in a 2-year-old Thoroughbred racehorse. The problem was of sudden onset during exercise and manifested as acute respiratory distress. The rupture is of a chorda (C) extending from the right papillary muscle (rpm) to the right commissural cusp (RC). There was no evidence of chronic valvular disease. Note the characteristics knotting of the retracted chorda (large arrow). LA = left atrium. LV = left ventricle. (Courtesy of Dr. S. Green)

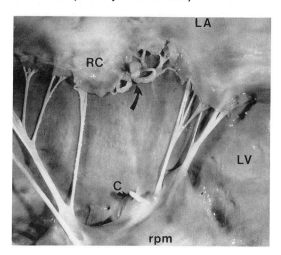

distress has been described in adults and foals.[349,373,374] In 3 horses, all ruptures involved chordae arising from the right papillary muscle and inserting on or supporting the right commissural cusp (Fig 66).[349,629] In other cases, chordae supporting the septal or free wall (caudal) cusp were variously involved. Rupture appears to have occurred close to the papillary muscle in most cases; no consistent underlying cause was detected. In particular, no consistent association with intense exercise was established. Retraction of the ruptured corda results in a characteristic "knot" at the margin of the affected cusp (Fig 66).

Clinical Signs: It cannot be determined with any certainty how frequently AV valve lesions occur without generating a murmur. If valve changes are associated with insufficiency of sufficient degree to cause a sound auscultable at the body surface, the murmur typically is pansystolic, band shaped and blowing in character (Fig 31). It generally starts with, or directly after, S1 and has its point of maximum intensity close to the anatomic location of the left AV valve, on the left side of the thorax about two-thirds of the way between the elbow and the point of the shoulder at the fifth intercostal space.[152,198,350,609] From the point of maximum intensity, the murmur can radiate locally or can be widespread. Mild murmurs tend to radiate back toward the left apex rather than dorsally.[155]

In most cases of chordal rupture with left AV valve insufficiency, the murmur was intense and noisy, and radiated so as to extend the area of auscultation dorsally and caudally.[349,373,374] The point of maximum intensity thus may be found at the level of the shoulder in the sixth intercostal space. Such intense murmurs are widespread on the left, easily heard on the right, and frequently accompanied by palpable thrills.[348] Intense, noisy murmurs are found not only with chordal rupture, but also with generalized signs of heart failure.[350,372]

Change in tension on the chordae, pressure differential across the valve, or the relationship of the valve margins through systole can cause variation in intensity and character of the murmur.[350] Thus, a murmur may be mid-systolic or may begin well after S_1 because the valve cusp prolapses or everts after systole has commenced.[350,623] Eversion of valve margins may only develop as ventricular contraction moves the papillary muscles or at peak systolic pressure. Decrescendo murmurs also have been described in left AV valve sufficiency and may reflect a rapidly falling pressure differential across the valve in cases of severe insufficiency with left atrial/pulmonary venous hypertension.[349,373] Finally, a coarse, variable, mid-systolic, low-frequency "brr" has been described in left AV valve insufficiency and ascribed to vibration of the valve margin.[350]

An intense S_3, which may be accompanied by or take on the characteristics of an early diastolic murmur, often is encountered in moderate to severe left AV valve insufficiency.[198,349,350,372,609] This is thought to reflect rapid filling of the left ventricle in early diastole consequent to increased filling of, and pressure in, the left atrium and pulmonary veins due to regurgitation. The early diastolic murmur then reflects increased and rapid flow across the valve.[349,350]

Variation in intensity of the murmur associated with arrhythmia, with the murmur becoming more intense with successive close-coupled beats then subsiding in the first beat after a pause, strongly suggests left AV valve insufficiency.[162,350] The finding may raise particular difficulties when atrial fibrillation also is present.

Whether there are any systemic consequences of left AV valve insufficiency depends upon the speed of onset and the extent to which compensation is possible.[349, 350] In mild to moderate and slowly progressive cases, volume overload on the left ventricle is associated with eccentric hypertrophy of the chamber. The proportion of stroke volume that flows backward into the left atrium may be small, however, despite the fact that the pressure gradient across the AV valve is much greater than that across the aortic valve. In most cases, regurgitation into the left atrium occurs from onset of systole, before the aortic valve opens, because there is a pressure gradient throughout this period, hence the pansystolic murmur. Where the valve is insufficient for only part of systole, as in cases of prolapse, the murmur may be mid-systolic.

The left atrium progressively dilates in response to the increased volume it must accommodate and effectively protects the pulmonary circulation from the regurgitant flow; thus, other than the murmur, there are no clinical consequences at rest. However, exercise can induce problems, either because of elevation in systemic pressure or reduced myocardial reserve. The former is likely to lead to increased regurgitation, while the letter reflects limiting pumping capacity of the hypertrophied myocardium. This effect may be difficult to measure without sophisticated measurement techniques (see discussion of Exercise Testing).

Horses with acute onset or severe left AV valve insufficiency may exhibit sudden onset of distress, with predominantly respiratory signs, a loud, widespread pansystolic murmur loudest over the left AV valve, extension of the area of cardiac auscultation and a loud S_3.[349,350,373,374] Affected horses may show severe dyspnea, tachypnea, cough, flaring of the nostrils, tachycardia and severe exercise intolerance. A profuse, frothy, occasionally blood-stained nasal discharge is observed in the most acute cases. These signs are the result of rapid onset of severe pulmonary edema secondary to severe pulmonary venous hypertension.

Despite the severity of the acute signs, most horses described in the literature survived for several days, probably as a result of symptomatic treatment, and most went on to develop further fulminating signs of biventricular failure, including jugular pulsation and extensive ventral edema. Signs of right heart failure may be seen within 24 hours of the acute episode and reflect pressure overload as a result of pulmonary hypertension. More protracted cases exhibit weight loss and apathy.[198,609] Though peracute onset of heart failure may be seen in acutely stressed animals with chronic valvular insufficiency, chordal rupture always should be considered as a differential diagnosis. In peracute cases manifesting severe respiratory signs, differential diagnoses would include acute pulmonary edema secondary to septicemia or toxemia. Differentiation from acute bronchospasm should not be difficult because of the relatively dry, wheezing lung sounds in the latter and the absence of a systolic murmur.

Diagnosis: The extent of compensatory change can be evaluated most easily by M-mode echocardiography and Doppler ultrasonography.[374,623,630] Cardiac catheterization and phonocardiography can confirm the clinical impression of failure and help localize the murmur, though they may be more of academic interest than practical utility. Electrocardiography has been used with left AV valve insufficiency but is of undetermined utility.[198,349,350,609]

Treatment: Treatment of horses with mild left AV valve insufficiency is not indicated, and no treatment options exist. Horses exhibiting atrial fibrillation may be cardioverted, though the prognosis is not good because there is likely to be a cause-effect relationship between the arrhythmia and the valvular insufficiency.[162,163] Acute cases may be treated symptomatically with total rest and diuretics, though the prognosis generally is poor. Where insufficiency is due to progression of a chronic valve lesion and myocardial failure, digitalization may result in considerable improvement.[372] However, in cases of chordal rupture, positive inotropes can increase the regurgitant volume by enhancing myocardial performance and may not improve respiratory signs. The greatest response is likely to be seen with diuretics. Afterload reducers theoretically should increase forward flow and reduce regurgitant flow, though this therapeutic approach has not received any attention in horses.

The prognosis for cases of left AV valve insufficiency is difficult to determine because the natural history of most of the lesions is unknown and followup studies have not been performed. The results of an abattoir study would suggest that many horses with left AV valve lesions and valvular insufficiency live long lives.[116,160,595] The potential for progression in AV valve abnormalities is always present, however, particularly with left AV valve lesions. Left AV valve insufficiency in association with atrial fibrillation carries a guarded to poor prognosis. In young horses, particularly those used for intense exercise, left AV valve insufficiency should be viewed with suspicion and the horse reexamined frequently. Endocarditis or acute chordal rupture warrants a poor prognosis because of the nature of the underlying abnormality and/or the speed of onset.

Acute onset of heart failure in cases of chronic left AV valve insufficiency may reflect further deterioration in the valve, though postmortem descriptions of the valves themselves do not differ greatly from those detected incidentally, found in association with arrhythmia, or observed in animals killed simply because they had exercise intolerance.[116,162,350] Thus, other factors probably are necessary to cause acute decompensation and may include acquired myocardial disease. Hypervolemia and hypertension as a result of chronically reduced left heart output and fluid retention also may occur, as observed in people.[190] This outcome may be more likely to develop in horses with left AV valve insufficiency that continue in work.[350,372]

Left Atrioventricular Valve Stenosis

Stenosis of the left AV valve is rarely diagnosed in horses. Damage to the extent that the valve has become anatomically stenotic has not been demonstrated. The murmur of AV stenosis is biphasic, and loudest in early diastole during rapid filling and in late diastole after atrial contraction. Because the pressure gradients are likely to be low in most cases, an intense sound would not be expected and the murmur, where it occurs, is of low frequency and intensity.

Reduction in the size of a valvular orifice to the extent that it is truly stenotic is very uncommon and only likely to be encountered as a congenital defect and in severe cases of vegetative endocarditis. When an early and/or late diastolic, soft, blowing murmur is encountered in the region of the left AV valve, relative or functional stenosis is the most likely cause. This occurs when the orifice is relatively small in relation to flow volume. The early diastolic sound heard in severe cases of left AV insufficiency is generated in this manner.

Right Atrioventricular Valve Insufficiency

Acquired insufficiency of the right AV valve is reported occasionally, though the problem is recorded most often secondary to generalized cardiac failure caussed by left AV insufficiency, as a consequence of bacterial endocarditis, or as a complication of ventricular septal defect.[17,152,163,198,592,609,631] Only infrequently is it an isolated, primary finding.[595,630]

Clinical Signs: A low-grade but typical murmur has been encountered in a large number of horses presented at the University of Guelph clinic with a history of poor performance. It has been an incidental finding in many others presented for elective procedures. Doppler ultrasonography confirmed insufficiency of the right AV valve in a high percentage of these animals. Though some of the horses had clinical and laboratory evidence of low-grade small airway disease and/or exercise-induced pulmonary hemorrhage, the significance of these clinical observations is unclear. Damage secondary to transient, exercise-associated pulmonary hypertension is a possible explanation in some cases, though a slight degree of valvular incompetence at rest could also be normal. The murmur frequently is absent after exercise.

The same spectrum of valve changes is seen on the right AV valve as identified for the left AV valve and include fibrous thickening, nodularity with distortion, endocarditis and hematocysts.[116,160,162,188,198,592,609] The septal cusp appears involved most often. Rupture of the right AV valve chordae has not been described. Right AV valve insufficiency in cases of right heart failure secondary to left heart failure may not be associated with obvious lesions, espe-

cially if the problem is of recent onset.[372] Jet lesions in the right atrium may be anticipated in chronic cases.

The murmur of right AV insufficiency is similar to that of left AV insufficiency, though rarely of the same intensity. It is soft, blowing, band shaped and pansystolic and only infrequently radiates widely. It is best heard from the second to fourth intercostal space just dorsal to the elbow on the right side of the thorax. Where there is pulmonary hypertension, the murmur may reach grade IV/VI in intensity but still rarely radiates widely. Right AV valve insufficiency murmurs are very unlikely to demonstrate the extensive caudal and dorsal extension on the right side of the thorax seen on the left with severe left AV valve insufficiency. In an abattoir study of 1557 horses, only 6 cases of right AV valve insufficiency were noted, and none occurred in conjunction with any other valve lesion.[152] The resultant murmur was described as loudest on the left over the right AV valve in 4 horses. Murmurs of AV insufficiency heard on the right were more often a result of radiation to the right in left AV valve insufficiency than a result of right AV valve insufficiency.

That sounds originating from the right AV valve can be heard on the left, cranially and more ventrally over the second and third intercostal spaces is unquestioned. However, the right AV valve is relatively isolated from the chest wall at this site (Fig 2). Right AV valve murmurs rarely achieve significant intensity. The reasons for the murmur distribution in the animals examined in the abattoir study are thus unclear. In animals I have examined exhibiting a murmur confirmed by Doppler ultrasonography as originating in the right AV valve, the point of maximum intensity has consistently been located on the right as described above.

Clinical signs in right AV valve insufficiency depend upon the severity of the insufficiency and accompanying cardiac abnormalities. Acute right AV valve insufficiency as a clinical syndrome is not recognized except insofar as it may accompany acute left AV valve insufficiency and decompensation. Recognition of right AV valve insufficiency in racehorses with limited performance raises the possibility that there may be a causative association though the valve lesion could itself be secondary. Right AV valve insufficiency may accompany myocardial failure when the signs are those of congestive heart failure. Endocarditis of the right AV valve also may be encountered.

Regurgitant flow to the extent that jugular pulsation develops is rare. Elevation of central venous pressure (as from right heart failure, right AV valve stenosis induced by endocarditis or volume overload) is a far more potent factor in causing jugular filling and pulsation than right AV valve insufficiency. These possibilities should be ruled out before assuming that valvular insufficiency is the primary culprit. Right AV valve insufficiency has been associated with atrial fibrillation as with left AV valve insufficiency, though a left AV valve insufficiency appears to be most common in such cases.

Diagnosis: Right AV valve insufficiency is diagnosed as for left AV valve insufficiency. Where there is a similar murmur on the left side, radiation of a murmur of left AV valve insufficiency to the right cannot always be ruled out. Echocardiographic examination must be performed to confirm right AV valve insufficiency. Where the point of maximum intensity is detected on the right, auscultation cranially and ventrally on the left should be performed to detect radiation to this side. Though generally responsible for a harsher, more intense murmur, a ventricular septal defect sometimes may generate a similar softer sound. Ventricular septal defect always is a differential diagnosis with a harsh intense murmur. In general, murmurs associated with simple ventricular septal defects radiate cranially and toward the right on both sides, and become louder the further cranially you go. Right AV valve insufficiency murmurs, on the other hand, peak and then start to fade as the stethoscope is advanced cranially and rarely radiate as widely as those associated with ventricular septal defect.

The prognosis cannot be assessed accurately on the basis of the information available. Based on clinical experience alone, the prognosis appears to be better than for left AV valve insufficiency in that affected horses may continue to perform satisfactorily. Deterioration in the valve is probable in horses performing maximally and those with respiratory disease. Frequent reexami-

nations are indicated. Development of atrial fibrillation is always a possibility. A poor prognosis should be given if right AV valve insufficiency is detected in association with other signs of cardiac disease. Increase in the intensity of the murmur of right AV insufficiency during inspiration has been noted in horses. Respiration appeared to have a greater effect on benign than on significant murmurs.[152]

Right Atrioventricular Valve Stenosis

This is an infrequently diagnosed condition. It has been only identified in association with endocarditis and once as a congenital lesion.[129,623]

Aortic Valve Insufficiency

Lesions of the aortic valve are more common than lesions of any other valve in horses.[116,160,593] With the possible exception of abnormalities that promote valvular insufficiency, clinical signs are uncommon and not always accompanied by a murmur. Left ventricular volume overload and eccentric hypertrophy have been thoroughly documented in moderate to severe aortic insufficiency.[17] In animals showing obvious signs of cardiovascular insufficiency, such additional conditions as myocardial disease, atrial fibrillation, left AV insufficiency or endocarditis have been present most often.[17,163,188,371,623,628] Though the sequence of events in most of these cases can only be guessed at, uncomplicated aortic insufficiency rarely appears to lead to clinical signs. However, the hemodynamic consequences of the abnormality can be expected to result in exercise intolerance in performance horses irrespective of other findings.[17]

Lesions: Lesions detected on the aortic valve at necropsy have variously been described as nodules, bands, plaques and fenestrations.[116,160,593,594] The last, usually consisting of small holes in the margin of the valve cusp, generally are considered of little or no clinical significance.[116,593,597,606] Their location places them in apposition with opposing valve cusps during diastole, which would preclude regurgitant flow through the defect in most cases. They may, on occasion, be responsible for musical systolic murmurs. Fibrous bands and the distortion that they can cause when extensive or accompanied by many nodules generally are regarded as responsible for most clinical cases of aortic insufficiency.[116,594,632] The bands form on the peripheral half of the valve along the line of closure.[593]

Nodules are less frequently associated with valvular dysfunction yet are the most commonly encountered lesion.[116,593] They may form anywhere on the valve but are found most often on the ventricular surface, and may arise on the edge or toward the middle of the cusp. They vary from one to several millimeters in diameter. In their mildest form, they are covered by endothelium and have an amorphous core with minimal fibrous tissue. Larger lesions are associated with fibrosis and may coalesce to form the plaques, with resultant valve distortion. They also may exhibit ulceration and have been equated to a form of nonbacterial thrombotic endocarditis observed in people.[593]

There is unequal involvement of the 3 aortic valve cusps. The cranial (right coronary or right cusp) is most frequently diseased, though in many cases, especially where regurgitation is severe, all 3 cusps are involved.[116,593,597] This may reflect the relationship between blood flow and curvature of the outflow tract; the cranial cusp is subject to the most trauma.[116,593,597] The remaining valves are affected equally often. Jet lesions may be encountered in the left ventricular outflow tract and on the base of opposing cusps (Fig 67), as well as on the ventricular surface of the septal cusp of the left AV valve.[594] Aortic dilatation often accompanies aortic insufficiency, though the significance of this change is unclear.

Band lesions are composed largely of amorphous ground substance with varying degrees of collagen and elastic fiber formation as the lesion becomes more extensive. The endothelium is intact and inflammatory cells usually are absent. Nodules more frequently exhibit erosion of endothelium and fibrin accumulation, though without inflammatory cells.[593] Though older literature frequently refers to parasitic lesions of the aortic valve (Fig 54), these are not reported often in recent literature, possibly reflecting improved parasite control. Endocarditis of the aortic valve is encountered and, as with severe fibrosis and distortion, may be associated with insufficiency and stenosis.

Cause: The cause of the valvular lesions is undetermined in most cases but is thought to reflect trauma during normal function. This interpretation is supported by the tendency for most lesions to be found on the ventricular surface of the cusps, where the valve cusps contact each other during diastole. While the frequency of lesions appears to be related to age, aortic valve changes may be encountered even in young horses.[116]

Clinical Signs: Clinical signs of uncomplicated aortic insufficiency are generally limited to the murmur. Reflux of blood into the left ventricle results in increased end-diastolic volume and volume overload.[17] Fractional shortening is typically increased, as is stroke volume. The increased stroke volume, allied with the rapid runoff during diastole as blood flows back into the ventricle, results in a prominent, bounding pulse. The presence of this pulse in association with the typical murmur has been described as adequate for diagnosis of aortic insufficiency.[17] However, in my experience, only moderate to severe aortic insufficiency causes such an obviously abnormal pulse.

The murmur of aortic insufficiency is typically pandiastolic, starting immediately after S_2 and often lasting until the next S_1.[17,33,34,188,371,594,609,623,633,634] It usually is decrescendo, best heard over the aortic valve at the left heart base, and radiates toward the apex of the left ventricle. The sound can vary in intensity from barely perceptible to grade V/VI, with an associated thrill and may radiate to the right side. A systolic murmur may accompany the diastolic sound, and reflects increased stroke volume and volume rate of flow during ventricular ejection (Fig 33).

Variation may be encountered. One author has divided the murmur of aortic insufficiency into 2 types.[633,634] In Type I the sound is as described above and may be quite harsh and noisy, varying in intensity and typically associated with more severe hemodynamic consequences and a poorer prognosis. In Type II the murmur starts up to 0.2 seconds after S_2 and may only commence with atrial systole of the next cycle. The sound being quite soft but of relatively low frequency. A higher-frequency, musical but separate component may be detected in early diastole.[633,634]

The significance of these observations has been questioned, however, as indicative only of 2 extremes in a continuum of sounds that may be encountered in progression of valve changes.[597] That numerous variations can be encountered is true. In some cases, the sound is of high frequency and blowing throughout diastole; in others, it starts at a high frequency but becomes coarse and of lower frequency in later diastole.[594] Late diastolic (pre-systolic) accentuation of the murmur has been commented upon.[594] The origin of the apparently separate late component is postulated to be vibration of the septal cusp of the left AV valve as it contends with 2 flows of blood, 1 from the insufficient aortic valve and the other from the left atrium during atrial systole.[634] Other investigators favor an everted valve cusp as the probable source of both the early and late components of the sound.[594]

In cases I have observed, the louder and coarser murmurs of aortic insufficiency usually were of clinical significance, particularly if they radiated widely, persisted for only the early part of diastole or were associated with an obvious, bounding pulse. Soft and high-frequency decrescendo sounds, particularly those lasting through to S_1 and those that can last throughout a double diastolic interval when a beat is dropped, appeared to be of limited clinical significance. In such cases, however, a tendency not to do a detailed workup biases interpretation.

Care should be used in attempting to define prognosis on the basis of auscultatory findings alone. In an echocardiographic study of aortic insufficiency, subjective evaluation of murmur intensity did not provide guidance to left ventricular internal diameter in diastole (an index of chamber failure) or shortening fraction.[17] The extent to which aortic insufficiency limits exercise tolerance and the probability of progression to more severe valvular dysfunction has not been investigated.

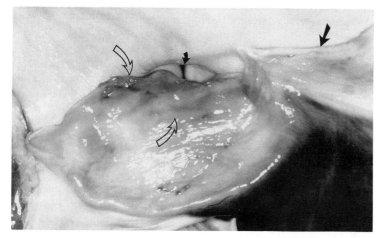

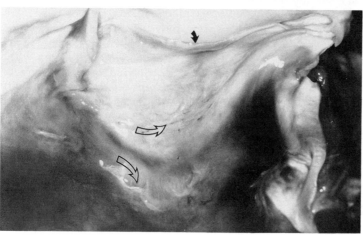

Figure 67. Aortic valve of a 17-year-old Thoroughbred gelding with an aortic insufficiency of 3 years' duration. Top: The principal damage is to the left caudal (left coronary) cusp, which is thickened at the margin and in its middle (open arrows). The cranial (right coronary) cusp (large solid arrow) is unaffected. Small solid arrow = left coronary artery. Bottom: There is endocardial scarring (open arrows) of the outflow tract just distal to the right caudal (noncoronary) cusp and of the base of the cusp itself. The margin of the valve cusp is marked by a solid arrow. See Figure 33 for murmurs detected in this case.

Complications involve changes to the left AV valve as a result of trauma from the regurgitant stream of blood. Thickening of the septal cusp of the left AV valve may thus be observed. Though this may theoretically lead to left AV insufficiency, this has not been conclusively demonstrated in horses.

Diagnosis is by auscultation and by palpation of peripheral pulses. Diagnosis is aided by phonocardiography, particularly if the heart rate is elevated. The diagnosis can be confirmed by M-mode, 2-dimensional or Doppler echocardiography.[17] Even in the absence of Doppler echocardiography, diastolic vibration of the septal cusp of the left AV valve may be demonstrated in an M-mode echogram, as well as thickening or distortion of aortic valve cusps. There is no specific treatment.

Aortic and Pulmonic Valve Stenosis

Describing a valve as stenotic implies to many that there is significant narrowing of the valve orifice. In fact, such structural stenosis only rarely occurs as an acquired lesion and then most often as a consequence of active or healing endocarditis. Most aortic "stenoses" involve either minor disruptions of valvular structure that do not reduce the cross-sectional area of the valve but do cause disturbance of flow during systole, or relative stenosis in which volume flow during all or part of systole exceeds the flow capacity of the valve, resulting in flow disturbance and a murmur. It has been suggested that as much as one-half of the available orifice area is not used at rest, implying considerable reserve flow capacity.[597] Many of the sounds described are functional and benign, and their origin cannot be determined with any certainty. In recognition of this, both aortic and pulmonic valves are discussed together.

True Stenosis: The murmur of true, anatomic outflow tract stenosis is classically crescendo-decrescendo in shape, starts after S_1 and ends before S_2, and occupies *most* of systole, peaking shortly after S_1 (Fig 30). It varies in quality from musical to harsh and vibrant, and is best heard over the heart base on the left. The higher-frequency components of the sound have a tendency to radiate backward toward the apex of the chamber being drained and also may radiate along the outflow tract.[155] The intensity of the sound may increase with exercise.

Other than in relation to endocarditis and congenital heart disease, stenosis of outflow tract (semilunar) valves is very rare. In an abattoir study of 1557 horses, 70% of the lesions identified involved the aortic valve while only 3% involved the pulmonic valve (Table 8).[116] Severe lesions of the pulmonic valve were not identified, whereas the aortic valve often showed severe distortion. All 3 cusps were involved in 60 horses. A systolic murmur with lesions restricted to the aortic valve was described in only 21 horses, while a further 53 exhibited concurrent involvement of a second valve and/or both systolic and diastolic murmurs. In these cases, the murmur tended to be loud and widespread, and the origin of the systolic component not always clear. The role played by the aortic valve could thus not be determined in most cases.

In none of the reports of aortic or pulmonic stenosis is a significantly stenosed valve described, though valve cusp distortion and systolic murmurs of up to grade IV/VI are discussed.[116,162,188,198,609,623,631] Similarly, in none of the reports is true stenosis associated with other signs of cardiovascular dysfunction in the absence of other valve abnormalities, such as vegetative endocarditis. Thus, while distortion of the aortic valve and resultant intense, midsystolic murmurs are encountered, these are not usually associated with clinical signs.

The diagnosis is suggested by the characteristics of the murmur and can be confirmed by echocardiographic examination and cardiac catheterization. Poststenotic dilatation of the artery can be anticipated. In moderate to severe stenosis, pressure overload on the ventricle leads to concentric hypertrophy. The primary differential diagnosis is a congenital heart lesion in which there is outflow tract stenosis and/or a ventricular septal defect just proximal to the outflow tracts. Outflow tract stenosis has not been described as an isolated congenital lesion in horses; thus the coexistence of a ventricular septal defect can be anticipated. In such cases, the murmur is harsh and loud and tends to be heard from S_1 to S_2, sometimes appearing to extend into early diastole. Functional sounds also should be considered in some cases, especially if the horse is stressed from colic or excitement. Further auscultation at a later time is recommended in such cases.

Functional Stenosis: Early to mid-systolic murmurs of short duration and variable intensity often can be detected over the left heart base. The sound is crescendo-decrescendo and has no predictable relationship with heart rate or degree of arousal. It may disappear with exercise, for instance, or may become very loud during excitement. The source of these so-called "innocent" sounds is undetermined (Fig 32). Catheterization studies have identified systolic ejection murmurs in both the left and right heart outflow tracts in horses without valvular stenosis, though these sounds could not be heard at the thoracic surface.[33,34] Flow disturbance in the left heart appears to have been most easily detected in this study. Earlier observational studies have assumed that the pulmonic valve was the source of the murmur.[598]

Regardless of anatomic source, the sound is thought to reflect disturbances of blood flow that in turn can be precipitated by functional factors, such as increases in stroke and flow volumes. Short, localized ejection murmurs in the region of outflow tracts usually can be disregarded, especially if they are of low grade. Intense sounds should be subjected to reevaluation under different circumstances to rule out accentuation of innocent sounds by excitement.

Pulmonic Insufficiency

This condition is rarely diagnosed.[631] The normally low pressure in pulmonary circulation would not lead to a loud murmur, though quality of the sound could be expected to be similar to aortic insufficiency.

DISEASES OF THE MYOCARDIUM

P.W. Physick-Sheard

Diagnostic and Therapeutic Considerations

Acquired Myocardial Disease

General Observations: It has been stated that inflammatory or degenerative changes in the myocardium are the most common cardiac lesions in horses.[156] The full significance of this statement is not immediately obvious from the literature, as few myocardial changes in the species have been fully characterized and, until recently, no systematic studies had been performed. The authors of a comprehensive review of myocardial disease in animals state, "The myocardial diseases represent the largest group in the spectrum of spontaneous cardiac diseases in animals."[635] Yet it is apparent that our knowledge and understanding of myocardial disease in horses is rudimentary. In view of the dependence of performance horses upon the structural and functional dimensions of the cardiovascular system, this lack of information is of some concern.[91]

Studies suggest that degeneration of the equine myocardium and its vasculature, and also the intrinsic nervous system, may be relatively common processes. The full etiologic and clinical significance of these findings remains unclear. In many cases, myocardial involvement could be an unrecognized component of systemic disease and might only be adequately characterized by biopsy. However, a great deal of evidence suggests that the clinician should pay greater attention to subclinical myocardial involvement in many systemic disease conditions and cardiac arrhythmias.

Clinical Signs: The clinical signs of myocardial disease consist of tachycardia, arrhythmias and heart failure. Compromise of the myocardium causes some reduction in functional capacity. If this compromise is generalized or involves a large percentage of myocardial tissue, there may be an elevation in heart rate at any particular level of activity over that before the injury. If the damage is mild, especially if the changes are essentially metabolic and temporary, the outcome may be total resolution. If the damage is structural and/or involves loss of myocytes, the consequence is fibrosis and compensatory hypertrophy. In either case, slight elevation of heart rate may be temporary. More severe and persistent elevation of heart rate, out of proportion to the apparent severity of other clinical signs and environmental factors, accompanies extensive myocardial damage and/or persistent insult. Here, arrhythmias may or may not be detected. Cardiac hypertrophy may occur as a chronic consequence of the myocardial damage, and insufficiency of the AV valves may result from damage to papillary muscles or from cardiac dilatation.

However, if myocardial damage is focal, tachycardia and signs of failure may not be seen. Yet arrhythmias are quite likely, especially if the damage is acute or inflammatory and involves a zone of progression from normal to essentially necrotic tissue. The transitional zones are likely sites for genesis of ectopic activity. Such arrhythmias may be persistent or transient, requiring ongoing monitoring in some cases. Essentially, any arrhythmia may be encountered, though the ventricular myocardium is the most likely source of ectopic activity in inflammatory and infarctive processes. Premature ventricular contractions, ventricular bigeminy and ventricular tachyarrhythmias are encountered. Severe myocardial damage leads to heart failure, signs of which may develop surprisingly rapidly, possibly within 1-2 days after acute toxic insult (*eg*, ionophore intoxication). Extensive left ventricular involvement can result in respiratory distress as the most obvious indication of heart failure.

Diagnosis: Myocardial damage is diagnosed by clinical signs, echocardiography, electrocardiography and enzymology. Even with application of all 4 modalities, the clinical diagnosis may be difficult to confirm. Myocardial function has been characterized by catheterization, but the procedure does not present a realistic option for clinical diagnosis.[636,637]

Clinical signs are as discussed above. Echocardiography can be used to demonstrate deterioration in functional indices, such as fractional shortening, and end-diastolic and end-systolic dimensions. Results may be somewhat equivocal if there was not a pre-insult echocardiogram or if deterioration is mild. The technique for making these determinations is covered elsewhere in this chapter.

Electrocardiography may be useful for detecting and/or characterizing arrhythmias, and for demonstrating other changes. Electrocardiographic abnormalities in myocarditis have been described as ST-segment and T-wave deviations, slurring and prolongation of QRS complex, electrical alternans and prolongation of the PR and QT intervals.[376] Similar abnormalities occur in a wide range of myocardial disturbances, and

the signs thus are nonspecific. The sensitivity and specificity of such ECG changes have not been determined.

Isoenzyme analysis has been used to characterize myocardial damage.[137,638-640] However, the value of isoenzyme analysis in differentiating skeletal muscle damage from cardiac damage and damage in other tissues (*eg*, red cells) has not been investigated fully. Accurate detection is likely to require serial enzyme profiles.

Congenital and Familial Diseases

Ventricular Septal Defect

Ventricular septal defect is the most commonly reported congenital cardiac anomaly in horses, whether alone (about 38 cases reported, see references in Table 4) or as a component of more complex developmental anomalies. The following discussion considers the ventricular septal defect as an isolated anomaly only.

Lesions: A ventricular septal defect can form in several locations in the septum (Figs 50 and 51). Defects located just distal to (beneath) the septal cusp of the right AV valve represent abnormalities of the septum membranaceum.[422] Large defects in this region involve both septum membranaceum and the smooth septum. Those separated from the very base of the valve but still adjacent to the valve and its chordae are defects of the smooth septum. Though not strictly correct, in the interests of simplicity and in view of the fairly uniform clinical signs, defects in this entire region are referred to below as *membranous* defects (Fig 68).

Defects involving the crista supraventricularis (ridge of muscle separating the inflow and outflow tracts of the right ventricle, see Figs 50, 51) are referred to as *infundibular* defects. These range from discontinuity of the crista adjacent to the right AV valve, to defects near the pulmonic valve and aortic valves (Fig 69). The entire crista may be absent in some cases. Finally, defects of the trabeculated septum (ventral part of the septum where the muscular bands or trabeculae carneae are prominent) are called trabecular or *apical* defects and may be multiple.

Some defects have been described as "high" or "subaortic" while the location of others is not given.[426,641] These terms are vague. The term "subaortic" is not helpful because on the *left* side of the septum most membranous and infundibular defects open just proximal to (below) the aortic valve (Fig 51). No conclusion can be drawn as to the precise position if photographic evidence is not presented and terminology is used loosely. If an adequate description is provided, most defects appear to be membranous. Apical defects are very rare in horses. One case, in which 2 defects were present, has been described as part of a complex anomaly.[642] In a Thoroughbred foal, I observed a 2-cm defect at the very apex of the septum at necropsy.

Location of the murmur can be used to gain insight into the position of the defect, which may influence the prognosis. Membranous defects shunting blood left to right tend to generate a murmur with a point of maximum intensity on the right side.[592,643] The murmur becomes progressively louder as one auscultates farther cranially. The sound usually can be heard cranially on the left, but is often less intense. If the flow of blood through the shunt reverses, the murmur is most intense over the left ventricle on the left thorax. Membranous defects tend to be isolated anomalies or associated with only limited additional findings.

At the other extreme are infundibular defects that involve the crista close to the base of the pulmonic valve. The murmur associated with such defects tends to be loudest at the left heart base over the outflow tracts. Ventricular septal defects associated with anomalies of the great vessels usually are infundibular. A shunt-type murmur at the left heart base should alert the clinician, therefore, to the possibility of a complex congenital anomaly. Isolated infundibular defects near the pulmonic/aortic valves may be relatively uncommon in horses, though

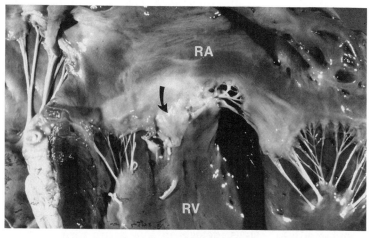

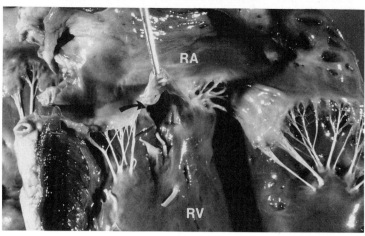

Figure 68. Membranous ventricular septal defect in a 3-year-old Standardbred gelding viewed from the right side. Top: The septal cusp of the right AV valve is thickened and distorted. Bottom: The cusp has been elevated to reveal the underlying defect. RA = right atrium. RV = right ventricle.

this information is difficult to extract from the literature. Other infundibular defects may produce a jet stream that radiates cranially, creating a sound that is equally loud on both sides of the thorax. In the isolated apical defect described above, the point of maximum intensity was at the apex of the heart on the right thorax.

The characteristics of a ventricular-level shunt murmur have been reviewed earlier in this chapter. Regardless of the location of the defect, the murmur of a ventricular septal defect tends to be intense and harsh, and to radiate widely. Both first and second heart sounds may be obliterated (Fig 20). There is only inconstant correlation between intensity and significance. Small defects can produce intense sounds but may have minimal clinical consequences. Even with isolated ventricular septal defects, a secondary acquired valvular abnormality is likely to be found, especially in older animals, and more than one murmur may be encountered. Diastolic sounds may be heard with aortic valve damage. Attendant murmurs attributable to AV insufficiency are likely to be detected in horses showing signs of heart failure.

Clinical Signs and Diagnosis: The clinical signs and consequences of an isolated ventricular septal defect vary enormously. Affected foals may be cyanotic and distressed at birth, or the defect may be an incidental finding in a mature asymptomatic animal. There are several reasons for this variability. Clinical signs are most likely to be seen with a large (several centimeters) defect. This is true of all defects regardless of location but is a more common consequence in membranous defects. Failure is likely to occur before the right heart can compensate, while severe pulmonary overcirculation leads to pulmonary congestion, dyspnea and cyanosis secondary to respiratory embarrassment. Cyanosis also may be a direct consequence of mixing at the ventricular level in larger defects. The ultimate defect is a common ventricle, of which 1 equine case has been reported.[367]

Defects of the infundibular type may have limited immediate effect if the shunted blood is directed along the conus arteriosus and out of the pulmonic valve, aiding rather than compromising right ventricular function. Such defects may produce only mild volume overload (eccentric) hy-

Figure 69. Infundibular defect in a 9-year-old Standardbred mare. The presenting history was of poor response to training as a 3-year-old. Top: Viewed from the right side, the defect (arrow) opens just below the pulmonic valve and between that structure and the crista supraventricularis (CS). The prolapsing left caudal cusp of the aortic valve can be clearly seen through the defect. RA = right atrium. RV = right ventricle. PA = pulmonary artery. Bottom: Viewed from the left side, the defect (large arrow) opens just below the aortic valve. The valve cusps are indicated by small arrows. Note the hyperplasia of the left caudal (left coronary) cusp. This region is shown in more detail in Figure 70. A = aorta. LV = left ventricle.

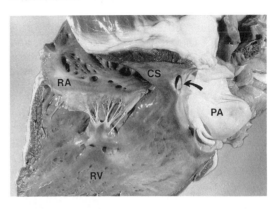

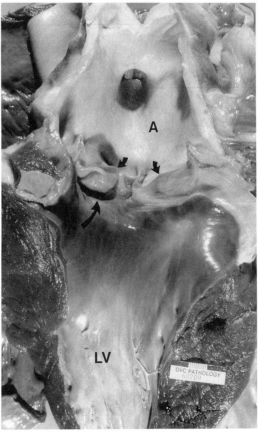

pertrophy of the left heart. Small defects may be associated with very limited shunting and may allow a normal lifespan. In performance horses, the finding is likely to limit maximal aerobic rate of working but still may be compatible with work, depending upon use.

Even with relatively small defects, constant overcirculation in the lungs can lead to a progressive, protective, pulmonary hypertensive response. This puts a pressure overload on the right heart, leading to right ventricular hypertrophy and possibly failure. Whether failure occurs or whether the pressure in the right heart eventually rises to exceed left ventricular systolic pressure, promoting a reversed, right-to-left or bidirectional shunt (Eisenmenger's syndrome) depends upon many factors, principally the volume of shunt flow and the health of the respiratory system.[422,643] Animals with chronic airway disease may develop pulmonary hypertension for 2 reasons. In horses I have observed, reversal of blood flow through the shunt has occurred only infrequently and then only in association with moderate to large defects (4-7 cm).

Other, secondary complications involve heart valves. With membranous defects shunting blood left to right, trauma to the right AV valve may result in thickening of the septal cusp, and thickening and shortening of the chordae. This can lead to right AV insufficiency.[592] If an infundibular defect is large or positioned just proximal to the pulmonic valve, there may be a lack of support for the base of the cranial (right coronary) cusp of the aortic valve, which may prolapse through the defect during diastole.[607] Such a lesion in a 9-year-old Standardbred mare is shown in Figure 70. The base of the hyperplastic right coronary cusp had developed a hard, necrotic, hemorrhagic plaque as a result of constant trauma. Eventual rupture of the plaque would have led to acute aortic insufficiency.

A ventricular septal defect should be suspected if the typical murmur is detected in a neonate or young foal. Signs of decompensation may not become evident for several months, even with large defects. The abnormality may be associated with clinical signs in adults, especially those with complaints of failure to thrive or exercise intolerance, or may be an incidental finding.[159,592,607,641,643] A shunt-type murmur should always prompt thorough investigation to define the prognosis. Thorough auscultation often reveals the probable site of the defect in uncomplicated cases. Systemic signs and determination of arterial oxygen tension can be used to rule out a right-to-left shunt and may help differentiate a complex congenital abnormality from a simple ventricular septal defect.

Definitive diagnosis may involve thoracic radiography, angiocardiography, blood pressure studies, blood gas analysis and echocardiography. Electrocardiography is of limited value. Thoracic radiography may reveal cardiomegaly and overcirculation in the lungs, with prominence of pulmonary vasculature.[641] Angiocardiography can be used to reveal a shunt and the direction of blood flow, and usually necessitates catheterization of both sides of the heart. Blood pressure studies may require only right-sided catheterization in left-to-right shunts.[159,357,641] If the defect is small, there may be little or no pressure change in the right ventricle unless there is secondary pulmonary hypertension. Allowing the catheter to flow deep

Figure 70. Closeup of the infundibular defect shown in Figure 69 and viewed from the left side. The hyperplastic left caudal (left coronary) cusp of the aortic valve (AV) has been reflected. Repeated prolapse of the cusp through the defect (open arrow) has resulted in a necrotic, thick plaque (solid arrow) at the valve base. LV = left ventricle. A = aorta.

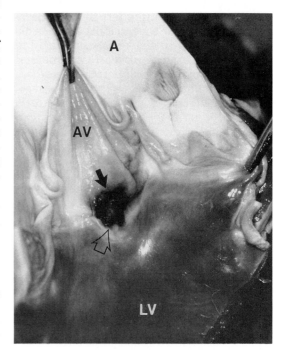

into the pulmonary artery and collecting blood samples provide confirmation of the shunt in most cases, however, by demonstrating higher oxygen tension in the pulmonary artery than in the right ventricle or right atrium. Multiple samples should be taken at each of several sites, as there may be incomplete mixing and streaming of the shunted blood. Single samples from 1 location may result in incorrect interpretation. A peripheral arterial sample also should be collected for comparison. If pressures are elevated in the right ventricle, the catheter must be passed into the pulmonary artery to rule out pulmonic stenosis and confirm pulmonary hypertension.

Echocardiography is very useful but may not clearly demonstrate a small defect, especially of the infundibular type.[643] Bubble studies, in which sterile saline that has been shaken before administration is deposited by catheter upstream of the shunt, may be used to demonstrate direction of flow. First-pass nuclear angiocardiography shows promise in diagnosis of ventricular septal defects.[644]

The prognosis varies. With a small defect and no other abnormal cardiovascular findings, the prognosis is very good. Defects tend to enlarge less rapidly than the heart during normal growth. Some in the trabecular region may close or may become much smaller during systole.[422] Large defects and those complicated by other congenital abnormalities of the heart associated with extensive secondary valve damage or in animals with concurrent respiratory disease have a guarded prognosis, as decompensation eventually develops.

Atrial Septal Defects and Persistent Foramen Ovale

During embryologic development of the interatrial septum, 3 communications between the left and right atria develop sequentially.[422,645] The first, the ostium primum, represents the initial discontinuity of the septum as the primitive atrium first begins to septate by development of the septum primum. The opening closes as the endocardial cushions come together. Its persistence is a reflection of endocardial cushion defects during septation of the atrioventricular canal. During closure of the ostium primum, the ostium secundum

forms in the developing septum primum, initially by development of multiple fenestrations. This allows systemic venous blood to bypass the lungs and support development of the left ventricle by entering the left atrium.

A partition (septum secundum) that develops in the craniodorsal wall of the right atrium forms a flap over the ostium secundum and directs caudal vena caval blood into the left atrium. Septum secundum and the ostium secundum collaborate to form the foramen ovale, while the free margin of ostium secundum develops into the sleeve-like valve of the foramen. The latter partially fenestrated sleeve lies in the left atrium.[646] The combined structures form a tube running from the junction between the caudal vena cava and the right atrium into the left atrium. The structure of the valve discourages left atrial blood from flowing into the right atrium. The valve's fine structure has been described.[647]

Developmental anomalies can involve any of these 3 stages and may be referred to as true atrial septal defects (ostium primum defect and ostium secundum or fossa ovalis defect) and persistent foramen ovale. More than one atrial defect may be present in affected individuals. Though all have been described in horses, they are not common.

True Atrial Septal Defects: An ostium primum defect has been described in a Welsh pony foal with a hypoplastic right ventricle and dysplasia of the AV valves.[603] This foal also had a persistent foramen ovale. Ostium secundum defects may be more common, though inconsistent use of terminology in the literature causes some confusion. One review suggests that many defects described as persistent foramen ovale would be described more accurately as atrial septal defects.[603] Large defects or multiple fenestrations are encountered in tricuspid atresia.[362,368,413,599] Atrial septal defect also has been observed with a hypoplastic left heart and in Lutembacher's syndrome (atrial septal defect with left AV stenosis).[365,604] However, atrial septal defects accompany complex congenital heart disease far less frequently than, for example, patent ductus arteriosus. Atrial septal defect as an isolated finding is very uncommon and may have been described once.[648]

Persistent Foramen Ovale: Persistent foramen ovale is often diagnosed at necropsy in neonatal foals. A more accurate description would be probe patency of the foramen, because anatomic closure is delayed for several days after functional closure and may not occur for several weeks.[646] Small fenestrations may persist into adulthood. Unless the opening is unusually large, therefore, the term "probe-patent foramen ovale" should be used. While persistent foramen ovale is reported in the equine literature rather frequently, most of the cases appear to represent atrial septal defects, though the complex structure of the opening may defy precise definition in some cases. True persistence of the foramen ovale (persistence and patency of the sleeve-like structure described above) appears to be very uncommon.

Functional Consequences of Atrial Septal Defects: For small defects, the consequences are minimal, with small volumes of blood shunted in either direction. Pressure differentials are very low and the lesion is essentially asymptomatic. Larger defects are associated with flow from left to right, volume overload of the right heart and over- circulation in the lungs. In time, pulmonary hypertension and secondary pressure overload on the right heart lead to reduced distensibility of the ventricular chamber and some elevation in right atrial pressure, reversing the shunt. Systemic hypoxemia and volume overload of the left heart follow.

Any disturbance promoting elevation of atrial pressure (*eg*, AV valve insufficiency, chamber failure) may induce a significant shunt before the pulmonary vascular response develops. The consequences will depend upon the direction of the shunt. Until blood flow through the shunt reverses or limitation of pumping capacity becomes evident, the condition is asymptomatic. There is no auscultable murmur. Too few cases have been described in the equine literature to comment further. In the case of complex anomalies, the role played by the atrial discontinuity depends upon the nature of the other anomalies.

Other Congenital Myocardial Abnormalities

Single cases of hypoplastic right heart syndrome, hypoplastic left heart syndrome and cor triloculare biatriale (single ventricle) have been reported.[365,367,603] An un-usual anomaly that included defects in the right AV valve, a double apical ventricular septal defect and abnormal development of the crista supraventricularis has been reported.[642]

Infectious, Inflammatory and Immune Diseases

Myocarditis

It is stated that myocarditis is relatively common in horses.[376,496] Yet the disorder is reported infrequently and characterized inadequately. Most references to the condition are found in reviews. Myocarditis implies an active inflammation of the heart muscle of parasitic, viral or bacterial origin.[455] It is rarely primary, and usually secondary to extension of pericardial or endocardial processes, or secondary to hematogenous spread of infection. Lesions usually are focal and widely scattered, and may not be obvious at necropsy unless necrosis is severe. Histologically, the reaction is typically interstitial and perivascular, with a cellular infiltrate notably devoid of neutrophils in most cases. It is rarely considered the primary cause of death in affected animals.[455]

Viral myocarditis has been associated with influenza A-equi 2.[192,649] Myocardial inflammation with degeneration and necrosis is seen in African horse sickness.[650] Purulent myocarditis may result from septic embolization in acute endocarditis of the left heart. In a review of the literature in an earlier edition of this text, cases of acute and chronic bacterial myocarditis secondary to a primary focus elsewhere in the body were described.[18] Reference was made to allergic myocarditis and sudden death in horses recently recovered from strangles or influenza. Most of the references quoted, however, predated development of the first antibiotics; such cases are uncommon today.

Horses manifesting ECG abnormalities suggestive of myocardial disease after outbreaks of strangles have been reported.[651] Myocarditis may accompany any condition associated with a septicemia. Diagnosis may be difficult because of spontaneous recovery (and thus lack of postmortem material) and the clinician's preoccupation with the primary infection.[376] It is advisable, therefore, to consider the possibility of active myocardial inflammation in any horse with systemic consequences of a local infection or septicemia. The implications for performance are obvious.

The clinical signs of myocarditis are nonspecific and could reflect cardiac insufficiency of any cause.[376] They include exercise intolerance, dyspnea on exertion, syncope, tachycardia disproportionate to fever, murmurs, gallop sounds, arrhythmias, ST-segment abnormalities, signs of generalized congestive failure and sudden death. Diagnosis is aided by enzymology and echocardiography, but findings are not specific. Definitive diagnosis of myocarditis is by postmortem examination during the active disease.

Nutritional Diseases

Nutritional Myopathy

Selenium and/or vitamin E deficiency is associated with degeneration and necrosis of muscle in several domestic species, including horses, and can involve extensive myocardial damage.[455] Nutritional myopathy is seen at all ages.[652-654] Details are provided in the chapter on Diseases of the Musculoskeletal System. In horses with extensive myocardial involvement, there may be sudden death, often with exercise, or rapid onset of weakness with tachycardia. In these cases, dyspnea may reflect heart failure and pulmonary edema. Arrhythmias are not uniformly present and should not be depended upon for diagnosis. Postmortem findings in the heart consist of pale streaking of the myocardium and, occasionally, calcification. Histologically there is myocardial degeneration and necrosis with replacement fibrosis in horses that survive the acute episode.

Toxic Diseases

Ionophore Toxicity

Ionophores are monocarboxylic polyether antibiotics that facilitate transport of cations across biological membranes (cell or mitochondrial membranes). They are used in agriculture primarily as coccidiostats in poultry and to enhance feed conversion in cattle. The skeletal and cardiac muscle toxicity of a related compound, A204, was recognized in rats as early as 1971.[655] The first report of toxic effects in horses appears to be a letter published in 1975.[656] Since that time, there have been numerous reports of intoxication in horses, most often by monensin, but also by salinomycin.[348,657-661] A fourth agent, lasalocid, also is toxic in horses though no reports of accidental intoxication have been published.[662] While the acute toxic effects of ionophores in horses involve renal and hepatic damage, intravascular hemolysis and skeletal and cardiac myopathy, the principal consequences appear to relate primarily to myocardial damage.

Pathophysiology: The mode of toxicity of ionophores is assumed to be their ability to transport alkali cations across cell membranes. This compromises mitochondrial function and interferes with the behavior of excitable tissue.[639,663,664] The cation affinity of different ionophores varies. Monensin has the greatest affinity for sodium, for example, and salinomycin for potassium.[663,665] Toxicity also varies. The estimated LD_{50} for salinomycin, monensin and lasalocid is 0.6 mg/kg, 2-3 mg/kg and 21.5 mg/kg, respectively.[191,662,666] Horses appear to be especially sensitive to ionophores, as compared with other species.[384]

The proposed pathophysiology of monensin intoxication involves an acute effect described as hypovolemic shock secondary to loss of plasma water through acutely nephrotic kidneys, complicated by hypokalemia induced by movement of potassium into cell organelles, and intravascular hemolysis due to changes in red cell fragility.[639,667] Later changes reflect compromised mitochondrial function, which may be progressive and cumulative in low-dose intoxication without preliminary acute signs.[638] This influences primarily skeletal and cardiac muscle. Muscles that are active constantly appear predisposed.[655] Findings in natural outbreaks of intoxication are not entirely consistent with experimental studies, however. Factors that probably influence clinical manifestations include ingested dose, period over which intoxication occurred, level of the ionophore in the feed, preexisting health and electrolyte status, and the ionophore involved.

Cause: Circumstances of intoxication vary but have involved the conscious feeding of treated cattle or poultry rations or premixes to horses and accidental contamination of horse feeds during their compounding.[348,658,661] This may occur as a result of retention in hoppers of concentrated premixes and failure to clean equipment adequately between batches, or from accidental use of the wrong premix.[657] Entire batches of feed may be affected or perhaps only 1-2 bags, necessitating careful sampling when attempting to confirm a tentative diagnosis by feed analysis and perseverance if initial assays are negative.[384]

Clinical Signs: A change in diet (new diet or new batch of feed) within the preceding 1-10 days is a consistent finding. Acutely intoxicated horses may show muscle weakness, ataxia, intermittent, profuse sweating, difficulty rising, and finally recumbency.[191,657,662,664] These signs have been likened to the tying-up syndrome.[656] Abdominal pain, ileus and/or diarrhea may initially be the prominent finding in less severely affected horses.[384,657,658,661,664] Severe dyspnea reflecting cardiogenic pulmonary edema and/or compromised diaphragmatic function may be observed.[661] Cardiac arrhythmias may occur, and sudden death at work has been described in acutely intoxicated performance horses.[661] With the exception of anorexia and depression, the onset of signs does not appear to occur at any consistent interval after poisoning. The above signs generally are evident within 2-3 days. Death may occur from 12 hours to several days after ingestion of the ionophore, though most deaths occur within 24-36 hours.[639,668,669]

Peracute experimental ionophore poisoning in ponies caused intense sweating with increased urine output and hematuria, followed by oliguria and hypovolemic shock.[639] Bladder distension, which might have reflected increased urine output combined with ataxia or muscle damage and failure to adopt a urination posture, was observed in acutely affected horses.[661]

Horses that survive the acute episode and milder cases show less severe and often more insidious signs that primarily reflect the effect of the drugs on skeletal and cardiac muscle metabolism.[639] Subacute and chronic intoxication also may be due to ingestion of small quantities over a long period. However, the anorexia that ionophores usually induce in horses tends to make in-

gestion self-limiting and is probably responsible for moderation of clinical consequences in all episodes except those in which the agent is present in feed at high concentrations.

Subacute signs include depression, reduced feed intake, cardiac arrhythmias, tachycardia, heart failure and respiratory signs with hyperventilation. Sudden death may occur without prodromal signs, presumably due to cardiac arrhythmias.[639,657,660]

A particularly disturbing observation in cases of ionophore intoxication has been the apparent tendency to chronic disability, especially in terms of unthriftiness, cardiac dysfunction and reduced exercise tolerance.[385,668] In some cases, specific clinical signs were lacking and the association between the historical episode of ionophore intoxication and subsequent poor performance was presumptive. In others, findings have included tachycardia, cardiac arrhythmias (including ventricular ectopic activity and atrial fibrillation), ST-segment changes and heart failure. Reports suggest that deaths and onset/recurrence of clinical signs may occur weeks after the acute episode.[668]

The full significance of these observations for long-term prognosis requires further investigation. Postmortem findings support the probable presence of chronic myocardial damage in some horses, while the acute changes can reasonably be expected to have a permanent influence on cardiac functional capacity and aerobic performance. However, the extent to which such chronic sequelae vary with pattern of intoxication, agent and dosage is unclear.

Serum biochemical and enzymatic changes in acute experimental intoxication in ponies have been thoroughly documented.[639] These include transient (<24 hours) dereases in serum calcium and potassium levels, and elevation of serum urea, creatinine and unconjugated bilirubin levels. Decreased serum magnesium and phosphorus levels have also been observed.[670] Serum sodium levels show little change. Serum gamma glutamyl transferase activity does not change, indicating minimal hepatic damage. Elevation in serum alkaline phosphatase activity, primarily of bone origin, also is seen. Changes in serum AST, CPK and LDH occur, with isoenzyme patterns in CPK and LDH indicating skeletal and cardiac muscle and red cell damage, though in the acute picture the enzymatic contribution from myocardium appears to be minimal.[639] Changes in serum CPK and AST activities may be massive. Hemoconcentration is evident by elevation in PCV and serum protein levels.

These experimental observations are essentially mirrored in spontaneous cases of poisoning, though the transient changes in electrolyte levels may be missed by the time veterinary attention is sought.[385,661] Also, muscle enzyme elevation may not always be detectable in chronic ambulatory cases.[385] Muscle enzyme changes in animals in recumbency and thrashing are difficult to interpret. Muscle enzyme ratios and acute serial samples may prove of diagnostic value in affected horses.

ECG changes are nonspecific and may develop progressively the first 24 hours.[639] A decrease in serum potassium levels initially is associated with flattening of the T wave, though subsequent changes are likely to reflect a combination of factors, including stress. Thus, a large T wave may be observed.[657] Extensive myocardial damage may lead to ST segment depression. Cardiac arrhythmias occur but are nonspecific.

Postmortem findings vary widely among different outbreaks and experimental studies, in part because of different dosage regimens and agents. Acute experimental intoxication with single doses of monensin given at 2-3 mg/kg caused toxic tubular nephritis and hepatitis, but myocardial and skeletal lesions were not mentioned.[191] Smaller doses in subacute feeding experiments were not associated with any lesions. Single doses of lasalocid at 15-26 mg/kg also affected the kidneys and liver but caused no myocardial changes. In contrast, in another experimental study in which ultrastructural lesions were examined, the most significant changes observed were in the myocardium, while only minimal lesions were found in the liver, skeletal muscles and diaphragm.[664] No abnormalities were observed in the kidneys of any of these latter horses.

While similar renal and hepatic damage occasionally has been seen in cases of natural exposure, myocardial lesions and changes secondary to circulatory embarrassment have been far more consistent. Gross findings have included paleness or streaking of the myocardium, subcutaneous and pulmonary edema, congestion and hemorrhage, and increased pleural, abdominal and pericardial fluid.[348,384,385,657,661,668] Histologic lesions in the myocardium consist of vacuolation, separation of myofibrils, hyaline and granular degeneration, loss of cross striation and, ultimately, myocardial necrosis.[455] Changes tend to be focally intense by replacement with collagenous and fatty tissue in chronic cases.[385] Increased cellularity (suggesting attempts at regeneration) also has been seen.[657] In an experimental study of monensin intoxication in ponies, ultrastructural lesions in the myocardium included pronounced enlargement of mitochondria. It was concluded that mitochondria were the primary targets of the poisoning.[664]

Diagnosis: Diagnosis is based upon the combination of clinical signs, including the pattern of herd involvement, clinical laboratory findings and history of recent diet change. Failure of several horses to consume all of their concentrate ration should cause immediate dietary evaluation and analysis. The ration should be immediately withdrawn until it is established to be safe. Detection of arrhythmias and other signs of cardiovascular dysfunction may guide diagnosis, but signs of cardiac disease may appear later in the clinical course so that the horse may die before myocardial involvement is well established.[384] Demonstration of an ionophore in the feed or in stomach contents confirms the diagnosis.

Treatment: Treatment is largely symptomatic. Use of activated charcoal or mineral oil has been suggested to delay absorption and to promote expulsion of the contaminated feed from the gastrointestinal tract.[639,671] Volume replacement to counteract hypovolemia and shock in acute cases has been recommended.[639] Intravenous supplementation with magnesium and phosphate, together with balanced electrolyte solutions, has been investigated experimentally in acute intoxication ponies with some apparent response.[670] Stall rest and minimization of stress are essential in view of the compromised cellular metabolism represented by extensive mitochondrial damage, so as to limit tissue loss and allow repair. Digoxin should *not* be used in animals with suspected monensin poisoning because the 2 agents are synergistically toxic to myocardial cells.[672]

The prognosis depends upon several factors, including the ionophore involved and the amount consumed. Intoxication with small quantities of feed containing high concentrations of monensin or salinomycin warrants the worst prognosis. Accidental poisoning with premixes, contamination of compounded horse rations and exposure to poultry feeds pose the greatest risk. If the ionophore is present in lower concentrations and the horses have a low intake and/or stop eating the feed, the prognosis for survival is fair to guarded, especially for performance horses, which conceivably may not return to their previous level of performance because of myocardial damage.

Other Toxic Myopathies

Though myocardial damage can occur in association with any nonspecific toxemia, myocardial necrosis has been specifically associated with intestinal clostridiosis and cantharidin poisoning. In intestinal clostridiosis, changes usually are appreciated only histologically and may not be obvious in horses dying after a short clinical course.[673] Arrhythmias are encountered, though ECG abnormalities may reflect electrolyte and acid-base disturbances as well as specific toxic myocardial damage.

Cantharidin (blister beetle) poisoning results from ingestion of hay contaminated with dead blister beetles.[674] Clinical signs include oral ulceration, colic, depression, pollakiuria, and occasionally hematuria and synchronous diaphragmatic flutter. In rare cases, there are signs of heart failure. Postmortem findings include necrosis and sloughing of intestinal mucosa, renal tubular damage and myocardial necrosis.[675] The last may be a direct effect of the cantharidin and a consequence of hypocalcemia and hypomagnesemia. Myocardial mitochondrial damage may be detectable even if lesions are not grossly obvious.[676]

Neoplastic Diseases

Myocardial Neoplasia

While primary neoplasia of the heart is rare in domestic animals, secondary myocardial involvement is not.[455] However, myocardial neoplasia of any type is ex-

tremely unusual in horses. Reported cases include melanoma, infiltrative lipoma, and hemangiosarcoma.[188,481,677]

Multifactorial Diseases

Fibrosis, Infarction and Coronary Arterial Disease

Myocardial fibrosis represents the end stage of loss of myocardial tissue, regardless of the primary insult. It reflects a loss of cells and subsequent coalescence of stroma in cases of degeneration of myocytes, or actual proliferation of fibrocytes and collagenous tissue at the site of an inflammatory process or acute necrosis. It is discussed separately here, not as an implication that it constitutes a distinct clinical and pathologic entity, but because it represents a common end-point of myocardial disease.

Incidence and Distribution of Lesions: Fibrosis is encountered frequently at necropsy of horses. Lesions often are grossly detectable on the surface of the heart or on cut section. Areas of scarring commonly range up to 3 cm in diameter and may appear as discrete to irregular pale areas or as linear streaks presenting a "tigroid" appearance (Fig 71). Whether or not these more obvious lesions are present, histopathologic examination frequently reveals focal fibrosis. The lesions have commonly been regarded as a reflection of age, parasitism or previous episodes of inflammation or infarction.[56,188,189,678-681]

In a study of 2076 equine hearts obtained from an abattoir, 296 (14.3%) exhibited macroscopically visible focal zones of myocardial fibrosis, but no age association was found.[189] This is the only study specifically interested in myocardial disease in which cases were selected for further examination solely on the basis of the presence of myocardial lesions. Findings in other studies indicated an increase in frequency with age. A study in which the extent of grossly fibrosed tissue was determined morphometrically in a selected abattoir population of 68 horses revealed a distinct direct age association.[340,496-498] Scars were observed in the ventricles in 77% of the horses and in the atria in 7% (age range of subjects 6 months to 25 years, mean 11 years). No indication was given as to how the animals were selected for inclusion in the study. In contrast, in an abattoir study of 1557 horses, myocardial scarring was infrequently observed except in horses over 20 years of age, in which lesions were confined to the epicardium and immediately adjacent myocardium.[116] The main emphasis in this study, however, was on valve changes. Other authors do not describe any endocardial vs epicardial predilection. Lesions of myocardial fibrosis have been encountered even in very young animals.[189,497] A greater incidence of inflammatory reaction in such cases led to the suggestion that infarction was the most frequent cause in young animals.[189]

There is some disagreement as to the areas of the myocardium most severely affected. The differences in published studies probably reflect varying populations and methods of investigation. Early studies suggested the right atrium and auricular appendage as a predilection site for age-related fibrosis, perhaps because changes in this area of relatively thin myocardium are easily seen.[188,679,682] Gross and microscopic fibrosis of both atria is particularly prominent in cases of atrial fibrillation.[162,272,683] Some horses show almost total replacement of the atrial myocardium with scar tissue.

The exact relationship between atrial arrhythmias and atrial myocardial disease has been examined. A high frequency of focal atrial myocardial fibrosis, together with changes in microvasculature and both intrinsic and extrinsic cardiac nerves, has been found in horses exhibiting arrhythmias ranging from second-degree heart block and wandering pacemaker to atrial fibrillation.[182,194,196,197,226,272] Similar lesions were encountered but with much lower frequency in horses not exhibiting such arrhythmias.[228] The ventricles were not examined in all of these horses.

Others have found the ventricles, mainly the proximal one-third (base) to be most frequently involved.[498] While one study suggested no predilection for either ventricle, other workers report predominant involvement of the septum and left heart.[188,189,498] Using a morphometric approach, one study describes a distinctly regional distribution.[498] Changes were detected most often in the septum and, in particular, that region supplied by the right coronary artery. Unfortunately, in that investigation the atrial myocardium was not subjected to histologic examination, though scarring of the atria was observed. There is general consensus that the free wall of the right ventricle is involved infrequently. Most reported observations, it must be remembered, were made in abattoir populations.

The picture for grossly inapparent lesions remains unclear. The distribution of intramural coronary vascular lesions detected in one study suggests that microscopic fibrosis may often be found in the cranial papillary muscle of the left ventricle, with the frequency of lesions increasing as one approaches the endocardium.[498] However, all areas, particularly of the septum and left ventricle, appear to be affected, with the right ventricle affected minimally.[188,189] Overall incidence of macroscopic and microscopic lesions was strongly correlated in one study.[498] While the entire myocardium was surveyed for gross lesions,

Figure 71. Myocardial fibrosis in a 3-year-old Thoroughbred gelding. The horse had a history of myositis and recent cardiac arrhythmia (atrial fibrillation) and syncopal episodes. Clinically both left and right AV insufficiency were evident. At necropsy there was severe cardiomegaly with eccentric hypertrophy of all 4 chambers. Valves were unremarkable and there were no congenital abnormalities. The myocardium, especially of the subepicardial one-third, showed extensive degeneration and replacement fibrosis (note streaking of myocardium). It was not possible to determine whether this case represented primary cardiomyopathy, nutritional myopathy or unusually severe myocardial involvement in repeated episodes of rhabdomyolysis.

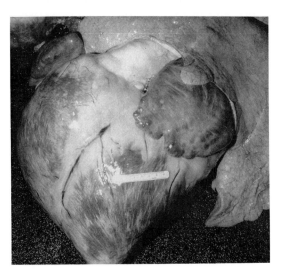

only selected areas were subjected to histologic examination. Other authors did not differentiate between gross and microscopic lesions.[188,189]

Cause: The cause of myocardial fibrosis in horses remains contentious. Great interest has been shown in changes in coronary arteries. Lesions variously described as arteriosclerosis, atherosclerotic stenosis, medial proliferation, fibrosis of media and adventitia, and intimal proliferation have been identified in fetuses and neonatal foals, as well as adults.[188,189,495,498,681,684] Extramural and intramural vessels have been identified as abnormal, though changes in intramural vessels are more frequently described. In one study, areas of fibrosis were consistently related to obstructed vessels.[189] A strong correlation between the incidence of fibrosis and that of parasitic thromboendarteritis of the proximal aorta was found. It was concluded that the damage to intramural coronary arteries (and thus myocardial fibrosis) reflected frequent embolic episodes and incorporation of emboli into the vessel wall. A similar association between arterial changes and fibrosis has been speculated upon by other workers.[188,678,679,681,685]

In a more recent study, however, no relationship between vascular change or myocardial fibrosis and parasitic thromboendarteritis of the proximal aorta could be demonstrated, neither was there any apparent relationship between total area of *grossly* detectable fibrosis and coronary arterial obstruction.[498] These authors did note correlation between fibrosis detected on tissue sections and the overall degree of intramural coronary arterial stenosis but concluded that other factors in addition to vascular insufficiency/infarction must be involved in development of myocardial fibrosis. They found a correlation between age and degree of arterial obstruction. It appears that evidence of inflammation in these areas of fibrosis is uncommon, except perhaps in younger animals, tending to rule out ongoing infarction or myocarditis as common causes.

In addition to narrowing of arteries in the study cited above, some related fibrosis of the media and/or adventitia of vessels was noted.[498] It was suggested that the reduced distensibility of these vessels may be of significance. The vasodilator reserve of the coronary vasculature is not exhausted at maximal effort in ponies.[686] It is possible, however, that areas of myocardium supplied by vessels with reduced vasodilator reserve may be subject to acute hypoxia at maximal exertion. Such damage may be cumulative with repeated exercise.

Atrial myocardial fibrosis in horses with arrhythmias has been ascribed to changes in intramural vessels, which, in turn, were assumed to be the result of primary degeneration in intrinsic autonomic nerves.[228] Overexertion in racehorses was suggested as one possible cause of the neural degeneration, though use of electrocution for destruction in some of these cases might have caused such lesions. Temperament has been suggested as a possible factor in coronary artery disease with secondary fibrosis.[495] Myocardial damage may accompany disease of the nervous system and is characterized as myocardial necrosis.[455,687] The most probable mechanisms are overactivity of the sympathetic nervous system and local catecholamine release or parasympathetic overactivity. Catecholamines and endotoxin can precipitate myocardial degeneration;[688,689] potassium deficiency also has this potential.[690] While these factors may act to varying degrees and synergistically in performance horses to promote myocardial degeneration, satisfactory evidence that performance horses are more prone to myocardial fibrosis than more sedentary animals is lacking.[498]

These data suggest that myocardial fibrosis, both gross and presumably microscopic, is relatively common, and the incidence and degree of fibrosis increase with age. Coronary arterial disease also is common, age-related and of probable etiologic significance in many cases. Parasitism, temperament and intense exercise may represent additional risk factors, as well as any other cause of myocardial degeneration. Neural factors, principally involving the autonomic nervous system, may play a role in the vascular changes that appear to underlie fibrosis in at least some affected areas of myocardium. The absence of inflammation and the histologic findings suggest chronic, ongoing, focally diffuse myocardial degeneration, possibly in addition to infrequent, acute episodes in most cases. Regional distribution of lesions suggests a predilection for the septum and left ventricle, and possibly the right atrium. In any case, postmortem evaluation of the equine myocardium must include both gross and histologic examination and must be thorough. The absence of grossly obvious lesions of fibrosis cannot be taken to exclude the presence of such changes at the histologic level.

Gross Infarction: Notwithstanding the above discussion, while the cause of myocardial fibrosis in horses is generally undetermined, gross infarction is observed occasionally. However, gross changes in the extramural coronary arteries are rare.[684] Horses are not subject to severe disease of the larger coronary arteries. Massive myocardial infarction, as occurs in people, is not seen. Cases of infarction reported in the earlier veterinary literature appear most often to have been secondary to obstruction of the right coronary artery, with the right atrial myocardial branches affected, leading to fibrosis.[18,682] Parasitic thromboendarteritis of the proximal aorta with embolism appears to have been the most common cause.[338,465] Ventricular infarction in equine infectious anemia has been described, though myocardial lesions are probably more frequently microscopic in these cases.[691] Myocardial infarction can be anticipated in endocarditis involving the left side of the heart, and has also been related to hyperlipemia in ponies.[692]

Equine Rhabdomyolysis Syndrome

Equine rhabdomyolysis syndrome (tying-up, azoturia, exertional rhabdomyolysis) is discussed in depth in the chapter on Diseases of the Musculoskeletal System.[693] It is mentioned here because of the myocardial involvement found in some cases.[694-696] Myocardial involvement is of minor importance, rarely contributing to death,[697] though progressive loss of myocardial functional capacity as a consequence of repeated milder episodes may be a more significant complication for most affected horses.[696] Limited myocardial involvement probably reflects the tendency for the condition to affect cell types primarily dependent upon anaerobic glycolysis, whereas the myocardium functions aerobically.[696]

The possibility that the myocardial degeneration observed in clinical cases was due to coexisting vascular disease raises questions as to the significance of lesions.[696]

However, ECG changes, including arrhythmias, tachycardia and ST segment changes, were described in most horses with exercise-related muscle disease in 1 report.[181] Because of functional similarities between skeletal and cardiac muscle and current theories as to the pathogenesis of myopathy, it is improbable that the myocardium is entirely spared, particularly in severe cases and possibly those experiencing repeated episodes (Fig 71).[693] Further work must be performed to evaluate the extent of myocardial involvement in equine rhabdomyolysis syndrome.

Nonspecific Degeneration and Concurrent Systemic Disease

Aside from the possibility that factors causing or resulting from systemic disease may have a direct effect upon myocardial structure or metabolism, such disturbances of homeostasis as dehydration and electrolyte imbalance or increased metabolic rate with fever create a further demand for cardiac output. If the insult is mild or short lived, the myocardium may be able to meet demands yet remain within the limits of its reserve capacity. However, that reserve can be drastically reduced by structural damage to heart muscle or compromised mitochondrial function. If the heart functions for any time beyond its current functional capacity, myocardial degeneration and necrosis are likely consequences. Additionally, direct toxic effects of therapeutic agents and drug hypersensitivity may further compromise the myocardium.[698] Most of these effects are poorly quantified.

Any damage that results from this increased load may be overshadowed by the presenting problem; it may be several days into the clinical episode before cardiovascular signs become obvious and can be differentiated. In many cases, no specific evidence of myocardial compromise is detected and recovery appears complete. For example, Figure 72 shows an ECG from a 7-year-old mare that had an acute episode of abdominal hemorrhage. The PCV was 14% and the resting heart rate was 70 bpm. A financial decision was made not to transfuse the horse. Over the next 3 days, her condition stabilized, with no further fall in PCV. However, on day 7, the heart rate was still 70 bpm and the mare began to show runs of ventricular ectopic beats, jugular filling and edema. The clinical signs were interpreted as indicating damage to the myocardium and incipient myocardial failure due to hypoxia and the anemia-induced high-output state.[699] Slow digitalization or a concurrent increase in PCV led to a fall in heart rate, and the arrhythmia subsided. Isoenzyme studies were inconclusive, though signs suggested that myocardial damage had occurred and could perhaps have been avoided by transfusion.

The significance of all these concerns is open to conjecture. Few adverse, secondary myocardial responses have been documented, though early signs of myocardial

Figure 72. ECG recorded from a 7-year-old Thoroughbred mare with a history of colic. A clinical diagnosis of intraabdominal hemorrhage was established, with the PCV reaching a low of 14%. During persistent tachycardia associated with the anemia, the mare developed cardiac arrhythmias. The ECG shows a run of closely coupled ventricular ectopic beats (onset marked by arrow), suggesting secondary myocardial damage.

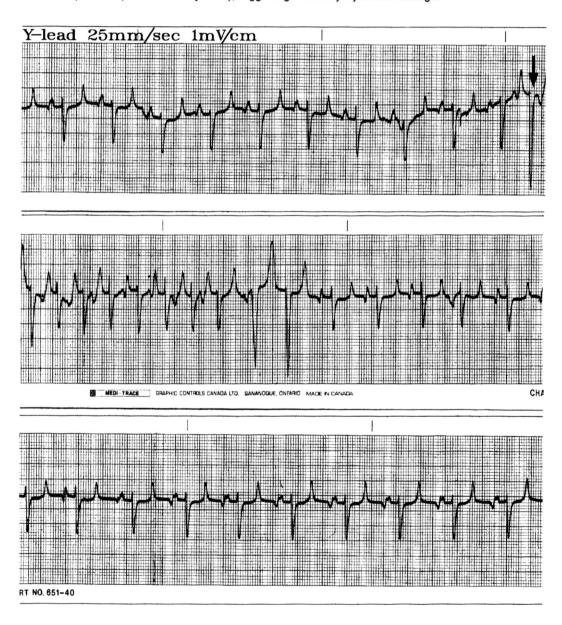

compromise, such as intermittent arrhythmias, slight elevation of jugular venous pressure, increased respiratory rate and ventral edema, might be ascribed secondary significance in light of the severity of the primary disease process and resultant homeostatic disturbances. Postmortem findings are likely to be nonspecific. Degeneration is the main finding, with frank necrosis if the insult was massive. It is, of course, a moot point whether death in all cases is not in fact due to cardiac failure. When it occurs after a short clinical course, myocardial lesions at other than the ultrastructural level are likely to be absent.

Cardiomyopathy

A definition of "cardiomyopathy" is elusive. In its broadest interpretation, the term connotes "any structural and/or functional abnormality of ventricular myocardium."[698] A tendency has developed, however, to use cardiomyopathy in a more restricted sense to describe myocardial disease in the absence of any extrinsic or extracardiac problem, such as a defective valve or chronic respiratory disease.[698] Reference to the term "idiopathic" in any definition is confusing, as "cardiomyopathy" still tends to be used even when the cause is understood.

For our purposes, cardiomyopathy may be regarded as myocardial disease arising spontaneously and in the absence of any obvious predisposing cause, such as valve dysfunction, congenital abnormality, respiratory disease, or direct toxic or infectious insult to the heart. The condition might thus be regarded as primary, though the mechanism causing the myocardial change may affect several tissues simultaneously. Clinical signs thus may reflect cardiac insufficiency or may be primarily referable to some other body system, and myocardial involvement may be overlooked.[700]

In people, numerous different cardiomyopathies are described, and some of these are genetically or nutritionally determined.[700] Cardiomyopathies have been described in many animals.[635] The disease in cats is associated with low plasma taurine levels in some cases.[701] Cardiomyopathy has also been described in cattle.[702,703] However, primary cardiomyopathy has not been characterized in horses.[635] Reference has been made to cases of idiopathic heart failure in which necropsy revealed symmetric cardiac dilatation.[704] In 2 cases of biventricular failure in 3-year-old Thoroughbred geldings examined at our hospital, histopathologic examination revealed only diffuse, generalized myocardial degeneration and early fibrosis (Fig 71, 73). Characteristically, review of the history failed to reveal any predisposing cause.

Myocardial Hypertrophy

Myocardial hypertrophy has been discussed in the section on Heart Failure. It is, however, relevant to reemphasize that a hypertrophied myocardium is not normal and that cardiac reserve is reduced. Episodes of myocardial insult and loss of tissue are accompanied in the compensatory phase by hypertrophy of remaining myocardium, the extent of which depends upon the degree and rate of development of the damage and the nature of the ongoing load placed on the heart. Horses undergoing repeated episodes

Figure 73. Cardiomegaly in a 3-year-old Thoroughbred gelding presented in an emaciated condition. Clinical signs were of biventricular failure. The photograph shows severe dilatation of the right atrium and ventricle. Necropsy revealed ongoing myocardial degeneration and early fibrosis. AV valvular insufficiency appeared to be recent and secondary to dilation of the valve annulus as the valve cusps were normal. No other lesions were found and the history revealed no explanation for findings.

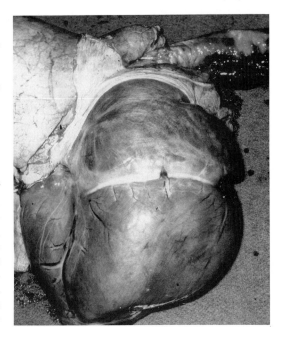

of myocardial damage may go through cycles of compensation, each episode leaving the heart less able to accommodate the next insult or the demands of exercise. The frequency with which such events occur is unknown and is only implied by such postmortem findings as myocardial fibrosis.

Myocardial Calcification

Calcification of the myocardium is a frequent finding in acute myocardial degeneration, though horses do not appear particularly predisposed to this complication.[455] Severe calcification of the heart and pulmonary vasculature has been described in horses exposed to hay contaminated with plants containing vitamin D analogs.[595] The underlying cause frequently is tuberculosis or parasitism; hence its current rarity.

DISEASES OF THE PERICARDIUM AND THORACIC CAVITY

P.W. Physick-Sheard

Neoplastic Diseases

Pericardial Neoplasia

Though the pericardium may become secondarily involved in any thoracic neoplastic process, with resultant effusion, pericardial neoplasia is extremely rare in horses.[455] Two cases of primary pericardial mesothelioma have been reported.[705,706] In the first case, there was extensive thoracic involvement. In the second, the horse was 27 years old and was killed because of weight loss and old age. The neoplasm was an incidental postmortem finding and was restricted to the pericardial sac; moderate effusion was present. Fluid accumulation in such cases is likely to be a transudate or modified transudate; the cytologic picture may be diagnostic.

Pericardial hemangiosarcoma with a short clinical course has been described in a 22-year-old heavy horse.[482] Death was due to thoracic hemorrhage. While involvement of the heart in cases of lymphosarcoma is likely, direct involvement of the pericardial sac is uncommon and signs in such cases appear to be limited to an increase in fluid

secondary to irritation caused by neoplastic involvement of the heart.[707]

Multifactorial Diseases

Pericardial Effusion and Pericarditis

Though not a common problem in horses, clinically significant pericardial effusion has long been recognized.[708] Benign pericardial effusion in the form of a transudate may occur in any disorder of tissue fluid balance, such as congestive heart failure or hypoproteinemia, but hydropericardium as a discrete clinical entity is not common.

Cause: Most cases of pericardial fluid accumulation involve inflammation. Pericarditis secondary to trauma, extension from myocardial/endocardial infection, neoplasia and as a probable complication of systemic viral or bacterial disease has been reported.[318,709-712] Pericardial effusion in cases of viral respiratory disease and arteritis also has been referenced;[713,714] however, it probably is only occasionally clinically significant.

Most cases of spontaneous pericardial effusion in horses are idiopathic and appear to consist of primary fibrinous pericarditis.[318,715-718] The literature refers to extension of pleural and pulmonary inflammatory processes as a common cause of pericarditis, though the direct evidence for this interpretation is limited.[18,156,719]

Trauma may be direct and caused by rib fractures, laceration of the pericardium secondary to penetrating wounds, and foreign bodies, such as pieces of wire.[709,716] Involvement of the pericardium in other forms of cardiac trauma, such as rupture of the aorta or heart, also may be encountered.[330,720,721] Foreign bodies have included pieces of metal or hard plant stems migrating from the esophagus, stomach or duodenum.[710,719,722] A simple transudate may be encountered in heart failure and severe hypoalbuminemia but fluid accumulation is unlikely to progress to the extent of causing clinical signs specifically related to pericardial effusion.

Clinical Signs: Clinical findings in pericardial effusion reflect pressure on the heart and cardiac displacement, causing obstruction to venous return and reduced cardiac output. The result is the classic triad of tachycardia with weak rapid pulse, muffled heart sounds and venous obstruction.[723] Systemic venous, right atrial, ventricular and pulmonary arterial diastolic pressures all are elevated.[718] Elevated venous pressure leads to extensive ventral edema and jugular venous distention. Development of edema may be enhanced initially by maintenance of systemic arterial pressure, as left ventricular function is influenced less rapidly than right ventricular function, and later by salt and water retention secondary to reduced cardiac output. In the early stages, pulsation may be evident in the jugular furrows though severe distention of the pericardial sac (cardiac tamponade) later may result in fully distended, nonpulsatile veins. The heart rate is elevated and the pulse weak. Peripheral circulation is compromised, as indicated by prolonged capillary refill time and cool periphery. Clinical signs thus are those of congestive heart failure, though the myocardium is essentially normal.

Auscultation usually reveals muffling and occasionally dorsal displacement of heart sounds. Splashing sounds are likely to be heard only if a mixed bacterial population with putrefactive organisms is present or if prior pericardiocentesis has allowed entry of air. Very early in the disease, when little effusion is present and after pericardiocentesis and drainage of the sac, clear heart sounds and friction rubs may be heard. These may be soft or quite loud and harsh, and must be differentiated from murmurs. It is improbable that they will be detected at presentation in most cases, as effusion is likely to develop rapidly.[718] Fever is not a consistent finding. The horse's demeanor depends somewhat upon the underlying cause, but depression and lethargy usually are observed. Colic has been described in some cases.[318,716,718] In people, pericarditis can be very painful, which could explain some of the signs seen in horses.

Several authors describe congestion/hyperemia of mucous membranes or cyanosis.[318,710,716] Dyspnea is observed in most cases. Mucosal congestion and cyanosis are not typical signs of heart failure, and probably reflect toxemia due to sepsis and/or respiratory compromise. Respiratory involvement and findings upon thoracic percussion

are somewhat dependent upon duration of the problem, rate of pericardial fluid accumulation and the extent of coexisting pleural effusion. The pericardial sac is fibrous in nature and does not distend readily. However, if fluid accumulation has been slow, quite remarkable distention can develop, with the sac containing up to 12 L of fluid.[716] This volume can cause significant distress and respiratory embarrassment.

The relationship between pleural and pericardial effusion, and their relative contribution to respiratory signs are unclear. In horses I have treated, primary pleural/pneumonic processes infrequently led to clinically significant pericardial effusion, even with extensive local tissue necrosis. In a review of 37 cases of pleuritis and pleural effusion, significant pericardial involvement was not discussed.[724] Pericardial effusion, when it occurs in such cases, usually involves slight increase in quantity of normal fluid or mild pericarditis that may result from septicemia rather than direct local spread.

Diagnosis: The diagnosis is based upon clinical signs and is best confirmed by echocardiographic examination.[623,717,718] This demonstrates the increased pericardial fluid and differentiates pericardial from pleural disease. The procedure also can confirm the location of the heart within the fluid-filled cavity and provide insight into the type of process by detecting fibrin masses. Diagnosis is further aided by pericardiocentesis which is essential if the nature of the effusive process is to be fully explored.[725,726] However, differentiation between pericardial and pleural effusion is not necessarily achieved by this method unless the tap is performed directly over the heart at the fourth or fifth intercostal space, which is potentially dangerous (see below). If primary pleuritis is a strong differential diagnosis, there is the danger of spreading the infection to the pericardial sac. Thoracentesis at the ninth or tenth intercostal space is advisable to evaluate pleural fluid first. Use of diagnostic ultrasound largely resolves these dilemmas.

The nature of the pericardial fluid depends upon the primary insult. With bleeding into the pericardial sac, whether traumatic or iatrogenic, the fluid is bloody to serosanguineous.[725,727] In idiopathic cases, a range of findings have been described, including aseptic but mildly inflammatory effusions, sometimes containing significant numbers of eosinophils or histiocytes.[718] Effusion also may be septic, though in most published cases, bacterial culture was negative.[318,711,712] If bacteria have been isolated, they have been nonspecific and, with the possible exception of one report, not indicating involvement of any particular pathogen.[711,712]

Failure to isolate causative organisms may reflect treatment with antibiotics before culture and/or failure to culture sufficiently early in the clinical syndrome. Implication of *Mycoplasma felis* in pleurisy suggests that attempts to isolate these organisms should be pursued in cases of idiopathic pericarditis, particularly if macrophages and healthy-looking neutrophils are found on centesis.[728,729] Culture for *Mycoplasma*, assuming they are present, is likely to be successful only early in the clinical course of the disease. If a heavy, especially a mixed, bacterial population is cultured a penetrating wound, either from the exterior or from the digestive tract, must be considered as a cause. This is especially true when splashing sounds on auscultation suggest gas-producing organisms are present. With the exception of such cases and those in which cytologic examination indicates neoplasia, the prognosis cannot be determined from results of cytologic examination.

Radiography may not be very revealing, as accumulation of large quantities of fluid in the pericardial sac or pleural space obliterates detail and produces a similar radiographic picture.[318] Rounding of the cardiac silhouette may be detectable in early cases. Though electrocardiography has been used diagnostically and consistent ECG changes described, patterns detected are not sufficiently specific to diagnose pericardial effusion.[156,318,716-718,730,731] Findings usually consist of tachycardia, reduced amplitude of the QRS complex, and nonspecific ST-segment and T-wave changes. Electrical alternans, in which amplitude of waveforms varies from beat to beat as a result of movement of the heart in the distended pericardial sac, also is observed in some cases.

Hematologic and serum biochemical findings are nonspecific and of limited value in diagnosis. Elevated serum globulin levels and/or mature neutrophilia may be detected in cases associated with sepsis. Eosinophils have been detected in pericardial fluid in some cases and associated with transient eosinophilia. Elevated serum fibrinogen levels can be anticipated.

Treatment: Treatment is aimed primarily at draining the pericardial sac by pericardiocentesis, and controlling inflammation. This appears to be sufficient in many cases.[717,718] Pericardiocentesis can be performed with a needle but is most safely done with a polyethylene (intravenous) catheter so that once the sac is penetrated, the sharp trocar can be withdrawn. A 14-ga catheter usually is adequate, though drainage of the sac through this size of tube may be slow. Rapid drainage is contraindicated, especially in acute cases, because this can cause a rapid fall in cardiac output. The catheter must be at least 5 inches long to allow for the thickness of the chest wall and up to several centimeters of fibrin on the inside of the pericardium. There also is a tendency for the catheter to move in and out of the tissue as the animal shifts its weight. Aseptic technique must be employed even if a septic process is suspected; introduction of a second pathogen into the sac may lead to rapid deterioration.

The pericardial sac can be entered directly over the heart at the fourth or fifth intercostal space at a level halfway between the elbow and the shoulder.[725] However, this can be dangerous because laceration of a coronary artery can lead to fatal cardiac tamponade. When this site must be used, the procedure must be performed with extreme caution, particularly if only a small volume of pericardial effusion is suspected.

If significant pericardial effusion is present, the distended sac is easily entered farther caudally at the sixth to seventh intercostal space on either side of the thorax with less chance of tamponade.[156,726] Chances of lacerating a coronary artery also can be reduced by staying ventral on the thorax, 2-3 inches dorsal to the level of the elbow; in some cases, sedimented debris may continually occlude the catheter at this level.

Echocardiographic examination should be performed whenever possible to differentiate between pleural and pericardial effusion and to guide pericardiocentesis. Separation of the pericardium from the ventricular wall by a fluid-density interspace usually can be clearly seen. An ECG also should be recorded at the same time. Accidental contact with the heart during pericardiocentesis usually leads to ventricular ectopic beats.

The intercostal space should be infiltrated with local anesthetic and the needle introduced in the direction indicated by the results of ultrasound examination. In the absence of ultrasonographic guidance, the needle should be introduced at the sixth intercostal space, with the needle oriented in a horizontal plane and pointing approximately 30 degrees cranial to the transverse plane. The bevel should point cranially. The needle is advanced cautiously, taking care to avoid the intercostal artery on the caudal border of the rib, and is withdrawn slightly if it grates against the heart. It should be withdrawn completely if an initially yellowish fluid becomes bloody, especially if this fluid clots.

If the diagnosis is correct, fluid flows as soon as the sac is penetrated because pericardial effusions usually are fairly serous. Repositioning of the catheter may be necessary if fibrin obstructs the tip. Placement of an indwelling 20-Fr catheter at the fifth intercostal space facilitates drainage and flushing of the pericardial sac, and may be necessary if fluid accumulates rapidly after drainage.[717] However, because of the possibility of introducing infection and stimulating fibrin formation by tissue irritation secondary to catheter placement, it may be advisable to attempt only drainage initially. In some cases, a single draining of the sac may suffice.[718]

Antiinflammatory therapy may help control fluid accumulation. Corticosteroids have been used and are not contraindicated if cultures are negative and antibiotics are used. The relative value of nonsteroidal antiinflammatory drugs cannot be determined on the basis of the small number of cases reported. Similarly, there have been an insufficient number of bacterial isolates to make specific recommendations regarding antibiotic therapy. Pericardiectomy or pericardiotomy are employed frequently in people to relieve constrictive pericardial disease. Surgical treatment has been described in cattle.[732] However, this procedure has not been described in horses and may not be indicated either in terms of need or prognosis.

The clinical course is variable but usually short. In a study of 10 cases, the mean duration of illness before examination was 9 days (range 1-21).[718] This is consistent with findings in other reported cases, though histories of weeks to months have been documented. It is significant that, even in cases of only a few days' duration, ventral edema may be extensive. Ascites may be clinically detectable, which is a rather unusual finding in horses. This assists in differential diagnosis because in congestive heart failure, the clinical course is more prolonged and edema does not develop so rapidly. In venous obstruction secondary to a thoracic mass, the edema usually is not generalized but restricted to the cranial thorax, neck and head.

The disease course depends upon the presence or absence of sepsis, rate of accumulation of fluid, and response to therapy. Death may occur within days or the disease may follow a protracted course of weeks to months. The prognosis for recovery is likely to be greatly improved by early diagnosis and appropriate therapy, including drainage and, if necessary, lavage of the pericardial sac, along with antiinflammatory and antibiotic therapy. If a foreign body or mixed bacterial infection is involved, the prognosis is poor.

The long-term prognosis partly depends upon the extent to which fibrin has been laid down and organizes. In other species, scar tissue contraction leads to constriction and low-output failure. Too few cases have been described in horses to determine the probability of this consequence, though survival of months to years after treatment of pericarditis has been reported.[717,718] Whether this reflects limited fibrin deposition and fibrous tissue formation or the cardiovascular reserve in horses is unclear. Regardless, rapid resolution of the inflammation can be expected to enhance chances of survival and return to work.

Postmortem findings depend somewhat upon the underlying cause. Pericarditis usually is fibrinous and the inside of the pericardium and epicardium are covered by a layer of fibrin, with degrees of organization reflecting the chronicity of the process. Along with a pericardial sac containing many liters of fluid, pleural and peritoneal effusion usually are present with extensive ventral edema. Lesions in other organs are then essentially those caused by congestive heart failure.

DISEASES OF THE THORACIC CAVITY

P.W. Physick-Sheard

Problems in the thoracic cavity of direct importance in the context of cardiovascular diseases are chronic respiratory disease and thoracic masses. Chronic respiratory disease can lead to severe pulmonary hypertension and right heart failure, a syndrome referred to as cor pulmonale. The latter is discussed in the section on Heart Failure, while chronic respiratory disease is discussed in the chapter on Diseases of the Respiratory System.

The most common thoracic masses are pulmonary abscesses and tumors, of which lymphosarcoma is by far the most common cause.[707,733-735] Pulmonary abscesses most often form in the ventral or cranioventral lung, particularly on the right side. Unless the mass is particularly large and interferes with cardiac filling, involvement of the heart is limited to variable degrees of caudal cardiac displacement and some difference in the relative intensity of heart sounds on the 2 sides of the chest. Heart sounds may not be muffled and may even be heard over a wider area than normal.

Cardiovascular involvement in lymphosarcoma takes 2 forms: infiltration of the myocardium and pressure from a heart-base mass. Neoplastic masses in the mediastinum can be very large and can impinge on the great veins, atria and major airways. Interference with cardiac filling and/or venous return causes venous hypertension and reduced cardiac output, a clinical syndrome not obviously distinguishable from right heart failure.[707,733,735,736] The onset of clinical signs can be very rapid (2-3 days), though usually the course is a matter of weeks. Though all degrees of involvement can occur, masses most often form in the cranial mediastinum and initially cause selective obstruction of cranial venous drainage, resulting in marked distention of the jugular veins and edema in the breast and pectoral region; veins in the caudal half of the body are normal. Filling of the thoracic inlet may be an early sign. A tendency for

edema to involve the forelimbs is characteristic. Caudal displacement of the heart may be detected.

Mediastinal lymphosarcoma may be accompanied by pleural and pericardial effusion. Affected horses may be anemic because of bone marrow involvement; chronically affected horses may have weight loss. Peripheral lymphadenopathy is common but not invariably present. With severe mediastinal lymphadenopathy there may be little or no involvement of other lymphoid tissues. Horses of all ages can be affected, including foals, though the mean age of involvement varies from 6 to 10 years.[707,733, 736,737] There is no sex predilection.

The diagnosis is based upon clinical signs and cytologic examination. Fluid can be obtained by thoracentesis (or abdominocentesis if abdominal masses are detected) or by fine-needle aspiration of lymphoid masses if they are accessible. Typically the fluid is sanguineous and contains lymphocytes with marked variation is size and morphology, together with immature, large pleomorphic lymphoid cells. However, neoplastic masses may be entirely intrathoracic, with enlargement of superficial nodes (caudal cervical nodes) reflecting only local congestion. Thus, fine-needle biopsy and centesis may be unrewarding. Peripheral blood changes are inconsistent, though leukemia and atypical lymphocytes are found in some cases.[706] Short-term improvement may be achieved with corticosteroid therapy, but the prognosis for recovery is poor.

References

1. Guyton AC: *Textbook of Medical Physiology.* Saunders, Philadelphia, 1981.

2. Persson SGB: On blood volume and working capacity in horses. *Acta Vet Scand* 19:1-189, 1967.

3. Physick-Sheard PW: Cardiovascular response to exercise and training in the horse. *Vet Clin No Am* (Equine Pract) 1:383-417, 1985.

4. Quiring DP and Baker RJ: The equine heart. *Am J Vet Res* 13-14:62-67, 1953.

5. Ghoshal NG, in Getty R *et al: Sisson and Grossman's The Anatomy of the Domestic Animals.* Saunders, Philadelphia, 1975. pp 554-618.

6. Brown CM and Holmes JR: Haemodynamics in the horse. 1. Pressure pulse contours. *Equine Vet J* 10:188-194, 1978.

7. Brown CM and Holmes JR: Haemodynamics in the horse: 2. Intracardiac, pulmonary arterial and aortic pressures. *Equine Vet J* 10:207-215, 1978.

8. Beltran LE: *A critical evaluation of right heart catheterisation in the horse.* Dissertation. Royal Veterinary College, London, 1975.

9. Holmes JR and Darke PGG: Foetal electrocardiography in the mare. *Vet Record* 82:651-655, 1968.

10. Colles CM *et al:* Foetal electrocardiography in the mare. *Equine Vet J* 10:32-37, 1978.

11. Matsui K *et al:* Alterations in the heart rate of Thoroughbred horse, pony and Holstein cow through pre- and post-natal stages. *Jpn J Vet Sci* 46:505-510, 1984.

12. Buss DD *et al:* Limitations in equine fetal electrocardiography. *JAVMA* 177:174-176, 1980.

13. Matsui K *et al:* Changes in the fetal heart rate of Thoroughbred horse through the gestation. *Jpn J Vet Sci* 47:597-601, 1985.

14. Amada A and Senda T: Fetal electrocardiogram of horses.. *Jpn J Vet Sci* (Suppl) 26:431-432, 1964.

15. Too K *et al:* Fetal and maternal electrocardiograms during parturition in a mare. *Jpn J Vet Res* 15:5-13, 1967.

16. Rossdale PD: Clinical studies on the newborn Thoroughbred foal II. Heart rate, ausculation and electrocardiogram. *Brit Vet J* 123:521-532, 1967.

17. Reef VB and Spencer P: Echocardiographic evaluation of equine aortic insufficiency. *Am J Vet Res* 48:904-909, 1987.

18. Detweiler DK and Patterson DF, in Catcott EJ and Smithcors JF: *Equine Medicine and Surgery.* American Veterinary Publications, Goleta, CA, 1972. pp 277-347.

19. Miklausic B and Dolinar Z: Die digito-digitale Perkussion und topographische Grenzbestimmung der Hertzdampfung beim Pferd. *Veterinarski Archiv* 36:284-290, 1966.

20. Miklausic B and Vulinec M: Ein neuer topographischer Orientierungspunkt zur Grenzbestimmung der Herzdampfung bei Pferd und Rind. *Zbl Vetmed* 17A:592-597, 1970.

21. Holmes JR: *Equine Cardiology. Vol I.* University of Bristol, Bristol, 1986.

22. Rushmer RF: *Cardiovascular Dynamics, a Physiologic Approach.* Saunders, Philadelphia, 1970.

23. Luisada AA *et al:* Changing views on the mechanism of the first and second heart sounds. *Am Heart J* 88:503-514, 1974.

24. Rushmer RF: *Cardiovascular Dynamics.* Saunders, Philadelphia, 1976.

25. Neumann-Kleinpaul K and Steffan H: Zur graphischen Darstellung der Herztone bei Tier und Mensch. *Arch wiss prakt Tierheilk* 65:629-642, 1932.

26. Charton A *et al:* Les bruits normaux de coeur du cheval; Etude phonocardiographique. *Bull Acad Vet Fr* 16:215-224, 1943.

27. Smetzer DL and Smith CR: Diastolic heart sounds of horses. *JAVMA* 146:937-944, 1965.

28. Patterson DF *et al:* Heart sounds and murmurs of the normal horse. *Ann NY Acad Sci* 127:242-305, 1965.

29. Smetzer DL *et al:* The fourth heart sound in the equine. *Ann NY Acad Sci* 127:306-321, 1965.

30. Holmes JR: Equine phonocardiography. *Med Biol Illus* 26:16-25, 1966.

31. Senta T and Kubo K: Clinical phonocardiography in the racehorse. I. The first and the second heart sounds recorded by thermal stylus type direct recording phonocardiograph. *Exp Rep Equine Hlth Lab* 9:44-54, 1972.

32. Vanselow B *et al:* A phonocardiographic study of equine heart sounds. *Aust Vet J* 54:161-170, 1978.

33. Brown CM and Holmes JR: Phonocardiography in the horse: 1. The intracardiac phonocardiogram. *Equine Vet J* 11:11-18, 1979.

34. Brown CM and Holmes JR: Phonocardiography in the horse. 2. The relationship of the external phonocardiogram to intracardiac pressure and sound. *Equine Vet J* 11:183-186, 1979.

35. Littlewort MCG: The clinical auscultation of the equine heart. *Vet Record* 74:1247-1256, 1962.

36. Littlewort MCG, in Hickman J: *Equine Surgery and Medicine, Vol 2.* Academic Press, London, 1986. pp 1-87.

37. Meyling HA and Ter Borg H: The conducting system of the heart in hoofed animals. *Cornell Vet* 47:419-447, 1957.

38. Getty R, in Getty R *et al: Sisson and Grossman's The Anatomy of the Domestic Animals.* Saunders, Philadelphia, 1975. pp 168-169.

39. Hamlin RL *et al:* Atrial activation paths and P waves in horses. *Am J Physiol* 219:306-313, 1970.

40. Muylle E and Oyaert W: Atrial activation pathways and the P wave in the horse. *Zbl Vetmed A* 22:474-484, 1975.

41. Hamlin RL *et al:* P wave in the electrocardiogram of the horse. *Am J Vet Res* 31:1027-1031, 1970.

42. Bishop SP and Cole CR: Morphology of the specialized conducting tissue in the atria of the equine heart. *Anat Record* 158:401, 1967.

43. McKibben JS and Getty R: Innervation of heart of domesticated animals: horse. *Am J Vet Res* 30:193-202, 1969.

44. Miller PJ and Holmes JR: Beat-to-beat variability in QRS potentials recorded with an orthogonal lead system in horses with second degree partial A-V block. *Res Vet Sci* 37:334-338, 1984.

45. Miller PJ and Holmes JR: Interrelationship of some electrocardiogram amplitudes, time intervals and respirations in the horse. *Res Vet Sci* 36:370-374, 1984.

46. Holmes JR and Darke PGG: Studies on the development of a new lead system for equine electrocardiography. *Equine Vet J* 2:12-21, 1970.

47. Holmes JR and Else RW: Further studies on a new lead system for equine electrocardiography. *Equine Vet J* 4:81-88, 1972.

48. Holmes JR: Spatial vector changes during ventricular depolarisation using a semi-orthogonal lead system-a study of 190 cases. *Equine Vet J* 8:1-16, 1976.

49. Muylle E and Oyaert W: Equine electrocardiography. The genesis of the different configurations of the "QRS" complex. *Zbl Vetmed A* 24:762-771, 1977.

50. Muylle E: *Experimenteel onderzoek naar het verloop van de depolarisatiegolf in het hart van het paard. De genesis van het electrocardiografisch P- en QRS-complex.* Dissertation. Rijksuniversiteit Ghent, Belgium, 1975.

51. Castellanos A and Myerburg RJ, in Hurst JW: *The Heart, Arteries and Veins.* McGraw-Hill, New York, 1986.

52. Norr J: Das Elektrokardiogramm des Pferdes. Seine Aufnahme und Form. *Zeitschr Biol* 61:197-229, 1913.

53. Lalezari K: *Evaluation and use of the equivalent generator of the equine heart. Dissertation.* Rijksuniversiteit te Utrecht, The Netherlands, 1984.

54. Physick-Sheard PW, in Robinson NE: *Current Therapy in Equine Medicine 2.* Saunders, Philadelphia, 1987. pp 147-151.

55. Dezobry JM: *Contribution a l'etude clinique et electrocardiographique chez le cheval de l'action d'un cardiotonique: la pentaformylgitoxine. Dissertation.* Ecole Nationale Veterinaire d'Alfort, Paris, 1972.

56. Detweiler DK and Patterson DF, in Bone JF: *Equine Medicine and Surgery.* American Veterinary Publications, Goleta, CA, 1963. pp 338-397.

57. Shaffer CA and Gabel AA: Photographic recording of cardiovascular data in horses during exercise. *Biological Photography* 54(2):51-53, 1986.

58. Baron M: *Vectorcardiogram of the sporting horse. Its use in examination before surgery. Dissertation.* Ecole Nationale Vetrinaire d'Alfort, Paris, 1970.

59. Grauerholz H: Eine Methode zur vektoriellen Auswertung des Elektrokardiogramms beim Pferd. *Zbl Vetmed A* 21:188-197, 1974.

60. Lalezari K and Kroneman J: Comparison of different lead systems in the horse. *Proc 5th Mtg Acad Soc for Large Anim Vet Med,* 1980. pp 65-75.

61. Lalezari K and Kroneman J: Distribution of the heart potentials on thoracic surface of the horse. *Proc 5th Mtg Acad Soc for Large Anim Vet Med,* 1980. pp 171-189.

63. Hanak J and Jagos P: Electrocardiographic lead system and its vector verification. *Acta Vet Brno* 52:67-75, 1983.

63. Holmes JR: A method of vectorcardiogram loop portrayal. *Equine Vet J* 2:27-34, 1970.

64. Grauerholz H: Untersuchungen uber den QRS-Komplex im EKG des Pferdes. *Berl Münch Tierärztl Wochenschr* 93:301-309, 1980.

65. Physick-Sheard PW and Hendren CM, in Snow DH *et al: Equine Exercise Physiology.* Granta Editions, Cambridge, 1983. pp 121-134.

66. Tschudi PR: *Das Vektorkardiogramm des Pferdes und seine diagnostische Bedeutung. Dissertation.* Veterinaermedizinischen Fakultaet der Universitaet Bern, Switzerland, 1982.

67. Matthiesen TH and Deegen E: Untersuchungen zum EKG des Fohlens. I. Untersuchungen zur Entwicklung des Massenverhaltnisses der Herzmuskulatur bei Fohlen im Zusammenhang mit der postnatalen Kreislaufumschaltung. *Zbl Vetmed A* 23:709-716, 1976.

68. Deegen E and Matthiesen TH: Untersuchungen zum EKG des Fohlens. II. Entwicklung des QRS-Komplexes in den Standard-Extremitaten-Ableitungen innerhalb des ersten Lebensjahres. *Zbl Vetmed A* 24:799-816, 1977.

69. Hanak J: Angle of the electrical cardiac axis and magnitude of the ventricular vector in thoroughbred foals. *Acta Vet Brno* 50:207-212, 1981.

70. Hanak J: The angle of electrical cardiac axis in trained Thoroughbred race horses. *Acta Vet Brno* 49:205-210, 1980.

71. Hanak J: Changes of ventricular vector during training of Thoroughbred race horses. *Acta Vet Brno* 49:211-216, 1980.

72. Hanak J: Effect of training Thoroughbred foals on the angle of their electrical cardiac axis and magnitude of the ventricular vector. *Acta Vet Brno* 51:69-73, 1982.

73. Fister D *et al:* Konfigurationsanderung der QRS-Gruppe im EKG bei Rennpferden im ersten Trainingsjahr. *Zbl Vetmed A* 28:102-112, 1981.

74. Fister D and Deegen E: Verhalten der QRS-Gruppe im EKG bei Rennpferden im zweiten Trainingsjahr. *Zbl Vetmed A* 29:721-727, 1982.

75. Fregin GF: The equine electrocardiogram with standardized body and limb positions. *Cornell Vet* 72:304-324, 1982.

76. Fregin GF: Electrocardiography. *Vet Clin No Am* (Equine Pract) 1:419-432, 1985.

77. Sporri H: Untersuchungen uber Systolen- und Diastolendauer bei verschiedenen Haustierarten und ihre Bedeutung für die Klinik und Beurteilungslehre. *Schweiz Arch Tierheilk D* 96:598-604, 1954.

78. Mill J: Die Zeitwerte und der Diastolen-Systolenquotient im Elektrokardiogramm des Sportpferdes und ihre Beziehung zur Leistung. I. Mitteilung: Untersuchungen ohne physische Belastung. *Monatshefte Vetmed* 32:861-866, 1977.

79. Ischikawa K *et al:* Electrocardiographic changes due to cardiac enlargement. *Am Heart J* 81:635-643, 1971.

80. Steel JD: *Studies on the Electrocardiogram of the Racehorse.* Australian Medical Publishing, Sydney, 1963.

81. Holmes JR and Rezakhani A: Observations on the T wave of the equine electrocardiogram. *Equine Vet J* 7:55-62, 1975.

82. Rose RJ and Davis PE: Treatment of atrial fibrillation in three racehorses. *Equine Vet J* 9:68-71, 1977.

83. Rose RJ and Davis PE: The use of electrocardiography in the diagnosis of poor racing performance in the horse. *Aust Vet J* 54:51-56, 1978.

84. Stewart JH *et al,* in Snow DH *et al: Equine Exercise Physiology.* Granta Editions, Cambridge, 1983. pp 135-143.

85. Irvine CHG: Clinical electrocardiography in the horse. *Proc 12th Ann Mtg AAEP,* 1967. pp 305-314.

86. Dohmen EG and Zaccardi EM: Electrocardiogram of a horse with chronic pulmonary emphysema. *Rev Fac Cienc Vet* 6:195-197, 1964.

87. Parkes RD and Colles CM: Fetal electrocardiography in the mare as a practical aid to diagnosing singleton and twin pregnancy. *Vet Record* 100:25-26, 1977.

88. Matsui K: Fetal and maternal heart rates in a case of twin pregnancy of the Thoroughbred horse. *Jpn J Vet Sci* 47:817-821, 1985.

89. Fregin GF and Thomas DP, in Snow DH *et al: Equine Exercise Physiology.* Granta Editions, Cambridge, 1983. pp 76-90.

90. Evans DL and Rose RJ: Method of investigation of the accuracy of four digitally-displaying heart rate meters suitable for use in the exercising horse. *Equine Vet J* 18:129-132, 1986.

91. Persson SGB and Ullberg LE: Blood volume in relation to exercise tolerance in trotters. *J So Afr Med Assn* 45:293-299, 1974.

92. Persson SGB, in Snow DH *et al: Equine Exercise Physiology.* Granta Editions, Cambridge, 1983. pp 441-457.

93. Maier H: *Messung der Herzschlagfrequenz bei Pferden mit Lungen- Herz- und Kehlkopferkrankungen wahrend einer definierten Belastung. Eine Moglichkeit zur Objektivierung der Leistungsminderung.* Dissertation. München: Fachbereich Tiermedizin, 1976.

94. Beglinger R *et al:* Herz-und Kreislaufdiagnostik beim Pferd im Institut für Veterinär-Physiologie (Direktor: Prof. Dr. Dr. h.c.H. Sprri) der Universitat Zurich. *Schweiz Arch Tierheilk* 122:533-539, 1980.

95. Littlejohn A *et al:* Cardiopulmonary function studies in saddle horses during exercise. *J So Afr Vet Med Assn* 49:269, 1975.

96. Ehrlein H-J *et al:* Die Herzschlagfrequenz während standardisierter Belastung als Mass für die Leistungsfahigkeit von Pferden. *Zbl Vetmed A* 20:188-208, 1973.

97. Rose RJ and Hodgson DR: Haematological and plasma biochemical parameters in endurance horses during training. *Equine Vet J* 14:144-148, 1982.

98. Rose RJ, in Snow DH *et al: Equine Exercise Physiology.* Granta Editions, Cambridge, 1983. pp 505-509.

99. Senta T *et al:* Effects of exercise on certain electrocardiographic parameters and cardiac arrhythmias in the horse. A radiotelemetric study. *Cornell Vet* 60:552-569, 1970.

100. Holmes JR and Alps BJ: The effect of exercise on rhythm irregularities in the horse. *Vet Record* 78:672-683, 1966.

101. Holmes JR: An investigation of cardiac rhythm using an on-line radiotelemetry/computer link. *J So Afr Vet Med Assn* 45:251-261, 1974.

102. Glendinning ESA: Significance of clinical abnormalities of the heart in soundness. *Equine Vet J* 4:21-26, 1972.

103. Holmes JR *et al:* Paroxysmal atrial fibrillation in racehorses. *Equine Vet J* 18:37-42, 1986.

104. Physick-Sheard PW *et al,* in Gillespie JR and Robinson NE: *Equine Exercise Physiology.* ICEEP Publications, Davis, CA, 1987. pp 102-116.

105. Karras: Demonstration of heart sounds of army horses by means of a simple adjustment to an ordinary wireless receiving set. *Z Veterinark* 56:304-308, 1944.

106. Essler WO and Folk GE Jr: Determination of physiological rhythms of unrestrained animals by radiotelemetry. *Nature* 190:90-91, 1961.

107. Nomura S *et al:* Adaptation of radiotelemetry to riding horses and jockeys. I. Radiotelemeter and its performance. *Exp Rep Eq Hlth Lab* 2:29-47, 1964.

108. Banister EW and Purvis AD: Exercise electrocardiography in the horse by radiotelemetry. *JAVMA* 152:1004-1008, 1968.

109. Amada A and Koike N: A specially made transmitter for recording of exercise electrocardiograms in the racehorse by radiotelemetry. *Bull Eq Res Inst* 17:32-38, 1980.

110. Veletzky S: Methodische Untersuchungen zur Belastungselektrokardiographie beim Pferd mit telemetrischer Ubertragung und rechnergestutzter Aus-

wertung (Abstract). *Wien Tierärztl Mschr* 72:61, 1985.

111. Holmes JR: Equine electrocardiography: some practical hints on technique. *Equine Vet J* 16:477-479, 1984.

112. Hall MC *et al:* Cardiac monitoring during exercise tests in the horse. 1. Magnetic tape recording in preference to radio-telemetry. *Aust Vet J* 51:547-553, 1975.

113. Bitter G: Die telemetrische Übertragung des Belastungs-Elektrokardiogramms beim Trabrennpferd, eine vergleichende methodische Arbeit. *Wien Tierärztl Mschr* 67:380, 1980.

114. Parks CM: *Exercise in ponies: a study of myocardial blood flow, coronary vasodilator reserve, regional distribution of cardiac output and effects of heart rate on coronary flow.* Dissertation. College of Veterinary Medicine, University of Illinois, Urbana, 1983.

115. Azzie MAJ: Aortic/iliac thrombosis of Thoroughbred horses. *Equine Vet J* 1:113-115, 1969.

116. Else RW and Holmes JR: Cardiac pathology in the horse (1). Gross Pathology. *Equine Vet J* 4:1-8, 1972.

117. Wilson FN and Herrmann G: Relation of QRS interval to ventricular weight. *Heart* 15:135-140, 1930.

118. Steel JD: The equine electrocardiogram and the heart score concept. *Victorian Vet Proc* 25:84-85, 1967.

119. Gross DR *et al:* Reevaluation of the equine heart score. *Southwest Vet* 27:231-233, 1974.

120. Moodie EW and Sheard RP: The use of electrocardiography to estimate heart weight and predict performance in the racehorse. *Aust Vet J* 56:557-558, 1980.

121. Hörnicke H *et al,* in Snow DH *et al: Equine Exercise Physiology.* Granta Editions, Cambridge, 1983. pp 7-16.

122. Tenney SM, in Swenson MJ: *Dukes' Physiology of Domestic Animals.* 9th ed. Cornell University Press, Ithaca, 1982. pp 175-202.

123. Swenson MJ, in Swenson MJ: *Physiology of Domestic Animals.* Cornell University Press, Ithaca, 1982. pp 14-35.

124. McKusick VA *et al:* Spectral phonocardiography: Clinical studies. *Johns Hopk Hosp Bull* 95:90-110, 1954.

125. Bornert D and Bornert G: Untersuchungen zur Phonokardiographie in der Veterinärmedizin 2. Mitteilung: Theoretische Grundlagen der Phonokardiographie. *Arch Expt Vetmed* 25:565-579, 1971.

126. Koblik PD and Hornof WJ: Diagnostic radiology and nuclear cardiology: Their use in assessment of equine cardiovascular disease. *Vet Clin No Am (Equine Pract)* 1:289-309, 1985.

127. Farrow CS, in Thrall DE: *Textbook of Veterinary Diagnostic Radiology.* Saunders, Philadelphia, 1986. pp 339-355.

128. Scott EA *et al:* Closure of ductus arteriosus determined by cardiac catheterization and angiography in newborn foals. *Am J Vet Res* 36:1021-1023, 1975.

129. Bayly WM *et al:* Multiple congenital heart anomalies in five Arabian foals. *JAVMA* 181:684-689, 1982.

130. Carlsten J *et al*: Method of selective and non-selective angiocardiography for the horse. *Equine Vet J* 16:47-52, 1984.

131. Carlsten J: *Imaging of the equine heart. An angiocardiographic and echocardiographic investigation.* Dissertation. Faculty of Veterinary Medicine, Swedish University of Agricultural Sciences, Uppsala, Sweden, 1986.

132. Koblik PD *et al*: Left ventricular ejection fraction in the normal horse determined by first-pass nuclear angiocardiography. *Vet Radiol* 26:53-62, 1985.

133. Douglas SW *et al*: *Principles of Veterinary Radiography.* Ballière Tindall, London, 1987.

134. Colles CM and Cook WR: Carotid and cerebral angiography in the horse. *Vet Record* 113:483-489, 1983.

135. Boyd JW: The mechanisms relating to increases in plasma enzymes and isoenzymes in diseases of animals. *Vet Clin Path* 12(2):9-24, 1983.

136. Fujii Y *et al*: Analysis of creatine kinase isoenzymes in racehorse serum and tissue. *Bull Equine Res Inst* 17(20):21-31, 1980.

137. Fujii Y *et al*: Serum creatine kinase and lactate dehydrogenase isoenzymes in skeletal and cardiac muscle damage in the horse. *Bull Equine Res Inst* 20:87-96, 1983.

138. Nuytten J *et al*: Heart failure in horses: hemodynamic monitoring and determination of LDH1 concentration. *J Eq Vet Sci* 8:214-216, 1988.

139. Bonagura JD *et al*: Echocardiography. *Vet Clin No Am (Equine Pract)* 1:311-333, 1985.

140. Lescure F and Tamzali Y: Valeurs de référence en échocardiographic TM chez le cheval de sport. *Rev Méd Vét* 135:405-418, 1984.

141. Pipers FS and Hamlin RL: Echocardiography in the horse. *JAVMA* 170:815-819, 1977.

142. Tithof PK *et al*: Ultrasonographic diagnosis of aorto-iliac thrombosis [in a horse]. *Cornell Vet* 75:540-544, 1985.

143. Reef VB *et al*: Pulsed wave doppler evaluation of intracardiac blood flow in 30 clinically normal Standardbred horses. *Am J Vet Res* 50:75-83, 1989.

144. Eberly VE *et al*: Cardiovascular parameters in the Thoroughbred horse. *Am J Vet Res* 25:1712-1716, 1964.

145. Parry BW *et al*: Influence of head height on arterial blood pressure in standing horses. *Am J Vet Res* 41:1626-1631, 1980.

146. Parry BW *et al*: Correct occlusive bladder width for indirect blood pressure measurement in horses. *Am J Vet Res* 43:50-54, 1982.

147. Latshaw H *et al*: Indirect measurement of mean blood pressure in the normotensive and hypotensive horse. *Equine Vet J* 11:191-194, 1979.

148. Parry BW *et al*: Survey of resting blood pressure values in clinically normal horses. *Equine Vet J* 16:53-58, 1984.

149. Johnson JH *et al*: Ultrasonic measurement of arterial blood pressure in conditioned Thoroughbreds. *Equine Vet J* 8:55-57, 1976.

150. Lombard CW *et al*: Blood pressure, electrocardiogram and echocardiogram measurements in the growing pony foal. *Equine Vet J* 16:342-347, 1984.

151. Parry BW *et al*: Prognosis in equine colic: A comparative study of variables used to assess individual cases. *Equine Vet J* 15:211-215, 1983.

152. Holmes JR and Else RW: Cardiac pathology in the horse. (3) Clinical correlations. *Equine Vet J* 4:195-203, 1972.

153. Bruns DL: A general theory of the causes of murmurs in the cardiovascular system. *Am J Med* 27:360, 1959.

154. Rushmer RF and Morgan C: Meaning of murmurs. *Am J Cardiol* 21:722, 1968.

155. Criscitiello MG, in Levine HJ: *Clinical Cardiovascular Physiology.* Grune & Stratton, New York, 1976. pp 259-302.

156. Fregin GF, in Mansmann RA and McAllister ES: *Equine Medicine and Surgery.* 3rd ed. American Veterinary Publications, Goleta, CA, 1982. pp 645-704.

157. Machida N *et al*: Auscultatory and phonocardiographic studies on the cardiovascular system of the newborn Thoroughbred foal. *Jpn J Vet Res* 35:235-250, 1987.

158. Glendinning SA: A distinctive diastolic murmur observed in healthy young horses. *Vet Record* 76:341-342, 1964.

159. Critchley KL: The importance of blood gas measurement in the diagnosis of a intraventricular septal defect in a horse: a case report. *Equine Vet J* 8:128-129, 1976.

160. Else RW and Holmes JR: Cardiac pathology in the horse (2). Microscopic pathology. *Equine Vet J* 4:57-62, 1972.

161. Brown CM: Acquired cardiovascular disease. *Vet Clin No Am (Equine Pract)* 1:371-382, 1985.

162. Else RW and Holmes JR: Pathologic changes in atrial fibrillation in the horse. *Equine Vet J* 3:56-64, 1971.

163. Reef VB *et al*: Factors affecting prognosis and conversion in equine atrial fibrillation. *J Vet Int Med* 2:1-6, 1988.

164. Norr J: 100 Klinische Fälle von Herz-und Pulsarhythmien beim Pferde. *Monats prakt Tierheilk* 34:177-232, 1924.

165. Spörri H: Über die Genese und klinische Bedeutung des partiellen Herzblockes beim Pferd. *Schweiz Arch Tierheilk* 94:337, 1952.

166. Brooijmans AWM: *Electrocardiography in horses and cattle. Theoretical and clinical aspects.* Dissertation. Rijksuniversiteit te Utrecht, Netherlands, 1957.

167. Glendinning SA: Heart disease in the horse and electrocardiography. *Vet Record* 75:871, 1963.

168. Deegen E: Diagnostik und Bedeutung von Reizbildungsstörungen beim Pferd. II. Zur Klinischen Bedentung der Reizbildungsstörungen. *Dtsch Tierärztl Wochenschr* 83:483-489, 1976.

169. Deegen E: Diagnostik und Bedeutung von Reizbildungsstörungen beim Pferd. I. EKG-Diagnostik der Reizbildungsstörungen. *Dtsch Tierärztl Wochenschr* 83:361-367, 1976.

170. Ghergariu S and Danielescu N: Sur quelques problèmes de l'électrocardiographie en clinique èquine. *Zbl Vetmed A* 24:566-574, 1977.

171. Hilwig RW: Cardiac arrhythmias in the horse. *JAVMA* 170:153-163, 1977.

172. Holmes JR: Cardiac rhythm irregularities in the horse. *In Practice* 2(6):15, 25, 1980.

173. Lekeux P et al: Comparaison du type et de la frequence relative des principales arythmies cardiaques observees chez les chevaux en fonction de leurs performances en course: une etude radiotelemetrique. *Ann Med Vet* 126:205-208, 1982.

174. Muir WW and McGuirk SM: Pharmacology and pharmacokinetics of drugs used to treat cardiac disease in horses. *Vet Clin No Am (Equine Pract)* 1:335-352, 1985.

175. McGuirk SM and Muir WW: Diagnosis and treatment of cardiac arrhythmias. *Vet Clin No Am (Equine Pract)* 1:353-370, 1985.

176. Hilwig RW, in Robinson NE: *Current Therapy in Equine Medicine 2*. Saunders, Philadelphia, 1987. pp 154-164.

177. Arnsdorf MF: Membrane factors in arrhythmogenesis: concepts and definitions. *Prog Cardiovasc Dis* 19:413, 1977.

178. Singer DH et al: Cellular electrophysiology of ventricular and other dysrhythmias: studies on diseased and ischemic heart. *Prog Cardiovasc Dis* 24:97, 1981.

179. Byrne MJ: Coronary thrombosis leading to auricular fibrillation in a Thoroughbred gelding. *Irish Vet J* 4:90-92, 1950.

180. Detweiler DK: Auricular fibrillation in horses. *JAVMA* 126:47-50, 1955.

181. Grodzki K: The electrocardiogram in horses with paralytic myohemoglobinaemia. *Polskie Archwm Wet* 8:505-512, 1964.

182. Kiryu K et al: Uniformity of cardiac lesions in incomplete atrioventricular block in the horse. *Exp Rep Equine Hlth Lab* 16:30-36, 1979.

183. Button C et al: Multiple atrial dysrrhythmias in a horse. *JAVMA* 177:714-719, 1980.

184. Satoh A et al: Histopathological studies on cardiac disturbances in racehorses with special reference to myocardial fibrosis and scar formation. *J Fad Agric Iwate Univ* 18:21-32, 1986.

185. Buchanan JW: Spontaneous arrhythmias and conduction disturbances in domestic animals. *Ann NY Acad Sci* 127:224-238, 1965.

186. Dhillon KS and Smith CR: Incidence of heart block in horse. *Orissa Vet J* 6:9-11, 1971.

187. Amada A: Atrial fibrillation in the horse, a review. *Adv Anim ECG* 11:1-16, 1978.

188. Marcus LC and Ross JN Jr: Microscopic lesions in the hearts of aged horses and mules. *Path Vet* 4:162-185, 1967.

189. Cranley JJ and McCullagh KG: Ischaemic myocardial fibrosis and aortic strongylosis in the horse. *Equine Vet J* 13:35-42, 1981.

190. Silber EN: *Heart Disease*. MacMillan Publishing, New York, 1987.

191. Matsuoka T: Evaluation of monensin toxicity in the horse. *JAVMA* 169:1098-1100, 1976.

192. Gerber H and Löhrer J: Influenze A/equi-2 in der Schweiz 1965. III Symptomatologie. 2. Komplicationen, Folgekrankheiten und pathologisch-anatomische Befunde. *Zbl Vetmed B* 13:517, 1966.

193. Kiryu K et al: Cardiopathological observation on a case of paroxysmal ventricular tachycardia in a Thoroughbred colt: formal pathogenesis. *Exp Rep Equine Hlth Lab* 12:74-88, 1975.

194. Kiryu K et al: Histopathogenesis of atrial fibrillation in the horse: cardiopathology of an additional case. *Exp Rep Equine Hlth Lab* 14:54-63, 1977.

195. Kiryu K: Cardiopathology of arrhythmias in the horse. *Proc Ann Mtg AAEP*, 1986. pp 457-468.

196. Kiryu K et al: Cardiopathological observations on histopathogenesis of wandering pacemaker in horses. *Jpn J Vet Sci* 40:131-140, 1978.

197. Kiryu K et al: Cardiopathology of sinoatrial block in horses. *Jpn J Vet Sci* 47:45-54, 1985.

198. Deegen E: Provokation von Extrasystolen und paroxysmalen Tachykardien bei Pferden mit Herzklappenerkrankungen durch Belastung. *Dtsch Tierärztl Wochenschr* 81:532-537, 1974.

199. Toyoshima H et al: The nature of normal and abnormal electrocardiograms. VIII. Relation of ST segment and T wave changes to intracellular potentials. *Arch Intern Med* 115:4, 1965.

200. Watsabaugh C et al: Second degree atrio-ventricular block in the horse. *The Physiologist* 7:280, 1964.

201. Senta T et al: A case report on ventricular paroxysmal tachycardia (permanent type) in a Thoroughbred colt. *Exp Rep Equine Hlth Lab* 8:61-71, 1971.

202. Amada A et al: Atrial fibrillation in the horse: clinical and histopathological studies of two cases. I. Clinical study. *Exp Rep Equine Hlth Lab* 11:51-69, 1974.

203. Brown CM: *A micromanometer study of intracardiac pressure and sound in horses*. Dissertation. Bristol University, Bristol, England, 1980.

204. Miller PJ and Holmes JR: Effect of cardiac arrhythmia on left ventricular and aortic blood pressure parameters in the horse. *Res Vet Sci* 35:190-199, 1983.

205. Miller PJ and Holmes JR: Relationships of left side systolic time intervals to beat-by-beat heart rate and blood pressure variables in some cardiac arrhythmias of the horse. *Res Vet Sci* 37:18-25, 1984.

206. Muir WW and McGuirk SM: Hemodynamics before and after conversion of atrial fibrillation to normal sinus rhythm in horses. *JAVMA* 184:965-970, 1984.

207. Holmes JR and Alps BJ: Observations on partial atrioventricular heart block in the horse. *Can Vet J* 7:280-290, 1966.

208. Grauerholz H: Untersuchungen uber ST-Strecke und T-Welle im EKG des Pferdes. *Berl Münch Tierärztl Wochenschr* 94:71-76, 81-85, 1981.

209. Deegen E and Buntenkötter S: Behaviour of heart rate of horses with auricular fibrillation during exercise and after treatment. *Equine Vet J* 8:26-29, 1976.

210. Amada A and Kurita H: Treatment of atrial fibrillation with quinidine sulfate in the racehorse. *Exp Rep Equine Hlth Lab* 15:47-61, 1978.

211. Rezakhani A: Equine electrocardiography. *J So Afr Vet Med Assn* 46:207, 1975.

212. Spörri H: Der respiratorisch induzierte Herzblock des Pferdes. *Cardiologia* 20:180-187, 1952.

213. Spörri H: Partial atrioventricular block in horses. *Wien Tierärztl Mschr* 94:347-356, 1952.

214. Smetzer DL et al: Second-degree atrioventricular block in the horse. Am J Vet Res 30:933-946, 1969.

215. Watsabaugh CJ: Second degree heart block in the horse. Dissertation. Ohio State Univ, Columbus, Ohio, 1963.

216. Kroneman J: Het Electrocardiogram van het getrainde Paard. Dissertation. Rijksuniversiteit te Utrecht, Netherlands, 1965.

217. Glazier DB: Electrocardiography in veterinary medicine. Irish Vet J 12:230-252, 1958.

218. Vibe-Petersen G and Nielsen K: Electrocardiography in the horse. (A report on findings in 138 horses). Nord Vet Med 32:105-121, 1980.

219. Nicholson JA et al: Sino-atrial heart block in the horse. Irish Vet J 13:168-172, 1959.

220. Holmes JR: Clinical examination of the equine heart. Proc 17th Intl Vet Cong, 1963. pp 1195-1199.

221. Lannek N and Rutqvist L: Normal area of variation for the electrocardiogram of horses. A statistical examination of extremity leads and unipolar leads. Nord Vet Med 3:1094-1117, 1951.

222. Smetzer DL: Equine sino-atrial and second-degree atrioventricular heart-block. Dissertation. Ohio State University, Columbus, Ohio, 1967.

223. Watanabe Y and Dreifus LS: Second-degree atrioventricular block. Cardiovasc Res 1:150-168, 1967.

224. Smetzer DL et al: High-grade second-degree atrioventricular block in a horse. Am J Vet Res 30:337-343, 1969.

225. Obel N: Fjsiologiska synpunkter pa det habiuella atrioventrikulärblocket hos höst. Skand Vet Tidskr 32:200-208, 1942.

226. Kiryu K et al: Cardiopathological observations on histopathogenesis of incomplete atrioventricular block in horses. Jpn J Vet Sci 39:425-436, 1977.

227. Fister D: Wandlund der QRS-Gruppe in EKG bei Rennpferden im ersten Trainingsjahr. Dissertation. Tierärztliche Hochschule, Hannover, Germany, 1980.

228. Kiryu K et al: Microscopic observations on the heart in horses which exhibited no arrhythmias. Bull Equine Res Inst 18:141-147, 1981.

229. Bang O et al: Two cases of bradycardia in horses. Adams-Stokes disease. Sinus bradycardia. Heart 6:199-205, 1915.

230. Domracev G: A case of Adams-Stokes disease in horse. Ucenie Zap Kazan Vet Inst 37:157-166, 1926.

231. Marek J and Mocsy J: Zwei Falle von Adams-stokesscher Krankheit infolge von Herzdissoziation beim Pferd. Prag Arch Tiermed vergl Path 6:43, 1926.

232. Kozma I and Szekely EG: A case of Stokes-Adams disease in a horse. Allatorvosi Lapok 50:299, 1927.

233. Wirth D: Adams-Stokes'sche Krankheit bei zwei Pferden, bedingt durch Herzblock. Wien Tierärztl Mschr 14:1-8, 1927.

234. Krinizin DJ: Adams-Stokesscher Symptomenkomplex bei partiellem Herzblock beim Pferde. Arch Tierheilk 60:444-463, 1929.

235. Hamerski E: Difficulty in atrioventricular conductibility in the horse in a case of complete blockage. Rozprawy Biol 11:46-86, 1933.

236. Dukes HH: A case of heart-block in a horse. Cornell Vet 30:248, 1940.

237. Bosnic L and Rapic S: Adams-Stokes sindrom kod Parcialnoga bloka Knoja. Vet Arhiv 11:1-17, 1941.

238. Bosnic L and Rapic S: Two further cases of Adams-Stokes syndrome in horses. Vet Archiv 11:166-179, 1941.

239. Martincic M: Pathology of changes in the atrioventricular system of a horse with the Adams-Stokes syndrome. Vet Arhiv 11:76-99, 1941.

240. Moretti B: Sindrome di Morgagni-Adams-Stokes in un cavallo determinata da blocco totale del cuore. Atti Soc Ital Sci Vet 2:1, 1948.

241. Desliens: Cardiac arrhythmia in the horse (cerebral anaemia and Adams-Stokes syndrome). Bull l'Acad Nat'l Med (Paris) 133:327-330, 1949.

242. Taylor DH and Mero MA: The use of an internal pacemaker in a horse with Adams-Stokes syndrome. JAVMA 151:1172-1176, 1967.

243. Mihaljevic K: Prilog poznavanju Adams-Stokesove bolesti u konja. Veterinarski Archiv 41:59-66, 1971.

244. Dugardin F et al: Observation d'un syndrome de Stokes-Adams chez le cheval. Pratique Veterinaire Equine 12:265-267, 1980.

245. Volckart W and Loeffler K: Atrioventrikuläre Herzblockbildungen bei einem Pferd mit Lymphosarkomen in der Milz. Dtsch Tierärztl Wochenschr 78:446-449, 1971.

246. Berg et al: Anwendung eines implantierbaren Herzschrittmachers bei einem Esel mit Adams-Stokes-Syndrom. Tierärztl Umschau 28:616-618, 1973.

247. le Nihouannen JC et al: Implantation d'un stimulateur cardiaque chez le cheval. I. Presentation du materiel et description des techniques. Rev Méd Vét 135:91-95, 1984.

248. Detweiler DK: Experimental and clinical observations on auricular fibrillation in horses. Proc 89th Ann Conv AVMA, 1952. pp 119-130.

249. Bertone JJ: Atrial fibrillation in the horse; diagnosis, prognosis, treatment. Equine Pract 6(8):6-12, 1984.

250. Deem DA and Fregin GF: Atrial fibrillation in horses: a review of 106 clinical cases, with consideration of prevalence, clinical signs, and prognosis. JAVMA 180:261-265, 1982.

251. Lewis T: Irregularity of the heart's action in horses and its relationship to fibrillation of the auricles in experiment and to complete irregularity of the human heart. Heart 3:161-171, 1911.

252. Deem-Morris D and Fregin GF: Atrial fibrillation in horses: Factors associated with response to quinidine sulfate in 77 clinical cases. Cornell Vet 72:339-349, 1982.

253. Amada A and Kurita H: Five cases of paroxysmal atrial fibrillation in the racehorse. Exp Rep Equine Hlth Lab 12:89-100, 1975.

254. Glendinning SA: The use of quinidine sulphate for the treatment of atrial fibrillation in twelve horses. Vet Record 77:951-960, 1965.

255. Iida M et al: Quinidine therapy of atrial fibrillation in a horse. Adv Anim ECG (Japan) 6:44-50, 1973.

256. Hurst JW: The Heart, Arteries and Veins. McGraw-Hill, New York, 1986.

257. Moe GK and Abeldskov JA: Atrial fibrillation as a self-sustaining arrhythmia independent of focal discharge. *Am Heart J* 58:61-70, 1959.

258. Boswell SH *et al*: Body size in the maintenance of experimental atrial fibrillation in the dog. *Cardiovasc Res Ctr Bull* 6:99, 1968.

259. Rytand DA: The circus movement (entrapped circuit wave) hypothesis and atrial flutter. *Ann Intern Med* 65:125, 1966.

260. Kroneman J and Breukink HJ: Treatment of atrial fibrillation in the horse with digitalis tincture and quinidine sulfate. *Tijdschr Diergeneeskd* 91:223-229, 1966.

261. Fregin GF and Deem D: Epistaxis in horses with atrial fibrillation. *Proc 26th Ann Mtg AAEP*, 1980. pp 431-433.

262. McGuirk SM *et al*: Pharmacokinetic analysis of intravenously and orally administered quinidine in horses. *Am J Vet Res* 42:938-942, 1981.

263. Ebert PA: Relationship of myocardial potassium content and atrial fibrillation. *Circulation* 151/152 Suppl II:137-141, 1970.

264. Braunwald E *et al*, in Harrison TR: *Principles of Internal Medicine*. McGraw-Hill, New York, 1970. pp 1148-1149.

265. Gerber H *et al*: Treatment of atrial fibrillation in the horse with intravenous dihydroquinidine gluconate. *Equine Vet J* 3:110-113, 1971.

266. Gerber H *et al*: Intravenöse Behandlung des Vorhofflimmerns beim Pferd. *Schweiz Arch Tierheilk* 114:57-72, 1972.

267. Deegen E and Buntenkotter S: Intravenöse Behandlung des Vorhofflimmerns beim Pferd mit Chinidinsulfat. Vorläufige Mitteilung. *Dtsch Tierärztl Wochenschr* 81:161-162, 1974.

268. Lekeux P *et al*: Comparison of different treatments of atrial fibrillation in the horse. *Zbl Vetmed A* 28:475-480, 1981.

269. Roos J: Vorhofflimmern bei den Haustieren. *Arch wiss prakt Tierheilk* 51:280-293, 1924.

270. Batt HT: Three cases of heart disease in horses. *Cornell Vet* 31:70-76, 1941.

271. Fregin GF: Atrial fibrillation in the horse. Proc Ann Mtg AAEP, 1970. pp 383-388.

272. Kiryu K *et al*: Atrial fibrillation in the horse: clinical and histopathological studies of two cases. II. Formal pathogenesis. *Exp Rep Equine Hlth Lab* 11:70-86, 1974.

273. Rivard G: Un cas de fibrillation auriculaire chez un cheval de competition. *Can Vet J* 18:122-126, 1977.

274. Glazier DB and Kavanagh JF: An unusual case of atrial fibrillation in a racing Thoroughbred filly. *Irish Vet J* 21:107-110, 1967.

275. Rose RJ and Davis PE: Paroxysmal atrial fibrillation in a racehorse. *Aust Vet J* 53:545-549, 1977.

276. Miller MS *et al*: Paroxysmal atrial fibrillation: a case report. *J Eq Vet Sci* 7:95-97, 1987.

277. Machida N *et al*: Three cases of paroxysmal atrial fibrillation in the Thoroughbred newborn foal. *Equine Vet J* 21:66-68, 1989.

278. Detweiler DK: Electrocardiographic and clinical features of spontaneous auricular fibrillation and flutter (tachycardia) in dogs. Comparison with spontaneous auricular fibrillation and flutter in other species and with experimentally induced arrhythmias in dogs. *Zbl Vetmed A* 4:509-556, 1957.

279. Robertson BT: Correction of atrial flutter with quinidine and digitalis. *J Small Anim Pract* 11:251-255, 1970.

280. Van Zijl WJ: Electrocardiografische opmerkingen over het boezemfibrilleren bij het paard. *Tijdschr Diergeneeskd* 76:553-555, 1951.

281. Holzmann M: *Klinische Elektrokardiographie*. Thieme, Stuttgart, 1955.

282. Glazier DB and Dukes HH: Atrial premature beats in a horse. *Irish Vet J* 17:87-88, 1963.

283. Amada A and Kurita H: A case of atrial premature beats in the horse. *Adv Anim ECG* (Japan) 9:18-27, 1976.

284. Wolff L *et al*: Bundle branch block with short PR-interval in healthy young people prone to paroxysmal tachycardia. *Am Heart J* 5:685, 1930.

285. Landgren S and Rutqvist L: Electrocardiogram of normal cold-blooded draft horses after work. *Nord Vet Med* 5:905-914, 1953.

286. Delahanty DD and Glazier DB: The Wolff-Parkinson-White (atrio-ventricular conduction) syndrome. *Irish Vet J* 13:205-207, 1959.

287. Cooper SA: Ventricular pre-excitation (Wolff-Parkinson-White syndrome) in a horse. *Vet Record* 74:527-530, 1962.

288. Senta T and Amada A: Wolff-Parkinson-White (ventricular pre-excitation) syndrome in a Thoroughbred. *Exp Rep Equine Hlth Lab* 4:129-136, 1967.

289. Glazier DB: The Wolff-Parkinson-White (pre-excitation) syndrome in a racing Thoroughbred – a case report. *Irish Vet J* 22:214-217, 1968.

290. Amada A and Kaneko T: Ventricular parasystole in a racing Thoroughbred: a case report. *Exp Rep Equine Hlth Lab* 7:84-93, 1970.

291. Muir WW and McGuirk SM: Ventricular pre-excitation in two horses. *JAVMA* 183:573-576, 1983.

292. Bonagura JD and Miller MS: Common conduction disturbances. (ECG in the horse). *J Eq Vet Sci* 6:23-25, 1986.

293. Tschudi P: Elektrokardiographie beim Pferd (2) Erregungsbildungs- und Erregungsleitungsstorungen. *Tierärztl Prax* 13:529-539, 1985.

294. Schoon H-A and Deegen E: Autopsiebefunde bei zwei Pferden mit paroxysmaler Tachykardie. *Dtsch Tierärztl Wochenschr* 89:293-295, 1982.

295. Littlewort MCG *et al*: Symposium on practical aspects of equine cardiology. *Equine Vet J* 9:172-185, 1977.

296. Too K: Abnormal electrocardiograms in the horse. *Jpn J Vet Res* 8:29-34, 1960.

297. Bohn FK and Zoller A: Befunde bei einer polytopen Kammerextrasystolie eines Pferdes. *Berl Münch Tierärztl Wochenschr* 79:307-309, 1966.

298. Hilwig RW: ECG of the month (parasystole in a horse). *JAVMA* 171:168-169, 1977.

299. Krinitzin J and Philippoff JJ: Die kombinierte Form der extrasystolischen ventrikularen Arrhythmie und der sinus Arrhythmia beim Pferde. *Arch wiss prakt Tierheilk* 64:281, 1931.

300. Glazier DB and Nicholson JA: Premature ventricular beats. *Irish Vet J* 13:82-86, 1959.

301. Pfister R *et al:* Die Bestimmung des Ursprungsortes ventrikularer Extrasystolen beim Pferd. *Schweiz Arch Tierheilk* 126:165-172, 1984.

302. Norr J: Paroxysmale Tachykardie und partieller Vorhof-Hammerblock bei einem Reitpferd mit Aorteninsuffizienz. *Arch wiss prakt Tierkeilk* 63:103-119, 1931.

303. Steffan H: Das sternbende Herz des Pferdes im Elektrokardiogramm. *Arch wiss prakt Tierheilk* 78:32, 1942.

304. Schuzler G: Belastungeselektrokardiogramm des Pferdes. *Arch wiss prakt Tierheilk* 78:40-55, 1944.

305. Wirth D: Vorhofflimmern und flattern beim Pferde. *Wien Tierärztl Mschr* 29:241-251, 1942.

306. Witzel DA *et al:* Electrical defibrillation of the equine heart. *Am J Vet Res* 29:1279-1285, 1968.

307. van Zijl WJ: Een geval van rechten bundeltakblock bij het paard. *Tijdschr Diergeneeskd* 77:417, 1952.

308. Ettinger SJ and Suter PF: *Canine Cardiology.* Saunders, Philadelphia, 1970.

309. Alfredson BV and Sykes JF: Studies of the bovine electrocardiogram. *Proc Soc Exp Biol Med* 43:580, 1940.

310. Pruitt RD: Electrocardiogram of bundlebranch block in the bovine heart. *Circ Res* 10:593-597, 1963.

311. Bonagura JD and Miller MS: Electrocardiography: What is your diagnosis? Junctional and ventricular arrhythmias. *J Eq Vet Sci* 5:347-350, 1985.

312. Klein L, in Mansmann RA and McAllister ES: *Equine Medicine and Surgery.* American Veterinary Publications, Goleta, CA, 1982. pp 282-300.

313. Goodman LS and Gilman AZ: *The Pharmacological Basis of Therapeutics.* MacMillan, London, 1970.

314. Bertone JJ *et al*: Arial fibrillation in a pregnant mare: treatment with quinidine sulfate. *JAVMA* 190:1565-1566, 1987.

315. Wallace AG *et al*: Electrophysiologic effects of isoproterenol and beta blocking agents in awake dogs. *Circ Res* 18:140-148, 1966.

316. Muir WW and Sams R: Clinical pharmacodynamics and pharmacokinetics of beta-adrenoreceptor blocking drugs in veterinary medicine. *Compend Cont Ed Pract Vet* 6:156-167, 1984.

317. Davis RH and Fisch C: Potassium and arrhythmias. *Geriatrics* 25:108-116, 1970.

318. Dill SG *et al*: Fibrinous pericarditis in the horse. *JAVMA* 180:266-271, 1982.

319. Vitums A and Bayly WM: Pulmonary atresia with dextroposition of the aorta and ventricular septal defect in three Arabian foals. *Vet Pathol* 19:160-168, 1982.

320. Reef VB *et al*: Echocardiograhic detection of tricuspid atresia in two fals. *JAVMA* 191:225-228, 1987.

321. Platt H: Sudden and unexpected deaths in horses: a review of 69 cases. *Brit Vet J* 138:417-429, 1982.

322. Gelbert HB *et al*: Sudden death in training and racing Thoroughbred horses. *JAVMA* 187:1354-1356, 1985.

323. Magnin ML: Rupture del'artere cardiaque droite. *Rec Med Vet* 10:693-695, 1903.

324. Kiryu K *et al*: A supplementary contribution to formal pathogenesis of so-called idiopathic rupture of the aorta in the horse. *Jpn J Vet Sci* 31 (Suppl):115, 1969.

325. Allen JR *et al*: Spontaneous rupture of the great coronary vein in a pony. *Equine Vet J* 19:145-147, 1987.

326. Petit MG: Rupture de l'aorte, aneurisme disséquant et mort subite, chez un cheval. *Bull Société Méd Vét* 59:299-300, 1905.

327. Shuja J: Sudden death of a mare from rupture of the heart. *Vet Record* 57:465, 1945.

328. Faccincani F: Spontaneous rupture of the right auricle of the heart in a horse and in a mule. *Atti Soc Ital Sci Vet* 7:739-748, 1954.

329. Haaland MA and Davidson JP: Spontaneous left atrial rupture with associated chronic fibrotic myocarditis in a stallion. *VM/SAC* 78:1284, 1288, 1983.

330. Brunet ME: Note sur un cas de déchirure du péricarde et de rupture incomplète du ventricule gauche. *Rec Méd Vét* 7:464-475, 1900.

331. Sigl: Herzruptur bei einem Pferd. *Wschr Thierheilk Viehzucht* 49:181, 1905.

332. Fregin GF *et al*: Case presentation (rupture of pulmonary artery in a colt). *JAVMA* 164:813-816, 1974.

333. van der Linde-Sipman JS *et al*: Necrosis and rupture of the aorta and pulmonary trunk in four horses. *Vet Pathol* 22:51-53, 1985.

334. Lesbre MC: Un cas de mort subite par rupture de la veine cave antérieure chez un cheval. *J Méd Vét Zoot* 22:271-273, 1897.

335. Roger M: Hypertrophie cardiaque et déchirure de la veine cave postérieure. Kyste de l'ovaire. *Rev Vét* 26:168-170, 1902.

336. Rooney JR: Internal hemorrhage related to gestation in the mare. *Cornell Vet* 54:11-17, 1964.

337. Monolux WS: Sudden death in the horse due to myocarditis. *Iowa State Univ Vet* 29:40, 1961.

338. Cronin MTI and Leader GH: Coronary occlusion in a Thoroughbred colt. *Vet Record* 64:8, 1952.

339. Gunson DE *et al*: Sudden death attributable to exercise-induced pulmonary hemorrhage in racehorses: nine cases (1981-1983). *JAVMA* 193:102-106, 1988.

340. Dudan F *et al*: Etude cardiovasculaire chez le cheval: Relation entre les altérations vasculaires et tissulaires du myocarde: Troisième Partie: Suite et Fin. *Schweiz Arch Tierheilk* 127:369-378, 1985.

341. Young JR, in Hurst JW: *The Heart, Arteries and Veins.* McGraw-Hill, New York, 1982. pp 1339-1354.

342. Maxie MG and Physick-Sheard PW: Aorticiliac thrombosis in horses. *Vet Pathol* 22:238-249, 1985.

343. Physick-Sheard PW and Russell M: Career profile of the Canadian Standardbred. III. Influence of temporary absence from racing and season. *Can J Vet Res* 50:471-478, 1986.

344. Glazier DB: Congestive heart failure and congenital cardiac defects in horses. *Compend Cont Ed Pract Vet* 8:20-23, 1986.

345. Katz LN *et al*: Hemodynamic aspects of congestive heart failure. *Circulation* 21:95, 1960.

346. Fisher EW: Cardiac failure. *J Small Anim Pract* 8:137-141, 1967.

347. Johne: *Endocarditis verrucosa acuta und Myocarditis acuta bei einem Pferde.* Bericht über das

Veterinärwesen im Königreich Sachsen für das Jahr 1881, 1882. pp 44-46.

348. Ordidge RM et al: Death of horses after accidental feeding of monensin. *Vet Record* 104:375, 1979.

349. Holmes JR and Miller PJ: Three cases of ruptured mitral valve chordae in the horse. *Equine Vet J* 16:125-135, 1984.

350. Miller PJ and Holmes JR: Observations on seven cases of mitral insufficiency in the horse. *Equine Vet J* 17:181-190, 1985.

351. Mölbert E and Iijima S: Beitrag zur experimentellen hypertrophie und insuffizienz des Herzmuskels im elktrohenmikroskopischen bild. *Naturwissenschaften* 45:322, 1958.

352. Linzbach AJ: Heart failure from the point of view of quantitative anatomy. *Am J Cardiol* 5:370, 1960.

353. Bache RJ and Vrobel TR: Effects of exercise on blood flow in the hypertrophied heart. *Am J Cardiol* 44:1029-1033, 1979.

354. Marcus ML et al: Effect of cardiac hypertrophy secondary to hypertension on the coronary circulation. *Am J Cardiol* 44:1023-1028, 1979.

355. Wagenaar G and van Nie CJ: Een merkwaardige hartafwijking bij het paard. *Tijdschr Diergeneeskd* 88:950-954, 1963.

356. Carmichael JA et al: Diagnosis of patent ductus arteriosus in a horse. *JAVMA* 158:767-775, 1971.

357. Buchanan JW et al: Clinico-pathologic conference. *JAVMA* 160:451-460, 1972.

358. Knauer KW et al: Diagnosis of an interventricular septal defect in a horse *VM/SAC* 68:75-78, 1973.

359. Vitums A et al: Transposition of the aorta and atresisa of the pulmonary trunk in a horse. *Cornell Vet* 63:41-57, 1973.

360. Daniels H: Drei Falle einer komplexen Herzmissbildung beim Fohlen (Klinische Kurzmitteilung). *Dtsch Tierärztl Wochenschr* 81:622-623, 1974.

361. Critchley KL: An interventricular septal defect, pulmonary stenosis and bicuspid pulmonary valve in a Welsh pony foal. *Equine Vet J* 8:176-178, 1976.

362. Button C et al: Tricuspid atresia in a foal *JAVMA* 172:825-830, 1978.

363. Gross DR et al: Congestive heart failure associated with congenital aortic valvular insufficiency in a horse. *Southwest Vet* 30:27-34, 1977.

364. Scott EA et al: Interruption of aortic arch in two foals. *JAVMA* 172:347-350, 1978.

365. Musselmann EE and LoGuidice RJ: Hypoplastic left ventricular syndrome in a foal. *JAVMA* 185:542-543, 1984.

366. Hughes PE and Howard EB: Endocardial fibroelastosis as a cause of sudden death in the horse. *Equine Pract* 6(6):23-26, 1984.

367. Zamora CS et al: Common ventricle with separate pulmonary outflow chamber in a horse. *JAVMA* 186:1210-1213, 1985.

368. Honnas CM et al: Tricuspid atresia in a Quarter Horse foal. *Southwestern Vet* 38:17-20, 1987.

369. Sojka JE: Persistent truncus arteriosus in a foal. *Equine Pract* 9(4):19-20, 24-26, 1987.

370. Ostermann J: Beitrag zur Beurtheilung der Dilatation und Hypertrophie des Herzens nach chronischer Endocarditis und Klappeninsufficienz bei Pferden. *Berl Tierärzt Wschr* 35:275-277. 1889.

371. Deegen E et al: Klinische und kardiologische Untersuchungsbefunde bei 3 Deckhengsten mit Aortenklappeninsuffizienz. *Tierärztl Prax* 8:211-222, 1980.

372. Brumbaugh GW et al: Medical management of congestive heart failure in a horse. *JAVMA* 180:878-8983, 1982.

373. Brown CM et al: Rupture of the mitral chordae tendineae in two horses. *JAVMA* 182:281-283, 1983.

374. Reef VB: Mitral valvular insufficiency associated with ruptured chordae tendineae in three foals. *JAVMA* 191:329-331, 1987.

375. Berthelsen H: A case of arotic rupture as a result of acute mycarditis. *Vet J* 91:362-366, 1935.

376. Fregin GF: Acquired cardiovascular diseases affecting exercise performance-diagnosis, therapy, and prognosis. *J So Afr Vet Med Assn* 45:269-271, 1974.

377. Lorscheid: Herzkrankheiten bei Truppenpferden. *Dtsch Tierärztl Wochenschr* 26:136, 1918.

378. Petersen G: Nogle Tilfaelde af Hjertelidelser hos Heste. *Maanedsskr Dyrlaeger* 39:579-585, 1928.

379. Rubarth SL: Plotsliga dodsfall hos häst och deras samband med fokalinfektioner. *Svenska Militär-veterinär-sallskapet Kvartalsskrift* 30:1, 1943.

380. Burger LL: Ein Fall von Arrhythmia absoluta beieinem Pferde. *Wein Tierärztl Mschr* 42:904, 1955.

381. Corhs P: *Nieberle's und Cohrs', Lehrbuch der speziellen pathologischen Anatomie der Haustiere*. Fischer, Stuttgart, 1962.

382. Kraft H: Folgeerscheinungen nach Virusinfektionen der Luftwege beim Pferd. *Tierärztl Umschau* 30:422-424, 1975.

383. Peet RL et al: Fungal myocarditis and nephritis in a horse. *Aust Vet J* 57:439-440, 1981.

384. Beck BE and Harries WN: The diagnosis of monensin toxicosis: a report on outbreaks in horses, cattle and chickens. *Proc Amer Assn Vet Lab Diag*, 1979. pp 269-282.

385. Muyelle E et al: Delayed monensin sodium toxicity in horses. *Equine Vet J* 13:107-108, 1981.

386. Holmes JR et al: Rupture of a dissecting aortic aneurysm into the left pulmonary artery in a horse. *Equine Vet J* 5:65-70, 1973.

387. Derksen FJ et al: Aneurysm of the aortic arch and bicarotid trunk in a horse. *JAVMA* 179: 692-694, 1981.

388. Rooney JR et al: Aortic ring rupture in stallions. *Path Vet* 4:268-274, 1967.

389. Sirotkin VA: Cardiovascular insufficiency in pulmonary emphysema of horses. *Sbornik Rabot Leningradskogo Veterinarnogo Instituta* 19:87, 1959.

390. Deegen E; *Klinische Elektrokardiographie beim Pferd mit Berücksichtigung der Muskelmassenverteilung am Herzen. Dissertation.* Tierärztliche Hochschule, Hannover, Germany, 1976.

391. Stratman: Enormous distension of the right auricle and ventricle of the heart in a two-year-old colt. *The Veterinarian* 24:54-56, 1851.

392. Wirth D: Action of chinin on two horses with heart failure. *Wien Tierärztol Mschr* 21:689-692, 1934.

393. Drieux H et al: Malformation du coeur chuz un poulain. *Rec Méd Vét* 122:491-500, 1946.

394. Velasquez QJ: "Altitude" disease. (Cardiac insufficiency in horses imported into Colombia caused by high altitude). *Rev Med Vet* (Bogota) 16:53-70, 1947.

395. Tashjian RJ and McCoy JP: Acquired mitral stenosis resulting in left atrial dilatation with thrombosis. A case report. *Cornell Vet* 50:485-493, 1960.

396. Vitums A: Origin of the aorta and pulmonary trunk from the right ventricle in a horse. *Path Vet* 7:482-491, 1970.

397. Glazier DB: Some aspects of heart failure. *Irish Vet J* 25:125-129, 1971.

398. Prickett ME *et al*: Tetralogy of Fallot in a Thoroughbred foal. *JAVMA* 552-555, 1973.

399. Lekeux P *et al*: Un cas de decompensation cardiaque bilaterale chez le cheval. *Ann Med Vet* 125:561-565, 1981.

400. Labe J: De la sémiologie au diagnositic d'insuffisance cardiaque: notions pratiques. *Point Vét* 19:343-352, 1987.

401. Bayly WM and Vale BJ: Intravenous catheteriztion and associated problems in the horse. *Compend Cont Ed Pract Vet* 4:S227-S237, 1982.

402. Eberly VE *et al*: Cardiovascular parameters in emphysematous and control horses. *J Appl Physiol* 21:883-889, 1966.

403. Dixon PM *et al*: Chronic obstructive pulmonary disease; anatomical cardiac studies. *Equine Vet J* 14:80-82, 1982.

404. Muylle E *et al*, in Snow DH *et al*: *Equine Exercise Physiology*. Granta Editions, Cambridge, 1983. pp 366-370.

405. Detweiler DK, in Jones LM *et al*: *Veterinary Phamacology and Therapeutics*. Iowa State University Press, Ames, 1977. pp 496-542.

406. Francfort P and Schatzmann HJ: Pharmacological experiments as a basis for the administration of digoxin in the horse. *Res Vet Sci* 20:84-89, 1976.

407. Button C *et al*: Digoxin pharmacokinetics, bioavailability, efficacy, and dosage regimens in the horse. *Am J Vet Res* 41:1388-1395, 1980.

408. Brumbaugh GW *et al*: A pharmacokinetic study of digoxin in the horse. *J Vet Pharmacol Therap* 6:163-172, 1983.

409. Pedersoli WM *et al*: Pharmacokinetics of a single, orally administered dose of digoxin in horses. *Am J Vet Res* 42:1412-1414, 1981.

410. Pearson EG *et al*: Digoxin toxicity in a horse. *Compend Cont Educ Pract Vet* 9:958-961, 963-964, 1987.

411. Bartels JE and Vaughan JT: Persistent right aortic arch in the horse *JAVMA* 154:406-409, 1969.

412. Ippolitova TV: Electrocardiography in horses, using precardiac and modified standard leads. *Sbornik Nauchnykh Trudov Moskovskaya Veterinarnaya Akademiya* 100:38-40, 1978.

413. Gumbrell RC: Atresia of the tricuspid valve in a foal. *N Zeal Vet J* 18:253-256, 1970.

414. Hadlow WJ and Ward JK: Atresia of the right atrioventricular orifice in an Arabian foal. *Vet Pathol* 17:622-637, 1980.

415. Borst GHA: Tetralogie van Fallot bij een koudbloed veulen. *Tijdschr Diergeneeskd* 103:968-970, 1978.

416. Reynolds DJ and Nicholl TK: Tetralogy of Fallot and cranial mesenteric arteritis in a foal. *Equine Vet J* 10:185-187, 1978.

417. Hare T: Patent ductus arteriosus in an aged horse. *J Pathol Bacteriol* 34:124, 1931.

418. Rooney JR and Franks WC: Congenital cardiac anomalies in horses. *Path Vet* 1:454-464, 1964.

419. Glazier DB *et al*: Patent ductus arteriosus in an eight-month-old foal. *Irish Vet J* 28:12-13, 1974.

420. Lowe JS: Patent ductus arteriosus in a donkey foal. *N Zeal Vet J* 20:15, 1972.

421. van der Linde-Sipman JS *et al*: Persistent right aortic arch associated with a persistent left ductus arteriosus and an interventricular septal defect in a horse. *Vet Quarterly* 1:189-194, 1979.

422. Bankl H: *Congenital Malformations of the Heart and Great Vessels*. Urban & Schwarzenberg, Baltimore, 1977.

423. Petrick SW *et al*: Persistent right aortic arch in a horse. *J So Afr Vet Med Assn* 49:355-358, 1978.

424. Vitums A: Development and transformation of the aortic arches in the equine embryos with special attention to the formation of the definitive arch of the aorta and the common brachiocephalic trunk. *Z Anat Entwickl Gesch* 128:243-270, 1969.

425. Bryden MM: Vascular ring anomalies associated with persistent right aortic arch. *Aust Vet J* 46:513-514, 1970.

426. Lilleengen K: Hjürtmissbildningar hos djuren. *Skand Vet Tidskr* 24:493-555, 1934.

427. Greene HJ *et al*: Two equine congenital cardiac anomalies. *Irish Vet J* 29:115-117, 1975.

428. Rang H and Hurtienne H: Persistierender Truncus arteriosus bei einem 2 jährigen Pferd. *Tierärztl Prax* 4:55-58, 1976.

429. Wensvoort P: De Tetralogie van Fallot, met atresie van de arteria pulmonalis, bij het hart van een Shetland pony. *Tijdschr Diergeneeskd* 84:939-942, 1959.

430. Rittenbach PV: Zwei Falle kongenitaler Herzmissbildung beim Pferd. *Monats Vet Med* 18:61-63, 1963.

431. Keith JC Jr: Tetralogy of Fallot in a Quarter horse foal. *VM/SAC* 76:889-895, 1981.

432. Amend JF *et al*: Systolic time intervals in domestic ponies: alterations in a case of coarctation of the aorta. *Can J Comp Med* 39:62-66, 1975.

433. Fröhner: Angeborene Aortenstenose als Ursache des intermittirenden Hinkens. *Monat Prakt Tierheil* 16:553-558, 1905.

434. Cupps TR and Fauci AS, in Smith LH: *Major Problems in Internal Medicine*. Saunders, Philadelphia, 1981. p 1.

435. Easley JR: Nectrotizing vasculitis: an overview. *JAVMA* 15:207-211, 1979.

436. Fauci AS, in Wyngaarden JB: *Cecil's Textbook of Medicine*. 17th ed. Saunders, Philadelphia, 1985. pp 1937-1941.

437. Schalm OW and Carlson GP, in Mansmann RA and McAllister ES: *Equine Medicine and Surgery*. 3rd ed. American Veterinary Publications, Goleta, CA, 1982. pp 410-411.

438. Morris DD: Cutaneous vasculitis in horses: 19 cases (1978-1985). *JAVMA* 191:460-464, 1987.

439. Gunson DE and Rooney JR: Anaphylactoid pupura in a horse. *Vet Pathol* 14:325-331, 1977.

440. Morris DD et al: Chronic necrotizing vasculitis in a horse. *JAVMA* 183:579-582, 1983.

441. Werner LL et al: Acute necrotizing vasculitis and thrombocytopenia in a horse. *JAVMA* 185:87-90, 1984.

442. Mackel SE: Treatment of vasculitis. *Med Clin No Am* 66:941-954, 1982.

443. Caciolo PL et al: Michele's medium as a preservative for immunofluorescent staining of cutaneous biopsy specimens in dogs and cats. *Am J Vet Res* 45:128-130, 1984.

444. Galan JE and Timoney JR: *Streptococcus equi* associated immune complexes in the sera of horses with purpura hemorrhagica. *Proc Ann Conf Res Work Anim Dis*, 1984.

445. Roberts MC and Kelly WR: Renal dysfunction in a case of purpura hemorrhagica in a horse. *Vet Record* 110:144-146, 1982.

446. Gillespie JH and Timoney JF: *Hagan and Bruner's Infectious Diseases of Domestic Animals*. Cornell Univ Press, Ithaca, New York, 1981. pp 685-687.

447. Cole JR et al: Transmissibility and abortigenic effect of equine viral arteritis in mares. *JAVMA* 189:769-771, 1985.

448. Traub-Dagartz JL et al : Equine viral arteritis. *Compend Cont Ed Pract Vet* 7:S450-S496, 1985.

449. Tashjian RJ: Transmission and clinical evaluation of an equine infectious anemia herd and their offspring over a 13-year period. *JAVMA* 184:282-288, 1984.

450. Issel CJ and Coggins L: Equine infectious anemia: Current knowledge. *JAVMA* 174:727-733, 1979.

451. Coggins L: Carriers of equine infectious anemia. *JAVMA* 184:279-281, 1984.

452. Gribble DH: Equine ehrlichiosis. *JAVMA* 155:462-469, 1969.

453. Madigan JE and Gribble D: Equine ehrlichiosis in northern California: 49 cases (1968-1981). *JAVMA* 190:445-448, 1987.

454. Ziemer EL et al: *Ehrlichia equi* infection in a foal. *JAVMA* 190:199-200, 1987.

455. Robinson WF and Maxie MG, in Jubb KVF et al: *Pathology of Domestic Animals*. Vol III. Academic Press, San Diego, 1985. pp 2-81.

456. Kiryu et al: *Dirofilaria immitis* from the right ventricle of an equine heart. *Exp Rep Equine Hlth Lab* 7:58-64, 1970.

457. van Knapen F et al: Experimental *Trichinella spiralis* infection in two horses. *Veterinarski Archiv* 57:123-132, 1987.

458. Hilali M and Nassar AM: Ultrastructure of *Sarcocystis* spp from donkeys (*Equus asinus*) in Egypt. *Vet Parasitol* 23:179-183, 1987.

459. McCraw BM and Slocombe JOD: *Strongylus vulgaris* in the horse: A review. *Can Vet J* 17(6):150-157, 1976.

460. Duncan JL and Pirie HM: The life cycle of *Strongylus vulgaris* in the horse. *Res Vet Sci* 13:374-379, 1972.

461. Duncan JL and Pirie HM: The pathogenesis of single experimental infections with *Strongylus vulgaris* in foals. *Res Vet Sci* 18:82-93, 1975.

462. Aref S: A random walk model for the migration of *Stronglus vulgraris* in the intestinal arteries of the horse. *Cornell Vet* 72:64-75, 1982.

463. Wright AI: Verminous arteritis as a cause of colic in the horse. *Equine Vet J* 4:169-174, 1972.

464. Greatorex JC: Diarrhoea in horses associated with ulceration of the colon and caecum resulting from *S vulgaris* larval migration. *Res Vet Sci* 97:221-225, 1975.

465. Farrelly BT: The pathogenesis and significance of parasitic endarteritis and thrombosis in the ascending aorta of the horse. *Vet Record* 66:53-61, 1954.

466. Johne: *Thrombose der linken Kranzarterie des Herzens*. Bericht über das Veterinärwesen im Königreich Sachsen für das Jahr, 1880, 1881. pp 37.

467. Cadiot M: Thrombose parasitaire de l'artère coronaire gauche chez l'ane. *Bull Société Méd Vét* 11:57-58, 1893.

468. Little PB et al: Verminous encephalitis of horses: experimental induction with *Strongylus vulgaris* larvae. *Am J Vet Res* 35:1505-1510, 1974.

469. Slocombe JOD and McCraw BM: Controlled tests of ivermectin against migrating *Strongylus vulgaris* in ponies. *Am J Vet Res* 42:1050-1051, 1981.

470. Drudge JH and Lyons ET: The chemotherapy of migrating strongyle larvae. *Proc 2nd Intl Conf Equine Infect Dis*, 1970. pp 310-332.

471. Slocombe JOD and McCraw BM: Controlled tests of fenbendazole against migrating *Strongylus vulgaris* in ponies. *Am J Vet Res* 47:541-542, 1982.

472. Slocombe JOD et al: Effectiveness of oxfendazole against early and later 4th-stage *Strongylus vulgaris* in ponies. *Am J Vet Res* 47:495-500, 1986.

473. Platt H: Vascular malformations and angiomatous lesions in horses: A review of 10 cases. *Equine Vet J* 19:500-504, 1987.

474. Murray DR et al: Granulomatous and neoplastic diseases of the skin of the horse. *Aust Vet J* 54:338-341, 1978.

475. Cannon SRL and Loh H: Treatment of a cavernous hemangioma-like lesion in a polo pony. *Equine Vet J* 14:254-255, 1982.

476. Hargis AM and McElwain TF: Vascular neoplasia in the skin of horses. *JAVMA* 184:1121-1124, 1984.

477. Johnstone AC: Congenital vascular tumours in the skin of horses. *J Comp Pathol* 97:365-368, 1987.

478. Ferwerda S: Haemangio-endotheliomen bij een paard. *Tijdschr Diergeneeskd* 65:374-376, 1938.

479. Waugh SL et al: Metastatic hemangiosarcoma in the equine: Report of 2 cases. *J Equine Med Surg* 1:311-315, 1977.

480. Reinacher M: Hamangioendotheliome in der Skelettmuskulatur eines Pferdes. *Berl Münch Tierärztl Wochenschr* 91:121-123, 1978.

481. Frye FL et al: Hemangiosarcoma in a horse. *JAVMA* 182:287-289, 1983.

482. Birks EK and Hultgren BD: Pericardial haemangiosarcoma in a horse. *J Comp Pathol* 99:105-107, 1988.

483. Webster JE and McDonald DA: Coronary flow patterns in the horse. *Fed Proc* 29:653, 1970.

484. Hoffmann V: die Blutgefassversorgung des Pferdeherzens, zugleich auch eine vergleichende

Betrachtung der Topographie der herzeigenen Blutgfasse der Haussauger (Fleischfresser, Schwein und Wiederkauer). *Anatomischer Anzeiger* 137:79-109, 1975.

485. Reddy VK et al: Regional coronary blood flow in ponies. *Am J Vet Res* 37:1261-1265, 1976.

486. Rawlings CA: Coronary arterial anatomy of the small pony. *Am J Vet Res* 38:1031-1035, 1977.

487. Amend JF et al: Xeroradiographic observations of coronary arterial distribution in domestic ponies. *Microvascular Research* 20:151-155, 1980.

488. Manohar M et al: Blood flow in the hypertrophied right ventricular myocardium of unanesthetized ponies. *Am J Physiol* 240:H881-H888, 1981.

489. Parks CM and Manohar M, in Snow DH et al: *Equine Exercise Physiology*. Granta Editions, Cambridge, 1983. pp 105-120.

490. Manohar M: Transmural coronary vasodilator reserve and flow distribution during maximal exercise in normal and splenectomized ponies. *J Physiol* 387:425-440, 1987.

491. Reg JD: Some cases of abnormality in the source of the coronary artery in horses. *Vlaams Diergeneesk Tijdschr* 11:213-216, 1942.

492. Van Nie CJ: Anomalous origin of the coronary arteries in animals. *Path Vet* 5:313-326, 1968.

493. Mieog WHW and van Londen JG: Afwijkende oorsprong van de arteria coronaria sinistra. *Tijdschr Diergeneeskd* 94:1370-1372, 1969.

494. Pauli B and Alroy J: Veränderungen and Herzkranzgefässen bei Pferdeföten und wenige Tage alten Saugfohlen. *Schweiz Arch Tierheilk* 114:83-88, 1972.

495. Pauli B: Koronarsklerose beim Pferd. *Schweiz Arch Tierheilk* 115:517-526, 1973.

496. Dudan F and Luginbuhl H: Etude cardiovasculaire chez le cheval: relation entre les altérations vasculaires et tissulaires du myocarde. Première partie. *Schweiz Arch Tierheilk* 126:277-286, 1984.

497. Dudan F et al: Etude Cardiovasulaire chez le cheval: Relation entre les altérations vasculaires et tissulaires du myocarde. Deuxième partie. *Schweiz Arch Tierheilk* 126:527-538, 1984.

498. Dudan F et al: Etude cardiovasulaire chez le cheval: Relation entre les altérations vasulaires et tissulaires du myocarde: Troisième Partie: Résultats. *Schweiz Arch Tierheilk* 127:319-338, 1985.

499. Colombo S and Marazza V: Coronary aneurysm in cattle and horses. *Clinica Veteromaroa e rassegna di Polizia Sanitaria di Igiena* 84:209-225, 1961.

500. Kiryu K et al: Coronary aneurysm accompanied by rupture in a colt: its formal pathogenesis. *Exp Rep Equine Hlth Lab* 5:35-44, 1968.

501. Hübner: *Ruptur der Aorta beim Pferde*. Bericht über das Veterinärwesen im Königreich Sachsen für das Jahr 1888, 1889. pp 63.

502. Schmidt: Aneurysma und Ruptur der Aorta eines Pferdes. *Arch wiss prakt Tierheilk* 15:295-296, 1889.

503. Sequens F: Drei Fälle von Aortenruptur beim Pferde. *Veterinarius Allatorvosi havi folyoirat*, 8:1892.

504. Schade: *Zerreisung der Aorta an ihren Ursprunge*. Bericht über das Veterinärwesen im Königreich Sachsen für das Jahr, 896, 1897. pp 199.

505. Engelen: Ruptur der aorta und der halbmondförmigen Klappen beim Pferd. *Dtsch Tierärztl Wochenschr*, 1898. pp 228.

506. Caparini: Spontaneous rupture of the aorta and its primary branches. *Archivo scientifico dell reale società ed accademia vetinerina italiana*, 1903. p 87.

507. Marcato A: Two new cases of spontaneous rupture in the aorta in the horse. *Nuova Vet* 19:135-138, 1941.

508. Winterhalter M: Spontane rupture aorte kod konje. Medionecrosis aorte. *Vet Archiv* 8:471-497, 1938.

509. Joest E; *Handbuch der speziellen pathologischen Anatomie der Haustiere*. Paul Parey, Berlin, 1963. pp 258-260, 390-392.

510. Meyer O: Bursting of blood vessels in mares. *Dtsch Tierärztle Wochenschr* 55:8-9, 1948.

511. Cook WR: Epistaxis in the racehorse. *Equine Vet J* 6:45-58, 1974.

512. Pascoe JR et al: Exercise-induced pulmonary hemorrhage in racing thoroughbreds: A preliminary survey. *Am J Vet Res* 42:703-707, 1981.

513. Raphel CF and Soma LR: Exercise-induced pulmonary hemorrhage in Thoroughbreds after racing and breezing. *Am J Vet Res* 43:1123-1127, 1982.

514. O'Callaghan MW et al: Exercise-induced pulmonary hemorrhage in the horse: results of a detailed clinical, post mortem, and imaging study. IV. Changes in the bronchial circulation demonstrated by CT scanning and microradiography. *Equine Vet J* 19:405-410, 1988.

515. Hirsch EA: Rupture of the pulmonary artery leading to sudden death in a Thoroughbred foal. *Irish Vet J* 6:565, 1952.

516. Dedrick P et al: Treatment of bacterial endocarditis in a horse. *JAVMA* 193:339-442, 1988.

517 Buergelt CD et al: Spontaneous rupture of the left pulmonary artery in a horse with patent ductus arteriosus. *JAVMA* 157:313-320, 1970.

518. Schrulle: Verblutung infolge von Zerreissung der Arteria axillaris. *Arch wiss prakt Tierheilk* 13:362, 1887.

519. Pröger: *Zerreissung der Arteria thoracica externa*. Bericht über das Veterinärwesen im Königreich Sachsen für das Jahr 1888, 1889. p 63.

520. Schwarzmaier: Gefässzerreissung. *Wschr Thierheilk Viehzucht* 41:13-14, 1897.

521. Lehnert: *Zerreissung der Achselarterie bei einem Pferde*. Bericht über das Veterinärwesen im Königreich Sachsen für das Jahr 1899, 1900. p 86.

522. Hübner: Seltener Fall einer Blutgefassruptur. *Mitt Ver bad Tierärzte* 27:70, 1927.

523. Danelius G: Fatal hemorrhage caused by rupture of the anterior mesenteric artery due to excessive aneurysm, thrombi, and abscesses of the mesenteric trunk in a colt. *Cornell Vet* 31:307, 1941.

524. Berg R et al: Beitrag zu den Plötzlich auftretenden Gefässrupturen beim Pferd unter besondere Berucksichtigung der Pathogenese der Ruptur der Vena Portae. *Monat Vetmed* 25:314-316, 1970.

525. Litt WE: Rupture of renal vein. *Vet Record* 17:327, 1904.

526. Garbe W: Rupture of caudal vena cava in a troop horse. *Dtsch Tierärztl Wochenschr* 46:133-135, 1938.

527. Martin: Thrombose der linken Achselarterie. *Wschr Thierheilk Viehzucht* 29:278-279, 1891.

528. Wollmann: Thrombose de Achselarterie. *Zeitschr Vet Berücks Hyg* 1:24-26, 1900.

529. Durieux J: Thrombosis of the humeral artery in a horse. *Bull Acad Vét Fr* 25:355-360, 1952.

530. Wagenaar G and Kroneman J, in Wintzer H-J: *Equine Diseases*. Paul Parey, Berlin, 1986. pp 47-88.

531. de Toledo Piza E *et al*: Marlforma cao ossea congenite levando a trombose arteriovenosa tardia em equino. *Arqulvos Fluminenses de Med Vet* 2(2):39-42, 1987.

532. Spier S: Arterial thrombosis as the cause of lameness in a foal. *JAVMA* 187:164-165, 1985.

533. Colles CM and Hickman J: The arterial supply of the naviular bone and its variations in navicular disease. *Equine Vet J* 9:150-154, 1977.

534. Colles CM: Ischaemic necrosis of the navicular bone and its treatment. *Vet Record* 104:133-137, 1979.

535. Bibrack B: Uber die formale und kausale Genese der Zehenarterien-obliterationen beim Pferd. *Zbl Vetmed A* 10:67-84, 1963.

536. Fricker CH *et al*: Verschluss der Digitalarterien beim Pferd. *Tierärztl Prax* 10:81-90, 1980.

537. Fricker CH *et al*: Occlusion of the digital arteries. A model for pathogenesis of navicular disease. *Equine Vet J* 14:203-207, 1982.

538. van Kraayenburg FJ *et al*, in Snow DH *et al*: *Equine Exercise Physiology*. Granta Editions, Cambridge, 1983. pp 144-154.

539. Burkert LH: Brachiocephalic thrombosis and aortic arteriosclerosis in a horse. *Vet Med* 38:156-157, 1943.

540. Yamagiwa S *et al*: Morbid anatomy of serum horse. V. On the pathogenesis of the thrombosis in pulmonary artery. *Jpn J Vet Sci* 13:169-181, 1951.

541. Gabel AA: Intravenous injections-Complications and their prevention. *Proc Ann Mtg AAEP*, 1977. pp 29-33.

542. Spurlock SL *et al*: Long term jugular vein catheterization in the horse. *JAVMA*. In press, 1990.

543. Basset MJ: Phlébite purulente de al veine cave, thromboses secondaires dans les divisions de l'artère pulmonaire, pneumonie systématique consecutive. *Rec Méd Vét* 82:609-615, 1905.

544. Jones RS *et al*: Pulmonary micro-embolism following orthopaedic surgery in a Thoroughbred gelding. *Equine Vet J* 20:382-384, 1988.

545. Dungworth DL, in Jubb KVF *et al*: *Pathology of Domestic Animals*. Vol II. Academic Press, San Diego, 1985. pp 413-556.

546. Collin M de W: Du traitement de al boiterie par suite d'oblitération artérielle. *J Méd Vét Zoot* 10:122-129, 1882.

547. Eligio: Paralisi consecutiva all'obliterazione delle arterie illiache in un cavallo Morete. Reporto cadaverico. *Gior med vet practica dell scuola vet* (Turino), 1882. pp 598-603.

548. Johne: *Thrombose des hinteren Endes der Aorta, der Schenkel- und Beckenarterien*. Bericht über das Veterinärwesen im Königreich Sachsen für das Jahr 1881, 1882. pp 47-48.

549. Gratia: Oblitération incomplète de l'extrémité terminale de l'aorta posteriéure et des artères iliaques internes par thrombose. *Ann Med Vet*, 1884. p 57.

550. Cadéac and Malet: Thrombose der Oberschenkelarterie beim Pferde; Embolien in den Verästelungen dieser Gefässe; Arteritis; Venenthrombose; Gangrän der Bliedmassen. *Rev Vét* 9:350, 1885.

551. Roy and Guneu: Thrombose de l'aorte postérieure sue une jument. *Rev Vét* 23:286-289, 1899.

552. Merillat LA: *The Principles of Veterinary Surgery*. Alexander Eger, Chicago, 1906.

553. Dollar JAW, in Dollar JAW: *Regional Veterinary Surgery and Operative Technique*. Hartz, Toronto, 1912. pp 947-949.

554. Hoare EW: *A System of Veterinary Medicine*. Vol II. Balliere, Tindall & Cox, London, 1915.

555. Cartwright CW: Iliac thrombosis. *Vet Record* 15:1068, 1935.

556. Maqsood M: Traumatic iliac thrombosis in a race-horse. *Indian Vet J* 20:133-136, 1943.

557. Savage A: Iliac thrombosis in a Thoroughbred. *Can J Comp Med* 8:117-118, 1944.

558. Merillat LA: Thrombosis of the iliac arteries in horses. *JAVMA* 104:218-220, 1944.

559. Azzie MAJ: Clinical diagnosis of equine aortic-iliac thrombosis and its histopathology as compared with that of the strongyle aneurysm. *Proc 18th Ann Mtg AAEP*, 1972. pp 43-50.

560. Azzie MAJ: *Some observations on equine aortic iliac thrombosis*. Dissertation. University of Zurich, Switzerland, 1973.

561. Damodaran S *et al*: Thrombosis in animals. *Indian Vet J* 52:52-55, 1975.

562. Crawford WH: Aortic-iliac thrombosis in a horse. *Can Vet J* 23:59-62, 1982.

563. Physick-Sheard PW and Maxie MG, in Robinson NE: *Current Therapy in Equine Medicine*. Saunders, Philadelphia, 1983. pp 153-155.

564. Physick-Sheard PW and Maxie MG, in Robinson NE: *Current Therapy in Equine Medicine 2*. Saunders, Philadelphia, 1987. pp 173-176.

565. Mayhew IG and Kryger MD: Aortic-iliac-femoral thrombosis in a horse. *VM/SAC* 70:1281-1284, 1975.

566. Reef VB *et al*: Use of ultrasonography for the detection of aortic-iliac thrombosis in horses. *JAVMA* 190:286-288, 1987.

567. Edwards GB and Allen WE: Aorto-iliac thrombosis in two horses: Clinical course of the disease and use of real-time ultrasonography to confirm diagnosis. *Equine Vet J* 20:384-387, 1988.

568. Tillotson PJ and Kopper PH: Treatment of aortic thrombosis in a horse. *JAVMA* 149:766-767, 1966.

569. Branscomb BL: Treatment of arterial thrombosis in a horse with sodium gluconate. *JAVMA* 152:1643-1644, 1968.

570. Moffett FS and Vanden P: Diagnosis and treatment of thrombosis of the posterior aorta or iliac arteries. *VM/SAC* 73:184, 1978.

571. Merkt H *et al*: Impotentia coeundi beim Hengst infolge Thrombose der Arteria iliaca externa. *Pferdeheilkunde* 3:97, 1987.

572. Hilbert BJ and Rendano VT: Venous aneurysm in a horse. *JAVMA* 167:394-396, 1975.

573. Baker JR and Ellis CE: A survey of post mortem findings in 480 horses 1958-1980 1: Causes of death. *Equine Vet J* 13:43-46, 1981.

574. Livesey MA *et al*: Rupture of the portal vein in epiploic foramen entrapment. *Can Vet J*. In press, 1990.

575. Postiglione E: Malformations of the left common iliac vein with anastomosis with the corresponding artery in a horse. *Nuova Vet* 14:57-61, 1936.

576. Neal PA: Aneurysmal varix in the horse: a sequel to the perivascular injection of thiopentone sodium. *Vet Record* 75:289-291, 1963.

577. Bouayad H *et al*: Peripheral acquired arteriovenous fistula: a case report of four cases and literature review. *JAAHA* 23:205-211, 1987.

578. Gerhards H: Untersuchungen zur Entstehung der Thrombophlebitis beim Pferd - der Beitrag der erworbenen Hyperkoaguloabilitat. *Dtsch Tierärztl Wochenschr* 94:173-174, 1987.

579. Taylor AW: Traumatic duodenitis with subsequent thrombosis of the posterior vena cava in a horse. *Aust Vet J* 46:281-283, 1970.

580. Deem DA: Complications associated with the use of intravenous catheters in large animals. *Calif Vet* 6:19-24, 1981.

581. Burrows CF: Techniques and complications of intravenous and intra-arterial catheterization in dogs and cats. *JAVMA* 180:747-749, 1982.

582. Stillman RM *et al*: Etiology of catheter-associated sepsis. Correlation with thrombogenicity. *Arch Surg* 112:1297-1299, 1977.

583. Righter J *et al*: Infection and peripheral venous catheterization. *Diag Microbiol Infect Dis* 1:89-93, 1983.

584. Bishop R and Boles CL: An indwelling venous catheter for horses. *VM/SAC* 67:415-420, 1972.

585. Welch GW *et al*: The role of catheter composition in the development of thrombophlebitis. *Surg Gynec Obstet* 138:421-424, 1976.

586. Spanos HG and Heckler JF: Thrombus formation in indwelling venous canulae in sheep: Effects of time, size and material. *Anaesth Intens Care* 4:217, 1976.

587. Curelaru I *et al*: Material thrombogenicity in central venous catheterization. III. A comparison between soft polyvinylchloride and soft polyurethane elastomer, long antebrachial catheters. *Acta Anesth Scand* 28:204-208, 1984.

588. Hoshal VL *et al*: Fibrin sleeve formation on indwelling central venous catheters. *Arch Surg* 102:352-358, 1971.

589. Peters WR *et al*: The development of fibrin sheath on indwelling venous catheters. *Surg Gynec Obstet* 137:43-47, 1973.

590. Michel L *et al*: Microbial colonization of indwelling central venous catheters: Statistical evaluation of potential contaminating factors. *Am J Surg* 137:745-748, 1979.

591. Burrow CF: Inadequate skin preparation as a cause of intravenous catheter related infection in the dog. *JAVMA* 180:747-749, 1982.

592. Muylle E *et al*: An interventricular septal defect and a tricuspid valve insufficiency in a trotter mare. *Equine Vet J* 6:174-176, 1974.

593. Bishop SP *et al*: Functional and morphologic pathology of equine aortic insufficiency. *Path Vet* 3:137-158, 1966.

594. Smetzer DL *et al*: Diastolic murmur of equine aortic insufficiency. *Am Heart J* 72:489-497, 1966.

595. Kohler H: Zur Kalzinose in Osterreich. IX. Kalzinose beim Pferd? *Zbl Vetmed A* 28:187-200, 1981.

596. Marr CM *et al*: Clinical, ultrasonographic and pathological findings in a horse with splenic lymphosarcoma and pseudohyperparathyroidism. *Equine Vet J* 21:221-226, 1989.

597. Littlewort MCG: Cardiological problems in equine medicine. *Equine Vet J* 9:173-175, 1977.

598. Niemetz E: Über das funktionelle systolische Geräusch an der Pomonalis bei Pferden. *Wien Tierärztl Mschr* 11:321-327, 1924.

599. Wilson RB and Haffner JC: Right atrioventricular atresia and ventricular septal defect in a foal. *Cornell Vet* 77:187-191, 1987.

600. Brandt A: Misselbildung des Herzens eines neugeborenen Fohlen. *Rev Tierheilk Tierzucht (Wien)* 7:65-69, 83-93, 1884.

601. van der Linde-Sipman JS and van den Ingh TS: Tricuspid atresia in a foal and a lamb. *Zbl Vetmed A* 26:239-2452, 1979.

602. van Nie CJ and van der Kamp JS: Atresie van het ostium atrioventriculare dextrum (tricuspidalis) bij een te vroeg geboren veulen. *Tijdschr Diergeneeskd* 104:411-416, 1979.

603. Physick-Sheard PW *et al*: Atrial septal defect of the persistent ostium primum type with hypoplastic right ventricle in a Welsh pony foal *Can J Comp Med* 49:429-433, 1985.

604. Grunberg W and Jaksch W: Lutembacher-Syndrom bei einem alten Lipizzaner-Hengst. *Wien Tierärztl Mschr* 59:211-216, 1972.

605. Clark ES *et al*: Aortic valve insufficiency in a one-year-old colt. *JAVMA* 191:841-844, 1987.

606. Mahaffey LW: Fenestration of the aortic and pulmonary semilunar valves in the horse. *Vet Record* 70:415-418, 1958.

607. Glazier DB *et al*: Ventricular septal defect in a 7-year-old gelding. *JAVMA* 167:49-50, 1975.

608. Buergelt CD *et al*: Endocarditis in six horses. *Vet Pathol* 22:333-337, 1985.

609. Deegen E: Formveränderungen de P-Welle im Elektrokardiogramm des Pferdes bei Herzklappenerkrankungen. *Dtsch Tierärztl Wochenschr* 79:532-537, 1972.

610. Davies GO: Mitral endocarditis in a five-month-old foal. *Vet Record* 14:1446-1447, 1934.

611. Miller JK: Meningococcal endocarditis in immunized horses. *Am J Pathol* 20:269, 1944.

612. Innes JRM *et al*: Subacute bacterial endocarditis with pulmonary embolism in a horse associated with *Shigella equirulis*. *Brit Vet J* 106:245-250, 1950.

613. Wagenaar G *et al*: Endokarditis beim Pferde. *Blauen Hefte den Tierärztl* 12:38-45, 1967.

614. Reef VB: Cardiovascular disease in the equine neonate. *Vet Clin No Am (Equine Pract)* 1:117-129, 1967.

615. Stünzi H: Zur Pathogenese der Endocarditis valvularis. *Schweiz Arch Tierheilk* 104:135-146, 1962.

616. Angrist AA and Oka M:. Pathogenesis of bacterial endocarditis. *JAVMA* 183:249, 1963.

617. Weinstein L and Schlesinger JJ: Pathoanatomic, pathphysiologic, and clinical correlations in endocarditis. *N Eng J Med* 291:832-836, 1974.

618. Kay ND: *Infective Endocarditis*. University Park Press, Baltimore, 1976.

619. Weinstein L, in Braumwald E: *Heart Disease: A Textbook of Cardiovascular Medicine*. Saunders, Philadelphia, 1980. pp 1166-1184.

620. Weidlich N: Beitrag zur Biologie des Rotlaufserumtieres. *Berl Münch Tierärztl Wochenschr* 30:135-140, 1943.

621. Yamagiwa S et al: Morbid anatomy of serum Horse. III On thrombosis in the pulmonary artery. *Jpn J Vet Sci* 13:145-155, 1951.

622. Anonymous: Van een goede, maar niet perfecte diagnose. *Tijdschr Diergeneeskd* 94:380-388, 1969.

623. Pipers FS et al: Echocardiographic detection of cardiovascular lesions in the horse. *Equine Med Surg* 3:68-77, 1979.

624. McCormick BS et al: *Erysipelothrix rhusiopathiae* vegetative endocarditis in a horse. *Aust Vet J* 62:392, 1985.

625. Winqvist G: Topografisk och etiologisk sammanstälining av de fibrinösa och ulcerösa endokaditerna hos en del av våra husdjur. *Skand Vet Tidskr* 35:575-585, 1945.

626. Schaff AV der: Bacteriologische aspecten van endocarditis. *Tijdschr Diergeneeskd* 95:939-946, 1970.

627. Svenkerud RR and Iversen L: *Shigella equirulis (B viscosum equi)* som arsak til klappe-endocarditis hos hest. *Nord Vet Med* 1:227-232, 1949.

628. Shaftoe S and McGuirk SM: Valvular insufficiency in a horse with atrial fibrillation. *Compend Cont Ed Pract Vet* 9:203-208, 1987.

629. Miller PJ and Holmes JR: Observations on structure and function of the equine mitral valve. *Equine Vet J* 16:457-460, 1984.

630. Wingfield WE et al: Echocardiography in assessing mitral valve motion in 3 horses with atrial fibrillation. *Equine Vet J* 12:181-184, 1980.

631. Mill J and Hanak J: Abnorme Herzbefunde bei Vollblutrennpferden. *Monat Vetmed* 33:508-511, 1978.

632. Bishop SP et al: Functional and morphologic pathology of equine aortic insufficiency. *Lab Invest* 15:1124, 1966.

633. Spörri H: Two clinical types of aortic insufficiency in horses. *Ann NY Acad Sci* 127:358-363, 1960.

634. Spörri H and Leemann W: Zur Pathophysiologie der Aortenklappeninsuffizienz des Pferdes. *Berl Münch Tierärztl Wochenschr* 85:441-448, 1972.

635. van Vleet JF and Ferrans VJ: Myocardial diseases of animals *Am J Pathol* 124:98-178, 1986.

636. Brown CM and Holmes JR: Assessment of myocardial function in the horse 1. Theoretical and technical considerations. *Equine Vet J* 11:244-247, 1979.

637. Brown CM and Holmes JR: Assessment of myocardial function in the horse 2. Experimental findings in resting horses. *Equine Vet J* 11:248-255, 1979.

638. Blässing E-M et al: Enzymaktivitatsbestimmungen in Organen des Pferdes. *Berl Münch Tierärztl Wochenschr* 95:281-284, 1982.

639. Amend JF et al: Equine monensin toxicosis: Some experimental clinicopathologic observations. *Compend Cont Ed Pract Vet* 11:S173- S183, 1983.

640. Dobin MA and Epschtein JF: Myokardinfarkte und Thrombose bei Tieren. *Monat Vetmed* 23:666-669, 1968.

641. Lombard CW et al: Ventricular septal defects in the horse. *JAVMA* 183:562-565, 1983.

642. van der Luer RJT and van der Linde-Sipman JS: A rare congenital cardiac anomaly in a foal. *Vet Pathol* 15: 776-778, 1978.

643. Pipers FS et al: Echocardiographic detection of ventricular septal defects in large animals. *JAVMA* 187:810-816, 1985.

644. Koblik PD and Hornof WJ: Use of first-pass nuclear angiocardiography to detect left-to-right cardiac shunts in the horse. *Vet Radiol* 28:177-180, 1987.

645. Vitums A: The embryonic development of the equine heart. *Zbl Vet Med C Anat Histo Embryol* 10:193-211, 1981.

646. Ottaway CW: The anatomical closure of the foramen ovale in the equine and bovine heart: A comparative study with observations on the foetal and adult stages. *Vet J* 100:111-118, 1944.

647. MacDonald AA et al: The foramen ovale of the foetal and neonatal foal. *Equine Vet J* 20:255-260, 1988.

648. Wilson AP: Persistent foramen ovale in a foal. *Vet Med* 38:491-492, 1943.

649. Rooney JR: The pathology of respiratory diseases of foals. *Proc 1st Intl Conf Equine Inf Dis*, 1966. pp 70-75.

650. Reid NR: African horsesickness. *Brit Vet J* 118:137-142, 1961.

651. Bergsten G and Persson S: Studies on the ECG in horses with acute strangles. *Proc 1st Intl Conf Eq Inf Dis*, 1966. pp 76-81.

652. Kroneman J and Wensvoort P: Muscular dystrophy and yellow fat disease in Shetland pony foals. *Neth J Vet Sci* 1:42-48, 1968.

653. Wilson TM et al: Myodegeneration and suspected selenium/vitamin E deficiency in horses. *JAVMA* 169:213-217, 1976.

654. Owen R ap R et al: Dystrophic myodegeneration in adult horses. *JAVMA* 171:343-349, 1977.

655. Todd GC et al: Acute reversible myopathy produced by compound A204. *Proc 10th Interscience Conf Antimicrobial Agents Chemotherapy*, 1970. pp 361-365.

656. Stoker JW: Monensin sodium in horses. *Vet Record* 97:137-138, 1975.

657. Whitlock RH et al: Monensin toxicosis in horses. Clinical manifestations. *Proc 24th Ann Mtg AAEP*, 1978. pp 473-486.

658. van de Kerk P: Monensin-intoxicatie bij paarden. *Tijdschr Diergeneeskd* 103:699-700, 1978.

659. Nava KM: Mysterious horse deaths at Bonita Valley farms. *Calif Vet* 32:27-28, 1978.

660. Nuytten J *et al*: Acute en subacute verschijnselen bij monensin intoxicatie bij paarden. *Vlaams Diergeneesk Tijdschr* 50:242-249, 1981.

661. van Amstel SR and Guthrie AJ: Salinomycin poisoning in horses: case report. *Proc 31st Ann Mtg AAEP*, 1985. pp 373-382.

662. Hanson LJ *et al*: Toxic effects of Lasalocid in horses. *Am J Vet Res* 42:456-61, 1981.

663. Mitani M *et al*: Salinomycin effects on mitrochondrial ion translocation and respiration. *Antimicrob Ag Chemother* 9:655-660, 1976.

664. Mollenhauer HH *et al*: Ultrastructural observations in ponies after treatment with monensin. *Am J Vet Res* 42:35-40, 1981.

665. Sutko JL *et al*: Direct effects of the monovalent cation ionophores monensin and nigericin on myocardium. *J Pharmacol Exp Ther* 203:685-700, 1977.

666. Anonymous: *Verträgglichkeit von Salinomycin beim Pferd*. Versuchsbericht Hoescht Pharmaceuticals, 1978.

667. Lewis L and Amend J: Osmotic fragilities of erythrocytes in ponies and horses: Effects of monensin exposure. *Proc 65th Ann Mtg Conf Res Workers Anim dis*, 1984. p 47.

668. Nava KM: Mysterious horse deaths caused by rumensin. *AAEP Newsletter* 2:46-49, 1979.

669. Amend JF: Cardiovascular disturbances in monensin sodium (rumensin) intoxication in ponies. *Proc Ann Mtg Am Coll Vet Int Med*, 1980. p109.

670. Gast AM and Amend JF: Specific electrolyte replacement protects against lethal experimental monensin toxicosis in ponies. *Proc 64th Ann Mtg Conf Res Workers Anim Dis*, 1983. p 174.

671. Lloyd WE, in Mansmann RA and McAllister ES: *Equine Medicine and Surgery*. 3rd ed. American Veterinary Publications, Goleta, CA, 1982. p 198.

672. Burt JM and Burns MW: Effects of monensin on electrical and contractile activity of cultured heart cells. *Fed Proc* 39:298, 1980.

673. Wierup M: Equine intestinal clostridiosis: An acute disease in horses associated with high intestinal counts of *Clostridium perfringens* type A. *Acta Vet Scand* 61 (Suppl 62):1-182, 1977.

674. Schoeb TR and Panciera RJ: Blister beetle poisoning in horses. *JAVMA* 173:75, 1978.

675. Schmitz DG and Reagor JC, in Robinson NE: *Current Therapy in Equine Medicine 2*. Saunders, Philadelphia, 1987. pp 120-122.

676. Rabkin SW *et al*: A model of cardiac arrhythmias and sudden death: Cantharidin-induced toxic cardiomyopathy. *J Pharmacol Exp Therap* 210:43, 1979.

677. Baker D and Kreeger J: Infiltrative lipoma in the heart of a horse. *Cornell Vet* 77:258-262, 1987.

678. McCunn J: Remarks on heart disease in the horse. *Vet Record* 14:780-792, 1934.

679. Miller WMC: Cardiovascular disease in horses. *Vet Record* 74:825-827, 828, 1962.

680. Else RW, in Phillipson AT *et al*: *Scientific Foundation of Veterinary Medicine*. Heinemann Medical Books, London, 1980. pp 328-349.

681. Fassi-Fehri N *et al*: Aspects of lesionnels cardio-vasculaires chez les equides au Maroc. *Rec Méd Vét* 156:721-728, 1980.

682. Urman HK: Atlarda trial cardiomyofibrosis. *Veteriner Fakultesi Dergisi Ankara Universitesi* 12:264-274, 1965.

683. Glazier DB *et al*: Atrial fibrillation in the horse. *Irish Vet J* 13:47-55. 1959.

684. Rothenbacher HJ and Tufts S: Coronary arteriosclerosis in a horse. *JAVMA* 145:132-138, 1964.

685. Kiryu K: Cardiopathology of arrhythmias in the horse. *Proc 26th Ann Mtg AAEP*, 1981. pp 457-468.

686. Manohar M and Parks C, in Snow DH *et al*: *Equine Exercise Physiology*. Granta Editions, Cambridge, 1983. pp 91-104.

687. King JM *et al*: Myocardial necrosis secondary to neural lesions in domestic animals. *JAVMA* 180:144-148, 1982.

688. Palmerio C *et al*: Cardiac tissue response to endotoxin. *Proc Soc Exp Biol Med* 109:773-776. 1962.

689. Ron G: Catecholamine cardiotoxicity. *J Molec Cell Cardiol* 17:291-306, 1985.

690. Tate CL *et al*: Morphologic abnormalities in potassium-deficient dogs. *Am J Pathol* 93:103-116, 1978.

691. Dobin MA and Epschtein JF: Myokardinfarkete bei Pferden mit Infektiöser Anamie. *Monat Vetmed* 23:627-630, 1968.

692. Gay CC *et al*: Hyperlipaemia in ponies. *Aust Vet* 54:459-462, 1978.

693. Harris P: Equine rhabdomyolysis syndrome. *In Practice* 11(11):3-4, 6-8, 1986.

694. Lindholm A *et al*: Acute rhabdomyolysis ("tying up") in standardbred horses: A morphological and biochemical study. *Acta Vet Scand* 15:335-339, 1974.

695. Bartsch RC *et al*: A review of exertional rhabdomyolysis in wild and domestic animals and man. *Vet Pathol* 14:314-324, 1977.

696. McEwen SA and Hulland TJ: Histochemical and morphometric evaluation of skeletal muscle from horses with exertional rhabdomyolysis (tying up). *Vet Pathol* 23:440-410, 1986.

697. Hulland TJ, in Jubb KVF *et al*: *Pathology of Domestic Animals*. Vol III. Academic Press, San Diego, 1985. pp 176-177.

698. Wenger NK *et al*, in Hurst JW: *The Heart, Arteries and Veins*. McGraw-Hill, New York, 1986. pp 1181-1248.

699. Martin AM *et al*: Mechanisms in the development of myocardial lesions in hermorrhagic shock. *Ann NY Acad Sci* 156:79-90, 1969.

700. Taylor WJ, in Hurst WJ: *The Heart, Arteries and Veins*. McGraw-Hill, New York, 1986. pp 566-579.

701. Pion PE *et al*: Myocardial failure in cats associated with low plasma taurine: a reversible cardiomyopathy. *Science* 237:764-768, 1987.

702. Watanabe S *et al*: Evidence for a new lethal gene causing cardiomyopathy in Japanese black calves. *J Hered* 70:255-258, 1979.

703. Martig J *et al*: Gehäufte Falle von Herzinsuffizienz beim Rind: Vorläufige Mitteilung. *Schweiz Arch Tierheilk* 124:69-82, 1982.

704. Rooney RJ: *Autopsy of the Horse–Technique and Interpretation*. Williams & Wilkins, Baltimore, 1970.

705. Rocken H and Bohn FK: Malignes Mesotheliom im Perikard eines Pferdes. *Prakt Tierärztl* 56:584-587, 1975.

706. Carnine BL *et al*: Pericardial mesothelioma in a horse. *Vet Pathol* 14:513-515, 1977.

707. Neufeld JL: Lymphosarcoma in the horse: A review. *Can Vet J* 14(6):129-135, 1973.

708. Shawcross A: Observations on cases of cardiac and pericardiac disease in horses with special reference to their diagnosis and etiology. *The Veterinarian* 58:548-550, 1885.

709. Bradfield T: Traumatic pericarditis in a horse. *Southwest Vet* 23: 145-146, 1970.

710. Bertone JJ *et al*: Traumatic gastropericarditis in a horse. *JAVMA* 187:742-743, 1985.

711. Ryan AF and Rainey JW: A specific arthritis with pericarditis affecting horses in Tasmania. *Aust Vet J* 21:146-148, 1945.

712. Rainey JW: A specific arthritis with pericarditis affecting young horses in Tasmania. *Aust Vet J* 20:204-206, 1944.

713. Manninger R and Mocsy J: *Spezielle Pathologie und Therapie der Haustiere*. 10th ed. Gustav Fischer, Jena, Germany, 1954.

714. Doll ER *et al*: Isolation of a filterable agent causing arteritis of horses and abortion by mares. *Cornell Vet* 47:3-41, 1957.

715. Stevens G *et al*: Pericarditis. *Cornell Vet* 28: 254-256, 1938.

716. Wagner PC *et al*: Constrictive pericarditis in the horse. *J Eq Med Surg* 1:242-247, 1977.

717. Reef VB *et al*: Successful treatment of pericarditis in a horse. *JAVMA* 185:94-98, 1984.

718. Freestone JF *et al*: Idiopathic effusive pericarditis with tamponade in the horse. *Equine Vet J* 19:38-42, 1987.

719. Ackerknecht E, in: *Joest's specielle pathologische Anatomie der Haustiere*. Schoetz, Berlin, 1925.

720. Anonymous: Statistischer Veterinarbericht über das deutsche Reichseer für das Jahr 1923. *Jahresber Vet Med* 43:317, 1923.

721. Hughes W: Rupture of the pericardium in a horse. *Vet J* 79:266, 1923.

722. Jaehnke: Traumatische Perikarditis bei einem Pferd. *Zeitschr Veterinärkunde* 3:130-131, 1918.

723. Foss RR: Effusive-constrictive pericarditis; diagnosis and pathology. *Vet Med* 80:79, 89, 1985.

724. Smith BP: Pleuritis and pleural effusion in the horse: A study of 37 cases. *JAVMA* 170:208-211, 1977.

725. Wagner PC, in Robinson NE: *Current Therapy in Equine Medicine*. Saunders, Philadelphia, 1983. pp 149-151.

726. Dill SG, in Robinson NE: *Current Therapy in Equine Medicine 2*. Saunders, Philadelphia, 1987. pp. 171-172.

727. Maqsood M: Hemopericardium in a mare. *Indian Vet J* 20:266-268, 1944.

728. Ogilvie TH *et al*: *Mycoplasma felis* as cause of pleuritis in horses. *JAVMA* 182:1374-1376, 1983.

729. Rosendahl S *et al*: Detection of antibodies to *Mycoplasma felis* in horses. *JAVMA* 188:292-294, 1986.

730. Gross DR: Possible electrocardiographic diagnosis of pericarditis in a horse. *VM/SAC* 64:1077-1079, 1969.

731. White NA and Rhode EA: Correlation of electrocardiographic findings to clinical disease in the horse. *JAVMA* 164:46-56, 1974.

732. Nigam JM and Manohar M: Pericardectomy as treatment for pericarditis in a cow. *Vet Record* 92:202-203, 1973.

733. Schalm WO: Lymphosarcoma in the horse. *Compend Cont Ed Pract Vet* 3:23-27, 1981.

734. Rebhun WC and Bertone JJ: Equine lymphosarcoma. *JAVMA* 184:721-721, 1984.

735. Neufeld JL: Lymphosarcoma in a mare and review of cases at the Ontario Veterinary College. *Can Vet J* 14:149-153, 1973.

736. Dewes HF and Blakeley JA: Lymphosarcoma in a thoroughbred filly. *N Zeal Vet J* 28:82, 1980.

737. Theilen GH and Madewell BR, in Theilen GH and Madewell BR: *Veterinary Cancer Medicine*. Lea & Febiger, Philadelphia, 1979. pp 273-279.

738. Leinati L: Su di un caso raro di malformazione del cuore in un puledro. *Clin Vet* (Milano) 52:6-10, 1928.

739. Johnson JW *et al*: Diaphragmatic hernia with a concurrent cardiac defect in an Arabian foal. *J Eq Vet Sci* 4:225-226, 1984.

740. Wathue LB: Persistent foramen interventricular in a horse. *Norsk Vet Tidsskr* 49:21, 1937.

741. Gavrashanski P and Dyakov L: Interventricular foramen in a horse. *Naus Trud Viss Vet Med Inst* 10:321-323, 1962.

742. Nielsen K: Et tilfaelde af ventrikel-septumdefekt hos hest. *Dan Vet Tidsskr* 63:885-888, 1980.

743. Evans DL: Cardiovascular response to exercise and training. *Vet Clin No Am* (Eq Pract) 1:513-531, 1985.

This page is intentionally left blank.

Diseases of the Respiratory System

F.J. Derksen

Examination of the Respiratory System

F.J. Derksen

History

Evaluation of the respiratory system starts with taking a history. The history, probably one of the most important aspects of a general physical examination, can be tailored to the problem for which the horse is presented. Questions regarding the respiratory system include the time when the presenting problem was first observed, the amount and character of nasal discharge, the presence or nature of a cough, exercise tolerance, and any observation regarding pattern of breathing. In addition, the vaccination history, especially vaccinations against *Streptococcus equi*, rhinopneumonitis virus and equine influenza virus, should be ascertained.

Physical Examination at Rest

The next step in evaluation of the respiratory system is observation. Observation of horses with respiratory disease should include an evaluation of general condition. Horses with such chronic debilitating conditions as pleuritis, weight loss and a dull haircoat. Horses with acute disease may be depressed, but their general condition is usually satisfactory.

The horse should be observed in a quiet surrounding to evaluate the pattern of breathing. Most horses have a respiratory rate of 10-40 breaths per minute at rest.

The inspiratory and expiratory times are approximately equal in length. Inhalation is accomplished actively by contraction of the diaphragm and intercostal muscles. The first part of exhalation is passive, followed by an active phase involving recruitment of expiratory abdominal muscles. Respiratory disease may manifest itself by an increased respiratory rate (tachypnea) or increased effort of breathing (dyspnea). The latter is evidenced by flaring of the nostrils, exaggeration of the abdominal push on exhalation, or both.

When observing the pattern of breathing, it is important to note whether dyspnea occurs on inspiration or expiration. Inspiratory dyspnea usually is associated with upper airway disease, while expiratory dyspnea usually is the result of lower airway or pulmonary disease. Thus, careful observation of the breathing pattern of horses at rest may give valuable clues regarding the site of the respiratory problem. Tachypnea in horses may be the result of respiratory disease causing hypoxemia or hypercapnia. However, anxiety and pain also cause tachypnea. Airway disease in horses may activate pulmonary receptors, with vagal afferent fibers causing bronchoconstriction and marked tachypnea.[1] By this mechanism, tachypnea may be a prominent sign of respiratory disease without arterial hypoxemia, pain or anxiety. In foals with increased respiratory effort, the pattern of breathing may become paradoxical. That is, on inhalation the abdomen may expand, with concomitant collapse of the very pliable thoracic cage. When severe, this pattern of respiration can lead to respiratory failure and is a sign of significant respiratory disease.

A detailed physical examination of the horse with respiratory disease should start at the head. The clinician can evaluate the amount of air exiting the nares by cupping the nostrils with the hands. In many cases of upper airway obstruction restricted to one nasal passage, a decrease in air flow through the affected nostril is appreciated. Subsequently, careful attention should be paid to any discharge around the nares and eyes. In some cases, the discharge is fresh and may be characterized as purulent, mucoid or serous. In other cases, the discharge may have dried up and is no longer obvious.

Next, muscular tone of the external nares should be evaluated. Horses with neuromuscular disease may have respiratory obstruction because of collapse of the external nares. The paranasal sinuses can be evaluated by percussion. Clinicians should have a clear understanding of the anatomy of the head and be able to outline paranasal sinuses on the surface of the head.

Evaluation of the lymph nodes of the head and neck is an important part of a detailed physical examination of the respiratory system. Those that can be evaluated include the mandibular and retropharyngeal lymph nodes. These may not be obvious in a normal animal but may be greatly enlarged in horses with disease of the upper respiratory system.

Palpation of the larynx can yield substantial information. In horses with atrophy of the intrinsic laryngeal musculature, the muscular process of the arytenoid cartilage is readily palpated. In addition, space-occupying lesions around the larynx can be evaluated by palpation in this manner. When evaluating the laryngeal adductor, the *slap test* may be used. This test involves palpating the dorsolateral aspect of the larynx while slapping the horse's wither on the contralateral side. In normal horses, this procedure causes palpable movement of the dorsolateral musculature in synchrony with adduction of the arytenoid cartilage. This should be confirmed with an endoscope when any question arises about the presence or absence of the response. A negative response may result from neurologic dysfunction or dysfunction of the laryngeal cartilage and associated musculature.

A detailed physical examination of the respiratory system of the horse is not complete without a thorough oral examination. Roots of the upper teeth protrude into the paranasal sinuses, and oral cavity diseases can be responsible for lesions in the paranasal sinuses. Following examination of the head, the cervical trachea should be evaluated. This can be done by palpation and auscultation. Palpation may reveal space-occupying lesions, as well as deformities of the trachea. While palpating the trachea, the jugular furrows should be evaluated carefully. Respiratory disease may be caused by dysfunction of the recurrent laryngeal nerve, vagus nerve and/or sympathetic trunk that course in this region.

Auscultation and Percussion

Lung Auscultation: Evaluation of the lung is the most challenging part of examination of the respiratory system. First, the clinician must be aware of the lung field that can be evaluated by auscultation. The lung field is bordered cranially by the heavy musculature of the shoulder and dorsally by the back muscles. The caudoventral border is marked by the 17th intercostal space at the level of the tuber coxae, the 11th intercostal space at the level of the point of the shoulder, and the point of the elbow (Fig 1). One of the limitations of auscultation and percussion is that a large portion of the

Figure 1. The lung field is bordered cranially by the heavy musculature of the shoulder and dorsally by the back muscles. The caudoventral border is marked by the 17th intercostal space at the level of the tuber coxae, the 11th intercostal space at the level of the point of the shoulder, and the point of the elbow.

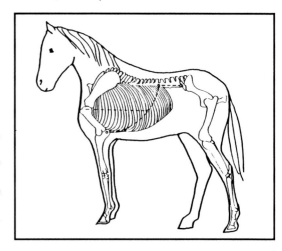

cranioventral lung region cannot be evaluated using these techniques because of the shoulder and its associated musculature. In spite of its limitations, auscultation is still one of the most sensitive qualitative methods of evaluation available to the equine clinician.

Auscultation should be carried out using a quality stethoscope that fits the operator's ears tightly and comfortably. Because respiratory sounds originating from a horse's thorax are not very loud, the environment in which auscultation is performed must be quiet. The clinician should not allow loud noises or talking while the examination is being conducted. Breath sounds are produced by turbulent air flow in the large airways and are conducted through the lung parenchyma and thoracic wall to the stethoscope. The intensity of breath sounds varies directly with air flow velocity. Therefore, breath sound production may be enhanced by increased ventilation and ventilation through partially obstructed airways.

In a normal horse, breath sounds may be accentuated by exercising the horse before auscultation or by use of a rebreathing bag. Breath sounds may be decreased or eliminated by complete obstruction of the airways. Conduction of breath sounds from the site of production to the stethoscope is enhanced by lung consolidation or atelectasis and reduced by lung inflation or pleural fluid accumulation. Interestingly, heart sounds often appear to be carried over a wide area on the thoracic wall when excessive pleural fluid is present. Thus, the intensity of breath sounds heard at the thoracic wall in disease is a combination of changes in sound production and transmission. Pulmonary disease can result in increased or decreased intensity of breath sounds, and auscultation should be considered a qualitative test only.

Auscultation should not be used to specifically diagnose diseases or to quantitate the severity of disease. Abnormal lung sounds or adventitious sounds may be superimposed on normal breath sounds. Adventitious sounds are classified as crackles or wheezes.[2] Crackles are short, nonmusical, sharp, explosive sounds, while wheezes are musical, high-pitched sounds of variable duration. Wheezes and crackles can be further described by evaluating their loudness, pitch and timing in the respiratory cycle (Fig 2). The primary mechanism of crackles production is through equalization of pressure when a collapsed region of lung is reinflated. Crackles are uncommon in horses and associated with restrictive lung disease, including pulmonary edema, atelectasis, diffuse fibrosis and interstitial pneumonia. Crackles are most commonly heard in foals with bacterial pneumonia. Wheezes are produced by vibrations of airway walls and associated with obstructive lung diseases, including bronchopneumonia and chronic obstructive pulmonary disease.

The term "friction rub" cannot be used when discussing lung sounds. Certainly, crepitus or thumping may be palpable on the thoracic wall, but even these findings more often originate from the airways than the pleural space. From the above description it should be apparent that lung sounds are not pathognomonic for any disease, and conclusions based on auscultation findings regarding etiology or pathologic should be drawn with caution.

Tracheal Auscultation: Auscultation of the trachea is important when evaluating the respiratory system. Tracheal sounds are transmitted through a small amount of tissue and reflect the sounds generated in central airways without the attenuation caused by transmission through pulmonary parenchyma. Thus, comparison of lung sounds with tracheal sounds may provide useful information regarding transmission of lung sounds through lung parenchyma.

Figure 2. Nomenclature used to describe respiratory sounds.

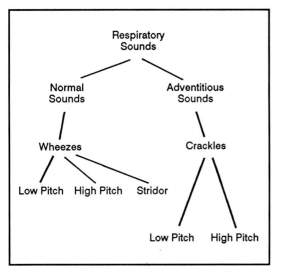

Thoracic Percussion: Percussion is accomplished using a rubber hammer (plexor) and a flat instrument (pleximeter) or, conveniently, using the first 2 fingers of one hand as the plexor and one finger of the other hand, firmly pressed between ribs, as the pleximeter. The technique allows delineation of the boundaries of the aerated lung and detection of large space-occupying lesions, such as abscesses and pleuritis.

Examination after Exercise

Evaluation of the respiratory system is not complete without examination during or after exercise. Obviously, horses in respiratory distress should not be forced to exercise. Horses should be exercised in the manner in which they usually are used. Thus, Standardbred horses should be evaluated on the race track, while pleasure horses should be either ridden or lunged. Exercising horses with respiratory disease may yield valuable information regarding exercise tolerance, respiratory noise production, or pattern of breathing during exercise. In addition, the rate of recovery following exercise may help determine the extent of respiratory disease.

In many cases, respiratory disease can be diagnosed after detailed physical examination of the respiratory system. In other cases, ancillary aids are required.

Evaluating Foals for Respiratory Disease

M.R. Paradis

Respiratory disorders of the newborn foal represent some of the most common problems in equine neonatal care.[3] They also are some of the most underdiagnosed problems in the field. Clinical signs of pulmonary involvement may be subtle, and it takes experience in observing foals to recognize the problem.[4] Even so, the skills of history-taking and physical examination must be combined with diagnostic tests. This section discusses recognition of pulmonary disorders in the foal. Specific problems and their associated therapies are discussed later under their respective headings.

The history may indicate that the respiratory system is compromised. Premature birth or induced parturition can produce a foal with immature lungs. The lungs of foals delivered by cesarean section are likely to contain more fluid because during a normal delivery, lung fluids are expressed mechanically. Premature placental separation or rapid expulsion of the placenta after delivery suggests prenatal asphyxia. Meconium aspiration should be suspected if there is yellow staining of the amniotic fluid or the foal.[5] Prenatal colostrum leakage may be responsible for failure of passage of immunoglobulin and supports a diagnosis of septicemia or bacterial pneumonia.

Clinical signs of respiratory problems in the newborn foal can be very subtle. The normal foal's respiratory rate varies from an average of 70 bpm at birth to about 40 bpm by one hour postpartum.[6] Breathing should be quiet, without nostril flaring, exaggerated rib movements or obvious abdominal effort. Immediately after birth, soft wheezes and crackles may be auscultated over the lung fields. These sounds are due to the initial opening of the newborn's airways. However, there should be normal breath sounds within 15 minutes.[7]

An elevated respiratory rate and increased respiratory effort suggest pulmonary disease. Tachypnea can be caused by hypoxia, hypercapnia, fever or metabolic acidosis. A paradoxical medial movement of the pliable rib cage with expansion of the abdomen on inspiration is a sign of severe respiratory disease in the neonate.[4]

Auscultation of the lung fields of the foal is important but does not correlate well with the severity of the pulmonary problem. Quiet breath sounds may be auscultated in spite of severe interstitial disease or a consolidated lung lobe. Abnormal lung sounds, such as crackles and wheezes, may be present in disease but also may be the result of hypostatic congestion of the dependent lung in a foal that has been in lateral recumbency. Foals have a compliant thoracic wall that can prevent lung expansion if it is compressed in any way.[4]

The foal's mucous membranes should be carefully examined. A blue-tinged membrane indicates cyanosis, which may be associated with severe arterial hypoxemia. It usually does not become clinically evident until the arterial oxygen tension (PaO_2) is <40 torr.[4] A cardiovascular examination should be performed to rule out congenital heart defects as a cause of cyanosis and signs of respiratory disease.

Ancillary Diagnostic Aids

F.J. Derksen

Endoscopy

Fiberoptic endoscopic examination of the respiratory system is a valuable aid in diagnosis of upper and lower respiratory disease.[8] It is the most effective method to evaluate the upper respiratory tract. It allows identification of the source of nasal discharge and, in many instances, the source of respiratory noise. If possible, horses should not be tranquilized before evaluation because tranquilization may affect function of upper respiratory musculature.[9] Fiberoptic endoscopy of the upper and lower airways should be performed before and after exercise. In many cases, exudate is not present at rest but may be seen following exercise.

When evaluating the respiratory system through the fiberoptic endoscope, a systematic approach should be used to avoid overlooking lesions. Both nasal passages should be used. Using the standard 11-mm-diameter fiberoptic endoscope, the nasal opening of the maxillary sinus may not be viewed directly. However, abnormal secretions may be present at this opening and drain into the caudal part of the middle meatus. The ethmoid turbinates should be inspected, especially when the source of hemorrhage is being sought.

The pharyngeal openings to the guttural pouches may be examined next. A discharge often exits these openings when the horse is made to swallow; this can be done by placing some water in the pharynx. The fiberoptic endoscope also may be used to evaluate the guttural pouches, with the help of a Chambers catheter or by using the guidance of the fiberoptic biopsy instrument inserted into the openings of the pouches. The guttural pouches may be examined for foreign bodies, protruding masses, mycotic plaques, secretions, purulent material, chondroids and blood.

The pharyngeal area then is evaluated for color and abnormal secretions. In addition, the anatomy of the pharyngeal region should be evaluated carefully.

Next, the laryngeal cartilages are assessed. Function of the arytenoid cartilage may be evaluated by observing the horse at rest, after occluding both its nostrils for 20-40 seconds, and during swallowing. This allows evaluation of symmetry of movement of the arytenoid cartilage as well as its ability to be fully abducted or adducted. This examination may be repeated following exercise because tiring of intrinsic laryngeal muscles may lead to dysfunction that is not present at rest. Using the fiberoptic endoscope, laryngeal function has been evaluated in horses exercising on a treadmill. Horses generally tolerate this procedure well, and it has allowed definitive diagnosis of laryngeal dysfunction in horses appearing normal at rest.

The fiberoptic endoscope also may be used to evaluate the trachea for strictures, granulomas or foreign bodies. The amount and color of secretions also should be noted. Ochre-colored secretions suggest the presence of hemosiderin and indicate bleeding several days before the examination. The fiberoptic endoscope may be inserted as deeply as possible into the trachea, allowing visualization of the trachea as it enters the thoracic inlet.

Radiography and Ultrasonography

The extrathoracic portion of the respiratory system lends itself well to examination by radiography. The head and trachea may be radiographed with portable equipment. Radiographic examination is helpful when evaluating the nasal passages, perinasal sinuses, guttural pouches, pharynx, larynx and trachea. In contrast, radiographic examination of an adult horse's thorax can only be performed in a clinic. Even with the powerful radiographic equipment available, radiographic detail is poor because of the sheer mass of tissue to be penetrated by the x-ray beam. In addition, such factors as the horse's size, the point in the respiratory cycle at which the radiograph is made, and the distance between the x-ray head and the film plate are difficult to control. The clinical usefulness of radiography of the adult horse's thorax is further limited because only lateral views can be obtained readily and because several films are needed to evaluate the entire thorax. Radiographic evaluations of the thorax may be used to detect large or extensive lesions, such as pneumonia, pleuritis and lung abscesses (Fig 3). In contrast, radiographic evaluation of the foal lung is possible with commonly available radiographic equipment. Lung radiography is a valuable diagnostic aid when evaluating infectious lung disease in young horses because it can determine the extent of lung injury.

Ultrasonography is useful in evaluation of the pleural space. Ultrasound is reflected at the lung parenchyma-air interface; therefore, in the normal horse, ultrasound does not penetrate lung tissue. Because the thoracic wall is relatively thin, small portable ultrasound units may be used to evaluate the equine thorax. Obtaining high-quality sonograms requires clipping the hair over the region to be examined. Using ultrasonography, small amounts of fluid may be detected in the pleural space, and fibrinous material in pleural fluid may be visualized. In addition, any lung abscesses or areas of lung consolidation contiguous with the pleural space may be detected and evaluated.

Collection of Airway Secretions

Bacteriologic and cytologic evaluation of airway secretions may be useful in diagnosis of infectious respiratory disease. When a purulent nasal discharge is noted, it is tempting to culture this material. However, bacteriologic interpretation of cultures obtained from the nares, pharynx or guttural pouch is difficult because the upper airway has an extensive normal flora. It often is not possible to distinguish between normal flora and pathogens. In many cases, the number of normal organisms in the upper airway exceeds the number of pathogenic organisms. However, when collecting upper airway secretions for virus isolation, pharyngeal or nasal swabs may be useful, especially when obtained using a guarded collection device. Material from the guttural pouch intended for bacterial evaluation may be obtained by percutaneous puncture through Viborg's triangle. The preferred method is via a gas-sterilized fiberoptic endoscope using a sterilized catheter.

Transtracheal Aspiration: Transtracheal aspiration of airway secretions has been used extensively as a diagnostic aid in bacteriologic and cytologic evaluation of the equine lung.[10] A 5-cm-square area is clipped on the ventral midline of the midcervical region, where the trachea is easily palpable. The area is prepared for surgery, and 2 ml of local anesthetic solution are injected subcutaneously. A stab incision is made through the skin, and a trocar is inserted between adjacent tracheal rings into the trachea. A catheter inserted through the cannula is directed down the trachea, and 50 ml of physiologic saline solution are injected into the catheter and aspirated immediately. The aspirate is submitted for bacteriologic culture and cytologic evaluation. Even when secretions are obtained in this manner, results of bacterial cultures must be interpreted with caution. The equine trachea normally contains microorganisms reflecting those present in the horse's environment.[11] Interpretation of bacterial cultures is aided by quantitation.

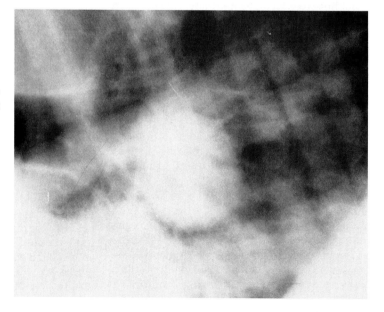

Figure 3. Lung abscess caused by *Streptococcus zooepidemicus* in a 4-year-old Thoroughbred.

Less than 10 colony-forming units likely reflects environmental contamination, whereas ≥100 colony-forming units probably is clinically significant. In addition, bacterial cultures always must be interpreted in light of other clinical data.

When evaluating transtracheal aspirates, it has been assumed that tracheal cytologic findings in some manner reflect the pulmonary or airway cell population. Though this assumption may be valid in some diseases, in normal horses and in horses with chronic obstructive pulmonary disease, there is no significant correlation between tracheal cell populations and the airway cell population as determined by histopathologic examination or bronchoalveolar lavage.[12] In addition, the variability in tracheal cell population of normal horses is very large, further limiting the clinical usefulness of cytologic evaluation of transtracheal aspirates.[12]

Bronchoalveolar Lavage: In contrast to transtracheal aspiration, the variability in cell population obtained by bronchoalveolar lavage is relatively small, and cell counts obtained by this method correspond well with histopathologic evaluations.[13] To obtain bronchoalveolar lavage fluid, the horse is tranquilized, and a 180-cm-long fiberoptic endoscope or commercially available bronchoalveolar lavage tube (Bivona, Gary, IN) is passed via the nostrils into the trachea. Lidocaine solution (5 ml of 0.5% lidocaine) is used to desensitize the carina and airways beyond. The instrument is wedged gently in a lower lobe bronchus, and 3 100-ml aliquots of saline at body temperature (37 C) are infused and aspirated gently. The recovered fluid may be filtered through a single layer of gauze and the volume measured. A differential count of 500 consecutive cells is performed using a Wright's-Giemsa-stained preparation. The procedure appears safe and is tolerated well by most horses. Normal values used in our laboratory are shown in Table 1.

Thoracentesis

Thoracentesis is indicated when pleural disease is suspected. In the right hemithorax, thoracentesis may be performed at the level of the point of the elbow in the seventh intercostal space. In the left hemithorax, thoracentesis is performed 4-6 cm dorsal to the point of the elbow at the eighth or ninth intercostal space. Alternatively, a site is chosen by evaluation of pleural or lung abscess fluid using ultrasonography. A 5-cm-square area is aseptically prepared. Following desensitization of the skin and underlying musculature with 5 ml of local anesthetic solution, a stab incision is made through the skin. An 8-cm teat cannula or blunt catheter is attached to a 3-way stopcock. The catheter is inserted into the thoracic cavity along the cranial border of the rib, avoiding the intercostal artery (Fig 4). A distinct release of tension is felt when a normal pleural space is entered. In the normal horse, air rushes through the cannula into the thorax when the stopcock is opened. Aspiration yields 1-2 ml of straw-colored fluid. Because pleural disease commonly is bilateral, both left and right sides of the thorax should be tapped. In cases of pleuritis, pleural fluid usually drains freely through the cannula. Pleural drainage may be performed for diagnostic and/or therapeutic reasons. After the procedure is completed, the thoracentesis site is covered with an antiseptic cream and bandaged (Fig 4). Thoracentesis is a safe and simple technique, and complications are uncommon.

Lung Biopsy

Percutaneous lung biopsy is a simple technique, but it may have a variety of potentially serious complications, including hemoptysis, neurogenic shock and death. The procedure should be performed only if a pathologic diagnosis is essential in management of the case and when less invasive methods of evaluation have failed. A lung biopsy may be taken from the right hemi-

Table 1. Total white blood cell counts and differential counts in bronchoalveolar lavage fluid of normal horses.

	Mean	Range
Neutrophils	8.9% ± 1.2%	1-17%
Macrophages	45% ± 2.8%	28-63%
Lymphocytes	43% ± 2.7%	25-61%
Eosinophils	≤1.0%	<1.0%
Mast cells	1.2% ± 0.3%	0-3.2%
Epithelial cells	3.5% ± 0.7%	0-8%
Total WBC/L (x10^6)	182 ± 35	0-390
Volume recovered (ml)	150 ± 24	50-250

thorax at the level of the point of the shoulder in the eighth intercostal space or from a site determined by ultrasonography. The biopsy site is prepared aseptically and desensitized using 5 ml of local anesthetic solution. A stab incision is made through the skin, and a 14-ga biopsy needle is advanced into the parenchyma. The needle's obturator is pushed forward into the lung parenchyma and stabilized. The cannula then is advanced to procure the specimen. The external site is covered with an antiseptic ointment and bandaged.[14]

Pulmonary Function Tests

Tests of pulmonary function include those that assess the mechanical properties of the lung, lung volumes and gas exchange.[15] Pulmonary function tests allow quantitative assessment of several aspects of pulmonary function. However, most of the tests require specialized equipment and personnel, and are not useful in detecting subclinical lung disease. Therefore, with the exception of measurement of arterial blood gas tensions, pulmonary function tests are used only rarely in equine practice.

Blood Gas Analysis

Measurement of arterial blood gas tension is the simplest quantitative test of pulmonary function available to equine practitioners. In addition, the test evaluates the most important aspect of pulmonary function: gas exchange. Arterial blood from the facial, carotid or greater metatarsal artery is collected in a syringe coated inside with heparin. Blood gas tensions in arterial blood samples remain constant for several hours if air is expelled from the syringe immediately after collection, the syringe is sealed, and the sample stored on ice. The normal arterial carbon dioxide tension ($PaCO_2$) is 40-45 torr. An increase in $PaCO_2$ suggests hypoventilation, while $PaCO_2$ is decreased with hyperventilation. Thus, the $PaCO_2$ is an indicator of alveolar ventilation but provides little information about gas exchange in the lung. At sea level, the normal arterial oxygen tension (PaO_2) is >85 torr. At higher elevations, a lower PaO_2 may be normal. In the absence of cardiovascular shunts or hypoventilation, a decreased PaO_2 indicates pulmonary disease. Thus, evaluation of PaO_2 allows quantitative assessment of the severity of pulmonary disease, and this often is helpful in formulating a prognosis or when evaluating the response to therapy.

Diagnostic Tests for Neonatal Foals

M.R. Paradis

A more accurate assessment of a foal's respiratory system can be made using thoracic radiographs and arterial blood tensions. With the advent of new radiographic screens, thoracic radiography of the neonatal foal can be performed by veterinarians under field conditions. Foals can be placed in lateral recumbency or restrained in the standing position. Ventrodorsal views can be obtained by placing the foal on its back, with 2 assistants restraining the patient. Though foals resent this procedure, ventro-

Figure 4. A. A teat cannula is inserted through a stab incision in the skin. B. The cannula is pulled dorsally and forced through the thoracic wall. C. The overlying skin seals the wound in the thoracic wall after retraction of the cannula.

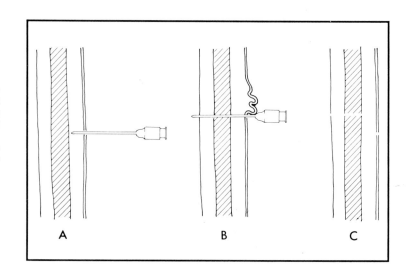

A   B   C

dorsal views may help further evaluate the heart and lung fields.

Thoracic radiographs of equine neonates >4 hours old show a clear air density in the caudodorsal lung fields. The heart, caudal vena cava, aorta and pulmonary vasculature should be clearly defined. A thymic shadow may be seen cranioventral to the heart (Fig 5).[7] Circular 0.5- to 2.0-cm lucencies appear to be clinically inconsequential. Abnormalities seen in radiographs of foals with respiratory disease include loss of vascular clarity, consolidation of one or more lung lobes, increased interstitial patterns, and edema with air bronchograms.

Arterial blood gas tensions are important in defining the severity of the respiratory problem and the mode of therapy needed to resolve the problem. Samples can be obtained by direct puncture of the great metatarsal, femoral, brachial, carotid or facial artery.[4] The great metatarsal artery is located on the lateral side of the metatarsus between the third metatarsal bone and the flexor tendons. It is the most stable of the arteries, and there are no veins nearby to contaminate the sample with venous blood. Because of its small size, however, it is difficult to locate in hypotensive or hypovolemic animals. The femoral artery is located deep in the inguinal region. Palpation of the pulse is necessary to ensure that an arterial and not a venous sample is obtained. The brachial, carotid and facial arteries tend to roll away from the needle and are difficult to sample in an active foal.

A heparinized 3-ml syringe and a small-gauge needle (25-ga, 5/8-inch) are used to obtain the arterial sample. First anesthetizing the puncture site with a small bleb of lidocaine (1% without epinephrine) can greatly facilitate sample collection. After the arterial sample has been collected and the needle is withdrawn, pressure should be applied to the area to prevent hematoma formation. If the sample is sealed with a rubber cork and placed in an ice slush, it can be stored up to 6 hours without significant changes in the P_aO_2.

The arterial blood gas values of normal-term foal vary considerably and depend on the position and excitement of the patient. The P_aO_2 ranges from 60 to 100 torr, and the P_aCO_2 may be 31-55 torr.[6] The average values at 4 hours of age are P_aO_2 of 80 torr and P_aCO_2 of 45 torr (Table 2). A laterally recumbent foal has a decrease in P_aO_2 as compared to one in sternal recumbency.[4]

Pathophysiology of Upper Airway Disease

F.J. Derksen

The upper airway is a complex structure with many functions, including olfaction, phonation, and conditioning and filtering of inspired air. In addition, the upper airway helps in thermoregulation and serves as a conduit for air during respiration. The upper airway is lined by a contiguous mucous membrane enveloping not only the air passages but also the paranasal sinuses and

Figure 5. Thoracic radiographs of a normal 24-hour-old foal.

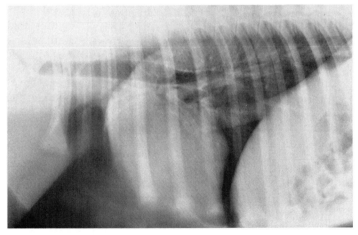

guttural pouches. Therefore, it is not surprising that, in cases of upper airway infection, sinusitis and guttural pouch empyema are possible sequelae.

The upper airway of horses is unique because horses can only breathe efficiently through the nares and use mouth breathing a last resort. Obligate nasal breathing is the result of the tight seal formed between the soft palate and laryngeal cartilages. This implies that upper airway obstruction involving the nasal passages is particularly critical in horses because such an obstruction cannot be bypassed easily by mouth breathing.

The upper airway contributes significantly to total resistance to air flow in the respiratory system. Upper airway resistance in resting horses constitutes about 30-40% of total resistance to air flow. Therefore, even small changes in upper airway caliber may add significantly to the total work of breathing and result in clinical signs of exercise intolerance or dyspnea.

On inhalation, pressure within the upper airway is negative relative to atmospheric pressure; on exhalation, the pressure in the upper airway lumen is positive.[9] Most upper airway structures are rigidly supported by cartilage or bone and are unaffected by these pressure swings. However, structures supported by muscle, such as the external nares, pharyngeal wall and arytenoid cartilages, are moved into the lumen on inhalation. This explains why, in the resting horse, upper airway resistance on inhalation is about 50% greater than on exhalation.[16] During exercise, pressure changes in the upper airway are much greater than at rest. Therefore, during heavy exercise, total inspiratory resistance may be 2 times higher than total expiratory resistance.[16]

Table 2. Findings of arterial blood gas analysis in neonatal respiratory problems.

	Normal	Respiratory Distress Syndrome
pH	7.4	< 7.2
PaO_2 (torr)	60-100	< 60
$PaCO_2$ (torr)	31-55	> 55
HCO_3 (mEq/L)	22-26	24

When a horse starts to exercise, air flow through the upper airway increases from about 4 L per second at rest to more than 75 L per second during exercise.[17] Flow through the upper airway is turbulent. Increasing turbulent flow through a fixed conduit increases resistance to flow. However, when the horse starts to exercise, the upper airway dilates, keeping resistance constant. This dilation is achieved by dilation of the nostrils and other unsupported structures, straightening of the upper airway and vasoconstriction within the vascular mucosa.

Upper airway obstruction may be fixed or dynamic. Fixed obstructions, such as pharyngeal cysts, cause dyspnea on inhalation as well as exhalation, while dynamic obstructions, such as left laryngeal hemiplegia, cause only inspiratory dyspnea.

In normal horses, the tendency of soft tissues to collapse into the lumen of the upper airway is counteracted by muscular activity. In diseases that decrease this muscular tone, such as left laryngeal hemiplegia or facial paresis, dynamic collapse of unsupported soft tissue structures may cause inspiratory dyspnea and flow limitations. Thus, flow rates remain constant despite increasing inspiratory efforts. In horses with left laryngeal hemiplegia, upper airway luminal pressure swings are insufficient to cause dynamic collapse at rest. However, galloping horses with left laryngeal hemiplegia generate tracheal pressures up to 60 cm of water on inhalation, resulting in severe inspiratory dyspnea and flow limitation (Fig 6). Similarly, many horses with dorsal displacement of the soft palate are asymptomatic at rest or during moderate exercise. However, during heavy exercise, the soft palate-epiglottis seal is broken, and the soft palate is sucked dorsally into the pharyngeal lumen. A characteristic rattling sound is heard as air moves over the free end of the soft palate.

Pulmonary Physiology and Pathophysiology

N.E. Robinson

The athletic prowess of horses demands efficient functioning of the respiratory system. The major function of the respiratory system, which is gas exchange, normally occurs at minimal energy cost to the animal.

Figure 6. Inspiratory resistance (Ri) in normal horses (–·––·–), horses with left laryngeal hemiplegia (—·—), and after prosthetic laryngoplasty (—). Standing (A), walking (B), trotting 2.5 m/sec (C), trotting 4.3 m/sec (D), and immediately after exercise (E).[16] The treadmill had a 6-degree incline. Note that in normal horses Ri does not increase with exercise. In horses with a dynamic airway obstruction (left laryngeal hemiplegia), Ri is normal at rest but increases markedly (*) during exercise.[16]

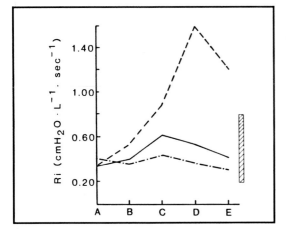

When the respiratory system is diseased, gas exchange is less efficient, and the horse's performance deteriorates. Adequate gas exchange requires ventilation of the lung, distribution of gas among lung lobules, perfusion of lobules, and diffusion of gases between air and blood. Because diffusion only occurs when air and blood are in close proximity, matching of ventilation and blood flow is an essential component of gas exchange. In addition to exchanging gas, the respiratory tract also filters inhaled air and the blood, and performs a variety of metabolic functions. All of these functions can be impaired in respiratory disease.

Mechanics of Ventilation

When a horse breathes, the respiratory muscles must overcome the frictional resistance of the air passages and stretch the elastic lung parenchyma to accommodate inhaled air. Respiratory disease can obstruct the airways or alter the elasticity of the lung parenchyma. Movement of gases through conducting airways into and out of the gas exchange region is known as *ventilation*. Gas exchange occurs in the acinus, which consists of respiratory bronchioles, alveolar ducts and alveoli. Conducting airways, which include the nasopharynx and tracheobronchial tree to the level of the re-

spiratory bronchioles, do not participate in gas exchange and are regarded as deadspace.

In most species at rest, inhalation is an active phenomenon and exhalation is a passive one. The resting horse exhibits biphasic inhalation and exhalation.[18] Inspiratory muscles enlarge the thorax during inhalation, thereby decreasing pleural pressure from its resting value of -5 cm H_2O to an end-inspiratory value of about -10 cm H_2O. This change in pleural pressure stretches the lung and generates flow through the conducting airways. During exhalation, the elastic recoil of the lungs and thorax forces air out of the respiratory system. A second peak-expiratory flow occurs late in exhalation and is due to forced exhalation brought about by contraction of abdominal muscles. In the resting horse, an accentuated abdominal effort during exhalation indicates severe airway obstruction, as in heaves.

Pulmonary Elasticity: The elasticity of the lungs is due to elastin and collagen fibers in the lung parenchyma, and surface tension forces provided by the air-liquid interface lining the alveoli. Surface tension, which tends to collapse the lung, is reduced by pulmonary surfactant. Surfactant, which contains dipalmitoyl lecithin, stabilizes the lung, slows development of atelectasis, and reduces the work of breathing. Sighing reactivates surfactant. Anesthesia and painful lesions of the thorax and abdomen can eliminate sighing and enhance development of atelectasis. Anesthetized horses should be given deep breaths (airway pressure of 25-35 cm H_2O) by positive-pressure ventilation every 5 minutes to prevent atelectasis and maintain adequate gas exchange.

Intracellular, lamellated, osmiophilic bodies representing intracellular surfactant are first observed in type-II alveolar epithelial cells at 150 days of gestation, but surfactant is not fully developed until 300 days or even later.[19] The conditions causing inadequate surfactant in some foals at term are not well understood, but inadequate surfactant is one cause of newborn respiratory distress.[19] Lack of surfactant results in atelectasis and increased work of breathing.

Pulmonary elasticity is evaluated by measurement of lung compliance. Decreased compliance ("stiff lungs") can result from surfactant deficiency, edema, consolidation (as in pneumonia), or increased connective tissue in lung parenchyma. Decreased lung compliance makes lung inflation more difficult and increases the work of breathing, which appears clinically as inspiratory dyspnea.[20] Other diseases that restrict inhalation include pleural effusion, intrathoracic masses and abdominal distention.

Airway Resistance: In addition to stretching the lungs, respiratory muscles cause air to flow through the nasopharynx and tracheobronchial tree. The resistance to air flow created by these conducting airways is determined primarily by their cross-sectional area, which varies with a variety of physiologic stimuli and disease processes (see Pathophysiology of Upper Airway Disease).

Moving distally, the tracheobronchial tree divides repeatedly from the trachea to the alveoli (10-24 times in people). The total cross-sectional area of the airways does not change in the first 4-7 divisions but increases dramatically at the level of the bronchioles. In people, the total cross-sectional area of the twentieth-generation airways is 1000 times the total cross-sectional area of the trachea.[21] If similar figures apply to horses, about 80% of the resistance of the tracheobronchial tree is in airways ≥2-3 mm in diameter. Because of the large total cross-sectional area of the bronchioles, bronchiolar obstruction must be extensive to produce respiratory distress. In contrast, modest decreases in the diameter of larger airways make breathing very difficult.

Airways >1-2 mm in diameter are known as bronchi and have cartilaginous plates to provide some support. Airways <1 mm in diameter (bronchioles) have no rigid support but are kept patent by the tethering action of surrounding lung parenchyma. Smooth muscle is found in the walls of airways from the trachea to the alveoli. Vagal parasympathetic fibers, which provide the primary excitatory innervation, preferentially innervate the larger airways but also extend into the bronchioles. Sympathetic innervation of smooth muscle is present in the trachea, and sympathetic nerves may modulate neural traffic at parasympathetic ganglia. Nonadrenergic, inhibitory nerves in the vagus, with vasoactive intestinal peptide as the mediator, also may oppose bronchoconstriction.

Airway resistance can change in response to a variety of causes. Because intrapulmonary airways are tethered by surrounding lung parenchyma, they dilate and narrow as lung volume increases and decreases, respectively. This narrowing of small airways explains why wheezes are loudest at the end of expiration. Because emphysema destroys lung parenchyma, the tethering of airways by adjacent tissue is reduced and airways narrow. However, "emphysema" in horses usually consists of bronchiolitis rather than the extensive tissue destruction observed in people.[22]

Increases in smooth-muscle tone increase airway resistance. Bronchoconstriction can result from a vagal reflex induced through stimulation of irritant receptors by physical agents, such as dust, or by chemical mediators, such as histamine. Chemical mediators also may stimulate smooth muscle directly. With inflammation, response of airway smooth muscle to bronchoconstrictor stimuli is accentuated, and airways then are said to be hyperreactive.[23] In horses with chronic obstructive airway disease, airway obstruction and hypoxemia occur when the animal is exposed to antigens barn environments (Fig 7). The importance of parasympathetic activity as a cause of airway obstruction in heaves is demonstrated by bronchodilation that follows administration of atropine.[24] Administration of such bronchodilators as atropine or beta-2 adrenergic agonists does not completely reduce the increased airway resistance to normal, indicating that such factors as secretions and airway edema are responsible for part of the airway obstruction. In heaves, bronchoconstriction is opposed by increased sympathetic activity. As a result, administration of a beta-adrenergic blocking drug, such as propranolol, causes bronchoconstriction.[25]

In horses, the bronchoconstrictor role of chemical mediators released from inflammatory cells is not well defined. In other species, mediator release is controlled by a variety of stimuli, including immune responses and stimulation of adrenergic or cholinergic receptors.[26] Agents capable of stimulating adenylate cyclase, such as beta-adrenergic agonists and certain prostaglandins, increase tissue concentrations of cyclic AMP. Cyclic AMP inhibits mediator release and results in bronchodilation. Phosphodiesterase metabolizes cyclic AMP, and substances that inhibit phosphodiesterase, such as aminophylline, cause accumulation of cyclic AMP and inhibit mediator release. In contrast, other prostaglandins, such as PGF_{2a}, decrease cyclic AMP levels and enhance mediator release. Cholinergic stimulation of mast cells results in accumulation of cyclic GMP, which enhances mediator release and causes bronchoconstriction.[26]

In addition to histamine, such chemical mediators as leukotrienes, kinins, prostaglandins and platelet-activating factor are released from target cells in antigen-antibody reactions. Many of these mediators are bronchoconstrictors.[26] Such drugs as cromolyn sodium, diethylcarbamazine and meclofenamic acid block synthesis and release of mediators and consequently can be used to prevent bronchoconstriction.

Clinical signs of increased airway resistance (airway obstruction) vary from reduced exercise tolerance to expiratory dyspnea at rest. In addition to bronchoconstriction resulting from mediator release and vagal stimulation of smooth muscle, airway obstruction can result from masses impinging on the airway (as in hilar lymphadenopathy), airway foreign bodies, and accumulation of secretions.

Figure 7. The effect of environment on ventilatory mechanics and gas exchange in horses with chronic airway disease (heaves, COPD) and in normal horses. When horses are at pasture, arterial oxygen tension (PaO_2) and airway resistance (R_L) do not differ between the 2 groups of horses. Housing horses in a barn causes hypoxemia (decreased PaO_2) and airway obstruction (increased R_L). Lung function returns to normal again within 2 weeks after returning horses to pasture.

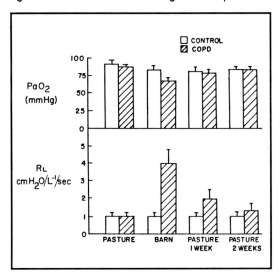

Intrathoracic airway obstruction prolongs exhalation, so the horse uses the abdominal muscles in an attempt to speed exhalation. The abdominal push raises intrathoracic pressure, which compresses the intrathoracic airways, further limiting expiratory air flow.

Gas Distribution

In an ideal lung, air and blood are distributed evenly to the many gas-exchange units. Due to gravity, healthy lungs have some uneven distribution of ventilation and blood flow, resulting in less than ideal gas exchange. In the standing horse, there is a vertical gradient of both ventilation and blood flow per unit lung volume, with dorsal regions receiving less ventilation and blood flow than more ventral regions.[27] In sternally recumbent horses, distribution of ventilation is much more uniform than in laterally or dorsally recumbent horses, probably because the sloping diaphragm of the horse prevents undue compression of the lungs by abdominal contents in the upright animal.[28]

In lung disease, regional variation in airway resistance and lung compliance results in uneven distribution of ventilation. Air is preferentially delivered to regions of high compliance served by airways with low resistance.

Airway obstruction by foreign bodies, exudate and bronchoconstriction results in regional variations in airway resistance. Uneven distribution of ventilation due to local increases in airway resistance is accentuated by increased respiratory frequency. Whereas regions served by partially obstructed airways have time to fill with air when the horse breathes slowly, there is insufficient time for filling when the horse ventilates rapidly. As a result, horses with bronchiolitis may show few signs of lung disease at rest but have poor exercise tolerance because of increasingly uneven distribution of ventilation.

Localized inflammatory processes, edema and fibrosis all result in local variations in lung compliance, which restrict delivery of air to affected parts of the lung. Pleural effusions and local restrictions in thoracic cage mobility also may cause uneven distribution of ventilation.

In species with unlobulated lungs, such as dogs, collateral ventilation may reduce some inequalities in ventilation distribution. Horses have poor collateral ventilation that may add little to gas exchange maintenance.[29]

Pulmonary Circulation

The lung has 2 systems of blood circulation. The pulmonary circulation delivers blood to the lungs for gas exchange, acts as a filter for venous blood, supplies nutrients to the lung parenchyma, acts as a reservoir for the left ventricle, provides a large surface area for absorption of liquids from the alveoli, and modifies many vasoactive agents. The bronchial circulation, a branch of the systemic circulation, supplies the bronchi and visceral pleura and subsequently drains into the pulmonary veins.[30] Proliferation of the bronchial circulation has been described in the dorsocaudal regions of the lungs with a history of exercise-associated pulmonary hemorrhage.[31]

Mean pulmonary arterial pressure averages 25 mm Hg and left atrial pressure is 8 mm Hg, to give a driving pressure for pulmonary blood flow of only 17 mm Hg, compared to the pressure differential of 100 mm Hg in the systemic circulation. Because blood flow in the pulmonic and systemic circulations is equal, it is apparent that the pulmonary circulation has very low resistance. In all species studied, pulmonary vascular resistance decreases even further during exercise because of distension of perfused vessels and recruitment of previously unperfused vessels. In this way, blood flow may increase greatly without doubling the pressure differential across pulmonary circulation.

Pulmonary vascular resistance can change in response to a variety of passive and active factors. Passive factors include changes in lung volume and intravascular pressure. One of the most potent pulmonary vasoconstrictors is alveolar hypoxia.[32] Hypoxic vasoconstriction directs blood away from poorly ventilated lung and may help maintain gas exchange with airway obstruction. Though this system works effectively in normal horses, it may fail to compensate in the presence of inflammatory lung disease, and high blood flow may be maintained to regions of lung receiving little ventilation. When alveolar hypoxia is diffuse, as occurs when horses are kept at high altitudes or in the presence of extensive lung disease, vasoconstriction throughout the pulmonary circulation may lead to right heart failure, ("cor pulmonale").

Blood flow through the pulmonary capillaries depends on the relative magnitudes of alveolar, pulmonary arterial and pulmonary venous pressures. As a result of gravity, intravascular pressures increase from the uppermost to the dependent portions of the lung, so that blood flow is least in the uppermost lung and greatest in dependent portions of the lung.

Increased pulmonary venous pressure (as with left heart failure) and increased pulmonary arterial pressure (as with exercise or patent ductus arteriosus) raise capillary pressure, which increases vascular volume throughout the lung. Vascular engorgement may be observed radiographically as arterial and/or venous enlargement. In contrast, decreased pulmonary venous pressure (as with shock), decreased pulmonary arterial pressure (as during anesthesia), and increased alveolar pressure (as during positive-pressure ventilation) produce a hypoperfused lung. Because both decreased vascular pressures and positive-pressure ventilation tend to hypoperfuse the lung, it is important to maintain vascular volume and to keep the inspiratory phase of ventilation as short as possible in surgical patients.

Gas Exchange

Evaluation of gas exchange by determination of arterial O_2 and CO_2 tensions (PaO_2, $PaCO_2$) shows the end result of gas-exchange processes, including alveolar ventilation, diffusion between the alveoli and capillaries, and matching of ventilation and blood flow.

Alveolar Ventilation: The volume of air breathed per minute is known as minute ventilation and is the product of tidal volume and respiratory rate. In a conscious horse, 40-70% of minute ventilation enters the exchange area of the lung and is involved in gas exchange. This portion is known as alveolar ventilation, while the remainder (deadspace ventilation) enters the conducting airways and does not participate in gas exchange. Alveolar ventilation normally is matched to the body's rate of CO_2 production so that, as tissue metabolism increases, there is a similar increase in alveolar ventilation, causing P_aCO_2 to remain at the normal 40 mm Hg.

The P_aCO_2 decreases when alveolar ventilation is large in relation to tissue CO_2 production. This hyperventilation occurs in cardiopulmonary disease in an attempt to compensate for low P_aO_2, in metabolic acidosis to help to return body pH to normal, and also, to a small degree, during exercise.[33]

The P_aCO_2 increases when alveolar ventilation fails to keep pace with the body's CO_2 production. This is known as *alveolar hypoventilation* and is observed in some horses with severe heaves.[34] It also occurs when ventilation is severely compromised by upper airway obstruction, abdominal distention, or trauma to the thoracic cage.[35] To prevent severe acidosis, alveolar ventilation should be restored by removing the cause of hypoventilation whenever possible. While O_2 administration elevates P_aO_2 depressed by hypoventilation, it does not aid elimination of CO_2 and correction of acidosis.

The surgeon should be aware that anesthetized horses frequently are acidotic due to hypoventilation. Therefore, a means of positive-pressure ventilation should be available for use in deeply anesthetized horses or when acid-base homeostasis is endangered by other disease processes, such as intestinal obstruction. It also is important to ensure that anesthetic equipment minimally contributes to deadspace. This is accomplished by using endotracheal tubes of proper length and a nonrebreathing system.

Deadspace ventilation may be an important method of heat loss in exercising horses. When horses are exercised at a fixed workload, there is a progressive increase in minute ventilation. Alveolar ventilation remains constant, but deadspace ventilation increases, primarily because of increased ventilation to the upper airway.[36,37]

Diffusion: When barometric pressure is 760 mm Hg, the 21% O_2 content of air results in inspired O_2 tension (PO_2) of 160 mm Hg. In the upper respiratory tract, water vapor is added to the air and, in alveoli, O_2 diffuses into the capillary bed and CO_2 diffuses into the alveoli so that alveolar O_2 tension averages 100 mm Hg and CO_2 tension averages 40 mm Hg. The PO_2 and PCO_2 of venous blood returning to the lungs averages 40 and 46 mm Hg, respectively, so that the pressure gradient for O_2

between the alveolus and capillary blood is 60 mm Hg and the pressure gradient for CO_2 between blood and the alveolus averages 6 mm Hg. Because CO_2 is so much more diffusible than O_2, about equal volumes of these 2 gases diffuse across the alveolar capillary membrane per minute despite differences in the pressure gradient.

The rate of gas diffusion across the alveolar capillary membrane is determined by available capillary surface area, pressure gradient, and physical properties of diffusing gas. In horses, a large alveolar surface area per kg of body weight satisfies the high maximum oxygen consumption attained during exercise.[38-40] The rate of gas diffusion can be reduced by diseases that reduce the alveolar surface area available for diffusion (as in atelectasis), or by reduction in capillary surface area resulting from hypoperfusion of the lung (as in shock). When blood containing a large amount of desaturated hemoglobin passes through the lungs at high velocity, as occurs during strenuous exercise, there may be insufficient time for equilibration of alveolar and blood O_2 tensions. This most probably is the cause of the hypoxemia seen in exercising horses.[41]

Because CO_2 is so much more diffusible than O_2, diffusion barriers cause hypoxemia but not hypercarbia (increased P_aCO_2).

Matching Ventilation and Blood Flow: The most common cause of low PaO_2 in horses probably is mismatched ventilation and blood flow. In healthy horses, most alveolar ventilation and pulmonary blood flow is delivered to gas-exchange units in which the ratio of ventilation:blood flow is close to 1.0. Though no vertical gradient of ventilation-perfusion ratios could be measured in standing horses by means of scanning techniques, use of multiple inert gases showed that up to 10% of blood flow goes to high ventilation-perfusion regions.[27,42] Some alveoli in the upper part of the lung may receive more ventilation than blood flow. This normal distribution of ventilation to blood flow ratios results in normal arterial blood gas values (P_aO_2 85-100 mm Hg, P_aCO_2 40 mm Hg).[34,43] In horses with lung disease, the normal distribution of ventilation and blood flow is severely disturbed so that some groups of alveoli receive very little ventilation but continue to receive blood flow, while others receive ventilation but no blood flow.

Bronchitis, bronchiolitis, bronchoconstriction, airway closure, and local restriction of lung movement result in reduced ventilation to portions of the lung. If these portions of lung continue to receive normal blood flow, they have a low ventilation:blood flow ratio, and the blood leaving such areas has a low O_2, high CO_2 content. The extreme case of a low ventilation:blood flow ratio is a right-to-left vascular shunt, in which blood passes from the right to the left ventricle without contacting ventilated alveoli. Such shunts occur in congenital cardiac defects, such as tetralogy of Fallot, and through areas of atelectasis and consolidation within the lung.

If areas of lung have reduced blood flow because of emboli or decreased pulmonary arterial pressures (as in shock) but continue to receive ventilation, these units are said to have a high ventilation:blood flow ratio. Blood leaving such units has a high PO_2 and a low PCO_2. However, because of the sigmoid shape of the oxyhemoglobin-dissociation curve, the high PO_2 produced by these units does not increase the O_2 content of blood significantly. In contrast, the low PO_2 produced by poorly ventilated lung units lowers O_2 content. Combining blood from high- and low-ventilation:blood flow ratio regions of the lung results in a low arterial O_2 content and low PaO_2. Because of the almost linear CO_2 dissociation curve, high ventilation:blood flow ratios compensate for low ventilation:blood flow ratios in CO_2 elimination so that $PaCO_2$ often is normal. If hypoxemia is stimulating ventilation, PaO_2 may be even lower than normal.

Hypoxemia from ventilation-perfusion inequalities can be corrected by administration of O_2, which increases the rate of O_2 delivery to poorly ventilated alveoli. However, O_2 administration does not increase PaO_2 significantly in horses or foals with extensive right-to-left shunts because poorly oxygenated blood bypasses the lung completely. When right-to-left shunts result from pneumonia, the response to oxygen therapy can be used to monitor the progress of the disease (Fig 8).

Gas Transport

Arterial O_2 tension averages 85-100 mm Hg, and alveolar O_2 tension 100-110 mm Hg in horses.[34,43] The difference between arterial and alveolar O_2 tensions results from admixture of venous blood from bronchial and coronary circulations into the oxygenated blood leaving the lungs, and also from ventilation-perfusion inequalities. Foals have a lower O_2 tension than older horses.[6,19]

Hemoglobin (Hb) is necessary for transport of O_2 because O_2 has low solubility in plasma. Each gram of Hb can carry 1.34 ml O_2, so that blood with an average of 15 g Hb/dl has an O_2 capacity of 21 ml/dl blood or 21 volumes percent. Because it is dependent on the amount of Hb in the blood, O_2 capacity decreases in anemia and increases with the polycythemia of exercise.

The combination of O_2 and Hb depends mainly on PO_2 but also is affected by pH, PCO_2, temperature, and the levels of 2,3-diphosphoglycerate (2,3-DPG) within the RBC. Hemoglobin is almost fully saturated with O_2 when blood PO_2 exceeds 85 mm Hg. Increasing PO_2 further by O_2 therapy adds little O_2 to Hb and only a small amount into solution in the plasma. This plateau in the oxyhemoglobin-dissociation curve allows saturation of Hb when PaO_2 is slightly reduced by altitude, cardiopulmonary disease or strenuous exercise.

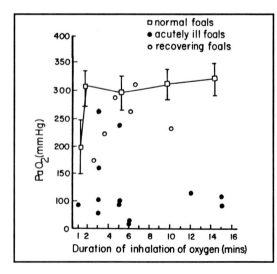

Figure 8. Effect of oxygen administration on arterial oxygen tension (PaO_2) in foals.[6,372] In normal foals (squares), oxygen administration rapidly increases PaO_2. In foals with lung disease (solid circles), oxygen administration fails to increase PaO_2, presumably because of right-to-left shunting of blood through unventilated diseased parts of the lung. As foals recover (open circles), oxygen therapy effectively increases PaO_2.[6,372]

The slope of the oxyhemoglobin-dissociation curve is steep in the range of tissue PO_2, allowing rapid unloading of O_2. Unloading of O_2 is enhanced by increased PCO_2 and decreased pH of tissues. About one-third of O_2 is removed from Hb by the tissues in a resting animal, which allows an O_2 reserve for increased metabolism. The unloading of O_2 also is enhanced by increasing RBC levels of 2,3-DPG, which occur with chronic hypoxemia and increased metabolic rates from thyroid activity.[44,45] The reduction in 2,3-DPG levels in stored blood prevents release of O_2 to the tissues when this blood is transfused into an animal. Twenty-four hours may be required to restore normal 2,3-DPG levels in transfused blood.

Observation of the oxyhemoglobin-dissociation curve reveals several clinically important facts. Administration of pure O_2 to normal animals does not provide a significant O_2 store because Hb is already saturated at a PO_2 of 100 mm Hg. The additional O_2 adds only a small amount in solution in plasma. This small O_2 reserve is rapidly depleted when O_2 administration is discontinued.

Anemic horses with healthy lungs have a normal PaO_2, and all available Hb is saturated. These horses need Hb, not treatment with O_2. Horses with lung disease have a low PaO_2 and usually have normal Hb levels. Low PaO_2 results in desaturation of Hb, and O_2 therapy is needed to elevate PaO_2. In many cases, pure O_2 is not necessary, and 40-60% O_2 will suffice. Though high levels of O_2 given over several hours can result in O_2 toxicity and lung damage, it is unlikely that oxygen toxicity will occur in horses when the usual O_2 therapy methods are used.

Because PaO_2 must decrease below 60 mm Hg to significantly reduce O_2 content or the percent saturation of Hb, PaO_2 is a better measure of gas exchange than is O_2 content or Hb saturation. Mixed venous PO_2 has little use as an indicator of gas exchange, as it is affected by tissue metabolism, blood flow and PaO_2. Cyanosis results from the presence of unsaturated Hb and is a sign of severely impaired gas exchange. It is important to remember that cyanosis also results from local decreases in the blood flow:metabolism ratio.

In contrast to O_2, CO_2 is very soluble, and large amounts are transported in solution in plasma or within the RBC. Carbon dioxide also is transported as bicarbonate ion and as carbamino compounds formed by combination of proteins and CO_2. The transport of CO_2 is accompanied by production of hydrogen ions, which are buffered by Hb, plasma proteins and phosphates. Because there are large reserves of buffer in the body, blood does not become saturated with CO_2.

Pulmonary Fluid Exchange

Many lung diseases are accompanied by changes in the rate of fluid filtration from the pulmonary capillaries into the interstitium and the alveoli. These changes occur as a result of changes in the relative magnitudes of vascular and osmotic pressures. Even in normal horses, there is fluid movement from the pulmonary microvasculature into the tissues. Normally this fluid is removed by lymphatics, and the alveoli remain dry.

Fluid filtration occurs between the microvasculature, arterioles, capillaries and venules, and the interstitial tissue. Transfer of fluid across the endothelium is governed by capillary permeability, vascular pressure, interstitial fluid pressure, and vascular and interstitial colloid osmotic (oncotic) pressures. Filtered fluid tracks toward peribronchial connective tissue, where lymphatics are located. Though fluid moves easily across the vascular endothelium, the alveolar epithelium is less permeable and thus more resistant to fluid movement.

Fluid flux varies with changes in vascular permeability and hydrostatic and oncotic pressures. Left heart failure increases fluid filtration because capillary hydrostatic pressure is increased. Hypoproteinemia, which occurs in starvation and severe parasitic infections, increases fluid filtration by decreasing plasma oncotic pressure. Vascular permeability is increased in inflammatory lung diseases, probably by the effects of neutrophil products on the endothelium.[46,47]

When fluid filtration rates increase, fluid does not immediately accumulate in the alveoli. Lymphatics accommodate quite large increases in fluid flux, particularly if the onset of increased fluid filtration is gradual.[48] Compliant peribronchial and perivascular spaces also provide intrapulmonary sinks for fluid accumulation. Alveolar flooding occurs once the peribronchial capacity is exceeded or when the alveolar epithelium is damaged. Once in the airspace, fluid fills the alveoli. The foaming seen clinically with pulmonary edema probably results from the mixing of air, edema fluid and surfactant within the larger airways.

Pleural Fluid Exchange

The pleural cavity contains a small volume of fluid distributed over the pleural surfaces in a 10- to 20-μ layer that couples the lungs to the chest wall and lubricates the pleural surfaces. Pleural fluid originates by filtration from capillaries in the visceral and parietal pleura. In horses, both pleural surfaces have a systemic blood supply; therefore, capillary pressures of visceral and parietal vessels should be similar. Even though the protein content of pleural fluid normally is low (1.5 g/dl), the net hydrostatic and osmotic forces favor filtration of fluid into the pleural space.[49] Fluid probably is removed by lymphatics, which communicate directly with the pleural space via stomata in the surface of the parietal pleura. Fluid accumulates in the pleural space when the rate of fluid filtration exceeds the rate of removal by the lymphatics. Filtration is increased by an increase in capillary hydrostatic pressure, as with right heart failure, a decrease in capillary oncotic pressure caused by hypoproteinemia, an increase in vascular permeability as during inflammation, or an increase in pleural fluid oncotic pressure that occurs when protein accumulates in the interstitial space. If the fluid filtration rate is high, the lymphatics may not be able to remove fluid as fast as it is filtered. Lymphatic obstruction by fibrin also may hinder fluid removal when the pleurae are inflamed.

Respiratory Tract
Defense Mechanisms

The resting adult horse inhales about 100,000 L of air daily. If the horse is grazing, the air contains few potentially harmful particles and little in the way of pollutant gases. If, however, the horse is stabled or being transported, the air may be rich with dust, spores, pollen, bacteria and viruses, and may have high levels of ammonia. Further, if the horse is transported by truck, it may be exposed to diesel fumes, oxides of nitrogen and sulfur, and ozone. The gas-exchange surface of the lung is a delicate but very extensive membrane that can be damaged by inhaled substances. Defense mechanisms of the respiratory membrane may provide adequate protection to a horse in its rural environment, but they frequently are overwhelmed by stresses of domestication.

Defense mechanisms are either specific or nonspecific. The former involve the immune system and will not be discussed herein. The latter are the subject of this section.

Particle Deposition: Potentially harmful material is inhaled either suspended in air as gas or as aerosols, the depth of penetration of the latter depending to a large degree on particle size. Particles are removed from the air when they contact the moist epithelial surface of the tracheobronchial tree. Particles >10 μ in diameter, and even smaller, contact the airway wall by inertial impaction at the bends in the larger airways. Sites of inertial impaction are provided with lymphoid tissue, such as pharyngeal and bronchus-associated lymphoid tissue. Particles 2-5 μ in diameter pass deeper into the lung, where they sediment onto the walls of the airways. The smallest particles, ≤ 0.5 μ, reach the alveoli where, by diffusion, they contact the epithelial surface.[50]

Particle deposition is influenced by the pattern of breathing. Slow, deep breathing enhances particle transport deep into the lung, while rapid, shallow breathing enhances inertial deposition in the larger airways.[51] Bronchoconstriction enhances deposition of particles in more central airways, while bronchodilation favors more peripheral distribution.

Distribution of toxic gases depends on their solubility and concentration. Very soluble gases, such as SO_2 in low concentrations, are removed by nasal mucosae; in higher concentrations, soluble gases penetrate deeper into the lung. Less soluble gases may reach down to the alveoli. Toxic gases may stimulate a variety of protective mechanisms, resulting in bronchospasm, mucus hypersecretion, coughing and sneezing.

The Mucociliary System: The respiratory tract is lined by an epithelium overlaid with a layer of mucus that is propelled by cilia. In the nasal cavity, the extensive epithelial surface warms and humidifies air. Though inhaling very cold air or increasing minute ventilation, as during exercise, may exceed the warming capacity of the upper airway, horses exercising at -20 C showed no abnormality of gas exchange.[52]

Particles deposited on the surface of the mucociliary system are transported in the mucociliary escalator and swallowed or are engulfed by macrophages or other cells recruited from the blood. The mucociliary system consists of the epithelial cells and the overlying sol and gel mucus layers. The epithelial cells are immediately overlaid by a periciliary fluid of low viscosity (the sol layer), in which the cilia beat in a coordinated fashion. The gel layer, which may be continuous or in plaques, consists of viscous mucus that protects the sol layer from desiccation and entraps inhaled particles.

Because the epithelial surface area decreases between the bronchioles and trachea, mucus should "pile up" as it approaches the larger airways. However, differential rates of mucus transport in small and larger airways and transport of ions and water across the epithelium keep the depth of the mucus layer similar throughout the respiratory tract.

The mucus layer originates from several sites. In respiratory bronchioles, secretion by the nonciliated Clara cells may be a major source of the airway lining fluid. In the terminal bronchioles and larger airways, goblet cells produce mucous secretions, with serous secretions coming from the less common serous cells. Goblet cells apparently increase in number in response to irritation of the respiratory tract. In the bronchi, most mucus originates from the submucosal bronchial glands. Secretion is under autonomic regulation via parasympathetic and sympathetic nerves. Mucociliary transport rates are highly variable between horses but relatively constant in an individual; for instance, clearance half times range from 8 to 35 minutes in the miniature donkey.[53]

Changes in the composition and rheologic (flow) properties of mucus occur in response to many stimuli and can be the cause or the result of respiratory disease. A change in the depth or viscosity of the sol layer impairs ciliary function, and changes in the viscoelastic properties of gel alter clearance rates. The effects on mucus properties of most environmental pollutants found in animal housing are unknown.

Coughing, which is part of the clearance mechanism of the respiratory tract, is initiated by stimulation of subepithelial irritant receptors most numerous in the larger bronchi.[54] Receptors are stimulated by the mechanical deformation that results either from material on the epithelial surface or from bronchoconstriction.

Alveolar Macrophages: Particles deposited on the alveolar surface are cleared by alveolar macrophages, which constitute 45-50% of cells in fluids washed from the lung periphery.[13] Macrophages have adapted to the high oxygen levels of the alveolus, their phagocytic ability being depressed by hypoxia. Complement, opsonins and lysozyme in respiratory tract secretions assist in killing and removing organisms.[55]

Once phagocytized, particles may be digested by the macrophage or transported out of the lung. Some macrophages enter the mucociliary system directly from the alveolus; others traverse the alveolar wall and enter the lymphoid tissues associated with the airways. They may be retained in the lymphoid tissue, return to the airway mucociliary system, or travel to lung lymphatics for removal. Suppression of alveolar macrophage function probably is important in the pathogenesis of respiratory disease. Corticosteroid release suppresses the bactericidal ability of macrophages and may be one cause of pleuropneumonia after transport.[56] Viral infections also suppress macrophage function, with maximal suppression occurring 7 days after virus inoculation and coinciding with secondary bacterial infections.[57]

Alveolar macrophages form the first line of defense against particles that reach the lung periphery. When large numbers of particles are inhaled, macrophages are assisted by other phagocytic cells that enter the alveolus from the blood under the influence of chemotactic stimuli. Polymorphonuclear leukocytes emigrate more quickly and in larger numbers than monocytes. Phagocytes break down particles by means of toxic oxygen radicals and proteolytic enzymes, both of which may leak from the cells and damage the lung tissue. Protease inhibitors, such as alpha-1 antitrypsin, and antioxidants, such as glutathione peroxidase, help protect the lung from its own potentially cytotoxic defense mechanisms.

Principles of Emergency Respiratory Therapy

C.M. Honnas & F.J. Derksen

Equine clinicians occasionally are asked to attend a horse with severe respiratory embarassment and blue mucous membranes. In these cases, immediate and decisive action is often required to save the animal's life. The most common therapies used in respiratory emergencies are oxygen, bronchodilators and tracheostomy. Bronchodilator therapy is discussed later in this chapter.

Oxygen Therapy

The most important function of the lung is exchange of oxygen for oxidative metabolism in tissues. Failure of this process leads to tissue hypoxia, anaerobic metabolism, acidosis and organ dysfunction. Therefore, emergency respiratory therapy should be aimed at relieving tissue hypoxia. Tissue hypoxia may be caused by pulmonary disease, but it also may result from upper air-

way obstruction, cardiovascular shunting, anemia and a decrease in cardiac output (Fig 9).[58] Oxygen therapy is only effective when tissue hypoxia is the result of pulmonary disease. Oxygen therapy is ineffective if tissue hypoxia is the result of upper airway obstruction, anemia or decreased cardiac output (as in shock).

In the field, compressed oxygen may be delivered via a tube placed in the horse's nose. In an adult horse, the oxygen flow rate should be no less than 10 L per minute. If the patient is recumbent, the trachea should be intubated; oxygen is delivered most efficiently using a demand valve.[59] If oxygen therapy is to be continued for an extended period, the oxygen should be administered in prescribed doses, and the response should be monitored. The ability of the lung to oxygenate the arterial blood may be assessed by measurement of arterial oxygen tension, while tissue oxygenation is evaluated by measuring mixed venous oxygen tension ($P\bar{v}_{O2}$). The normal value for $P\bar{v}_{O2}$ in the horse is 40 torr. When $P\bar{v}_{O2}$ is decreased to ≤ 25 torr, oxygen therapy may be indicated to prevent tissue hypoxia.

Temporary Tracheostomy

Tracheostomy usually is performed as an emergency procedure to relieve upper air-

Figure 9. Principles of emergency therapy for airway obstruction and severe lung disease.

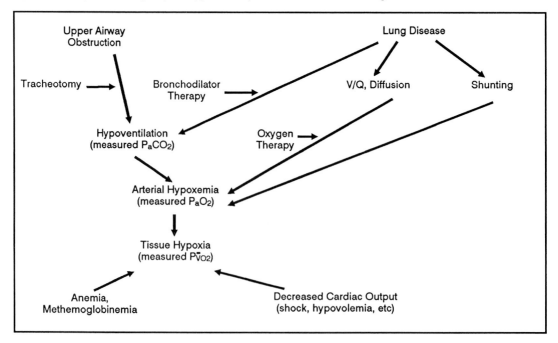

way obstruction. Partial or complete airway obstruction may occur with inhalation of foreign bodies, mechanical obstruction of the upper airways (as with arytenoid chondritis, laryngeal edema), lymph node abscessation, tumors, or swelling associated with snakebites. Elective tracheostomy may be indicated before induction of anesthesia to facilitate intubation if surgical access would be compromised by orotracheal intubation. In such cases, a tracheostomy tube often is maintained during the immediate postoperative period to divert air flow from the surgical site.[60,61]

Tracheostomy can be performed in either standing or recumbent horses. In a non-emergency situation, access to the trachea is easiest in the standing horse or the anesthetized horse in dorsal recumbency. In an emergency, it may be necessary to perform a tracheostomy on a laterally recumbent horse. The optimal site for tracheostomy is the midcervical ventral midline, where the sternocephalic muscles diverge and the omohyoid muscles converge. The trachea is superficial and easily palpated in this location. The site is clipped, shaved and surgically prepared, and the skin, subcutis and deeper tissues infiltrated with local anesthetic on the midline.[60] A 7-cm incision is made on the midline, through the skin and subcutis, to expose the paired bellies of the sternothyrohyoideus muscles, which are separated by sharp or blunt dissection to expose the underlying trachea. An annular ligament is identified between 2 consecutive tracheal rings and is incised transversely to allow separation of adjacent tracheal rings and placement of the tracheostomy tube.[60] Longitudinal incision through the tracheal rings is not recommended because healing often is associated with narrowing of the tracheal lumen, particularly in foals.[62,63]

Management of a tracheal stoma initially includes frequent inspection to ascertain whether the tube has been dislodged or obstructed by inspissated respiratory secretions. The tracheostomy tube should be changed and the surgical site cleaned at least once daily or more often, if indicated. The airway can be maintained in this manner for 7-10 days if needed.[60] Complications resulting from temporary tracheostomy increase in direct proportion to the time the tracheostomy tube is left in place.[61]

Once the airway rostral to the tracheostomy is patent, the tracheostomy tube should be removed and the wound allowed to heal by second intention. In most instances, healing is complete within 14-21 days. Primary closure usually is not recommended because of complications, such as infection or subcutaneous emphysema.[60]

Three different types of tracheostomy tubes are available commercially: a Dyson self-retaining tube (Intermountain Vet Supply), a McKillip J-tube (Intermountain Vet Supply), and a cuffed tube (Bivona) (Fig 10). The Dyson self-retaining tube consists of interlocking male and female cannulae, which are self-retaining when inserted into the trachea. Though this tube is convenient to use, its intraluminal flanges may produce mucosal ulceration where they contact the tracheal wall. Swelling of soft tissue interposed between the extraluminal portion of the tube and the trachea may increase the risk of intraluminal pressure necrosis and subsequent tracheal stenosis.

Though the McKillip J-tube requires fixation to the skin, fewer long-term complications have been associated with its use. The J-tube is easy to insert and, when fitted correctly, does not exert pressure on the mucosal surface, even with long-term use. In thick-necked horses, the standard J-tube occasionally is not angled correctly, and pressure from the tip may produce tracheal ulceration dorsally. This complication can be avoided by obtaining a lateral radiograph of the trachea with the horse in a normal rest-

Figure 10. McKillip J-tube (A), Dyson self-retaining tracheotomy tube (B), and cuffed tracheotomy tube (C).

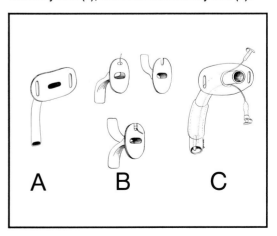

A   B   C

ing position. If the tube is impinging on the tracheal wall, then a tube of different shape or different dimensions should be used.

The cuffed silicone tube is flexible, and the cuff conforms well to the lumen of the trachea when inflated. Long-term use of the inflated cuff may result in mucosal damage and possibly tracheal scarring and/or stenosis.[64] Generally, the cuff is not inflated. The outside diameter of the cuffed tubes ranges in size from 14.7 to 41 mm. Though pliable, the relatively larger diameter of these tubes requires a longer transverse incision in the annular ligament to facilitate insertion. If maintained for long periods, this tube also may cause local deformation of the separated cartilage rings.

Medical Respiratory Therapy

F.J. Derksen

Inhalation Therapy

The respiratory system seems ideally suited for local application of therapeutic agents. The respiratory tract surface area is large and easily accessible. When delivered by aerosol, therapeutic agents may achieve high concentrations in the lung, with minimal systemic effects. In equine medicine, inhalation therapy is prescribed commonly, especially in performance horses. However, when the principles of aerosol therapy are not adhered to, inhalation therapy may be ineffective or, worse, detrimental to horses.

Principles of Inhalation Therapy: An aerosol is a group of particles that, because of their low settling velocities, remain suspended in air for a prolonged time.[65] In respiratory therapeutics, aerosols may be used to cause bronchodilation, to humidify inspired air, to change the consistency of secretions, and to carry therapeutic agents, such as antibiotics and corticosteroids, into the lung.[65] The objective of inhalation therapy is deposition of therapeutic aerosol deep within the lung. The mechanism of aerosol deposition on the respiratory mucosa depends on characteristics of the aerosol, patency of the airways, and the pattern of breathing.

Large aerosol particles $>10\,\mu$ in size settle as the result of inertial impaction and are filtered out primarily in the upper respiratory system or at divisions of the large airways.[66] Smaller particles settle by sedimentation, which occurs in the region of the respiratory tract where linear air velocity is decreased: the small airways and gas exchange regions of the lung. Particles $<0.5\,\mu$ in size generally remain suspended in the air and are exhaled. Thus, the particle size of a therapeutic aerosol should be 1-5 μ in diameter to obtain optimal aerosol deposition deep within the lung.[66]

Other physical characteristics of a therapeutic aerosol that affect deposition, and therefore efficacy of inhalation therapy, include droplet constituents, aerosol cloud density, aerosol temperature and electrostatic charge. Hypertonic aerosols containing salts or other osmotically active chemicals attract water molecules from the humid atmosphere in airways and increase in size.[66] This favors deposition of aerosols in larger airways and causes ineffective treatment of diseases in the distal lung. Conversely, particles of low tonicity tend to decrease in size and are likely to be deposited in the distal lung. The density of aerosol clouds determines the amount of therapeutic agent available for deposition on the respiratory mucosa. Generally, ultrasonic nebulizers produce a denser cloud than other nebulizers.[66] When the aerosol temperature is less or greater than body temperature, aerosol particles tend to evaporate or increase in size, making them less stable. However, air-conditioning capacity of the nose and upper airway ensures that aerosol reaching the lung usually is at body temperature. Finally, it has been suggested that negatively charged aerosol particles are more stable and deposited more distally in the lung. However, evidence is controversial and effects too small to justify the inconvenience of ensuring a therapeutic aerosol receives a negative charge.

The amount and site of deposition of therapeutic aerosols depend in large part on the physical characteristics of the airways and on the pattern of breathing. When airways subserving large portions of lungs are obstructed with mucus or exudate, inhalation therapy is ineffective. Because of this, in cases of suspected obstructive lung disease, bronchodilators should be administered before inhalation therapy is used. Rapid, shallow breathing favors deposition of aerosol in the upper airways, pharynx and conducting airways, while slow, deep breathing encourages aerosol delivery to the gas-exchange regions of the lung.[65] Even when aerosol characteristics are optimal and airways are not obstructed, rapid, shallow breathing results in deposition of up to 90% aerosol in the upper airways and pharynx.[67] Much of this aerosol is absorbed systemically, and benefits attributed to deposition of therapeutic agents in the lung may be because of such systemic drug administration. Thus, it is apparent that, in equine medicine, the clinical usefulness of inhalation therapy is limited. With uncooperative patients like horses, the clinician has little control over many factors that affect efficacy of inhalation therapy, including pattern of breathing and airway obstruction. In addition, when solutions to be aerosolized are homemade, the characteristics of the aerosol usually are unknown.

Water and saline are among the most commonly used solutions in inhalation therapy and serve to hydrate airway secretions, thereby promoting their removal. Water is more irritating than saline, and coughing or bronchospasm may result, especially if dense aerosols generated by ultrasonic nebulizers are used. The volume of solution that can be delivered to the respiratory system by aerosol is very small compared to the enormous surface area of the lung.[68] Though aerosolization of water or saline has been used for centuries, the efficacy of this therapy has not been documented in any disease. Systemically administered fluid therapy probably is much more effective than aerosol therapy in hydrating airway secretions in horses. Antibiotics, including gentamicin and kanamycin, have been used in inhalation therapy with suspected airway infection. Aminoglycosides are inactivated by purulent material; therefore, their use in inhalation therapy should be discouraged. In infectious pneumonia, antibiotics are best administered systemically.

Inhalation therapy probably is most suitable when bronchodilation is required. Administration of anticholinergic and sympathomimetic agents allows delivery of high concentrations in the lung while minimizing systemic effects of these drugs.[69]

Bronchodilator Therapy

Because airway obstruction resulting from airway smooth muscle contraction is a common mechanism in pulmonary disease in horses, bronchodilators are of major importance in respiratory pharmacology. In spite of the importance placed on bronchodilator therapy, little is known about the autonomic receptor populations in equine airways, the pharmacokinetics of bronchodilator drugs, or efficacy of bronchodilation therapy in clinical cases. Much investigation is needed before bronchodilator therapy may be used rationally in equine medicine.

Hypoxemia is a common complication of bronchodilator therapy by aerosol or other routes. This paradoxical problem is explained by ventilation-perfusion mismatching caused by preferential deposition of aerosol bronchodilator in well-ventilated lung regions while, in poorly ventilated regions, little bronchodilator drug is deposited. In addition, systemically absorbed bronchodilators may cause vasodilation (beta-2 effect) in poorly ventilated lung regions. Especially in patients with $PaO_2 < 64$ torr, as in foals with pneumonia, bronchodilator therapy may decrease PaO_2 to critically low levels. In these cases, oxygen therapy is indicated in conjunction with bronchodilator therapy.

Sympathomimetic Agents: Sympathomimetic agents with specific affinity for beta-2 receptors are the most common bronchodilators used in veterinary medicine. Beta-2 receptor bronchodilators include norepinephrine, isoproterenol, ephedrine and clenbuterol. Sympathomimetic agents cause bronchodilation by stimulation of beta-2 receptors present in the large and small airways. This, in turn, results in increased intracellular concentrations of cyclic AMP in airway smooth muscle cells, with resulting muscle relaxation. Sympathomimetic bronchodilators were developed for their specific affinity for beta-2 adrenergic receptors in the airways, vascular beds and uterus, thereby minimizing their side effects on other organs, including the heart, and on the CNS and GI tract. However, beta-2 receptor specificity is not complete, and large doses of beta-2 receptor agonists cause side effects, including trembling, excitement, sweating, ileus, colic and tachycardia. These effects can, in large part, be attributed to inadvertent stimulation of beta-1 receptors.

Ephedrine is a sympathomimetic bronchodilator present in several commercially available oral preparations. The drug is derived from the shrub *Ephedra sinica.* Ephedrine is a moderately active beta-2 receptor stimulant. However, its main mechanism of action is through release of stored norepinephrine. After a few days of therapy, stores of norephinephrine may become depleted and drug tolerance develops, so progressively more drug is needed to maintain bronchodilation. In addition, because norepinephrine does not have beta-2 receptor specificity, alpha and beta-1 receptors also are stimulated. In human medicine, use of ephedrine largely has been superseded by newer generations of more specific beta-2 receptor agonists. The empirically recommended dosage for ephedrine is 0.14 mg/kg of body weight BID.

Isoproterenol is one of the most potent sympathomimetic bronchodilators available. The drug is classified as a catecholamine and has a low affinity for alpha-adrenergic receptors but has marked beta-1 effects. The lack of beta-2 receptor specificity limits the clinical usefulness of this drug as a bronchodilator in lung disease because therapeutic doses given systemically cause serious side effects, including tachycardia, tremors, anxiety and sweating. These side effects are due mainly to beta-1 receptor stimulation. In addition, isoproterenol has a short half-life, and bronchodilation may last <1 hour. Isoproterenol may be useful in treatment of acute airway obstruction sometimes seen in foal pneumonia or acute exacerbations of chronic obstructive pulmonary disease. The drug is diluted in saline and given IV at 0.4 μg/kg of body weight. The infusion should be discontinued when the heart rate doubles. Isoproterenol at the same dosage may also be delivered by aerosol. Though this route of administration is less convenient, side effects are greatly reduced, and effective bronchodilation is achieved. Isoproterenol should not be given PO because absorption is erratic.

Clenbuterol is a specific beta-2 agonist, as well as an expectorant in horses. The drug is absorbed well when give PO and has >90% bioavailability. The half-life of clenbuterol is long, and a twice-daily oral or IV dosage regimen maintains blood levels in a therapeutic range. Because of its specificity for beta-2 receptors, clenbuterol at the recommended dosage of 0.8 μg/kg of body weight has little effect on the GI tract or heart; therefore, side effects are minimal. Several reports in the literature suggest that clenbuterol at 0.8 μg/kg of body weight is an effective bronchodilator in normal horses and in horses with chronic obstructive pulmonary disease.[70] In addition, clenbuterol has been used successfully in treatment of bronchospasm associated with infectious lung disease in foals. However, clenbuterol given at 1.6 μg/kg of body weight did not prevent histamine-induced airway obstruction in ponies, suggesting that it is not an effective bronchodilator in horses.[71] The drug has been on the market for several years in Europe and in Canada, but it is not available in the United States.

Anticholinergic Drugs: For centuries, extracts of the plant *Atropa belladonna* (deadly nightshade) have been used to treat asthma in people. The chief constituent of this plant is atropine. Some of the earliest remedies used in treatment of heaves in horses also contained anticholinergic agents related to atropine. Atropine is a potent parasympatholytic agent and, because of its competive antagonism of acetylcholine, blocks muscarinic neural transmission. However, when administered systemically, bronchodilation is only one of many possible effects. Other effects of atropine administration include ileus, tachycardia, mydriasis and excitation, especially in ponies. These many side effects preclude routine systemic use of atropine as a bronchodilator in horses. However, therapeutic selectivity may be obtained by local delivery of the drug. When administered by aerosol, atropine is an effective bronchodilator with few systemic side effects. New anticholinergic agents with more specific bronchodilator effects and fewer side effects presently are being evaluated in bronchodilator therapy in people.

Phosphodiesterase Inhibitors: Cyclic AMP promotes airway smooth muscle relaxation and bronchodilation. Cyclic AMP is metabolized to the inactive 5-AMP by phosphodiesterase. Thus, phosphodiesterase inhibitors, such as caffeine, thiobromine and theophylline, promote bronchodilation by inhibiting breakdown of intracellular cyclic AMP. Theophylline, the most commonly used bronchodilator in this group, is an effective bronchodilator in horses when blood concentrations reach about 10 μg/ml. However, excitement occurs at 15 μg/ml. Thus, in horses, as in other species, the therapeutic blood level of theophylline is close to the toxic level. In addition, absorption of theophylline is erratic after oral administration, making the drug difficult to use clinically. It is likely that theophylline or related phosphodiesterase inhibitors will play a larger role in bronchodilator therapy in horses as part of a combination of agents acting synergistically.

Postural Drainage

The aim of postural drainage is to help clear secretions from the airways. Drainage of secretions from the paranasal sinuses, guttural pouch and large airways is greatly facilitated by a head-down position. Horses with accumulated secretion in these regions may be encouraged to remain with the head down by feeding them off the ground or by tranquilization.

Positional drainage for intrathoracic airways can be achieved easily only in neonatal foals. Postural drainage is indicated in foals with a large amount of airway secretions. Foals are placed in the prone position and left and right lateral positions for about 5 minutes each. The hindquarters are elevated slightly, and drainage is encouraged by chest percussion using a cupped hand (coupage). The procedure usually is carried out twice daily after bronchodilator therapy.

Airway drainage also may be encouraged by modest exercise. Exercise causes the horse to breath deeper, thereby dilating the airways.

Principles of Therapy for Foals

M.R. Paradis

Once respiratory difficulty has been identified in the patient, the type of therapy is dictated by blood gas, radiographic and physical examination findings. A foal in respiratory failure with a persistent PaO_2 <50 torr and P_aCO_2 >60 torr may require mechanical ventilation and supplemental oxygen for survival. A hypoxemic foal with a normal $PaCO_2$ may need only supplemental oxygen via nasopharyngeal insufflation.

Mechanical ventilation of a foal is an extremely labor-intensive form of therapy and often is limited to intensive-care facilities. When a foal is placed on a respirator, it requires 24-hour attendance by a knowledgeable person. Manual restraint or sedation may be needed to protect the patient from self-inflicted trauma and disconnecting its tubing.

Short-term ventilation may be required when transporting an affected foal to an intensive-care facility. This can be accomplished in several ways. First, an artificial airway must be established by placing a 45- to 55-cm-long endotracheal tube through a nostril into the trachea. Most newborn foals can accommodate an 8- to 10-mm internal-diameter (large dog size) tube. The foal's neck is held in extension, and the tube is passed through the ventral meatus of the nasal turbinates. Then the tube is passed through the larynx into the trachea. The cuff is inflated. Care should be taken not to overinflate the cuff, as this will cause mucosal damage. After a patent airway has been established, increased ventilation can be accomplished by manual compression of a self-inflating, nonrebreathing, 1-L resuscitation bag (Ambu Bag: Draeger) or by use of a demand valve (Hudson Demand Valve, Hudson Oxygen Therapy, Orange Park, FL) attached to an oxygen source.[72]

Increasing the concentration of inspired oxygen is therapy specifically for hypoxemia. Oxygen can be administered via a face mask or an intranasal tube, which allows the foal more freedom of movement. A small feeding tube is inserted about 5 cm into the nasal turbinates of the foal and sutured to the nostril. Oxygen can be delivered initially at 5-10 L per minute. Blood gas monitoring allows adjustments of O_2 flow to maintain the P_aO_2 between 70 and 100 torr. Oxygen delivered in this manner should be humidified to prevent drying of the nasal and bronchial mucosae. This is done by bubbling the oxygen through a canister of sterile physiologic saline.[73-75]

General nursing care of a neonatal foal with respiratory problems can be labor intensive. Keeping the foal warm is of great importance. A decrease of 2 C in body temperature from the normal thermoneutral point decreases oxygen consumption in a sleeping, inactive human infant by 20%. Heat can be provided for the patient with radiant heat lamps, hot-water blankets and heating pads. Adequate hydration and nutritional status of the foal are important components of nursing care of foals. Adequate hydration helps loosen bronchial secretions, but care must be taken not to overhydrate a foal that is already at risk of developing pulmonary edema. In reference to the nutritional aspects of these foals, the stress of disease can increase the caloric needs of the patient 150-200%. The neonate in severe respiratory distress requires more energy for breathing. The necessary calories can be provided enterally or parenterally with calorie-dense solutions.[76]

Coupage is a technique used by physical therapists to attempt to loosen adherent bronchial secretions in their patients. In the foal, coupage is used by rapidly slapping the foal's chest with a cupped hand. The air trapped between the cupped hand and the chest wall produces a percussive effect without bruising the animal.[72]

In foals with bacterial pneumonia, broad-spectrum antibiotics are necessary to combat the infection. A beta-lactam antibiotic (such as penicillin), combined with an aminoglycoside, provides good coverage until a more specific regimen can be determined.

RESPIRATORY DISEASES AFFECTING MULTIPLE SITES

Inflammatory, Infectious and Immune Diseases

African Horse Sickness

R.C. Knowles

African horse sickness virus usually produces an acute and highly fatal disease in horses. The noncontagious seasonal infection is transmitted by night-flying insect vectors, and is characterized by fever, edema of the subcutaneous tissues and lungs, and hemorrhage of the heart and digestive organs.

Species Affected: Horses are highly susceptible, mules less so and donkeys much less so. Zebras may be inapparent carriers of the virus. Dogs fed infected horse meat have shown signs similar to those observed in horses. Dogs may also become transient virus carriers.

In the laboratory, mice are the most convenient host; baby mice are preferred for virus isolation from field samples. African

horse sickness virus also replicates in specific cell lines.

Cause: African horse sickness virus is similar in many respects to bluetongue virus and is classified as an arbovirus in the family Reoviridae. Both differ from classic arboviruses in mode of replication and resistance to lipid solvents. The virus of African horse sickness is quite durable at ambient temperatures and is stable between pH 6.2 and 10, but is rapidly inactivated in solutions of pH <6. The virus is not destroyed by temperatures <55 C.

Nine immunologically distinct virus types have been identified. Types 1 through 8 have been mainly confined to Africa. The most recently identified, type 9, was associated with the epizootic of African horse sickness in the Near East (1959-1961) and in Mediterranean North African countries and Spain (1965-1966).

Blood collected for submission to a laboratory for virus isolation should be shipped unfrozen as heparinized, oxalated or defibrinated blood. Organ or tissue samples can be preserved in buffered glycerol and submitted in this manner.

Geographic Distribution: African horse sickness is primarily a disease of Africa. The disease is prevalent in SubSahara Africa. Occasionally it progresses beyond the continent, as in 1959 into the Near East to Pakistan, India and Afghanistan, and the following year to other countries of the Near East and southern Turkey. The most recent case reported from Turkey was in September, 1961, in the vicinity of Manisa in western Turkey. The same year it also invaded Cyprus. In 1965 and 1966, an epizootic caused by type 9 appeared in North Africa and spread to southern Spain. The disease died out in this epizootic as in the Near East. African horse sickness invaded southern Spain in the summer of 1987 and there were outbreaks in the summers of 1988 and 1989, which caused the deaths of more than 1400 animals. Additional outbreaks were reported in 1989 in Saudi Arabia, Morocco and Portugal.[378] African horse sickness appeared in North Yemen in 1985 and has become enzootic in that area.

Transmission: The disease is transmitted by night-flying biting insects. Species of *Culicoides* have been conclusively identified as the major vector. In enzootic areas of Africa there is strong evidence that a nonequine host is a reservoir for survival of the virus between seasonal attacks. Observations suggest that donkeys may be the reservoir host. The disease appears seasonally following rains. Animals in low-lying areas are most severely affected and the disease disappears suddenly about 10 days after the first frost in temperate zones.

The last case of African horse sickness of the 1959-61 Near East epizootic occurred near Manisa, Turkey, in September, 1961, a region in which horses had not been vaccinated. Vaccination with a polyvalent vaccine began immediately. Clinical evidence of infection ceased 9 days following vaccination of the horse population of the region. At that time, no type-9 monovalent attenuated vaccine was available. Consequently polyvalent vaccine of attenuated virus types 107 was used successfully. Eventually the homologous monovalent vaccine was prepared and used equally successfully during the epizootic in North Africa.

The outbreak in Cyprus may have been associated with transportation of vectors in hay taken to the island for Turkish military horses. The mechanism of introduction from Africa to the Near East in 1959 is not known, nor is the means of introduction of the same virus type into Mediterranean countries of North Africa and Spain in the mid-1960s. The disease does not occur in the absence of night-flying biting insects. Transmission does not occur to susceptible horses in close physical proximity to a horse in the viremic stage without injection of blood.

Clinical Signs: African horse sickness is characterized by high fever and extensive edema. The edema is first apparent in the subcutaneous tissues of the head and neck (particularly supraorbital tissues), and is accompanied by hydrothorax and progressive edema of the lungs. Inflammatory changes in the heart and stomach are marked. In susceptible equine populations, mortality is very high but a few animals recover gradually.

Pulmonary edema may develop so rapidly that some animals die before other pathologic changes develop. In such peracute cases, the temperature may rise to about 41 C (105.8 F), the conjunctivae are infected, and acute dyspnea, tachypnea and coughing appear. As the disease progresses, coughing is accompanied by copious frothy nasal discharge, and breathing becomes increasingly difficult until the animal collapses and dies.

When lung involvement is less severe, eddema, high temperature, swelling of the supraorbital tissue and cyanosis of the tongue develop. Edema extends down the neck and along the brisket and abdominal wall. In spite of the high temperature and obvious severe illness, animals with advanced African horse sickness continue eating until a few hours before death.

Lesions: Because death occurs with the pulmonary form, subcutaneous edema is usually absent. In such cases there is massive pulmonary edema of gelatinous consistency and the trachea and bronchi are filled with froth. If the disease is more protracted, there is extensive edema. The edema seen clinically is confirmed at necropsy. It is mainly located in the head and neck region but may continue along the brisket and abdomen. There is considerable fluid in the pleural cavity and pericardial sac, and hemorrhages in the epicardium and endocardium. Myocardial lesions include severe hemorrhage, edema, myocarditis with multiple inflammatory cell types, and focal necrosis with partial replacement of cardiac muscle by proliferating connective tissue. The severity of the myocarditis is unique to horse sickness.

Reactions in lymph nodes do not reflect grossly or microscopically the acute inflammatory changes associated with this acute viral disease. Hemorrhage is rarely seen grossly and congestion is best seen microscopically. Gastritis is strikingly severe.

Diagnosis: Because of rapid dissemination by insects and high mortality, rapid diagnosis is important. To diagnose African horse sickness, it is necessary to establish that the local environment contains insect populations capable of transmitting the disease and to correlate the potential for insect transmission with the clinical signs observed. In areas where the disease is not enzootic, the clinician should identify any possible virus carriers, such as horses from enzootic areas, or insect vectors.

Isolation of the virus is necessary to confirm the diagnosis. Blood should be taken in the early stages of the disease in an anticoagulant container and kept on ice, but not frozen, until it reaches the laboratory. At the laboratory, virus isolation and neutralization tests identify the immunologic type causing the infection. It is possible that infection may be caused by a virus type other than the 9 known virus groups. In addition to blood, samples of spleen, kidney or lymph nodes may be submitted for virus isolation. These samples should likewise not be frozen but maintained in buffered glycerol.

The virus is isolated by inoculating suckling mice intracranially. The incubation period varies from 4 to 20 days. Mouse brain tissue is harvested for virus content and serial passage. Neutralization can be performed in mouse or tissue culture inoculations.

In serum, African horse sickness antibodies can be detected by complement-fixation, agar gel diffusion and fluorescent antibodt tests, but the virus strain cannot be identified. Complement-fixation antibody levels usually appear about a week after onset of fever, peaking in the second week, and decline rapidly after a month. Neutralizing antibodies may persist for years.

The appearance of the disease in a susceptible horse population causes considerable alarm among owners. Because the pulmonary form of African horse sickness can cause death in <12 hours, such diseases as anthrax must be considered in differential diagnosis. Consideration of other diseases with similar signs, such as babesiosis, equine infectious anemia and equine infectious arteritis, is also warranted.

Treatment: There is no known therapy specific for African horse sickness. Supportive treatment is considered beneficial.

Control: Because transmission of the disease depends on insecy vectors, control of those vectors prevents transmission of African horse sickness virus. This has been used for many years in parts of the world where the disease is enzootic. Stabling animals in screened buildings to protect them from night-flying biting insects and using smokes and smudges to discourage insect populations are common techniques. Likewise, disinfection of aircraft, stables and material used in conjunction with horses to prevent transportation of insect vectors or infected blood is considered essential.

Each of the 9 serologic types of African horse sickness has been attenuated through serial mouse brain passage and is used as an immunizing agent. Once attenuated through mouse brain passage, the virus is grown in tissue culture for vaccine production. Before type-9 virus had been attenuated, a polyvalent mouse brain vaccine containing types 1-7 was used and conferred immunity to type 9. In Turkey about 1 million horses were vaccinated with the polyvalent vaccine, some during severe field challenge, and good immunity was produced against type 9. Subsequently, a monovalent type-9 vaccine was prepared and used with satisfactory results to contain the epizootic. Limited trials using killed-virus vaccine have shown encouraging results. Where the disease is enzootic, it is routine practice to commence vaccination 2 months before the insect season.

The primary method of prevention in the United States is a 60-day quarantine of all horses imported from Africa, Asia and Mediterranean countries. Current research is aimed at improving the stored vaccines. There is a need for greater understanding of the epizootiology of this disease. Where the virus is harbored between epizootic outbreaks must be known before repeated outbreaks, as have occurred in Spain, can be prevented.[378]

Equine Influenza

L. Coggins

Equine influenza is an acute, highly contagious, febrile respiratory disease. It is a major cause of respiratory illness among horses in training areas, on racetracks and at shows. Commercial vaccines have reduced the problem somewhat, but the frequency of use required and level of protection provided remain unsatisfactory. There is evidence that antigenic variation has occurred with the possible disappearance of the earlier A/equi/1 subtype.

History: Enzootics of "influenza" in horses have been reported for centuries. Equine influenza was differentiated from other respiratory diseases when an orthomyxovirus virus was isolated from horses during an outbreak in Czechoslovakia in 1956. Subsequently, another equine influenza virus was isolated from horses in the United States in 1963. These viruses are commonly known as A/equi/1 and A/equi/2, respectively.[77] In recent years, the A/equi/2 subtype has been the only virus isolated from outbreaks, and antigenic variants have been found.[78] The A/equi/2 virus circulates enzootically among horses in almost all areas of the world where significant numbers of horses are assembled except in Australia and New Zealand.

Properties of the Virus: Two immunologically distinct subtypes of equine influenza virus have been recognized: A/equi/1/Prague/56(H7N7) and A/equi/2/Miami/63 (H3N8). An antigenic variant of the A/equi/2 subtype has been recognized as represented by A/equi/2/Fontainbleu/79 and A/equi/2/Saratoga/83. The significance of this variation has not been extensively documented but has caused most companies to incorporate one of the recent isolates in their vaccine.[78,79]

The equine influenza viruses are irregularly shaped, spherical particles containing a lipid envelope through which the rod-shaped hemagglutinin and mushroom-shaped neuraminidase glycoproteins project. The lipid envelope makes these viruses susceptible to inactivation by common detergents, most disinfectants, and most ordinary environmental conditions. Antibodies to hemagglutinin confer immunity to reinfection to viruses containing the homologous hemagglutinin. All influenza viruses contain an RNA genome composed of 8 distinct segments; one of these segments codes for the hemagglutinin and one for the neuraminidase. Reassortment of RNA segments during a mixed infection of a single cell results in the frequent genetic changes observed with influenza viruses. A major antigenic change in the hemagglutinin and neuraminidase is called an antigenic "shift," and a minor change in the hemagglutinin or neuraminidase molecule is known as antigenic "drift." Because the hemagglutinin and, to a lesser extent, the neuraminidase proteins are important in virus attachment and in neutralization, major changes in these antigens have important consequences on vaccine efficacy. Slight antigenic drift has been detected among A/equi/2 viruses since 1980.

Clinical Signs: In a typical outbreak of equine influenza, the disease may be diagnosed on the basis of clinical signs and pattern of spread. The onset is sudden and spread is very rapid, and there is a characteristic cough. When influenza is introduced into a stable, all susceptible horses become infected within 2-3 days. Usually there is a transient swelling of the pharyngeal lymph nodes before a sudden elevation of temperature to 39.5-41 C. The fever may be diphasic and usually persists for several days. The conjunctival and nasal mucosae quickly become red, and a watery nasal discharge is accompanied by a frequent, harsh, nonproductive cough. The cough may last 2-3 weeks. Horses that continue to be exercised may show muscular weakness, soreness and inappetence. In very young or very old horses, apparently uncomplicated cases of A/equi/2 infection may be followed by a more severe disease course leading to viral pneumonia. If fever persists and the discharge becomes purulent, secondary bacterial infection has probably caused guttural pouch infection, sinusitis or bronchopneumonia. Mildly affected horses recover completely within 2-3 weeks, but severely affected animals may convalesce for 1-6 months.

Influenza in partially immune horses is difficult to diagnose clinically and may be confused with equine herpesvirus, adenovirus and rhinovirus infections.

Laboratory Diagnosis: Clinical diagnosis of influenza may be confirmed by isolation of the virus from nasal swabs, which are collected during the early hours of illness and inoculated into embryonated chicken eggs, or by serologic testing of acute and convalescent serum samples. Swabs should be inserted into a transport medium and taken to the laboratory under cool conditions (not frozen). For the most successful isolations, specimens must be inoculated into eggs shortly after swab sample collection. Serum samples also are collected at the time of nasal swabbing and 2-3 weeks later. Development of complement-fixation or precipitating antibody indicates recent infection by influenza virus. A 4-fold increase or more in the hemagglutination inhibition antibody titer is used to identify the subtype of influenza virus involved. The virus isolate can be characterized further by neuraminidase inhibition tests.

Because many diagnostic laboratories do not offer equine influenza virus isolation and serologic testing, one should make arrangements beforehand.

Epizootiology: Equine influenza viruses spread rapidly in groups of susceptible horses. The short incubation period of 1-3 days and the frequent, hacking cough help spread the virus effectively by aerosol. Infected horses shed virus during the incubation period and for at least 5 days after clinical signs begin. Previously uninfected horses are the most efficient transmitters of the virus and are the horses from which the virus can be most easily isolated. Close contact between horses seems to be necessary for rapid transmission.

The pattern and nature of influenza spread among horses are determined by prior exposure and the level of existing immunity. Other factors that determine the outcome of an infection seem to be the virulence of the virus, amount of exposure, and environmental conditions. Generally, it has not been posssible to reproduce experimentally the raging clinical respiratory disease seen under field conditions. Part of the reason seems to be the rapid loss of virulence these viruses undergo when grown in the laboratory.

Because equine influenza is so widespread and occurs so frequently in mobile populations, most outbreaks are seen in young horses 2-3 years of age when they first are moved into training areas or onto racing and show circuits. It is common for such outbreaks to occur a few weeks after young horses are assembled. Currently, outbreaks usually are caused by A/equi/2; isolations of A/equi/1 have not been reported for nearly a decade. However, both subtypes can occur simultaneously. Influenza is not ordinarily seen on breeding farms.

Though major outbreaks of influenza tend to occur during cold weather, infections may occur at any time of the year. Seasonal prevalence probably is the result of commingling of susceptible young horses with adults at certain times of the year. Horses are the only known reservoir of equine influenza viruses.

Treatment: Rest and confinement are essential for affected horses. Training should not be resumed until at least a week after clinical signs abate; then, training should be resumed only if there is no coughing upon exercise. Horses exhibiting pulmonary signs, with fever lasting longer than 5 days or with purulent nasal discharge, should be treated with antibiotics to control secondary bacterial infection and prevent harmful sequelae. The importance of good stable hygiene, such as sufficient ventilation and freedom from drafts and dust, should be stressed.

Control and Prophylaxis: Stables and courses where equine influenza outbreaks occur should be put under quarantine for at least 4 weeks. Movement of persons associated with diseased horses also should be limited. After all horses have recovered, stalls, stables, equipment and transport vehicles should be cleaned and disinfected.

Clinical observations suggest that immunity following a natural infection with either equine influenza virus is quite solid and lasts at least a year. However, protection seems to depend to some extent upon a massive challenge dose of virus. Antibodies transferred from dam to foal via colostrum protect the newborn for 30-35 days after birth.

Equine influenza can be prevented by vaccination with a bivalent inactivated vaccine. Commercial vaccines contain the A/equi/1 and A/equi/2 influenza viral antigens, and most have incorporated a recent antigenic variant of the A/equi/2 subtype. These vaccines are available in the United States and Europe. Initially, 2 vaccinations are given 8-12 weeks apart, followed by a third given 6 months later. Revaccination is recommended every 6-12 months or just before possible exposure. They may be given at any age, but foals <6 months of age respond poorly to influenza antigens. In situations in which horses come in contact with massive virus challenge, serviceable immunity from vaccines may last only 3-4 months. Consequently, booster injections are recommended for race or show horses every 3 months. Unfortunately, a transient reaction occurs in a small percentage of vaccinates, and this has caused owners to resist vaccinating during the racing season. Such reactions may include fever, depression, and edema and pain at the site of injection.

Equine Herpesvirus Infections

Four types of equine herpesviruses have now been recognized.[78] The classic rhinopneumonitis equine herpesvirus historically has been regarded as a single entity but recently has been separated into 2 distinct but antigenically related viruses designated equine herpesvirus-1 and equine herpesvirus-4. Equine herpesvirus-2 is a slow-growing cytomegalovirus whose role as a cause of respiratory disease remains uncertain. Equine herpesvirus-3 is the causative agent of coital exanthema but does not cause any significant respiratory disease.

Equine herpesvirus-1 and -4 are the major causes of acute respiratory disease of foals on breeding farms. In mares, equine herpesvirus-1 infection may result in epizootics of abortion, often without any preceding signs of rhinopneumonitis. Equine herpesvirus-1 also is recognized as a cause of perinatal foal mortality, and some strains seem to have a predilection to produce encephalitis. Equine herpesvirus-4 is thought to be the most common cause of acute upper respiratory disease in foals during the first 1-2 years of life, and it also has been recovered in sporadic cases of abortion.

History: Though abortion as a sequel to infection with equine herpesviruses was described as long ago as 1932 and called "equine virus abortion," the respiratory syndrome was not recognized and distinguished from infections by equine influenza virus until the mid-1950s, when the influenza virus A/equi/1 first was isolated. More recently, equine herpesvirus-4 has been distinquished from equine herpesvirus-1 on the basis of lack of DNA homology. Equine herpesvirus-4 has been credited with causing much of the acute respiratory disease in foals worldwide in the absence of abortion in pregnant mares.[80] Most reports to date have not distinquished between respiratory disease caused by these 2 viruses. Furthermore, because these viruses are antigenically related, serologic tests may not differentiate between them. No comparative pathogenesis studies have been reported.

Properties of the Viruses: Equine herpesviruses-1 and -4 are typical alpha herpesviruses containing a DNA genome within a characteristic icosahedral capsid, as seen with the electron microscope. The viruses grow in a number of tissue culture systems, producing a characteristic rapid cytopathic effect and intranuclear inclusion bodies (Cowdry Type A). Certain strains of virus tend to cause cell fusion, leading to giant cells or syncytia. The outer membrane of the virus contains lipid that can be disrupted by detergents or weak acid solutions at about pH 3, which destroys infectivity. Restriction endonuclease analysis of the DNA can be used to differentiate between equine herpesvirus-1 and herpesvirus-4.

Clinical Signs: Clinical signs may take the form of respiratory disease, abortion, myeloencephalitis and perinatal disease. The respiratory form of equine herpesvirus-1 and -4 infection usually is mild, transient and confined to young foals. It is one of the most common upper respiratory diseases in weanlings and yearlings. The incubation period usually is 3-4 days. The infection often spreads rapidly and may affect most susceptible horses. The infection is characterized by high fever and a serous nasal discharge. Usually there is no cough. Fever commonly lasts 4-5 days. In many instances, the respiratory infection is mild and goes unnoticed unless the horses are under close supervision. Infection in older animals is mostly subclinical.

Infection may recur as early as 4-5 months but are asymptomatic. Virus usually is recoverable from leukocytes. Inapparent infection is a common form of equine herpesvirus-1 infection among pregnant mares, in which the virus invades the fetus and causes abortion. Abortion may occur as early as the fourth month of gestation, though it usually occurs during the last 4 months. It occurs without premonitory signs, and usually without complications. The infected fetus is expelled rapidly with little or no decomposition evident. Virus can usually be recovered from the fetus but not from the mare's leukocytes at this time (see Diseases of the Reproductive System.)

The paralytic syndrome may occur as an epizootic, usually associated with reintroduction of the virus in a group of horses. The initial signs are weakness and incoordination of the pelvic limbs, which may progress to recumbency. Affected horses often cannot void urine and have urinary incontinence. Mild forms of this syndrome probably go unrecognized. Virus usually can be recovered from blood leukocytes at this stage of the infection. (Also see Diseases of the Nervous System.)

Diagnosis: Clinical diagnosis of respiratory disease caused by equine herpesviruses-1 and -4 usually is very tentative because often the only signs are fever, slight nasal discharge and leukopenia. Infection may be confirmed by virus isolation from nasal swabs collected during the acute febrile period or by serologic tests on acute and convalescent serum samples from young horses. Fluorescent microscopy of infected material collected from the upper respiratory tract may reveal specific viral antigens.

Abortion due to equine herpesvirus-1 can be diagnosed tentatively when pulmonary edema, widespread petechiae, and grossly evident hepatic necrosis are present in a spontaneously aborted fetus. Immunofluorescent inclusions in hepatic cells and bronchiolar and alveolar epithelium can confirm the diagnosis quickly. Serologic examination of aborting mares is not helpful because the infection has been in progress too long. Likewise, virus usually cannot be recovered from the mare's leukocytes. However, circulating leukocytes are a good source of virus isolation in horses exhibiting the encephalitic form of infection.

Epizootiology: Respiratory disease caused by equine herpesviruses-1 and -4 occurs enzootically among young horses on breeding farms and at assembling points, such as sales and training areas.[81] Such outbreaks are common in the fall months, and older horses may be inapparently infected at this time.

Abortion, perinatal mortality and neurologic syndromes affecting a significant percentage of horses in a herd may follow recent introduction of an index case. Equine herpesvirus-1 is thought to be the major cause of abortion storms, though type 4 has been isolated from sporadic aborted fetuses.

Control and Prophylaxis: Much can be done with sanitary management to prevent the catastrophic consequences of abortion. Efficient quarantine measures should be imposed on outside horses arriving on a stud farm. On large farms, separation of mares into small bands, isolation, and strict sanitary precautions undertaken with all newly introduced horses can help avert an outbreak. However, after respiratory disease or abortions have begun within a band, little is accomplished by isolating individuals from the band, though the farm should be isolated. The source of virus for the respiratory infection in foals is thought to be from older horses, which shed virus after reactivation of latent virus. To date, however, evidence for such a carrier state remains circumstantial.

Inactivated and live attenuated equine herpevirus-1 vaccines are used to control both respiratory disease and abortion, but their efficacy, especially in preventing abor-

tion, is doubtful. A commercially available inactivated vaccine (Pneumabort-K: Fort Dodge) is reported to be quite effective in preventing abortion when given at 5-7 and 9 months of gestation. It is less effective in immunization against respiratory disease, presumably because of the predominance of equine herpesvirus-4 involved in this syndrome. A commercially available live-virus vaccine (Rhinomune: Norden) is reportedly effective in reducing respiratory disease, but its effectiveness in preventing abortion has not been documented.

Equine Arteritis

In 1953, a virus was isolated from horses with a disease clinically and pathologically distinguishable from equine rhinopneumonitis. The disease was called equine viral arteritis. Though serologic surveys indicate that viral arteritis is widespread, the clinical disease is recognized only rarely and has been reported only in the United States, Austria, Switzerland and Poland.[82] The significance of this virus as a cause of respiratory disease appears to be minor. It essentially is a systemic febrile disease that sometimes causes reproductive failures.

Clinical Signs: From serologic studies, it is presumed that most infections are subclinical. The virus apparently varies greatly in virulence, and some isolates can cause overt infection and death. Clinical signs include acute depression, fever, congestion of the nasal mucosa and conjunctiva, serous nasal discharge, excessive lacrimation, palpebral edema, anorexia, dyspnea, weakness, loss of weight, dehydration, and edema of the legs, genitalia and abdomen. Of pregnant mares at risk, 40-80% may abort.

Diagnosis: A diagnosis may be based on clinical signs, isolation of the virus in tissue culture, or demonstration of a 4-fold increase in neutralizing antibody in convalescent serum. The virus has characteristics of the RNA togaviruses and is enclosed in a lipid envelope. It grows in equine fetal kidney cell cultures and produces plaques, which are used in neutralization tests to identify the virus. The virus may be isolated in tissue culture from swabs of the nasal passages or conjunctival sac, and from the blood. An isolation was made by first inoculation of blood into an experimental horse, then subinoculation of this horse's blood into tissue culture. Virus can be isolated from the semen of carrier stallions. Because few laboratories work with this virus, consultation with a laboratory is suggested before collecting samples for virus isolation and serologic tests.

Transmission and Control: Transmission is via aerosol and contact with infected horses or aborted fetuses and placentae. Persistent infections of stallions are important in transmission of the virus.[83] Virus can be shed in the semen for months.

Immunization of horses with attenuated live-virus vaccine prepared in cell cultures produces lifelong immunity and no untoward effects. Vaccinated horses do not shed the virus. Immunization of valuable mares has become an accepted practice in some parts of the United States. However, at this time, certain countries do not admit antibody-positive horses.

Equine Adenovirus Infection

Equine adenovirus infection is widespread and usually inapparent, except in immunodeficient foals, in which it is invariably fatal.

The equine adenovirus was isolated first in 1969 in Pennsylvania from an Arabian foal with acute respiratory disease.[84] It since has been isolated from foals of other breeds with and without clinical disease.[85] The virus most likely persists latently in the pharyngeal lymphoid tissues of apparently healthy animals for long periods.

Equine adenovirus is a DNA-containing ether-resistant virus that can be cultured in a number of equine cells. It has a cytopathic effect and a characteristic hexagonal virion when observed by electron microscopy. All isolates thus far compared serologically belong to the same antigenic serotype.

Certain Arabian foals with a primary severe combined immunodeficiency disease, in which there is an almost total absence of both T- and B-lymphocytes, are particularly susceptible to adenovirus infection.[86] These foals are especially vulnerable during the first few weeks of life if they receive inadequate amounts of colostrum. The virus attacks the respiratory epithelium, in which it replicates, and may cause cell death, intranuclear inclusions and epithelial hyperplasia. In the lungs, the epithelial cells become swollen and hyperplastic, and slough into the lumen of the bronchioles and alveoli,

leading to pulmonary atelectasis and bronchopneumonia. In affected foals, lymph nodes, Peyer's patches and thymus often are depleted, but these do not appear to be a primary viral lesion. These lesions of insufficient lymphocytes exist before infection and are responsible for the immunologic defect that allows the virus to become established in the first place.

Equine adenovirus infection occurs throughout the world and in all major horse breeds. It has been reported more frequently in the Arabian breed because the infection has been more severe and fatal in foals with the inherited immunodeficiency in this breed. Serologic surveys indicate that the infection is common and that foals become infected at a few weeks of age.

Clinical Signs: Most adenovirus infections in horses produce an asymptomatic or mild upper respiratory tract disease. In susceptible Arabian foals, however, clinical signs are fever, mucous nasal and ocular discharges, coughing and bronchopneumonia, as evidenced by muffled normal airway sounds, and wheezes and crackles over affected portions of the lungs. The oral mucosa may be ulcerated and diarrhea may be present. Affected foals become unthrifty, develop a rough haircoat, and tire easily. A cardinal hematologic sign has been severe absolute lymphopenia and low levels or total lack of serum immunoglobulins.

Diagnosis: Diagnosis of adenoviral pneumonia may be based on clinical signs and isolation of the virus from nasal swabs or lung lesions at necropsy. Finding characteristic intranuclear inclusions in epithelial cells on a conjunctival or nasal smear is highly suggestive, but infection should be confirmed by virus isolation. Adenovirus isolation can be confirmed by hemagglutination inhibition or neutralization assays.

The fact that all equine adenoviruses belong to a single serotype greatly simplifies production of a vaccine for this infection. The need for a vaccine has yet to be demonstrated, however, because there is little evidence that equine adenovirus causes respiratory disease in most infected horses.

Equine Rhinovirus Infection

In nature, equine rhinovirus infection is widespread but causes little or no significant disease, though a mild upper respiratory disease has been attributed to the virus.[87] The first reported association of equine rhinovirus with respiratory illness was reported in 1962. Since that time, 3 types of equine rhinovirus have been identified; the significance of these agents as serious causes of respiratory illness still is questionable. The equine rhinoviruses are unrelated to the bovine or human rhinoviruses. Experimentally, clinical disease is rarely elicited, though neutralizing antibody is rapidly produced (7-14 days). Antibody titers persist for several years and appear to protect against further infection.

Most animals develop antibody during their second year of life. This suggests that most infections occur during the period of training and racing, though a few foals may become infected with rhinovirus quite early in life and while still on the breeding farm. About 60-80% of horses 5 years of age have antibody titers. It is thought that the infection spreads mainly by inhalation.

Rhinovirus infection produces viremia and can be isolated from the feces even after neutralizing antibody appears. A carrier state with a prolonged period of shedding is thought to explain why young horses become infected rapidly when mingled with adult horses.

Rhinoviruses are a group of small, ether-resistant RNA viruses that are inactivated rapidly in weak acid solutions. However, they are very resistant under ordinary stable conditions. The equine rhinoviruses differ from human rhinoviruses in that they grow in a number of cell cultures.

Diagnosis: Equine rhinovirus infection is diagnosed by isolation of the virus during clinical illness or by demonstration of a 4-fold increase in serum neutralizing antibody titer during convalescence. Virus may be recovered from nasopharyngeal swabs. Equine kidney cells are commonly used for virus isolation, in which the virus produces a cytopathic effect. Clinical signs include fever, anorexia and pharyngitis, with a copious serous and later mucopurulent nasal discharge. Some horses have a mild cough that may persist. Lymphadenitis of the submaxillary lymph nodes has been observed.

No vaccine is available to prevent equine rhinovirus infection, nor is it known if one is needed.

Viral Pneumonia in Neonates

M.R. Paradis

Viral pneumonia is recognized rarely in neonatal foals. Pneumonia caused by equine herpesvirus-1 has been reported in neonates as a result of *in-utero* infection during the last trimester of gestation. These foals were delivered at term and most were considered normal at birth. There was no history of failure of passive transfer of maternal antibodies. During the first week of life, these foals developed respiratory distress, reddened mucous membranes, and intractable diarrhea. Absolute lymphopenia and neutrophilic leukocytosis developed during the course of disease.[5]

Historical evidence of respiratory disease or recent abortions on the farm may aid diagnosis of equine herpesvirus-1 infection. A significant rise in acute and convalescent antibody titers to the virus in the mare or other horses on the farm suggests recent exposure. Postmortem findings of interstitial pneumonia, hypoplasia of the spleen and thymus, adrenocortical hyperplasia, and focal adrenocortical hemorrhages are consistent with viral infection.[5]

Bacterial infection or sepsis due to failure of passive transfer and combined immunodeficiency with failure of passive transfer must be differentiated from equine herpesvirus-1 infection. At this time, there is no specific therapy available for treatment of viral diseases in the foal. Supportive care with IV fluids, warmth and nutrition is necessary for survival. The prognosis is grave. Affected foals have an apparent virus-induced immunodeficiency and are more susceptible to bacterial infection.

DISEASES OF THE NASAL CAVITY AND PARANASAL SINUSES

J.P. Caron

Diagnostic and Therapeutic Considerations

Clinical Anatomy

Alar Folds and Nasal Diverticulum: The nose and rostral nasal cavity of horses differ from those of other domestic animals in several respects. At rest, each nostril (naris) is the shape of an inverted comma but is more or less circular in outline when dilated. The horse's unique ability for nostril dilation is related to the lack of lateral cartilaginous support rostral to the nasoincisive notch. Several muscles effect dilation of the nostrils, all of which are innervated by the facial nerve. Thus, facial nerve dysfunction can cause inability to dilate the nostrils and their collapse at rest. As the nares are considered a major site of upper airway resistance in horses, inability to dilate the nares may be of considerable significance to the equine athlete.

Medial support to the nostrils is provided by the alar cartilages, which are C-shaped structures oriented back-to-back, with loose connective tissue attachments to the nasal septum. This anatomic arrangement provides for mobility of the muzzle.

Another unique characteristic of the nasal anatomy is the presence of a "false nostril" or nasal diverticulum, a blind cavity formed by the external naris and alar fold. The external opening of the diverticulum is located in the dorsolateral aspect of the true nostril. The alar fold is a shelf of tissue covered by skin on its dorsolateral surface and respiratory mucosa on its ventromedial surface. The fold extends obliquely from the lateral extremity of the alar cartilage to its medial attachment on the ventral nasal concha. The medial attachment site envelopes the medial accessory cartilage.

Nasal Septum and Nasal Conchae: The nasal cavity is divided into halves by the nasal septum. The septum is composed mainly of hyaline cartilage, except at its most caudoventral extremity at the level of the ethmoturbinates. The septum extends from the rostral extent of the nasal cavity to the ethmoid labyrinth and is covered by respiratory epithelium.

The 2 nasal conchae, or turbinates, arise from the lateral walls of the nasal cavity and occupy much of its volume. There are dorsal and ventral nasal conchae. The remaining space, between the nasal septum and nasal conchae, comprises the air passages. Each of the potential routes that air may take is called a meatus. There are dorsal, middle and ventral nasal meati. The largest of these is the ventral nasal meatus, which lies on the ventromedial surface of

the nasal cavity and is the preferred route for passage of nasogastric and nasotracheal tubes and such diagnostic instruments as the fiberoptic endoscope. Inadvertent introduction of instruments into the middle meatus may cause trauma to the respiratory mucosa investing the ethmoid turbinate bones. This results in impressive but self-limiting hemorrhage. The nasal conchae contain air-filled sinuses that communicate with the other paranasal sinuses.

Paranasal Sinuses: There are essentially 4 pairs of paranasal sinuses: the frontal, maxillary, sphenopalatine and ethmoidal sinuses. However, the dorsal conchal (turbinate) part of the frontal sinus and the rostral, caudal and ventral conchal (turbinate) compartments of the maxillary sinuses may be considered as separate structures, giving 7 pairs of paranasal sinuses.

The maxillary is the largest of the paranasal sinuses. In the adult horse, its dorsal boundary is along a line from the infraorbital foramen caudally, parallel to the facial crest. The rostral limit is at a line from the facial crest to the infraorbital foramen, and its caudal limit at a transverse plane slightly rostral to the root of the orbital process of the zygomatic bone. In older individuals, the ventral limit of the sinus may extend ventral to the level of the facial crest. The ventral limit in a foal is considerably higher because of incompletely erupted teeth. The maxillary sinus is divided into rostral and caudal compartments by a complete, oblique septum. The septum usually lies about 5 cm caudal to the rostral extent of the facial crest, but its exact location is variable. Its presence should be considered when elevating facial bone flaps to avoid iatrogenic fractures during sinus surgery. The rostral maxillary sinus communicates with the ventral conchal (turbinate) sinus. The caudal maxillary sinus communicates with the frontal sinus through the fronto-maxillary aperture.

The rostral and caudal maxillary sinuses communicate with the nasal cavity via a common nasomaxillary aperture. The aperture, located in the middle nasal meatus, bears a dorsoventrally flattened duct that bifurcates to enter each of the sinus compartments individually.[88] Thus, either or both of the ducts or the common aperture can become occluded in disease, with consequent compromised drainage from the sinus. It is for this reason that openings into the nasal cavity are commonly created during surgical procedures involving the maxillary sinus. As mentioned, the nasomaxillary opening enters the nasal cavity via the middle nasal meatus, approximately at the level of the medial canthus of the eye. A small-diameter endoscope can be used to inspect the area of the aperture for discharges in suspected cases of sinus disease.

The frontal sinus is also paired, and each half of the structure separated by a bony septum. The rostral limit of the frontal sinus is a transverse plane through the skull, halfway between the infraorbital foramen and the orbit, which corresponds to the level of the fifth cheek tooth. A palpable landmark of the rostral limit of the sinus is the point at which the facial bones diverge. The caudal limit of the sinus is about at the level of the temporomandibular joint. The frontal sinus communicates with the nasal cavity via the nasomaxillary opening in the caudal maxillary sinus. Unique to the horse is a large communication with the dorsal conchal (turbinate) sinus. This sinus, therefore, may be known as the conchofrontal sinus.

The sphenopalatine sinus is a diverticulum of the caudal maxillary sinus. The sphenopalatine sinus seldom is affected in isolation from diseases involving the other sinus compartments. This sinus has several important vessels and nerves coursing through it, including the optic nerve, so that sphenopalatine sinusitis may produce striking clinical signs.

Clinical Examination and Diagnostic Aids

Many diseases of the nose, nasal cavity and paranasal sinuses can be diagnosed by physical examination. Thorough visual inspection of the nostrils and rostral nasal cavity can be conducted with no more than adequate lighting. Asymmetry, discharges, odors and mucosal abnormalities may herald disease of the upper airway. Septic sinusitis frequently is accompanied by fetid breath and unilateral nasal discharge. The adequacy and symmetry of air flow can be evaluated by cupping the hands over the external nares. Dissimilar air flow between the right and left nares suggests a lesion rostral to the nasopharynx. Digital palpation of the rostral portions of the nasal turbinates and nasal septum may reveal abnormalities. Similarly, passing a nasogastric tube may be of value in discovering and localizing space-occupying lesions of the nasal cavity.

Careful inspection of the horse's face may be of diagnostic value. Abnormal prominences, corresponding to the location of the paranasal sinuses, suggest a chronic, expansive lesion within a sinus compartment (Fig 11). Palpation of the area over an affected sinus may cause pain, and dullness on percussion is common. An ocular discharge and/or exophthalmos occasionally accompanies sinus disease. Chronic problems, especially aggressive neoplasms and certain mycoses, may result in formation of draining tracts in the facial region.

Diseases of the nasal septum and conchae are relatively uncommon. Diseases causing thickening or deviation of the nasal septum may result in upper airway obstruction. The causes vary but include trauma, congenital lesions, neoplasia, infection and deviation secondary to lesions of the paranasal sinuses. Exercise intolerance may not be evident with a congenital lesion until the horse begins training. Similarly, acquired

Figure 11. Facial deformity (arrows) associated with maxillary sinusitis. (Courtesy of Dr. J.A. Stick)

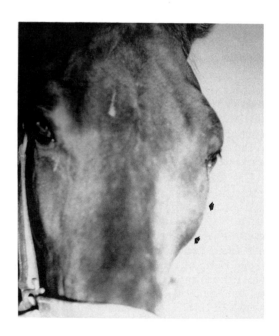

lesions may have an insidious onset of clinical signs.

The more caudal region of the nasal cavity and nasal septum may be directly inspected with fiberoptic endoscopic equipment. Use of the standard (11-mm) colonoscope is restricted to the ventral meatus. A pediatric bronchoscope (6-mm) may be used to examine the turbinates, middle nasal meatus and nasomaxillary opening.

Radiographs are useful in evaluating the nasal cavity and paranasal sinuses. The bones of the face are relatively thin, and the air-filled sinuses and nasal cavity provide excellent radiographic contrast. These anatomic characteristics make it possible to obtain films of diagnostic quality with standard equipment, especially if high-speed film and rare earth screens are used.

Structures usually evaluated include the nasal septum, facial skeleton, tooth roots, nasal conchae and paranasal sinuses. Abnormalities of the nasal septum include thickening and deviation, which may be primary or secondary to abnormalities of adjacent structures (Fig 12). Both thickening

Figure 12. Dorsoventral radiograph of a right-sided mass in the maxillary sinus producing marked lateral deviation of the nasal septum (arrows).

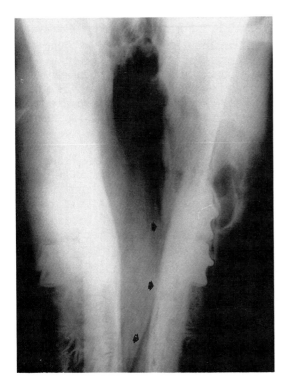

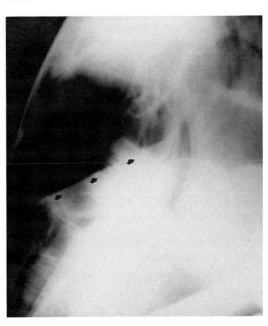

Figure 13. Lateral radiograph of the skull of an adult horse, depicting a fluid line (arrows) in the maxillary sinus.

and deviation of the septum are best evaluated with a true dorsoventral projection; oblique projections may be misleading. Radiographic abnormalities that accompany diseases of paranasal sinuses include fluid lines, and osteolysis or new bone production (Fig 13). When uncertain about the presence of a fluid line, a second film should be made with the horse's head in a slightly different position to change orientation of fluid in the sinus. Empyema of the maxillary sinus often is the sequel to dental disease, and radiographic appearance of tooth roots occupying the sinus should be evaluated carefully. Abnormalities include loss of the normal radiodense "halo" (lamina dura) surrounding the tooth root and loss of tooth crown detail.

Percutaneous centesis (Kral tap) of the maxillary and frontal sinuses is possible using local anesthesia, with or without prior sedation. Following an initial cutaneous stab incision, a sterile Steinmann pin is used to penetrate the bone overlying the sinus. A small sterile catheter is introduced into the lumen and a sample of the compartment's contents is obtained for culture and cytologic examination. Radiographic localization of sites of fluid accumulation before the tap frequently is helpful. It may be necessary to repeat the centesis at another site because abnormal contents may be compartmentalized by inflammatory debris.

Another alternative for characterization of diseases of the paranasal sinuses is endoscopic examination using an arthroscope; however, detailed protocols for use of this technique have not been published. The technique may prove useful in diagnosis and surgical treatment of sinus diseases.

Surgical exploration is the final and most radical diagnostic tool. The surgeon may use a trephined opening or a facial bone flap technique. Exposure afforded by the latter is much greater and, for that reason, is preferred. Adequate knowledge of the regional anatomy is imperative to avoid damage to important structures, such as the nasolacrimal duct and infraorbital nerve.

Surgery of the Nasal Septum and Nasal Turbinates

Surgery of the nasal cavity is indicated whenever a lesion causes a primary respiratory obstruction or when it is known to be progressive or invasive. Equine nasal surgery ranges from resection of a local lesion to removal of an entire nasal turbinate or the nasal septum.

Nasal Septum Resection: Resection of the nasal septum is indicated when air flow through the nasal passages is impaired by primary abnormalities or by lesions of adjacent structures that compromise the lumen of the nasal cavity. In a review of nasal septum resection, obstruction secondary to trauma was the most frequent reason for resection of the nasal septum.[89]

Commonly, the nasal septum has been removed by creating a trephine opening in the nasal cavity just rostral to the frontal sinus, where frontal bones begin to diverge. Through the trephine hole, forceps are used to stabilize the septum. A second vertical incision is made in the nasal septum, through the nostril, at a level immediately caudal to the alar cartilages. Subsequently, a guarded chisel or obstetric wire is used to separate the dorsal and ventral septal attachments between the 2 vertical incisions, and the septum is removed through the nostril. When necessary, a greater portion of the caudal septum may be removed by directing the caudal vertical incision at a more oblique angle. This modification of the standard technique is indicated when septal thickening or deviation includes the more caudal portion of the septum.

An alternative technique uses a dorsal bone flap. This procedure involves creation of a rectangular bone flap about the size of the portion of the septum to be removed. A 3-sided bone flap is elevated, and the dorsal attachment of the septum to the frontal and nasal bones is separated with a Stryker (oscillating) saw. Forceps are applied perpendicularly to the intended site of resection of the nasal septum, and vertical incisions are made with a hard-backed scalpel or osteotome. The remaining ventral attachment is broken by gripping the septum in 2 locations with forceps and rocking the septum back and forth until it comes free from the notch it occupies in the vomer bone. This method is preferred when resection of a portion of the turbinates or other lesion is to be performed concurrently.

Regardless of the method used to remove the septum, hemorrhage is profuse, and the surgeon is well advised to have compatible whole blood available should transfusion be required. Hemorrhage is controlled by packing the nasal cavity with sterile gauze; therefore, a temporary tracheostomy must be performed. The nasal packing and tracheostomy tube can be removed about 48 hours postoperatively. Horses with an uncomplicated convalescence may be returned to work in 4-6 weeks.

In addition to complications related to soft tissue healing, the most common complication of nasal septum resection is removal of an excessive amount of the rostral septum. This may result in a concave conformation to the nose and, if severe, may result in partial airway obstruction by the false nostrils. This problem may necessitate removal of the alar folds.[89] Other complications include removing an insufficient amount of abnormal septum, and chondroma formation at the incised edge of the septal cartilage.

Congenital and Familial Diseases

Choanal Atresia and Other Developmental Abnormalities

Congenital lesions of the nasal cavity are uncommon. One of the most frequently recognized is congenital thickening or deviation of the nasal septum. Cystic degeneration and congenital overgrowth of normal tissues of the nasal septum (hamartoma) are 2 reported causes of nasal septal thickening.[89,90] Longitudinal deviation of the nasal septum is another congenital malformation. Deviation may be restricted to the nasal septum or may accompany the lateral nasomaxillary deviation or "wry nose" syndrome, in which the entire rostral facial skeleton is deviated (Fig 14). Successful correction of this abnormality has been described.[91]

Successful management of bilateral choanal atresia has been reported.[92] This congenital malformation involves failure of perforation of the bucconasal membrane located at the caudal extent of the nasal cavity. The condition may be bilateral or unilateral. The result of bilateral congenital atresia is that the foal is born with a complete respiratory obstruction, requiring immediate tracheostomy. Definitive treatment involves resection of the occluding membrane, usually via a dorsal facial bone flap.

Figure 14. A foal with lateral nasomaxillary deviation or "wry nose."

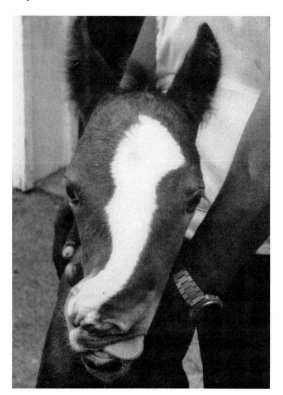

Diseases With Physical Causes

Redundant Alar Folds

Flaccid or redundant alar folds may compromise respiratory function by causing partial upper airway obstruction. The condition is rare as compared to other obstructive lesions of the upper respiratory tract in horses. For this reason, careful consideration should be given to the contribution of redundant alar folds to the overall performance of the horse before establishing the diagnosis of "false nostril noise." If the results of physical examination and endoscopic examination fail to disclose attendant or "primary" lesions, a diagnosis of false nostril noise may be considered. False nostril noise is characterized by a biphasic fluttering noise that is most pronounced on expiration, unlike that in idiopathic laryngeal hemiplegia, which results in a predominately inspiratory noise.[93]

Frequently there is no impairment of exercise capacity associated with redundant alar folds; however, excessive alar fold tissue may produce excessive upper airway resistance in horses that tend to have small nostrils or narrow nasal passages.[94]

To confirm that the source of the abnormal respiratory noise is redundant or flaccid alar folds, a mattress suture can be placed through the alar folds and over the bridge of the nose to attenuate the lumen of the nasal diverticulum. In horses with redundant alar folds, this procedure eliminates the abnormal respiratory noise. As the noise may only be evident with exercise, the horse should be exercised following suture placement.

Treatment of redundant alar folds consists of bilateral resection. This may be conducted with or without incision of the skin of the external nares (rhinotomy). When postoperative appearance is not an overriding consideration, the procedure should be conducted through an incision in the lateral wall of the true nostril (rhinotomy). Rhinotomy greatly facilitates alar fold resection, and attention to skin closure minimizes postoperative scarring. It is possible to perform the procedure without rhinotomy in show horses.

Regardless of the specific approach, resection involves incising the alar fold at its junction with the lamina of the alar cartilage and dissecting caudally to the caudal limit of the nasal diverticulum. A second incision is made caudally from the medial attachment of the alar fold to meet the previous incision. This results in resection of a portion of the cartilage of the ventral turbinate (medial accessory cartilage). One can anticipate copious hemorrhage at this stage of the dissection, and it may be difficult to control this hemorrhage without the exposure provided by a rhinotomy. If the procedure is conducted through an intact nostril, it is advisable to be conservative in removing the ventral turbinate cartilage (medial accessory cartilage). Several vessels in the submucosa contribute to the bleeding, and ligation is difficult. Closure and hemostasis are effected by placing a simple-continuous suture pattern in the incised skin and mucosa. Using absorbable material eliminates the need for suture removal. Healing of the incisions usually is complete in 7-10 days, at which time the horse may be returned to work.

Facial Trauma

Facial trauma can damage the nasal septum or conchae and cause fractures of facial bones. Treatment usually is directed at restoration of a normal facial contour, with little specific treatment of the nasal septum or conchae. Surgical management consists of elevation of depressed fragments with reduction maintained by wire or synthetic nonabsorbable sutures. Specific techniques are described in the literature.[95,96] In rare circumstances, excessive bony or soft tissue callus produced during healing causes respiratory embarrassment. This may necessitate resection of the exuberant fibrous tissue or bone or a portion of the nasal septum. Another complication of facial fractures is sinusitis resulting from contamination of a sinus. Fortunately, sinusitis is rare, probably due to the rich blood supply and free drainage of these structures.

Inflammatory, Infectious and Immune Diseases

Bacterial Rhinitis

Bacterial infections of the nasal cavity are uncommon; however, there have been isolated reports of bacterial infections of the equine upper airway. Staphylococcal granulomas occasionally are found on the nasal turbinates or nasal septum. These lesions may be secondary to respiratory mucosal trauma.

Bacterial Sinusitis (Empyema)

Bacterial infection of the paranasal sinuses most often involves the maxillary sinus. Empyema (sinusitis) often is secondary to dental disease (Fig 15). One report indicated that sinusitis was related to tooth abnormalities in 50% of reported cases.[97] In my experience, sinusitis unrelated to dental disease is uncommon.

Empyema may occur secondary to upper respiratory infections by *Streptococcus equi* and equine influenza virus, especially in young horses. Also, empyema of the paranasal sinuses may be a sequel to alveolar periostitis in growing horses. Sinusitis occasionally is observed without any apparent primary cause.

Clinical signs of sinusitis include unilateral nasal discharge, dullness on percussion and/or pain over the affected sinus, facial deformity (Fig 16) and, occasionally, an ocular discharge. The nasal discharge is of variable character but usually mucopurulent. Bacterial sinusitis may be accompanied by mandibular lymphadenopathy. Because sinusitis often is related to dental disease, a thorough oral examination is

Figure 15. Lateral radiograph of a horse with maxillary and frontal sinusitis, secondary to an abnormality of the third molar (arrows). The fifth cheek tooth (second molar) is numbered. Note the soft tissue density within the sinuses.

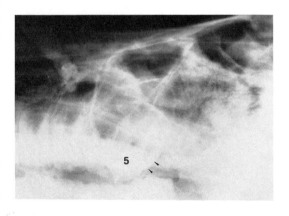

worthwhile. Frequently the involved tooth is the first molar (fourth cheek tooth). Primary dental abnormalities include patent infundibulum, caries, tooth fracture and periodontal disease. Endoscopic examination reveals purulent exudate draining from the nasomaxillary opening, unless the nasomaxillary ducts or foramen have been occluded by inflammatory debris.

Definitive diagnosis is by radiography and percutaneous centesis (Kral tap) of the sinus. Radiographic abnormalities associated with empyema include fluid lines (Fig 13) and signs of dental disease when a tooth problem is the underlying cause (Fig 15). Percutaneous centesis of the sinus is easily performed and usually done on a standing, sedated patient. Because the transverse septum between the rostral and caudal compartments of the maxillary sinus is complete, it may be necessary to tap each compartment. Sinus aspirate should be submitted for culture and sensitivity tests to select an appropriate antibiotic.

Treatment of bacterial sinusitis is directed at the underlying etiology. In the case of a primary dental problem, it is necessary to remove the offending tooth. Preservation of a diseased tooth invites recurrence of the sinus infection. In the case of empyema secondary to respiratory infection, treatment of the sinusitis usually is sufficient because the predisposing respiratory malady has resolved or has been treated.

Treatment of sinusitis involves the same principles as those for any closed-space infection, *ie*, adequate drainage and antimicrobial therapy based on known sensitivity data. Drainage often is accomplished at the time of removal of the diseased tooth. The most popular method for tooth removal is via a facial bone flap and subsequent repulsion of abnormal teeth. Following tooth repulsion, the sinus is debrided. Liberal lavage with isotonic fluids is advantageous because of the complex topography of the area. In chronic cases, it frequently is necessary to create a rostral nasomaxillary opening to ensure adequate postoperative drainage. This opening is best created at the conclusion of the procedure, as moderate hemorrhage results.

Lavage of the sinus, either as the primary treatment or as an adjunct to surgery, is indicated. For lavage to be employed as the sole treatment, the sinusitis must not be caused by dental disease, and the nasomaxillary opening must be patent to allow drainage of the irrigation solution.[98] Postoperative lavage is indicated when the debris encountered at the time of surgery is inspissated or particularly adherent. Also, in chronic cases, it may be difficult to perform optimal surgical debridement. Lavage may be accomplished using an indwelling catheter placed in the sinus through a stab incision adjacent to the primary surgical incision. A Steinmann pin of appropriate size is used to perforate the bone over the sinus. An IV extension tube can be attached to allow the lavage solution to be delivered at some distance from the entrance of the catheter into the skin. Once- or twice-daily irrigation of the sinus can be continued until the solution fails to dislodge a significant quantity of debris. Several recommendations have been made regarding the most appropriate lavage solution; however, satisfactory results may be obtained with sterile saline. Use of saline avoids the irritation of mucous membranes associated with use of many antiseptics.[99]

Antimicrobial therapy should be considered on an individual basis. With adequate drainage, the course of antimicrobial use

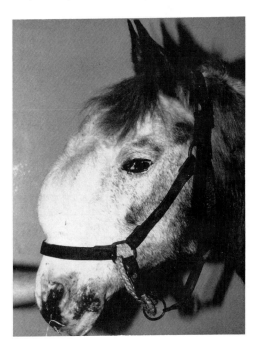

Figure 16. Advanced adenocarcinoma of the frontal sinus. (Courtesy of Dr. B. Darien)

can be relatively short, especially in acute sinusitis. In more chronic cases, a 3- to 4-week regimen or longer may be required.

The prognosis in bacterial sinusitis depends on the underlying cause. Sinusitis as a result of upper respiratory infection without involvement of bone generally has a good prognosis for complete resolution. Chronic empyema, with bony involvement and facial deformity, has a much less favorable prognosis.

Cryptococcosis

Fungal infections of the upper respiratory tract have a regional distribution, often restricted to the more southern portions of North America. In general, the mycoses produce granulomatous lesions that may reach size sufficient to cause partial obstruction of the upper airway. Certain mycoses are aggressive and may invade the paranasal sinuses or produce facial disfigurement. Treatment is directed at removing abnormal tissues, to relieve airway compromise and eliminate the inciting organism. Mycotic lesions may advance sufficiently that total extirpation is impossible, and the prognosis must be adjusted accordingly.

Cryptococcal infection may involve tissues of the upper respiratory tract. It is thought to be restricted to immunosuppressed or malnourished hosts.[100] A chronic form affects the nasal cavity and sinuses of horses. The causative organism (*Cryptococcus neoformans*) tends to be quite invasive, and disease often is accompanied by draining tract formation through facial bones.[101] Infection can be diagnosed by cytologic inspection of smears, and the organism is easily cultured. Cryptococcosis is considered of some public health significance, and it has been recommended that infected horses be destroyed.[100,101] Zoonotic potential is not great, as there is no aerosolization of infectious material either from infected animals or culture media.[102] Canine cryptococcosis has been treated with a combination of amphotericin B and flucytosine.[102]

Rhinosporidiosis

A second fungal infection of the sinuses and nasal cavity is caused by *Rhinosporidium seeberi*. Rhinosporidiosis is characterized by granuloma formation near the mucocutaneous junction of the nares.[103,104] The lesion tends to be located in the rostral and ventral portions of the nasal cavity and nasal septum. Granulomatous polyps may reach sufficient size to produce respiratory obstruction. Treatment is by surgical removal; unfortunately, masses frequently recur. Because the organism is difficult to culture, the infection is recognized by identification of the organism in biopsy specimens. The disease is not considered highly contagious.

Coccidioidomycosis

Coccidioides immitis has been reported to infect the nasal mucosa of the horse.[105] The disease has both localized and generalized forms. Coccidioidomycosis occurs in semi-arid climates but has been seen as far north as Canada. The diagnosis is based on demonstration of characteristic "spherules" in a biopsy. If the granuloma is accessible, treatment is by excision. The drug of choice for treatment in people is amphotericin B, but this drug has been replaced by ketoconazole in small animals.[106] Long-term treatment often is required, and use of either drug may be cost prohibitive in horses.

Phycomycosis

Phycomycosis is a general term for infections caused by the organisms *Hyphomyces destruens* (*Pythium* spp) or *Entomophthora coronata* (*Conidiobolus coronatus*). *Entomophthora* has an affinity for the tissues in and around the nares, producing a condition known as rhinophycomycosis.[107] The disease is most common in, but not restricted to, coastal lowland areas. It is characterized by a purulent nasal discharge and one or more areas of exuberant granulation tissue that frequently contain cores of necrotic material known as "leeches" or "kunkers." Lesions are pruritic and often are traumatized. The organism is quite invasive, and involvement of the lips and oral cavity may impair eating. A favorable prognosis is expected with early surgical removal. Ancillary treatment has involved use of amphotericin B, adding 100 mg in 250 ml of dimethyl sulfoxide solution applied topically twice daily for 8 weeks.[108]

Aspergillosis

Aspergillus has been reported to produce fungal plaques in the nasal passages of horses.[109] Affected animals have a slight purulent nasal discharge and may show intermittent epistaxis. Plaques are observed endoscopically, and definitive diagnosis is by microscopic examination of exudate or biopsies of the lesions. The condition has been successfully treated with daily topical natamycin (Natacyn: Alcon) irrigation (25 mg in 100 ml sterile water).[107]

Neoplasia

Nasal and Paranasal Neoplasms

Neoplastic conditions of the nasal septum and turbinates are rare. The abundance of tissue types in the upper respiratory tract explains the variety of tumor types affecting this area.[110-112] Both carcinomas and mesenchymal neoplasms have been reported. The most common neoplasms of the nasal passages are squamous-cell carcinoma and fibroma.[110] Squamous-cell carcinoma may occur in areas devoid of squamous epithelium, and it is thought that more specialized epithelia undergo squamous metaplasia before neoplastic transformation. In an extensive review of neoplasms in this part of the body, 68% of nasal cavity and paranasal sinus tumors were malignant.[110] Typical of neoplasms in this region in most species, the onset of clinical signs is insidious and many tumors are not detected until they are advanced (Fig 16). Late detection and the complex anatomy of the area complicate treatment of these lesions.[113]

Neoplasms of the paranasal sinuses are similar to those described for the nasal cavity and turbinates. One neoplasm of the upper airway that usually has its origin in the paranasal sinuses is the osteoma.[112,113] The tumor produces clinical signs similar to those of follicular cyst but is differentiated by its radiodensity. It is treated by surgical removal and has a favorable prognosis.

Idiopathic Diseases

Nasal Amyloidosis

The most common form of amyloidosis is the visceral form. Amyloid deposits in the nasal cavity may accompany the cutaneous form of the disease, the latter characterized by formation of nodules in the dermis. A second manifestation of amyloidosis is restricted to the rostral nasal cavity and is known as local or "tumor-like" amyloidosis.[114] This form is associated with single or multiple deposits of amyloid of various sizes. The deposits frequently are localized but may become extensive and involve the entire nasal cavity, nasopharynx, guttural pouches and larynx. The lymph nodes of the head and neck also may be involved. The specific cause of the disease is unknown, but it has been observed in conjunction with chronic suppurative diseases, including *Streptococcus equi* infection, and with hyperimmunization. The disease can be diagnosed by special staining of biopsy specimens. Treatment principles include excision of accessible focal lesions and removal of the primary cause, if it can be identified. Reports of successful treatment of amyloidosis are rare.

Atheroma
(Epidermal Inclusion Cyst)

An atheroma is a fluid-filled, cyst-like structure located at the caudal aspect of the nasal diverticulum or false nostril (Fig 17). Atheromas previously were thought to be sebaceous cysts, but microscopic examina-

Figure 17. Epidermal inclusion cyst (atheroma).

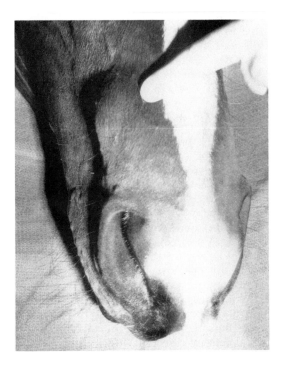

tion of these lesions has shown them to be of epidermal origin.[115] Inclusion cysts are most commonly located at the caudal fornix of the nasal diverticulum, but may occur at other locations. The exact etiology is unknown but they most likely represent a congenital ectopic sequestration of epithelium.[115] Sudden increases in size of the cysts in adults is thought to be due to the inflammation that attends leakage of keratinized material into surrounding tissues.

Inclusion cysts are easily identified by palpation of the caudal extent of the nasal diverticulum. Rarely are they associated with impaired athletic performance, and they need not be treated if they are small and not unsightly.

If objectionable for cosmetic reasons, cysts may be treated by drainage or surgical removal. Cysts may be lanced through the nasal diverticulum and allowed to heal by second intention. The cyst cavity may be obliterated using swabs soaked in counterirritants, such as 2% tincture of iodine. This technique avoids the necessity of incising the external nostril. An alternative treatment is to surgically extirpate the lesion through a dorsal approach. This may be done using regional (infraorbital) analgesia or with the horse under general anesthesia. Careful dissection allows complete removal of the cyst. The capsule of the lesion varies in thickness but usually is well differentiated from surrounding tissues. Use of a subcuticular pattern for skin closure may minimize postoperative fibrosis and scarring. *En-bloc* removal of a cyst lessens the likelihood of recurrence.

Nasal Septum Deformation

The nasal septum may be deformed congenitally or by trauma, infection or neoplasia. The signs of deformation may be obvious because air flow through one or both nostrils may be seriously restricted and cause dyspnea. Generally, however, the signs are subtle and evidenced only during strenuous exercise. Diagnosis may be by simply palpating the rostral septum, endoscopically observing the deformity or the narrowing of the ventral meatus the deformity causes, or by a dorsoventral radiograph of the head (Fig 12). Treatment of deformations restricting performance is by nasal septum resection.

Paranasal Sinus (Follicular) Cyst

Cyst-like lesions of the maxillary sinus are infrequent but well-recognized entities in horses. The etiology of the lesion is not known; however, it is thought that the cysts are congenital abnormalities, possibly of dental origin.[116] Despite the belief that the lesion may be congenital in origin, clinical signs in affected horses may not be apparent until adulthood.

The hallmark of the disease is facial deformity produced by enlargement of the cyst. Dyspnea is observed when the cyst expands to a size sufficient to compromise the lumen of the nasal meati. A nasal discharge may occur if the fluid volume in the sinus is sufficient to overflow into the nasal meatus. Percutaneous centesis of the affected sinus compartment yields a thick, honey-like fluid. Sometimes the cyst becomes secondarily infected, resulting in a purulent nasal discharge. In this case, the disease resembles septic sinusitis. Radiographs may show abnormalities of one or more tooth roots, in addition to a multiloculated cystic cavity within the maxillary sinus (Fig 18).

Treatment is aimed at drainage of the cyst's contents and removal of its lining.

Figure 18. Dorsoventral radiograph of a horse with a maxillary sinus cyst. Note the facial deformity and nasal septal deviation associated with the lesion (arrows).

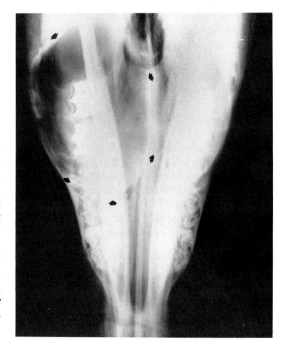

Generally this is performed using the facial bone flap approach to allow adequate exposure. The prognosis is fair to guarded. Persistent respiratory obstruction, chronic nasal discharge, and concomitant dental abnormalities complicate recovery.

Ethmoid Hematoma

Ethmoid hematoma, or progressive ethmoid hematoma, is a slowly progressive, expansive hematoma developing under the respiratory mucosa of the caudal nasal cavity or paranasal sinuses.[117,118] The cause and specific pathogenesis of the disease are unknown. It has been proposed that the condition is a congenital angiomatous lesion resulting from repetitive trauma. A neoplastic etiology also has been suggested; however, neoplastic cells have not been observed in the lesion. A third proposed etiology is chronic irritation and trauma.

The usual presenting complaint is a unilateral, sanguineous nasal discharge at rest. The volume of the discharge is small, which helps differentiate the disease from guttural pouch mycosis with arterial erosion, in which hemorrhage is profuse. The hematomata usually originate from the ethmoid labyrinth, though they may also arise within a sinus compartment. The hematoma is confined by respiratory mucosa, which stretches to accommodate its expansion. The lesion has a typical greenish coloration and enlarges along a path of least resistance, rostrally within the nasal cavity or caudally into the nasopharynx (Fig 19). Due to its progressive nature, surgical removal of the lesion is recommended. A good prognosis with surgical treatment has been suggested; however, recurrence of the lesion was observed in 38% (5 of 13) horses, many with a short followup.[108]

The specific surgical approach to be used for resection of the mass is dictated by its location and accessibility. Incipient lesions have been removed with a snare via the external nares. A frontal bone flap is used for more extensive hematomata. Preoperative considerations include obtaining crossmatched whole blood as intraoperative hemorrhage is often profuse. It would be advisable at least to have a compatible donor available. Cryosurgery has been advocated to minimize the hemorrhage associated with the procedure and to decrease the rate

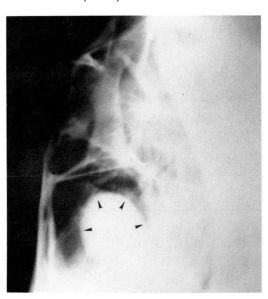

Figure 19. Lateral radiograph of a horse with an ethmoid hematoma (arrows).

of recurrence. Both sides of the nasal passages may be involved, necessitating packing of the nasal cavity and a temporary tracheostomy. Followup endoscopic examination is recommended, as recurrence has been observed as long as 3-4 years after surgical removal.[108]

Nasal Polyps

The term "nasal polyps" has been used to describe a number of polypoid masses of different etiology, including progressive ethmoid hematoma (discussed above). "True" nasal polyps are pedunculated masses of inflammatory origin, comprised of connective tissue covered by respiratory epithelium.[111] The lesions may be attached to either the conchae or the nasal septum and may occur bilaterally (Fig 20). Presenting signs include exercise intolerance or stertorous respiratory noise. Clinical signs are related to the space-occupying effect of the polyp. Affected horses also may have mild, intermittent epistaxis or mucopurulent nasal discharge. Treatment is by excision of the lesion, the specific approach dictated by the polyp's location. Electrosurgical removal is recommended because the superior hemostasis facilitates complete excision of the base of the lesion. Small polyps not directly accessible through the external nares may be removed by snare or transendoscopic

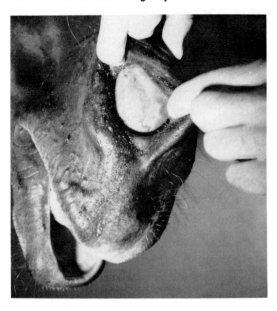

electrosurgery. Because other granulomatous lesions of different etiology and prognosis may have a similar appearance, histopathologic examination is advised. The most frequent postoperative complication following removal of polyps is recurrence.

DISEASES OF THE PHARYNX

G.J. Baker

Diagnostic and Therapeutic Considerations

Various papers have described the functional anatomy of the equine upper respiratory tract.[119,120] It has been emphasized that the integrity of the smoothly streamlined airway is vitally important to enable air flow rates to change from minute volumes of 100 L to over 1000 L during maximal exercise. From the external nares to the larynx, the conducting passages of the upper airway are composed of tubular structures with a mucosal lining designed to minimize air flow turbulence. Most of the nasal chambers have a rigid external skeletal support. However, the nasopharynx is a key segment linking the nasal chambers to the larynx and has rigid support only to its dorsal wall and not the ventral and lateral walls. The nasopharynx, therefore, can be regarded as a potentially weak link in this tubular system, a compliant tube between 2 rigid tubes.

The nasopharynx is separated from the oropharynx by the soft palate. The free border of the soft palate lies beneath the epiglottis, and the horse is unique in that it does not have a common pharynx (except during swallowing). The free border of the soft palate in the horse has a dorsal extension: the palatopharyngeal arch, which forms an important air-tight seal around the rostral margin of the larynx. This arrangement facilitates high-velocity air flow. When the larynx is withdrawn and raised during deglutition, the caudal pharynx and the laryngeal orifice are sealed to enable food to pass through the piriform recesses and enter the esophagus.

Blood supply to the nasopharynx or oropharynx is extensive and provided through the internal and external maxillary arteries. Lymph drainage is directed through the retropharyngeal and cranial cervical lymph nodes. Innervation of the soft palate comes from cranial nerves IX, X and possibly V.

Developmental abnormalities and acquired diseases of the pharynx result in clinical signs of abnormal airway function. In cases of palatine clefts, cysts, ulcers, inflammation, foreign bodies or neurologic disorders, there may be dysphagia, choking, and food exiting the nares.

An accurate history and complete physical examination are the first steps in diagnosis of pharyngeal disease. Fiberoptic endoscopy, radiography, contrast studies, cultures, biopsy and exercise tests yield valuable adjunct information in appropriate cases.

Congenital and Familial Diseases

Pharyngeal Cysts

In young horses, subepiglottic and pharyngeal developmental cysts may cause acute respiratory disease that necessitates emergency tracheostomy before an accurate diagnosis can be achieved. In less dramatic cases, however, subepiglottic and pharyngeal wall cysts cause intermittent respiratory obstruction and dysphagia associated with coughing. Clinical diagnosis can be made by physical, endoscopic and radiographic evaluation.

Such cysts may be developmental, arising from remnants of the thyroglossal duct or as inclusion (follicular) cysts within the fold of the aryepiglottic tissue or soft palate. Treatment should be carried out under general anesthesia. In some cases, resection may be achieved via the oral approach using fiberoptic endoscopy and diathermy. In other cases, a ventral midline pharyngotomy incision rostral to the thyroid cartilage provides access to the subepiglottic tissues for excision. Hemorrhage is controlled by ligation and diathermy.

Diseases With Physical Causes

Pharyngeal Foreign Bodies

Because horses usually are selective feeders, pharyngeal foreign bodies are not common. On occasion, horses that browse rather than graze have small foreign fragments impact within the walls of the oropharynx, soft palate or nasopharynx. Clinical signs follow development of a local obstructive inflammatory process and, in some cases, abscess formation.

As in all cases of obstructive pharyngeal disease, it is important for the clinician to evaluate the extent of airway obstruction and be ready to perform a temporary tracheostomy. Once the airway obstruction has been relieved, clinical signs associated with acute edema, pharyngitis and perilaryngitis can be treated medically with systemic antimicrobials, nonsteroidal anti-inflammatory drugs and diuretics. Subsequent evaluation includes endoscopic and radiographic examination and appropriate surgical exploration to remove foreign bodies or drain retropharyngeal or intrapharyngeal abscesses.

Iatrogenic Trauma

Pharyngeal and perilaryngeal trauma commonly results from overzealous use of nasogastric tubes, particularly in fractious patients. Repeated, overvigorous use of a nasogastric tube in attempting to dislodge an esophageal obstruction can cause the nasogastric tube to penetrate the roof of the nasopharynx, especially at the pharyngeal recess, with the tube entering the guttural pouch. This results in development of a nasopharyngeal-guttural pouch fistula. Similarly, the nasogastric tube may penetrate the laryngopharynx and traverse the structures of the neck parallel to the esophagus. In some cases, signs are not observed until the inflammatory process results in gross cervical cellulitis and obstruction of the thoracic inlet. In the presence of severely traumatized tissue, first-aid therapy is essential to restore airway patency and to achieve ventral drainage. Possible development of septic mediastinitis should be monitored, and high levels of broad-spectrum antimicrobial agents should be given.

Inflammatory, Infectious and Immune Diseases

Pharyngeal Lymphoid Hyperplasia

The more common diagnosis of this condition directly parallels the increasingly more common use of flexible fiberoptic endoscopic equipment on racetracks.[120] Environmental pollution, including that from bacterial and viral pathogens, results in antigenic stimulation of the oral and nasopharynx. The response to such stimulation is proliferation of lymphoid tissue within the pharyngeal recess, ie, the pharyngeal tonsil. From a clinical point of view, it may be of value to stage the severity of the lesion to both qualify and quantify the extent of the infection.[121,122] However, histopathologic evaluation of tissue biopsies from both low-grade pharyngeal lymphoid hyperplasia and extensive proliferative pharyngeal tonsillitis and dorsal pharyngeal wall vesicle formation show there to be only minor differences. Biopsies of both types of tissue show lymphoid hyperplasia, with development of germinative centers. In advanced disease, such changes are associated with mucosal vesicle formation, hemorrhage and ulceration (Fig 21).

It is normal for all horses to exhibit pharyngeal lymphoid hyperplasia during maturation. It perhaps is unfortunate that it is during these formative years that many horses are expected to perform competitively, from the ages of 2 to 4. Though studies have shown changes in the severity of lymphoid hyperplasia in relation to environmental challenges, the effect of these changes on performance of the horse has yet to be documented fully.[123] Endoscopic surveys of large numbers of horses of the same age in training and under the same environmental conditions clearly show individual variation. Some horses with lymphoid hyperplasia perform poorly, while others with similar degrees of pharyngeal inflammation enter the winner's circle. This individual variation may be a result of stimulation of pharyngobronchial reflexes that result in lower airway constriction. It also has been suggested that horses with marked pharyngeal lymphoid hyperplasia producing tenacious mucoid exudate may break stride during exercise (see Dorsal Displacement of the Soft Palate). Various treatments for pharyngeal lymphoid hyperplasia have been tried; these range from rest for 30-60 days in a clean environment, to aggressive surgical therapy.

Systemic and topical antimicrobial drugs have been used alone or in combination with antiinflammatory drugs, such as corticosteroids. However, no studies have been published that quantify the efficacy of these procedures. Immunostimulation and hyperimmunization, using frequent vaccination procedures against viral respiratory diseases, have purportedly reduced the prevalence of pharyngeal lymphoid hyperplasia in the racetrack population. It has been suggested that horses with severe exercise intolerance caused by pharyngeal lymphoid hyperplasia should be managed by pharyngeal cautery, curettage or cryotherapy. Though the efficacy of pharyngeal tonsillectomy, curettage and topical iodine cautery to control advanced pharyngeal lymphoid hyperplasia is being evaluated, no data support these therapies.

Idiopathic Diseases

Dorsal Displacement of the Soft Palate

Dorsal displacement of the soft palate occurs during normal deglutition. Thus, it is a normal phenomenon. If the external nares are occluded, all horses can be induced to displace their soft palate dorsally and produce the characteristic gurgling noise as the horse breathes over the free border of the soft palate obstructing the epiglottis (Fig 22). Numerous disease processes within the pharynx, larynx and lower airway can change the stability of the relationship between the palatopharyngeal arch and larynx. Normal horses running despite painful disorders, such as sore shins, ankles or hocks, also may displace the soft palate dorsally, perhaps in response to pain. During exercise, there may be a caudal retraction of

Figure 21. Endoscopic view of the nasopharyngeal wall shows extensive pharyngeal lymphoid hyperplasia and vesicle formation.

Figure 22. Dorsal displacement of the soft palate.

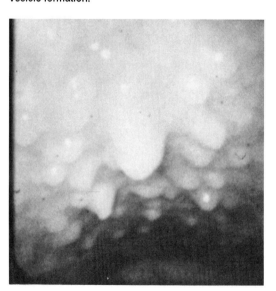

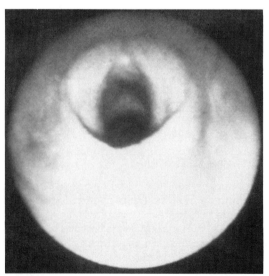

the larynx and dislocation of the larynx from the palatopharyngeal arch. Such diseases as epiglottic hypoplasia, rostral displacement of the palatopharyngeal arch, pharyngeal lymphoid hyperplasia, laryngeal chondroma and chondritis, subepiglottic cysts and epiglottic entrapment may lead to instability of the palatopharyngeal arch and larynx (Fig 23). Therefore, when treating dorsal displacement of the soft palate, all systems of the horse should first be evaluated thoroughly to eliminate specific diseases (Fig 23).

Where other specific disease, such as laryngeal hemiplegia, lower airway hemorrhage, musculoskeletal disease, epiglottic hypoplasia or pharyngeal cyst formation, also is diagnosed, treatment is directed at these diseases. However, an unpublished study showed that in 30% of horses in which exercise intolerance was attributed to dorsal displacement of the soft palate, no specific predisposing disease was found. Therefore, in these cases, management is directed at limiting the ability of the horse to dislocate the larynx.

The tongue tie limits, to a certain degree, caudal retraction of the larynx. Excision of portions of the free border of the soft palate via a midline ventral laryngotomy has been advocated. This may not reduce the ability of the horse to dislocate the larynx at times of maximum air flow, but excising the portion of the soft palate that interferes with air flow at the glottis prevents airway obstruction.

Combination surgery involving soft palate trimming and excision of the ventral neck muscles that cause caudal retraction

of the larynx has a place in treating this disease.[119] With the anesthetized horse positioned in dorsal recumbency and the airway intubated, a ventral midline 12-cm incision is made starting at the cricoid cartilage. By blunt dissection, the hyoid insertion of the ventral throat muscles are divided and retracted caudally. Care is taken to preserve the lingual facial and jugular veins. A 10- to 12-cm section of the sternothyrohyoideus and portions of the omohyoideus muscles are resected. The surgical site should be irrigated with warm saline and all bleeding controlled before skin closure. A 2-cm Penrose drain is placed to facilitate drainage postoperatively. In the postoperative period, the surgery site is hot-packed and massaged daily. Partial dehiscence of the skin wound is not uncommon because of the unavoidable deadspace and potential serum pocketing.

As in all surgical and medical conditions in which the precise significance and etiology of the disease are unknown, it is not surprising that the surgical results of such procedures are difficult to assess. In the author's case, followup was possible in only 48 of 64 cases and, of these, 52% returned to effective performance. This is comparible to results of another study, in which 71% of horses followed benefitted from the operation.[119] Following sternothyrohyoidmyectomy, the horse should be rested for at least 90 days in a clean environment. Thus, it is possible to speculate that the eventual success of surgery is a result of the rest, rather than the surgical procedure.

Pharyngeal Collapse

Pharyngeal collapse, distinct from dorsal displacement of the soft palate, is manifested not as intermittent airway obstruction but rather as permanent nasopharyngeal collapse and inability to swallow normally. Some cases can be caused by neurologic disorders, including complicated guttural pouch mycosis, protozoal encephalitis and botulism. The prognosis with cranial nerve damage is poor because even if the primary lesion is resolved, recovery of pharyngeal nerve function is delayed and incomplete. Aspiration pneumonia is common. (See the chapter on Diseases of the Nervous System for details of diagnosis and therapy.)

Figure 23. Etiopathogenesis of dorsal displacement of the soft palate (DDSP). (From *Current Therapy in Equine Medicine 2,* courtesy of W.B. Saunders)

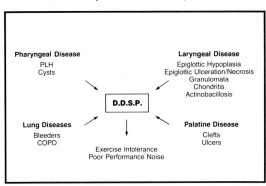

DISEASES OF THE GUTTURAL POUCHES

S.M. Barber

Diagnostic and Therapeutic Considerations

Anatomy

The guttural pouches are diverticula of the eustachian tubes and are unique to equids. The pouches do not communicate but contact one another medially, ventral to the rectus capitus ventralis muscles. Each guttural pouch has a capacity of about 300 ml and is partially divided by the stylohyoid bone. The medial compartment is 2-3 times the size of the lateral compartment and extends more caudal and ventral. Each pouch communicates with the pharynx through a slit-like opening rostroventral to the pharyngeal recess, along the pharyngeal wall. A thin plate of fibrocartilage is located on the medial aspect of the opening. The pharyngeal opening is located near the dorsal aspect of the guttural pouch, and drainage from the pouch is poor unless the head is lowered. The pouches are lined by ciliated epithelium containing glands that predominately produce mucus.[124]

The walls of the guttural pouch are thin and intimately associated with many vital structures, including the pharynx, larynx, esophagus, parotid and mandibular salivary glands and retropharyngeal lymph nodes. The associated neurovascular anatomy is complex (Fig 24). A fold of mucous membrane extending from the roof of the guttural pouch along the caudal aspect of the medial compartment contains the vagus, accessory and sympathetic nerves, cranial cervical ganglion and internal carotid artery. The hypoglossal and glossopharyngeal nerves are associated with the caudolateral aspect of the medial compartment, and the pharyngeal branch of the vagus with the ventral aspect. The external carotid artery and its branches and the facial nerve traverse over the lateral compartment.[124]

The eustachian tubes probably serve to equalize pressure on both sides of the tympanic membrane. The function of the diverticula remains unknown, but the pharyngeal orifice is known to dilate during swallowing.[125] Speculatively, inspired air

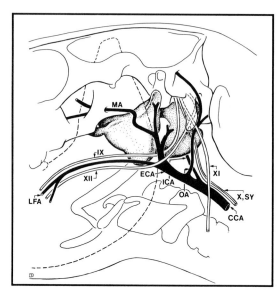

Figure 24. The relationship of the major neurovascular structures to the left guttural pouch. The guttural pouch is illustrated as the stippled area. The position of the left mandible is indicated by the dashed line. The stylohyoid bone partially divides the guttural pouch into a lateral and medial compartment. Common carotid artery (CCA), occipital artery (OA), internal carotid artery (ICA), external carotid artery (ECA), linguofacial artery (LFA), maxillary artery (MA), sympathetic nerve trunk (SY), vagus nerve (X), spinal accessory nerve (XI), hypoglossal nerve (XII), glossopharyngeal nerve (IX).

may be warmed by entering the guttural pouches during expiration or swallowing and may leave the guttural pouch during inspiration.

Surgical Approaches to the Guttural Pouches

The anatomy of the guttural pouch region is complex and may be altered by guttural pouch distention. Therefore, caution must be taken to avoid iatrogenic injury during a surgical approach to the guttural pouch. Once a skin incision is made, the subcutaneous dissection is done bluntly to minimize the risk of neurovascular injury. If the guttural pouch is not markedly distended, locating it may be rather difficult. Placing an endoscope or rigid catheter into the guttural pouch via the pharyngeal openings during surgery can help locate the guttural pouch by feel and illumination. The wall of the normal guttural pouch is thin but, in a diseased state, the wall may be greatly thickened. If the pouch is large and filled with purulent material, its identification is easy. Needle aspiration can be used to identify the pouch; however, care should be used not to perforate any important neurovascular structures, as thickening of the guttural pouch wall by the disease process may make identification of nerves and vessels difficult. The guttural pouch is opened cautiously with scissors at an area of the wall devoid of vessels and nerves, and the opening is enlarged gradually. The edges of the guttural pouch may be grasped with Allis tissue forceps, but caution must be used to prevent injury to local nerves. Likewise, broad-blade retractors, if used, should be applied gently.

The guttural pouches usually are approached surgically to permit removal of purulent material, provide ventral drainage, provide access to the medial septum for fenestration, or provide access to the pharyngeal orifice of the eustachian tube for surgical trimming of the mucosal flaps. There are 3 basic surgical approaches to the guttural pouches (Fig 25).[126] The approach selected depends on the objectives of the surgery, size of the patient and severity of the condition.

Hyovertebrotomy Approach: The hyovertebrotomy approach is a lateral approach to the guttural pouch (Fig 25). It also has been referred as Chabert's approach. If this approach is combined with a ventral approach through Viborg's triangle, it is referred to as Dieterich's approach.

The hyovertebrotomy approach has been used primarily for removal of chondroids and inspissated pus from the guttural pouch. Because the surgical anatomy is complex in this area, the procedure should be performed only with the horse in lateral recumbency under a general anesthetic. A 10- to 12-cm skin incision is made parallel and just cranial to the wing of the atlas and about 4 cm ventral to the base of the ear. The dense fascia over the parotid gland is incised, and the parotid gland and auriculocutaneous muscle are reflected rostrally. The areolar connective tissue deep to the parotid gland is bluntly dissected and the mandibular salivary gland is identified and reflected rostrally. The occipitomandibularis muscle is visible then in the rostral aspect of the incision. This muscle may be divided on the long axis of its muscle fibers or, preferably, retracted out of the surgical

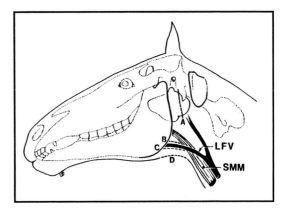

Figure 25. Surgical approaches to the guttural pouches. The hyovertebrotomy approach (A) is dorsolateral, cranial to the wing of the atlas. Viborg's approach (B) is ventrolateral, within the triangle formed by the linguofacial vein (LFV), sternomandibularis muscle (SMM), and vertical ramus of the mandible. The modified Whitehouse approach (C) is paramedian, while the Whitehouse approach (D) is on the ventral midline.

field. The guttural pouch is identified with its overlying internal carotid artery and associated glossopharyngeal, hypoglossal and vagus nerves. The guttural pouch is entered on the caudolateral aspect of the medial compartment rostral to these neurovascular structures.

The advantages of the hyovertebrotomy approach are good access to the guttural pouch for removal of chondroids and inspissated material, even when the guttural pouch is not enlarged very much, and good access to the medial septum. The major disadvantages are that surgery must be performed under general anesthesia, local neurovascular structures are easily damaged, there is poor access to the pharyngeal openings, and ventral drainage is not established.

Viborg's Approach: In Viborg's approach, 3 anatomic structures form triangular surgical borders (Fig 25). The tendinous insertion of the sternomandibularis muscle is located dorsally, the linguofacial vein ventrally and the vertical ramus of the mandible rostrally. A horizontal 6- to 8-cm skin incision is made dorsal to the linguofacial vein. The subcutaneous soft tissue is dissected carefully to avoid the parotid salivary gland and salivary duct. A plane of dissection is established immediately ventral to the external carotid artery until the guttural pouch is reached. The ventral aspect of the medial compartment of the guttural pouch is carefully entered.

The Viborg approach has the advantage of being relatively free of neurovascular structures, as compared to the hyovertebrotomy approach. There is good ventral drainage and, if the guttural pouch is enlarged greatly, this procedure can be done with the horse standing, though lateral recumbency provides greater safety. If the guttural pouch is not greatly enlarged, it may be difficult to locate. Accessibility of the pharyngeal openings and the medial septum is less than that afforded by a ventral Whitehouse approach (see below). In small horses, the triangular borders may limit accessibility to the interior of the guttural pouch. The guttural pouch is opened on the ventral aspect, where injury to the glossopharyngeal and hypoglossal nerves is a danger.

Modified Whitehouse Approach: The modified Whitehouse approach uses a ventral paramedian incision just ventral to the linguofacial vein. Following a 10- to 12-cm longitudinal skin incision, the plane of dissection is established between the sternothyrohyoideus and omohyoideus muscles and linguofacial vein. Blunt dissection is continued in a dorsal direction along the lateral side of the larynx until the enlarged guttural pouch is identified and the ventral aspect of the medial compartment is carefully entered. The dorsal aspects of the guttural pouch and the medial septum can be visualized easily.

The modified Whitehouse approach has the advantage of the best ventral drainage and excellent accessibility to the pharyngeal openings and medial septum. The surgical approach and manipulations are not limited by the size of the patient or regional anatomic structures. If the guttural pouch is very small, its identification may be difficult with this approach. Drainage can be established with the horse standing if the guttural pouch is greatly distended. However, when visualization of internal aspects of the guttural pouch is important, placing the horse in lateral or dorsal recumbency is recommended. Neurologic injury occasionally occurs with this approach.

A midline Whitehouse approach has also been described. Its major advantage is allowing accessibility to both guttural pouches via one ventral midline skin incision while still allowing good ventral drainage. The major disadvantage is that a midline approach necessitates splitting the sternothyrohyoideus and omohyoideus muscles along the midline and their subsequent retraction laterally, which greatly limits surgical access to the interior of the guttural pouch.

Incisions used to approach the guttural pouch are left to heal by second intention, with the exception of the hyovertebrotomy incision, which can be closed by primary intention if a ventral approach was concurrently used and left open for drainage. A catheter can be placed into the guttural pouch through the pharyngeal openings of the eustachian tube and the guttural pouch lavaged daily. Petroleum jelly is applied to surrounding skin to prevent scalding from the discharge. If primary closure of the guttural pouch is attempted in cases of guttural pouch tympany, it is important not to incorporate much of the guttural pouch wall in the closure to avoid incorporating branches of the glossopharyngeal or hypoglossal nerve, subsequently producing neurologic deficits.

In summary, the modified Whitehouse approach is the surgical approach of choice for drainage of the guttural pouch, fenestration of the medial septum, and trimming the mucosal flaps of the pharyngeal openings. If surgery must be performed in a standing horse, an approach via Viborg's triangle is recommended. The hyovertebrotomy approach rarely is useful.

Congenital and Familial Diseases

Tympany

Guttural pouch tympany is the accumulation of a large volume of air within the guttural pouch due to malfunctioning of the pharyngeal orifice of the eustachian tube. The pharyngeal orifice is thought to act as a 1-way valve, allowing air only to enter the guttural pouch.[127-130] The etiology of this condition remains unclear. It may occur secondary to upper respiratory tract infection because of scarring of the orifice, thickening of the mucous membrane, or altered function of the pharyngeal orifice. More commonly, it is considered a congenital abnormality, as it frequently is seen in young foals. There is a much higher incidence of this condition in fillies than in colts.[130] There may be an excessive amount of mucous membrane on the medial lamina of the eustachian tube cartilage, or the salpingopharyngeal fold may be large and redundant.[127,130,131]

A large fluctuant, resonant, nonpainful swelling occurs in the parotid laryngeal area (Fig 26). The location and nature of the swelling are characteristic of this condition. Unilateral involvement is more common, but the external swelling usually appears bilaterally and even can be symmetric with unilateral involvement.[132] Foals may appear normal otherwise, but if the swelling is severe, dyspnea and dysphagia can occur due to displacement of the pharyngeal roof, larynx and proximal trachea by the enlarged guttural pouch.[132] Dysphagia may be evidenced by milk or feed exiting the nares. Aspiration of food into the lungs results in septic pneumonia.

On endoscopic examination, the pharyngeal opening of the eustachian tube appears normal because the excessive plica salpingopharyngea cannot be seen from the pharynx. The dorsal pharynx may appear to be compressed asymmetrically in cases of unilateral tympany. Distortion and displacement of the proximal trachea and larynx are seen in severe cases. Catheterization of the guttural pouches, using a Chambers urinary cannula inserted through the pharyngeal openings, deflates the involved pouch. This helps differentiate a unilateral condition from a bilateral condition before surgical treatment. Alternatively, percutaneous centesis may be used to confirm the diagnosis and determine if the condition is unilateral. This technique carries with it some risk of iatrogenic injury to nerves and blood vessels and introduction of bacteria into the guttural pouch or surrounding tissues. Decompression by percutaneous centesis or catheterization is only transitory.

Radiographs of the guttural pouch show that they are enlarged and filled with gas. If the problem is unilateral, the outline of the normal guttural pouch may be seen. However, if the swelling is severe, the normal pouch may be compressed too severely to be identified. Placing a small amount of contrast material into a guttural pouch may help determine which pouch is involved. A fluid line may be seen in the ventral aspect of the pouch from accumulation of exudate and secondary empyema due to improper guttural pouch drainage. In severe cases, the radiographic silhouette of the nasal pharynx is compressed, and the larynx and proximal cervical trachea displaced.

Conservative treatment with antibiotics, antiinflammatory agents and decompression by indwelling guttural pouch catheters usually is not effective.[133] Surgical treatment is recommended. The method of surgical treatment chosen depends primarily on whether it is a unilateral or bilateral problem. Excision of excessive plica salpingopharyngea with scissors from the guttural pouch side of the pharyngeal opening was the initial treatment recommended for this condition.[132] This surgery is performed with the horse under general anes-

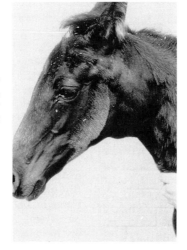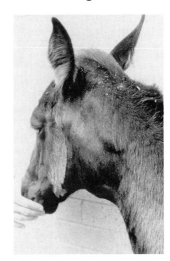

Figure 26. Guttural pouch tympany in a 4-month-old foal showing the characteristic swelling produced by enlargement of the guttural pouch with air.

thesia. Long-handled forceps and scissors are used to remove the excessive fold of mucous membrane. However, a modified Whitehouse approach with the horse in dorsal recumbency is preferred by the author for this procedure. Incomplete removal of the excessive tissue or scarring of the pharyngeal orifice postoperatively can result in recurrence of tympany.[134]

Establishing communication between 2 guttural pouches through the medial septum now is considered the most reliable method of treating unilateral guttural pouch tympany.[127,131] This procedure allows accumulated air to exit via the normal pharyngeal opening of the opposite guttural pouch. Resection of a 3- to 5-cm square portion of the medial septum between the guttural pouches is recommended to prevent closure of the stoma and recurrence.[127,129] A modified Whitehouse approach provides the best exposure. If bilateral tympany is present, fenestration of the medial septum and trimming the membranous flap of the pharyngeal orifice within one of the guttural pouches are recommended. This combined treatment eliminates the need to enter both guttural pouches. Once the membranous flap of the pharyngeal orifice has been trimmed, an indwelling catheter is left in place for several days in an attempt to prevent scarring and closure of the pharyngeal orifice. The surgical incision into the guttural pouch is left to heal as an open wound, and the guttural pouch is lavaged via the indwelling catheter or by introduction of a sterile catheter through the surgical wound. A technique of electrosurgically fenestrating the medial septum using endoscopic instrumentation eliminates the need for surgical exposure.[127]

The prognosis is good for unilateral problems treated by medial septal fenestration. Bilateral tympany has a worse prognosis because of the greater chance of recurrence of tympany following scarring of the pharyngeal opening. This also may predispose the foal to guttural pouch empyema. A guarded prognosis should be given for foals with aspiration pneumonia before surgical treatment. Neurologic injury occasionally occurs with approaches to the guttural pouch and can result in dysphagia and dyspnea. If these are not resolved a few days postoperatively, a grave prognosis is warranted.

Inflammatory, Infectious and Immune Diseases

Empyema

Empyema, the accumulation of exudate within the guttural pouches, is the most common guttural pouch disease. It may occur in horses of any age but is particularly common in younger individuals.[135] It usually occurs secondary to upper respiratory tract infections, especially those associated with beta-hemolytic streptococci.[135] Abscessation of lymph nodes adjacent to the guttural pouch by *Strep equi* (strangles) probably results in drainage of exudate into the guttural pouch in 50% of cases.[136] Accumulation of exudate usually is transitory but occasionally infection may become established, as drainage from the guttural pouch is poor.[127,136] Any disease or treatment that interferes with normal drainage of exudate from the guttural pouch contributes to persistent infection.

The most common clinical sign of guttural pouch empyema is a mucopurulent nasal discharge, often persisting after recovery from an upper respiratory tract infection. Guttural pouch empyema usually is unilateral but results in a bilaterally asymmetric nasal discharge, with a heavier discharge from the naris on the same side as the infected pouch. The discharge may be intermittent and usually increases when the horse lowers its head, allowing greater drainage from the guttural pouch. External pressure on the guttural pouch area when the horse's head is lowered frequently results in a marked increase in discharge.

External enlargement of the guttural pouch region is uncommon, as the guttural pouches can expand a great deal before external enlargement is seen. In chronic empyema, the exudate may become inspissated to develop a cottage cheese-like consistency. Such thickened exudate does not drain well from the guttural pouch, possibly leading to externally visible enlargement. Internal enlargement also can displace the pharynx and soft palate, resulting in dyspnea and dysphagia. In chronic infections, injury to the glossopharyngeal, vagus, accessory and hypoglossal nerves can result in pharyngeal paralysis, dyspnea and dysphagia. Rupture of the guttural pouch or abscessation of associated lymph nodes can produce regional swelling and cellulitis. Epistaxis is uncommon following guttural pouch empyema, but a few flecks of blood may be present in the discharge due to mucosal erosion or from injury to the guttural pouch wall at the site of abscess rupture.

Endoscopic examination of the pharyngeal openings of the eustachian tubes is an important part of the examination. A discharge of mucopurulent material from the pharyngeal opening strongly suggests guttural pouch empyema. However, a mucoid discharge at the pharyngeal openings can be seen with pharyngitis and upper respiratory tract infections in the absence of guttural pouch empyema. Guttural pouch empyema can occur without any discharge from the pharyngeal openings.

Discharge may be demonstrated by pressure applied externally over the guttural pouches, by lowering the horse's head with the aid of tranquilization, or by dilating the pharyngeal opening by introduction of a catheter into the guttural pouch. A small Chambers urinary cannula or an artificial insemination pipette with a bent end is useful for this purpose. Either of these can be placed into the guttural pouch blindly or with the aid of an endoscope. It is easiest to enter the guttural pouch opening at the most dorsal aspect of the cartilage flap. Aspiration of mucopurulent material from the pouch helps confirm the diagnosis and allows retrieval of material for culture, sensitivity tests and cytologic examination. If no material can be aspirated through the catheter, the sample may be obtained by lavage with a sterile solution.

Percutaneous centesis of the guttural pouch is also possible. The appropriate site is 5-8 cm ventral to the base of the ear and half the distance between the mandible and the wing of the atlas. A 5- or 8-cm needle is inserted perpendicular to the overlying skin. If the stylohyoid bone is contacted, the needle is moved caudally into the medial compartment of the guttural pouch. Aspiration of fluid or air confirms correct placement of the needle. This procedure can be used for diagnosis and to obtain exudate samples for culture and sensitivity tests. The complex anatomy of the region and possibility of displaced anatomic structures secondary to guttural pouch infection make

neurovascular injury a possible complication of this technique.

Radiographic examination of the guttural pouch can be an important diagnostic aid.[128] A standing lateral projection is most useful in evaluating general pouch size, shape and contents. The guttural pouch normally is filled with air, and exudate within the guttural pouch creates a distinct fluid line. If the guttural pouch is completely filled with exudate, it acquires the same density as soft tissue. Some irregularity to the density may occur dorsally due to mixing of gas with exudate. Chondroids are inspissated concretions that can form with chronic guttural pouch infection. Chondroids may produce an irregular pattern to the fluid line identified on radiographic examination. Because the guttural pouches are superimposed upon each other in a lateral radiographic projection, obtaining oblique views or instilling contrast medium occasionally is necessary to identify the involved pouch.

Acute empyema may respond rapidly to treatment with systemic antibiotics for several days. If drainage persists or the condition is chronic when identified, insertion of indwelling catheters into the guttural pouches for daily lavage is indicated. Lavage is performed 2-3 times per day with 500 ml of fluid. After the guttural pouch has been lavaged, the horse's head must remain in a lowered position to assist natural drainage; this can be expedited by tranquilizing the horse or by placing the horse's feed on the ground. Many lavage fluids have been used, including solutions of sterile saline, antimicrobials and antiseptics. Irritating solutions must not be used, as they may produce neurologic damage.[135] Culture and sensitivity tests of the exudate are important to select appropriate antimicrobials to use topically and systemically. Systemic antimicrobial therapy is indicated concurrently with lavage.

Surgical drainage of the guttural pouch is indicated if: the discharge persists several days after lavaging the guttural pouch; inspissated material or chondroids cannot be removed by lavage; dyspnea or dysphagia are present; or regional infection and cellulitis are present.

Exudate can be removed via several surgical approaches as discussed above. The objective of surgical treatment is complete removal of all exudate. Once the pouch is entered, a spoon or curette and liberal lavage are used to remove the foreign material. Retention of semi-solid material within the pouch may predispose to recurrence. Gentle handling of the pouch wall is important to prevent iatrogenic neurovascular injury. The surgical incision usually is left to heal as an open wound to provide drainage and because of contamination of regional soft tissues during removal of the exudate. After surgery, the guttural pouch should be lavaged daily through the surgical site or through a catheter placed into the guttural pouch via the pharyngeal opening. The prognosis is good if the condition is diagnosed early and treated aggressively. The prognosis is poor if neurologic signs are present, as reflux of water and ingesta from the external nares, coughing, aspiration pneumonia, reinfection of the guttural pouches, and chronic weight loss are likely.

Mycosis

Guttural pouch mycosis is a fungal infection of the guttural pouch wall that often interferes with various neurovascular structures closely associated with the wall (Fig 24).[127,137-139] There appears to be no breed or sex predisposition.[140] The condition is the most common guttural pouch abnormality seen in the United Kingdom.[127] It appears to be more sporadic in North America.

Mycotic infection of the guttural pouch usually is unilateral. The fungus *Aspergillus nidulans* commonly is incriminated as the cause; however, the specific etiologic agent sometimes is not identified.[140,141] The mycotic growth usually occurs on the roof of the medial compartment of the guttural pouch wall, over the petrous temporal bone and the distal segment of the internal carotid artery. The mycotic infection can spread from this location deeper into the guttural pouch wall to affect neurovascular structures, or it may extend over a larger area of the guttural pouch wall or to an alternate location within the guttural pouch. The mycotic lesion appears as a necrotic diphtheritic membrane that is raised from the surface of the guttural pouch wall and is brown, yellow, green or black and white.

The pathogenesis of this condition remains unclear. Guttural pouch mycosis probably is an opportunistic infection requiring appropriate environmental conditions or predisposing factors for its development. In the United Kingdom, this condition occurs almost exclusively in horses housed indoors;[138] this environment may play a role in development of guttural pouch mycoses.[140] It is interesting that the lesion typically has a very discrete and specific location over the internal carotid artery. An aneurysm of the internal carotid artery at the site of mycotic development may provide a suitable environment for infection.[142] The pathogenesis for development of an aneurysm within the distal aspect of the internal carotid artery is unknown.

Some cases of guttural pouch mycosis are asymptomatic.[127] A wide range of clinical signs can be seen, depending on which neurovascular structures are involved.[137] Epistaxis, the most common clinical sign, usually occurs at rest and may be preceded by a slight mucoid nasal discharge.[138] Mycotic infection usually is unilateral but causes bilateral epistaxis, with most of the hemorrhage exiting the nostril on the affected side. The degree of epistaxis can vary from mild, with a few trickles of blood from the nostril, to very severe bleeding leading to exsanguination. The blood usually is bright red, suggesting arterial origin.

Several bouts of epistaxis usually occur over several days to several weeks. A large percentage of affected horses die of fatal hemorrhage if the condition is untreated; however, death does not usually occur during the first episode of epistaxis. With severe hemorrhage, the guttural pouch occasionally becomes filled with blood, resulting in external enlargement. Drainage of large amounts of blood into the pharynx can cause the horse to swallow blood or aspirate blood into the lower respiratory tract, resulting in foamy blood at the nostrils. Severe acute blood loss leads to hypovolemic shock. The origin of the hemorrhage almost always is from the internal carotid artery, which has been eroded by the fungal lesion at the roof of the guttural pouch, where the internal carotid artery enters the petrous temporal bone. The external carotid artery or other arteries associated with the guttural pouch wall are involved occasionally.

Dysphagia is the second most common clinical sign of guttural pouch mycosis. This results from loss of function of pharyngeal branches of the vagus and glossopharyngeal nerves. Dysphagia may occur suddenly or develop slowly after a period of coughing and nasal discharge.[138] Injury to the nerves results from inflammation and infiltration by the fungal mycelia or from the nerves' becoming entrapped in scar tissue. Other clinical signs seen, in order of decreasing frequency, are parotid pain, abnormal head posture, nasal catarrh, head shyness, abnormal respiratory noise, sweating and shivering, Horner's syndrome, colic and facial paralysis.[138] Signs can be explained by erosion of blood vessels, local pain, paralysis of cranial nerves, and paralysis or stimulation of the sympathetic trunk. (See the chapter on Diseases of the Nervous System for further discussion of this subject.)

Endoscopic examination is important in confirming guttural pouch mycosis. Laryngeal hemiplegia, dorsal displacement of the soft palate or collapse of the pharyngeal roof caused by neurologic injury may be seen. The absence of hemorrhage at the pharyngeal openings does not rule out the guttural pouch as a source of hemorrhage. Blood exiting the eustachian tube openings strongly suggests guttural pouch mycosis, but a definitive diagnosis can be made only by endoscopic examination of the interior of the guttural pouch. This examination should not be performed until the bleeding stops and the horse's condition stabilizes. Then it is safe to introduce the endoscope into the guttural pouch without great risk of inducing further hemorrhage.

Passing a uterine infusion catheter or small Chambers urinary catheter with a bent tip into the eustachian tube opening provides dilation for introduction of the endoscope. Alternatively, biopsy forceps within the endoscope can be extended through their portal on the endoscope tip and inserted into the pouch ahead of the endoscope, thus acting as a guide wire. The guttural pouch usually is only partially filled with blood. The walls of the pouch should be examined thoroughly for the source of the hemorrhage and any mycotic lesion. Mycotic lesions usually are fairly distinct, diphtheritic growths located on the dorsal roof of the medial compartment over the internal carotid artery. The external carotid artery as it passes over the lateral compartment should be examined as a possible source of arterial bleeding.[143]

Radiographs of the guttural pouches may show partial or complete filling of the guttural pouch with a fluid density. Radiographs usually are not necessary for diagnostic purposes, but bony lesions have been reported.[137,140] Angiography can be used to demonstrate aneurysms of the internal and external carotid arteries.[140,142]

Stabilization of the patient is the most important facet of treatment for acute guttural pouch hemorrhage. Usually the initial hemorrhagic episode is not fatal. The horse should be confined and observed closely while awaiting spontaneous remission of bleeding. If blood loss is severe, the horse may become markedly hypovolemic and anemic. Volume replacement with fluids or blood may be necessary, particularly if anesthesia and surgical treatment are anticipated. Antibiotics are indicated if dysphagia is present and feed or blood has been aspirated into the lungs. Aspiration of feed or blood predisposes to septic pneumonia. Blood clots in the guttural pouch also predispose to secondary infections.

Numerous medications have been used in treatment of guttural pouch mycosis. Topical and systemic antifungal agents, topical enzymes and corticosteroids, dilute organic iodine compounds and other agents have been used in various treatment regimens.[127,142-147] The effectiveness of these compounds remains controversial, based on subjective evaluation. Part of the problem in evaluating the response to treatment of guttural pouch mycosis is that some horses have spontaneous resolution of the disease.[138] The location of the mycotic mass and the type of organism involved pose difficulties in medical management. The lesions are infiltrative, and topical agents alone usually are not effective in resolving the infection. Also, the lesion is located in the dorsal aspect of the guttural pouch, limiting contact of any topical agent with the mycotic mass. Placing the horse in dorsal recumbency at periodic treatment intervals has been suggested as a means of increasing contact time. Powders have been recommended, as they may be sprayed onto the mycotic mass and may adhere better than solutions. Also, nebulization of antifungal agents has been suggested as a means of better topical contact.

Aspergillus has been reported to be the most common fungus isolated from guttural pouch mycosis, but other fungi have been isolated.[139] The choice of antifungal agent should be based on identification of the specific fungus involved. When epistaxis is of major concern, biopsy of the mycotic mass should be discouraged for fear of initiating fatal hemorrhage.[143]

Most of the drugs commonly recommended are not effective against *Aspergillus* or are very expensive and may be quite toxic. Amphotericin B and ketoconazole are effective against *Aspergillus*, but the former is relatively toxic and both are rather expensive. Griseofulvin can be absorbed from the GI tract and is excreted and deposited in keratin but is not effective against mycelial fungi, such as *Aspergillus*. Nystatin is not absorbed from the GI tract but can be used topically. However, it is not effective against *Aspergillus*. Thiabendazole also has been used but without evidence of efficacy against *Aspergillus*.[148,149]

Aspergillus may be a secondary invader when predisposing conditions occur within the guttural pouch. Therefore, the need for topical or systemic antifungal agents is questionable. Recently, the use of systemic antifungal agents has been thought to be inappropriate. When aneurysm of the internal carotid artery is not present, ventilation of the guttural pouches is thought to be important in eliminating the predisposing factors that result in mycotic infection.[140] Placement of a catheter within the eustachian tube opening may lead to remission of the mycotic infection.

Surgical treatment of guttural pouch mycosis can be challenging due to the location and nature of the lesion. Surgical treatment has been attempted primarily because of the high incidence of fatal hemorrhage. Surgical removal of the mycotic mass via entry into the guttural pouch has resulted in fatal hemorrhage following rupture of the internal carotid artery.[150] Removal of the mycotic mass is not recommended, as spontaneous remission of the mycotic lesion appears to occur following occlusion of the underlying carotid artery.[141] Ligation of the internal carotid artery on the cardiac side of the lesion has been inadequate in preventing fatal hemorrhage, as retrograde bleeding can occur via collateral circulation from the circle of Willis.[143,147,151,152] The location

of the mycotic lesion at the base of the skull virtually prevents surgical access to the distal segment of the internal carotid artery via intradiverticular or extradiverticular approaches. Neurologic damage and severe hemorrhage have been reported following attempts to ligate the internal carotid artery distal to the mycotic mass.[145,151] Occlusion of the internal carotid artery on both sides of the lesion currently is considered necessary to prevent retrograde bleeding.[143,145,151,153,154]

A technique of intravascular occlusion has been developed for occlusion of the internal carotid artery on both sides of the arterial lesion.[153,154] An incision is made at the wing of the atlas, similar to that for the hyovertebrotomy approach (see above). The origin of the internal carotid artery is identified and ligated, and a balloon-tipped catheter is passed distally in the internal carotid artery until the balloon tip lies distal to the mycotic lesion. The catheter's balloon tip is inflated, and the catheter is secured and left in place for several days. This causes permanent thrombosis of the internal carotid artery. This technique has been successful in eliminating fatal postoperative hemorrhage.[141] Single ligation of the artery proximal to the lesion has a higher incidence of single or repeated postoperative hemorrhage and a significant incidence of fatal hemorrhage.[147,152]

Mycotic lesions also can occur over the external carotid artery, and this artery may be a source of arterial hemorrhage.[143] Identification of the specific vessel involved in hemorrhage should be attempted endoscopically or with angiography. The external carotid artery is not an end artery, and retrograde hemorrhage may occur following ligation on the cardiac side of the lesion.[143] Access to the distal aspect of the external carotid artery for distal ligation is very difficult. The technique of proximal ligation and distal occlusion by intravascular balloon-tipped catheter has been adapted to lesions of the external carotid artery.[141,143] The central retinal artery arises from the external ophthalmic artery, a branch of the maxillary artery. Blindness has been reported following occlusion of the external carotid artery.[143] Determining the appropriate location and depth of insertion of the intravascular catheter intraoperatively is difficult.[141] A new technique using dual occlusion of the external carotid artery by 2 balloon-tipped catheters has been reported.[155] This technique should eliminate much of the uncertainty involved in proper placement of a catheter down the external carotid artery.

When epistaxis is associated with a guttural pouch mycotic lesion, occlusion of the affected artery both proximal and distal to the lesion is indicated to prevent fatal hemorrhage. When this has been achieved, prognosis for survival is good. However, in patients that exhibit signs of cranial nerve dysfunction before or after surgical treatment, the prognosis for complete recovery is poor. The severity of the neurologic deficit may necessitate humane destruction.

DISEASES OF THE LARYNX

J.I. Cahill and B.E. Goulden

Congenital and Familial Diseases

Rostral Displacement of the Palatopharyngeal Arch

Rostral displacement of the palatopharyngeal arch is a recently recognized disease of the equine upper respiratory tract.[8,156,157] The palatopharyngeal arch is a fold of mucous membrane that extends from the caudal pillars of the soft palate along the lateral pharyngeal wall, uniting immediately dorsal to the esophageal opening. In the normal horse, the arch lies just caudal to the apices of the arytenoid cartilages. In the condition known as rostral displacement of the palatopharyngeal arch, this fold of mucous membrane is displaced rostrally to overlie the apices of the arytenoid cartilages (Figs 27, 28).

Clinical Signs: Clinical signs vary considerably between individual horses with rostral displacement of the palatopharyngeal arch. An abnormal inspiratory noise and exercise intolerance appear to be consistent features of the disease, while dysphagia, regurgitation of food, and persistent coughing also may be observed.[8,156,157]

Diagnosis: Endoscopic examination of the larynx reveals the rostrally displaced palatopharyngeal arch, obscuring the normal view of the apices of the arytenoid cartilages (Figs 27, 28). The fold of tissue may cover the apex of one or both cartilages and may appear larger than normal.[156,158] While the arytenoid cartilages move actively during respiration, the range of abduction appears to be limited.[156]

A slight fold of palatopharyngeal arch overlying the arytenoid apices is seen in some horses without any clinical evidence of disease. This situation is seen more commonly than the clinically evident condition and should not be misinterpreted as a cause of laryngeal dysfunction.[158]

Pathogenesis: Bilaterally symmetric abnormalities of laryngeal anatomy are present in this condition.[156,157] The cricopharyngeal muscles are absent and the

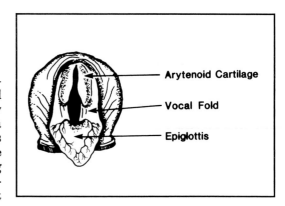

Figure 27. Line drawing of the equine larynx, showing the normal endoscopic appearance of the arytenoid cartilages and vocal fold. (From *Practice of Large Animal Surgery,* courtesy of W.B. Saunders)

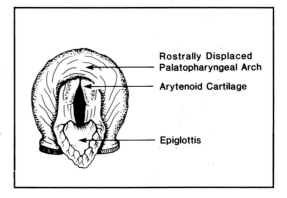

Figure 28. Line drawing of the endoscopic view of the equine larynx, showing rostral displacement of the palatopharyngeal arch, obscuring the apices of the arytenoid cartilages. (From *Practice of Large Animal Surgery,* courtesy of W.B. Saunders)

thyroid cartilage is deformed. No crico-thyroid articulations exist.

The etiology of the condition remains obscure, though it has been suggested that the anomaly is due to aberrant development of the fourth branchial arch.[156]

The abnormal respiratory noise associated with this disorder does not result from recurrent laryngeal nerve disease.[156, 157] Apparently it is caused by mechanical limitations on arytenoid abduction by the abnormally shaped thyroid cartilage or the overlying fold of palatopharyngeal arch.[156,157]

Treatment: While resection of a wedge of tissue from the displaced palatopharyngeal arch has been described as a possible method of correction of this condition, the associated anatomic abnormalities of the larynx make successful application of this procedure unlikely.[158]

Inflammatory, Infectious and Immune Diseases

Arytenoid Chondritis

Arytenoid chondritis is a chronic, progressive inflammatory disease of adult horses that results in laryngeal obstruction. The left and/or right arytenoid areas may be involved in what appears endoscopically as a diffuse, irregular swelling of the arytenoid cartilage and surrounding mucosa.

Clinical Signs: Horses with arytenoid chondritis usually have a history of persistent excessive respiratory noise at rest and/or at exercise. The signs are often gradual in onset and progressively worsen with time. Dyspnea and heaving respiration are seen in advanced cases. Chronic nonproductive coughing also may be present. The clinical signs, particularly in earlier stages of the disease, may be very similar to those of laryngeal hemiplegia.

Diagnosis: Endoscopic examination of the laryngeal area is the primary aid in diagnosis of arytenoid chondritis (Fig 29). There usually is medial displacement of a swollen arytenoid, with little or no respiratory movement. The affected area often is misshapen, and the normal roughened appearance of the mucosa overlying the corniculate portion of the arytenoid cartilage may appear smooth.[159] Often, however,

there are focal lesions projecting into the laryngeal lumen from the mucosal surface.[160] Contact lesions may be seen on the apposing cartilage, generally appearing as mucosal erosions.[160] In advanced cases, there may be almost complete occlusion of the glottis, making visualization of the lesions difficult. It is important, particularly in early left-sided cases, not to confuse the endoscopic findings with those of laryngeal hemiplegia. Features that help differentiate the 2 diseases are the mucosal projections and distortion of the arytenoid cartilages in arytenoid chondritis.

Diagnosis of arytenoid chondritis can be aided by palpation of the larynx and radiography. On palpation, the larynx may be firmer than normal. Also, firm compression of the larynx may produce dyspnea and an abnormal respiratory noise at rest.[161] Radiography frequently reveals calcification of the area over the dorsum of the larynx and of the arytenoid cartilages.[159,161] This calcification appears to be a characteristic change in chronic disorders involving the laryngeal cartilages and their surrounding tissues. This should not be confused with calcification of the thyroid cartilage that occurs as a consequence of aging.

Pathogenesis: The pathogenesis of arytenoid chondritis is unknown. A traumatic origin, such as inhaled or swallowed foreign bodies, has been suggested.[162] This is supported by an association between other inflammatory disorders of the nasopharynx and this disease.[162,163] However, a

Figure 29. Line drawing of the endoscopic view of the equine larynx in arytenoid chondritis. Note the swollen, distorted right arytenoid cartilage.

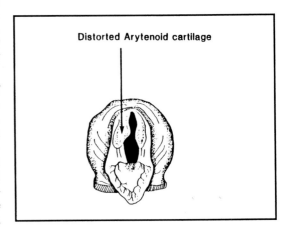

Distorted Arytenoid cartilage

traumatic cause does not explain why the disease is not observed in young horses.

Pathologic findings in affected larynges are consistent with a chronic inflammatory process involving the arytenoid cartilage and surrounding tissues, including the laryngeal mucosa and dorsal muscular structures.[159,160,164] Recurrent inflammation apparently leads to irregular enlargement and fibrous tissue infiltration of the affected cartilage, resulting in the space-occupying lesion of the laryngeal airway.[160]

Treatment: Two techniques have been described for treatment of arytenoid chondritis, the choice of treatment depending on the severity of obstruction to the airway and future use of affected horses.

The first, less invasive approach involves excision of projecting lesions on the arytenoid cartilages, curettage of sinus tracts within the cartilage, and ventriculectomy.[160] This procedure is said to be transiently and moderately successful in mildly affected animals with dyspnea only during exercise, limited airway compromise and only partial interference with arytenoid function.[165]

The operation is performed with the horse in dorsal recumbency and under general anesthesia. A ventral laryngotomy incision is made through the cricothyroid ligament to expose the affected arytenoid cartilage. Any firm projections of cartilage are removed by sharp dissection to a level below the mucosal surface. Granulating lesions, including contact lesions of the opposite cartilage, are examined for sinus tracts. Any such tracts are curetted with a small bone curette, and surrounding granulation tissue removed. In addition, a ventriculectomy is performed on the affected side.[160] The ventral laryngotomy is not closed, and the wound is cleaned daily. The horse is returned to work after endoscopic examination confirms healing of the surgical sites, usually 45-60 days postoperatively. One investigator reported a 50% success rate with this technique in selected cases, though he qualified the claim by stating that it is only transiently effective due to the progressive nature of arytenoid chondritis.[165]

The surgical treatment of choice for arytenoid chondritis is subtotal or partial arytenoidectomy. This procedure is indicated in horses that are dyspneic at rest or in which athletic performance is required.

This more extensive technique has been described by many authors.[160,165-168] Arytenoidectomy is not a new procedure, and methods for total, partial and subtotal arytenoidectomy have been described. Total arytenoidectomies were first performed late in the 19th century but were associated with unacceptable complications of dysphagia and pneumonia; thus, the partial and subtotal modifications were devised.

In partial arytenoidectomy, all of the cartilage is resected except for the muscular process. In the subtotal method, the corniculate portion of the cartilage is retained but the muscular process may or may not be preserved. Results of subtotal arytenoidectomies apparently are the most satisfactory, as they produce the least complications and least respiratory noise postoperatively.[160,167] Coughing and dysphagia are seen postoperatively but, according to Haynes, are of no clinical significance.[165] However, the possible complication of subclinical aspiration pneumonia in association with these sequelae should not be ignored.[167]

Arytenoidectomy is recommended for individuals with a severely compromised airway. Even in bilateral cases, usually only a unilateral arytenoidectomy is performed.[165] Though generally only considered to be a salvage procedure, it allows some return of exercise capacity in some horses.[160,166,167]

To perform a subtotal arytenoidectomy, the horse is anesthetized, and a cuffed endotracheal tube is placed through a midcervical tracheotomy incision. In severe cases of arytenoid chondritis, a tracheotomy tube should be inserted in the midcervical trachea under local anesthesia before surgery. The horse is placed in dorsal recumbency with the neck extended. The affected arytenoid is approached through a ventral midline incision that transects the cricothyroid membrane and cricoid ring. If increased exposure is required, the body of the thyroid cartilage or the first 1-2 tracheal rings also may be divided. However, the least possible interference with the circumferential integrity of the larynx and trachea is desirable. The surgery can be performed in some horses through a simple laryngotomy incision. Self-retraining retractors are placed in the laryngeal wound and the trachea immediately caudal to the larynx is packed with a moist towel.

Once the arytenoid cartilage is adequately exposed, sterile saline may be injected submucosally to help elevate the mucosa over the part of the arytenoid cartilage to be removed. An L-shaped mucosal incision is made along the caudal and ventral margins of the cartilage and the mucosa is elevated by blunt dissection (Fig 30). Attachments on the lateral surface of the cartilage are freed using a combination of sharp and blunt dissection. The exposed cartilage is transected vertically, leaving a 4- to 6-mm rim of corniculate cartilage in place. Then the body of the arytenoid cartilage is grasped with tumor-holding forceps to assist in the final dissection. The muscular process is transected close to the cricoarytenoid articulation or, in some cases, disarticulated, and the arytenoid cartilage is removed. A ventriculectomy may be performed subsequently.

Hemorrhage is minimized by dissecting as close to the cartilage as possible and controlled with electrocautery. Primary closure of the mucosal incision has been recommended to minimize postoperative swelling, allow faster healing and avoid excessive granulation.[165,167] However, evidence suggests that other postoperative complications, including suture granulomas, wound breakdown, submucosal hematomas and upper airway obstruction, are less likely if the mucosa is not closed.[169] The incision in the cricoid cartilage and tracheal rings may be sutured, while the rest of the ventral laryngotomy is left to heal by granulation. The endotracheal tube is removed and a

Figure 30. Diagram showing the ventral approach to the larynx for subtotal arytenoidectomy. The cricoid cartilage and first tracheal rings have been incised. The solid black line indicates the site of the mucosal incision for dissection of the arytenoid cartilage.

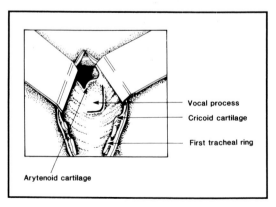

Vocal process

Cricoid cartilage

First tracheal ring

Arytenoid cartilage

tracheotomy tube inserted into the tracheotomy incision.

In the immediate postoperative period, feed is withheld. It is then offered at ground level to minimize feed's entering the larynx and trachea. Antibiotics and phenylbutazone are given for 5 days postoperatively and the tracheotomy tube changed daily or as required.[165] The wound and tracheotomy tube are cleaned and the tube is checked for patency once or twice daily. Endoscopic examination allows monitoring of healing and determines the time of removal of the tracheotomy tube, usually about 5 days after surgery.

Postoperative complications of dysphagia and aspiration pneumonia are not as common as in partial arytenoidectomies, probably because of the increased protection for the laryngeal opening provided by the retained corniculate cartilage.

While the prognosis for return to full exercise potential is very guarded, usually there is sufficient improvement of laryngeal diameter for increased usefulness of the horse.[159,160,170,171]

Neoplasia

Laryngeal neoplasms are covered fully in other sections of this chapter and in the chapter on Diseases of the Alimentary System.

Idiopathic Diseases

Laryngeal Hemiplegia

Cause: Laryngeal hemiplegia is an important and incurable condition caused by damage to the recurrent laryngeal nerve.[172,173] In a small percentage of cases, the underlying cause can be determined. These causes include irritant perivascular and perineural injections, cervical trauma, guttural pouch mycosis, neoplasia, organophosphate intoxication, lead poisoning and plant poisoning.[174-179] However, usually the cause remains unknown; the term idiopathic laryngeal hemiplegia describes these cases.

The idiopathic form of this disease is characterized by polyneuropathy.[172] What initiates the neuropathy is unknown, but it affects mainly large-diameter myelinated fibers in long nerves. The left recurrent laryngeal nerve is the longest nerve in horses; the distal end of this nerve is damaged initially. The neuropathy is chronic in nature and, as the disease progresses, more proximal regions of the left recurrent laryngeal nerve and distal regions of the next-longest nerve (right recurrent laryngeal) become affected. Other peripheral nerves and central long neural fibers eventually may become involved.[172]

The left recurrent laryngeal nerve provides motor innervation to the left intrinsic laryngeal muscles, with the exception of the cricothyroid. Nerve fiber damage at its distal end results in atrophy of these muscles. When sufficient nerve fibers become involved, atrophy of the dorsal cricoarytenoid muscle becomes significant. This, in turn, causes loss of muscular control of arytenoid cartilage movements. At exercise, abduction of this cartilage is compromised, and negative respiratory pressures may suck the uncontrolled cartilage into the laryngeal lumen. This increases airway resistance, creates turbulence and increases the workload of breathing. These impairments are manifested clinically as an abnormal respiratory noise at exercise and interference with athletic performance.

Because the main degenerative changes in the idiopathic form of this disease occur in the left recurrent laryngeal nerve, the hemiplegia always affects the left side of the larynx. Unilateral right-sided laryngeal hemiplegia is unrelated to the idiopathic form of the disease and usually is due to traumatic damage to the right recurrent laryngeal nerve or to right-sided guttural pouch mycosis.[174]

An important feature of laryngeal hemiplegia is that a substantial proportion of apparently normal horses have pathologic changes characteristic of the idiopathic form of the disease in their laryngeal muscles and nerves.[173,180] The significance of these changes in relation to asynchronous movements of the arytenoid cartilage is discussed in the section on diagnosis.

Incidence: Laryngeal hemiplegia, long referred to as "roaring," is of particular significance in young performance horses of the larger breeds. Though the clinical prevalence of the disease in these horses is not accurately known, histologic evidence of its existence in a substantial proportion of Thoroughbreds indicates that it must be one of the most common pathologic syndromes described in horses.[180]

The disease occurs about 6 times more frequently in males than females.[181,182] In Thoroughbred foals, the pathologic changes characteristic of laryngeal hemiplegia are minor and probably insufficient to cause clinical disease.[180] These changes, however, increase in prevalence and severity during adolescent life and become associated with clinical signs in the youthful animal.[180] Many veterinarians believe that clinical signs usually appear after 3 years of age.[174,176,178,182] However, a study in Thoroughbreds, which included a statistical comparison of the age distribution of the population from which affected horses were taken, indicated that the relative risk of laryngeal hemiplegia in this breed was greatest at their earliest racing age of 2 years.[181]

Over many years, veterinarians have considered long-necked and tall horses predisposed to the disease. Evidence of the close relationship between the pathologic changes characteristic of this disease and long nerve fibers in the recurrent laryngeal nerve supports this contention.[172] At present, there is no evidence that the idiopathic form of the disease exists in ponies.

A hereditary predisposition to laryngeal hemiplegia has long been suspected. While the majority of evidence implicating inheritance is anecdotal, some scientific reports support an inherited basis for the disease.[183] At the present time, there is insufficient evidence to deduce the exact mode of inheritance of laryngeal hemiplegia. Its prevalence in certain family lines strongly suggests that inherited factors play an important role in this disease. However, the possibility of this occurring as a result of heritable conformational characteristics, such as long neck length and large body size, cannot be dismissed.[184]

Clinical Signs: Most horses with laryngeal hemiplegia are presented because of increased respiratory noise at exercise.[174,181,185] The loudness and pitch of the respiratory sound vary considerably between affected horses. In some, a coarse sawing noise can be heard, while others make a soft whistling sound.

The other major presenting sign of laryngeal hemiplegia is poor performance or exercise intolerance. Coughing, choking or gasping is seen in some affected horses.[176,181] Whether these signs result from medial displacement of the arytenoid cartilage or laryngopalatal dislocation is not known.

Some affected horses have impaired vocalilization. The neigh may become quieter or more hoarse.[181,185]

The onset of clinical signs is extremely variable, from sudden abnormal respiratory noise in some exercising horses, to an almost imperceptible increase in the inspiratory noise occurring over several weeks or months. It is interesting that the first signs of laryngeal hemiplegia frequently are noticed when a horse is put into training initially or when it returns to training after a period of inactivity.[181,186]

Diagnosis: A meticulous and methodical diagnostic routine is required to differentiate this disease from other obstructive respiratory disorders, many of which have similar clinical signs. An adequate history should be obtained. This should include the age at which the abnormality was first noted, the horse's activity at the onset of signs, whether the respiratory noise is progressively worsening with time, any adverse effect on athletic performance, any other health problems the horse may have had in the past, and any changes in the voice.

Horses with suspected laryngeal hemiplegia should be examined at rest and, if the diagnosis is still in doubt, during and immediately after exercise.

At rest, a thorough physical examination should be done to rule out other disorders that may affect performance and detect signs of injury along the course of the recurrent laryngeal nerve. This should be followed by examination of the respiratory system, as roaring is frequently complicated by other respiratory diseases.[181] Finally, the larynx should be thoroughly examined by endoscopy and palpation.

Endoscopy is the most useful diagnostic aid for detection of this disease. In laryngeal paresis or hemiplegia, there usually is displacement of the arytenoid cartilage toward the midline (Figs 27, 31), shortening of the vocal fold and kinking of the aryepiglottic fold. Abduction of the arytenoid cartilage may be completely absent or reduced when compared with that on the other side. Some affected horses have a compensatory increase in the degree of abduction on the unaffected side.[174,185] Unfortunately, similar endoscopic changes may occur in other diseases of the larynx, such as arytenoid chondritis and congenital malformations.[156,187,188] In the case of chondritis, careful endoscopic examination may reveal arytenoid distortion and mucosal erosions, but most congenital conditions may only be differentiated from laryngeal hemiplegia by biopsy, surgery or necropsy.

The diagnosis of idiopathic laryngeal hemiplegia becomes uncertain when degrees of partial paralysis of the intrinsic laryngeal muscles are present. In normal horses, the degree or timing of arytenoid movements should be similar on both sides. Unfortunately, many horses show very little movement of the arytenoid cartilages at rest, fixing their arytenoids during both inspiration and expiration. These horses can be made to abduct their arytenoids by inducing them to swallow and adduct the arytenoids by applying the laryngeal adductor (slap) test.[189] Swallowing can be induced by introducing several milliliters of fluid into the area via an endoscope. Swallowing causes brief but full abduction of the arytenoids in normal horses. Similarly, slapping the withers on alternate sides during expiration may stimulate instantaneous arytenoid adduction.

Because a substantial proportion of horses have pathologic evidence of left-sided laryngeal paresis, it could be expected that endoscopically obvious inefficient left arytenoid movements would be common. This certainly is the case in Thoroughbreds, in which the inability to hold the left arytenoid in the abducted position as long as the right and fluttering of the cartilage during abduc-

Figure 31. Line drawing of the equine larynx illustrating the characteristic endoscopic appearance of laryngeal hemiplegia during maximal inspiratory effort. The left arytenoid cartilage is displaced toward the midline, and there is hyperabduction of the right cartilage.

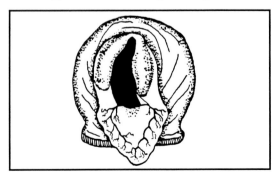

tion may indicate possible left dorsal crico-arytenoid muscle damage.

Palpation of the larynx is a useful diagnostic procedure in some horses. In advanced cases of laryngeal hemiplegia, the muscular process of the arytenoid cartilage on the affected side is more obvious because of atrophy of the attached dorsal and lateral cricoarytenoid muscles. Scars or swellings around previous laryngeal operation sites also may be detected, though scars may be extremely difficult to discover unless the hair is removed from the area.

Other external manipulations of the larynx, which attempt to produce an abnormal inspiratory noise, have been described. The most common is the "arytenoid depression maneuver."[174] In this procedure, pressure is placed on the muscular process of the arytenoid cartilages with 1 or 2 fingers. The characteristic inspiratory noise sometimes can be produced with much less force applied on the affected side.

Another clinical aid to diagnosis of advanced cases of the disease is referred to as "grunting to the stick" or Valsalva's maneuver. The horse is threatened with a strike to the abdomen. When so threatened, horses with laryngeal hemiplegia, produce a long grunt, resulting from failure to completely close the glottis due to adductor paralysis.

If the diagnosis remains uncertain, examination during and immediately after exercise may be helpful. Horses with suspected abnormal respiratory noises at exercise are best examined by having the horse ridden in a circle around the observer. Once in each cycle, the rider should bring the horse close to the examiner so that the respiratory noises can be heard very clearly. In some horses, abnormal noises are made only at the gallop or in competitive situations. When this occurs, examination should be performed in a situation as close as possible to that in which the history indicates the noise is made.

At the canter and faster paces, there is a precise time relationship between breathing and stride. Each time the foot of the leading forelimb strikes the ground, the horse exhales. As this foot is lifted from the ground, the horse inhales. This is helpful when considering whether the noise is made on inspiration or expiration. Unfortunately, it can be used without confusion only when ob-serving a horse near at hand because, if the horse is galloping about 100 meters from the observer, the sound produced at the horse's nostrils will take about half the time occupied by one stride to reach the examiner. Thus, the inspiratory sound is heard at approximately the time that expiration is taking place, and confusion results.[176]

Immediately after the horse has completed the prescribed amount of exercise, it should be returned quickly to the examiner, who can listen to any noise still present. A healthy horse will be making a loud expiratory noise at this time. In horses with laryngeal hemiplegia, however, the abnormal inspiratory noise gradually decreases over a series of respirations. At this time, the examiner may place a stethoscope over the horse's larynx or trachea to detect fremitus (increased turbulence) and also may perform an arytenoid depression maneuver.

Once exercise is completed, the horse should be placed in a nearby stall and examined endoscopically. The laryngeal asymmetry may be more obvious at this time.

Treatment: The aim of treatment of laryngeal hemiplegia is to reduce exercise-induced stridor and allow affected horses to perform efficiently.

Numerous horses with this disease are required to perform over short distances or using submaximal efforts, as with show jumpers, dressage horses and hunters. Many of these horses can perform successfully despite their airway obstruction.[190] Laryngeal hemiplegia has its most devastating effects in horses required to apply maximal efforts over reasonable distances, such as Thoroughbreds performing ≥1400 meters. Because the demands for proficient gaseous exchange are rigorous in these horses, effective surgical relief of the laryngeal obstruction usually is required for an individual to reach its true potential.

The ideal surgical treatment for laryngeal hemiplegia is one that creates a larynx with minimal air flow turbulence and resistance at fast exercise over a long period, is simple to perform and is free of complications. Unfortunately, no operation meets these requirements. For this reason, several operations are being used to ameliorate the effects of laryngeal hemiplegia on performance horses. By far, the most common of these is the combined abductor muscle prosthesis and left ventriculectomy technique.[174,191-193] Other surgical procedures also are used, such as ventriculectomy alone or partial arytenoidectomy.[167,176,190,194] Because all of these operations are associated with a substantial percentage of failures, particularly when applied to Thoroughbreds performing over middle or long distances, additional techniques are being evaluated.[195,196]

Combined Abductor Muscle Prosthesis (Laryngoplasty) and Ventriculectomy: The aim of this operation is to prevent intrusion of the arytenoid cartilage and vocal fold into the laryngeal lumen during exercise. Many variations in surgical technique have been described.[197] In all, one or more sutures (prostheses) are placed between the cricoid and arytenoid cartilages in such a way as to mimic the action of the contracted dorsal cricoarytenoid muscle. The prosthesis material commonly used is a double strand of #5 Dacron or Lycra.[174,187]

Under general anesthesia, the horse is placed on its right side with its neck extended. The surgical area over the left side of the larynx is prepared, and a 10-cm skin incision is made about 1 cm ventral to the linguofacial vein, immediately cranial to its junction with the jugular vein. This exposes the pale fascia associated with the linguofacial vein in the upper part of the wound and the omohyoid muscle below. Between these structures lies a plane of dissection through which, by blunt dissection and digital manipulation, the caudal border of the cricoid lamina is exposed. Across the plane of dissection lies the neurovascular pedicle supplying the omohyoid and sternothyrohyoid muscles. This can be ligated and transected or retracted and avoided.

The loose fascia is dissected from the caudal border of the cricoid cartilage, using care to avoid the cranial thyroid vessels in this area. The caudal border of the cricoid cartilage is easily recognized and is distinguishable from the tracheal rings by a small but obvious prominence that can be palpated 1-2 cm from the midline. To facilitate correct placement of the prosthesis through the cricoid cartilage, a towel clamp may be placed on the cricoid arch and the cartilage rotated outward.

A strong needle to which the prosthesis is attached is inserted behind the caudal border of the cricoid cartilage. It is advanced immediately under the medial surface of this cartilage to avoid penetrating the laryngeal lumen and is positioned to penetrate the lamina of the cartilage at least 1.5-2 cm rostral to its caudal margin (Fig 32). A flat spatula should be placed above the dorsal cricoarytenoid muscle, which overlies the cricoid cartilage, before the sharp point of the needle penetrates this structure. This precludes the possibility of penetrating the carotid artery or esophagus, which overlie the area.

Occasionally the cranial thyroid blood vessel is penetrated during placement of the prosthesis through the cricoid cartilage. Bleeding from this vessel can be controlled by packing the area with sponges, which are removed after the prosthesis has been positioned in the muscular process of the arytenoid and tied.

A second prosthesis then is placed in the cricoid cartilage. To assist in its placement, the towel clamp is removed and the larynx rotated outward by applying traction to the first prosthesis.

The septum between the thyropharyngeal and cricopharyngeal muscles is then identified and opened with scissors. This exposes the muscular process of the arytenoid, which can be felt as a knuckle-like structure caudal to the septum. The muscular process is freed by sharp dissection from the surrounding fascia. Identification and dissection around the muscular process can be expedited by placing a hook (*eg,* a spay hook) over the dorsal lamina of the thyroid cartilage and, by ventral traction, rotating the larynx outward.

A curved (cholecystectomy) forceps then is introduced close to the muscular process and passed caudally over the surface of the

Figure 32. Diagram of the left lateral aspect of the larynx illustrating approximate positioning of the prosthesis in the cricoid cartilage.

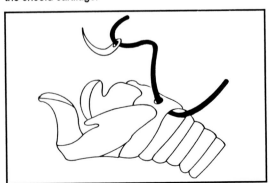

cricoid lamina to the point of emergence of the prosthesis from the cricoid. Both ends of the prosthesis are placed in the jaws of the forceps and retrieved. The procedure is repeated for the second prosthesis. Care is taken to avoid crossing or twisting of the prostheses during retrieval. A hole is then drilled transversely in the muscular process using a 14- or 16-ga hypodermic needle that, for convenience, is attached to a syringe. Once the needle has penetrated the medial surface of the muscular process, the syringe is removed and a length of twisted wire is pushed through the lumen of the needle. The end of the twisted wire can be recovered from the medial side of the muscular process by grasping it with curved artery forceps and pulling it gently toward the skin wound. The prostheses are placed through the end of the twisted wire, which, by traction on the other end, are pulled through the muscular process in a medial to lateral direction (Fig 33). Some surgeons prefer to make individual holes in the muscular process for each prosthesis.

Tension is applied to both prostheses and the ends of one are tied with a square knot and additional throws (Fig 34). The second prosthesis is tied in a similar manner. The redundant ends of the prostheses are removed with scissors.

The degree of tension required to pull the arytenoid laterally can be determined during endoscopic examination of the larynx by an assistant after removal of the endotracheal tube.

The gap between the thyropharyngeal and cricopharyngeal muscles is closed using an absorbable suture. After removal of sponges and any clotted blood that may

Figure 33. Diagram of the lateral aspect of the larynx illustrating placement of the prosthesis through the muscular process of the arytenoid cartilage using a length of twisted wire.

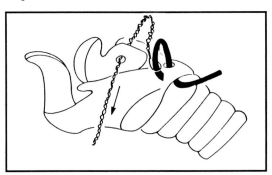

Figure 34. Diagram of the dorsal aspect of the larynx illustrating approximate positioning of the prosthesis in the arytenoid (A) and cricoid (C) cartilages. T=thyroid, E=epiglottis.

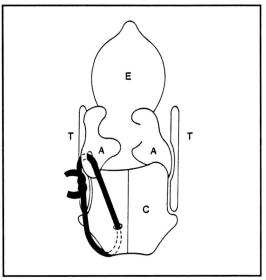

have accumulated in the depth of the incision, the fascia adjacent to the linguofacial vein is sutured to the omohyoid muscle with absorbable suture material. The skin is sutured with nonabsorbable material in a vertical mattress pattern.

Immediately following completion of the laryngoplasty, the horse is repositioned in dorsal recumbency with its neck outstretched. After suitable skin preparation, an 8-cm skin incision is made in the midline, proceeding caudally from the caudal border of the mandible. The underlying muscles are parted on the midline and a retractor placed in the wound. The triangular cricothyroid membrane is identified by palpating the laryngeal prominence of the thyroid cartilage rostrally and the circular cricoid arch caudally. A stab incision is made through the cricothyroid membrane and laryngeal mucosa, and the incision is lengthened to the limiting cartilages. A self-retaining retractor is then placed in the wound. The left vocal fold is identified visually and a Blattenburg bur inserted deeply into the left ventricle. By rotating, lifting and twisting the bur in a rostromedial direction, the mucous membrane surrounding the bur is withdrawn. The mucosa is held with forceps and the bur removed. Traction is applied until all the mucosa is removed from the ventricle. The mucosa then is excised by sharp dissection. The wounds are left open to heal.

Postoperative Care: If the animal's mane is long, it is plaited to prevent its covering the laryngoplasty wound. Petroleum jelly is applied daily to the areas around the wounds and the intermandibular space to prevent irritation of the skin. Iodine is applied over the laryngoplasty wound for the first few postoperative days. Antibiotics are administered immediately before and for a few days after the operation. The ventral laryngotomy wound is cleaned with moist gauze swabs daily until it is healed.

Stall rest is recommended for 6 weeks after surgery. The horse should be reexamined endoscopically before resumption of training.

Variations in Technique: Many variations in the surgical technique of both laryngoplasty and ventriculectomy operations have been described. In the laryngoplasty procedure, elastic and nonelastic prostheses have been used.[187] The technique of inserting the prosthesis through the muscular process of the arytenoid differs widely among surgeons.[191,198] In the ventriculectomy procedure, some surgeons excise part of the vocal fold or suture the excision site. Others remove the mucosa from both ventricles.

If the design of the table and padding permit, laryngotomy and ventriculectomy can be done with the horse in lateral recumbency, reducing risk to the horse and the effort of repositioning in dorsal recumbency.

Results: The reported success rate of this operation varies markedly between 5% and 95%.[197] Short-term improvement of both respiratory flow mechanics at submaximal exercise and arterial blood gas tensions after fast exercise has resulted from this surgery.[16,35] This probably reflects the adequate degree of arytenoid abduction achieved in most horses in the initial postoperative period.[197] However, because of the propensity of the prostheses to pull out of the cartilages, this degree of abduction often is not maintained.[197] For this reason, a significant proportion of Thoroughbred horses treated by this surgery and subsequently raced over middle to longer distances make an obvious abnormal inspiratory noise to the trained ear and do not perform successfully at the level achieved before surgery.[198]

Complications: The most common complication of this procedure is postoperative coughing that persists a variable time, from a few days to a few months.[197] Most often it is associated with eating or exercise and may be related to the inability of the larynx to function effectively as a sphincter during deglutition and perhaps obstruction of the left pharyngeal food channel by the constantly abducted arytenoid.[189] Coughing also may result from complicating pharyngitis or bronchitis.

The second most common complication of this surgery is a nasal discharge or reflux of food or water through the nostril. The cause of this is not known but may be related to interference with normal function of the lateral food channels. Whatever its cause, it apparently does not cause serious harm, as many of the animals with this complication perform successfully.

Many other complications have been recorded and include sinus formation from the prosthesis, dysphagia or choking, dislocation of the prosthesis into the lumen of the larynx, chondritis of the cricoid cartilage, granuloma formation, development of right-sided laryngospasm at exercise, laryngeal edema, pneumonia, inhalation tracheitis, extensive seroma formation, rejection-like phenomena of the prosthesis material, and death due to asphyxia or postoperative complications, including diarrhea and laminitis.[197]

Ventriculectomy: Though this operation, first described in 1845, seemingly has stood the test of time, it has been displaced by the combined laryngoplasty/ventriculectomy procedure as the treatment of choice in laryngeal hemiplegia.[199]

The aim of the operation is abduction of the arytenoid cartilage by adhesions between the arytenoid and thyroid cartilages and reduced filling of the ventricle during inspiration.[187] However, endoscopic examination following ventriculectomy has revealed that neither arytenoid abduction nor lateral retraction of the vocal fold results from this surgery. The operation apparently does not influence the airway-restricting position of the paralyzed arytenoid cartilage and, therefore, only can have a minor beneficial effect at best on laryngeal air flow mechanics.[200]

Debate over the effectiveness of this operation has continued over the years. In a review of 4000 ventriculectomy operations, only 20% of treated horses showed sufficient improvement to pass a soundness examination.[186] This percentage may reflect the error in diagnosis of laryngeal hemiplegia during the early part of this century. In a more recent study, no horse treated by ventriculectomy was regarded as silent to the rider's ear.[190] Others are of the opinion that in racehorses, ventriculectomy has no significant effect on abnormal respiratory noise at exercise or on performance.[183]

The ventriculectomy operation is described above under Combined Abductor Muscle Prosthesis (Laryngoplasty) and Ventriculectomy Operation.

Arytenoidectomy: Before the 20th century, partial arytenoidectomy was considered the treatment of choice for laryngeal hemiplegia.[178] It was abandoned because of various serious complications, but it did allow some patients to return to competitive athletic activity.[187] Partial or subtotal arytenoidectomies have been used recently in cases of failed laryngoplasty, and there is some evidence that they may be of value in performance horses.[187] However, further evaluation of this technique is required before it can be recommended as a reasonably reliable method of relieving the respiratory distress in maximally exercising horses. The operative technique is detailed above in the section entitled Arytenoid Chondritis.

Epiglottic Entrapment

Epiglottic entrapment is a disease in which the freely movable mucosa on the ventrum of the epiglottis and on the adjacent floor of the oropharynx becomes folded or overlapped on itself and displaced over the dorsum of the epiglottis. In normal horses, the subepiglottic tissue is folded in a loose accordion-like fashion and provides a tissue reserve, allowing unhindered elevation of the epiglottis during deglutition.[201] Entrapment of the epiglottis takes place because a fold of this tissue becomes transposed over the dorsum of the epiglottis (Fig 35).[183]

The condition affects both male and female horses of all ages and is most commonly diagnosed in Standardbred and Thoroughbred horses.[202,203]

Cause: The cause is not yet clear.[183] On endoscopic examination, it occurs intermit-

tently during deglutition. Whether swallowing is the precipitating mechanism for displacement in most cases is not known.[204] The condition occurs quite frequently in association with palatine or epiglottic defects, such as persistent laryngopalatine dislocation, cleft palate, hypoplasia of the soft palate, hypoplasia of the epiglottis and epiglottic deformities.[8,162,202,205-207]

Epiglottic entrapment occurs as both a congenital and an acquired disease. Its association with hypoplasia of the epiglottis and occurrence with congenital cleft of the soft palate suggest that it is congenital in some animals. However, whether it is present in these animals at birth or develops later as a consequence of either a defective palate or epiglottis is not known.

In some horses it apparently is acquired because, on occasion, its presence coincides with a sudden loss of racing form and production of abnormal respiratory noises at exercise.[204]

Clinical Signs: Though entrapment of the epiglottis has been found incidentally during endoscopic examination of apparently normal horses, it frequently is associated with decreased exercise tolerance and abnormal respiratory noises made during fast work.[208] The abnormal noise may occur on inspiration and/or expiration.[94] An uneven respiratory pattern during exercise and coughing, either at exercise or after eating, also have been noted.[202,204,209]

Figure 35. Sagittal section of the larynx illustrating positioning of a fold of ventral epiglottic mucosa over the dorsum of the epiglottis in epiglottic entrapment.

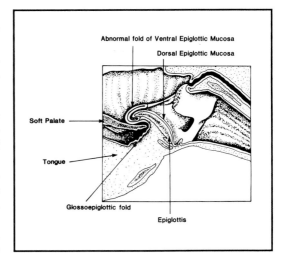

421

When entrapment is associated with palatine disorders, such as persistent dorsal displacement of the palate, cleft palate or hypoplasia of the soft palate, clinical signs frequently are indistinguishable from the signs characteristic of those anomalies.

Diagnosis: Definitive diagnosis of epiglottic entrapment can be made endoscopically or radiographically.

Endoscopically, the entrapping tissue obscures the normal serrated margin of the epiglottis and frequently its dorsal vascular pattern. The shape of the epiglottis can be appreciated, but the entrapment creates a tissue mass that is thicker, blunted at the apex, and more rounded on its lateral margins. The free margin of the entrapping tissue can be seen over the laryngeal surface of the epiglottis.[210] Occasionally the entrapping tissue may overlie only the lateral borders of the epiglottic cartilage, thus obliterating them visually. On other occasions, the borders and apex of the epiglottis are obscured (Fig 36).

Ulceration of the dorsal surface of the entrapping tissue in the area overlying the apex of the epiglottis is not uncommon. These ulcers should not be confused with the less common ulceration of the epiglottic apex.[203,210] Difficulty in diagnosing epiglottic entrapment endoscopically may be encountered with concurrent persistent dorsal displacement of the soft palate. In both these conditions, a free margin of tissue overlies the laryngeal surface of the epiglottis. However, with dorsal displacement of the soft palate, the shape of the epiglottis is completely obscured; in entrapment, the shape of the underlying epiglottis, though indistinct, can still be appreciated.

Persistent dorsal displacement of the soft palate may mask epiglottic entrapment during nasopharyngeal endoscopy. In these circumstances, endoscopic examination PO or lateral pharyngeal radiography may be required.

Radiography of the pharyngeal region is an important diagnostic aid in horses with entrapment of the epiglottis, as it provides information about the thickness, length and shape of the epiglottis that may not be evident on nasopharyngeal endoscopy.[203] It also allows measurement of the epiglottic length. Horses with a very short epiglottis have a poorer postsurgical prognosis.[162,202,211] In affected horses, the entrapping folds of tissue can be observed radiographically dorsal to the epiglottic cartilage. At the tip of the epiglottis, the radiodensity of the displaced folds often is increased. A radiolucent (air) shadow commonly is located between the tip of the epiglottis and the rostral portion of the displaced folds of tissue.[203]

To measure the length of the epiglottic cartilage, straight lateral radiographs should be obtained with the horse unsedated and the head in resting position.[203] Direct accurate measurement of the epiglottic cartilage is not possible because of the difficulty in determining the precise location of the base of the epiglottic cartilage on the radiograph. However, the epiglottic cartilage is attached to the body of the thyroid cartilage, which can be seen readily. Thyroepiglottic length (tip of epiglottis to the body of the thyroid cartilage) can be determined and, with radiographic magnification factors taken into account, correlates well with actual epiglottic length measured postmortem.[203] Thyroepiglottic length in adult Thoroughbreds, measured radiographically, averages between 8.76 cm and 9.35 cm.[194,203] Thus, normal adult Thoroughbreds can be expected to have a thyroepiglottic length of >8 cm. When this length is <7.5 cm, a guarded to poor prognosis for surgical correction of the entrapment is warranted.[194]

Treatment: Transection or removal of some of the entrapping tissue is the usual method of treatment for this condition. Approaches can be made through a ventral laryngotomy, ventral pharyngotomy or the oral cavity.

The most common approach is via a ventral laryngotomy incision. This allows adequate surgical exposure of the entrapped

Figure 36. Line drawing showing various degrees of epiglottic entrapment in horses.[183]

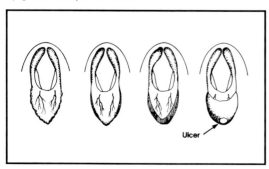

Ulcer

epiglottis. In experienced hands, the operation only takes a few minutes, so IV anesthesia alone can be used. Less experienced surgeons, however, should have inhalation anesthesia available.

The horse is positioned in dorsal recumbency, and the approach is made through the cricothyroid membrane. A self-retaining retractor is placed in the laryngotomy wound and an attempt is made to view the entrapping mucosa. This may be facilitated by placing the rounded tip of a cholecystectomy forceps beneath the body of the thyroid cartilage and applying upward traction or, in difficult cases, by placing a lighted endoscope in the pharynx to provide illumination to the epiglottic area. If an endotracheal tube has been used, it can be removed, though the operation can be performed while it remains in place.

The free margin of the entrapping mucosa lying immediately dorsal to the epiglottis usually can be distinguished from the free border of the soft palate. It can be grasped with tissue forceps and caudal traction applied. This retroflexes the epiglottic cartilage into the laryngeal lumen.

In some horses, particularly those with intermittent entrapment, the mucosa at the time of surgery may be in its normal position ventral to the epiglottis. In these cases, the loose mucosa lateral to the epiglottic cartilage is grasped with tissue forceps and caudal traction applied. A second pair of forceps then is attached to the most rostral mucosa exposed and traction applied again. This can be repeated until the epiglottic cartilage retroflexes into the laryngeal lumen. To assist this, a finger may be placed under the tip of the epiglottis and gradual posterior pressure applied until the cartilage retroflexes.

A sponge forceps then is placed on the mucosa attached to the tip of the epiglottis, using care not to damage the cartilage. At this stage, the cartilaginous tip of the epiglottis can be identified easily visually and by palpation.

Some controversy exists as to how the entrapping mucosa should be resected and the amount of tissue to be excised. Certainly, removal of too much tissue increases the chances of postoperative complications, particularly persistent dorsal displacement of the soft palate. Transection of the entrapping tissue at the tip of the epiglottis

may be sufficient for relief of the entrapment, but this technique frequently is complicated by reentrapment following surgery.[210,212] Removal of some entrapping tissue seems to be required to prevent reentrapment in many horses. Just how much to remove, however, is equivocal. Either a triangular (V-shaped) excision, with the apex of the V positioned immediately caudal to the apex of the epiglottis, or a crescentic excision 3-4 mm from the epiglottic margin, similar to that described for resection of the free border of the soft palate, can be used.

In either case, tissue forceps are placed centrally, immediately behind the retroflexed tip of the epiglottis, so that the midline is identified. A second pair of forceps then can be placed on one side and slight traction applied. The required amount of entrapping tissue is removed to the level of the epiglottic tip from one side. The procedure is repeated on the opposite side. Some surgeons using the crescentic excision remove a section of up to 8 cm of the entrapping mucosa, measured on a transverse plane, by 2 cm, measured on a sagittal plane.[210]

Once the entrapping mucosa is removed, the epiglottis is replaced in its normal position. Both the subepiglottic area and the laryngotomy incision are allowed to heal as open wounds.

The epiglottic area can be observed endoscopically before the horse's recovery from the anesthesia.

Postoperative Care: In the immediate postoperative period, the horse must be restrained from eating food or bedding to prevent contamination of the subepiglottic wound. Phenylbutazone and prophylactic antibiotics may be given for several days.[210] Stall rest is recommended, at least until the laryngotomy incision has healed. The length of this rest varies, but periods of up to 45 days are desirable. Endoscopic examination of the area is recommended before training is resumed.

Prognosis: The prognosis for this operation depends on any preoperative complications, such as palatal or epiglottal anomalies. Also, as mentioned, controversy exists as to the approach and method of sectioning or removal of the entrapping mucosa. This probably reflects the fact that all techniques are associated with some failures.

The prognosis for return to the competition before clinical signs arose cannot be accurately forecast but it may approach 75% in uncomplicated cases of entrapment.[210]

Alternative Procedures for Correction of Epiglottic Entrapment: Alternative surgical techniques include the oral or nasal approach to the entrapment, with splitting of the entrapping tissue on the midline using a long-handled scalpel and midline transendoscopic electrosurgical division of the entrapping mucosa.[209,212] A similar approach, using biopsy forceps to remove a notch of tissue, has been documented.[210]

The oral approach has the advantage of enabling surgery in the conscious horse and minimizing the amount of tissue damage. However, with this method, uneven healing of the cut edges of the entrapping mucosa sometimes causes recurrence.[210]

A ventral pharyngotomy approach to correct epiglottic entrapment has been reported.[210] It offers no advantage over the technically easier laryngotomy approach, which provides greater surgical exposure.[210] Microsurgery using a CO_2 laser also has been described and may become a valuable technique in the future.[213]

Complications: The most common complications of epiglottic entrapment surgery are recurrence of the entrapment and dorsal displacement of the soft palate.

Postoperative recurrence of entrapment appears to be associated with insufficient removal of the offending tissue. Certainly it is seen more frequently following incision than excision and sometimes can be corrected by removal of a small amount of the entrapping mucosa.

The most serious complication of this surgery is dorsal displacement of the soft palate. This may occur intermittently following surgery, especially in the first postoperative week, after which it may resolve spontaneously.[210] Persistent dorsal displacement of the soft palate can be anticipated in cases when it accompanies the entrapment before surgery, when there is a severely shortened epiglottic cartilage, or when an excessive amount of entrapping mucosa was removed during surgery.[194,212] The importance of this complication is that the patient is less useful after surgery than before.[210] The cause of this complication is unknown. In an attempt to minimize this postoperative complication, some surgeons recommend removal of a small portion of the free border of the soft palate when the entrapping mucosa is resected. However, the value of this soft palate surgery itself is shrouded in controversy, and there is little evidence that it lessens the chances of postoperative dorsal displacement of the soft palate.

Another but rarer complication of entrapment surgery is formation of a granulomatous lesion ventral to the epiglottis.[210] This probably results from infection of the exposed tissue. It frequently is associated with dorsal displacement of the soft palate, and its removal often results in persistent dorsal displacement of this structure.[210]

DISEASES OF THE TRACHEA

C.M. Honnas

Diagnostic and Therapeutic Considerations

Recognition of tracheal disease in horses has been facilitated by the availability of refined diagnostic procedures and an increased awareness of specific diseases involving the trachea. The ability to anesthetize horses routinely has allowed development of improved tracheal reconstructive techniques.

Surgery of the trachea may be necessary for relief of obstruction in the rostral airway, removal of foreign bodies, repair of traumatic injuries, and reconstruction of stenotic or collapsed segments of the trachea.

Permanent Tracheostomy

Permanent tracheostomy is indicated when the primary obstructive disease of the upper airway is irreversible or requires a protracted time for resolution. Traumatic collapse of the nasal passages and neoplastic disease of the upper respiratory tract are conditions that might require permanent tracheostomy.

The surgical site for permanent tracheostomy is the mid- to proximal cervical ventral midline, where the trachea is most superficial. A 15-cm area of the trachea is exposed, and the sternothyrohyoideus muscle bellies are transected at the proximal and distal limits of the incision. The ventral one-third of the circumference of the 3 most central tracheal rings are removed without penetration of the tracheal mucosa. The tracheal mucosa then is incised longitudinally on the midline and then transversely at the proximal and distal limits to form an I-shaped incision. To facilitate apposition of the tracheal mucosa and the skin and to minimize tension on the suture lines, crescent-shaped pieces are resected from the left and right omohyoid muscles adjacent to the tracheal incision. The tracheal mucosa and skin edges are apposed with simple-interrupted nonabsorbable sutures to produce a stoma of about 3 x 4 cm (Fig 37). A tracheostomy tube may be required in the immediate postoperative period and may be positioned through the surgical site.[61]

Permanent tracheostomy compromises respiratory defense mechanisms by reducing filtration and humidification of air in the nasal passages, and thus increases the risk of lower respiratory tract infection. Management of a permanent tracheostomy requires daily observation and cleaning to remove respiratory secretions deposited at the stoma by mucociliary action. Optimally, the environment should be dust free, such as permanent pasture or appropriate stall and paddock, to compensate for the altered defense mechanisms. With proper care, long-term survival is dictated by the primary condition necessitating permanent tracheostomy.[61]

Tracheal Resection and Anastomosis

Tracheal reconstruction by resection and end-to-end anastomosis is indicated in horses with segmental cervical tracheal stenosis or collapse involving <6 tracheal rings. The most common indication for tracheal resection in horses is impaired breathing associated with tracheal stenosis following tracheotomy.[63] Surgical success requires restricted head movement and maintenance of neck flexion to prevent disruptive tension on the tracheal anastomosis during healing. This can be achieved using a martingale-type harness with a line running from the ventral girth to the halter. Presurgical application facilitates postoperative acceptance of this harness. Maintaining neck flexion reportedly reduces suture line tension by about 50%.[63]

Tracheal resection and anastomosis are done under general anesthesia with the pa-

Figure 37. Permanent tracheostomy immediately after surgery (A) and 22 days postoperatively (B). (Courtesy of Dr. D.V. Hanselka)

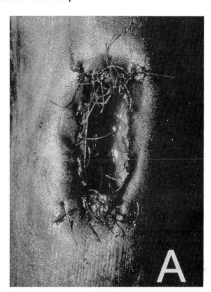

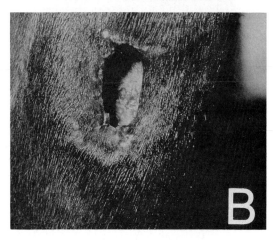

tient in dorsal recumbency. The surgical procedure requires a ventral midline cervical incision of sufficient length to permit mobilization of the trachea from the cricoid cartilage to the thoracic inlet.[63] This reduces tension on the resected ends of the trachea. The trachea is freed from the surrounding fascia, and blood vessels are ligated and transected as necessary. The diseased trachea is resected and special attention is given to creating a circumferential mucosal flap on the free ends of the remaining trachea. Gas anesthesia then is continued through an endotracheal tube placed in the distal tracheal segment. The freed mucosa of the proximal and distal segments are reflected over the tracheal ends and sutured to the adventitia with absorbable suture in a simple-continuous pattern. Reflection of mucosa in this manner directly apposes the mucosa and provides an airtight seal at the anastomotic site.

The endotracheal tube is removed from the surgical field and replaced through the oropharynx and proximal trachea into the distal tracheal segment. With the head flexed 90 degrees to the neck, the tracheal ends are held in apposition with a suitable instrument and the anastomosis performed with 25-ga stainless-steel wire in a simple-interrupted pattern. Each suture encompasses half the thickness of the tracheal rings, and care is taken not to penetrate the mucosa except where it has been reflected over the tracheal ends.[63] Tension sutures encompassing tracheal rings proximal and distal to those removed may be placed to relieve stress at the anastomotic site.[214]

The endotracheal tube is withdrawn into the proximal trachea, and the surgical field is flooded with saline to check for air leaks while positive pressure is applied. A suction drain is placed next to the trachea before closure of the incision. Recovery from anesthesia necessitates use of the martingale harness and judicious use of slings or other aids as indicated. Antibiotics are given for 10 days. The harness should remain on the horse for 3 weeks postoperatively.[63]

Tracheal collapse also has been treated by tracheal resection and replacement with a 45-cm reinforced polyvinyl chloride hose prosthesis. The horse survived for 9 1/2 months but was eventually euthanized due to complications.[215]

Diseases With Physical Causes

Tracheal Trauma

Clinical signs of trauma depend on the site of tracheal injury and the amount of air leakage.[64] Blunt injury resulting in tracheal perforation without disruption of the skin may not be recognized until regional or generalized subcutaneous emphysema develops. Tracheal injuries of this type may occur in mares separated from their foals by wire fences at weaning. Signs of subcutaneous emphysema include subcutaneous swelling that is nonpainful, soft, easily indented, mobile and crepitant.[216] Other causes of subcutaneous emphysema involving the neck and head include deep axillary wounds and injuries to the paranasal sinuses.

When tracheal perforation is suspected, thoracic radiographs should be made to check for pneumomediastinum.[217] Continued leakage of air into the mediastinum may predispose to pneumothorax. Generally, both the subcutaneous emphysema and pneumomediastinum resolve without special therapy.[217] Diagnosis of tracheal perforation or rupture usually can be confirmed by a complete clinical examination, endoscopy and radiography.

Treatment for cervical tracheal injuries depends on the extent of the injury. Small tears can be managed conservatively and generally form a fibrin seal within 24-48 hours.[214] Large tears, however, should be managed surgically as soon as the horse's condition allows. Generally, tears of the cervical trachea are approached through the wound after debridement of devitalized tissue. Wound margins are apposed with a simple-interrupted pattern of absorbable or nonabsorbable suture material.[214,218] Injuries involving the trachealis muscle and adventitia of the trachea can be repaired by rotating the trachea to expose the dorsal surface.[217] Closed-suction drains are recommended in the immediate postoperative period and should be removed after 48-72 hours, depending on the appearance of the wound and the amount of drainage.[214] Once the tracheal defect is closed, the subcutaneous emphysema often resolves in 7-10 days.[217]

Intrathoracic tracheal tears have not been reported in horses, but it is likely that trauma sufficient to result in thoracic injuries of this nature would warrant a poor prognosis for survival.

Tracheal Foreign Bodies

Horses with tracheal foreign bodies usually have a history of persistent, chronic coughing.[219] Inhaled objects of plant origin have been associated with chronic coughing, intermittent fever, fetid breath and intermittent bilateral purulent nasal discharge that is periodically blood tinged.[219] Tracheal endoscopy can be used to identify the foreign body. Complete examination of the trachea requires an endoscope longer than 100 cm. Alternatively, the distal trachea can be examined with a 100-cm endoscope passed through a tracheotomy. Foreign bodies often tend to lodge in the horizontal portion of the trachea near the tracheal bifurcation, and examination of this area via the nose requires a longer endoscope.[219] Occasionally it may be necessary to suppress the cough reflex by topical instillation of local anesthetic to facilitate tracheoscopy.[220]

While it may be possible to remove the foreign body using an endoscope biopsy instrument, tracheotomy generally is necessary to gain access to the site of obstruction. Attempts to remove objects in standing horses may be unsuccessful due to lack of patient cooperation, the size of the object, or inability to adequately view foreign bodies surrounded by granulation tissue.[220] In such cases, exploration and removal via tracheotomy are required. The site of the cervical tracheotomy should be as close to the foreign body as possible. A distal cervical tracheotomy is necessary for foreign bodies lodged near the tracheal bifurcation. Guidance and illumination with the endoscope facilitate removal of a foreign body using a suitable instrument introduced through the tracheotomy.[219] The tracheotomy should be allowed to heal as an open wound and appropriate antibiotics given on the basis of culture and susceptibility testing of transtracheal aspirates.

Tracheal Collapse

In large animals, tracheal collapse occurs most frequently as a result of trauma from ropes, fences, gates and gunshot wounds.[221] It also has occurred after emergency tracheotomy.[61,62]

Less commonly, tracheal collapse results from dorsoventral flattening of the trachea. Though the etiology of this condition is unknown, it appears to occur more frequently in ponies >10 years of age.[222] In this sense, it is similar to the syndrome reported in aged toy-breed dogs.[214,223] In affected horses and ponies, the tracheal rings form shallow arcs, and the dorsal tracheal membrane is stretched, creating an elliptic lumen, rather than a circular cross section.[224] The entire trachea may be affected or the condition may be limited to cervical or thoracic segments.

Clinical signs vary. Most affected horses exhibit inspiratory stridor, exercise intolerance, respiratory distress and cyanosis, while others may be asymptomatic.[222] Diagnosis can be confirmed by auscultation, palpation, endoscopy and radiography. Auscultation may identify the site of maximal air flow turbulence. Palpation of the cervical trachea may reveal the lateral edges of the flattened trachea in the jugular groove.[215] Endoscopy reveals an abnormal shape to the tracheal lumen, as well as flaccid dorsal musculature (Fig 38). Lateral radiographs show a narrow tracheal outline.[224]

Treatment of tracheal collapse depends on the etiologic factors, length of trachea involved, and accessibility of the affected trachea.[225] The primary goal of surgery is to restore tracheal diameter without affecting the mucociliary apparatus. This can be accomplished with an extraluminal prosthetic device, which restores tracheal diameter by eliminating redundant dorsal tracheal membrane and by providing rigid support for the tracheal wall.[214,226] Various tracheal prostheses, such as polypropylene syringe cases, have been used successfully in small and large animals.[227] Partial chondrotomy may be required on the ventral aspect of each collapsed tracheal ring to correct some deformities managed with a prosthesis.[221] Cervical dorsoventral tracheal collapse in a 2-month-old Shetland pony was corrected via chondrotomy of alternate tracheal rings

Figure 38. Dorsoventral collapse of the cervical trachea in a 14-year-old pony. The dorsal fibroelastic membrane (arrows) sags into the airway, creating an elliptic tracheal lumen.

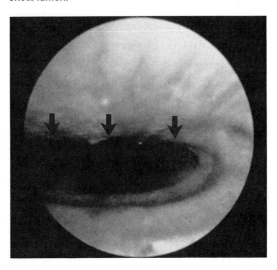

and fixation of the trachea to a steel spring spiralled around the trachea. The pony was clinically normal for 3 1/2 years before clinical signs recurred when dorsoventral collapse progressed to the thoracic trachea.[227] Similar techniques using extraluminal prostheses fashioned from polypropylene syringe cases have been used.[62,225,228] Identification and preservation of the recurrent laryngeal nerves is important in all cases managed by surgical implantation of a prosthesis.

Surgical aftercare consists of antimicrobial therapy and stall rest. Suction drains should be used when warranted for dead-space management. Long-term prognosis for horses with tracheal collapse is variable. Involvement of only short segments of the trachea that are accessible surgically improves the long-term prognosis. Horses with dorsoventral collapse have a poorer prognosis, especially if the thoracic trachea is involved.

Tracheal Stenosis

Tracheal stenosis is a narrowing or stricture of the tracheal lumen. In foals, tracheal stenosis may occur during healing of a tracheotomy made by longitudinal incision through the tracheal rings (Fig 39).[62,63] Other causes of tracheal stenosis include *Streptococcus equi* abscesses in the peritracheal mediastinal lymph nodes and trauma.[62,221,229-231] Tumors occur infrequently in this region, but tracheal collapse and stenosis secondary to a lipoma have been reported.[225] Prolonged endotracheal intubation has been associated with severe mucosal hemorrhage corresponding to the position of the endotracheal tube cuff. Though many of these lesions resolve without untoward sequelae, similar lesions have been seen with circumferential fibrous tracheal stenosis in human patients.[64]

The site and extent of an obstructive tracheal lesion in a horse can be determined by auscultation, radiography and endoscopy. On auscultation, wheezing may be detected directly over the area of stenosis during inspiration and expiration. An intraluminal mass or luminal narrowing may be seen on radiographs of the trachea, and it may be possible to confirm narrowing or partial occlusion of the tracheal lumen using an endoscope.[63]

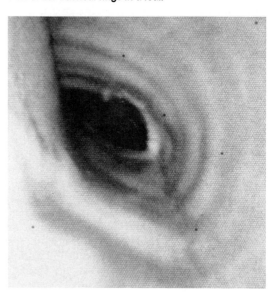

Figure 39. Tracheal stenosis following longitudinal incision of the tracheal rings in a foal.

Numerous surgical procedures have been used in the treatment of tracheal stenosis, including tracheal resection and anastomosis, extraluminal polypropylene prostheses, surgical drainage of peritracheal abscesses and multiple tracheal ring chondrotomies with placement of retention sutures anchored to the skin.[62,63,221,224,225,230,231]

Inflammatory, Infectious and Immune Diseases

Granulomas

Granulomatous nodules are occasionally observed in the trachea during endoscopic examination. Often these nodules are in the proximal trachea near the larynx, but occasionally granulomas are associated with healing tracheotomy incisions. The etiology of granulomas not associated with healing incisions is unknown, but they may result from foreign body irritation (*eg,* grass awn) or inappropriate passage of a stomach tube that damages the tracheal mucosa.[232] Similar lesions in the rostral nasal passages have contained plant material.[232]

Tracheal granulomas are usually an incidental finding and often not associated with clinical signs. Granulomas of sufficient size to create air flow obstruction are removed using a snare guided endoscopically or via tracheotomy. Alternatively, cryotherapy via endoscopy may be indicated for smaller granulomatous lesions.[232] Generally the prognosis is good, provided the granuloma does not continue to enlarge and encroach on the tracheal lumen, resulting in compromised air flow.

DISEASES OF THE LUNG

Congenital and Familial Diseases

Neonatal Respiratory Distress Syndrome

M.R. Paradis

Neonatal respiratory distress syndrome is a condition characterized by failure of pulmonary gas exchange. Atelectasis becomes progressive, and pulmonary edema develops.[233] Respiratory distress syndrome usually is seen in premature foals, particularly those delivered by cesarean section. In human infants, the major cause of respiratory distress syndrome is immature or no surfactant.[233] Preliminary data suggest that this deficiency also may be present in affected foals.[7]

Surfactant is a complex phospholipid essential to reduce surface tension between the air and fluid lining the alveoli. Without surfactant, the alveolar walls become unstable and collapse, resulting in atelectasis and respiratory failure. As this process continues, pulmonary microvascular permeability increases, and proteins and fluid leak into the alveolar space. The protein gives rise to hyaline membranes seen lining the alveolar spaces of these foals on histopathologic examination.[73]

Foals with respiratory distress syndrome generally show physical signs of prematurity, including low birth weight, short silky haircoat and soft pliant ears. For the first 30 minutes of life, they may be as active as a normal foal, but they quickly tire and become distressed. The respiratory rate is elevated, but the most obvious sign of distress is increased respiratory effort. A marked degree of abdominal effort and rib retraction can be observed with paradoxical breathing movements. The normal soft, moist wheezes and crackles auscultated in the first 5-10 minutes of life may be absent in affected premature foals. This may be due to areas of atelectasis.[7]

Thoracic radiographs of premature foals with respiratory distress syndrome generally show a diffuse, alveolar pattern identified by air bronchograms. As the disorder progresses, there is edema and increased lung density (Fig 40).[7]

Hypoxemia, hypercapnia and respiratory acidosis are characteristic of respiratory distress syndrome. The P_aO_2 usually is <60 torr, while the P_aCO_2 is >60 torr. The pH ranges from 6.9 to 7.3, depending on the degree of metabolic compensation and degree of hypercapnia (Table 2).[7]

A diagnosis of respiratory distress syndrome in foals is based on the history of prematurity, combined with the radiographic and blood gas findings of respiratory failure. Other causes of respiratory failure

Figure 40. Thoracic radiograph of a 310-day-gestation foal at 24 hours of age. This foal was born prematurely after induced parturition and had clinical signs of respiratory distress syndrome.

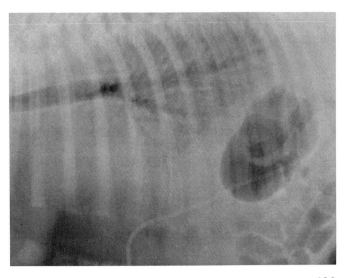

must be ruled out. Congestive heart failure secondary to a congenital heart defect, severe meconium aspiration, or *in-utero* bacterial or viral pneumonia must be considered in the differential diagnosis.

The primary objectives in supporting these foals is to provide an increased percentage of inspired O_2 and decreased CO_2 in the blood. Mechanical ventilation with supplemental oxygen is the most effective way. Early diagnosis and use of ventilators have markedly reduced mortality in human infants with respiratory distress syndrome.[233] Premature foals with respiratory distress syndrome have a grave prognosis with our present technology. The future holds a great deal of promise with development of new treatments, such as high-frequency ventilation and surfactant replacement.

Meconium Aspiration

Meconium is the first fecal material found in the intestine of the full-term neonate. It is composed of inspissated intestinal secretions and some amniotic fluid. Fetal stress, such as *in-utero* asphyxia or umbilical cord compression, can result in expulsion of the meconium into the amniotic fluid before birth. If the fetus gasps while *in utero,* this material is aspirated into the lungs. Airway obstruction and chemical irritation of the lung tissue result if this material is not removed.[5]

Foals stained with yellowish-brown amniotic fluid at birth are likely to suffer from meconium aspiration. Lung sounds may be normal or harsh. Respiratory rate and effort increase, depending on the severity of the aspiration. A brown-tinged nasal discharge that is bilirubin-positive on testing with a urinary reagent test strip also may be noted.

Blood gas abnormalities vary from normal to those of hypoxia or respiratory acidosis. A caudal granular infiltrate is seen radiographically.

The diagnosis of meconium aspiration is based on the history of dystocia, appearance of the foal at birth, and clinical and radiographic findings. The therapeutic plan should include an attempt to suction the foreign material from the lungs. It is best if the problem is recognized immediately so that suction is performed early in the foal's life. Suctioning of the lungs should be performed carefully. Continuous strong suction results in tissue trauma and pulmonary atelectasis. A small feeding tube or suction catheter can be inserted through the foal's nose and into the trachea. Mild suction is applied to the tube as it is withdrawn from the trachea.

Appropriate respiratory supportive therapy should be determined by blood gas analysis. Treatment with antibiotics and corticosteroids in human infants with meconium aspiration is considered controversial. There is no evidence to support their usefulness.[5]

Persistent Pulmonary Hypertension

Persistent pulmonary hypertension or persistent fetal circulation has been recognized in human neonates for many years. These infants have cyanosis and marked elevation of pulmonary arterial pressure. Radiographically, the lung fields are normal. Often there is right-to-left shunting of blood through the foramen ovale and ductus arteriosus.[234]

Persistent pulmonary hypertension should be differentiated from other causes of cyanosis, such as cardiac anomalies, respiratory distress syndrome and meconium aspiration. Thoracic radiographs and cardiac ultrasonography aid in differentiation.

Persistent pulmonary hypertension has been observed in a foal.[235] The foal had severe cyanosis that was unresponsive to nasal oxygen administration. Ultrasonic cardiography demonstrated a right-to-left shunt at the atrial level, without evidence of other heart disease.

Persistent pulmonary hypertension has been associated with prenatal antiprostaglandin therapy, chronic hypoxia, *in-utero* infection and meconium aspiration. The most consistent stimulus for pulmonary vasoconstriction is hypoxia. Acidosis and hypothermia also contribute to pulmonary hypertension. Therapy for this syndrome involves reversal of these factors. Because persistent pulmonary hypertension can be rapidly fatal, it should be treated as an emergency. Correction of metabolic acidosis, hypotension and hypothermia is necessary for survival of the foal. A good outcome requires a fully staffed and well-equipped intensive care unit.[234,235]

Diseases With Physical Causes

P.J. Provost and F.J. Derksen

Smoke Inhalation

Horses that survive a barn fire may sustain life-threatening respiratory tract injury and extensive skin burns. Reports describing smoke inhalation injury are limited, but much information can be gleaned by reviewing the comparative literature.

Smoke inhaled into the airways can cause both thermal and chemical injury.[236] Smoke includes products of combustion, particulate matter and gases. Combustion products and their toxicity vary with the type of flammable material involved.[237] Most inhalation injury results from inhalation of these gaseous and particulate materials, and rarely from heat alone.[238] Direct heat causes edema and obstruction of the upper airway but, due to the efficient heat-exchange capacity of the upper airway, even very hot air is cooled before entering the lower respiratory tract.[239] The edema progresses over the first 18-24 hours and is accentuated by release of vasoactive amines from thermally injured tissues. Thus, continual patient reassessment is necessary.[240]

Two distinct mechanisms are involved in inhalation injury. One mechanism is carbon monoxide poisoning, and the other is direct lung injury caused by toxic combustion products. Carbon monoxide intoxication is a frequent cause of acute death from fire.[240] Toxic concentrations of this gas accumulate in poorly ventilated areas. As oxygen in the air decreases from 21% to $\leq$10% during a fire, the concentration of carbon monoxide rises.[241] Carbon monoxide has a greater affinity than oxygen for hemoglobin, causing carboxyhemoglobin formation, tissue hypoxia and death.

Toxic combustion products may injure the respiratory tract directly. Upper airway damage is common; damage to the distal airways and parenchyma depends on the amount of smoke inhaled and its composition.[238] In combustion, carbon particles become coated with a variety of organic acids and aldehydes, depending on the parent compound. When inhaled, these particles attach to the airway mucosa, where they can remain and cause chemical injury for extended periods.[240] Therefore, pulmonary damage is often underestimated initially.

Pulmonary infection is a potential complication in every smoke inhalation patient. Alveolar macrophages are important in clearing inhaled bacteria from the lung. Though alveolar macrophage numbers increase in the lung after smoke inhalation, phagocytic and bactericidal activity are decreased.[242] In addition, mucociliary clearance is depressed.[241] These findings may partially explain the enhanced susceptibility of smoke inhalation patients to pulmonary infection.

Major skin burns also may cause pulmonary dysfunction in the absence of smoke inhalation.[243] Several mechanisms may be involved, including the activation of serum complement and the coagulation cascade caused by release of denatured proteins from burned tissue, and pulmonary edema secondary to release of vasoactive mediators.[244-246]

Therapy for smoke inhalation depends upon severity of the condition and presence of other injuries, especially skin burns. A patent airway must be maintained. Because upper airway obstruction may develop over several days, the patient must be watched closely for signs of impending obstruction that necessitates tracheostomy. Oxygen therapy may be needed to reduce tissue hypoxia caused by carbon monoxide poisoning. Pain is controlled with nonsteroidal antiinflammatory agents and, in some instances, narcotics. Broad-spectrum antibiotics may reduce likelihood of pulmonary infection.

The prognosis varies from case to case, but owners should be warned that smoke inhalation causes progressive and, in many instances, permanent damage. In 20 horses that survived a barn fire, tachypnea and coughing developed 1-7 days after the fire.[247] Wheezes were auscultated for the first week after injury, but auscultation findings were normal within a week. Persistent lung injury may have resulted, as several of these horses developed a chronic cough and never returned to their previous level of performance. Thus, with severe skin burns and sepsis, the prognosis for return to full function is guarded.

Aspiration Pneumonia

F.J. Derksen

When liquid or solid substances enter the tracheobronchial tree, an instantaneous and vigorous protective response is evoked in most mammalian species. This response includes coughing and bronchospasm. In contrast, horses allow entrance of liquid and solid materials into the trachea without coughing. Only when foreign materials reach the carina is a cough response elicited. For example, after racing in muddy conditions, dirt and grass commonly are present in the horse's trachea, and coughing is not observed. The clinician can place a fiberoptic endoscope in the trachea without a cough response. Though most of the foreign material in the airways is removed from the tracheobronchial tree within a few hours, the poorly developed protective response against aspiration may predispose horses to pulmonary injury.

Several diseases may cause aspiration of food material by interfering with swallowing. These conditions include esophageal obstruction, guttural pouch mycosis and tympany, pharyngeal foreign bodies, pharyngeal cysts and cleft palate. In addition, aspiration of food material is a common sequel to laryngeal surgery (Fig 41). The type of pulmonary injury caused by aspiration depends, for the most part, upon the pH of the material and its microbial flora.[248] Aspiration of gastric content with a low pH causes severe tissue injury including epithelial injury, pulmonary edema and hemorrhagic

Figure 41. Radiograph after a barium swallow 3 days after laryngotomy shows aspiration of barium. The mandible (M), guttural pouches (GP) and trachea (T) can be seen, with barium in the esophagus (open arrow) and floor of the trachea (solid arrow).

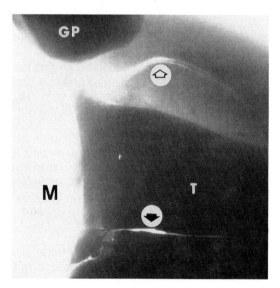

pneumonia.[249] However, because vomiting does not occur in horses, this type of injury is uncommon. In addition, gastric reflux fluids associated with colic usually have a near neutral pH because the reflux fluid usually is a mixture of acidic gastric secretions and basic duodenal fluids.

Pulmonary infection is the most important complication of aspiration in horses. Because the bacterial flora in the oral cavity is mixed, the type of organism causing aspiration pneumonia cannot be predicted accurately. However, because anaerobic organisms are common in the oral cavity, anaerobic infections are likely. Horses that aspirate foreign material into the lungs may remain asymptomatic, but combined with such stresses as racing or anesthesia and surgery, aspiration may cause fulminating pneumonia and pleuritis.

Therapy first is directed against preventing further aspiration of material. Antimicrobials used should have a broad antibacterial spectrum. Because of its activity against anaerobic organisms, penicillin or metronidazole should be included in the antimicrobial regimen.

Inadvertent deposition of mineral oil into the lungs can occur when a nasogastric tube is misplaced or if the oil is given as an oral drench. In the latter situation, because of the bland nature of the oil, no protective coughing occurs. If oil is thought to have reached the lungs, xylazine sedation should be used to lower the horse's head and promote drainage. Antiinflammatory drugs should be given for several days to weeks and any possible secondary bacterial disease monitored using thoracic radiographs, hemograms and transtracheal aspirate culture. The prognosis usually is unfavorable because of the chronic and progressive granulomatous reaction initiated by mineral oil.

Silicosis

See the section on Granulomatous Pneumonia under Diseases of the Lung for information on silicosis.

Pneumothorax

See the sections on Pneumothorax under Diseases of the Pleura, Mediastinum, Diaphragm and Chest Wall for a complete discussion of this subject.

Inflammatory, Infectious and Immune Diseases

J. Beech

Viral Respiratory Diseases

See the section on Diseases Affecting Multiple Sites in this chapter for a full discussion of this topic.

Streptococcus zooepidemicus Infection

Streptococcus zooepidemicus probably is the most common bacterium isolated from the lower respiratory tract of horses with respiratory disease, and it has been isolated occasionally from the respiratory tract of healthy horses. In a study of 86 healthy horses, hemolytic streptococci were isolated from the tracheobronchial aspirates of 2.[11] A higher isolation rate has been reported from samples obtained from the trachea at necropsy.[250] Also, *Strep zooepidemicus* has been one of the most common bacteria isolated from horses with pleuritis and pleuropneumonia.[251,252] Because *Strep zooepidemicus* cannot invade intact mucous membranes, it probably is most important as a secondary invader in horses with increased susceptibility because of viral infection or such stresses as transport. Long-distance transport decreases the number of alveolar macrophages, neutrophils and lymphocytes recovered from bronchoalveolar lavages of horses; this could alter disease resistance. This may be the reason that severe respiratory diseases, such as pleuritis, often occur after transport or other stress.[252,253]

Inhalation of the organism by a susceptible host can result in infections of the upper respiratory tract, such as sinusitis and abscessation of lymph nodes. Subsequently the lower respiratory tract can become infected; resulting pneumonia may be diffuse or focal. Abscesses and pleuritis can result. Clinical signs depend on the severity of infection, whether it affects the upper or lower respiratory tract more adversely, and the horse's immune status.

Depression, fever, anorexia and mucopurulent nasal discharge are common reasons for clients to request veterinary attention for their horse. A complete physical examination can reveal whether there is lymphadenopathy, whether sinuses are dull on percussion indicating fluid therein, and whether the character of lung sounds suggests pneumonia with consolidation or pleural fluid. Dullness on thoracic percussion and decreased audible air movement suggest intrathoracic fluid or lung consolidation. Wheezes may be heard when airways are narrowed; wheezes and crackles occur when there is fluid or exudate in the airways. The pattern of respiration usually gives some information about the severity of the disease.

The diagnosis is based on isolation of the organism from the site(s) of infection. Sensitivity testing of streptococci is advisable, especially because organisms have become increasingly resistant to penicillin. In a 6-month report from the author's hospital, 80% of beta-hemolytic streptococci tested were sensitive to penicillin, 20% were moderately sensitive, and 100% were sensitive to erythromycin. Other drugs that may be effective are chloramphenicol, trimethoprim-sulfa combinations, and synthetic penicillins. An advantage of erythromycin, in addition to the sensitivity pattern, is that it apparently achieves high lung and pleural fluid levels and penetrates neutrophils. Erythromycin, penicillin and many of its synthetic forms, and trimethoprim-sulfa all are available for oral use. Diarrhea occasionally may accompany oral antibiotic use but usually ceases when the drug is discontinued or the dose is reduced.

In addition to medical therapy with appropriate antibiotics, any areas amenable to drainage should be drained. Flushing of the sinuses or guttural pouches also may be helpful. Isotonic sterile saline is suitable. Potentially irritating solutions should be avoided. Persistent streptococcal sinus or guttural pouch infections may require multiple lavages and long-term antimicrobial therapy. Whether such drugs as levamisole or other immunostimulants serve any purpose in boosting the immune response and shortening the treatment period has not been proven. Local hot pack application may aid resolution of abscesses.

Stress, including transport, should be avoided in affected horses. Though nonsteroidal antiinflammatory drugs may improve the horse's attitude and appetite, their antipyretic action complicates monitoring body temperature as a guide to therapeutic efficacy of selected antimicrobials. Duration of therapy depends on the severity and location of the disease. It may exceed several months in persistent infections or when there is pleuritis and pneumonia. Nursing care and maintenance of the patient's appetite and good attitude all are important in contributing to a favorable outcome.

Streptococcus equi Infection

Streptococcus equi is commonly known to cause strangles; however, infection does not always result in grossly obvious cranial lymphadenopathy. The organism is highly contagious and young horses 1-5 years old are predisposed. Clinical signs usually appear 2-20 days after infection, but usually within 10 days.[254,255] Feed, water buckets and areas contaminated with secretions from infected horses facilitate spread of the infection. The bacterium enters the host via the upper respiratory tract, especially the nasopharynx.

Clinical signs are variable, and expression of the disease is greatly affected by the horse's immune status and antibodies from earlier exposure. In a susceptible horse, the organism can survive in neutrophils following phagocytosis.[256] Milder forms of the disease involve strains with decreased antiphagocytic capacity.[257]

Fever, depression, anorexia, a serous nasal discharge that becomes mucopurulent, and abscessed submaxillary, mandibular and retropharyngeal lymph nodes characteristically are seen in affected horses. Neck pain may be apparent, and lymph node enlargement may obstruct respiration and affect swallowing. The retropharyngeal lymph nodes may rupture and drain externally or internally. When the latter occurs, aspiration pneumonia or guttural pouch empyema may result. The recurrent laryngeal nerve and nerves passing near the guttural pouch may be affected. Myocarditis has been reported. Lactating mares may become agalactic. Clinical signs may last from <1 week to >2 months.[254,255] Purpura hemorrhagica and disseminated internal abscesses ("bastard strangles") may be sequelae of this or other streptococcal infections.

The diagnosis is based on culture of the organism. Direct smears of exudate frequently reveal chains of streptococci. Though there is great variation in nasal shedding patterns with regard to both numbers of organisms and duration of shedding, nasal swabs are more likely to yield positive cultures from infected horses than are pharyngeal swabs. Lymph node swabs are the most likely specimens to culture positive. In one study, lymph node swabs were positive 50% of the time, in contrast to nasal and pharyngeal swab specimens, which cultured positive only 24% of the time.[254,255] A selective transport medium, such as Strepswab (Medical Wire and Equip, Cleveland), reduces contamination by other nonstreptococcal organisms and aids the laboratory in handling such samples. However, the prevalence of isolation was the same as when a Culturette (Marion Scientific) was used.[254,255]

When a source of exudate is not readily available for culture, diagnosis becomes more difficult. Inspissated pus in the guttural pouches may not produce a nasal discharge, and internal abscesses may be impossible to diagnose, even with radiographs and internal palpation per rectum. An elevated serum fibrinogen or globulin level, anemia of chronic disease, and possible leukogram changes may give nonspecific indications of infection. Historical exposure to "strangles" often is used for tentative diagnosis of *Strep equi* infection in horses with these laboratory abnormalities.

Control of the disease requires quarantine of affected animals and preventing exposure of unaffected horses. Because the degree of nasal shedding is not directly related to the severity or presence of clinical signs, inapparently infected horses may spread the disease. A horse may have repeated attacks months after apparent recovery.[258] The infection may be maintained for at least 8 months in a group of horses.[256] Premises are said to harbor the infection for up to a year.[258] However, the duration of survival of the organism has not been clearly defined. Because attendants may transmit the disease among horses, those caring for sick horses should not work with other horses. If this is impossible, then these people should conscientiously and rigorously wash their hands and use disposable gowns and footwear that can be disinfected after contact with affected horses.

Treatment of exposed horses or foals with antibiotics can prevent infection during therapy, but these horses can develop clinical signs if they are exposed after antibiotic use is discontinued. One study showed a significant decrease in foal morbidity when benzathine penicillin was given (900,000 IU IM every 48 hours for 21 days).[254,255]

The decision to use antibiotics depends on the severity of clinical signs, and numbers and ages of exposed horses. Mild infections localized to the lymph nodes or upper respiratory tract usually do not require systemic antibiotic treatment. Pneumonia, pleuritis, sinusitis, synovitis, guttural pouch empyema and other systemic manifestations of the infection may require long-term therapy. Pneumonia has been the most common fatal complication, and horses with suspected lower respiratory tract infections should be treated rigorously. Antibiotic sensitivity testing of the *Strep equi* isolate should be performed to choose the appropriate drug. Comments made previously on antibiotics elected for streptococci apply to *Strep equi*. Current evidence indicates that use of antibiotics does not predispose horses to "bastard strangles," and one should not avoid using them because of this potential sequel to the disease.[254,255]

Purpura hemorrhagica can be a severe complication, often requiring long-term therapy with antibiotics and antiinflammatory drugs. Relatively large doses of dexamethasone (Azium: Schering) are required. If other factors deter use of corticosteroids, one could try flunixin meglumine (Banamine: Schering). Surgical drainage occasionally is needed for guttural pouch empyema, sinusitis or retropharyngeal lymph node abscessation.

Other important contributions to recovery from *Strep equi* infection are nursing care, hot packing abscessed lymph nodes, providing palatable and easily swallowed food and, with animals unable or unwilling to eat, feeding by nasogastric tube. Dyspneic horses may require tracheostomy. Handlers always should be alerted to check for respiratory difficulty that could indicate an impending need for tracheostomy.

Commercial vaccines are available. None is completely effective in preventing the disease, but both M-protein extract (Strepvax: Coopers) and adjuvanted concentrated purified enzyme extract (Strepguard: Haver) reduce the frequency of clinical disease. Very large challenge doses may overcome immunity. Yearly booster vaccinations are recommended. However, immunity may not persist this long, as clinical signs of strangles were reported in yearlings within 6 months of vaccination with M-protein vaccine or bacterin.[259] It is not clear how long immunity persists following natural infection. Some clinicians claim that it is several years, while others believe it is <6 months.[254,255,258] Measurement of bactericidal antibodies is not helpful in evaluating whether a horse is protected, as there is no correlation between serum antibodies and protection.[260] Protection correlates with the levels of antibodies in the pharyngeal mucosa, but this provides no useful diagnostic application for the practitioner.[261]

Streptococcus pneumoniae Infection

This alpha-hemolytic streptococcus is a recognized pathogen of the upper respiratory tract in people. From 5% to 60% of people are carriers, depending on season and environmental conditions.[262] Though it has sporadically been isolated from horses, its importance in this species remains unknown.[263-265] Pneumococcal septicemia was reported in a foal, and a single serotype of the organism also has been isolated from tracheobronchial aspirates from adult horses and a foal, and from an adult horse's pleural fluid.[263,265] Of these last horses, 3 had pneumonia, and 1 also had pleuritis and pericarditis. Other pathogens, (*Streptococcus, Pasteurella, Actinobacillus*) were concurrently isolated from these animals. Two others had a chronic cough, 3 had decreased exercise tolerance, and 1 had exercise-induced pulmonary hemorrhage. In only 2 was *Strep pneumoniae* the sole isolate, and its role in the disease was unknown. Horses recovered after treatment with antibiotics appropriate for all involved pathogens isolated.[263]

In an English study, when 26 2- to 3-year-old Thoroughbred horses had sequential tracheobronchial aspirates obtained via endoscope over 1-18 months, *Strep pneumoniae* (capsule type 3) was recovered on ≥1 occasions from 18 horses, and 1 horse cultured positive 13 of 17 times sampled. In none of the horses was the organism clearly documented as a cause of clinical disease.[264] However, clinically ill horses from which *Strep pneumoniae* was cultured showed a rise in antibody titers to *Strep pneumoniae* type 3 for 2-4 weeks after onset of clinical signs. *Streptococcus pneumoniae* was isolated in pure culture from only 1 of these horses. *Streptococcus zooepidemicus* and other bacteria also were isolated in all the other horses. Seroconversion also was seen in asymptomatic horses; some horses never seroconverted.

In none of these cases was the source of infection identified, and it is not known if infected horses pose a hazard to people. Though no association was made between infected horses and people with *Strep pneumoniae* infections, horses potentially could transmit the organism to susceptible people. Therefore, people with increased risk of infection should not expose themselves to known infected horses.

As the organism never has been demonstrated as a primary cause of respiratory disease in horses, infected horses usually are treated for coexisting pathogens.

Rhodococcus equi Infection

This organism, formerly called *Corynebacterium equi*, is an important cause of pneumonia in foals, primarily those 1-6 months of age.[266-268] Most show signs at 2-4 months of age.[266-268] It rarely causes pneumonia in older horses.[269]

Rhodococcus equi can survive in soil for at least a year and withstand drying and direct sunlight.[266,270] On some farms it is isolated in large quantities from the soil, independent of whether horses are present; on other farms it has been isolated only from areas with horses.[271,272] In one study, 65% of 106 horses had the organism in their feces.[273] In another study, there was a significant difference in culture results from different sites on the same farm. The number of foals with clinical *R equi* infection correlated with the number of bacteria cultured from the stable area but not from elsewhere. Also, there was a correlation between soil contamination at all sites (paddocks, stables, pastures) and the presence of horses.[272]

Dusty environments and dry weather appear to increase the prevalence of the disease. Even when numbers of *R equi* in pasture soil are high, foals grazing these grass pastures seem to be at less risk than foals around stables, where there is more chance of environmental dust.[272] The importance of inhalation as the route of infection for the respiratory form also is substantiated by the fact that ingestion of *R equi* usually results in self-limiting intestinal infection.[274]

Clinical Syndromes: Clinical signs of *R equi* respiratory tract infection vary. Some foals apparently are asymptomatic until found dead in the field; necropsy reveals diffuse lung abscessation. Other foals suddenly develop respiratory distress, with a rapid respiratory rate, flared nostrils, heaving respiratory pattern and fever. Auscultation may reveal wheezes and crackles in the lungs or there may only be an increase in coarseness and loss of soft vesicular sounds. Cyanosis is common. Usually there is no nasal discharge despite exudate in the lower airways. These foals often die within several days, even if treatment is initiated. Necropsy reveals lung abscesses and diffuse pneumonia.

Other foals have a more chronic course over weeks to months. Systemic signs (*eg*, synovitis and uveitis) may accompany pneumonia. Pleural effusion is rare. These foals are febrile and often dyspneic, and usually lose condition and look unthrifty. Nasal discharge and coughing are variable. When present, the cough is usually soft and deep. Auscultation may reveal only coarse sounds or large airway sounds, suggesting loss of aeration of lung parenchyma, or there may be wheezes and crackles. It may be possible to percuss areas of dullness when consolidated areas are extensive and superficial in the lungs. Affected foals usually are severely exercise intolerant, and even minor stresses can worsen their dyspnea and precipitate collapse. Blood gas determinations often reveal severe hypoxemia and hypercarbia. The intestinal form of *R equi* infection rarely accompanies the pulmonary disease in North America, but it may be present in up to half the cases in other countries. Diarrhea and weight loss can occur with intestinal disease.

Adult horses with *R equi* have shown weight loss, fever, coughing and dyspnea.[269] Rapidly progressive pneumonia and pleuritis occurred in one horse, and another had ulcerative lymphangitis. The former horse was 18 years old and had polyuria, polydipsia and glucosuria, signs suggestive of an underlying pituitary adenoma, which may cause increased susceptibility to infections.

Diagnosis: Results of clinical laboratory tests are nonspecific for *R equi* infection and usually include leukocytosis and increased serum fibrinogen concentration. One study showed no difference between the leukogram or serum fibrinogen concentration of survivors vs nonsurvivors,[275] but another study showed nonsurvivors had significantly higher values.[276] Thoracic radiographs and analysis of the tracheobronchial aspirates are most helpful in diagnosing this disease. Direct microscopic evaluation of a transtracheal aspirate often reveals Gram-positive pleomorphic rods. Tracheobronchial aspirates from infected foals usually are culture positive for *R equi* but false-negative results may occur. The organism may be shed only periodically and often is intracellular and may not grow in culture.[277] Multiple other pathogens may be isolated along with *R equi*.[275,276]

Radiographs often are most helpful when cultures are negative. A prominent alveolar pattern with ill-defined regional consolidation is a common radiographic finding.[276] Nodular lesions in the lungs and lymphadenopathy are almost pathognomonic in foals in this age range; however, they may not be present on initial examination. Lesions may become cavitary, demonstrating air-fluid interfaces within circumscribed lesions. Pleural effusion is very rare, even in chronic cases. Acutely or mildly affected foals may have a prominent interstitial pattern alone. Tracheobronchial lymphadenopathy reportedly is useful prognositically because it is more common in foals that do not recover.[276] However, some foals with severe radiographic changes do recover; therefore, radiographs should not be used as the sole criterion to establish a prognosis or to recommend euthanasia of an infected foal.

Lymphocyte immunostimulation tests are useful diagnostically in foals ≤2 months of age, as these foals have a very high stimulation ratio compared to normal foals. In foals >2 months old, the test is helpful only when negative (stimulation rate ≤0.6), as this rules out *R equi* as the cause of pneumonia. Some normal foals >2 months old have higher stimulation ratios than infected foals, and positive responses are not diagnostic.[278] An enzyme-linked immunosorbent assay was useful in detecting specific *R equi* antibodies;[279] however, other studies showed no correlation between titers and infection.[280,281] In the future, immunologic

tests useful in identifying and monitoring infected foals will likely be developed.

Treatment: Sensitivity patterns for the organism may vary slightly in different geographic regions. The organism usually is sensitive to gentamicin, often to trimethoprim-sulfonamide combinations and chloramphenicol, and occasionally to tetracycline. Often it is resistant to penicillin. Erythromycin, usually combined with rifampin, is widely recommended as the treatment of choice;[282,283] this therapy has resulted in decreased mortality.[275] Most isolates are sensitive to erythromycin, and the minimal inhibitory concentration is low. The minimal inhibitory concentration for gentamicin also is low but considerably higher for kanamycin and amikacin, making the last 2 drugs less useful.[276] In terms of minimum inhibitory concentrations, rifampin is 5 times as potent as gentamicin and erythromycin is almost twice as potent as gentamicin. The reported minimal inhibitory concentration for trimethoprim-sulfonamide combinations (<4.75 μg/ml) suggests this combination may not be effective because required therapeutic concentrations may not be achieved with current regimens. However, clinical successes have been reported.[275]

In-vitro studies have shown antagonism when gentamicin is combined with erythromycin or rifampin; therefore, this combination should be avoided. Synergy was reported for erythromycin and rifampin or penicillin.[282] Gentamicin reportedly has been used successfully, but another survey comparing different treatments showed that none of 17 foals treated with penicillin and gentamicin survived, while all of 12 foals treated with erythromycin and/or rifampin survived.[275] The reported *in-vitro* synergism of penicillin and gentamicin in killing *R equi* seems to have had no beneficial clinical effect in this survey.

The usual dosage of erythromycin is 25-30 mg/kg PO 4 times daily and of rifampin is 5 mg/kg PO twice daily.[282,285] There appears to be no clinical advantage to IV use unless oral medication is contraindicated in a patient. The low minimum inhibitory concentrations and good cellular penetration probably are responsible for the success of these drugs. Because they seem to act synergistically and because rifampin resistance can occur if this drug is used alone, rifampin always should be combined with another drug. Oral erythromycin may cause diarrhea but usually it is not severe and does not preclude use of the drug.

Nursing care, adequate nutrition and excellent ventilation are very important. In the author's experience, bronchodilators or drugs to decrease the work of breathing, such as aminophylline, have no definite clinical benefit. Aminophylline should be used cautiously in patients receiving erythromycin because erythromycin delays clearance and elevates blood levels of aminophylline, thus potentiating its toxicity. Excitement and seizures may occur. If the drugs are used simultaneously, blood levels always should be monitored. Some clinicians also use cimetidine or ranitidine plus sucralfate as prophylaxis for gastric ulcers.

Prevention and Control: The disease is difficult to prevent and control. Its insidious nature hampers early detection and isolation of affected foals. Poor ventilation and dusty conditions probably are major contributory factors, and often are the most difficult to correct. Attempts should be made to house foals in well-ventilated, dust-free areas and avoid dirt paddocks and crowded conditions, especially around stable areas where animal movement is heavy. Stress and drugs that decrease immune function should be avoided. Monitoring the rectal temperature may be one of the best means of early detection of infections in foals, but normal fluctuations, particularly in hot climates, can limit the usefulness of this. Complete blood counts may be abnormal before overt signs of pneumonia occur but, on a practical basis, usually they are not helpful.

Bacterial cultures of respiratory tract secretions inconsistently reveal the organisms, and finding *R equi* in the feces is not particularly helpful diagnostically. *Rhodococcus equi* has been cultured from feces of foals and mares and occasionally from tracheal secretions from healthy foals. In some cases, the foal's value may warrant thoracic radiography, as radiographic evidence of infection usually precedes development of clinical signs.

Any foals that die should be necropsied. Findings vary, depending on severity of infection and whether the infection was confined to the lungs. One form was described as diffuse, multiple, enlarging lung abscesses, another as multiple, small parenchymal foci of inflammation, with intervening areas of alveolar emphysema and edema, and a third as a mixture of these 2.[267] Tracheobronchial lymph nodes usually are enlarged and abscessed or edematous.

Histologically, the lymph nodes and spleen have hyperplasia of the T-dependent paracortical areas, suggesting stimulated cell-mediated immune processes. In the lungs, macrophages and neutrophils fill airways and alveoli, and necrosis and granulomatous reactions are evident. Organisms are often numerous and found primarily within macrophages.

Miscellaneous Bacterial Infections

The Gram-negative bacterium *Bordetella bronchiseptica* is a respiratory pathogen in several species, but its role in equine respiratory diseases has yet to be defined. In species in which it has recognized pathogenicity, it attaches to airway surfaces, causing acute inflammation, mucus secretion and altered mucociliary clearance. It is cultured only rarely from transtracheal aspirates and even more rarely is a pure isolate.[287] The low frequency of isolates is unlikely to be due to unusual culture requirements because though growth may require 48 hours' incubation, it grows easily on commonly used media. In some geographic areas, it has been isolated more commonly both as a pure isolate and with other bacteria.[288,289]

Bordetella bronchiseptica was isolated in a hospital outbreak of respiratory disease in 9 horses.[288] In a survey of 80 foals <6 months of age with pneumonia, *B bronchiseptica* was isolated from up to 28% of the aspirates from which respiratory pathogens were cultured.[289] Of 61 foals from which 1-2 pathogens were cultured, *B bronchiseptica* was the third most common isolate. All isolates were sensitive to gentamicin, 90% were sensitive to amikacin, kanamycin, ticarcillin and chloramphenicol, and 75% to trimethoprim-sulfadiazine and tetracycline. The same authors also reported that erythromycin was effective.[289]

When the organism is isolated from clinically ill horses, appropriate antimicrobial therapy should be started and should also be effective against any other pathogens isolated.

Other bacteria that can cause pneumonia include *Klebsiella, Escherichia coli, Pasteurella, Actinobacillus equuli* and *Staphylococcus. Pseudomonas* spp have been isolated commonly from horses with pleuropneumonia. *Salmonella* rarely may cause pneumonia. Septicemic foals may have pneumonia as a component of their generalized infection.

Anaerobes also may be important pathogens in infections of the lower respiratory tract, especially in necrotizing pneumonia, lung abscesses or pleuritis and pneumonia. Because normal horses have anaerobes in their pharynx, positive anaerobic cultures from this site are not significant. Successful isolation of anaerobes requires special culture techniques, and samples should be transferred to the laboratory using special medium (Port-A-Cul: Becton-Dickinson). This medium is suitable for both aerobic and anaerobic cultures. Routine culture swabs are not suitable. Anaerobes most commonly isolated are *Bacteroides* spp, followed by *Clostridium* spp.[290] Though a putrid odor is characteristic of anaerobic infections and warrants poor prognosis in horses with pleuropneumonia, the absence of odor does not exclude the presence of anaerobes. Of 21 horses that had anaerobes cultured from a tracheobronchial aspirate or pleural fluid, 8 had no evidence of putrid odor to the breath or fluid sample.[290] Anaerobic infections of the lower respiratory tract have a poorer prognosis than aerobic infections.

Antimicrobial treatment of these miscellaneous bacterial infections should be based on Gram stain and sensitivity test results, and knowledge of which drugs are most likely to reach therapeutic levels at the site of infection. Gram stains of aspirates help in choosing an antimicrobial before culture results are available. An antimicrobial with broad antibacterial activity should be selected initially. When an anaerobic infection is suspected, penicillin is a good choice and often is combined with a drug effective against Gram-negative bacteria.

Resistance of many Gram-negative bacteria seems to have increased, and selection of appropriate drugs, especially aminoglycosides, is likely to vary among different clinics or in different areas. Metronidazole is excellent for treating anaerobic infections and is effective against beta-lactamase-producing anaerobes that are penicillin resistant. It can be given IV or PO; current dosage recommendations are 15-25 mg/kg PO 4 times daily.[291] The same supportive care, including maintenance of hydration, drainage of exudate when it is accessible, and providing a warm environment with good ventilation, is required in all respiratory infections, regardless of cause.

Melioidosis

R.C. Knowles

Melioidosis is an acute, febrile disease characterized by pneumonitis, a rapid course and high mortality.

Species Affected: This bacterial disease occurs in horses, cattle, sheep, goats, pigs, kangaroos, rodents, orangutans and people.

Cause: Melioidosis is caused by *Pseudomonas pseudomallei*, a Gram-negative bacillus that closely resembles *Pseudomonas aeruginosa*.

Transmission: The disease occurs naturally in rodents. Transmission among those animals by biting insects, such as mosquitoes and fleas, has been reported. The microorganism does not require the rat or any other animal as a maintenance host. In Malaysia, *Pseudomonas pseudomallei* is a normal inhabitant of soil and water.

In a Parisian zoo, 7 species were infected with melioidosis: Przewalski's horse (*Equus przewalskii*), oryx (*Oryx beisa*), zebu (*Bos indicus*), cercopithecus (*Cercopithecus aethiops sabaeus*), muntjac (*Muniacus muntjac*), sika (*Sika nippon*) and wild sheep (*Ovis musimon*). Manure from the zoo was spread on nearby pastures, causing an outbreak of melioidosis in horses.

Geographic Distribution: Early descriptions of the disease were principally from southeast Asia. However, it has also been reported in Australia and occasionally in Europe and the western hemisphere.

Clinical Signs: A salient feature of melioidosis is pneumonitis and fever. The course of the disease is short and mortality is high.

Lesions: Characteristic lesions are small (2-3 mm) caseous nodules. While most often found in lung tissue, such nodules may be found in almost any tissue, including the brain.

Diagnosis: Diagnosis of melioidosis depends upon demonstration and isolation of the causative organism in characteristic lesions.

Treatment and Control: Though *Pseudomonas pseudomallei* is susceptible to many antibiotics *in vitro*, it frequently develops *in-vivo* drug resistance. In people, chloramphenicol alone or combined with kanamycin has been the treatment of choice.

Recent episodes of melioidosis in people and animals indicate that this disease has likely spread from southeast Asia with the movement of animals and people. One should remember this when considering preventive measures, such as disposition of manure from zoologic parks.

Glanders

R.C. Knowles

Glanders is a contagious bacterial disease of equidae that also affects other animals, including people. It is characterized by formation of nodular lesions in the mouth, upper respiratory tract and skin.

Species Affected: The horse is the most commonly affected animal. Frequently the disease in this species is chronic, while in donkeys and mules it may be acute. Carnivores fed infected meat can acquire the disease. The disease affects people, frequently fatally. Cattle and swine are not susceptible, but guinea pigs and mice are highly susceptible.

Cause: The disease is caused by the non-spore-forming Gram-negative bacterium *Pseudomonas mallei*. The organism is isolated directly from lesions or tissues when cultured on peptone agar with 5% defibrinated sheep or rabbit blood incubated aerobically at 37 C (98.6 F). Care must be taken to differentiate glanders from *Pseudomonas pseudomallei* infection (melioidosis), as the clinical signs are similar.

Transmission: The bacterium is transmitted primarily by fomites, such as contaminated utensils or grooming equipment, or through direct contact.

Geographic Distribution: Glanders is not uncommon in countries of the Middle East, the Indian subcontinent and southeast Asia. It is reported in African countries and probably exists in many other countries where no systematic attempts at identification or control are conducted.

Clinical Signs: The incubation period varies from as short as 2 weeks to as long as several months. Clinical signs may be pulmonary, nasal or cutaneous, or concurrent combination of these signs. In the acute form there is fever, coughing and nasal discharge. The more common chronic form is characterized by general malaise, coughing, unthriftiness, intermittent fever and enlargement of the mandibular lymph nodes. Nodules on the nasal septum rupture to produce ulcers that leave star-shaped scars on the nasal septum. In the cutaneous form, commonly called farcy, nodules occur along the lymph nodes or subcutaneous vessels, usually on the rear legs. The nodules rupture, discharge a yellow-gray, oily pus and chronically ulcerate.

Diagnosis: An association with horses from affected areas or exposure to contaminated materials used in handling horses is significant.

Diagnosis and control of glanders are based on testing using the intradermal or intrapalpebral inoculation of mallein, an extract of *Pseudomonas mallei* cells. A positive reaction produces swelling, hyperemia, congestion or discharge with hyperthermia at the site of inoculation. The complement-fixation test is a reliable means of identifying antibodies.

The organism is readily cultured from exudates or affected organs. The material should be maintained under refrigeration until culture and bacterial examination are done. Direct examination of exudates is of little value.

Because of human susceptibility to infection, great caution must be taken in conducting physical examinations and particularly in collecting specimens for bacterial examination. Samples must be clearly marked "suspected glanders."

Evidence of respiratory disease with high fever, nasal discharge, coughing and stellate lesions on the nasal septum are presumptive evidence of glanders. Such conditions as melioidosis and infections of lymphatic vessels and glands, as observed with epizootic strangles or ulcerative lymphangitis, should be considered differential diagnoses.

Treatment: Some sulfa drugs have been used to arrest the disease. However, because treated animals can become carriers, treatment is contraindicated and is incompatible with the objectives of the eradication program. There is no effective immunization against glanders.

Control: Because transmission is mainly by contact or ingestion of contaminated food or water, disinfectants must be thoroughly applied in stables and on stable equipment. Materials that may harbor the organism should be destroyed following an outbreak of the disease.

Control has been effected by testing for active infection using the allergic mallein test at about 1-month intervals and slaughtering reactors. The complement-fixation test provides surveillance after the active phase of the eradication program has been carried out.

Bacterial Pneumonia in Neonates

M.R. Paradis

Bacterial pneumonia in neonatal foals is usually associated with septicemia. The newborn may be infected *in utero*, or during or following parturition. Complete or partial failure of transfer of maternal antibodies to the foal is common in foals infected postpartum. Bacteria enter the lungs by inhalation or via the circulation. The most common pathogens involved are *E coli, Klebsiella pneumoniae* and *Actinobacillus equuli*.[292]

Clinical signs in septicemic foals with pneumonia may be vague. The respiratory rate and effort can be normal. Lung sounds can range from quiet to harsh. A cough rarely is present. Some septic foals are normothermic on presentation.[292] The most common clinical sign in foals with septicemia is some degree of weakness and lethargy.[292]

Because the signs may be subtle in the early stages, the diagnostic plan should include a CBC, arterial blood gas analysis, thoracic radiographs, blood cultures and determination of blood glucose concentration. Serum immunoglobulin G (IgG) levels should be used to detect failure of passive transfer. An increased number of total band neutrophils and toxic changes in the neutrophils on the CBC are suggestive of septicemia in newborn foals. Hypoglycemia is common in septicemic foals <24 hours old. Some degree of failure of passive transfer almost always is present in septicemic foals infected after birth.[292]

The most definitive method to determine if septicemic foals also have pneumonia is thoracic radiography. Radiographic findings are similar to those in foals with immature lungs, including increased interstitial patterns and loss of vascular clarity. Consolidation of individual lung lobes (accessory lobe) may be evident.[293]

Arterial blood gas measurements often are helpful in evaluating foals with pneumonia. Septicemic foals with pulmonary involvement may have a mixed metabolic and respiratory acidosis, combined with hypoxemia (Table 2). Sodium bicarbonate ($NaHCO_3$) is a common buffer used in treatment of metabolic acidosis. Unfortunately, HCO_3 is metabolized to produce water and carbon dioxide (CO_2). This production of CO_2 may slightly worsen the respiratory component of such a mixed acidosis. In addition to bicarbonate administration and ventilatory therapy, an increase in the inspired oxygen concentration is needed to correct hypoxemia.

Additional therapy should be directed at resolving septicemia, hypoglycemia, failure of passive transfer and possible shock. A broad-spectrum combination of antimicrobials should be used until culture results are obtained. Fluid therapy should consist of 5% dextrose for hypoglycemia, plasma transfusions to correct failure of passive transfer and lactated Ringer's solution for volume expansion. General nursing care is paramount in successful treatment.

Pneumocystis carinii Infection

J. Beech

Pneumocystis carinii is a ubiquitous sporozoan that causes interstitial pneumonia in human infants and aged people, or people with primary or secondary immunodeficiency. There have been sporadic reports of infection in foals, usually in association with *Rhodococcus equi* but also with *Bordetella bronchiseptica*. Clinical signs reflect the bacterial pneumonia.

Diagnosis has been at necropsy, though in people, lung and endobronchial brush biopsies and tracheobronchial aspirates have provided the diagnosis. Silver staining (Gomori methenamine silver) is needed to reveal the organism, as it is not easily recognized using routine hematoxylin and eosin staining. It is seen as a cup- or crescent-shaped structure in alveoli and is associated with acidophilic material and mononuclear-cell infiltration.

The antimicrobial choice for treatment and prophylaxis of *Pneumocystis carinii* infection is trimethoprim-sulfamethoxazole, probably at high dosages, such as 30 mg/kg BID. In people, aerosolized pentamidine has been effective and could be used in affected foals. It is very important to treat the primary or coexistent disease with appropriate drugs, and combinations of antimicrobials may be necessary. If primary immunodeficiency is suspected, it is important to confirm or negate this suspicion, as this greatly alters the prognosis and treatment.

Parascaris equorum Infection

Though larvae of this parasite migrate through the lungs of foals and young horses, the clinical significance never has been well defined. Clinical respiratory disease has been reported in foals at 2-4 weeks of age and in horses 8-10 months old after experimental infection.[294,295] The idea that the parasite may be a clinically important pathogen is supported by clinical cases of mild pneumonia and coughing, characterized by the presence of eosinophils and no evidence of sepsis in transtracheal aspirates, no exposure to donkeys and response to fenbendazole (15 mg/kg) used for 5 days, in 2- to 4-month-old foals.

When parascarid eggs are ingested, larvae can be found 7-14 days later in the lungs, where they incite an eosinophilic reaction in the airways and alveoli, mucus exudation and focal hemorrhage.[295] The transitory eosinophilic reaction probably occurs because the larva's cuticle or excreted fluids cause degranulation of mast cells, releasing eosinophilic chemotactic factor. Within 3 weeks, lymphocytes replace eosinophils; these lymphocytic nodules usually regress by 73 days of age.

Foals infected at a young age cough, have a mucoid or mucopurulent nasal discharge for about 10 days, and sometimes have an increased respiratory rate. They remain afebrile unless secondary infections occur. Copious exudate may be seen on endoscopic examination of the trachea. When horses are infected at 8-10 months of age, within 2 weeks they develop a cough, hyperpnea, inappetence, depression and a serous or somewhat mucous nasal discharge, and they lose condition. Signs may persist for 3-4 weeks, and affected foals may fail to gain weight.

Diagnosis is difficult and often based on ruling out other causes of respiratory disease. The presence of eosinophils in transtracheal aspirates and lack of evidence of sepsis support the diagnosis. Though eosinophils may be found in transtracheal aspirates from clinically normal foals, it has not been determined whether this is due to ascarid migration.[296] Fecal examination for ascarid eggs may not be helpful, as clinical signs occur early in the prepatent period, before egg laying.

As the disease usually is self limiting, treatment may not be necessary. However, larvicidal doses of fenbendazole (60 mg/kg) may be helpful. The efficacy of ivermectin has not been studied.

Dictyocaulus arnfieldi Infection

The equine lungworm, *Dictyocaulus arnfieldi*, generally is thought to be uncommon in horses in North America. However, clinical disease indistinguishable from chronic obstructive pulmonary disease may be seen in horses pastured with donkeys, mules or asses, the usual reservoir hosts. In horses, signs have been seen in autumn following midsummer exposure to mules.[297] The reservoir hosts are asymptomatic, even when infected with large worm burdens.

After second-stage larvae are ingested, they migrate through the lymphatics to the lungs, mature there and, after 13 weeks, commence egg laying in equids with patent infections. The eggs are transported via mucociliary clearance to the pharynx, swallowed and then passed out in the manure. In the horse or pony, infection usually is nonpatent. First-stage larvae can live up to 7 weeks in warm soil but cannot withstand cold or live through the winter.

The infrequency of patent infections makes the Baermann fecal flotation technique unreliable for use in horses, though it usually is reliable in donkeys, mules and asses. Diagnosis usually is based on clinical signs of severe coughing and obstructive lung disease, and a history of signs starting in late summer or autumn after the horse is exposed to donkeys, mules or asses, or housed in an area where donkeys, mules or asses had been kept without an intervening winter to kill any infective larvae. Eosinophils may be seen on a transtracheal aspirate but are not diagnostic of parasitism. Rarely the larvae or adults may be found in a transtracheal wash; occasionally they have been seen on endoscopic examination. In one report, a fifth-stage larva was seen on direct examination of the centrifuged mucus but none could be found on fixed and stained slides.[297] The authors suggested that direct cytologic evaluation of unstained, unfixed mucus always should be performed. However, use of iodine to stain the larvae may be helpful. Other authors also have reported finding the larvae in tracheobronchial aspirates.[298] The Baermann fecal flotation technique should be performed on samples from the patient and any potential reservoir hosts (donkeys, mules or asses). Negative findings do not rule out infection; even in hosts with patent infections, egg laying may be variable. Even if a fecal examination is negative for a horse in contact with donkeys, mules or asses that are shedding larvae, the horse should be considered infected.

The usefulness of radiographs has not been determined. Calves with *Dictyocaulus viviparus* infections have diffuse mottling and loss of translucency around the terminal portions of the diaphragmatic bronchi.[299] At necropsy of infected horses, the adult parasite may be found in the peripheral bronchi, and larvae may be found when lung tissue is subjected to the Baermann flotation method. Circumscribed, pale, overinflated areas may be found in lung parenchyma, particularly in the caudal lung regions.

Prophylaxis requires housing horses where donkeys, mules or asses are (or were) present only when the weather is very cold. Thiabendazole, given on 2 consecutive days at 440 mg/kg, has been claimed to be effective in the horse.[297,300] Following such therapy in infected horses, no inflammatory cells or lungworms were recovered on subsequent tracheal lavage.[297] Side effects of thiabendazole treatment have included transient anorexia and fever. Studies on treated and control donkeys showed that oral mebendazole for 5 days at 15-20 mg/kg/day decreased worm burdens and larval counts.[301] Fenbendazole (15 mg/kg PO) reportedly has caused a remission of coughing but, at least in donkeys, fecal larval counts were suppressed only transiently.[301] It is claimed that ivermectin is effective.[302,303] To the author's knowledge, there has been no good comparative study on the efficacy of these various treatments in horses with clinical signs of *Dictyocaulus* infection but, at present, ivermectin would appear to be the drug of choice.

Chronic Obstructive Pulmonary Disease

F.J. Derksen

Chronic obstructive pulmonary disease (COPD) is a complex syndrome with clinical signs ranging from exercise intolerance in performance horses to expiratory dyspnea, chronic purulent nasal discharge, cough and weight loss in chronic respiratory cripples.[304] Between these extremes, a range of clinical signs is recognized. At present it is unclear whether this range of clinical signs can be explained by an orderly progression of clinical signs from mild to severe, or by multiple etiologic agents all causing the syndrome of chronic obstructive pulmonary disease.

There are many synonyms for chronic obstructive pulmonary disease in the literature. These include heaves, chronic emphysema, chronic bronchitis, chronic bronchiolitis, recurrent airway obstruction, broken wind and hay sickness.[22,305] In a clinical setting, such pathologic descriptions as chronic bronchitis, bronchiolitis or emphysema probably are not warranted because in individual cases the underlying pathologic process is unknown. In this discussion we will use the term COPD because it indicates the chronic nature of the disease and because the name suggests the presence of airway obstruction.

Epizootiology: Chronic obstructive pulmonary disease is a disease of domestication. The condition is rare in climates where horses are housed outside all year round and is common in climates where horses are stabled and fed hay for long periods. The disease is uncommon in young horses, and the incidence increases with age.[306] There is no apparent breed or sex predisposition and no evidence for genetic predisposition.[306]

Lesions and Etiology: Though COPD was recognized in antiquity, the lesions of the disease have not been described clearly.

In part, this is due to the fact that the severity and type of lesions vary and because, at the level of the bronchioles and the gas exchange region of the lung, the lesions are not distributed homogeneously. In some areas of the lung, airways may appear nearly normal while, in an adjacent region, lesions may be severe. Thus, careful sampling and quantitation of lesions are required to accurately describe COPD.

The main lesion of COPD is bronchiolitis characterized by diffuse epithelial hyperplasia, mucous plugging of airways, and neutrophilic, lymphocytic and plasmacytic infiltrates.[307] Commonly, the lesion extends into the peribronchiolar tissues, and peribronchiolar fibrosis is also present. The alveoli subserved by obstructed or partially obstructed bronchioles are overinflated (alveolar emphysema). In some cases, eosinophils are an important constituent of the cellular infiltrate; in others, eosinophils are rare. This suggests that different etiologic agents may be involved in the disease or that the lungs of individual horses respond differently to injurious stimuli.

Emphysema, defined as destruction of alveolar walls that creates abnormally large air spaces, has been described by some authors as an important feature of COPD.[308] However, it is now clear that emphysema is rare in horses with COPD.[22] In severe cases, emphysema may be found near the pleural surface; however, even in these cases, bronchiolitis and not emphysema is the dominant pathologic feature. In other species, chronic lung disease commonly causes increased pulmonary vascular resistance, resulting in right ventricular hypertrophy and right heart failure. Though right ventricular hypertrophy has been described in horses with COPD, congestive heart failure resulting from cor pulmonale is uncommon in these cases.

It appears unlikely that clinical signs of COPD in all horses are caused by one etiologic agent. Several different lung insults may result in a stereotypical response of the lung to these injuries and clinical signs of COPD. However, in a large subgroup of horses with COPD, the disease clearly has an allergic etiology.

The evidence for an allergic etiology of COPD comes from several immunologic, physiologic and epidemiologic studies. In horses with COPD, there is a greater prevalence of serum antibody titers against antigens commonly found in the horse's environment.[309] These antigens include such Actinomycetes as *Micropolyspora faeni* and *Thermoactinomyces vulgaris*, and such molds as *Aspergillus fumigatus, Alternaria, Penicillium* and *Rhizopus*. Many affected horses also have a positive intradermal allergy skin test against these antigens.[310] However, many horses without clinical signs of COPD also have serum antibody titers and positive skin tests using the same antigens. Conversely, some affected horses do not have serum antibody titers or positive skin tests. Thus, as a group, horses with COPD have serum antibody levels and positive skin tests against several environmental antigens more commonly than control horses. Because considerable overlap exists between normal and affected horses, serum antibody titers and skin testing cannot be used to diagnose COPD in individual horses.

Bronchial provocation tests also suggest an allergic etiology for COPD in horses.[310] Challenge of affected horses with *Micropolyspora faeni, Aspergillus fumigatus* or hay dust results in airway obstruction, hypoxemia, gas exchange impairment and clinical signs of COPD. Bronchoprovocation using these agents has no effect on control horses. Additional evidence suggesting an allergic etiology stems from a group of horses and ponies with COPD, in which airway obstruction and gas exchange impairment were repeatedly induced by placing these animals into a barn and feeding them dusty hay. These animals with COPD consistently went into clinical remission within 2 weeks after removal from the barn and pasturing without exposure to hay or straw.[23,311,312] These studies confirm epidemiologic observations that COPD is common in climates where horses are housed indoors and fed hay for long periods, while the disease is rare in climates where animals are kept on pasture.

Many of the epidemiologic data incriminating exposure to hay or straw as an important factor in the etiology of COPD may also be interpreted to suggest that hay or straw contains substances injurious to the lung. When 3-methylindol is fed to horses, clinical signs of lung disease indistinguishable from COPD result.[313] In addition, the pulmonary lesions induced by 3-methylindol in the horse also are characterized by bronchiolitis. A metabolite of L-tryptophane, 3-methylindol is an amino acid commonly found in some hay. However, preliminary evidence suggests that L-tryptophane, when fed to horses, is not metabolized to 3-methylindol. Under appropriate conditions, it may be possible that an oral pneumotoxin like 3-methylindol could be ingested and be responsible for pulmonary injury characterized by brochiolitis and clinical signs of COPD in a subgroup of horses.

Many authors report that COPD commonly follows viral respiratory tract infections.[314] A similar correlation exists between viral respiratory disease and chronic respiratory diseases including asthma in people.[315] Many human infants with severe viral bronchiolitis have chronic respiratory illness in later life.[316] The mechanism whereby viruses may induce long-term pulmonary injury is unknown, but viral infections may alter the ratio of alpha- and beta-adrenergic receptors in the airways in favor of alpha-receptors.[317] This causes airway narrowing in response to adrenergic agonists that normally cause airway dilation. This could explain in part the airway hyperresponsiveness observed in asthmatic people and in horses with COPD. Though the role of previous viral infections in the pathogenesis of COPD in horses awaits further investigation, it is clear that viruses may induce long-term pulmonary dysfunction; consequently, measures aimed at reducing the incidence of viral infections (*eg*, frequent vaccination) appear appropriate.

A genetic predisposition for COPD has been suspected for many years. It is based on the observation that, of horses kept under identical environmental conditions, some develop COPD while others do not. In addition, it has been suggested that COPD is more common in ponies and draft horses. The latter observation could be explained by the lower economic values of ponies and heavy horses and the resulting poor management conditions to which these animals may be subjected.[306]

Inherited deficiency of serum antiprotease-1-antitrypsin predisposes to emphysema in people. Antiprotease-1-antitrypsin protects the lung against lysosomal proteases. Preliminary evidence suggests that horses with COPD have normal serum levels of antiprotease-1-antitrypsin;[318] therefore, deficiency of this enzyme does not appear to be a likely cause of COPD in horses. Thus, though individual horses may be predisposed to COPD, a genetic predisposition to the disease remains unproven.

Chronic obstructive pulmonary disease is characterized by hypoxemia, decreased dynamic compliance, increased pulmonary resistance and prolongation of nitrogen washout, findings compatible with diffuse airway obstruction.[43] In part, airways are obstructed with mucus, cellular debris and exudate. Also, in most horses with COPD, airway obstruction may be substantially reduced by administration of atropine, an antimuscarinic bronchodilator. Therefore, airway obstruction in COPD cases also is caused by airway smooth muscle contraction. Understanding the mechanism of airway obstruction is important because it suggests that therapy of horses with COPD should be directed at reducing airway inflammation and relieving smooth muscle contraction. The mechanisms responsible for airway inflammation in COPD are unclear. In ponies with COPD, there is an increase in bronchoalveolar lavage IgG concentration a week after acute disease exacerbation induced by exposure to hay dust.[13] In addition, there is a marked increase in neutrophil numbers in bronchoalveolar lavage fluid of affected ponies.[13] This suggests that a type-III reaction of Gell and Coombs' may be involved in pathogenesis of the disease. The large number of neutrophils recruited into the lung may release toxic oxygen radicals or enzymes exacerbating lung injury. Such mediators as histamine, eicosanoids or platelet-activating factor also could play a part in the inflammatory response and result in airway smooth muscle contraction.

It ponies with COPD, there is an increased number or activity of alpha-adrenergic receptors.[25] The cause of this increased alpha-receptor activity is unknown but has been reported in asthmatic persons and several models of experimental lung disease. Because alpha-receptor stimulation results in bronchoconstriction, this change in airway receptors could in part explain the bronchoconstriction observed in horses with COPD.

Clinical Signs: Historical information is most important when evaluating horses with COPD. In many cases, the disease is seasonal and associated with housing horses indoors.[23] In other cases, clinical signs develop 1-2 weeks after feeding a new batch of hay or moving the horse to a new barn. In some cases, COPD has been associated with birds in the barn where the affected animals are housed. In many instances, the onset of the disease is insidious, and the owner is unaware as to exactly when clinical signs started. In some horses, clinical signs of lung disease became apparent following a viral respiratory tract infection from which the horse never fully recovers. This is particularly common in racehorses with COPD because racehorses commonly suffer from virus infections and because economic pressures often do not allow adequate time for recovery following viral infections in these animals.

Clinical signs of COPD may be apparent only during exercise. Affected horses show no clinical signs at rest but do not perform adequately. Other clinical signs include chronic intermittent dry or productive cough, intermittent purulent nasal discharge, especially after exercise, and expiratory dyspnea. Clinical signs usually are intermittent but, as the disease progresses, clinical signs may become continuous. The increased expiratory effort eventually results in hypertrophy of abdominal musculature, and a heave line becomes apparent.

The airways of horses with COPD are hyperreactive to nonspecific stimuli.[311,312] Thus, exposure of diseased horses to aerosolized irritants, such as ammonia fumes, dust or pollutants, causes airway obstruction. Airways of horses with COPD are hyperresponsive only during the time horses show clinical signs of disease but not during periods of clinical remission. Airway hyperresponsiveness also is characteristic of human asthma, in which the mechanism of airway hyperresponsiveness is unknown. Airway hyperresponsiveness in horses with COPD has important clinical implications because inhalation of irritants may exacerbate or prolong clinical signs of COPD in affected horses. Thus, when treating horses with COPD, careful attention should be paid to barn ventilation and air quality.

Diagnosis: In severe cases, a presumptive diagnosis of COPD may be based on the history and clinical signs. However, to confirm a diagnosis of COPD or in mild cases of disease, diagnostic aids may be helpful.

When COPD is clinically apparent only by a decrease in exercise tolerance, auscultation findings often are normal. However, the chance of finding abnormal lung sounds on auscultation may be increased by use of a rebreathing bag, by temporarily occluding the nares, or by exercising the horse just before auscultation. The earliest auscultation abnormality that may be appreciated is loud or harsh breath sounds. Wheezing may be apparent at the end of exhalation, when airways are narrowest. In more severely affected animals, a variety of adventitious lung sounds may be heard, including wheezes throughout the respiratory cycle and, rarely, crackles. It is important to understand that auscultation is only a qualitative test and does not reveal the severity of lung disease present.

Percussion is thought to be useful in the hands of some clinicians, while others minimize its importance. In mild cases of COPD, percussion of the thorax usually is normal. In advanced cases, it may reveal caudoventral enlargement of the percussible lung field and more resonant sounds suggestive of pulmonary hyperinflation.

Endoscopic examination of the upper airway, trachea and central airways is an important diagnostic aid when evaluating horses with COPD. Endoscopy is especially useful in mildly affected horses. In horses with COPD, the upper airway usually is normal, though exudate arising from the trachea may coat the pharynx. Most normal horses allow passage of the fiberoptic endoscope through the larynx into the trachea without coughing. In horses with COPD, introduction of the endoscope into the trachea may induce coughing, suggesting a hyperirritable airway. In affected horses, a variable amount of yellow viscous material is present in the trachea. Cytologic evaluation confirms that this material is an exudate and not primarily mucous in nature. In some horses, tracheal exudate only is apparent immediately following exercise. With the longer fiberoptic endoscopes now available, the clinician may evaluate airways beyond the carina. In COPD, central airways do not appear inflamed, but exudate is present in their lumen.

Radiography of the adult horse's thorax requires radiographic equipment not generally available to the equine practitioner. Even with the most powerful radiographic equipment, radiographic detail is poor. In horses with COPD, thoracic radiographs reveal a mixed pattern of radiodensity throughout the lung field. In experimental lung disease in horses, extensive pathologic lesions must be present in the lung before radiographic abnormalities are apparent. Thoracic radiographs are helpful in detecting focal or miliary lesions in the lung and distinguishing these cases from COPD. Thoracic radiographs have not been helpful in detection of early or subclinical cases of COPD.

Transtracheal aspiration has been used in evaluation of airway cell populations in horses with COPD.[319] The percentage of neutrophils in transtracheal aspirate fluid is increased in horses with COPD. When interpreting cytologic preparations of transtracheal aspirate, the assumption is made that the cytologic findings in some manner reflect the pulmonary airway cell population. Recent evidence suggests that this assumption is not valid in horses with COPD and that transtracheal aspirate cytologic findings correlate poorly with the airway cell population as assessed by histopathologic examination and bronchoalveolar lavage.[320] In addition, the variability in the percentage of neutrophils in transtracheal aspirate fluid of normal horses ranges from 0% to 83%.[320] This large variability in tracheal cell population of normal horses further limits the clinical usefulness of cytologic examination of transtracheal aspirates in chronic lung disease. However, transtracheal aspirates may have some value in distinguishing COPD from parasitic lung disease, in which the tracheal cell population contains a large percentage of eosinophils or even lungworm larvae.

In contrast, the variability in neutrophils observed in bronchoalveolar lavage fluid of normal horses ranges from 0% to 17%. In addition, there is a good correlation between bronchoalveolar lavage cytologic findings and histopathologic score in horses with COPD.[321] Thus, bronchoalveolar lavage appears to be a more useful technique than transtracheal aspiration when evaluating horses with COPD. The cytologic findings of bronchoalveolar lavage of ponies with COPD is normal when ponies are in disease remission. However, during periods of disease exacerbation, there is a marked and consistent increase in the percentage of neutrophils in bronchoalveolar lavage fluid.[13] In some horses with COPD, the number of eosinophils in bronchoalveolar lavage fluid also increases.[13] Though an increase in bronchoalveolar lavage neutrophils is not pathognomonic for COPD, pulmonary neutrophilia in bronchoalveolar lavage fluid may help detect COPD or, in conjunction with clinical data, confirm a diagnosis of COPD.

Chronic obstructive pulmonary disease is characterized by airway obstruction. This results in decreased dynamic compliance, increased pulmonary resistance and prolongation of nitrogen washouts.[43] Pulmonary function tests allow quantitative assessment of the severity of the lung disease and document airway obstruction. However, these tests require equipment not generally available to the equine practitioner. In addition, these tests are not particularly sensitive and not helpful in early detection of subclinical COPD. Therefore, they rarely are used in clinical practice.

The primary function of the lung is gas exchange; in horses with COPD, this function is impaired, resulting in hypoxemia. Measurement of arterial blood gas tension (PaO_2) is the simplest and often the most helpful test of pulmonary function. This test can be performed easily in the field. Arterial blood may be collected in a syringe coated with heparin and stored in ice for up to an hour before blood gas analysis. At sea level, a PaO_2 <83 torr is considered abnormal. Because in normal animals PaO_2 decreases with altitude, at higher elevations a lower PaO_2 may be normal.

Treatment: In most cases of COPD, lung injury is the result of exposure of the sensitized respiratory system to organic dust. Therefore, the most important aim of therapy is to prevent this exposure. Damp, dusty barns with poor ventilation tend to exacerbate clinical signs of COPD; the optimal environment is a pasture with a modest shelter against inclement weather. If pasture is not available, horses with COPD should be housed in a well-ventilated barn with access to the outside. Animals should be bedded on moist wood shavings or clay. Pelleted feed should be substituted for hay. Established management practices are often so ingrained that the veterinarian may have difficulty convincing owners to keep their horses out of their poorly ventilated barns. Consequently, therapy of horses with COPD often is centered around drug therapy with inevitably poor results.

No therapeutic effort can be successful unless the horse's environment is altered and exposure to offending aerosol antigens is eliminated. This fact must be emphasized to owners who might otherwise be reluctant to follow recommendations. A complete change of environment, such as hospitalization, with no therapy given, can result in a dramatic, temporary cure in 3-7 days. In mild COPD involving racehorses, rest appears to be an important part of therapy. Exercise to keep the horse in racing shape could delay resolution of the inflammatory response and may eventually lead to exercise-induced pulmonary hemorrhage.

Chronic obstructive pulmonary disease is characterized by airway inflammation. Reducing the inflammatory response with corticosteroids resolves clinical signs of the disease. However, it is important to emphasize that airway inflammation will return following cessation of therapy if exposure to offending irritants and antigens is not prevented. Corticosteroids reduce the inflammatory response by a variety of mechanisms. These include the inhibition of phospholipase A, thereby preventing production of metabolites of arachidonic acid, such as prostaglandins and leukotrienes. Corticosteroids also inhibit cellular migration, including migration of neutrophils into the lungs of horses with COPD. In addition, corticosteroids potentiate the action of beta-2-receptor stimulants, resulting in bronchodilation and inhibition of mediator release from inflammatory cells. Corticosteroids are powerful inhibitors of the inflammatory response. However, the undesirable side effects of corticosteroids also are potentially serious and may become apparent weeks after initiation of therapy. Thus, corticosteroids should be used with caution.

Therapy should be aimed at an optimal therapeutic response with minimal side effects. Corticosteroids in large doses suppress the immune response, resulting in respiratory or other infections. Prolonged use of corticosteroids may result in Cushingoid signs, such as depression, muscle wasting, a long dry haircoat, hyperglycemia, polydipsia and polyuria. Corticosteroids depress release of ACTH from the posterior pituitary, resulting in adrenal cortical atrophy. Therefore, sudden withdrawal of corticosteroids may result in adrenal insufficiency.

The risk of complications associated with corticosteroid usage may be minimized by a proper therapeutic regimen. To prevent dependence, prednisone is administered PO every other morning at 1-2 mg/kg. Endogenous plasma corticosteroid concentrations peak in the morning and decline to their lowest level in the early evening. When the drug is given every other day, the adrenal cortex is stimulated enough to prevent corticosteroid dependence. After 2 weeks of therapy, response to treatment is assessed and the dosage gradually reduced until a mimimum effective dosage is reached.

Chronic obstructive pulmonary disease is characterized by airway obstruction in part caused by constriction of airway smooth muscle. Therefore, a reasonable objective of therapy is to reduce airway narrowing using bronchodilators. Unfortunately, no clinically useful bronchodilators are licensed for use in horses in North America. In other species, bronchodilators are most effective when delivered by aerosol because, when delivered directly into the airways, drug concentration is highest at the intended site. Drug concentration is lowest in the systemic circulation, thereby minimizing undesirable side effects. Bronchodilator therapy is described in detail in the first part of this chapter in the section entitled Pathophysiology and Principles of Therapy.

Cromolyn sodium prevents mast-cell degranulation and is effective in treatment of human asthma.[322] The drug has no direct effect on airway smooth muscle and no direct antagonist activity against mediators of inflammation. Therefore, cromolyn sodium is effective only prophylactically and is not in established disease. Anecdotal reports suggest that 200-300 mg of cromolyn sodium, when insufflated into the pharynx before exercise or exposure to antigen, can prevent clinical signs of COPD in some horses.[323] The drug's effects last 3-4 hours, and side effects have not been reported.

Immunotherapy has been used to treat allergic lung disease in people for many years. Desensitization starts with skin testing to identify the offending antigen. Once the antigen is identified, allergens with adjuvant are injected SC at increasing concentrations at weekly intervals. Therapy is continued indefinitely. Production of blocking IgG antibodies, decreased levels of IgE and induction of T-suppressor cells have been proposed as mechanisms whereby immunotherapy exerts its effect. In horses, interpretation of skin tests is difficult because the skin of many clinically normal horses responds vigorously to a large number of antigens. Nonetheless, immunotherapy may be effective in treatment in some horses.[324]

Summer Pasture-Associated Obstructive Pulmonary Disease

F.J. Derksen

Summer pasture-associated obstructive pulmonary disease is a recurrent disease condition described in the southern United States.[325] Affected horses develop clinical signs of chronic obstructive pulmonary disease (COPD), including coughing, purulent nasal discharge, exercise intolerance and expiratory dyspnea. These signs are indistinguishable from those of COPD or heaves. (See the discussion under Chronic Obstructive Pulmonary Disease.) While heaves occurs predominantly in horses housed in barns and fed improperly cured hay, summer pasture-associated obstructive pulmonary disease occurs in pastured horses during the summer months.

There does not seem to be a sex or breed predisposition for the condition, but affected horses are at least 3 years old. Clinical signs of disease improve markedly during winter months whether horses are fed hay or remain on pasture. Clinical signs of disease are likely to recur each summer. The cause of summer pasture-associated obstructive pulmonary disease is unknown but an immunologic etiology appears likely.

The diagnosis is based on the history, clinical signs and exclusion of other causes of chronic pulmonary disease. Treatment is directed toward preventing exposure of affected animals to the offending environment. Horses should be stabled and fed a diet of hay or pelleted feed. Clinical signs abate 7-10 days after removal from pasture.

Granulomatous Pneumonia

R.A. Mansmann

In people, granulomatous pneumonia is seen with tuberculosis, brucellosis, leprosy, histoplasmosis, coccidioidomycosis, berylliosis, bagassosis, silicate pneumonoconiosis, farmer's lung and bird fancier's lung. Pulmonary sarcoidosis with accompanying skin nodules also is considered a granulomatous pneumonia in people.[326,327]

In horses, clinical signs of granulomatous pneumonia may be similar to those of chronic obstructive pulmonary disease (COPD). Affected horses may or may not have weight loss and fever. Careful auscultation reveals wheezes. There may be other auscultatory findings, such as dull areas due to large fibrotic masses or ventral pleural effusion. If affected horses are given a bronchodilating agent, such as glycopyrrolate (Robinul-V: Robins) IV at 2.0 mg/450 kg, the wheezes persist and do not decrease, as they do in horses with COPD. In addition, the clinical course of granulomatous pneumonia usually is more rapid than in COPD. Thoracic radiography is most helpful in diagnosis of granulomatous pneumonia and shows focal increases in lung density. Generally, treatment of granulomatous pneumonia is unrewarding.

Silicate Pneumonoconiosis: Nine horses of various breeds from the Monterey-Carmel peninsula in California, ranging from 2 1/2 to 20 years of age, had weight loss, increased respiratory rate and exercise intolerance caused by silicate granulomatous pneumonia.[328] Granulomas consisted primarily of large, foamy macrophages with occasional associated lymphocytes and plasma cells. The degree of fibrosis varied but was most severe in horses with large, confluent lesions. Refractile particles 1 μ in diameter and smaller were discernible within macrophages, which occasionally were birefringent. Using energy dispersive x-ray analysis and x-ray diffraction, these particles were identified as cristobalite, a fibrogenic and cytotoxic silica. A high concentration of cristobalite was found in the environment of affected horses. It was thought that cases of silicate pneumoconiosis seen since 1978 were due primarily to increased construction of homes and small ranches in areas with soils containing cristobalite. Silicate pneumoconiosis has been reported in zoo animals in San Diego, California. Though ungulates were involved, none was a horse.[329] Radiographs and postmortem lung specimens from a horse with silicate pneumoconiosis are shown in Figures 42 and 43.

Tuberculosis: Tuberculosis is rare in horses. Horses seem more resistant to tuberculosis than other species; tuberculosis was rare during the early part of this century when bovine and human tuberculosis was common. It is a multisystemic disease primarily involving the lung, cervical vertebrae and gastrointestinal tract. Clinical signs range from weight loss and neck stiffness to occasional diarrhea.

Antemortem diagnosis of tuberculosis is difficult. Chest and cervical radiographs may be useful to detect cervical osteolysis and osteoporosis (Fig 44). Tuberculin testing is unreliable in horses. Many apparently normal horses are tuberculin (avian) positive. A specific culture technique may help diagnose tuberculosis in horses.[330] Tissues obtained at necropsy were grouped and homogenized. The tissue was cultured using Stonebrink and modified 7H11 media. After 6 weeks' incubation at 37 C, smooth cream-colored, domed colonies grew on both media and were identified as *Mycobacterium avium*. The authors cautioned against a specific diagnosis of tuberculosis based on culture of tracheal secretions alone, as *Mycobacterium avium* may be an environmental contaminant.[330]

Figure 42. Chest radiograph of a 10-year-old Thoroughbred broodmare with silicate pneumoconiosis (referred by Dr. Morgan Patterson). The mare had lived in the Monterey peninsula of California before developing clinical signs about 4 weeks after being shipped to a breeding farm. The film shows a marked diffuse, patchy, interstitial density in the caudal lung region.

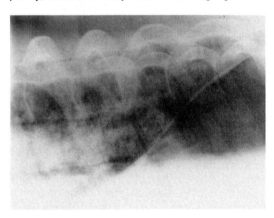

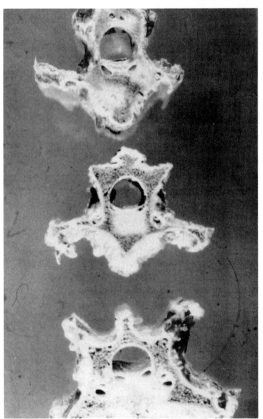

Figure 44. Vertebral osteoporosis and osteolysis caused by tuberculosis.

Figure 43. Postmortem lung specimens from the horse in Figure 42 with pneumoconiosis. The disease was histologically confirmed as silicate pneumoconiosis. Four longitudinal sections from the left apical (LA), left cardiac (LC), middle and diaphragmatic lung regions demonstrate fibrosis.

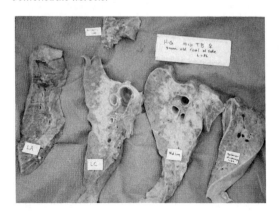

Chronic Fungal Infections: Chronic fungal infections, including coccidioidomycosis, histoplasmosis, cryptococcosis and aspergillosis, may cause chronic pulmonary disease and cachexia but are not common in horses.

Coccidioidomycosis appears to be the most common of these infections in horses in the United States. Coccidioidomycosis is a multisystemic disease of the desert areas of the southwestern United States and areas of South America. In a review of 15 cases of coccidioidomycosis, the most common clinical signs were weight loss and chronic cough. Other signs were musculoskeletal pain, superficial abscessation, intermittent febrile episodes and abdominal pain. The most common finding on thoracic radiography was increased interstitial density, pleural fluid accumulation and, in some cases, irregular pulmonary infiltrates or displacement of airways by soft tissues masses. Serum titers were demonstrated in all affected horses using complement-fixation tests or immunodiffusion.

The mean age of the horses was 6.3 years, with a range of 6 months to 12 years. One patient died naturally and 14 were euthanized. The mean duration of clinical signs before euthanasia was 7.3 months, with a range of 2 days to 2 1/2 years. Disseminated infection was apparent in most cases. The tissues most commonly involved, in order of decreasing frequency, were lung, thoracic lymph nodes, spleen, liver, bone or periosteum, pleura and peritoneum. In 4 cases, specific antifungal therapy for 20-96 days was unsuccessful.[331,332]

Other Granulomatous Pneumonias: A single case of granulomatous pneumonia has been reported in a yearling grazing on hairy vetch. Necropsy revealed severe weight loss, bilateral corneal ulcers and cutaneous edema. Multifocal to diffuse granulomatous inflammation involved the lungs, skin and several other organs.[333]

Neoplasia

Pulmonary Neoplasia

F.J. Derksen

Primary lung tumors are extremely rare in horses. The most prevalent primary lung tumor is the myoblastoma (granular-cell tumor), found in 3 of 200,000 slaughtered horses in one study and 3 of 40,000 in another.[334,335] The cell line from which this tumor originates is unknown but may be Schwann cells, smooth muscle cells or fibroblasts.[336] On endoscopic examination of the airways, a myoblastoma may appear as a nodular mass (Fig 45).[337] These masses are not restricted to the airway but are present throughout the lung parenchyma. Other tumors that may metastasize to the lung include squamous-cell carcinoma, lymphosarcoma and hemangiosarcoma.[338-340]

Clinical signs of pulmonary neoplasia may not be apparent or may be nonspecific and include weight loss, coughing, purulent nasal discharge and dyspnea.[337] These clinical signs are indistinguishable from those of chronic obstructive pulmonary disease. Thoracic radiographs, bronchoscopy and lung biopsy may be required for definitive diagnosis. Treatment of pulmonary neoplasms is usually unrewarding, and most affected horses are euthanized.

Idiopathic Diseases

Exercise-Induced Pulmonary Hemorrhage

J.R. Pascoe

Cause: Exercise-induced pulmonary hemorrhage (EIPH) is defined as bleeding from the lungs as a consequence of exertion.

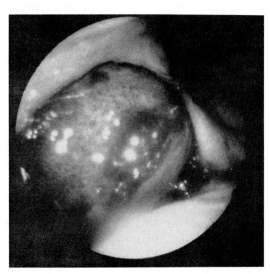

Figure 45. Endoscopic view of a myoblastoma in a mainstem bronchus of a 14-year-old Thoroughbred mare. (Courtesy of Dr. C.M. Brown)

Clinically, EIPH is diagnosed by endoscopic observation of blood within the tracheobronchial airways after exercise or by cytologic identification of hemosiderophages (macrophages containing hemosiderin) in tracheobronchial secretions.[336] Epistaxis is a relatively infrequent clinical sign of EIPH, and additional diagnostic tests, such as endoscopy, are necessary to differentiate EIPH from other causes of epistaxis. In racing parlance and clinical practice, horses experiencing EIPH often are referred to as "bleeders." This colloquial term refers to the historical association of epistaxis or "nose bleeds" with this condition and is not indicative of a defect in hemostasis.

Most horses involved in competitive racing experience EIPH. The incidence of EIPH ranges from about 30% for Standardbreds and polo ponies to >60% for Thoroughbreds, Quarter Horses and Appaloosas.[337] The minimal level of exertion needed to induce EIPH is unknown. Though it has been observed in some Thoroughbred horses after trotting, cantering and slow training gallops, it generally is associated with more strenuous exertion, such as competitive flat racing, pacing, trotting, jumping or barrel racing.[338]

Pulmonary hemorrhage usually is first noted in 2-year-olds when they commence training. Though some studies have suggested that the frequency of EIPH may be higher in older horses, exercise intensity appears to be a more consistent factor than age or sex. It generally is believed that, in Thoroughbreds, speeds of >14 meters/sec are required to induce EIPH. There appears to be no clear relationship between performance and EIPH as judged by race finishing position, though studies to determine the effect of EIPH on an individual horse's performance must be conducted. However, others have suggested, based on retrospective reviews of racing times, that continued episodes of EIPH may be associated with declining performance.[339] So far, no correlation has been shown between EIPH and such factors as track surface, trainer, stable location or bedding.[340]

Diagnosis: Definitive diagnosis requires recognition of blood within the airways, either by endoscopic observation or later identification of hemosiderophages in aspirates of respiratory secretions. Though endoscopy can be performed immediately after exercise, clinical experience suggests that delaying the examination until 30-90 minutes after exercise increases the likelihood of observing blood in the airways. When EIPH is strongly suspected, based on the horse's performance, but blood is not seen, reexamination 30 minutes later is recommended. If bleeding has occurred, the presence of blood in the trachea depends on a number of factors, including the interval between onset of bleeding and observation, the location of bleeding within the lung, the volume of extravasated blood, and the rate of mucociliary clearance. Recognizing the important influence these variables can have on a positive or negative result, it also should be apparent that it is difficult if not impossible to objectively assess the degree of bleeding that has occurred.

The repeatability of observations of EIPH for an individual horse are of interest because of their importance in designing studies to evaluate the efficacy of medication used to treat EIPH. Taking the variables listed above into consideration, it would seem that observations made from at least 4 consecutive exercise periods are necessary to establish the repeatability of EIPH for an individual horse.[341] In general, however, once a horse starts experiencing EIPH, it continues to do so for the remainder of its racing career.

Recognition of epistaxis alone is not sufficient evidence for definitive diagnosis of EIPH. While the probability of association is high in horses in race training, a thorough clinical examination is necessary to preclude other causes of epistaxis. If endoscopic examination is not possible, cytologic examination of a tracheobronchial aspirate might be considered. Observation of macrophages containing intracytoplasmic droplets of hemosiderin suggests recent pulmonary hemorrhage.[293] In some racing jurisdictions in North America, an affidavit attesting to recognition of these cells in airways secretions is acceptable proof that the horse has experienced EIPH and legally can receive "prophylactic or preventive" prerace medication. The temporal relationship between an episode of EIPH and initial recovery of hemosiderophages is unknown. Similarly, the duration of recovery relative to a single episode of EIPH is unknown. Hemosiderophages can be recovered for several weeks after a known episode of EIPH.[293] Recognition of these cells within alveoli at least 150 days after retirement from racing suggests that hemosiderophages may be recovered from aspirates of airway secretions for many months.[342] Because hemosiderophages contain iron pigment, their identification on smears can be enhanced by use of special stains.[293]

Thoracic radiographs also provide useful information but are not necessarily diagnostic for EIPH. Though earlier studies ascribed a regional pattern in the thoracophrenic angle on lateral radiographs as indicative of EIPH, recent studies suggest that this is relatively uncommon and probably indicative of more serious pulmonary disease.[343]

Lungs from horses with a confirmed history of EIPH have bilateral, symmetric subpleural staining of the lung parenchyma. This discoloration, which is blue brown in the collapsed lung and light brown in the inflated lung, is distributed primarily in the dorsocaudal region on the caudal lung lobe.[344] In more severely affected lungs, the discoloration is distributed cranially along the dorsal surface of the lung, toward the hilar region. The subpleural bronchial arteries also are more prominent in these discolored regions of the lung.[344] On cut section, the brown staining of the parenchyma extends ventrally from the dorsal surface beyond the level of the principal bronchus. These brown or rust-colored regions of the lung parenchyma appear to be preferentially supplied by the bronchial arterial circulation, rather than the normal pulmonary arterial circulation.[31] Radiographic imaging techniques also have highlighted distribution of bronchial arterial networks centered around small airways within the stained parenchyma.[345] On microscopic examination, the brown staining of the parenchyma resulted from massive deposition of hemosiderin, mostly contained within macrophages, within airspaces and connective tissue septa.[342] Airways in these sections show hyperplasia of the respiratory epithelium and peribronchiolar fibrosis.

These findings suggest that horses with a history of EIPH have specific lung regions with small airway disease, interstitial fibrosis and neovascularization. Though the genesis of these changes is not known with certainty, it has been suggested that small airway disease precedes interstitial fibrosis

and neovascularization.[346] Further, it is likely that the neovascularization occurs as a repair response within the lung and that the bronchial arterial circulation, which provides this neovascular response, is the most likely source of hemorrhage during exercise.[346] Whether or not this reflects the chronology of the histologic changes, it is clear that the lesions are chronic and unlikely to resolve during the racing life of the horse.

Though recognition of these pathologic features has improved our knowledge of the probable source of bleeding, the temporal development of the lesion or its cause(s) remain to be determined. Until this sequence of events is defined more accurately, mechanisms explaining the pathophysiology of EIPH remain speculative.

Etiopathogenesis: Several hypotheses have been suggested as possible explanations of EIPH.[337,347] Based on the limited information available, the most tenable hypothesis suggests that small airway disease may predispose to EIPH.[347] Because equine lungs have poor collateral ventilation, partial or complete airway obstruction from small airway disease might result in uneven expanding forces on segments of lung subtended by these airways. Vessels within these lung segments may be subjected to tremendous increases in local perivascular pressure because of the interdependence of lung tissue. Such distending pressure may be sufficient during exercise to produce tissue tearing or vessel rupture and subsequent hemorrhage.[347] Continued damage to tissue with progressive local tearing or disruption of the lung eventually could produce grossly visible lesions within the lungs. The primary dorsal distribution of the lesions also suggests that some mechanical phenomenon, such as regional changes in pleural pressure, may play an important role in development of lesions.

Unfortunately, these ideas do not explain why small airway disease occurs initially or if, in fact, it is the initial predisposing factor. An equally plausible hypothesis could suggest that mechanical stresses applied to the dorsocaudal lung during maximal exertion may cause tearing of lung tissue and hemorrhage that predispose to small airway disease, subsequent airway obstruction and its possible sequelae. The apparent bronchial arterial neovascularization of these abnormal areas of lung probably is a normal repair response to lung injury. To the extent that is this is part of the systemic circulation and that it is supplying developing vessels, it is not difficult to see why, once initiated, hemorrhage recurs with continued training and racing.[346]

Because there are no studies on development of airway disease in horses, factors contributing to such changes remain speculative. Considering the relatively common occurrence of juvenile respiratory disease in weanlings, viral respiratory disease in young horses in training, the dusty environment of stalls, inhalation of dust and dirt when racing, and the location of racetracks in major metropolitan centers with air pollution problems, it is not unreasonable to expect that small airway disease might be a common finding in racing horses. Though it might be anticipated that such lesions would be distributed randomly throughout the lung, certain anatomic considerations in equine lungs (such as the relatively straight principal bronchus) could predispose to the predominantly dorsocaudal distribution of these changes. Studies of aerosol and particle disposition within equine lungs are needed to answer these questions.

Treatment: The relatively chronic nature of the lung lesions, combined with our poor understanding of their development, makes it difficult to recommend rational therapeutic guidelines or a management plan for EIPH. Further, because clinical recognition of "bleeders" and EIPH predated an improved understanding of the pathologic changes, a plethora of treatments are in common use.[348] The variety of attested "treatments" further highlights the general level of frustration experienced by trainers and veterinarians in dealing with EIPH. Similarly, it should be recognized that efficacy data for many of these preparations used specifically for EIPH are lacking.

Limited data are available for furosemide, which has been the most controversial of the "approved" prerace medications for EIPH. Testimonial evidence indicates that furosemide originally was used in the early 1960s on the presumption that bleeding occurred because of pulmonary edema. Early endoscopic studies indicated that at least 50% of horses treated with furosemide still experienced EIPH.[336] Subsequently it was shown that furosemide may reduce

bleeding but is not effective in preventing EIPH.[341] Others have reported that furosemide appears to improve performance, based on racing time, of horses with declining performance attributed to EIPH.[339] If performance improves as a result of premedication with furosemide, it does not appear to increase beyond the pre-EIPH performance level recorded for the horse. Physiologic studies have documented only small transient improvements in cardiovascular performance; based on available data, it is difficult to explain why furosemide might have a beneficial effect on EIPH.[349] Where racing legislation permits, current use is restricted to 0.5 mg/kg IV or IM not less than 3 hours before racing.[348]

Other therapies include prerace administration of conjugated estrogens and feed supplementation with a variety of compounds, including bioflavonoids and vitamins C and K. With the exception of the hesperidin-citrus bioflavonoids, none of the other preparations have been critically evaluated for efficacy in treatment of EIPH.[348] The bioflavonoid feed supplement was not effective in preventing EIPH.[350] Claims for prevention of EIPH by intermittent therapy with heated humidified air have been discounted in a controlled study.[351]

The preceding comments summarize the paucity of knowledge about efficacy of currently used therapeutic regimens. Nonetheless, it is important to recognize that management of the horse with EIPH should begin with a thorough physical and clinical examination to detect other possible causes of hemorrhage and to evaluate the extent of preexisting pulmonary disease. Once this is established, palliative and possibly therapeutic steps can be taken to alleviate the condition. Attention also should be focused on management procedures, such as ventilation and air quality control in stables and regular prophylactic immunization against viral respiratory diseases. Improved understanding of the pathophysiology of EIPH ultimately will improve our ability to manage this condition.

Interstitial Pneumonia in Foals

F.J. Derksen

Interstitial lung disease primarily affects foals between 3 days and 6 months of age, though the disease also can occur in adult horses.[357] Interstitial pneumonia is characterized by marked respiratory distress. Foals have both inspiratory and expiratory dyspnea but appear bright and alert. There is no purulent nasal discharge. The heart rate, respiratory rate and rectal temperature are elevated, and auscultation reveals loud breath sounds but few adventitial sounds. Thoracic radiography shows a modest, diffuse increase in interstitial lung density. Transtracheal lavage yields fluid with low cellularity and a normal differential cell count. Bacterial culture fails to consistently yield pathogenic organisms.

Interstitial pneumonia can be distinguished from bacterial pneumonia on clinical grounds because affected foals are bright and alert, and have few adventitious lung sounds on auscultation and no purulent nasal discharge. In addition, radiographic lung changes are diffuse and sometimes modest, considering the severity of dyspnea. Transtracheal wash culture and cytologic examination do not support the diagnosis of bacterial pneumonia.

At necropsy, the lungs of affected horses fail to collapse and have a firm texture. Histologically, acute cases are characterized by coagulation necrosis of alveolar walls, with extensive focal alveolar hemorrhage and formation of hyaline membranes. In more chronic cases, there is diffuse proliferation of pneumocytes so that alveoli are lined with cuboidal epithelium. Intralobular septa are widened by proliferating fibroblasts and inflammatory cells.[357]

The etiology of interstitial pneumonia in foals is unknown, but the disease may be caused by viral infections, pneumotoxins or allergic disease.[358-362] Several reports in the literature incriminate equine influenza or equine herpesvirus in the pathogenesis of interstitial pneumonia in foals.[358-360] Experimentally, such toxic plants as *Perilla frutescens* containing perilla ketones cause interstitial pneumonia, with proliferation of alveolar or epithelial cells and formation of hyaline membranes.[361] Similarly, pyrrolizidine alkaloids may induce pulmonary lesions characterized by proliferation of bronchiolar and alveolar cells, with megalocytosis, interstitial fibrosis and inflammatory-cell infiltrates.[362] Paraquat, an herbicide, also causes interstitial inflammation and fibrosis in laboratory animals.[363] Finally, because endotoxins can cause vascular endothelial damage, it has been suggested that endotoxemia may result in interstitial pneumonia.[364]

Therapy of foals with interstitial pneumonia mainly is supportive in nature. Corticosteroids and bronchodilator therapy may be used but usually are ineffective.[357] Some foals require oxygen therapy or mechanical ventilation. Significant secondary bacterial pathogens must be identified by culture of tracheobronchial fluid and treated specifically. The prognosis for interstitial pneumonia in foals is unfavorable. Those that survive tend to be older foals with a more gradual onset of signs.

Hypoxemia in Foals

M.R. Paradis

Some newborn foals have mild to moderate tachypnea and increased respiratory effort. Normal inspiratory and expiratory breath sounds are heard on auscultation of the lungs. The foal's activity level may range from normal to lethargic.

The prominent finding of arterial blood gas analysis is hypoxemia. Thoracic radiographs may show loss of vascular clarity in the caudoventral region of the lungs and an increased interstitial pattern (Fig 46).

Several different causes for this decreased oxygenation warrant investigation. Cardiopulmonary shunting and pulmonary disease secondary to infection must be in-

Figure 46. Thoracic radiograph of a 300-day-gestation foal at 72 hours of age. This foal was one of twins. Hypoxemia was evident on blood gas analysis.

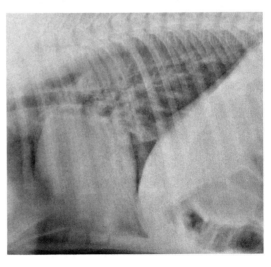

cluded in the differential diagnosis. Because hypoxemia frequently is seen in foals that appear immature (small size, silky haircoat, gestation <320 days), insufficient mature surfactant may be part of the pathogenesis. However, this problem is different than respiratory distress syndrome in that the foals are not in respiratory failure and are normocapneic and generally not acidotic. Radiographically, these foals do not have air bronchograms, which usually characterize the respiratory distress syndrome.

Oxygen administration is the specific therapy. Oxygen can be administered via a face mask or an intranasal tube. The prognosis is good if this condition is not complicated by infection. Supportive care generally is needed for 2-5 days.[19]

DISEASES OF THE PLEURA, MEDIASTINUM, DIAPHRAGM AND THORACIC WALL

R.E. Beadle

Diagnostic and Therapeutic Considerations

Adequate alveolar ventilation depends upon the thoracic wall, diaphragm and lung functioning properly and in concert. Any disease that interferes with the proper function of these structures may decrease alveolar ventilation and thereby adversely affect transfer of oxygen and carbon dioxide across the alveolar-capillary membrane. Hypercarbia and hypoxemia result if compensatory mechanisms cannot overcome the impairment of normal respiratory function. Though life can be sustained with some degree of hypercarbia and hypoxemia, more severe conditions are not compatible with life. The following discussion deals with diseases that interfere with the ability of the lung, thoracic wall and diaphragm to act in concert. For the most part these diseases and conditions deform the pleural space and/or uncouple the lung from the thoracic wall.

Diseases With Physical Causes

Thoracic Wall Trauma

Thoracic wall trauma may result in serious complications, including pleuritis, pneu-

mothorax, hemothorax and diaphragmatic hernia. Deformation of the thoracic wall due to multiple rib fractures can be seen and palpated. Multiple fractures of the same rib or several ribs destabilize the thorax. During inspiration, the affected region of the thorax may become depressed and then bulge outward during exhalation; this is termed "flail chest."

Skin and muscle lacerations are cared for using standard surgical techniques, but deeper wounds require more intensive therapy. Patient stabilization is the primary consideration with deeper wounds that enter the pleural cavity and/or cause copious hemorrhage. Air already in the pleural space must be removed and entrance of additional air prevented. Thoracic wounds must be closed quickly, as they may cause tension pneumothorax. Air must be immediately removed from the pleural space after the wound is closed because of the potential for fatal bilateral pneumothorax.

Ideally the pleural space should be surgically explored and flushed with balanced electrolyte solutions to remove bacteria and debris following a blunt wound that penetrates the thorax. Such surgery requires general anesthesia and use of positive-pressure ventilation. If surgical exploration and flushing are not possible, flushing the pleural space in the standing horse is an alternative. Broad-spectrum antibiotics should be given for at least 7-10 days after thoracic wall penetration.

Diaphragmatic Hernia

Diaphragmatic hernia is an infrequent finding in horses. By 1981, only 19 cases were available for review in the literature.[360] Both congenital and acquired diaphragmatic hernias have been documented in horses.[361]

Of 18 cases of diaphragmatic hernia, affected horses had a mean age of 8.6 years, with a range of 12 weeks to 19 years.[361] There did not seem to be a sex predilection. Abdominal pain was the primary presenting complaint in most affected horses. Often the history revealed a previous bout of strenuous exercise, such as jumping, striking a stationary object while running, being struck by an automobile or taking a hard fall. Pregnant or recently parturient mares also are at risk for diaphragmatic hernias.

In some cases, there is no history of any of the above factors.

Auscultation of the thorax does not always reveal ventral dullness or borborygmi. Even when borborygmi are heard in the thorax, this finding must be interpreted with caution because it is common even in normal horses. Heart sounds may be dramatically louder on one side than the other.

Percussion of the thorax may or may not reveal abnormalities. Hernias allowing large amounts of viscera to enter the thorax lateral to the lungs more often are associated with abnormalities detectable by percussion.

Radiography is an excellent way to detect viscera in the thorax. However, the procedure generally is only possible in foals unless specialized radiographic equipment is available. When appropriate radiographic equipment is available, films often show fluid or ingesta-filled loops of intestine, with overlying gas caps in the thoracic cavity. Ultrasound scan of the thoracic contents is likely to be very rewarding only if viscera or liver or spleen are against the parietal pleura.

Thoracentesis can be diagnostic in diaphragmatic hernia in which viscera have entered the thoracic cavity and become trapped and devitalized. In these cases, pleural fluid has an increased number of neutrophils and protein. There may also be large numbers of red blood cells in the pleural fluid. Fluid from abdominocentesis often shows no abnormalities.

Diaphragmatic hernia does not have a good prognosis if the condition is producing clinical signs. Diaphragmatic herniorrhaphy is difficult to perform in adult horses. Inability to adequately ventilate these patients while under anesthesia worsens the prognosis. The literature shows that only 1 foal and one mature horse have been successfully treated by herniorrhaphy.[362,363]

Pneumothorax in Adult Horses

Unilateral pneumothorax can be tolerated quite well in most horses. However, horses may develop bilateral pneumothorax due to their thin, fenestrated caudal mediastinal membrane. When this occurs, lung function is severely impaired and death may ensue. Therefore, pneumothorax is more of a cause for concern in horses than in most other species. However, puncture of the thoracic cavity does not always lead to bilateral pneumothorax.

Air may gain access to the pleural space by traversing either the lung or thoracic wall. Severely diseased lung, as with gangrenous pneumonia, may develop bronchopleural fistulas. Rupture of emphysematous bullae also allows air into the pleural space. Air also may be introduced into the pleural space as a result of various diagnostic procedures or trauma.

Horses with pneumothorax show signs of varying severity. Those with small amounts of air on one side of the thorax may not show any signs. Horses with larger amounts of air in the pleural space(s) show respiratory distress. Tachypnea and nostril flaring are most readily apparent, and cyanosis can occur if arterial oxygenation is sufficiently impaired.

Auscultation of the thoracic wall reveals less pronounced sounds on the affected side than expected. Bubbling sounds may be heard if air is escaping ventral to a fluid line. Diagnostic ultrasonography fails to detect lung tissue against the thoracic wall and shows no structures beyond the thoracic wall, as the sound beams are reflected by air in the pleural space. Thoracic radiographs reveal collapse of the lung.

Pneumothorax can be confirmed most easily by thoracentesis. Severe pneumothorax is an emergency, and air should be removed from the pleural space as quickly as possible. This can be accomplished with a needle, stopcock and syringe, or by using a vacuum device attached to a large-diameter trocar catheter (Argyle) introduced into the pleural space through the thoracic wall. Catheter placement is described below (Inflammatory, Infectious and Immune Diseases). Less severe cases can be treated by attaching a unidirectional air flow device to a thoracic drainage tube. Unidirectional air flow devices most commonly used include Heimlich valves (Bard-Parker) and water traps. Both of these devices allow air to escape from the pleural space during exhalation but not to reenter during inspiration.

Pneumothorax in Neonates

M.R. Paradis

Pneumothorax is uncommon in neonatal foals. It probably is a sequel to trauma during birth. Bruising or palpable fractures of the ribs may be found on examination of the foal's thorax. Or there may be no external evidence of trauma. The foal can appear normal at birth, and stand and nurse without difficulty.

An increased respiratory rate and effort may be the first clinical signs of distress. The foal's breathing pattern may become irregular, and it may take several shallow breaths, followed by a prolonged pause. Auscultation may reveal increased harshness over the cranioventral areas of the lungs because of atelectasis. Sounds over the dorsal regions of the chest may be absent due to free air.

Pneumothorax is diagnosed by radiographic and auscultative findings. Radiographs show retraction of the lungs away from the vertebral column and diaphragm. The lungs appear dense, most likely due to partial atelectasis.

Therapy to correct pneumothorax is directed at decreasing the amount of free air in the thoracic cavity. This is accomplished by thoracentesis in the caudodorsal corner of the lung field in the standing foal. A 5 x 5-cm area is shaved and surgically prepared and 1 ml of lidocaine is injected SC for local anesthesia. A 2-in, 18-ga needle, connected to extension tubing and a 3-way stopcock, is inserted into the pleural space, and the air is aspirated. This procedure may need to be repeated every 12-24 hours until the problem resolves.

If the air leak is small, it should seal within a few days. Each day less air can be aspirated from the chest. The prognosis is good if the condition is uncomplicated by other problems, such as laceration of the lung by a fractured rib.

Hydrothorax

R.E. Beadle

Hydrothorax can be caused by any condition that increases hydrostatic pressure in the postcapillary venules of the pleura or decreases plasma oncotic pressure. Specific conditions associated with hydrothorax include congestive right heart failure, hypoproteinemia, rupture of the thoracic duct, and thoracic wall trauma.

Horses with hydrothorax may show no clinical signs. Auscultation and percussion reveal a fluid line if the effusion is voluminous. Thoracentesis reveals an increased amount of pleural fluid with low cellularity and a low protein content. Hydrothorax is treated by draining excess fluid from the pleural space. Additionally, the inciting cause should be determined and treated.

Hemothorax

Hemothorax is an infrequent finding in horses. When it does occur, compression atelectasis of the ventral portions of the lungs may result. Hemorrhagic shock can also occur if large amounts of blood are lost into the pleural space over a short period. Hemothorax is caused by frank bleeding into the pleural space. Such bleeding can result from rupture of a damaged vessel or trauma to the thoracic wall and/or lung. Additionally, tearing of adhesions between the visceral and parietal pleural surfaces can produce hemothorax.

Clinical findings depend upon the rate and amount of blood loss. Horses with a ruptured major vessel, such as the aorta, have massive amounts of blood in the pleural space (and/or pericardium) and die acutely. Involvement of other vessels usually produces slower bleeding and lesser amounts of blood in the pleural space.

Tachycardia and tachypnea are seen in affected horses with inadequate oxygen-carrying capacity in the arterial blood. Tachypnea without tachycardia can be produced by pooling of enough blood in the pleural space to compress the ventral regions of the lungs and cause atelectasis. Auscultation and percussion of the thorax reveals a fluid line when moderate to large amounts of blood have pooled in the pleural space. Thoracentesis can confirm hemothorax after clinical findings suggest its presence.

Treatment should be directed toward correcting the cause of hemorrhage, if possible. Intravenous balanced electrolyte solutions can be used to treat hypovolemic shock, given at a volume of 2-7 times the blood volume lost. If large volumes of blood are lost, with hematocrit readings approaching 10%, blood transfusion is necessary. Uncontaminated blood removed from a sterile pleural space and treated with an anticoagulant may be used to autotransfuse the patient.

Inflammatory, Infectious and Immune Diseases

Bacterial Pleuritis

Pleuritis is inflammation of the pleural membrane. Pleural effusion is associated with pleuritis, but it is not invariably present. Likewise, pleural effusion does not necessarily signify pleuritis. Pleuritis may be acute or chronic and unilateral or bilateral.

Early cases of pleuritis are characterized by pain due to inflammation of the parietal pleura, and affected horses have restricted thoracic wall movement. As pleural effusion develops, pain subsides but compressive atelectasis of the lung interferes with ventilation and gas exchange. As the condition progresses, a fibrinopurulent exudate accumulates in the pleural cavity. If fibrin organizes, adhesions develop between the lung and parietal pleura, preventing the pleural linings from moving independently.

Chronic bacterial pleuritis warrants a poor prognosis and is expensive to treat. In addition, affected horses tend to develop secondary complications, such as laminitis and thrombophlebitis, that worsen the prognosis. All of the above factors can lead to a dissatisfied owner if they are not properly advised initially about the estimated cost and poor prognosis for life and future usefulness.

Etiology: Horses with infectious pleuritis usually have a history of a recent stressful event. Such stress can be caused by long-distance hauling or by a vigorous athletic endeavor, such as racing. General anesthesia also seems to predispose some horses to pleuritis. Mechanisms whereby such stressful events can cause pleuritis are presently undetermined. Possible mechanisms include interference with normal function of the mucociliary escalator and alveolar macrophages. Most cases of pleuritis result from pneumonic conditions and are, therefore, referred to as pleuropneumonia. Some cases of infectious pleuritis are primary and involve only the pleural membrane. Such cases are unusual in horses, but when they do occur, viral and bacterial infections are the most likely causes. Viral etiologies for primary pleuritis are recognized in people but have not received much attention in horses. Such conditions may occur but go unnoticed in horses due to the insidious nature of some viral infections. *Mycoplasma felis* was reported to be the etiologic agent in naturally occurring pleuritis in a horse. The organism subsequently was used to induce pleuritis in an experimental pony.[364]

Most cases of pleuritis are secondary to and an extension of pneumonia or lung abscesses, and thus are referred to as pleuropneumonia.[252] Viruses and/or bacteria can cause the primary pneumonic insult. Some cases of pleuritis are idiopathic. No causative organism or primary disease process could be determined in 14 of 37 (37%) horses with pleuritis.[251]

Clinical Findings: Clinical signs of pleuritis depend upon the severity and duration of the disease. Some cases are so mild that evidence of pleuritis can be detected only after careful examination of the respiratory system and thoracic wall. Severely affected horses show clear clinical signs, not only in the respiratory system but in other organ systems as well. Careful visual observation of an affected horse often provides valuable information. Severely affected individuals are depressed and have an anxious facial expression. They often avoid attempts by the examiner to touch them in the thoracic region. Some affected horses are cachectic and have edema in the pectoral region that occasionally extends to the ventral abdomen.

Respiratory rate, rhythm and character are variable. Mildly affected horses with no pleural effusion may show no respiratory signs. Horses with intense pleuritic pain but no pleural effusion may have rapid, shallow respiration marked by limited thoracic wall movement and an enhanced abdominal component. These horses may grunt while breathing. Horses with marked pleural effusion also have rapid, shallow respiration but usually have freer thoracic wall movement and fewer signs of respiratory pain. Their nostrils also flare markedly during inspiration, but abdominal breathing is not so marked.

Horses with intense pleuritic pain may stand with their elbows abducted and are reluctant to move. Their signs may cause the examiner to suspect laminitis, but examination of the feet with hoof testers usually fails to reveal painful foci. Laminitis may develop later in the disease, however. Horses with intense pleuritic pain may also show signs of colic, probably due to referred pain from the parietal pleura.

Mucous membrane color and perfusion usually are not changed in early cases of pleuritis. As the condition progresses, the mucous membranes can become either cyanotic or injected, and capillary refill time increases. Changes in the mucous membranes are probably the result of hypoxemia, toxemia or dehydration.

Pulse rates usually are increased in horses with pleuritis. Pain probably is responsible for reflex increases in heart rate in noneffusive cases, while ventilation-perfusion mismatching and resultant hypoxemia are more likely causes in affected horses with pleural effusion and resultant compression atelectasis.

Most horses with clinical signs of pleuritis have a fever. This is expected, as most cases of pleuritis have an infectious etiology.

Auscultation of the thorax is necessary when examining horses with suspected pleuritis. Horses without significant pleural effusion may have no abnormal lung sounds, or lung sounds may be louder than normal. Wheezes and/or coarse crackles may or may not be detectable in these early cases. Pleural friction sounds are very uncommon but are most likely in noneffusive cases. Their absence certainly does not rule out pleuritis. Thoracic auscultation of horses with effusive pleuritis usually provides significant diagnostic information. Lung sounds are heard quite distinctly dorsal to the fluid line but are not easily heard ventral to this line. Crackles and/or wheezes may or may not be detectable dorsally. Pleural friction sounds become diminished as effusion volumes increase and finally are no longer detectable.

Percussion often is helpful when evaluating horses with pleuritis. Pain and pleural fluid are the most common findings. Pain may be most readily elicited in the dorsal lung field of affected horses.[365]

Hematologic examination may show neutropenia in peracute cases. Subacute and chronic cases show neutrophilia with or without a left shift. The packed cell volume may be normal, elevated or decreased, depending upon the presence or absence of dehydration and anemia of chronic disease. Plasma fibrinogen content and monocyte counts usually are elevated.

Diagnostic Aids: Thoracentesis is an indispensable aid in diagnosis of infectious pleuritis in horses. Fluid can be collected through the sixth or seventh intercostal space, just dorsal to the costochondral junction. Aseptic surgical technique is employed when obtaining the sample. Local anesthetic is used to desensitize the skin, intercostal space and parietal pleura. No skin incision is required if a Quik-Cath (Travenol) or similar intravenous catheter is used. If a teat cannula or bitch catheter is used, a small skin incision is necessary. A syringe and/or 3-way stopcock (Pharmaseal) should be attached to the catheter or cannula, either directly or with an extension set (Travenol), before the catheter is inserted into the pleural space. The catheter should be placed just cranial to the rib to avoid intercostal vessels and the accompanying nerve. Both sides of the thorax should be tapped, using care not to transfer bacteria from one side to the other.

Collected fluid should be observed for color, turbidity and odor. Normal pleural fluid is yellow and clear. Increased turbidity suggests increased numbers of WBC and the presence of fibrin. A fetid odor suggests anaerobic infection, necrotizing pneumonia or abscessation. Harvested pleural fluid should be Gram stained and cultured for bacteria. Culture for both aerobic and anaerobic bacteria for each side of the thorax is essential.[285] Antibiotic sensitivities should be determined for all isolates.

Cytologic examination and a protein determination should be performed on the fluid. Total WBC counts and protein concentrations of pleural fluid from normal horses are $<10,000/\mu l$ and <2.5 g/dl, respectively.[366] Infectious pleuritis causes these values to rise. Neutrophils are the predominant cell and may be degenerate or contain bacteria. A transtracheal aspirate should be cultured at the time of thoracentesis, as sometimes it is possible to recover organisms from the transtracheal aspirate when they cannot be recovered from the pleural fluid.

Ultrasonography recently has become popular for evaluating the pleural space of horses with pleuritis. This technique is not limited to sector-scanning machines; less expensive ultrasound machines, such as those used for pregnancy diagnosis in mares, also can be used. Such information as pleural fluid volume, number and size of fibrin tags and amount of loculation can be determined. Ultrasonography also is useful to identify sites for thoracic drainage.

Radiography also can be used to evaluate the thorax of a horse with pleuritis. Much more information can be obtained if excess pleural fluid is drained before radiography, as all structures ventral to the fluid line will be obscured. Radiography offers additional information about the lung that cannot be obtained by ultrasonography. Lung radiographs can be assessed for signs of pulmonary disease, such as interstitial infiltrate, peribronchial infiltrate, alveolar filling, and abscessation. Bullae on the pleural surface of the lung and air in the pleural space are also detectable with lung radiographs.

Pleuroscopy should be reserved for evaluation of horses with chronic pleuritis and extensive areas of organized fibrin in the pleural space.[367] A sterilized or disinfected endoscope is used for the procedure. The thoracic wall should be entered in a sterile manner at the tenth intercostal space at the widest point on the thoracic wall. This procedure is not without hazard. Complications described include infection, pneumothorax, lung laceration and postexamination pleural pain.

Treatment: Treatment of pleuritis is determined by the severity and duration of the disease. Pain can be diminished using nonsteroidal antiinflammatory agents, such as phenylbutazone and flunixin meglumine. If pain appears to be causing anorexia, these agents should be used. However, these drugs mask fever and may cause renal damage if the horse is not properly hydrated.

Antimicrobial agents should be used when bacterial infection is present in the lungs or the pleural cavity or if secondary bacterial invasion is anticipated following a primary viral insult. Oral and IV routes are recommended over the IM route. Penicillin and trimethoprim-sulfonamide or penicillin-gentamicin combinations give a good spectrum of coverage initially. Final selection of antimicrobial drugs should be based on culture and sensitivity results. If specific therapy is needed for anaerobes, metronidazole can be given PO at 7.5-15 mg/kg QID. Long-term therapy with gentamicin usually is not rewarding in horses with large amounts of fibrin in the pleural space, even though sensitivity tests indicate gentamicin

to be appropriate for the organism(s) present. Probably this is because of the drug's decreased activity in the presence of proteinaceous substances, which bind and inactivate gentamicin. Though expensive, ticarcillin and third-generation cephalosporins deserve consideration in treating horses with pleuritis. For both Gram-positive cocci and Gram-negative organisms, rifampin at 5-10 mg/kg BID is worth considering, though it must be used in conjunction with other antimicrobial drugs.

Drainage of fluid from the affected pleural space is extremely important. If pleural fluid and fibrin are allowed to accumulate, fibrin plaques form on the surface of the lung and thoracic wall. Such plaques protect bacteria from antimicrobial agents, form loculations of fluid that inhibit proper drainage, and result in adhesions of the lung to the thoracic wall. Drainage can be accomplished by inserting a 28-Fr trocar catheter (Argyle) into the pleural space using the same techniques described for thoracentesis. Care must be taken to avoid the lateral thoracic vein and major structures in the thorax when placing this catheter. Insertion of a Heimlich chest drain valve (Bard-Parker) into the end of the catheter allows drainage and prevents aspiration of air through the catheter. Intermittent drainage of pockets of fluid with an appropriately sized catheter or cannula, using ultrasound guidance, is helpful when a permanent cannula stops draining fluid.

Intravenous fluid therapy is mandatory in many horses with pleuritis. The type of fluid used is dictated by serum electrolyte values, but lactated Ringer's solution and normal saline are common choices. Such fluid therapy helps correct prerenal azotemia, rehydrates horses that are dehydrated due to massive fluid losses into the pleural space, and helps replace fluid drained from the thorax. This also helps remove bacteria, fibrin and inflammatory mediators from the pleural space through drainage devices, such as cannulae and catheters.

Systemic heparin can be used to treat pleural effusion at 20,000 units BID. Beneficial effects are thought to be decreased fibrin formation in the pleural space and protection from laminitis. Controlled studies have not been performed to document the efficacy of this therapy. Heparin doses may have to be decreased or discontinued in treated horses that become anemic. Discontinuation of heparin use results in a quick rebound of the hematocrit.

Injection of such enzymes as fibrinolysin into the pleural fluid has been advocated to help natural processes of fibrin degradation. Appropriate dosages, routes of administration and frequency of administration have yet to be determined

Lavage of the pleural space may be attempted if the pleural fluid contains large numbers of bacteria and large amounts of free fibrin. Fluid can be introduced through a sterile 28-Fr trocar catheter (Argyle) in the ventral aspect of the thoracic wall. The rate of administration should not be so rapid that horses are uncomfortable during the procedure; the volumes administered are best determined from changes induced in the respiratory pattern. When the horse achieves a respiratory rate >40 breaths per minute and has inspiratory nostril flare, fluid administration should be discontinued and fluid in the thorax allowed to drain by gravity flow. Fluids used for thoracic lavage should be warm, isotonic and pH buffered, and should not contain calcium. Calcium-containing fluids appear to enhance fibrin formation in pleural fluid.

Thoracotomy has been suggested as a salvage procedure for horses with chronic pleuritis and associated abscesses in the pleural space. One report described rib resection and thoracotomy in the standing horse.[368] Removal of necrotic debris and establishment of surgical drainage are the goals of this procedure. Removal of the right sixth or left seventh rib is advocated on the respective affected side. Hydrotherapy with isotonic sterile saline and gentle manual massage are recommended for the first few postoperative days. After granulation tissue starts to form, tap water can be substituted for sterile saline solution. Wound closure occurs in 2-3 months. Bilateral pneumothorax can be a hazard with this procedure, so horses should be examined for this eventuality before the procedure is performed. Pneumothorax should be created intentionally on the hemithorax scheduled for surgery. If the horse does not experience respiratory distress, then a communication does not exist between the 2 halves of the thoracic cavity and surgery may be performed. If respiratory distress does occur, air must be removed from the thorax, and the surgery not performed.

Good supportive care is essential to the successful outcome of pleuritis. This includes providing good-quality feed and water. Leg wraps should be used to prevent swelling in the distal limbs, and frog supports should be applied to the front feet. Once frog supports are in place, the horse may be taken for short walks several times a day. Silastic catheters (Baxter) can be used in an attempt to decrease the incidence of thrombophlebitis.

Prognosis: Horses with pleural pain but no pleural effusion have a good prognosis if they are rested appropriately. The prognosis with pleural effusion is guarded. Therapy of severe pleuritis involves prolonged use of antimicrobials costing thousands of dollars; often this is the limiting factor in the prognosis. A grave prognosis should be given to horses that are toxemic and have developed laminitis as a secondary complication.

Mediastinal Abscesses

Mediastinal abscesses are the result of bacterial seeding of mediastinal lymph nodes. Routes by which such seeding occurs are not known but probably are through lymphatics that drain the lungs and cervical region. No studies have been reported to determine which organisms are most frequently isolated from these nodes, but clinical impression suggests that beta-hemolytic streptococci frequently are involved in young horses.

Horses with mediastinal abscesses usually show fever, inappetence, neutrophilia and an elevated plasma fibrogen level. Some affected individuals are in good condition, while others become very unthrifty. Clinical examination often reveals no additional abnormalities if the abscesses involve lymph nodes in the middle and caudal mediastinum. Radiographs of the thorax reveal enlarged lymph nodes, which can be mistaken for lung abscesses. Mediastinal abscesses produce soft tissue densities of equal size when viewed on radiographs made from both the left and right sides of the thorax. Lung abscesses, however, demonstrate the lesion to be larger in one lateral view than the other.

Abscesses in the cranial mediastinal space often cause swelling at the thoracic inlet and may impinge upon the trachea, esophagus and great vessels in this region. Horses with a narrowed trachea show respiratory distress during both inspiration and expiration. The severity of signs seen is determined by the degree of tracheal narrowing. Horses in which the abscess exerts pressure on the esophagus have difficulty swallowing and may show signs of choke. Aspiration pneumonia with its accompanying findings also may be seen. Apparent right heart failure, with distended jugular veins and pectoral, thoracic limb, neck and head edema, may occur as the mass decreases venous return to the heart from the cranial body.

Involved lymph nodes should be drained surgically if possible. Culture and sensitivity results should be used to determine which antimicrobials to use postsurgically. Broadspectrum antimicrobials should be used to treat horses in which surgical drainage and culture are not possible. A combination of procaine penicillin G and gentamicin provides a good spectrum of activity against both Gram-positive and Gram-negative bacteria.

Neoplasia

Thoracic Lymphosarcoma

Lymphosarcoma is not a common disease in horses. In a retrospective study involving 687 equine necropsies and 635 biopsies, 236 neoplasms were diagnosed and only 3 of these (1.3%) were lymphosarcomas.[369] Lymphoid tumors are, however, the most common type of hematopoietic neoplasm in horses.[370]

Various anatomic forms of equine lymphosarcoma have been described. These include mediastinal (thymic), alimentary, multicentric, cutaneous and generalized forms.[370] In addition to having signs of tumor impingement on other thoracic structures, most horses with thoracic lymphosarcoma develop pleural effusion.

Mechanisms that trigger development of lymphosarcoma in the horse are not understood. Viral, genetic and immune factors may be involved.[334]

Weight loss, anorexia, depression, pectoral edema, respiratory distress and exercise intolerance are common clinical signs. Progression of the disease usually is quite rapid once signs appear. Primarily middle-aged horses are affected, but the condition has been reported in horses as young as 2 years of age. There appears to be no sex or breed predilection. Examination often reveals pleural effusion and distended jugular veins. Thoracic auscultation may reveal wheezes and crackles in the dorsal lung fields. Other findings that are variably present include fever, dysphagia, colic and diarrhea.

Thoracentesis usually reveals copious fluid amounts in the pleural space; the fluid may be blood tinged. Pleural fluid from horses with thoracic lymphosarcoma is characterized as a modified transudate. Protein levels are elevated, though lower than those seen in pleuritis, and lymphocytes usually are the predominant cell rather than neutrophils. Many of the lymphocytes may be bizarre and have mitotic figures. Abdominocentesis should be attempted if a diagnostic sample cannot be obtained from the thoracic cavity. Lymphoblasts sometimes can be obtained from the abdominal cavity and not from the pleural space in horses with thoracic lymphosarcoma. Hematologic examination results usually do not provide evidence of lymphocytosis or abnormal circulating lymphocytes. Other changes may include anemia, leukopenia and neutrophilia. Hypercalcemia has been reported in a horse with lymphosarcoma.[371] Repeated determinations of serum calcium levels are warranted, as they may rise abruptly.

Glucocorticoids and chemotherapy offer potential avenues for therapy, but recommended drugs and dosage regimens are not available.

Idiopathic Diseases

Synchronous Diaphragmatic Flutter

Synchronous diaphragmatic flutter is discussed in the chapter on Diseases of the Musculoskeletal System.

References

1. Derksen FJ *et al*: Ovalbumin induced allergic lung disease in the pony: Role of vagal mechanisms. *J Appl Physiol* 53:719-725, 1982.
2. Kotlikoff MI and Gillespie JR: Lung sounds in veterinary medicine. Part I. Terminology and mechanisms of sound production. *Compend Cont Ed Pract Vet* 5:634-639, 1983.

3. Dubielzig RR: Pulmonary lesions of neonatal foals. *J Eq Med Surg* 1:419-425, 1977.

4. Kosch PC et al: Developments in management of the newborn foal in respiratory distress. 1: Evaluation. *Equine Vet J* 16:312-318, 1984.

5. Beech J: Respiratory problems in foals. *Compend Cont Ed Pract Vet* 8:S284-S290, 1986.

6. Stewart JH et al: Respiratory studies in foals from birth to seven days old. *Equine Vet J* 16:323-328, 1984.

7. Paradis MR: Lecithin/sphingomyelin ratios and phosphatidylglycerol in term and premature equine amniotic fluid. *Proc 5th Ann Vet Med Forum*, 1987. pp 789-792.

8. Cook WR: Some observations on the ear, nose and throat in the horse and endoscopy using a flexible fibreoptic endoscope. *Vet Record* 94:533-541, 1974.

9. Robinson NE and Sorensen PR: Pathophysiology of airway obstruction in horses: A review. *JAVMA* 172:299-303, 1978.

10. Mansmann RA and Knight HD: Transtracheal aspiration in the horse. *JAVMA* 160:1527-1529, 1972.

11. Sweeney CR et al: Bacterial isolates from tracheobronchial aspirates of healthy horses. *Am J Vet Res* 46:2562-2565, 1985.

12. Larson VL and Busch RH: Equine tracheobronchial lavage: comparison of lavage cytology and pulmonary histopathologic findings. *Am J Vet Res* 46:144-146, 1985.

13. Derksen FJ et al: Bronchoalveolar lavage in ponies with recurrent airway obstruction (heaves). *Am Rev Resp Dis* 132:1066-1070, 1985.

14. Raphel CF and Gunson DE: Percutaneous lung biopsy in the horse. *Cornell Vet* 71:439-448, 1981.

15. Derksen FJ et al: Pulmonary function tests in ponies: Reproducibility and effect of vagal blockade. *Am J Vet Res* 43:598-602, 1982.

16. Derksen FJ et al: Effect of laryngeal hemiplegia and laryngoplasty on airway flow mechanics in exercising horses. *Am J Vet Res* 47:16-20, 1986.

17. Hornicke H et al, in Gillespie JR and Robinson NE: *Equine Exercise Physiology 2*. ICCEP Publications, Davis, CA, 1987. pp 216-224.

18. Koterba AM et al: The breathing strategy of the adult horse (*Equus caballus*) at rest. *J Appl Physiol* 64:337-346, 1988.

19. Rossdale PD: Neonatal respiratory problems of foals. *Vet Clin No Am* 1:205-217, 1979.

20. Derksen FJ et al: Chronic restrictive pulmonary disease in a horse. *JAVMA* 180:887-89, 1982.

21. Weibel ER: *Morphometry of the Human Lung*. Springer-Verlag, Berlin, 1963.

22. Breeze RG: Heaves. The problem of disease recognition. *Vet Clin No Am* 1:219-230, 1979.

23. Derksen FJ et al: Airway reactivity in ponies with recurrent airway obstruction (heaves). *J Appl Physiol* 58:598-604, 1985.

24. Broadstone RV et al: Effects of atropine recurrent airway obstruction in ponies with chronic airway disease (heaves). *J Appl Physiol* 65:2720-2725, 1988.

25. Scott JS et al: B-Adrenergic blockade in ponies with recurrent obstructive pulmonary disease. *J Appl Physiol* 65:2324-2328, 1988.

26. Drazen JM and Austen KF: Leukotrienes and airway responses. *Am Rev Resp Dis* 136:985-998, 1987.

27. Amis T et al: Topographic distribution of pulmonary ventilation and perfusion in the horse. *Am J Vet Res* 45:1597-1601, 1984.

28. Sorensen PR and Robinson NE: Postural effects on lung volumes and synchronous ventilation in anesthetized horses. *J Appl Physiol* 48:97-103, 1980.

29. Robinson NE and Sorenson PR: Collateral flow resistance and time constants in dog and horse lungs. *J Appl Physiol* 44:63-68, 1978.

30. McLaughlin RF et al: A study of the subgross pulmonary anatomy in various mammals. *Am J Anat* 108:149-165, 1961.

31. O'Callaghan MW et al: Exercise-induced pulmonary haemorrhage in the horse: Results of a detailed clinical, post mortem and imaging study. III. Subgross findings in lungs subjected to latex perfusion of the bronchial pulmonary arteries. *Equine Vet J* 19:394-404, 1987.

32. Bisgard GE et al: Hypoxic pulmonary hypertension in the pony. *Am J Vet Res* 36:49-52, 1975.

33. Pan LG et al: Hyperventilation in ponies at onset of and during steady state exercise. *J Appl Physiol* 54:1394-1402, 1983.

34. Gillespie JR et al: Blood pH, O2 and CO2 tensions in exercised control and emphysematous horses. *Am J Physiol* 207:1067-1072, 1964.

35. Bayly WM et al: Arterial blood gas tension during exercise in a horse with laryngeal hemiplegia, before and after corrective surgery. *Res Vet Sci* 36:256-258, 1984.

36. Pelletier N et al, in Gillespie JR and Robinson NE: *Equine Exercise Physiology 2*. ICCEP Publications, Davis, CA, 1987. pp 225-234.

37. Forster HV et al: Changes in breathing when switching from nares to tracheostomy breathing in awake ponies. *J Appl Physiol* 59:1214-1221, 1985.

38. Gehr P and Erni H: Morphometric estimation of pulmonary diffusion capacity in two horse lungs. *Resp Physiol* 41:199-210, 1980.

39. Gehr P et al: Design of the mammalian respiratory system. V. Scaling morphometric diffusing capacity to body mass: wild and domestic animals. *Resp Physiol* 44:61-86, 1981.

40. Taylor CR et al: Design of the mammalian respiratory system. III. Scaling aerobic capacity to body mass: wild and domestic animals. *Resp Physiol* 44:25-37, 1981.

41. Wagner PD et al: Mechanism of exercise-induced hypoxemia in horses. *J Appl Physiol* 66:1227-1233, 1989.

42. Hedenstierna G et al: Ventilation-perfusion relationships in the standing horse: an inert gas elimination study. *Equine Vet J* 19:514-519, 1987.

43. Willoughby RA and McDonell WN: Pulmonary function testing in horses. *Vet Clin No Am* 1:171-196, 1979.

44. Pelletier N et al, in Gillespie JR and Robinson NE: *Equine Exercise Physiology 2*. ICCEP Publications, Davis, CA, 1987. pp 485-493.

45. Bunn HF and Kitchen H: Hemoglobin function in the horse: The role of 2, 3-diphosphoglycerate in modifying the oxygen affinity of maternal and fetal blood. *Blood* 42:471-479, 1973.

46. Heflin AC and Brigham KL: Prevention by granulocyte depletion of increased vascular permeability of sheep lung following endotexemia. *J Clin Invest* 68:1253-1260, 1981.

47. Slocombe RF et al: Importance of neutrophils in the pathogenesis of acute pneumonic pateurellosis in calves. *Am J Vet Res* 46:2253-2258, 1985.

48. Erdmann AJ et al: Effect of increased vascular pressure on lung fluid balance in anesthetized sheep. *Circ Res* 37:271-284, 1975.

49. Staub NC et al, in Chretien J et al: *The Pleura in Health and Disease*. Marcel Dekker, New York, 1985. pp 169-193.

50. Clarke AF: A review of environmental and host factors in relation to equine respiratory disease. *Equine Vet J* 19:435-441, 1987.

51. Brain JD and Valberg PA: State of the art. Deposition of aerosol in the respiratory tract. *Am Rev Resp Dis* 120:1325-1373, 1979.

52. Dahl LG et al, in Gillespie JR and Robinson NE: *Equine Exercise Physiology 2*. ICEEP Publications, Davis, CA, 1987. pp 235-242.

53. Albert RE et al: The characteristics of bronchial clearance in miniature donkey. *Arch Environ Hlth* 17:50-58, 1968.

54. Robinson NE: Pathophysiology of coughing. *Proc 32nd Ann Mtg AAEP*, 1987. pp 291-298.

55. Brain JD, in Fishman AP et al: *Handbook of Physiology*. American Physiological Society, Bethesda, MD, 1985. pp 447-471.

56. Huston LJ et al, in Gillespie JR and Robinson NE: *Equine Exercise Physiology 2*. ICEEP Publications, Davis, CA, 1987. pp 243-252.

57. Jakab GT, in Loan RW: *Bovine Respiratory Disease: A Symposium*. Texas A&M University Press, College Station, 1984. pp 223-286.

58. Wetmore LA et al: Mixed venous oxygen tension as an estimate of cardiac output in anesthetized horses. *Am J Vet Res* 48:971-976, 1987.

59. Reibold TW et al: Evaluation of the demand valve for resuscitation of horses. *JAVMA* 176:623-626, 1980.

60. Krpan MK: Tracheotomy in the horse: a photo essay. *MVP* 65:9-12, 1984.

61. Hynes PF, in Jennings PB: *The Practice of Large Animal Surgery*. Saunders, Philadelphia, 1984. pp 470-479.

62. Robertson JT and Spurlock GH: Tracheal reconstruction in a foal. *JAVMA* 189:313-314, 1986.

63. Tate LP et al: Tracheal reconstruction by resection and end-to-end anastomosis in the horse. *JAVMA* 178:253-258, 1981.

64. Holland M et al: Laryngotracheal injury associated with nasotracheal intubation in the horse. *JAVMA* 189:1447-1450, 1986.

65. Iourenco RV, in Fishman AP: *Pulmonary Diseases and Disorders*. McGraw-Hill, New York, 1980. pp 1596-1606.

66. Ferron GA et al: Properties of aerosols produced with three nebulizers. *Am Rev Resp Dis* 114:899-908, 1976.

67. Davies RS: Pharmacokinetics of inhaled substances. *Postgrad Med J* 51:69-75, 1975.

68. Asmundson T et al: Efficiency of nebulizers for depositing saline in human lungs. *Am Rev Resp Dis* 108:506-512, 1973.

69. Ziment I: *Respiratory Pharmacology and Therapeutics*. Saunders, Philadelphia, 1978. pp 21-34.

70. Sasse HL and Hajer R: NAB365, a beta-2 receptor sympathomimetic agent: Clinical experience in

horses with lung disease. *J Vet Pharmacol Therap* 1:241-244, 1978.

71. Derksen FJ et al: Effect of clenbuterol on histamine induced airway obstruction in ponies. *Am J Vet Res* 48:423-426, 1987.

72. Webb AI et al: Developments in management of the newborn foal in respiratory distress. 2: Treatment. *Equine Vet J* 16:319-323, 1984.

73. Sonea I: Respiratory distress syndrome in neonatal foals. *Compend Cont Ed Pract Vet* 7:S462-S468, 1985.

74. Rose RJ et al: Effect of intranasal oxygen administration on arterial blood gas and acid base parameters in spontaneously delivered, term induced and induced premature foals. *Res Vet Sci* 34:159-162, 1983.

75. Stewart JH et al: Response to oxygen administration in foals: effect of age, duration and method of administration on arterial blood gas values. *Equine Vet J* 16:329-331, 1984.

76. Koterba AM and Drummond WH: Nutritional support of the foal during intensive care. *Vet Clin No Am* 1:35-40, 1985.

77. Bryans JT and Gerber H, in Catcott EJ and Smithcors JF: *Equine Medicine and Surgery*. American Veterinary Publications, Goleta, CA, 1972. pp 17-22.

78. Fenner F et al: *Veterinary Virology*. Academic Press, Orlando, FL, 1987.

79. Baker K: Rationale for the use of influenza vaccines in horses and the importance of antigenic drift. *Equine Vet J* 18:93-96, 1986.

80. Campbell TM and Studdert MJ: Equine herpesvirus type 1 (EHV1). *Vet Bull* 53:135-146, 1983.

81. Allen GP and Bryans JT, in Pandey R: *Progress in Veterinary Microbiology and Immunology*. S Karger, Basel, 1986. pp 78-144.

82. McCollum WH and Bryans JT: Serological identification of infection by equine arteritis virus in horses in several countries. *Proc 3rd Intl Conf Eq Infect Dis*, 1973. pp 256-263.

83. Timoney PJ and McCollum WH: Equine viral arteritis-Epidemiology and control. *Proc 23rd World Vet Cong*, 1987. p 270.

84. Todd JD: Comments on rhinoviruses and parainfluenza viruses of horses. *JAVMA* 155:387-390, 1969.

85. McChesney AE et al: Adenoviral infection in foals. *JAVMA* 162:545-549, 1973.

86. McGuire TC et al: combined (B- and T-lymphocyte) immunodeficiency: A fatal genetic disease in Arabian foals. *JAVMA* 164:70-76, 1974.

87. Burrows R: Equine rhinoviruses. *Proc 2nd Intl Conf Eq Infect Dis*, 1970. pp154-164.

88. Schummer A et al: *The Viscera of the Domestic Animals*. 2nd ed. Springer-Verlag, New York, 1973.

89. Tulleners EP and Raker CW: Nasal septum resection in the horse. *Vet Surg* 12:41-47, 1983.

90. Servantie J and Sautet JY: Hamartoma of the nasal septum in a yearling. *Equine Pract* 8(6):11-14, 1986.

91. Valdez H et al: Surgical correction of a deviated nasal septum and premaxilla in a colt. *JAVMA* 173:1001-1004, 1978.

92. Goring RL et al: Surgical correction of congenital bilateral choanal atresia in a foal. *Vet Surg* 13:211-216, 1984.

93. Foerner JJ: The diagnosis and correction of false nostril noises. *Proc 13th Ann Mtg AAEP*, 1967. pp 315-327.

94. Boles CL: Abnormalities of the upper respiratory tract. *Vet Clin No Am* 1:89-111, 1979.

95. Levine SB: Depression fractures of the nasal and frontal bones of the horse. *J Equine Med Surg* 3:186-190, 1979.

96. Turner AS: Surgical management of depression fractures of the equine skull. *Vet Surg* 8:29-33, 1979.

97. Mason BJE: Empyema of the equine paranasal sinuses. *JAVMA* 167:727-731, 1975.

98. Kral F: Equine sinusitis - a new therapeutic approach. *JAVMA* 124:373-376, 1954.

99. Wilson JH: Effects of indwelling catheters and povidone iodine flushes on the guttural pouches of the horse. *Equine Vet J* 17:242-244, 1985.

100. Roberts MC *et al*: A protracted case of cryptococcal nasal granuloma in a stallion. *Aust Vet J* 57:287-291, 1981.

101. Scott EA *et al*: Cryptococcosis involving the postorbital area and frontal sinus on a horse. *JAVMA* 165:626-627, 1974.

102. Barsanti JA, in Greene CE: *Clinical Microbiology and Infectious Diseases of the Dog and Cat.* Saunders, Philadelphia, 1984. pp 700-709.

103. Myers DD *et al*: Rhinosporidiosis in a horse. *JAVMA* 145:345-347, 1964.

104. Smith HA and Frankson MC: Rhinosporidiosis in a Texas horse. *Southwestern Vet* 15:22-24, 1961.

105. Reed SM *et al*: Localized equine nasal coccidiodomycosis granuloma. *J Equine Med Surg* 3:119-123, 1979.

106. Macy DW, in Kirk RW: *Current Veterinary Therapy IX*. Saunders, Philadelphia, 1986. pp 1076-1079.

107. Hutchins DR and Johnston KG: Phycomycosis in the horse. *Aust Vet J* 48:269-278, 1972.

108. Hanselka DV: Equine nasal phycomycosis. *VM/SAC* 72:251-253, 1972.

109. Greet TRC: Nasal aspergillosis in three horses. *Vet Record* 184:487-489, 1981.

110. Madewell BR *et al*: Neoplasms of the nasal passage and paranasal sinuses in domesticated animals as reported by 13 veterinary colleges. *Am J Vet Res* 37:851-856, 1976.

111. Moulton JE: *Tumors in Domestic Animals*. 2nd ed. University of California Press, Berkeley, 1978.

112. O'Connor JP and Lucey MP: Osteoma in the maxillary sinus of a yearling Thoroughbred colt. *Irish Vet J* 30:81-83, 1976.

113. Peterson FB *et al*: Surgical treatment of an osteoma in the paranasal sinus of a horse. *J Equine Med Surg* 2:279-283, 1978.

114. Jakob W: Spontaneous amyloidosis of mammals. *Vet Pathol* 8:292-306, 1971.

115. Gordon LR: The cytology and histology of epidermal inclusion cysts in the horse. *J Equine Med Surg* 2:371-374, 1978.

116. Cannon JH *et al*: Diagnosis and surgical treatment of cystlike lesions of the equine paranasal sinuses. *JAVMA* 169:610-613, 1976.

117. Cook WR and Littlewort MCG: Progressive haematoma of the ethmoid region of the horse. *Equine Vet J* 6:101-108, 1974.

118. Platt H: Haemorrhagic nasal polyps of the horse. *J Pathol* 115:51-55, 1975.

119. Cook WR: Some observations on form and function of the equine upper airway in health and disease. I. The pharynx. *Proc Ann Mtg AAEP*, 1981. pp 355-391.

120. Baker GJ, in Robinson NE: *Current Therapy in Equine Medicine 2*. Saunders, Philadelphia, 1987. pp 607-611.

121. Raker CW, in Mansmann RA and McAllister EW: *Equine Medicine and Surgery*. American Veterinary Publications, Goleta, CA, 1987. pp 747-756.

122. Raker CW and Boles CR: Pharyngeal lymphoid hyperplasia in the horse. *J Equine Med Surg* 2:202-207, 1978.

123. Clarke AF *et al*: The relationship of air hygiene in stables to lower airway disease and pharyngeal lymphoid hyperplasia in two groups of Thoroughbred horses. *Equine Vet J* 19:524-530, 1987.

124. Sisson S, in Getty R: *Sisson and Grossman's The Anatomy of Domestic Animals*. 5th ed. Saunders, Philadelphia, 1975. pp 723-725.

125. Heffron CJ and Baker GJ: Fluoroscopic investigation of the pharyngeal functions in the horse. *Equine Vet J* 11:148-152, 1979.

126. Freeman DE: Diagnosis and treatment of diseases of the guttural pouch (Part II). *Compend Cont Ed Pract Vet* 2:S25-S32, 1980.

127. Cook WR, in Grunsell CSG: *The Veterinary Annual*. John Wright and Sons, Bristol, 1971. pp 12-43.

128. Cook WR: The auditory tube diverticulum (guttural pouch) in the horse: its radiographic examination. *J Am Vet Rad Soc* 14(2):51-71, 1973.

129. Cook WR: Clinical observations on the anatomy and physiology of the upper respiratory tract. *Vet Record* 79:440-446, 1966.

130. Freeman DE: Diagnosis and treatment of diseases of the guttural pouch (Part I). *Compend Cont Ed Pract Vet* 2:S3-S11, 1980.

131. Raker CW: Diseases of the guttural pouch. *MVP* 57:549-552, 1976.

132. Wheat JD: Tympanitis of the guttural pouch of the horse. *JAVMA* 140:453-454, 1962.

133. Mason TA: Tympany of the eustachian tube diverticulum (guttural pouch) in a foal. *Equine Vet J* 4:153-154, 1972.

134. Milne DW and Fessler JR: Tympanitis of the guttural pouch in a foal. *JAVMA* 161:61-64, 1972.

135. McAllister ES: Guttural Pouch disease. *Proc 24th Ann Mtg AAEP*, 1978. pp 251-256.

136. Knight AP *et al*: Experimentally induced *Streptococcus equi* infection in the horse with resultant guttural pouch empyema. *VM/SAC* 70:1194-1199, 1975.

137. Cook WR: Observations on the aetiology of epistaxis and cranial nerve paralysis in the horse. *Vet Record* 78:396-406, 1966.

138. Cook WR: The clinical features of guttural pouch mycosis in the horse. *Vet Record* 83:336-345, 1968.

139. Cook WR *et al*: The pathology and aetiology of guttural pouch mycosis in the horse. *Vet Record* 83:422-428, 1968.

140. Cook WR, in Robinson NE: *Current Therapy in Equine Medicine 2*. Saunders, Philadelphia, 1987. pp 612-618.

141. Caron JP et al: Balloon-tipped catheter arterial occlusion for prevention of hemorrhage caused by guttural pouch mycosis: 13 cases (1982-1985). *JAVMA* 191:345-349, 1987.

142. Cook WR: Carotid angiography. *Proc ACVS Surgical Forum*, 1978.

143. Smith KM and Barber SM: Guttural pouch hemorrhage associated with lesions of the maxillary artery in two horses. *Can Vet J* 25:239-242, 1984.

144. Jacobs KA and Fretz PB: Fistula between the guttural pouches and the dorsal pharyngeal recess as a sequel to guttural pouch mycosis in the horse. *Can Vet J* 23:117-118, 1982.

145. McIlwraith CW: Surgical treatment of acute epistaxis associated with guttural pouch mycosis. *VM/SAC* 73:67-69, 1978.

146. Owen R: Ligation of the internal carotid artery to prevent epistaxis due to guttural pouch mycosis. *Vet Record* 104:100-101, 1979.

147. Church S et al: Treatment of guttural pouch mycosis. *Equine Vet J* 18:362-365, 1986.

148. Weinstein L, in Goodman LS and Gilman A: *The Pharmacological Basis of Therapeutics*. 5th ed. MacMillan, New York, 1975. pp 1235-1241.

149. Huber WG et al, in Jones LM et al: *Veterinary Pharmacology and Therapeutics*. 4th ed. Iowa State University Press, Ames, 1977. pp 972-978.

150. Johnson JH et al: A case of guttural pouch mycosis caused by *Aspergillus nidulans*. *VM/SAC* 68:771-774, 1973.

151. Owen R: Epistaxis prevented by ligation of the internal carotid artery in the guttural pouch. *Equine Vet J* 6:143-149, 1974.

152. Greet TRC: Outcome of treatment in 35 cases of guttural pouch mycosis. *Equine Vet J* 19:483-487, 1987.

153. Freeman DE and Donawick WJ: Occlusion of the internal carotid artery in the horse by means of a balloon-tipped catheter: Evaluation of a method designed to prevent epistaxis caused by guttural pouch mycosis. *JAVMA* 176:232-235, 1980.

154. Freeman DE and Donawick WJ: Occlusion of the internal carotid artery of the horse by means of a balloon-tipped catheter: Clinical use of a method to prevent epistaxis caused by guttural pouch mycosis. *JAVMA* 176:236-240, 1980.

155. Freeman DE and Ross MW: Occlusion of the external carotid artery and its branches in the horse to prevent epistaxis from guttural pouch mycosis. *Proc Ann Mtg ACVS*, 1987.

156. Goulden BE et al: Rostral displacement of the palatopharyngeal arch: a case report. *Equine Vet J* 8:95-98, 1976.

157. Wilson RG et al: Rostral displacement of the palatopharyngeal arch in a Thoroughbred yearling. *Aust Vet J* 63:99-100, 1986.

158. Haynes PF, in Jennings PB: *The Practice of Large Animal Surgery*. Saunders, Philadelphia, 1984. pp 430-431.

159. Goulden BE: Less common diseases of the pharynx and larynx. *Proc Symp Aust Eq Vet Assn*, 1981. pp 58-62.

160. Haynes PF et al: Chronic chondritis of the equine arytenoid cartilage. *JAVMA* 177:1135-1142, 1980.

161. Haynes PF: Arytenoid chondritis in the horse. *Proc 27th Ann Mtg AAEP*, 1981. pp 63-69.

162. Koch C: Diseases of the larynx and pharynx in the horse. *Compend Cont Ed Pract Vet* 2:573-579, 1980.

163. Schumacher J and Hanselka DV: Nasopharyngeal cicatrices in horses: 47 cases (1972-1985). *JAVMA* 191:239-242, 1987.

164. MacLean AA and Robertson-Smith RG: Chronic chondritis of the arytenoid cartilages in a pony mare. *Aust Vet J* 61:27-28, 1984.

165. Haynes PF, in Jennings PB: *The Practice of Large Animal Surgery*. Saunders, Philadelphia, 1984. pp 450-455.

166. White NA and Blackwell RB: Partial arytenoidectomy in the horse. *Vet Surg* 9:5, 1980.

167. Spiers VC: Partial arytenoidectomy in horses. *Vet Surg* 15:316-320, 1986.

168. Donawick WJ: Partial arytenoidectomy. *Proc Univ Sydney Postgrad Comm Vet Sci, Refresher Course 54*. pp 164-166.

169. Harrison I et al: Assessment of partial arytenoidectomy without mucosal closure in the horse. *Vet Surg* 15:44, 1986.

170. Haynes PF et al: Subtotal arytenoidectomy in the horse: An update. *Proc 30th Ann Mtg AAEP*, 1984. pp 21-33.

171. Tulleners EP et al: Arytenoidectomy in the horse. *Vet Surg* 15:102, 1986.

172. Cahill JI and Goulden BE: Equine laryngeal hemiplegia. Parts I-V. *N Zeal Vet J* 34:161-175, 181, 193, 1986.

173. Duncan ID et al: A light and electron microscopic study of the neuropathy of equine idiopathic laryngeal hemiplegia. *Neuropath Appl Neurobiol* 4:483-501, 1978.

174. Marks D et al: Observations on laryngeal hemiplegia in the horse and treatment by abductor muscle prosthesis. *Equine Vet J* 2:159-167, 1970.

175. Gilbert GH: Laryngeal hemiplegia following jugular injury. *JAVMA* 161:1686-1687, 1972.

176. Cook WR: Idiopathic laryngeal paralysis in the horse; a clinical and pathological study with particular reference to diagnosis, aetiology and treatment. PhD Thesis, University of Cambridge, 1976.

177. Rose RJ et al: Laryngeal paralysis in Arabian foals associated with oral haloxon administrations. *Equine Vet J* 13:171-176, 1981.

178. Hoare EW: *A System of Veterinary Medicine*. Balliere Tindall, London, 1915. pp 825-840.

179. Kral F: Examination by endoscope. *No Am Vet* 32:91-95, 1951.

180. Anderson LJ: A study of some muscles of the equine larynx and soft palate. PhD Thesis, Massey University, 1984.

181. Goulden BE and Anderson LJ: Equine laryngeal hemiplegia. Part 1: Physical characteristics of affected animals. Part 2: Some clinical observations. *N Zeal Vet J* 29:150-153, 194, 198, 1981.

182. Williams WL: Clinical observations on roaring. *Am Vet Rev* 25:811-815, 1901.

183. Cook WR: Some observations on form and function of the equine upper airway in health and disease. II: Larynx. *Proc 27th Ann Mtg AAEP*, 1981. pp 393-451.

184. Cahill JI and Goulden BE: The pathogenesis of equine laryngeal hemiplegia. *N Zeal Vet J* 35:82-90, 1987.

185. Cook WR: The diagnosis of respiratory unsoundness in the horse. *Vet Record* 7:516-527, 1965.

186. Hobday F: The surgical treatment of roaring in horses. *Vet Record* 47:1535-1539, 1935.

187. Haynes PF, in Jennings PB: *The Practice of Large Animal Surgery*. Saunders, Philadelphhia, 1984. pp 435-444.

188. Kannegieter NJ et al: Right sided laryngeal dysfunction in a horse. *N Zeal Vet J* 34:66-68, 1986.

189. Greet TRC et al: The slap test for laryngeal adductory function in horses with suspected cervical spinal cord damage. *Equine Vet J* 12:127-131, 1980.

190. Baker GJ, in Robinson NE: *Current Therapy in Equine Medicine*. Saunders, Philadelphia, 1983. pp 496-500.

191. Spiers VC: Treatment of laryngeal hemiplegia with abductor muscle prosthesis. *Proc Univ Sydney Postgrad Comm Vet Sci, Refresher Course*, 1981. pp 61-64.

192. Spiers VC et al: Assessment of the efficacy of an abductor muscle prosthesis for treatment of laryngeal hemiplegia in horses. *Aust Vet J* 60:294-299, 1983.

193. Baker GJ: Laryngeal hemiplegia in the horse. *Compend Cont Ed Pract Vet* 5:561-567, 1983.

194. Haynes PF: Obstructive disease of the upper respiratory tract: Current thoughts on diagnosis and surgical management. *Proc 32nd Ann Mtg AAEP*, 1986. pp 283-289.

195. Ducharme NG et al: Nerve-pedicle transplants in an attempt to restore abduction of the paralysed equine arytenoid cartilage. *Vet Surg* 15:26, 1986.

196. Tate LP et al: Laser partial arytenoidectomy and ventriculectomy in horses. *Vet Surg* 15:104, 1987.

197. Goulden BE and Anderson LJ: Equine laryngeal hemiplegia. Part III: Treatment by laryngoplasty. *N Zeal Vet J* 30:1-5, 1982.

198. Goulden BE and Anderson LJ: Laryngeal hemiplegia-treatment by laryngoplasty. *Proc Symp Aust Eq Vet Assn*, 1983. pp 70-76.

199. Fleming G: *Roaring in Horses*. Balliere Tindall, London, 1889.

200. Derksen FJ: In search of the best surgical method to treat roaring in horses. *J Equine Vet Sci* 7:238, 1987.

201. Haynes PF: Dorsal displacement of the soft palate and epiglottic entrapment. Diagnosis, management and interrelationship. *Compend Cont Ed Pract Vet* 5:S279-S289, 1983.

202. Boles CL et al: Epiglottic entrapment by arytenoepiglottic folds in the horse. *JAVMA* 172:338-342, 1978.

203. Linford RL et al: Radiographic assessssment of epiglottic length and pharyngeal and laryngeal diameters in the Thoroughbred. *Am J Vet Res* 44:1660-1666, 1983.

204. Goulden BE: Some unusual cases of abnormal respiratory noises in the horse. *N Zeal Vet J* 25:389-390, 1977.

205. Boles CL: Epiglottic entrapment and follicular pharyngitis. Diagnosis and treatment. *Proc 21st Ann Mtg AAEP*, 1975. pp 29-33.

206. Bertone JJ et al: bilateral hypoplasia of the soft palate and aryepiglottic entrapment. *JAVMA* 188:727-728, 1986.

207. Raker CW, in Mansmann RA and McAllister ES: *Equine Medicine and Surgery*. American Veterinary Publications, Goleta, CA, 1982. pp 764-766.

208. Raphel CF: Endoscopic findings in the upper respiratory tract of 479 horses. *JAVMA* 181:470-473, 1982.

209. Wheat JD: Surgery of the larynx. *Proc Surg Forum ACVS*, 1979.

210. Haynes PF, in Jennings PB: *The Practice of Large Animal Surgery*. Saunders, Philadelphia, 1984. pp 444-450.

211. Haynes PF: Surgical failures in upper respiratory surgery. *Proc 24th Ann Mtg AAEP*, 1978. pp 223-249.

212. Jann HW and Cook WR: Transendoscopic electrosurgery for epiglottis entrapment in the horse. *JAVMA* 187:484-491, 1985.

213. Montgomery TC: CO_2 laser and microsurgery in the horse. *Proc 31st Ann Mtg AAEP*, 1985. pp 399-407.

214. Vasseur P: Surgery of the trachea. *Vet Clin No Am* 9:231-243, 1979.

215. Carrig CB et al: Dorsoventral flattening of the trachea in a horse and its attempted surgical correction: A case report. *J Am Vet Rad Soc* 14:32-36, 1973.

216. Caron JP and Townsend HGG: Tracheal perforation and widespread subcutaneous emphysema in a horse. *Can Vet J* 25:339-341, 1984.

217. Fubini SL et al: Tracheal rupture in two horses. *JAVMA* 187:69-70, 1985.

218. Scott EA: Ruptured trachea in the horse: a method of surgical reconstruction. *VM/SAC* 73:485-489, 1978.

219. Brown CM and Collier MA: Tracheobronchial foreign body in a horse. *JAVMA* 182:280-281, 1983.

220. Urquhart KA and Gerring EL: Tracheobronchial foreign body in a pony. *Equine Vet J* 13:262-264, 1981.

221. Boyd CL and Hanselka DV: Prosthesis for correction of collapsed trachea. *JAAHA* 12:829-830, 1976.

222. Martin JE: Dorsoventral flattening of the trachea in a pony. *Equine Pract* 3(2):17-22, 1981.

223. Bojrab MJ: Surgical reconstruction for collapsed tracheal rings. *Proc Ann Mtg AAHA*, 1973. pp 710-714.

224. Raker CW, in Mansmann RA and McAllister ES: *Equine Medicine and Surgery*. American Veterinary Publications, Goleta, CA, 1982. pp 768-770.

225. Yovich JV and Stashak TS: Surgical repair of a collapsed trachea caused by a lipoma in a horse. *Vet Surg* 13:217-221, 1984.

226. Delahanty DD and Georgi JR: A tracheal deformity in a pony. *JAVMA* 125:42-44, 1954.

227. DeMoor A et al: Surgical correction of a dorsoventral collapse of the trachea in a pony. *Vlaams Diergeneeskundig Tijdschrift* 50:32-37, 1981.

228. Hobson HP: Total ring prosthesis for the surgical correction to a collapsed trachea. *JAAHA* 12:822-828, 1976.

229. Hanselka DV: Tracheal collapse and laryngeal hemiplegia in the horse. *VM/SAC* 68:859-862, 1973.

230. Rigg DL *et al*: Tracheal compression secondary to abscessation of cranial mediastinal lymph nodes in a horse. *JAVMA* 186:283-284, 1985.

231. Randall RW and Myers VS: Partial tracheal stenosis in a horse. *VM/SAC* 68:264-266, 1973.

232. Hanselka DV: Personal communication, 1987.

233. Hallman M and Gluck L: Respiratory distress syndrome - update 1982. *Pediat Clin No Am* 29:1057-1071, 1982.

234. Drummond WH: Neonatal pulmonary hypertension. *Equine Vet J* 16:169-177, 1987.

235. Cottrill CM *et al*: Persistance of fetal circulatory pathways in a newborn foal. *Equine Vet J* 19:252-255, 1987.

236. Trunkey DD: Inhalation injury. *Surg Clin No Am* 58:1133-1140, 1978.

237. Zikria BA *et al*: The chemical factors contributing to pulmonary damage in smoke poisoning. *Surgery* 71:704-709, 1972.

238. Walker HL *et al*: Experimental inhalation injury in the goat. *J Trauma* 21:962-964, 1981.

239. Peter WJ: Inhalation injury caused by the products of combustion. *Can Med Assn J* 125:249-252, 1981.

240. Cahalane M and Demling RH: Early respiratory abnormalities from smoke inhalation. *JAVMA* 251:771-773, 1984.

241. Fein A *et al*: Pathophysiology and management of the complications resulting from fire and the inhalation products of combustion: A review of the literature. *Crit Care Med* 8:94-98, 1980.

242. Fick RB *et al*: Impaired phagocytic and bactericidal functions of smoke exposed rabbit alveolar macrophages. *Chest* 78:516, 1980.

243. Demling RH *et al*: Effects of major thermal injury on the pulmonary microcirculation. *Surgery* 83: 746-751, 1978.

244. Heiderman M: The effect of thermal injury on hemodynamic respiratory and hematologic variables in relation to complement activation. *J Trauma* 19: 239-243, 1979.

245. Demling RH *et al*: Early lung dysfunction after major burns: Role of edema and vasoactive mediators. *J Trauma* 25:959-966, 1985.

246. Anderson RR *et al*: Documentation of pulmonary capillary permeability in the adult respiratory dress syndrome accompanying human sepsis. *Am Rev Resp Dis* 119:869-877, 1979.

247. Mansmann RA, in Mansmann RA and McAllister ES: *Equine Medicine and Surgery*. American Veterinary Publications, Goleta, CA, 1982. pp 776-777.

248. Epstein PE, in Fishman AP: *Pleural Diseases and Disorders*. McGraw-Hill, New York, 1980. pp 1152-1163.

249. Greenfield LJ *et al*: Pulmonary effects of experimental graded aspiration of hydrochloric acid. *Ann Surg* 170:74-86, 1969.

250. Kamada M and Akujama Y: Studies on the distribution in the equine respiratory tract. *Exp Rep Eq Hlth Lab* 12:53-63, 1975.

251. Smith BP: Pleuritis and pleural effusion in the horse: A study of 37 cases. *JAVMA* 170:208-211, 1977.

252. Raphel CF and Beech J: Pleuritis secondary to pneumonia or lung abscessation in 90 horses. *JAVMA* 181:808-810, 1982.

253. Bayly WM *et al*: Stress and its effect on equine pulmonary mucosal defenses. *Proc 32nd Ann Mtg AAEP*, 1986. pp253-262.

254. Sweeney CR *et al*: *Streptococcus equi* infection in horses. Part I. *Compend Cont Ed Pract Vet* 9:689-695, 1987.

255. Sweeney CR *et al*: *Streptococcus equi* infection in horses. Part II. *Compend Cont Ed Pract Vet* 9:845-852, 1987.

256. Timoney JF: Recent field and laboratory observations on the epizootiology and pathogenesis of *Streptococcus equi* infections. *Proc 5th Int Conf Eq Inf Dis*, 1987.

257. Woolcock JB: Studies in atypical *Streptococcus equi*. *Res Vet Sci* 19:115-119, 1975.

258. Clabough D: *Streptococcus equi* infection in the horse: A review of clinical and immunological considerations. *J Equine Vet Sci* 7:279-283, 1987.

259. Sweeney CR *et al*: Complications associated with *Streptococcus equi* infection on a horse farm. *JAVMA* 191:1146-1148, 1987.

260. Timoney J and Eggers D: Serum bactericidal responses to *Streptococcus equi* of horses following infection or vaccination. *Equine Vet J* 17: 306-310, 1985.

261. Galan J *et al*: Expression of the *Streptococcus equi* M protein gene in *E coli* and *S typhimurium*. *Proc 5th Intl Conf Eq Inf Dis*, 1987.

262. Austrian R and Torn G, in Harrison TR: *Principles of Internal Medicine*. McGraw-Hill, New York, 1979. pp 802-808.

263. Benson CE and Sweeney CR: Isolation of *Streptococcus pneumoniae* Type 3 from equine species. *J Clin Microbiol* 20:1028-1030, 1984.

264. Mackintosh ME *et al*: Evidence of *Streptococcus pneumoniae* as a cause of respiratory disease in young Thoroughbred horses in training. *Proc 5th Intl Conf Eq Inf Dis*, 1987.

265. Harms FR: *Pneumokokkeninfektion beivn Rohlen*. *Dtsch Tierrztl Wockenschr* 49:10-13, 1941.

266. Ellenberger MA and Genetzky RM: *Rhodococcus equi* infections: Literature review. *Compend Cont Ed Pract Vet* 8:S414-S424, 1986.

267. Rooney JR: *Corynebacterium* infections in foals. *MVP* 47:43-45, 1986.

268. Bain AM: *Corynebacterium equi* infection in the equine. *Aust Vet J* 39:116-120, 1963.

269. Roberts MC *et al*: *Corynebacterium equi* infection in an adult horse. *Aust Vet J* 56:96, 1980.

270. Robinson RC: Epidemiological and bacteriologic studies of *Corynebacterium (Rhodococcus) equi*. Isolates from California farms. *J Reprod Fertil* 32:477-480, 1982.

271. Smith BP and Robinson RC: Studies of an outbreak of *Corynebacterium* pneumonia in foals. *Equine Vet J* 13:223-228, 1981.

272. Prescott JF *et al*: Epidemiologic survey of *Corynebacterium equi* infections on five Ontario horse farms. *Can J Comp Med* 48:10-13, 1984.

273. Woolcock JB *et al*: Epidemiology of *Corynebacterium equi* in horses. *Res Vet Sci* 28:87-90, 1980.

274. Prescott JF *et al*: Experimental studies on the pathogenesis of *Corynebacterium equi* infection in foals. *Can J Comp Med* 44:280-288, 1980.

275. Sweeney CR *et al*: *Rhodococcus equi* pneumonia in 48 foals: response to antimicrobial therapy. *Vet Micro* 114:329-336, 1987.

276. Falcon J *et al*: Clinical and radiographic findings in *Corynebacterium equi* pneumonia of foals. *JAVMA* 186:593-599, 1985.

277. Martens RJ *et al*: Experimental subacute foal pneumonia induced by aerosol administration of *Corynebacterium equi*. *Equine Vet J* 14:111-116, 1982.

278. Prescott JF *et al*: Lymphocyte immunostimulation in the diagnosis of *Corynebacterium equi* pneumonia in foals. *Am J Vet Res* 41:2073-2075, 1980.

279. Takai S *et al*: Enzyme linked immunosorbent assay for diagnosis of *Corynebacterium (Rhodococcus) equi* infection in foals. *Am J Vet Res* 46:2166-2170, 1985.

280. Ellenburger MA *et al*: Equine humoral immune response to *Rhodococcus equi*. *Am J Vet Res* 45:2428-2430, 1984.

281. Hietala SK *et al:* Detection of *Corynbacterium equi*–specific antibody in horses with enzyme-linked immunosorbent assay. *Am J Vet Res* 46:13-15, 1985.

282. Prescott JF and Sweeney CR: Treatment of *Corynebacterium equi* pneumonia in foals: a review. *JAVMA* 187:725-728, 1985.

283. Hillidge CJ: Use of erythromycin-rifampin combination in treatment of *Rhodococcus equi* pneumonia. *Vet Microbiol* 14:337-342, 1987.

284. Prescott JF and Nicholson VM: The effects of combinations of selected antibiotics on the growth of *Corynebacterium equi*. *J Vet Pharmacol Therap* 7:61-64, 1984.

285. Prescott JF *et al*: Pharmacokinetics of erythromycin in foals and adult horses. *J Vet Pharmacol Therap* 6:67-74, 1983.

286. Burrows GE *et al*: Rifampin in the horse: comparison of intravenous, intramuscular and oral administration. *Am J Vet Res* 46:442-446, 1985.

287. Knight HD and Hietala S: Transtracheal aspiration revisited. *Proc Ann Mtg Coll Int Med*, 1978. pp 120-131.

288. Bayly WM *et al:* Equine bronchopneumonia due to *Bordetella bronchiseptica*. *Equine Pract* 4(7): 25-32, 1982.

289. Darien BJ *et al*: Is *Bordetella bronchiseptica* a significant respiratory pathogen in foals and weanlings? *Proc 5th Intl Conf Inf Dis*, 1987.

290. Sweeney CR *et al*: Anaerobic bacteria in 21 horses with pleuropneumonia. *JAVMA* 187:721-724, 1985.

291. Sweeney RW *et al*: Pharmacokinetics of metronidazole given to horses by intravenous and oral routes. *Am J Vet Res* 47:1726-1729, 1986.

292. Koterba AM *et al*: Clinical and clinicopathological characteristics of the septicaemic neonatal foal: review of 38 cases. *Equine Vet J* 16:376-382, 1984.

293. Lamb CR *et al*: Thoracic radiography in the neonatal foal: A preliminary report. Unpublished report.

294. Clayton HM and Duncan J: Clinical signs associated with *Parascaris equorum* infection in worm free pony foals and yearlings. *Vet Parasitol* 4:69-78, 1978.

295. Nichols JM *et al*: A pathological study of the lungs of foals infected experimentally with *Parascaris equorum*. *J Comp Pathol* 8:261-274, 1978.

296. Crane S *et al*: Unpublished data.

297. George LW *et al*: Chronic respiratory disease in a horse infected with *Dictyocaulus arnfieldi*. *JAVMA* 179:820-822, 1981.

298. Whitwell KE and Greet TRC: Collection and evaluation of tracheobronchial washes in the horse. *Equine Vet J* 16:499-508, 1984.

299. Head JR *et al*, in Ettinger SJ: *Textbook of Veterinary Internal Medicine*. Saunders, Philadelphia, 1975. pp 661-723.

300. Round MC: A study of the natural history of lungworm infection of the Equidae. PhD Thesis, University of Cambridge, 1972.

301. Clayton HM, in Robinson NE: *Current Therapy in Equine Medicine*. Saunders, Philadelphia, 1983. pp 520-522.

302. Lyons ET *et al*: Ivermectin: Treating for naturally occurring infections of lungworms and stomach worms in equids. *Vet Med* 80:58-64, 1985.

303. Britt DP and Preston JM: Efficacy of ivermectin against *Dictyocaulus arnfieldi* in ponies. *Vet Record* 116:343-345, 1985.

304. Cook WR: Chronic bronchitis and alveolar emphysema in the horse. *Vet Record* 99:448-451, 1976.

305. Asmundson T *et al*: Haysickness in Icelandic horses: Preciptin tests and other studies. *Equine Vet J* 15:228-232, 1983.

306. McPherson EA *et al*: Chronic obstructive pulmonary disease (COPD): Factors influencing occurrence. *Equine Vet J* 11:167-171, 1979.

307. Thurlbeck WM and Lowell FC: Heaves in horses. *Am Rev Resp Dis* 89:82-88, 1964.

308. Gillespie JR and Tyler WS: Chronic alveolar emphysema in the horse. *Adv Vet Sci Comp Med* 13:59, 1969.

309. Halliwell REW *et al*: The role of allergy in the chronic pulmonary disease of horses. *JAVMA* 174:277-281, 1979.

310. McPherson EA *et al*: Chronic obstructive pulmonary disease (COPD) in horses: Aetiologic studies: Response to intradermal and inhalation antigen challenge. *Equine Vet J* 11:159-166, 1979.

311. Armstrong PJ *et al*: Airway response to aerosol methacholine and citric acid in ponies with recurrent airway obstruction (heaves). *Am Rev Resp Dis* 133:357-361, 1986.

312. Derksen FJ *et al*: Intravenous histamine administration in ponies with recurrent airway obstruction (heaves). *Am J Vet Res* 46:774-777, 1985.

313. Derksen FJ *et al*: 3-methylindole induced pulmonary toxicosis in the horse. *Am J Vet Res* 43:603-607, 1982.

314. Gerber H: Chronic pulmonary disease in the horse. *Equine Vet J* 5:26-33, 1973.

315. Witting HJ *et al*: The relationship between bronchiolitis and childhood asthma: A follow-up study of 100 cases of bronchiolitis in infancy. *J Allergy* 30:19-22, 1959.

316. Rooney JC and Williams HE: The relationship between proven viral bronchiolitis and subsequent wheezing. *J Pediat* 79:744-747, 1971.

317. Burse WW: Decreased granulocyte response to isoproterinol in asthma during upper respiratory infections. *Am Rev Resp Dis* 115:783-789, 1977.

318. Matthews AG: Identification and characterization of the major antiproteases in equine serum and

an investigation of their role in the onset of chronic obstructive pulmonary disease (COPD). *Equine Vet J* 11:177-182, 1979.

319. Beech J: Cytology of tracheobronchial aspirates in horses. *Vet Pathol* 12:157-164, 1975.

320. Larson VL and Busch RH: Equine tracheobronchial lavage: Comparison of lavage cytology and pulmonary histopathologic findings. *Am J Vet Res* 46:144-146, 1985.

321. Viel L: Structural Functional Correlations of the Lung in Horses with Small Airway Disease. PhD Thesis, University of Guelph, 1983.

322. Eggleston PA et al: A double blind trial of the effect of cromolyn sodium on exercise-induced bronchospasm. *J Allergy Clin Immunol* 50:57, 1972.

323. Beech J: Treatment of chronic obstructive pulmonary disease in horses. *Proc Symp Coll Vet Int Med*, 1978. pp 61-71.

324. Beech J and Perryman L: Immunotherapy for equine respiratory disease. *J Equine Vet Sci* 6:6-10, 1986.

325. Beadle RE, in Robinson NE: *Current Therapy in Equine Medicine*. Saunders, Philadelphia, 1983. pp 512-516.

326. Spencer H: *Pathology of the Lung*. 4th ed. Pergamon Press, Oxford, 1985. pp 413-510.

327. Weill H: Occupational lung diseases. *Chest* 80:545-575, 1981.

328. Schwartz LW et al: Silicate pneumoconiosis and pulmonary fibrosis in horses from the Monterey-Carmel peninsula. *Chest* 80:825-855, 1981.

329. Brambilia C et al: Comparative pathology of silicate pneumoconiosis. *Am J Pathol* 96:149-170, 1979.

330. Mair TS et al: Generalized avian tuberculosis in a horse. *Equine Vet J* 18:226-230, 1986.

331. Ziemer EL et al: Equine coccidioidomycosis. *Proc 5th Ann Vet Forum*, 1987. pp 455-458.

332. Mansmann RA and Pappagianis D: Unpublished data, 1987.

333. Anderson CA and Divers TJ: Systemic granulomatous inflammation in a horse grazing on hairy vetch. *JAVMA* 183:569-570, 1983.

334. Parodi AL et al: Myoblastoma cellules granuleuses. Trois noewelle observations localisation pulmonaire chez le cheval. *Rec Med Vet* 150:489-494, 1974.

335. Misdorp W and Mauta van Gelder HL: Granular cell myoblastoma in the horse. *Pathol Vet* 5:385-394, 1968.

336. Sobel HJ et al: Is schwannoma related to granular cell myoblastoma? *Arch Pathol* 95:396-401, 1973.

337. Nichels FA et al: Myoblastoma: Equine granular cell tumor. *MVP* 61:593-596, 1980.

338. Tennant B et al: Six cases of squamous cell carcinoma of the stomach of the horse. *Equine Vet J* 14:238-243, 1974.

339. Neufeld JL: Lymphosarcoma in a mare and review of cases at the Ontario Veterinary College. *Can Vet J* 14:149-153, 1973.

340. Valentine BA et al: Intramuscular hemangiosarcoma with pulmonary metastasis in a horse. *JAVMA* 6:628-629, 1986.

341. Pascoe JR and Raphel CR: Pulmonary hemorrhage in exercising horses. *Compend Cont Ed Pract Vet* 4:S411-S416, 1982.

342. Clarke AF: Review of exercise-induced pulmonary haemorrhage and its possible relationship with mechanical stress. *Equine Vet J* 17:166-172, 1985.

343. Burrell MH: Endoscopic and virological observations on respiratory disease in a group of young Thoroughbred horses in training. *Equine Vet J* 17:99-103, 1985.

344. Soma LR et al: Effects of furosemide on the racing times of horses with exercise-induced pulmonary hemorrhage. *Am J Vet Res* 46:763-768, 1985.

345. Mason DK et al: Effect of bedding on the incidence of exercise-induced pulmonary haemorrhage in racehorses in Hong Kong. *Vet Record* 115:268-269, 1984.

346. Pascoe JR et al: Efficacy of furosemide in the treatment of exercise-induced pulmonary hemorrhage in Thoroughbred racehorses. *Am J Vet Res* 46:2000-2003, 1985.

347. O'Callaghan MW et al: Exercise-induced pulmonary haemorrhage in the horse: Results of a detailed clinical, post mortem and imaging study. V. Microscopic observations. *Equine Vet J* 19:411-418, 1987.

348. O'Callaghan MW et al: Exercise-induced pulmonary haemorrhage in the horse: Results of a detailed clinical, post mortem and imaging study. VI. Radiological/pathological correlations. *Equine Vet J* 19:419-422, 1987.

349. O'Callaghan MW et al: Exercise-induced pulmonary haemorrhage in the horse: Results of a detailed clinical, post mortem and imaging study. II. Gross lung pathology. *Equine Vet J* 19:389-393, 1987.

350. O'Callaghan MW et al: Exercise-induced pulmonary haemorrhage in the horse: Results of a detailed clinical, post mortem and imaging study. IV. Changes in the bronchial circulation demonstrated by CT scanning and microradiography. *Equine Vet J* 19:405-410, 1987.

351. O'Callaghan MW et al: Exercise induced pulmonary haemorrhage int the horse: Results of a detailed clinical, post mortem and imaging study. VIII. Conclusions and implications. *Equine Vet J* 19:428-434, 1987.

352. Robinson NE and Derksen FJ: Small airway obstruction as a cause of exercise associated pulmonary haemorrhage: An hypothesis. *Proc 26th Ann Mtg AAEP*, 1980. pp 421-430.

353. Sweeney CR, in Robinson NE: *Current Therapy in Equine Medicine 2*. Saunders, Philadelphia, 1986. pp 603-605.

354. Manohar M: Effect of furosemide administration on systemic circulation of ponies during severe exercise. *Am J Vet Res* 47:1387-1394, 1986.

355. Sweeney CR and Soma LR: Exercise-induced pulmonary hemorrhage in Thoroughbred horses. Response to furosemide and hesperidin-citrus bioflavonoids. *JAVMA* 185:195-197, 1984.

356. Sweeney CR et al: Efficacy of water vapor-saturated air in the treatment of exercise-induced pulmonary hemorrhage in Thoroughbred racehorses. *Am J Vet Res* 44:1705-1707, 1988.

357. Buergelt CD et al: A retrospective study of proliferative interstitial lung disease of horses in Florida. *Vet Pathol* 23:750-756, 1986.

358. Turk JR et al: Diffuse alveolar damage with fibrosing aveolitis in a horse. *Vet Pathol* 18:560-562, 1981.

359. Hartley WJ and Dixon RJ: An outbreak of foal perinatal mortality due to equine herpes virus type I: pathologic observations. *Equine Vet J* 11:215-218, 1979.

360. Bryans JT *et al*: Neonatal foal disease associated with perinatal infection by equine herpes virus I. *Equine Vet J* 1:20-25, 1971.

361. Breeze RG *et al*: Perilla ketone toxicity: a chemical model for the study of equine restrictive lung disease. *Equine Vet J* 16:180-184, 1984.

362. Breeze RG and Carlson JR: Chemical-induced lung injury in domestic animals. *Adv Vet Sci* 26:201-227, 1982.

363. Murray RE and Gibson JE: A comparative study of paraquat intoxication in rats, guinea pigs, and monkeys. *Exp Mol Pathol* 17:317-325, 1972.

364. Moore JN *et al*: Equine endotoxemia: an insight into cause and treatment. *JAVMA* 179:473-477, 1981.

365. McGrath CJ *et al*: Diaphragmatic hernia in the horse. *VM/SAC* 76:733-737, 1981.

366. Wimberly HC *et al*: Diaphragmatic hernias in the horse: A review of the literature and an analysis of six additional cases. *JAVMA* 170:1404-140, 1977.

367. Spiers VC and Reynolds WT: Successful repair of a diaphragmatic hernia in a foal. *Equine Vet J* 8: 170-172, 1976.

368. Scott EA and Fishback WA: Surgical repair of diaphragmatic hernia in a horse. *JAVMA* 168:45-47, 1976.

369. Ogilvie TH *et al*: *Mycoplasma felis* as a cause of pleuritis in horses. *JAVMA* 182:1374-1376, 1983.

370. Arthur RM: Subacute and acute pleuritis. *Proc 29th Ann Mtg AAEP*, 1983. pp 65-69.

371. Wagner AE and Bennett DG: Analysis of equine thoracic fluid. *Vet Clin Pathol* 11:13-17, 1981.

372. Mansmann RA and Bernard-Strother S: Pleuroscopy in horses. *MVP* 66:9-17, 1985.

373. Shearer DC *et al*: Rib resection and thoracotomy as a treatment for chronic pleuritis. *Proc 31st Ann Mtg AAEP*, 1985. pp 393-397.

374. Sundberg JP *et al*: Neoplasms of equidae. *JAVMA* 170:150-152, 1977.

375. Theilen GH and Madewell BR: *Veterinary Cancer Medicine*. Lea & Febiger, Philadelphia, 1979.

376. Esplin DJ and Taylor JL: Hypercalcemia in a horse with lymphosarcoma. *JAVMA* 170:180-182, 1977.

377. Rossdale PD: Some parameters of respiratory function in normal and abnormal newborn foals with special reference to levels of PaO2 during air and oxygen inhalation. *Res Vet Sci* 11:270-276, 1970.

378. Brown CC and Dardiri AH: African horse sickness: a continuing menace. *JAVMA* 196:2019-2021, 1990.

7 Diseases of the Alimentary System

S.B. Adams

EXAMINATION OF THE ALIMENTARY SYSTEM

S.B. Adams

Physical examination for detection of diseases of the alimentary system often is very rewarding. Visual inspection, auscultation and percussion of the abdomen, nasogastric intubation, and rectal examination are the methods of examination performed most commonly.

Visual Inspection

Many abnormalities can be detected by visual inspection. These abnormalities can provide a definitive diagnosis or may indicate that another section of the alimentary system is diseased. The presence of an undershot or overshot jaw warrants more thorough inspection of the mouth and teeth, especially when quidding occurs during consumption of food. Complete methods of oral inspection are described in the section on Diseases of the Teeth and Gums. The conjunctiva and sclera of the eye should be inspected, as icterus may be caused by liver disease or by not eating. Parotitis is uncommon but, when present, causes a warm, painful swelling just caudal to vertical ramus of the mandible. Cervical esophageal choke and cervical esophageal diverticulitis may cause a firm swelling in the left jugular furrow.

Abdominal contours should be evaluated by observing the horse from each side and from behind. Bloated horses have distention of the flanks and paralumbar fossae. In adult horses, bloat usually is caused by gas within the large colon or cecum and occasionally by gas within the abdominal cavity. Bloat is not commonly caused by distention of the small intestine except in foals, as they have thinner abdominal walls and a relatively smaller abdominal cavity. Rapid onset of severe bloat in adult horses and signs of moderate to severe pain suggest large colon displacement or volvulus, whereas slow progressive bloat suggests obstruction of the small colon. Nephrosplenic ligament entrapment of the left colon may cause diffuse fullness over the left lumbar region in thin horses. A pendulous abdomen may be due to pregnancy, liver failure with ascites, peritonitis, or intake of large amounts of poor-quality feedstuffs ("hay belly"). Edema on the ventral abdomen may be caused by peritonitis, hypoproteinemia and abdominal trauma. Edema also is not uncommon following ventral midline laparotomy.

The anal sphincter and caudal rectum can be examined by inspection and palpation. The tone of the anal sphincter should be checked. A flaccid anal sphincter may be caused by cauda equina neuritis, spinal cord tumors, exhaustion, rabies, spinal cord trauma, equine herpesvirus infection and Sudan grass toxicity. Disruption of the anal sphincter and perineal body, with communication of the rectum and vestibule, occurs in mares with third-degree perineal lacerations. Neoplasms may occur around the anus and are not uncommon under the tail of gray horses. Clumps of *Oxyuris equi* eggs

473

and debris from ruptured adult parasites occur as grayish-white deposits around the anal region. Eversion of pink edematous rectal mucosa through the anal sphincter indicates rectal prolapse. Watery feces often cause staining of the perineal region and the tail. The frequency of defecation and the consistency of the feces should be determined. Diarrhea is considered to be caused primarily by diseases of the large or small colon.

Oral Examination

Oral examination provides information about the mouth, gums, lips, teeth, tongue and oropharynx. Thorough examination of the oral cavity requires a speculum, flashlight and probes. Indications for a complete oral examination include obvious oral abnormalities, facial or mandibular swellings, quidding, excessive salivation, dysphagia, hemorrhage from the mouth, headshaking, and malodorous breath suggestive of sinusitis. The technique for oral examination is discussed in the section on Diseases of the Teeth and Gums.

Auscultation

Auscultation and percussion of the abdomen are helpful when evaluating the parts of the alimentary system within the abdominal cavity. The functional activity of the intestines may be assessed on a general basis from peristaltic sounds and borborygmi. The abdomen of horses exhibiting colic, diarrhea, bloat, anorexia, weight loss or any other sign referable to diseases of the alimentary system should be auscultated. At least 3 areas on each side of the abdomen should be examined (Fig 1) and 3-5 minutes should be spent on the entire procedure. Many clinicians auscultate additional areas.

Intestinal sounds usually are not continuous but occur in intervals of 10-20 seconds.[1] Intestinal sounds created by normal propulsive and segmental motility can be described as gurgling, murmuring and rumbling. Sounds emanating from the large intestine are duller and deeper than sounds from the small intestine. The gurgling sounds of the small intestine can be heard on the dorsal left side of the abdomen. On the right side, a tinkling or splashing sound caused by fluid entering the cecum from the ileum may be heard 1-3 times per minute over the base of the cecum. Auscultation of the ileocecal valve is important because lack of the periodic squirts of fluid suggests small intestinal obstruction or cecal impaction. The rumbling sounds from the large colon can be heard over the entire ventral abdomen on both sides. High-pitched tinkling sounds in the colon indicate tympany.

Auscultation is important for monitoring the intestinal activity in horses with colic and may be useful for determining prognosis and methods of treatment, and for monitoring progress. Diagnoses seldom are made based solely upon auscultation. Intestinal sounds can be classified as increased (hyperactive), active or absent. Loud rumbling borborygmi audible at some distance from the horse are associated with spasmodic colic. Increased borborygmi may be auscultated during the early stages of enteritis. Hypermotility proximal to obstructed bowel occurs initially but subsides as the disease progresses and the horse deteriorates systemically. Absence of peristaltic sounds may be caused by adynamic ileus, irreversible morphologic damage to the intestine, shock and poor intestinal perfusion, high sympathetic nervous system tone, or administration of drugs that inhibit motility. However, even with bowel infarction or adynamic ileus, a complete absence of sounds does not occur. The interaction of gas and liquid in-

Figure 1. Lateral view of a horse's thorax and abdomen. At least 3 areas on each side of the abdomen should be auscultated for intestinal sounds.

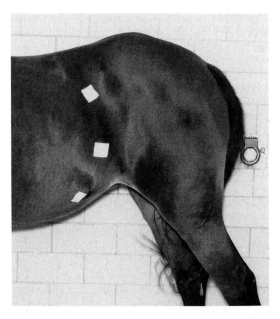

gesta as exercise or respiration causes movement of the abdominal wall results in isolated tinkles and blips.[2] These sounds are quite different from the sounds produced by normal intestinal motility.

Simultaneous auscultation and percussion of the abdominal wall can identify tympanitic (gas-filled) viscera that are in contact with the abdominal wall. A tympanitic cecum produces a high-pitched resonant ping not unlike the sound associated with a displaced abomasum in cattle.

Auscultation may be used to determine trends in intestinal activity. Repeated auscultation is particularly useful in horses with colic. Decreasing abdominal sounds indicate failure to respond to treatment and suggest a poor prognosis. The absence of intestinal sounds in horses with colic has been correlated with a poorer survival rate than for horses with intestinal sounds.[3] Auscultation following surgery may be misleading when ingesta has been removed from the bowel during the surgery. Though motility may return, intestinal sounds are hard to hear because gas and fluid have been removed, making borborygmi faint.

Nasogastric Intubation

Passage of a nasogastric tube can be used to detect obstruction of the pharynx and esophagus. The approximate level of obstruction can be determined by the length of tube that can be passed. A nasogastric tube should be passed in all horses exhibiting colic to remove fluid and gas accumulated within the stomach. Because horses rarely regurgitate to relieve gastric pressure, gastric distention causes pain and may result in gastric rupture. Infrequent regurgitation may be due to compression of the cardia when the stomach is dilated.[4]

Distention of the stomach does not ensure that fluid or gas will readily pass through the tube. Feed material may plug the distal end of the tube or the end of the tube may lie against the mucosa of the stomach. Persistent efforts to remove gas and fluid should be made when gastric dilatation is suspected. The nasogastric tube should have multiple ports or fenestrations at the distal end and the clinician should select a tube as large as can be safely passed through the nasal meatus. A common technique to induce gas and fluid flow is to fill the tube with water and gently aspirate with a large dose syringe (Fig 2). Alternatively, 1 L of water can be pumped into the horse's stomach, followed by detachment of the pump and positioning of the proximal end of the tube ventral to the level of the stomach to induce siphoning. This procedure can be repeated several times. The clinician should recover a minimum amount of fluid equal to what was pumped into the stomach. The tube should be moved back and forth several times to increase the chances that the end within the stomach is positioned in fluid or gas pockets. Though these procedures may take several minutes to complete, gastric rupture has occurred in horses with indwelling nasogastric tubes, thus underscoring the necessity for persistent efforts to remove fluids.[5]

There are numerous causes of gastric distention. Ingestion of large amounts of grain or other highly fermentable feedstuffs provides substrate for bacterial fermentation and gas production that causes dilation of the stomach. Obstructions of the pylorus with delayed gastric emptying occurs in foals with pyloric and duodenal ulcers, and in adult horses with gastric neoplasms. Gastric impaction may occur in adult horses.[6] Gastric distention is caused most commonly by retrograde reflux of fluids from the small intestine. Usually the small intestine is ob-

Figure 2. Excessive fluid in the stomach is removed with a nasogastric tube. Repeated efforts to prime the tube with water and aspirate with a stomach pump or dose syringe may be necessary to establish flow of fluid, even if the stomach is greatly distended.

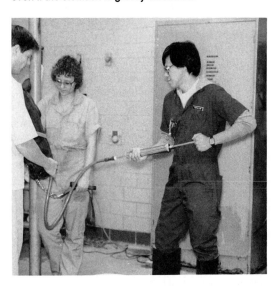

structed by mechanical lesions or because of inadequate motility. Large colon torsions, volvulus or displacements, or severe cecal dilatation may compress the duodenum and cause secondary gastric reflux in some horses. The pH of fluids in the stomach that have refluxed from the small intestine often is as high as 6 due to bicarbonate-rich pancreatic secretions.[7] Normal pH of gastric fluid is 2-4.

Rectal Examination

Rectal examination is one of the most important and rewarding procedures for evaluation of the alimentary system in horses. This examination provides an excellent means of evaluating the caudal abdominal cavity and its contents. Rectal examination should be performed when diseases of the alimentary tract are suspected or when confirmed diseases require evaluation beyond routine physical examination. Horses with colic, chronic diarrhea and weight loss should undergo rectal examination.[8]

The value of the rectal examination is dependent on the experience of the examiner and cooperation of the patient.[9] Findings on rectal examination always should be evaluated with all other clinical findings in mind to gain a proper perspective. The rectal examination may, however, be the single most important diagnostic procedure for evaluation of horses with colic.[10]

Technique

Rectal examination is not without risk to the examiner and the horse. Examiners should take precaution to avoid tearing the animal's rectum or distal small colon, and to avoid injury to themselves or to handlers. All horses should be placed in examining stocks when possible. When examining stocks are not available, the use of Dutch stall doors, hay bales or hobbles may protect the examiner from kicks. Alternatively, the horse may be placed alongside a wall or partition so the examiner may stand to one side of the barrier. Fractious or nervous horses should be sedated; a twitch usually is used for restraint and to reduce straining.

A well-lubricated examining glove is recommended to decrease the force necessary for insertion of the arm into the rectum. Rectal examination should never be done forcefully; peristaltic waves in the small colon and rectum should not be resisted but, rather, examiners should allow their hand to be swept out of the rectum behind the wave. Instillation of up to 30 ml of lidocaine or other suitable local anesthetic into the rectum can help reduce straining in horses irritated by the presence of the hand and arm. An epidural anesthetic to anesthetize the anus and rectum is useful for horses that resist rectal examination vigorously. Circumstances that dictate against rectal examinations include animals with a small anal sphincter and rectum that are difficult to enter, and extremely fractious patients that present a danger to themselves or the examiner.

The abdomen up to the level of the first lumbar vertebra may be palpated in a horse of average size by an examiner with an average-length arm (Fig 3). Structures that usually can be palpated in healthy horses include the rectum, female genital organs, male accessory sex organs, bladder, inguinal canals, small colon, left ventral and left dorsal colons, pelvic flexure, spleen, nephrosplenic ligament, caudal pole of the left kid-

Figure 3. Abdominal organs palpable during rectal examination of a normal horse as viewed from the top: 1. bladder; 2. inguinal rings; 3. pelvic flexure; 4. caudal margin of the spleen; 5. caudal margin of the left kidney; 6. root of the mesentery; 7. cecum; 8. small colon; 9. small intestine (not usually palpable in the normal horse).

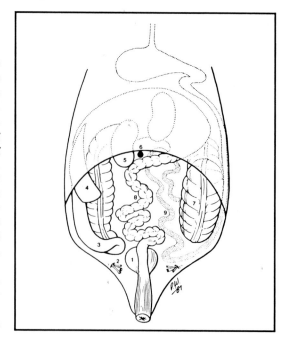

ney, root of the mesentery containing the cranial mesenteric artery and its branches, aorta and iliac arteries, the ventral band of the cecum, and dorsal attachment of the base of the cecum. Loops of small intestine are not palpable in normal horses. The bowel is identified by noting the position of the bowel and the presence or absence of bands and sacculations.

Rectal examination should be performed systematically to avoid missing abnormalities. All segments of bowel that can be palpated should be assessed for position, size, mobility, wall tension, thickness, edema, presence of taut attached mesentery and distention with gas, fluid or ingesta. Abnormalities may be classified as definitive or supportive findings. A definitive rectal finding is an abnormality that can be palpated and gives the definitive diagnosis. For instance, palpation of nephrosplenic entrapment of the large colon is a definitive rectal finding. Supportive rectal findings are abnormalities that indicate disease is present but do not directly identify the disease. Tightly distended loops of small intestine support a diagnosis of obstruction of the small intestine. A taut, painful mesenteric band suggests displacement of the attached bowel.

Abnormalities Detected by Rectal Examination

Rectal examination as it relates specifically to examination of the alimentary system is described in this section. The reader is referred to the chapters on the Diseases of the Reproductive System and Diseases of the Urinary System for discussions of rectal abnormalities noted with diseases of those systems.

The anus should be checked for lacerations, injuries, neoplasms, parasites and rectal prolapse. Third-degree rectovestibular lacerations cause complete disruption of the anal sphincter and perineal body. The rectum and vestibule have a common opening. Tone of the anal sphincter can be assessed as the examiner's hand is inserted into the rectum. The anal sphincter should provide a moderate amount of resistance unless an epidural anesthetic has been given. The examiner should remove all feces from the ampulla of the rectum. Soft, readily fragmented fecal balls are normal.

The feces should be examined for blood, mucus and sand. If fresh blood is noted, the rectum and small colon should be examined carefully for tears or other trauma. Hemorrhage from the proximal alimentary tract may be observed as melena. Intestinal obstruction delays passage of feces and allows fecal balls to become coated with dry, tacky, white mucus. Inspissated mucus may be felt on the rectal walls when no feces are present. Sand in the feed predisposes to sand impactions and sand-induced diarrhea. These diseases should be considered when sand is found in the feces and clinical signs of colic or diarrhea are present. Pneumorectum caused by removal of feces makes further examination more difficult.

Normal rectal mucosa should be smooth and folded. Careful palpation for rectal tears is possible after removal of the feces. Tears are found most often in the dorsal rectum or dorsal small colon. Perirectal abscesses may cause distortion of the tubular shape of the rectum and collapse of the pelvic canal. A tightly constricted rectum has been associated with obstruction or strangulation-obstruction of bowel proximal to the rectum.[8]

The inguinal rings are located about one hand's breadth lateral to midline and ventral to the brim of the pelvis. Incarceration of jejunum or ileum in the inguinal canal may occur in stallions. This can be determined rectally by palpation of loops of small intestine entering the vaginal ring. The small colon is readily palpable in the central abdominal cavity and is identified by the presence of fecal balls. The small colon is normally 5-8 cm in diameter, has prominent sacculations, is quite mobile due to a long mesocolon, and has a prominent antimesenteric band. Obstruction of the small colon results in dilation of the small colon proximal to the site of obstruction. These dilated loops may be located in the pelvic inlet. Enteroliths and fecoliths may be palpable per rectum. Blood-tinged, tar-colored mucus or rectal mucosa noted upon withdrawal of the arm from the rectum suggests necrosis of the small colon that can occur secondary to a ruptured mesocolon. Volvulus of the mesocolon prevents the examiner from fully inserting an arm into the rectum and small colon. In pregnant mares, uterine torsion may constrict the small colon and also prevent full insertion of an arm. Identification of crossed broad ligaments confirms a diagnosis of uterine torsion.

Normally the small intestine is not palpated in healthy horses. However, the examiner may be aware of an indefinite mass in the middle of the abdominal cavity that cannot be grasped but that gives the impression that the abdomen is not empty. Small intestine distended with gas or fluid can be identified via rectal examination. Moderate fluid distention with no evidence of a taut or painful mesentery suggests enteritis. Obstruction or strangulation-obstruction of small intestine causes distention proximal to the obstruction. Infarcted sections of bowel often are thickened and edematous. Long segments of distended small intestine may cause loops to be pushed into the pelvic inlet, making complete abdominal exploration difficult. Strangulated sections of small intestine may be identified by thickened edematous bowel wall, and pain may be elicited during palpation. The thickness of bowel wall and the amount of distention may be determined by pressing the bowel together between the thumb and forefinger or pushing the loop of bowel in question against the abdominal wall. When intussusceptions can be palpated, the bowel is thick and turgid and has been described as feeling like a sausage. Incarceration of bowel through internal hernias, volvulus of jejunum, and intussusceptions may have taut mesenteric bands that are painful when traction is applied. Small intestine is incarcerated infrequently in the epiploic foramen or in the chest through a diaphragmatic hernia. The examiner may get the impression of an empty abdomen in these instances.

The pelvic flexure may be identified in the left caudoventral abdomen or on the midline of the abdominal floor. This structure is soft and compressible normally. The left ventral colon can be identified by sacculations and bands. The dorsal colon often is medial to the ventral colon.[8] The left colon and pelvic flexure may be full of watery ingesta in horses with acute profuse diarrhea or in horses that will soon exhibit diarrhea.

Impactions of the pelvic flexure are noted as firm, doughy masses that can be indented with finger pressure. Massive impactions may fill the left colon, causing enlargement and moving the flexure to the pelvic inlet or over to the right side of the abdomen. Sand impactions often have a gritty texture when palpated. Obstruction of the large colon usually results in tympany of the bowel proximal to the obstruction. Extreme distention of the large colon with gas, accompanied by taut bands that are painful upon traction, suggests volvulus, torsion or malposition of the large colon. Tightly distended segments of large colon may push caudally against the pelvic inlet and make examination of the abdominal cavity impossible. Edematous and jelly-like colonic mesentery is caused by strangulation of vessels and usually is associated with torsion or volvulus. Infarction often can be noted as thickening of the wall of the colon. This is caused by blood and edema and makes detection of sacculations and bands easy. The dorsal and ventral colon may be severely distended and positioned horizontally across the abdomen just cranial to the pelvic inlet. The bands on the colon should be followed to the left and right in an attempt to identify the pelvic flexure. Right dorsal displacement of the large colon causes part of the large colon to be found between the cecum and right abdominal wall.[11]

The spleen is identified on the left side of the abdomen against the abdominal wall at the level of the last rib. The caudodorsal aspect of the spleen can be palpated per rectum on most horses and has a firm distinct shape with a sharp caudal edge. Nodules and irregularity of the surface of the spleen suggest neoplasia. An enlarged spleen may be the result of neoplasia, splenomegaly or secondary to administration of barbiturates or tranquilizers. The spleen may be displaced caudally when gastric distention is present. The examiner's hand should pass unimpeded from the spleen across the nephrosplenic ligament to the caudal pole of the kidney. The nephrosplenic space is large enough to admit several fingertips. Entrapment of the left ventral and dorsal colon, also called left dorsal displacement of the colons, can be palpated as the colon sweeps up to and over the nephrosplenic ligament.[12] In some horses with this condition, the spleen may be pushed medially away from the abdominal wall.

The root of the mesentery is to the right and slightly cranial to the caudal pole of the left kidney. In normal horses, the ileocecocolic artery and its branches pulsate, and fremitus is absent. Enlarged lymph nodes in the mesentery may be due to neoplasia, lymphadenitis or lymph node abscessation. Chronic mesenteric abscesses causing colic, weight loss and diarrhea may be palpated in this area. Verminous mesenteric arteritis can cause thickening and enlargement of the arteries and fremitus. These changes may be detected in some horses but have poor correlation with clinical signs of disease.[13]

The right dorsal colon may be palpable in small horses directly cranial to and to the right side of the mesenteric root. Distention of the right dorsal colon caused by impactions and large enteroliths may be palpated in average-size horses. Palpation requires full extension of the arm into the abdomen. Enteroliths in the transverse colon sometimes may be bumped with the fingertips but not grasped with the hand.

The ventral band of the cecum sweeps from caudodorsal to cranioventral in the abdomen on a slightly diagonal path. The ventral band seems to run on a line drawn from the right tuber coxae to the left olecranon. In small horses, the medial cecal band also can be identified. The dorsal attachment of the cecum can be identified along the right dorsal abdominal wall. The base and body of the cecum may be palpated when the cecum is distended with gas or ingesta. Cecal impactions are noted upon rectal examination as firm, doughy masses. Chronic cecal impactions may cause diarrhea. The ileum is difficult to palpate unless impacted or unless there is an intussusception of the ileum on itself or into the cecum. An impacted ileum feels like a firm tube that sweeps to the medial base of the cecum. Traction on ileal mesentery just medial to the cecum causes severe pain with ileocecal or ileoilial intussusceptions.[9] Though the duodenum normally cannot be palpated, distended duodenum may be palpated around the caudal base of the cecum.

Before completion of the rectal examination, the peritoneum should be evaluated for adhesions, nodules, roughening and response to pain. Multiple nodules suggest a neoplasm. Horses with ruptured bowel often have roughened, gritty, sandpaper-textured peritoneal surfaces. Emphysema also may be noted. Peritonitis may cause roughened peritoneal surfaces when fibrin tags are present. In all instances of suspected peritoneal disease, abdominocentesis should be performed. The section on peritoneal diseases contains more specific information on this procedure.

ANCILLARY DIAGNOSTIC AIDS

S.B. Adams and J.E. Sojka

Endoscopy

Endoscopy for examination of the gastrointestinal tract is limited by the length and diameter of the equipment and the expertise of the operator. Flexible fiberoptic endoscopes are used most commonly for endoscopy, though videoendoscopes have become available recently. Standard endoscopes for human use are 100 cm (gastroscope) or 180 cm (colonoscope) in length. These lengths allow viewing of the pharynx and proximal esophagus in the adult horse; the distal esophagus and stomach may be viewed in ponies or foals. Custom-made 300-cm long endoscopes allow examination of the stomach and proximal duodenum in all horses.[14,15] A fiberoptic endoscope with a length of 275-310 cm and diameter of 11-13.5 mm has been suggested as being satisfactory for use in adult horses and foals.[15] However, this diameter will not fit through the nasal passages of most young foals. The newer videoendoscopes have the same length but are 6-7 mm in diameter and so can be passed nasally in most neonatal foals.

Before endoscopy, the horse should be restrained adequately. A twitch or tranquilization usually is required in adult horses. If the stomach is to be examined, the horse should be held off feed for 24-48 hours to ensure that the that stomach is empty. Water should be withheld for 2 hours before the procedure.

Nasopharynx

Endoscopy of the nasopharynx is indicated in instances of dysphagia or abnormal nasal or oral discharge. The soft palate, larynx and dorsal pharyngeal recess can be seen and abscesses or foreign bodies may be noted. Dorsal displacement of the soft palate prevents the examiner from seeing the epiglottis. This condition is observed in normal horses occasionally, and they can reposition the soft palate correctly if they are stimulated to swallow. The guttural pouches should be examined for evidence of chronic infection in horses with dysphagia.

Esophagus

The normal esophageal mucosa is pale tan and arranged in linear folds. Air must be insufflated into the esophagus before it can be examined fully. Endoscopy can be used to identify foreign bodies, ulceration, areas of inflammation, diverticula or perforations.[15] Endoscopy is variably useful in identifying strictures. If the mucosa is intact, strictures are not appreciated easily and contrast radiography may be more beneficial.

Stomach

Endoscopy has been used to diagnose gastric ulceration, parasitic infection, neoplasia and pyloric stenosis.[14] The glandular and nonglandular regions of the stomach may be identified. They are separated by the margo plicatus, which looks like a raised ridge. Fluid often is present in the ventral portion of the stomach, making examination of the antrum and duodenum impossible. This fluid is a combination of gastric secretions, saliva and refluxed intestinal contents. The nonglandular portion of the stomach is pale tan to white.[14,15] The glandular region is a darker pink or red.[14,15]

Duodenum

Insertion of the endoscope into the duodenum is difficult and requires practice. This procedure cannot be performed in all horses, even by experienced practitioners.[14,15] The duodenal wall is pale pink. The opening of the common bile duct may be visible within the duodenal ampulla, and duodenal biopsies may be taken.[14,15]

Rectum and Terminal Colon

Fiberoptic endoscopy has not proven as useful for examining the terminal digestive tract as in the proximal tract. This is because it is virtually impossible to remove all fecal material from the area. The gas distention within the gut lumen necessary for thorough evaluation may produce colic. The procedure is potentially useful to obtain a biopsy or for direct examination of a mass,

rectal tear or diseased area that has been palpated per rectum.

Radiography

Radiography is most useful in evaluating the oral cavity and esophagus. Because of patient size, abdominal radiographs are of limited value in horses but may be helpful in foals. Positive (barium) and negative (air) contrast materials increase the diagnostic ability. The head and neck can be radiographed using portable radiographic equipment. A machine with a capacity of 25-300 mA and 85-125 kV is sufficient to obtain diagnostic images.[16] Radiography of the distal esophagus and stomach requires more powerful equipment in all but the smallest horses. Diagnostic films usually may be obtained with the horse standing. Tranquilization may be necessary. Placing portable x-ray machines on hay bales or other structures aids radiography by keeping the machine still and at the correct height for skull and neck films.

Radiographs can be used to diagnose a variety of tooth and skull problems, such as tooth root abscess, phosphorus-calcium imbalance and congenital anomalies. Trauma, such as maxillary or mandibular fractures, can be diagnosed, as can bony tumors such as osteomas, adamantinomas and bone cysts.[16] Pharyngeal or retropharyngeal abscesses can be imaged if a typical gas cap is present. In the absence of a gas cap, abscesses are suggested by compression of surrounding structures.

Conditions of the esophagus that can be detected radiographically include megaesophagus, choke secondary to foreign material, stenosis, traumatic rupture and diverticula.[16] These lesions can be best imaged if barium sulfate is given to delineate the esophageal margins. Barium should be mixed 1:1 with water and may be administered either in grain or via a nasogastric tube with a stomach pump. Gastric conditions that have been diagnosed radiographically include stenosis, ulceration and partial torsion. As with the esophagus, positive- and negative-contrast contrast studies increase the ability of the clinician to make a diagnosis. Despite using contrast material, radiography is a relatively poor way to diagnose gastric ulceration; endoscopic assessment of the stomach is the method of choice. Prolonged gastric retention of barium in the stomach suggests pyloric or duodenal stenosis.

Radiographs of the small and large intestine are of limited value. In neonatal foals, intestinal distention can be seen due to atretic areas of bowel or to generalized ileus. A body weight of 350 kg has been reported as an upper limit for diagnostic films of the abdomen.[16] Barium, administered either per os or per rectum, may be used to identify an area of intestinal atresia.

In larger horses, abdominal radiographs have been used to identify enteroliths that are located in the ventral abdomen and that have a mineral density.[17] Multiple views with both right- and left-sided exposures increase the likelihood of diagnosis.[16] Machines with a capacity of 600-800 mAs and 120 kVp are necessary.[16] This technique has been reported to correlate well with surgical findings. Candidates for radiology are horses over 4 years of age with signs of acute or intermittent colic that persist despite passage of mineral oil and feces. The main advantage of radiography is that the presence of enteroliths provides an immediate indication for surgical exploration and obviates the need for additional diagnostic tests. The main differential diagnosis for enterolithiasis is fecal impaction that usually responds to medical management. Using radiography, enteroliths in the large colon may be diagnosed more easily than those in the small colon.[18]

Ultrasonography

Ultrasonography is the science of using high-frequency sound waves to image tissue. The reader is referred to specialized texts for a complete review of the theory and general principles involved in ultrasound examination.[19,20]

Use of ultrasonography in evaluation of equine gastrointestinal disease is limited by that fact that it is not possible to image through bone or air, or to image structures beyond the range of the probe. In most instances, this limits the operator to a depth of 20 cm or less.

A sector scanner is recommended for abdominal ultrasonography due to its versatility in scanning different-sized structures. The scanhead design allows a small contact surface, which is ideal for imaging between costal margins, and it provides better resolution than with linear-array scanners.[20] When sector scanners are not available, a 3-MHZ linear-array scanner allows imaging of many abdominal structures. The liver, spleen and gut wall may be imaged percutaneously and evaluated for location, size, shape and texture.[21] The presence of fluid or fibrin in the abdomen can be determined and abnormal masses may be identified. Ultrasonic guidance may be used to facilitate abdominocentesis, liver biopsy and percutaneous biopsy of abdominal masses. Intestinal motility may be observed.[21] To obtain high-resolution images, the haircoat should be clipped and shaved to allow optimal contact between the skin and scanhead.

Liver

The liver may be imaged from both the right and left sides. From the left side, it is seen caudal to the heart around the seventh intercostal space. The diaphragm is visible immediately cranial to the liver. From the right side, the liver is ventral to the right lung and cranial to the right kidney. Though the entire liver is not accessible to ultrasonographic evaluation, one can get an overall impression of its size by noting the location of the caudal border of the liver margins. Tumors on the liver surface may be imaged, as may intrahepatic tumors, abscesses, dilated bile ducts and choleliths.[22]

Spleen

The spleen is on the left side just caudal and medial to the liver. It usually extends ventrally up to the left lung border and caudally to an area lateral to the left kidney, though it may be found along the ventral midline or medial to the left kidney. Metastatic masses may be imaged on the spleen. With tranquilization, the spleen may engorge and can reach thicknesses up to 15 cm.[21]

Intestinal Tract

Because ultrasound waves cannot penetrate gas, ultrasonography of the intestines is limited. Neoplasms, particularly gastric squamous-cell carcinoma, may be appreciated.[21,23] Gastric squamous-cell carcinoma appears as an area of homogeneous tissue that separates the spleen and liver from the lumen of the stomach. In foals, the duodenum may be imaged between the right liver lobe and the right dorsal colon. It may appear enlarged and fluid filled in foals with gastric ulcer disease. Normally the intestine is motile and ingesta can be imaged moving within the lumen. Ileus results in a lack of movement of either the intestinal wall or ingesta. If a localized segment of intestine is immobile in relation to the body wall or other internal structures, intestinal adhesions may be present.[21]

Peritoneal Cavity

Ascites is identified easily using ultrasonography as the borders of organs that normally are touching are separated by ascitic fluid. Ascitic fluid may be anechoic or contain numerous acoustic interfaces. All horses have a small volume of abdominal fluid, but excessive amounts are abnormal. Fibrin strands on serosal organ surfaces suggest inflammation and peritonitis.[21]

Clinical Pathology Tests

It is not our intent to cover all clinical pathologic tests in depth. Rather, this section describes tests that can help identify the alimentary system as the origin of disease. A more in-depth discussion of indicators for specific damage to organs of the alimentary system is given within the sections describing diseases of each organ. Unfortunately, there are very few clinical pathologic findings that are specific for intestinal disease. Clinical pathologic tests must be integrated with the history, physical examination and clinical course before a specific diagnosis can be made.

Complete Blood Count

Changes in the complete blood count (CBC) usually indicates general processes, such as inflammation or sepsis, and are not specific for the intestinal tract. Packed cell volume (PCV) is increased if dehydration is present or splenic contraction has occurred and is decreased with anemia. Other indices, such as hemoglobin level and red cell numbers, generally mirror the PCV. Because horses have a large splenic reserve of erythrocytes, splenic contraction may increase red cell numbers, and thus PCV, by

30% or more over baseline values.[24] Blood protein concentrations should be taken into account when deciding the significance of the PCV.

Increases in PCV occur commonly with dehydration. This most often is secondary to diarrhea, dysphagia or extravascular fluid losses during endotoxic shock. Anemia may be due to gastrointestinal blood loss, parasitism and neoplastic disease. In addition, chronic disease from any cause may produce a nonregenerative anemia. The presence of occult blood in the feces may implicate the gut as a source of blood loss. Blood in the gastrointestinal tract may not result in a positive occult blood test, however, if a sufficient volume of blood is not present. Local irritation and bleeding into the rectum following rectal examination may cause a positive test. Thus, assessment of fecal occult blood should be determined before a rectal examination is performed and a negative fecal occult blood does not absolutely rule out the gastrointestinal tract as a site of blood loss in horses.

Table 1 presents some CBC changes in various diseases.

Leukogram

Generally, increases in the white blood cell count are due to inflammation, sepsis, circulating corticosteroids (stress response) or leukemic neoplastic states. Inflammatory or necrotic lesions often result in a regenerative neutrophilia.[25] Lymphocyte and monocyte numbers usually are normal. High levels of corticosteroids increase the numbers of mature neutrophils in circulation by stimulating release of neutrophils from storage pools in the bone marrow and by decreasing margination of intravascular neutrophils. Increased corticosteroid levels also induce lymphopenia and eosinopenia. The net result is a "classic" stress leukogram with mature neutrophilia, lymphopenia and eosinopenia.

White blood cell counts are low when peripheral demand exceeds the ability of the bone marrow to produce new cells or when endotoxin causes increased margination of circulating cells. Diseases of the gastrointestinal tract that cause neutropenia include severe enteritis caused by salmonellosis or equine monocytic ehrlichiosis, and overwhelming sepsis accompanying bowel rupture. Uptake of endotoxin by neutrophils stimulates release of intracellular enzymes and autolysis. This causes a grainy, vacuolated cell described as a toxic neutrophil.[25] Viral diseases also may cause transient leukopenia. The most common cause of severe leukopenia due to intestinal disease is infectious enteritis. Leukopenia in horses less than 2 years of age is defined as a white blood cell count less than 7,000/μl and less than 5,500/μl in horses older than 2 years of age.[26]

Increased eosinophil counts most commonly occur secondary to parasitic disease. However, parasitized horses may have normal circulating eosinophil counts. Eosinophilia may occur with eosinophilic granulomatous enteritis. Basophilia may be present in horses with basophilic granulomatous enteritis.

Protein Concentrations

The protein in blood is composed of individual components, such as albumin, globulin and fibrinogen. If the proportion of one component is increased and another decreased, the overall total protein concentration remains in the normal range. Thus, it is important to determine each protein constituent separately. Serum protein electrophoresis is the most accurate way to determine protein concentrations. Chemical determinations of total protein and albumin often are performed as part of a chemistry panel, and these determinations are adequate for interpretation in most instances.

Increased blood protein concentrations are seen commonly with dehydration and/or hemoconcentration. Hyperproteinemia also may be present due to increased globulin

Table 1. Complete blood count and clinical chemistry values in healthy horses and in various diseases.

Measurement	Units	Normal Values*	Liver Disease	Acute *Salmonella* Enteritis	Parasitism	Protein-Losing Enteropathy	Cantharidin Toxicity
PCV	%	35-50	30	63	29	31	50
RBC	x 10^6/μl	6-12	6	20	4.5	5.5	12
WBC	x 10^6/μl	6-12	10	3	12	6	15
Bands	#/μl	0-1000	0	450	0	0	0
Neutrophils	#/μl	3000-7000	6400	1000	7400	4400	11,000
Lymphocytes	#/μl	1500-5500	3000	1500	3500	1000	3900
Monocytes	#/μl	50-800	50	50	100	50	50
Eosinophils	#/μl	0-400	10	0	1000	50	50
Fibrinogen	mg/dl	100-400	400	600	400	300	800
Platelet Count	x 10^5/μl	1-6	3	3	3	3	3
Glucose	mg/dl	58-134	50	100	100	100	100
Urea Nitrogen	mg/dl	7-28	5	36	10	7	50
Creatinine	mg/dl	1.1-2	1.5	2.1	1.5	1.2	2.5
Phosphorus	mg/dl	1.7-3.9	2	2	2	2	3
Calcium	mg/dl	11-13	12	12	12	12	7
Sodium	mmol/l	132-140	135	125	135	135	135
Potassium	mmol/l	3.1-4.8	3.5	2.5	3.5	3.5	3.8
Chloride	mmol/l	95-104	100	90	100	100	100
Carbon Dioxide	mmol/l	20-33	25	36	25	25	30
Total Protein	g/dl	5.3-7.3	6	8	5	4	7
Albumin	g/dl	2.3-3.1	2	3.5	1.9	0.9	3
AST (SGOT)	U/L	134-643	1500	643	600	250	1000
Alk Phos	U/L	128-512	900	500	490	400	500
GGT	U/L	0-53	100	50	40	35	50
Total Bilirubin	mg/dl	0-4.1	10	2	2	2	2
SDH	U/L	0-7	50	7	5	5	7

* Purdue University Clinical Chemistry Laboratory

levels secondary to chronic antigenic stimulation. Hepatitis is a potential cause of hyperglobulinemia, as are other inflammatory and septic conditions (Table 1).[26] Hypoproteinemia may result from panhypoproteinemia (low levels of proteins) or a low level of a single protein constituent. Panhypoproteinemia may be due to protein-losing enteropathy, acute blood loss or parasitism. Hypoalbuminemia occurs as a component of panhypoproteinemia and also occurs with starvation and severe liver disease. See the section on Diseases of the Small Intestine for further discussion.

Serum IgG(T) assays have been advocated as a way of diagnosing occult parasitism. However, the serum IgG(T) level is increased in many conditions, and an increase is not associated with a specific diagnosis.

Fibrinogen is a protein produced by the liver and is an important mediator of the inflammatory response, as well as a constituent of the clotting cascade. Serum fibrinogen concentrations reflect the magnitude of an ongoing inflammatory reaction.[26] A high serum fibrinogen concentration (>1000 mg/dl) is a poor prognostic indicator for life regardless of the underlying disease. Serum fibrinogen levels may be low (<200 mg/dl) in severe liver failure due to lack of hepatic production or in disseminated intravascular coagulation due to increased consumption.

Chemistry Panel

With the advent of automated chemistry determinations, "panels" of chemistry values often have replaced specific enzyme and electrolyte determinations. Generally, a blood chemistry panel provides glucose, BUN, creatinine and electrolyte determinations and the activities of various serum enzymes (Table 1). Many tests in panels designed for people or small animals have little use for equine patients. These tests include serum lipid and cholesterol concentrations and amylase, lipase and SGPT activities. See the sections Diseases of the Liver and Diseases of the Pancreas for further discussion of biochemical evaluation of diseases in these organs.

Serum electrolyte changes are not specific for gastrointestinal disease. Hyponatremia, hypochloremia and hypokalemia due to intestinal losses of these electrolytes often are present in animals with diarrhea.

Hyperchloremia may be found in animals with diarrhea and severe acidosis.[27] Hypocalcemia and hypomagnesemia are common findings in cantharidin (blister beetle) toxicosis.

Blood glucose may be increased due to high serum concentrations of corticosteroids or epinephrine, cantharidin toxicity or diabetes mellitus (type II). It should be noted that hyperglycemia due to a tumor of the pars intermedia of the pituitary gland is much more common than diabetes in horses. Hyperglycemia also is a consistent finding in horses with severe intestinal strangulation obstruction. Blood glucose values over 250 mg/dl are associated with a poor prognosis for life in horses requiring colic surgery.

Hypoglycemia may be present in horses with advanced liver disease, beta-cell tumors of the pancreas and secondary septicemia. Because of low glycogen reserves, young foals are particularly susceptible to hypoglycemia secondary to sepsis.

Several cellular enzymes are measured routinely as part of a chemistry panel. Alkaline phosphatase, gamma glutamyl transferase, aspartate aminotransferase (glutamic oxaloacetic transaminase) and lactate dehydrogenase all are enzymes present in the liver. Increases in plasma activities of these enzymes are found in animals with liver disease. Only sorbitol dehydrogenase is specific for the hepatocellular component. The blood urea nitrogen (BUN) level may be low in horses with liver disease due to inability of the liver to incorporate ammonia into urea. The BUN level also may be decreased in horses with severe diarrhea or in severe catabolic states.

Increased serum bilirubin concentration indicates liver disease, hemolytic disease or both. The percentage of unconjugated bilirubin in horses always is higher than conjugated bilirubin. Conjugated bilirubin values that are 20% or more of the total bilirubin value suggest cholestatic disease. Delta bilirubin is the fraction of conjugated bilirubin that is covalently bound to albumin. A high percentage of delta bilirubin also indicates resolving cholestatic disease.

Acid-Base Balance

There are no acid-base changes that are specific for gastrointestinal diseases. Acidosis is the usual trend and may result from excessive intestinal bicarbonate loss during secretory diarrheal disease, from intestinal obstruction, or due to accumulation of excess lactic acid in horses with severe dehydration and endotoxic shock. Alkalosis may result from sequestration of hydrogen and chloride in the gut. This may occur secondary to gastric diseases, proximal enteritis and colonic disease. Alkalosis is generally mild with gastrointestinal disease.

Fecal Examination

Fecal examination is indicated in various diseases. Fecal flotation using hypertonic salt solutions is the classic method to detect parasite ova, though a negative finding does not rule out parasitic infection. Horses may be infected with larvae or immature adults. Special techniques may be used to identify *Eimeria* spp, *Cryptosporidium* or *Giardia* organisms (see Diseases of the Small Intestine.) Microscopic examination of the feces may reveal increased leukocyte numbers in horses with infectious enteritis. Electron microscopy may be used to identify virus particles. Bacterial isolation techniques can be used to identify specific pathogens, such as *Candida, Salmonella, Campylobacter* and *Clostridium* species.

Organ Function Tests

The liver and small intestine are commonly evaluated with function tests. Several normal serum constituents are produced by the liver; thus their concentrations are a crude measure of liver function. These constituents include albumin, clotting proteins, glucose and urea. Serum levels of these compounds may be low due to decreased hepatic synthesis in advanced disease. The dyes sulfobromophthalein (BSP) and indocyanine green are removed from the circulation and excreted by the liver. An increase in the serum half-life of these dyes suggests liver disease or conditions in which blood flow through the liver is low. The ability of the liver to metabolize ammonia may be assessed by oral administration of ammonia. Increased blood ammonia concentrations after oral loading indicates hepatic disease or shunting of portal blood away from the liver. See the section Diseases of the Liver for a complete discussion of liver function tests.

The absorptive capacity of the small intestine may be evaluated by determining the increase in serum concentrations of monosaccharides or disaccharides. The 3 sugars commonly used are glucose, D-xylose and lactose.

Lactose absorption depends on both the ability of the small intestinal enzyme lactase to digest lactose and on the small intestine to absorb the digested products. The lactose absorption test usually is performed to document lactose intolerance in suckling foals. Lactose is given PO at 1 g/kg to fasted foals and plasma concentrations of glucose are measured. Blood glucose values increase 30-90 minutes after oral lactose administration in normal foals. A rise in the blood glucose level of at least 35 mg/dl over baseline is expected.[28]

Oral glucose and D-xylose absorption tests may be used to test the ability of the small intestine to absorb these sugars. Decreased absorption may be a result of small intestinal disease or may be due to delayed gastric emptying, abnormal small intestinal transit, increased bacterial metabolism within the gut lumen, and a decreased blood supply to the small intestine. Increased blood levels of D-xylose may occur secondary to renal disease because D-xylose is excreted by the kidney. Stress or other physiologic causes of hyperglycemia may produce false elevations of glucose following oral glucose loading. Absorption of D-xylose changes with age, with younger animals reaching higher peak xylose concentrations.[29] The diet affects absorption of both glucose and xylose, as a high-energy diet decreases absorption of both sugars.[30,31] Consequently, the dietary history must be taken into account when evaluating test results. Oral dosages of glucose and D-xylose are 1 g/kg and 0.5 g/kg respectively. Both sugars should be given as a 10% solution through a nasogastric tube. Horses should be fasted for 12-18 hours before testing so that gastric emptying is not delayed by the presence of ingesta. The blood glucose level increases at least 50% over baseline values within 2-4 hours after oral administration in normal horses.[31] The blood glucose level often doubles. A serum D-xylose concentration of at least 15 mg/dl is expected 60 minutes after oral administration in normal horses.[31,32]

Abdominocentesis

The constitution of abdominal fluid reflects the condition of the peritoneal surfaces in the abdomen. Evaluation of abdominal fluid can provide valuable information about many abdominal diseases. Abdominocentesis is performed regularly on horses with colic, weight loss, diarrhea, abdominal masses and abdominal infections. The technique for retrieving abdominal fluid via percutaneous centesis is simple and associated with a very low incidence of complications.[33]

Technique

Abdominocentesis is performed on the ventral midline of the abdomen at the lowest point in horses with pendulous abdomens or 8-10 cm caudal to the sternum in horses with a taut, sloping abdominal contour (Fig 4). Hair at the site of the puncture should be shaved or clipped and a surgical preparation performed on the skin. An 18-ga, 1 1/2-inch needle is satisfactory for abdominocentesis in most horses; however, longer needles are required for draft horses and fat horses. Spinal needles work well for collection of abdominal fluid, as these needles have a stylette and a short beveled point that reduces the possibility of enterocentesis or laceration of the bowel during movement of the horse. An 18-ga, 3 1/2-inch spinal needle is satisfactory for abdominocentesis. Some veterinarians prefer to use teat canulas for abdominocentesis; a small skin incision made after local anesthesia is necessary so that the blunt cannula can be inserted into the abdomen.

The needle should be advanced slowly into the abdominal cavity, with the hub rotated intermittently to clear the bevel and position the needle so fluid is obtained. It may be difficult to determine when the point of the needle has entered the abdominal cavity. When the hub of the needle moves back and forth in synchrony with respiration, the point of the needle often is against bowel wall or has perforated the bowel. More than one needle can be inserted into the abdominal cavity when no fluid is obtained from the first needle. All needles are left in position until fluid is obtained. Not uncommonly, as the second or third needles are being positioned, fluid begins to drip from the first needle.

Abdominal fluid should be obtained by gravity flow. Occasionally injection of 1-2 ml of air into one needle, followed by removal of the syringe, may result in fluid flow from a previously unproductive needle. Aspiration of abdominal fluid by attaching a syringe seldom is productive when other methods have failed. Abdominal fluid may be difficult to retrieve in some horses but patience will be rewarded.

Contamination of the abdominal fluid sample with peripheral blood can be reduced when teat cannulas are used by placing the canula through a gauze sponge. This prevents blood from the skin incision from flowing down the outside of the canula and into the collection tube. Contamination of abdominal fluid in the collection tube by peripheral blood often causes streaking of the sample as drops of blood fall into the abdominal fluid. Conversely, red-colored abdominal fluid caused by intraabdominal hemorrhage usually is homogeneous in color as the fluid enters the tube. Hemorrhage from peripheral blood clots in the collection tube. Abdominal fluid collected from horses with hemoperitoneum does not clot, and erythrophagocytosis can be seen upon cytologic examination of the fluid. Splenic puncture produces dark red blood with a higher PCV than peripheral venous blood.

Figure 4. Peritoneal fluid is collected using sterile technique. The fluid is allowed to drip into the collection tube containing EDTA. This allows the person collecting the fluid to appreciate the rate of flow and observe if any discoloration of the fluid is homogeneous.

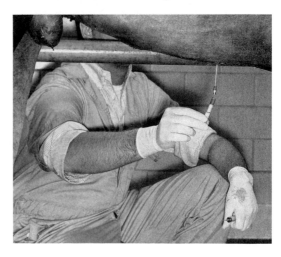

Interpretation of Abdominal Fluid

Normal abdominal fluid is yellow and clear or slightly turbid. Other characteristics of normal abdominal fluid are given in Table 2. Neutrophils are not degenerative but may exhibit hypersegmentation (Fig 5). Fluid from normal horses is sterile.

The generalized reaction of the peritoneum to trauma is inflammation. The peritoneum is capable of marked response, with elevations of total protein and white blood cell (WBC) counts. This response occurs with infection, exploratory laparotomy, enterocentesis, neoplasia and severely inflamed or infarcted bowel. Bacterial peritonitis can cause protein concentrations in the fluid to approach 7 g/dl and WBC counts as high as 600,000 cells/μl (Table 2). Fluid should be submitted for bacterial isolation in all horses with suspected bacterial peritonitis. White blood cell counts in excess of 400,000 cells/μl in healthy horses following

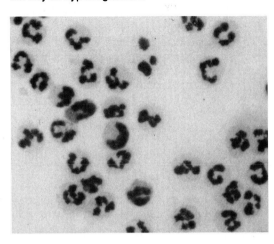

Figure 5. Stained smear of peritoneal fluid sediment from a normal horse. Neutrophils are not degenerative but may be hypersegmented.

enterocentesis or exploratory laparotomy have been recorded.[34,35] These high counts are transient but point out the difficulty in

Table 2. Characteristics of abdominal fluid in normal horses and in horses with various diseases.

Condition	Color	Turbidity	Total Protein (g/dl)	RBC Count (cells/μl)	WBC Count (cells/μl)	Cytologic Findings
1. Healthy horse (normal values).	Yellow	Clear to slightly opaque	<2	<8000	<8000	Neutrophils 40-90% of WBC population and no degeneration.
2. Strangulation/ obstruction of 3 meters of ileum.	Reddish-brown	Opaque	4.5	200,000	135,000	Neutrophils predominant and showing moderate degeneration. Many intracellular bacteria of varying morphologic forms.
3. Peritonitis secondary to abdominal abscess.	White with slight pink tinge	Opaque	6.1	120,000	175,000	Neutrophils predominant cell type with slight degeneration. Rare intracellular cocci observed.
4. Abdominal exploration for colic. No resection of bowel 24 hours after surgery.	Yellow	Cloudy	5.0	12,000	193,000	Mostly neutrophils with little evidence of degeneration.
5. Bowel necrosis and leakage at anastomotic site following resection and anastomosis of colon.	Orange	Opaque	6.3	3000	240,000	Very cellular, almost all neutrophils with moderate degeneration. Intracellular and extracellular bacteria of varying morphology.
6. Full-thickness rectal tear of 8 hours' duration.	Yellow	Cloudy	5.3	36,300	2100	Numerous yeasts, bacteria and protozoa. A few intact neutrophils with severe degeneration.

487

using elevated WBC counts alone for differentiating bacterial peritonitis, peritonitis associated with infarcted bowel, and normal peritoneal response to enterocentesis or exploratory laparotomy. However, a reliable correlation has been found between degenerative changes in neutrophils and the presence of toxin-producing microorganisms.[36] Degenerate neutrophils become pyknotic, karyolytic and karyorrhexic. The severity of degenerative changes is graded subjectively from mild, when few neutrophils show degeneration, to severe, when all neutrophils are degenerate. In Table 2, abdominal fluids from cases 4 and 5 have similar WBC counts and total protein levels. However, the horse in case 5 has degenerate neutrophils and microorganisms in the abdominal fluid indicative of intraabdominal sepsis.

White blood cell counts in exudative effusion should not be used to estimate severity of infection. This estimation is prone to error because neutrophils are fragile and lyse when exposed to high levels of toxins and neutrophils from exudative effusions tend to clump.[36] The WBC count of abdominal fluid in case 6 is extremely low because toxins caused lysis of neutrophils and could not be counted. Thus, the WBC count alone does not indicate the severe abdominal contamination in this horse. The presence of bacteria indicates, however, that contamination has occurred. White blood cell counts also may be misleading because WBCs are not distributed uniformly within the abdominal cavity. Following exploratory laparotomy, the ventral midline incision contributes to a localized elevation in the WBC count. Most abdominocenteses are performed close to the ventral midline incision.

The reaction of the peritoneum to neoplasia generally is much less marked than to bacterial peritonitis. Abdominocentesis may provide definitive diagnosis of neoplasia when a specific neoplastic cell type is identified in the fluid. Squamous-cell carcinoma, lymphosarcoma and mesothelioma have been identified by cytologic examination of abdominal fluid, but they may exist without causing changes in abdominal fluid.

Evaluating Fluid from Horses with Colic

Abdominocentesis is used most commonly for evaluation of horses with colic. Interpretation of abdominal fluid always should be made in light of all other clinical and laboratory findings. Analysis of abdominal fluid can be used prognostically and to aid selection of medical or surgical therapy. The color of abdominal fluid can provide valuable information.[37] Strangulation obstruction of intestine often occludes venous outflow but not arterial inflow. The resultant severe edema and capillary congestion causes movement of erythrocytes and free hemoglobin into the abdominal cavity. Free hemoglobin and red blood cells cause abdominal fluid to turn shades of pink and red. Serosanguineous fluid indicates the need for surgical intervention. Free hemoglobin, hemosiderin and other pigments are released into the abdominal cavity with necrosis of bowel, creating colors of abdominal fluid ranging from pink to brown.[37]

Discoloration of abdominal fluid in horses with colic is a reliable and useful indication of bowel necrosis.[38] Green and brown colors of abdominal fluid suggest the presence of bowel contents. Green or light brown fluid also is obtained by enterocentesis. Fluid obtained from enterocentesis may be difficult to differentiate from abdominal fluid.[34] Brown abdominal fluid suggests a very poor prognosis. Milky white abdominal fluid indicates a high WBC count and suggests that bacterial peritonitis is the cause of colic. Orange fluid may occur when yellow fluid is combined with moderate numbers of RBCs or hemoglobin. Orange fluid has been noted in nonstrangulating intestinal infarction.[39]

The total protein concentration in abdominal fluid often is elevated in horses with colic and indicates inflammation, vascular obstruction with protein leakage or necrosis of bowel. An elevation in total protein concentrations with normal or near normal WBC and RBC counts in horses with clinical signs of upper small intestinal obstruction suggests proximal enteritis as the cause of disease rather than strangulation obstruction of bowel. Abdominal fluid red blood cell counts may be used to help select medical versus surgical therapy. Horses with RBC counts of $\geq 20,000$ cells/μl in the abdominal fluid often require surgery.[40]

Cytologic examination of abdominal fluid can be a useful adjunct to evaluation of physical characteristics of the fluid. Abdominal fluid can be smeared on slides, air dried and stained in 5 minutes or less. Centrifugation of fluid may be necessary to concentrate cells in fluids with low cellularity. The slides should be examined for the presence of bacteria. Cell populations are defined and cell morphology, particularly neutrophil morphology, is determined.[41] Cytologic examination can confirm bowel rupture by the presence of plant material, numerous free bacteria, red blood cells and white blood cells in the abdominal fluid. Cytologic examination of bowel fluid obtained from enterocentesis reveals plant material and bacteria but no red blood cells or white blood cells. The presence of extracellular and intracellular bacteria with severe degeneration of neutrophils in abdominal fluid indicates loss of bowel integrity and suggests a poor prognosis for survival (Fig 6).

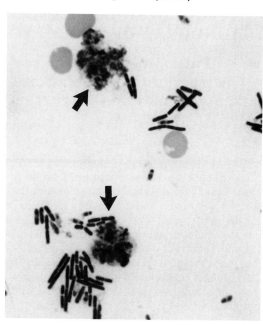

Figure 6. Stained smear of peritoneal fluid containing large numbers of intracellular and extracellular bacteria. The neutrophils are degenerate (arrows).

Exploratory Laparotomy

Laparotomy is a valuable diagnostic procedure for evaluation of the alimentary system. Laparotomy provides access to the abdominal cavity and its contents, allowing direct visual examination and palpation of many structures. Biopsies from the kidneys, liver, intestinal tract, abdominal masses and mesenteric lymph nodes are possible. Exploratory laparotomy is performed most frequently for evaluation of the gastrointestinal tract in horses with acute abdominal crises in which the specific diagnosis is not evident from physical examination and laboratory data. Indications for laparotomy on horses with acute abdominal crises are discussed in the section on Principles of Abdominal Surgery. Exploratory laparotomy also is useful for evaluation of horses with chronic colic of undetermined origin, chronic weight loss of undetermined origin, or masses identified by rectal examination or ultrasonography.

Exploratory laparotomy may be performed via a ventral midline celiotomy or via right or left flank celiotomy. The flank approaches may be performed on standing animals following tranquilization and instillation of a local anesthetic. Flank approaches allow limited visual assessment of abdominal organs, but jejunum, small colon and the mobile left ventral and dorsal colons can be partially exteriorized in the standing horse. Ventral midline celiotomy provides the best overall access to abdominal structures. This abdominal approach requires general anesthesia. Evaluation of the kidneys and other structures on the dorsal abdomen may be difficult due to the distance of the incision from these organs and interposition of intestines. Surgical techniques for exploratory laparotomy are discussed in the section on Principles of Abdominal Surgery.

Laparoscopy

Laparoscopy may be used for evaluation of abdominal diseases.[42,43] This procedure is less invasive than laparotomy, can be performed on the standing horse, and provides for direct viewing of some structures. Laparoscopy has been used to detect metastasis of primary neoplasms, evaluate rectal tears, and view masses in the dorsal abdomen. Laparoscopy also offers direct guidance to obtain biopsies. No reasonable view of the ventral abdomen can be obtained in the standing horse due to overlying bowel. Laparoscopy requires specialized equipment and experience by the surgeon. It is used most commonly for evaluation and manipulation of the reproductive tract. Increased use of laparoscopy for evaluation of diseases of the alimentary system is anticipated as equipment becomes more widely available to veterinarians.

PATHOPHYSIOLOGY AND PRINCIPLES OF THERAPY

Pathophysiology of Obstruction, Strangulation and Strangulation/Obstruction Ischemia

N.A. White

The pathophysiologic events that take place during an acute abdominal crisis include bowel distention, bowel ischemia, bacterial overgrowth and death, and changes in tissue perfusion. The responses to these events include changes in intestinal motility, secretion-absorption, permeability and morphology. These changes occur by stimulation of nervous reflexes and formation of chemical mediators that initiate pain, an increase in heart rate, pooling of blood, fluid sequestration, and alterations in tissue perfusion and oxygenation. Understanding the signs created by these changes helps the clinician determine the type of disease present and measure its severity.

Normal Function

The equine gastrointestinal tract is designed to digest and absorb carbohydrates and protein in the small intestine and to absorb volatile fatty acids from digestion of cellulose in the cecum and large colon. As most energy is derived from volatile fatty acids formed in the large intestine, the primary function of the stomach and small intestine is to hydrate the ingesta and move it into the cecum and large colon for fatty acid production.[44] This entails large fluid shifts from the extracellular fluid space into the intestine in the proximal gastrointestinal tract and subsequent resorption of fluid in the cecum and colon.

The secreted fluid is isotonic and contains mostly Na^+ and Cl^- or HCO_3^-.[44] Water follows Na^+ into the intestinal lumen and is partially resorbed in the cecum and large colon with volatile fatty acids.[44,45] The result is an enterosystemic cycle in which water is removed from extracellular fluid space and secreted into the proximal gastrointestinal tract, where it is used to liquefy and buffer the ingesta being delivered to the cecum and colon. The water is then returned to the extracellular space by absorption in the small intestine, cecum and large colon. The total water exchange is equivalent to 1.5 times the animal's total extracellular fluid volume in a 24-hour period.[45]

The digestive process of the equine stomach and small intestine is similar to that of other monogastric animals. Water absorption is linked to glucose absorption, and dipeptides, tripeptides and amino acids are absorbed. The cecum and colon function like the forestomach of the ruminant. These organs normally contain a variety of microorganisms, including Gram-negative and Gram-positive bacteria.[44] The breakdown of cellulose to volatile fatty acids (butyrate, propionate and acetate) can fluctuate with feeding.[44] Active absorption of these fatty acids enhances absorption of Na^+ and water. If horses are fed twice daily, rapid intraluminal production of acid lowers the luminal pH and causes a shift from absorption to secretion of fluid, which reduces the plasma volume. The systemic response is an increase in plasma renin and angiotensin concentrations.[46] This shift is due to the osmotic pressure from the fatty acids and lactate content within the intestinal lumen and secretion of HCO_3^- to buffer the increased acidity.[44] This is followed by a shift to absorption of fatty acids and water, producing relative dehydration of the ingesta.[44] If horses are fed at 2-hour intervals, plasma volume and renin-angiotensin response are unchanged.[46]

The intestinal motility that moves the ingesta and fluid aborally (distally) is cyclic and controlled by numerous factors within the intestine. The musculature of the duodenum, cecum and pelvic flexure responds to distention with ingesta by starting a peristaltic wave. A pacemaker in the pelvic flexure may start the electrical activity in this area, having a regular basal cycle that is increased with eating, increased fiber content and distention.[47-50] The small intestinal motor events can be measured as spiking activity that is classified as none, intermittent or regular.[47,48] These electrical spikes initiate muscular activity, some of which is transmitted aborally along the intestine. Distention increases this spike activity anywhere within the intestinal tract by activating peristalsis oral (proximal) to the distention and inhibition of peristalsis aborally.[44]

The cecum and colon produce haustral motility to mix and retain ingesta as well as propulsive motility to move the ingesta in both directions in the colon. Spike burst potentials may be short and produce local mixing contractions or may be long potentials that coordinate the oral (proximal) and aboral (distal) movements of the ingesta.[48] These movements also are increased by distention and by reflexes from other intestinal activities, including filling of the stomach, the gastrocolic reflex, filling of the ileum, and the enterocolic reflex.[50] The normal time required for fluid to travel from the stomach to the cecum is from 30-180 minutes. Total transit from the stomach to anus is as short as 12 hours for fluids and as long as 7-10 days for particulate matter.[44,47,51] Larger particulate matter is retained in the large colon for longer periods by mixing retropulsive movements that allow completion of fiber digestion.[47,51]

Intestinal blockage alters intestinal motility, initiates secretion of fluid into the intestinal lumen, and causes mucosal damage. Alteration in blood supply to the intestine causes ischemia that rapidly initiates cellular damage in the mucosa and serosa. Some of the diseases that produce these effects are categorized as obstruction (simple obstruction), strangulation obstruction, which can be divided into hemorrhagic strangulation obstruction and ischemic strangulation obstruction, and nonstrangulation infarction, which is synonymous with thromboembolic colic in the horse.

Obstruction

In the small intestine, obstruction of the intestinal lumen usually is due to intraluminal blockage from a dehydrated food mass or extraluminal pressure from adhesions, thickening of the intestinal wall or infection. Adynamic ileus may recur after surgery or may be associated with thromboembolism and cause functional obstruction due to lack of intestinal movement. Adynamic ileus is associated with peritonitis, ischemic intestinal insults, anesthesia, endoparasitism and electrolyte imbalances.[47] In the large colon or small colon, impaction by dry ingesta, concretions or sand most often cause blockage. The response to obstruction is increased motility of the segment of bowel oral (proximal) to the blockage due to distention and relaxation of the intestine

aboral (distal) to the blockage.[44,48,50] The muscular activity of the intestine is increased around the obstruction, increasing intraluminal pressure in this segment of intestine. Distention of the intestine stretches the wall of the intestine and combines with the reflex muscular spasm to initiate colic.[50]

When the small intestine is obstructed, the enterosystemic circulation of fluid is blocked and secreted fluid is prevented from passing to the large intestine for resorption (Table 3). Because normal secretion of fluid continues, the small intestine becomes distended oral (proximal) to the blockage. Once the luminal pressure becomes elevated, the tissue pressure compresses the capillaries and reduces venous drainage. Due to the increased capillary hydrostatic pressure, water moves into the lymphatic system or the intestinal lumen, or through the serosa.[44] The increased intraluminal hydrostatic pressure created by the enhanced secretion of fluid then initiates a cycle that increases secretion by continuing to elevate the intraluminal pressure.[52,53] Because the fluid secreted is isotonic, there is minimal acute change in serum electrolyte values. The consequences of intestinal distention are dehydration from third-space sequestration of the secreted fluid, mucosal injury, abdominal pain, and increased movement of protein across the serosa into the abdominal cavity.[53] The distention eventually reaches a level that inhibits motility in the affected

Table 3. Physiologic responses to small intestinal obstruction.

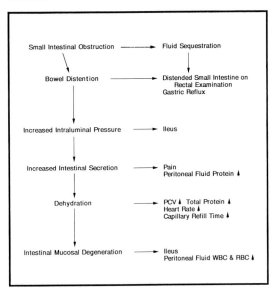

segment of intestine as well as other portions of the intestinal tract.[50] The clinical signs that result are colic, increased heart rate due to pain and decreased circulatory fluid volume, reduced borborygmi, gastric and intestinal fluid sequestration (gastric reflux), and increased protein concentration in peritoneal fluid (Table 3).

Obstruction of the cecum or large colon often blocks passage of ingesta but allows gas to pass. Exceptions to this include extremely dehydrated ingesta, sand impactions, enteroliths or entrapment displacements of the colon. Reflex muscular contractions increase in frequency, the intraluminal pressure increases and the intestine relaxes aborally.[49] Pain is intermittent and is associated with cyclic increase in intraluminal pressure proximal to the obstruction. Fluid entering from the small intestine continues to be absorbed in the cecum, which is normally oral to the blockage. The process slowly produces dehydration due to lack of water intake and also results in intermittent pain with an eventual reduction in borborygmi. Clinical signs seen with this type of obstruction include intermittent colic (usually mild to moderate), a slight increase in heart rate, mild dehydration, reduced borborygmi, and peritoneal fluid total protein levels ranging from normal to increased, depending on the duration of the obstruction (Table 4).

If the obstruction is complete, the gas no longer escapes, resulting in rapid distention of the proximal segments of the bowel. In many instances, this may include the entire colon and cecum. The massive distention creates other systemic effects. Severe stretching of the intestinal wall produces severe pain, and intestinal motility ceases due to intestinointestinal reflex.[50] Intraabdominal pressure also reduces diaphragmatic movement. As intraabdominal pressure increases, tidal volume is reduced and hypoxemia eventually may occur.

The increase in intraabdominal and intrathoracic pressures reduces venous return to the heart, causing reduced cardiac output and reduced arterial oxygenation, which can lead to severe shock and death. These advanced clinical signs include a very high heart rate, pale cyanotic mucous membranes, bloat, no borborygmi, and severe unrelenting pain.

Adynamic ileus can occur in the small or large bowel and produce signs similar to those of mechanical obstruction. Adynamic ileus in the stomach and/or small intestine can lead to signs identical to those of small intestinal obstruction, including gastric distention from fluid sequestration and eventual rupture of the stomach. Grain overload with volatile fatty acid production can cause stasis in both the stomach and small intestine. Chronic distention of the intestine secondary to a mechanical obstruction can stretch the musculature and injure the mucosa, causing adynamic ileus. This same sequence of events can occur in the cecum and large colon due to rapid distention of these segments of intestine with gas. The gas cannot escape as motility is reduced both from the by-products of rapid fermentation and massive distention of the bowel. This can lead to severe tympany with clinical signs similar to those in complete obstruction of the large bowel.

Reduced colonic motility also occurs in the large colon secondary to administration of atropine, alpha-2 receptor stimulation with such drugs as xylazine or detomidine, or opiate receptor agonists.[47,50] The stasis following administration of the last 2 types of drugs is normally short lived. Once the colon is not moving, both gas and fluid accumulate, creating the same problems seen

Table 4. Physiologic responses to large colon obstruction.

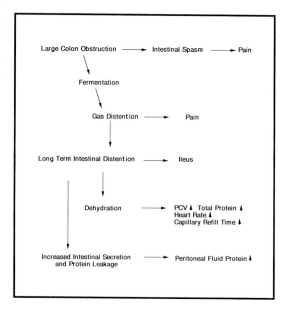

with an intraluminal obstruction or extraluminal compression.

Ileus also can be due to sympathetic stimulation in response to pain, or physical or ischemic trauma to the bowel. This form of functional obstruction is normally temporary and often not complete. Clinically this results in a lack of borborygmi on auscultation. Though mixing sounds from the colon may be present, long progressive sounds are absent until long spike burst activity returns.

Strangulation Obstruction

Strangulation obstruction is a combination of intestinal obstruction and ischemia. Strangulation is obstruction of the blood supply by vascular constriction and usually is due to intestinal torsion-volvulus or incarceration of the small intestine in a variety of intraabdominal sites, including the epiploic foramen, inguinal ring or rents in the mesentery. Depending upon the degree of constriction, venous return may be impeded without a loss of arterial inflow. This causes blood loss into the wall of the intestine, with most of the blood accumulating in the submucosa.[54] Arteriovenous constriction can occur acutely or may follow venous constriction. Both types of circulatory interruption result in development of lesions in the intestine. The underlying problem also is obstructive, as the torsion or incarceration also causes obstruction of the intestinal lumen.

Ischemia causes similar lesions in the large and small intestine. The lack of perfusion reduces oxygen delivery, which affects the mucosal cells first due to their high metabolic activity. The cells start to separate from the basement membrane from formation of extracellular edema at their attachment to the capillary tuft of the lamina propria. Thus, the cells slough before development of severe intracellular damage (Fig 7). Histologically, sloughing of the epithelial cells of the villi occurs in the small intestine and from the surface and into the crypts of the cecum and colon (Fig 8).[55,56] The slough is graded from 0 (normal) to 5 (total slough) with necrosis of the crypt cells.[55]

The loss of cells is sequential starting at the villus tip and progressing to the crypts. At the same time, the mesothelium of the

Figure 7. Epithelial cells lining the small intestine slough off the laminia propria during ischemia and reperfusion. The cells are loosened by edema between the cells at the basement membrane. Top: Histologic section of a grade-III lesion with loss of the mucosal-cell layer from the villus tip. (H&E stain, original magnification 292X) (Courtesy of *American Journal of Veterinary Research*) Bottom: Scanning electron photomicrograph of a grade-III lesion with mucosal-cell loss from the capillary folds of the laminia propria. (330X)

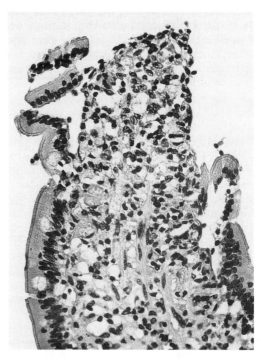

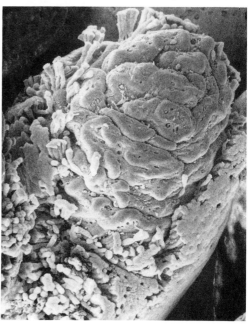

serosa also sloughs and the fibrous tissue layer becomes disrupted and infiltrated by inflammatory cells and edema (Fig 9). Ischemic changes continue as progressive necrosis unless blood flow resumes. Vascular damage initiates leakage of protein and erythrocytes out of the vascular space into the bowel lumen and peritoneal fluid.[41] Loss of the mucosal barrier allows bacteria and endotoxin to escape into the peritoneal cavity, causing increased neutrophil numbers in peritoneal fluid. With severe necrosis, bacteria are seen in the fluid or within the neutrophils, and the fluid itself may become serosanguineous.

If the strangulation is relieved, reperfusion produces a hyperemic reflex with an initial rush of blood throughout the injured intestinal segments. Ischemia initiates production of hypoxanthine via breakdown of ATP to AMP during the period of hypoxia. When oxygen is brought back to the tissue by reperfusion, xanthine oxidase, activated from xanthine dehydrogenase in the presence of calcium and a protease present in high concentration in the intestine, reacts with the hypoxanthine to make superoxide and hydrogen peroxide radicals, and subsequently hydroxyl radicals (Fig 10).[57] These oxygen and hydroxyl radicals cause tissue necrosis and progressive damage to the injured mucosa and capillary endothelium.[58] The loss of mucosal epithelial cells therefore continues down into the crypts.[55] If bowel necrosis is extensive, with total loss of the epithelium, and the capillaries are ob-

Figure 8. Scanning electron of photomicrograph of mucosal-cell loss on the large colon surface and the top of the crypts.

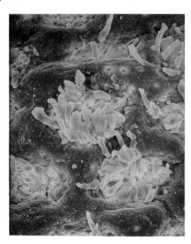

Figure 9. Top: Normal serosa with a single-cell mesothelial lining attached to a fibrous layer. Bottom: During ischemia and reperfusion, the serosa rapidly loses the mesothelial layer and becomes disrupted with edema, collagen separation and cellular infiltration. (H&E, original magnification 200X)

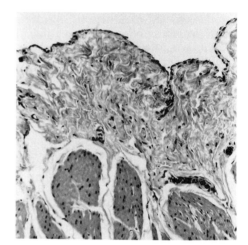

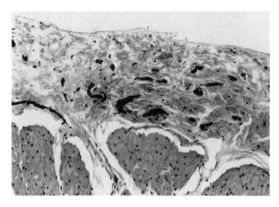

structed by swelling and thrombosis, there is no hyperemic reflex.

Initially strangulation obstruction causes clinical signs similar to those of simple obstruction. However, the abdominal pain is more severe due to necrosis, edema of the bowel wall and stretching of the mesentery seen with many of these diseases. Clinical signs that separate strangulating lesions from simple obstruction relate to disruption of the mucosal barrier and leakage of bacteria and endotoxin from the intestine.

Loss of the mucosal epithelium exposes the lamina propria and its capillary system to the contents of the bowel lumen. Bacteria and endotoxins invade the tissue, pass through to the peritoneal cavity and eventually enter the bloodstream. These events initiate shock by movement of fluid from the extracellular and intracellular compartments into the intestinal lumen, and by the response to endotoxemia.[59]

Hypovolemia causes a vascular response by increasing heart rate, influx of extracellular fluid from the tissue into the vascular space, intense vasoconstriction, and eventually a lack of perfusion of tissues, producing both an oxygen debt and a shift to anaerobic metabolism. The result is acidosis from lactate production, tachycardia, pale to cyanotic mucous membranes, hypotension and cold extremities.

Endotoxemia produces other effects that are dose-related and can be fatal. An immediate reaction is sloughing of the endothelium of the pulmonary vessels and formation of platelet aggregates.[59,60] Destruction of the cell wall causes release of fatty acids, including arachidonic acid. Enzymes throughout the body use arachidonic acid as a precursor to formation of prostaglandins. Levels of 2 of these metabolites of arachidonic acid, thromboxane and prostacyclin, increase dramatically in plasma during endotoxemia.[61,62] Thromboxane release is immediate, initiating pulmonary hypertension and causing vasoconstriction in other organs.[45] Prostacyclin is produced more slowly and appears to be responsible for many of the cardiovascular effects that occur during

Figure 10. Proposed scheme for superoxide and hydroxyl radical production during reperfusion. Excess hypoxanthine from AMP production during hypoxia is transformed to xanthine in the presence of xanthine oxidase. This reaction requires oxygen, which is provided from the renewed blood flow, and xanthine dehydrogenase, which is activated by protease and calcium. The resulting oxygen radical and hydrogen peroxide form hydroxyl radicals, which are toxic to the surrounding tissue.

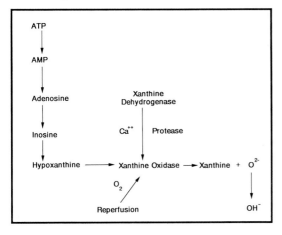

endotoxemia.[61] The effect is opposite that of thromboxane, with vasodilation and reduction of blood flow. Thus, generation of these vasoactive substances in response to endotoxemia causes initial vasoconstriction followed by vasodilation.[61,62] As the shock sequences progresses, there is compensatory vasoconstriction in response to the reduced blood pressure.[41] Specific vascular beds, including the splanchnic vasculature dilate, and blood pools peripherally in the face of reduced circulating blood volume.

Both of these mediators are responsible for production of pain. Both thromboxane and prostacyclin production can be partially or completely inhibited by nonsteroidal antiinflammatory drugs. Flunixin meglumine is the most potent of these drugs in horses and its application can totally obliterate the early responses to a nonlethal dose of endotoxin.[60,62] Other mediators are thought to be involved, including leukotrienes, interleukin-1 and tumor necrosis factor. Their effects have yet to be elucidated in horses in shock.

Endotoxin exerts a direct toxic effect on the cell by blocking the cytochrome oxidase system, shifting cellular metabolism to anaerobiosis and causing lactic acid production. Once a fatal dose of endotoxin has been absorbed, there is no antidote and the cellular metabolism will fail even if prostaglandin inhibitors have been administered or circulation volume is maintained.

During endotoxemia, white blood cells are sequestered in sites of vascular damage and in the peritoneal cavity. Therefore, colic can be accompanied by varying degrees of leukopenia. Neutrophils accumulate in the peritoneal cavity in response to bacterial migration and cause the inflammatory response in the serosa and peritoneal cavity. The combined effect of dehydration with reduced cardiac output and endotoxemia can be rapidly fatal, as seen in such diseases as large colon torsion or small intestinal volvulus.

Once shock has ensued, the intestinal lesions are not restricted to the strangulated segment. Intestine both proximal and distal to the strangulated segment is affected by distention or systemic shock.[56] This is predominantly a mucosal lesion, with mucosal cell loss and edema of the lamina propria. Thus, histologic lesions develop in bowel that appears viable to the surgeon. This bowel is prone to ileus, fluid secretion and eventual infarction unless the shock sequence can be reversed.[56]

When trying to relate all of the clinical signs that evolve from endotoxemia and bowel necrosis, the overlap of many reactions makes delineating specific causes and effects difficult. The signs of shock and pain from the intestinal lesion are amplified in severe cases by release of catecholamines. This causes sweating, tacky mucous membranes, poor membrane refill and tachycardia, and ileus becomes complete. Table 5 summarizes the pathophysiologic events and clinical signs that develop during strangulation obstruction.

These effects are dependent on the amount of intestine involved. Large colon torsion or small intestinal volvulus that involves a large portion of bowel induces more rapid systemic changes than conditions involving only small segments of intestine. Such conditions as intussusceptions or some inguinal hernias in which the strangulated bowel is separated from the abdomen do not produce the same acute signs of shock until endotoxins leak from the obstruction. Other than pain from stretching of the mesentery, these conditions may cause few other systemic signs or biochemical changes.

Nonstrangulation Infarction

Nonstrangulation infarction is a reduction of blood flow to the intestine due to an intravascular obstruction. This can be caused by blockage of a large artery or low flow through the capillaries. In horses, this is most often due to *Strongylus vulgaris* larval migration in the cranial mesenteric artery and its branches.[39] The degree of ischemia varies and usually does not cause clinical signs.[49] Blood flow to the intestine can be decreased more than 50% before the intestine is affected.[48] This is due to the ability of the intestine to increase oxygen uptake at lower blood flows and its ability to shunt blood to the mucosa, the area with the highest metabolic rate.

The migrating larvae cause an endothelial lesion and initiate thrombus formation. This appears to be a chronic process, with active coagulation taking place during the entire time the larvae are in the artery.[63] This process includes platelet aggregation and thrombus formation, and hypothetically

could lead to thromboxane production in the arterial system and thromboembolism (Fig 11). The resulting vasoconstriction could cause infarction similar to that seen in coronary artery disease in people. Often the intestinal lesions appear to have developed slowly due to chronic ischemia. The ischemic change is similar to that seen with strangulation except that with arterial obstruction there often is little trapping of blood in the lesions and the intestinal wall does not become thickened. The affected intestine first turns purple, then green brown, with subsequent necrosis.

The mucosal epithelium is lost and there may be simultaneous mural necrosis. Bacteria from the lumen leak through the degenerated tissue and seed the peritoneal cavity. The peritoneal lining responds with a massive accumulation of neutrophils and protein. The peritoneal fluid becomes serosanguineous. Bacteria often can be found in the fluid or within neutrophils. The horse responds with pain due to ischemia and endotoxemia. Depending on the size of the lesion, the horse develops peritonitis before severe signs of shock become apparent (Table 6). Once endotoxin leakage occurs, the sequence of events is similar to that of

Table 5. Physiologic responses to strangulation obstruction.

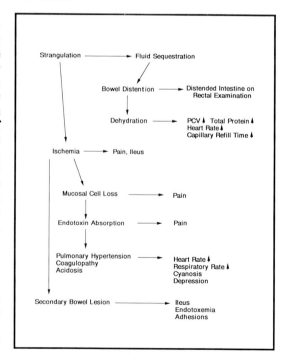

strangulation; however, the rate of bacterial and endotoxin diffusion seems to be dependent on the stage of intestinal degeneration. Fortunately, collateral circulation can rapidly allow such areas to heal.

Clinical signs of nonstrangulation infarction are variable and may resemble those of simple obstruction or severe strangulation obstruction.[39] Colic varies from mild to severe, as does the degree of dehydration. Absorption of endotoxin apparently can be slow, creating sublethal shock. The peritoneal fluid also can vary greatly but often has a large increase in neutrophils and protein when clinical signs are first noticed, rather than a progressive increase as occurs with prolonged obstruction or strangulation. Red blood cell numbers in the peritoneal fluid often are not as high as occurs with strangulating lesions.

Mucosal and Serosal Regeneration

Mucosal and serosal regeneration is a rapid and potentially totally reparative process that follows any of the intestinal injuries discussed. The mucosa can heal as long as viable enterocytes are present to migrate up the villus lamina propria. Though the villus is shortened by contraction and loss of the capillary tuft, it is covered by epithelium within 12-24 hours (Fig 12). Lack of healing leaves the lamina propria open to bacteria

Table 6. Physiologic effects of nonstrangulating bowel infarction.

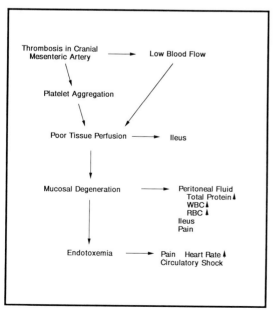

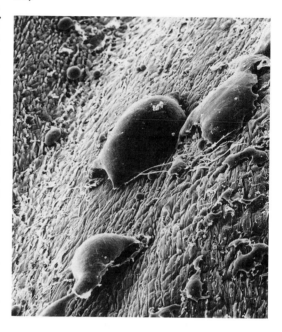

Figure 11. Thrombus formation with endothelial-cell disruption in the cranial mesenteric artery in the presence of *Strongylus vulgaris* larvae.[63] The thrombus is attached to the artery wall and can cause spontaneous embolus formation. (Courtesy of *Equine Veterinary Journal*)

Figure 12. The mucosal defect heals rapidly over the surface of the contracted laminia propria. The villus regenerates to normal length within 10 days if there is not permanent scarring of the laminia propria. (H&E, original magnification 200X)

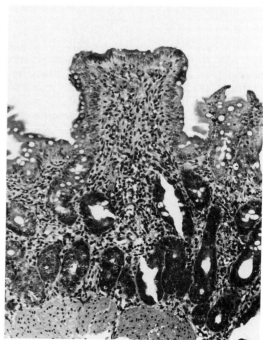

and endotoxin migration into the peritoneum. Within 10 days, the villus can regenerate to normal length and the intestine can return to its normal absorptive capacity.

Serosal responses to ischemia and bacterial invasion include edema, deposition of fibrin, and neutrophil and macrophage infiltration. Endothelial damage is severe and progresses during reperfusion. The serosal surface adheres to other peritoneal surfaces in the abdomen because there often is lack of normal movement in the abdomen and because the injured mesothelial surface is covered by a layer of fibrin. The response of the entire peritoneal cavity to leakage of bacteria depends upon the rate of healing and level of contamination. With severe contamination or bowel leakage, there is a massive influx of white blood cells and protein into the peritoneal cavity. Fibrin clots form diffusely and the omentum often is adhered to the site of leakage.

Healing of the serosal mesothelial surface occurs from the connective tissue layer of the serosa and is rapid unless the inflammatory response inhibits healing. Unfortunately, the mucosa may become normal after an insult while the serosa becomes fibrotic and causes chronic strictures, obstruction or mesenteric constriction, with a subsequent acute abdominal crisis.

Pathophysiology of Diarrhea

A.M. Merritt

The suggestion made more than 10 years ago that diarrhea is not manifested in an *adult* horse unless there is large intestinal malfunction has, to date, withstood the test of time.[32] That is, with regard to water fluxes, a healthy equine large intestine can compensate for any deficiency in small intestinal absorptive function. This probably is not true for foals, though such an opinion is presently based more upon deductive reasoning than on hard data.

The determining factor regarding colonic compensatory capacity may depend upon the degree of intraluminal fermentative activity, as absorption of volatile fatty acids across the large intestinal mucosa induces concomitant water absorption.[45,64-66] If this is a major determinant, the turning point in maturation of colonic function in young horses has yet to be established.

One argument against this theory is that extensive large colon resection in adult horses results in no change in the amount of fecal water. In this experiment, however, the cecum, from which the majority of water entering the large intestine is absorbed, was left in place (Fig 13).[65] Further, these horses were never challenged by a small intestinal malabsorptive condition. With that concept set forth, one can apply the classic "hypersecretory" and "malabsorptive" bases for diarrhea to neonatal and postnatal foals with some degree of confidence. There are surely some as-yet unrecognized differences in the pathophysiology of diarrhea in young equids versus other species.

Some organisms, such as certain *E coli*, adhere to small intestinal absorptive cells and elaborate an enterotoxin that evokes hypersecretion of water and electrolytes.[68-70] The excessive fluid leaving the ileum overwhelms any large intestinal compensa-

Figure 13. Water fluxes (L/day) across various portions of a pony's large bowel.[65] The cecum absorbs the largest amount of water leaving the ileum (net of 12.6 L/day in this 100-kg pony). The net absorption of 1.8 L/day from the small colon is necessary for formation of normal fecal balls.

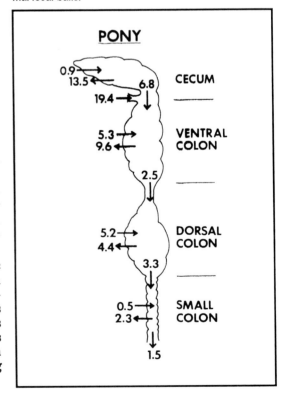

PONY

0.9
13.5   6.8   CECUM
19.4

5.3   VENTRAL
9.6   COLON

2.5

5.2   DORSAL
4.4   COLON

3.3

0.5   SMALL
2.3   COLON

1.5

tory capacity, and diarrhea results. There is evidence that enterotoxigenic colonic hypersecretion can also occur in some species, but this has yet to be established in horses. Mucosal damage is minimal with classic enterotoxigenic disease.[71]

However, some organisms, such as salmonellae, not only elaborate an enterotoxin but invade the submucosa to cause severe inflammation with mucosal/submucosal damage and sometimes endotoxemia.[72,73] The resultant combination of varying degrees of hypersecretion, tissue exudation and malabsorption results in the most serious and severe forms of diarrheal disease. Whereas both small and large bowel can be affected by such organisms, it probably is the degree of large bowel damage that is the major determinant of the severity of diarrhea and dehydration.

Other agents, including sand and a number of bacteria and parasites, can cause mucosal damage and enteritis but do not produce enterotoxin.[74-79] Chronic inflammatory bowel disease of unknown etiology also falls within this category of problems.[80-83] Whether there is diarrhea or not depends upon the extent of the lesions and especially on the degree of colitis. While the feces can be quite watery, they usually are not as liquid as those induced by enterotoxigenic/invasive organisms and the horse does not dehydrate rapidly. Any time there is enteritis, there also is some degree of plasma protein leakage into the bowel.

Primary mucosal damage, with minimal if any invasion and inflammation, can occur in the small and/or large intestine, the site(s) depending upon the pathogen. Many enteric viruses cause mucosal damage, the most notable in horses being the rotavirus.[84,85] It is reasonable to assume that diarrhea associated with rotaviral infection, where only the small intestine is involved, is manifested in foals but not in adults because of the "immaturity" of large intestinal function of foals. Poorly digested and malabsorbed soluble nutrients enter the large intestine in excessive amounts, where they trap water by osmotic effects and/or directly cause intestinal malfunction.

Diarrhea also can be seen in all ages of horses in which no gross or histologic lesions are evident. The presumption is that this is due to some functional deficiency that could be either congenital or induced.

In many cases, in both young and adult animals, the cause of the malfunction cannot be determined. If the animal is an adult, we assume the colon is involved.

Finally, foals are subjected to a unique problem called "foal heat diarrhea," so named because it occurs around the time of the mare's first postpartum estrus. The small amount of information regarding this self-limiting phenomenon is that it is a hypersecretory diarrhea, though the source and mechanism of hypersecretion have not been described.[86] Because protozoa are found in the feces only after cessation of the diarrhea, it has been suggested that this may be part of the normal maturation process of the foal's gut, signaling the initial establishment of colonic microflora.[86,87]

Medical Therapy for Gastrointestinal Diseases

C.W. Kohn

Control of Pain

Decompression: Horses with intestinal obstruction, ileus and occasionally acute enterocolitis may have nasogastric reflux. Because vomition does not occur readily in horses, gastric distention persists, resulting in severe pain. In such cases, a nasogastric tube should be placed immediately to evacuate the stomach and relieve pain. The nasogastric tube should be secured in place and vigorous, frequent priming efforts made to evacuate the stomach until reflux ceases.

Analgesics: Gastrointestinal obstruction and acute enterocolitis are frequently associated with severe abdominal pain. Relief of pain is sometimes a prerequisite to safe physical examination. Patients may require continual analgesic therapy until medical treatment is successful or surgical intervention becomes necessary. The choice of an appropriate analgesic should be based on analgesic efficacy and safety of the drug. Drugs with the least deleterious effects on a compromised cardiovascular system and on gut motility should be chosen. Drug effects vary with each patient, the quality of the pain, the degree of physiologic imbalance present, and the nature of underlying pathophysiologic processes. Minimal effective dosages of these drugs should be used in ill horses.

In the past, the choice of an appropriate analgesic was based largely on personal experience and on subjective assessment of response of patients to treatment. The clinical pharmacology of visceral analgesic drugs in horses has been investigated under controlled conditions. Analgesic potencies of drugs have been evaluated using visceral pain models of cecal distention with a balloon and by cecal impaction, and a superficial pain model by measuring the threshold to cutaneous heating.[49,88,89] *In-vivo* studies of electromyographic and mechanical activity of small and large bowel in healthy ponies and horses treated with pain-modifying drugs have demonstrated that analgesics may also alter gut motility. Changes in gut motility produced by these drugs may be deleterious to the patient, and these side effects should be considered when selecting drugs. In addition, adverse effects of some analgesics or sedatives on the cardiovascular system, especially in metabolically compromised horses, may preclude use of these drugs to control pain. Recommended dosages for the drugs and drug combinations discussed below are provided in Table 7.[90]

Most controlled studies indicate that the sedative-analgesic *xylazine* (Rompun: Bayvet) is the most effective analgesic available for visceral pain in horses.[88-92] Though this alpha-2 adrenergic agonist has a short duration of action, repeated small doses are tolerated well and may reduce visceral pain so effectively that the seriousness of the abdominal obstructive disease process is obscured. When xylazine is used for relief of abdominal pain, the patient must be monitored closely for evidence of progression of the disease.

Xylazine has some potentially deleterious effects on gut motility. Xylazine at 1.1 mg/kg decreased propulsive motility in the distal jejunum, cecum and pelvic flexure in healthy ponies.[93-95] Similarly, administration of lower dosages of xylazine has caused profound cessation of cecal mechanical activity and reductions in cecal arterial blood flow in healthy adult horses.[96] Administration of multiple large doses of this drug to a horse with an impaction might be contraindicated, as normal motility is essential to move ingesta aborally (distally). The effect of repeated doses of xylazine administered before anesthesia on development of postoperative ileus has not been assessed.

Other potential side effects of xylazine include initial transitory hypertension, followed by arterial hypotension resulting from decreases in cardiac output and peripheral vasodilation.[97] Bradycardia and second-degree atrioventricular block are also commonly encountered. Despite these side effects, xylazine is a relatively safe drug; healthy horses can tolerate up to 10 times the recommended dose.[98] Repeated small doses of xylazine usually provide excellent, relatively predictable, safe analgesia in volume-depleted, metabolically compromised colic or enterocolitis patients.

Detomidine (Domosedan: Farmos Group, Dormosedan: Norden), a more potent alpha-2 adrenergic agonist, produces dose-dependent sedation and visceral analgesia in horses. The drug is available for use by practitioners in most parts of the world. In experiments using the cecal balloon model for colic pain, detomidine at 20 μg/kg produced excellent analgesia of longer duration than that produced by xylazine at 1.1 mg/kg IV.[99] Higher dosages of detomidine produced excellent analgesia but sedation was too profound, as excessive swaying and ataxia were noted frequently. Though cecal contractions ceased after detomidine administration, none of the ponies had side effects from this interference with motility. The precise effects of this drug on bowel motility remain to be documented, and repeated doses may be constipating. Side effects following detomidine administration are dose dependent and include sweating, occasional tremors, increased urine production, ataxia, profound decreases in heart

Table 7. Dosages of drugs commonly used to provide visceral analgesia.[90] (Courtesy of *Journal of Veterinary Internal Medicine*)

Drug	IV Dosage (mg/kg)
Xylazine	0.6-1.0
Morphine	0.02-0.10
Meperidine	0.2-0.6
Oxymorphone	0.01-0.06
Pentazocine	0.4-0.8
Butorphanol	0.05-0.1
Flunixin meglumine	1.1
Dipyrone	11-22
Xylazine/morphine	0.6/0.2-0.6
Xylazine/meperidine	0.6/0.2-1.0
Xylazine/butorphanol	0.6/0.02-0.04
Xylazine/pentazocine	0.6/0.2-0.8

rate (as low as 10-15 bpm) and transient hypertension that persisted over 15 minutes and in some cases up to 60 minutes. Second-degree atrioventricular and sinoatrial block also were noted in some horses.[100-103]

Further research is required to determine the optimum dosage of detomidine. Preliminary studies suggest excellent visceral analgesia; sedation for standing diagnostic and minor surgical manipulations may be possible after treatment with this drug. The drug's prolonged duration of sedative and analgesic effects may make it an attractive alternative to xylazine in clinical practice. In a clinical trial performed in several universities, detomidine was consistently more effective than other analgesics in relieving abdominal pain.[104]

The opioids are centrally and peripherally acting analgesics that produce behavioral changes and increase the threshold to pain. The analgesic potency of opiate drugs varies. If morphine is arbitrarily assigned a visceral analgesic potency of 1, methadone has equal or slightly greater potency, with pentazocine 0.25 and butorphanol 7.[91,105] Though morphine has potent visceral analgesic effects as demonstrated in the cecal balloon colic model, the drug was not as effective as xylazine in that study.[91] Morphine and other opiate drugs have long been used as constipating agents.

Administration of *morphine* (Lilly) to healthy ponies decreases gut sounds, delays defecation and produces fecal drying, decreases overall mechanical and electrical activity in colonic muscle, and decreases propulsive activity from cecum to right ventral colon.[93,106,107] Whether use of morphine as a preoperative analgesic would potentiate postoperative ileus is unknown, but this possibility must be considered.

The narcotic agonist-antagonist *butorphanol* (Torbugesic: Bristol), a synthetic morphinan derivative, also has excellent visceral analgesic effects. In 66 equine patients with abdominal pain treated with butorphanol at 0.1 mg/kg, analgesic response was excellent (marked analgesic effect for a period adequate to permit specific therapy) or good (noticeable analgesic effect with minor indications of pain).[108] An IV dosage of 0.2 mg/kg produced good to excellent visceral analgesia, but this dosage also induced apprehension, increased locomotor activity and ataxia in some horses.[91,92] My personal experience suggests that total IV doses of 4-10 mg of butorphanol in a 450-kg horse provide safe analgesia alone or in combination with xylazine (0.6 mg/kg IV) in the clinical setting. Butorphanol has been reported to decrease jejunal but not pelvic flexure propulsive motility in ponies.[109]

Pentazocine (Talwin-V: Winthrop) is a synthetic narcotic agonist-antagonist with visceral analgesic effects inferior in intensity and duration to the effects of xylazine or butorphanol.[49,88-92] Pentazocine inhibits jejunal motility but not pelvic flexure motility in ponies.[109]

Meperidine (Demerol: Winthrop) is a synthetic narcotic analgesic that produces visceral analgesia inferior to that produced by xylazine.[88,89] Meperidine inhibits jejunal but not pelvic flexure motility in ponies.[109] *Oxymorphone* (Numorphan: DuPont) is a morphine analogue used successfully by some practitioners to manage colic pain.[105] This drug has not been tested in studies using colic pain models. *Methadone* (Dolophine: Lilly) is a synthetic narcotic reported to produce excellent analgesia without excitement in horses;[105] however, this drug is not readily available and has not been well studied.

In general, the narcotic agonists have minimal cardiovascular depressant effects in horses and ponies, and appear to be reasonably safe in animals with metabolic abnormalities associated with gastrointestinal obstructive diseases. However, these drugs may blunt the hemodynamic responses to obstructive diseases. They may increase blood pressure and therefore mask signs of worsening disease. Thus, horses with abdominal pain treated with these agents must be scrutinized carefully for indications that surgical intervention is necessary.[92]

Clinical use of opiates in treatment of colic has not become common practice. This is due, in part, to the dangers of maintaining a supply of these agents that have great potential for substance abuse and, in part, to the unpredictable behavioral side effects in horses and ponies. Behavioral changes seen after administration of these drugs to horses include apprehension, pawing and increased locomotor activity, such as pacing, restlessness, headshaking and shivering.[91,110,111] Improved analgesia with reduced behavioral side effects has been demonstrated after administration of xylaz-

ine and morphine, or xylazine and butorphanol.[111,112] Xylazine also provides improved, extended analgesia when combined
with fentanyl (Sublimaze: Janssen), meperidine, oxymorphone or pentazocine. Administration of these drug combinations has not
been associated with significant cardiopulmonary abnormalities in healthy horses.[112]
Safety at recommended dosages and synergistic analgesic effects of these drug combinations make them useful in restraint of
the equine colic patient.

Excitement or excessive depression
caused by narcotic agonists can be controlled by narcotic antagonists. This may be
particularly helpful before surgery on extremely ill patients. Because of its marked
agonistic effects, use of the narcotic agonist-antagonist nalorphine is not recommended. Naloxone is the antagonist of
choice.

The results of 1 study suggested that endogenous opiate-like substances might be
part of an inhibitory mechanism for controlling equine colonic motility.[107] Opiate antagonist drugs might, therefore, be useful in
countering potentially undesirable effects of
endogenous opiates in impactions and in
antagonizing the constipating effects of opiate analgesics. In this study, administration
of the opiate antagonist naloxone (Narcan:
DuPont) to healthy ponies produced propulsive colonic motility and defecation (see
below).[107] Further investigation is indicated
to explore the feasibility of administering
narcotic antagonists to prevent the constipating side effects of narcotic drugs employed to alleviate abdominal pain.

Dipyrone (Novin: BayVet), *phenylbutazone* (Butazolidin: Jensen-Salsbery) and
flunixin meglumine (Banamine: Schering)
are peripherally acting analgesics that prevent pain by inhibiting biosynthesis of prostaglandins in injured tissues. Flunixin is
considered to have the most potent visceral
analgesic effects of this group of drugs.
However, its analgesic effects have been inferior to those of xylazine, morphine and
butorphanol in several studies. In the cecal
balloon model, colic pain apparently results
from bowel distention and not, at least initially, from local synthesis of prostaglandins. Though these findings may be due to
limitations of the colic model used, in a clinical trial, the analgesic effects of flunixin

were clearly less than those of detomidine.[104]

Nonsteroidal antiinflammatory drugs are
especially useful for horses with moderate
or low-grade abdominal pain (impaction,
mild gas colic, diarrhea, peritonitis). However, flunixin may be such an efficient visceral analgesic in some colic patients that
the seriousness of the ongoing disease is obscured. Flunixin reduced pain associated
with colic in 68% of 118 horses tested in a
field study.[113] Flunixin and dipyrone have
no effect on mechanical or myoelectrical activity of pony jejunum and pelvic flexure.[49,94] In recommended doses, these drugs
do not cause significant hypotension and
are therefore safe for patients in shock.
Nonsteroidal antiinflammatory drugs are
well tolerated at recommended doses (Table
7); however, these drugs may be nephrotoxic if large doses are used. Usual
therapeutic doses may be nephrotoxic in dehydrated horses. Renal toxicity is characterized by renal papillary necrosis and tubular
nephrosis that may be associated with inappropriately dilute urine, hematuria and uremia. The attending clinician should make
every effort to ensure that the patient is
maintained in a state of adequate hydration, especially if a protracted course of
therapy with these drugs is anticipated, as
in a horse with laminitis that develops after
abdominal surgery.

Occasionally a colic patient exhibits severe, unrelenting pain that is not controllable with the analgesics mentioned previously. Severe pain can be controlled by a
slow intravenous drip of *guaifenesen* (Guai-
laxin: Robins) or 7% *chloral hydrate* (Hum-
co) given to effect. Chloral hydrate may be
administered slowly IV at 20-40 mg/kg; the
infusion should be stopped when the desired
level of sedation is achieved. Sedative doses
of chloral hydrate provide relief for 3 hours
or longer. Though the drug is relatively safe
for preoperative use if given in sedative
doses, anesthetic doses of chloral hydrate
cause significant hypotension. This drug
may be useful when affected horses must be
shipped to a hospital and to sedate horses
with persistent abdominal pain.

Some sedatives should be avoided in patients with shock, especially if general anesthesia is planned. Phenothiazine tranquilizers and ethaverine HCl, a smooth muscle

relaxant, cause marked hypotension, even in small doses. In severely dehydrated horses, sudden peripheral vasodilation enlarges the vascular space and compounds dehydration. Horses with peracute enterocolitis may have such marked fluid deficits that a sudden hypotensive episode may result in death.

Modifying Bowel Motility

Gastrointestinal diseases in horses may result in either delayed or rapid transit of ingesta. For patients with acute or chronic enterocolitis, clinicians search for pharmacologic means of slowing ingesta transit. For patients with simple, nonsurgical bowel obstruction or ileus, the attending veterinarian requires drugs that improve gut motility and speed transit of ingesta. The ability to pharmacologically manipulate gut motility depends on a clear understanding of gut motility in health and disease.

Drugs to Stimulate Gut Motility: Ileus is a major complication following intestinal resection or exploratory celiotomy, and may be a complication in medical intestinal diseases such as proximal enteritis. The search continues for methods to hasten return of gut motility to allow patients to return to voluntary intake of food and water as soon as possible. Though use of pharmacologic means to improve gut motility is an attractive strategy because it may be easiest, it is important to remember that return of gut motility usually depends on successful treatment of the underlying disease and its associated metabolic abnormalities. Bowel distention resulting from obstruction or stasis may potentiate ileus, and relief of distention by nasogastric intubation or surgical decompression is essential to successful therapy. Electrolyte disturbances, especially hypocalcemia and hypokalemia, may lead to gut stasis. Prompt adjustment of electrolyte and acid-base status of the patient may result in improvement of bowel motility without specific pharmacologic intervention. However, in some patients, particularly in the postoperative period, decreased motility or ileus persists despite adequate decompression of bowel and stable metabolic status. In such cases, pharmacologic attempts to stimulate motility become a necessity.

A model of postoperative ileus in ponies has been used to test potential methods of therapy.[110] Administration of metoclopramide, domperidone and cisapride to ponies with experimental postoperative ileus resulted in improvements in bowel motility.[114,115] In a small prospective clinical study, use of cisapride, an indirect cholinergic agent, reduced the incidence of serious postoperative ileus.[115] Studies of gut motility in healthy ponies have demonstrated that neostigmine and naloxone may increase motility. Because dosage regimens for these drugs have not yet been well established, many questions remain about the pathophysiology of ileus and the best method of treatment.

Neostigmine (Prostigmin: Roche), an anticholinesterase, allows acetylcholine to occupy and stimulate smooth muscle receptors.[102] Neostigmine also directly stimulates cholinergic receptors.[105] Experimentally, administration of neostigmine (0.022 mg/kg IV) increased the propulsive activity of the cecocolic area and the pelvic flexure, and increased the frequency of defecation.[93,94] Neostigmine decreased propulsive motility in healthy pony jejunum and delayed gastric emptying of particulate markers in horses.[94,116] The clinical importance of the effect of neostigmine on gastric emptying remains to be evaluated. This drug has been used clinically to promote colonic motility. Small intestinal motility might not be expected to improve after administration of this drug. It may cause abdominal discomfort and should be withdrawn if signs of abdominal pain follow its use. A clinically safe and dependable dose for this drug has not been documented.

Metoclopramide (methoxychloroprocainamide) (Reglan: Robins) stimulates and coordinates motility of the stomach and proximal small intestine but has little effect in the large intestine in people.[117] This drug has been studied in other species and has a parasympathomimetic effect; it also antagonizes the inhibitory neurotransmitter dopamine in gut smooth muscle.[114,117,118] In people and dogs, metoclopramide accelerates gastric emptying and shortens transit time through the small intestine via its ability to stimulate and coordinate gastric, pyloric and duodenal motor activity.[117,118] Metoclopramide restored normal stomach-to-anus transit time and restored coordinated gastric and small intestinal motility in the postoperative ileus model in ponies.[114] Use of metoclopramide within 4 days of bowel anastomosis in human patients is not recommended.[114] The safety of this drug in the early postoperative period in horses with bowel anastomoses must be investigated. Slow IV infusions at 0.5 mg/kg to ponies with experimental postoperative ileus caused periods of excitement. A dosage of 0.25 mg/kg administered IV over 30 minutes in the same experiments was associated with periods of restlessness, alternating with sedation and yawning.[114,119] Further investigation is required to develop a safe, effective therapeutic regimen.

Cisapride is an indirect cholinergic drug that promotes release of acetylcholine from nerve terminals. In a series of experimental trials and a small clinical trial, repeated IM administration of cisapride at 0.1 mg/kg appeared to enhance small intestinal motility.[115]

Naloxone (Narcan: DuPont), an opiate antagonist, when administered experimentally in a very high IV dosage of 0.5 mg/kg, elicited marked propulsive activity of the left ventral and dorsal colons lasting about 45 minutes. Defecation was observed but no untoward side effects were reported.[107] These results suggest that large doses of opiate antagonists may be useful in stimulating colonic motility, perhaps by antagonizing the effects of endogenous inhibitory opiate mediators of gut motility. These drugs also may be useful in antagonizing the inhibitory effects of previously administered opiate agonist analgesics. The clinical usefulness of this class of drugs requires further investigation.

Panthenol (Ilopan: Adria), a precursor of coenzyme A, is an alcohol analogue of pantothenic acid. Its use for stimulating intestinal motility has been advocated on the grounds that it increases formation of acetylcholine and thus has a parasympathomimetic effect. Panthenol had no effect on intestinal motility in a study of 6 ponies.[94] It has no known pharmacologic uses.

Drugs to Inhibit Gut Motility: Some cases of colic are thought to result from hypermotile, "spastic" bowel; hence the use of such "antispasmodic" drugs as *atropine* and *dipyrone* to normalize bowel motility. The efficacy of these agents as antispasmodics is a matter of debate. Dipyrone is discussed in the section on visceral analgesics.

Atropine sulfate (Elkins-Sinn) traditionally has been used to treat spasmodic colic in horses. This parasympatholytic drug is a competitive inhibitor of acetylcholine at the gut receptor site. Atropine administration (0.044 mg/kg SC or 0.176 mg/kg IV) to healthy ponies decreased auscultable gut motility within 30 minutes of drug administration at either dosage.[120] Cecal distention and abdominal pain were noted in some ponies given the higher dosage. Abdominal pain lasted for up to 4 hours. In another study, atropine (0.044, 0.125 or 0.2 mg/kg IV) caused dose-dependent reductions in gut sounds, discomfort, delayed defecation, fecal drying, and prolonged return to normal auscultable motility and defecation.[106] Administration of atropine to horses with abdominal pain may result in ileus that complicates antecedent obstructive disease and may obscure the diagnosis.[120] Thus, use of atropine as an antispasmodic for horses with abdominal pain is not recommended.

Some practitioners consider diarrhea an indication for use of drugs that depress gut motility. Unfortunately, decreasing propulsive gut motility does not necessarily slow ingesta transit. Abolition of mixing contractions, which retard movement of ingesta to maximize time for digestion, may actually speed ingesta transit. Thus, drugs that inhibit gut motility may worsen diarrhea in some cases. However, improvement of fecal character in horses has been reported after treatment with *loperamide* (Imodium: Janssen).[106] Though loperamide decreases gut motility in other species, its antidiarrheal effects in horses may be mediated through the antisecretory action of the drug (see Drugs that Modify Fecal Consistency). The efficacy of narcotic agonists, which decrease propulsive gut motility, in treating diarrhea has not been evaluated. These drugs have a constipating effect in healthy horses and ponies and have been used since antiquity to decrease diarrhea in people.

Modifying Fecal Consistency

Cathartics: These drugs are used most frequently in treatment of fecal impactions of the large colon. Cathartics have been classified by their mechanism of action as irritant (direct effect on the internal mucosa), bulk (hydrophilic agents that stimulate motility and help soften impactions by distending the bowel with fluid), emollient (bowel lubricants) and surfactants (detergent actions dissolve impaction) drugs (Table 8).[121]

Irritant cathartics should not be administered when the diagnosis of the type of bowel disease is uncertain, as these drugs are contraindicated in obstruction and enterocolitis. Bulk cathartics may be dehydrating because these hypertonic agents promote fluid shifts from the extracellular fluid into the bowel lumen. Emollient cathartics may interfere with absorption of fat-soluble vitamins, and foreign-body reactions may occur in the intestinal wall if lubricant particles are absorbed. The surface-active agents themselves are toxic if administered in excessive quantity. The daily dosage of dioctyl sodium sulfosuccinate (DSS) (Surfactant: Vetco) should not exceed 90 mg/kg. Mineral oil and DSS should not be used concurrently, as DSS may facilitate oil absorption.

Protectants: Mineral oil and bismuth subsalicylate may exert a coating, protective effect on irritated inflamed bowel.

Bulk Formers: Kaolin-pectin (Kaopectate: Butler) and bismuth subsalicylate (PeptoBismol: Norwich-Eaton) theoretically promote formation of fewer stools. In clinical practice, some horses respond to large (0.5-1 gallon) doses of Kaopectate, administered once to several times a day by nasogastric tube. However, in few cases does treatment with bulk formers result in immediate cure of diarrhea. Bismuth subsalicylate may be beneficial in some cases because of its antitoxic effect (see Antitoxic Drugs).

Loperamide: Loperamide (Imodium: Janssen) is a piperidine derivative related to meperidine. In species other than horses, it slows gut motility, probably in part by binding to intestinal opioid receptors. Loperamide has a low potential for abuse.[122] This drug has been studied infrequently in horses. One investigation of its effects on gut sounds, intestinal transit (as measured by transit of the soluble marker polyethylene glycol), and quality of feces indicated that loperamide (0.2 mg/kg IV or PO) decreased gut sounds and dried rectal and gut contents in horses.[106] This dosage did not delay defecation. The drying effect of this drug on feces was thought to be mediated through an antisecretory effect. Loperamide may be useful in some diarrheal diseases in horses. Further study and development of safe therapeutic regimens are needed.

Table 8. Types and dosages of cathartics.

Class	Active Ingredients	Site of Action	Dose/450 kg
Irritant	Cascara sagrada	Colon	–
	Danthron	Colon	–
	Aloe	Colon	–
	Castor oil	Small intestine	0.5 L
Saline	Sodium sulfate	Small intestine	–
	Magnesium sulfate	Small intestine	500 g
	Magnesium citrate	Small intestine	–
	Sodium phosphate	Small intestine	–
Bulk hydrophilic	Psyllium	Small intestine and colon	–
	Methylcellulose	Small intestine and colon	0.2-0.5 kg
	Bran	Small intestine and colon	1-2 kg
	Plantago	Small intestine and colon	
Emollient	Liquid petrolatum	Entire tract	2-4 L
	Raw linseed oil	Entire tract	1 L
Surfactant	Dioctyl sodium sulfosuccinate (7%)	Colon	0.2-0.4 L
	Dioctyl calcium sulfosuccinate (7%)	Colon	0.2-0.4 L

Phenoxybenzamine: Phenoxybenzamine (Dibenzyline: Smith, Kline and French) is an alpha-adrenergic antagonist reported to reduce diarrhea in a very limited number of clinical cases and to diminish the severity of diarrhea induced by experimental carbohydrate overload.[123] The mechanism by which this drug reduced or prevented diarrhea is unknown. Horses shedding *Salmonella* organisms in their feces were not improved. Hypotension may be a side effect of phenoxybenzamine therapy and its use in dehydrated horses is not recommended. Further experimental and clinical trials are needed to document the efficacy and safety of this drug as an antidiarrheal agent.

Modifying Gastric Acidity and Protecting the Gastric Mucosa

Cimetidine: Cimetidine (Tagamet: Smith, Kline and French) is a reversible, competitive histamine type-2 H2-receptor antagonist that blocks gastric acid secretion stimulated by histamine, acetylcholine and gastrin. Ranitidine (Zantac: Glaxo) is an H2-receptor antagonist estimated to be 5-12 times more potent than cimetidine in inhibiting gastric acid secretion in people. Ranitidine has a longer duration of action than cimetidine and causes fewer drug interactions and fewer side effects, but it is more expensive.[124] Cimetidine therapy may be associated with accumulation of concomitantly administered drugs that are metabolized by the cytochrome P-450 mixed-function oxidase system. Cimetidine has a greater affinity than ranitidine for cytochrome P-450 and binds tightly to it.[125] Theophylline, phenobarbital and diazepam, for example, may accumulate during cimetidine therapy.

Oral administration of cimetidine at 8.8 mg/kg or ranitidine at 2.2 mg/kg increased gastric pH of healthy young horses above 3.6 for about 8 hours.[126] An oral cimetidine dosage of 2.2 mg/kg increased gastric pH above 3.6 for only about 2 hours in the same study. In this study, samples of gastric juice were obtained via nasogastric tube. In another study of gastric acid output in young horses with a surgically implanted gastric cannula, cimetidine significantly decreased gastric acid output for 2 hours and ranitidine did so for 4 hours after treatment.[127,128] However, ranitidine given IV at 0.5 mg/kg did not significantly alter gastric pH.[128] The discrepancies in gastric pH measurement between these 2 studies remain to be resolved but may be related to the differences in gastric juice collection techniques.

Experimental demonstration of the efficacy of cimetidine and ranitidine in decreasing gastric acidity corroborates the clinical impression that their use in treatment of foals with gastroduodenal ulceration is commonly followed by cessation or marked diminution of anxiety, colic pain, bruxism and hypersalivation, especially when these drugs are given in conjunction with the mucosal protectant, sucralfate. Recommended dosages of cimetidine to a 150-kg foal range from 300 to 600 mg PO or IV QID.[129,130] An oral or IV dosage of 2 mg/kg QID also has been suggested.[131] Some clinicians prefer to use ranitidine because it can be given less frequently, and has fewer potentially detrimental drug interactions and fewer side effects. Foals that become refractory to cimetidine may respond to ranitidine. Recommended oral dosages for ranitidine are 150 mg BID or 2 mg/kg BID.[129-131] However, studies suggest that the oral dosage of ranitidine may need to be at least 4 mg/kg BID to have any clinically relevant effect on gastric acid secretion in horses.[126] Because absorption of cimetidine is blocked by antacid buffers, it should not be administered less than 1 hour after oral treatment with antacid preparations. The bioavailability of ranitidine is also decreased by antacids.[125]

It is important to note that though these agents relieve clinical signs of ulcer disease, withdrawal of medication may result in return of clinical signs. Relapse is particularly likely if the affected foal is still being stressed. For example, if the foal must wear a cast or be subjected to long-term antimicrobial therapy, the presumed stimulus to ulcer formation is still present.

Sucralfate: Sucralfate (Carafate: Marion Labs) is a sulfated disaccharide (sucrose) and polyaluminum hydroxide gel. When the gastric pH is less than 4, the compound is activated and extensively polymerized. This polymerized form of sucralfate is a viscid demulcent gel that adheres to intestinal epithelial cells and to the base the crater of ulcers, for which it has a particular affinity.[132] Antacids and foods do not affect the integrity of the adherent gel. The gel forms a protective barrier over the ulcer, prevents exudation of protein from the ulcer, and adsorbs pepsin, trypsin and bile acids. The therapeutic effect of sucralfate on ulcers may be related to the drug's ability to increase local prostaglandin production.[130]

Because the drug is activated by acid, in human patients it is recommended that antacids not be given 30 minutes before or after sucralfate. Because cimetidine (2.2 mg/kg PO) is reported to increase equine gastric pH to greater than 3.6 for 2 hours and ranitidine (2.2 mg/kg PO) for 8 hours, sucralfate should be administered 1 hour before either of these drugs.[126] Alternatively, sucralfate could be given 2 hours after cimetidine or 8 hours after ranitidine therapy.

It should be remembered that the effects of sucralfate on healthy or ulcerated equine gastric mucosa have not been studied. There are few side effects to sucralfate therapy reported in people and none yet attributed to use of this drug in foals. Sucralfate may be administered PO at 2 g QID to a 150-kg foal.[129,130]

Antacids: Antacids are basic compounds that neutralize gastric acid and usually are composed of aluminum and/or magnesium hydroxide. Magnesium hydroxide is the most rapidly acting insoluble antacid. Aluminum hydroxide is slower to neutralize gastric acid. Preparations that contain a combination of magnesium and aluminum hydroxide thus have both fast-acting and more sustained effects.[125] The acid-neutralizing capacities of various antacids are well documented in people but have not been studied in foals. A dose of 15 ml of an aluminum and magnesium hydroxide combination preparation has been used QID in foals.[130] One typical preparation contains 225 mg of aluminum hydroxide and 200 mg magnesium hydroxide per 5 ml (Maalox: Rorer). Content and acid-neutralizing capacities of commercially available antacids vary markedly. Antacids decrease the bioavailability of cimetidine and ranitidine when these histamine receptor blockers are administered concurrently.[125] Antacids should be given at least 1 hour after oral administration of H2 receptor blockers to avoid reducing bioavailability of the latter. In people, antacids are administered after eating, as the presence of food in the stomach delays gastric emptying and allows antacids more time to act. Though relationships between gastric emptying, feeding

and antacid administration have not been evaluated in horses, it seems wise to administer antacids 1 hour or so after feeding when possible.[130] Side effects of antacid therapy in foals have not been reported. Aggressive use of magnesium hydroxide might result in osmotic diarrhea.

Nutritional Support

Reviews of nutritional support for sick horses emphasize the importance of maintaining nitrogen balance in ill or recuperating equine patients.[133,134] Negative nitrogen balance adversely affects equine immune function and may delay wound healing and prolong recovery from debilitating diseases. Because metabolic demands increase substantially in sick animals, provision of adequate nutrition is critical.

Diets for sick horses should contain palatable, digestible feedstuffs rich in nutrients that are poorly stored and those needed to meet the demands of the metabolic stress of convalescence. Such nutrients include proteins, vitamins A and C, riboflavin, calcium, magnesium and potassium. Sources of protein are alfalfa hay, soybean meal, brewer's yeast and casein. If the horse has decreased feed intake but is still eating, it may be possible to tempt the patient to increase intake by providing a choice of fresh feeds. Changes in feed should be made slowly. A new grain concentrate should be introduced into the diet at the rate of about 0.5 kg/day for a 450-kg horse; a change in hay should be made over a 5-day period. Adding a protein supplement to the feed, such as 50 g of casein TID, has been suggested.[133,134]

Administration of anabolic steroids, including testosterone derivatives or preferably less androgenic compounds such as stanozolol (Winstrol V: Winthrop), may improve appetite; however, this effect may not be noticeable for 10 days after therapy. Benzodiazepines, such as diazepam (Valium: Roche), are reported to have appetite-stimulant effects in ruminants in limited studies.[135,136] The tranquilizing effects of these drugs in debilitated horses are undesirable, however, and their use is not recommended.[134] Supplementation with injectable B-complex vitamins may also improve appetite. Various preparations containing organic arsenical compounds and ginger are purportedly useful in promoting appetite. For a calming effect and to promote appetite, 50% ethanol in 10- to 20-oz oral doses may be tried.

Total nutritional support is indicated for horses unwilling or unable to eat due to pain, depression or incompetent bowel function, especially if anorexia persists for more than 5 days or if the horse is already thin and debilitated. For horses that require bowel rest (proximal enteritis, enterocolitis, persistent ileus), total parenteral nutrition may be indicated. Little information is available regarding response of such patients to total parenteral nutrition. Total parenteral nutrition is especially useful in septicemic young foals that frequently bloat if fed enterally. Healthy adult horses have been successfully maintained on total parenteral nutrition for 10 days, but this process is extremely expensive.[137] Suggested formulas for total parenteral nutrition solutions for foals and adults are presented in Tables 9 and 10.[133,137] Administration of such solutions requires careful, aseptic placement of a long intravenous catheter that reaches the cranial vena cava. Because these solutions are hypertonic and therefore irritating, slow administration into a large vein is required to decrease the incidence of

Table 9. Formulation of an intravenous feeding solution for foals.[133]

Ingredient	Amount
5% amino acid solution	1000 ml
50% dextrose	500 ml
Potassium chloride	30 mEq
Sodium bicarbonate	30 mEq
Injectable multivitamins	

These ingredients are mixed aseptically to yield a solution with a final volume of 1500 ml. The solution is hypertonic and is administered IV at 3 L/day to a 45-kg foal.

thrombophlebitis. Strict catheter asepsis must be maintained and all total parenteral nutrition solutions mixed under sterile conditions. A 1-day supply of total parenteral nutrition solution should be made each day and stored in a refrigerator until used. The reader is referred to other publications for a more complete discussion of total parenteral nutrition.[133,137]

Table 10. Formula for total daily parenteral nutrition.[137]

Sample Formulation for Foals	
Nutritional Source	**Amount**
50% dextrose (500 g/L)	15 g/kg/day
8.5% or 10% amino acid solution (85 or 100 g/L)	3 g/kg/day
10% or 20% lipid emulsion (100 or 200 g/L)	3 g/kg/day

Mix glucose and amino acid solutions together first, and then add lipid emulsion.

Start with glucose at 10 g/kg/day, amino acid at 2 g/kg/day and lipids at 1 g/kg/day. Increase to recommended amounts over a few days.

Sample Formulation for 450- to 500-kg horses[b]	
Nutritional Source	**Amount**
8.5% amino acid solution	4 L
50% dextrose	4 L
Polyionic electrolyte solution	11.2 L
10% fat emulsion	6 L
23% calcium gluconate[a]	0.5 L

a – Administer separately, before amino acid-glucose-electrolyte infusion.
b – Supplies 16,000 Kcal, 360 g amino acid, 2400 g glucose and 600 g fat per day.

In horses that can tolerate oral alimentation, provision of daily needs per os is preferred. Various alimentation solutions may be used. A complete pelleted feed may be soaked in water to make a slurry suitable for administration via nasogastric or, in carefully selected cases, esophagostomy tube. A maintenance electrolyte solution for horses is presented in Table 11.[133] A companion oral alimentation solution that provides daily nutritional needs for a 450-kg horse is outlined in Table 12.[133] A feeding schedule for this solution also is indicated in Table 12. To increase the energy content of this solution, corn oil may be added at 150 g/day. Because the electrolyte component of this solution is sodium poor, some horses may become hyponatremic when maintained on this solution. Addition of 15 g of sodium chloride per day to the solution is adequate to correct hyponatremia. This solution is not recommended for horses with laminitis or diarrhea. It is important not to administer more than 7 L of fluid by nasogastric tube at one time to a 450-kg horse to avoid gastric distention and abdominal pain. The reader is referred to published articles for a complete discussion of this alimentation solution[133,137]

Use of high-caloric-density alimentation solutions, designed for use in people, has been attempted in horses. One such solution contains a glucose polymer, medium-chain triglycerides and casein, and provides about 1 cal/ml (Osmolite: Ross). In limited clinical trials, this solution has been well tolerated by adult horses that received the solution via nasogastric or esophagostomy tube as their sole source of nutrition.[138] Development of such high-caloric-density solutions for use in horses may provide an effective means of maintaining nitrogen balance in inappetent individuals.

Table 11. One day's requirement for a maintenance oral electrolyte mixture for a 450-kg horse.[133]

Ingredient	Amount
Sodium chloride (NaCl)	10 g
Sodium bicarbonate (NaHCO₃)	15 g
Potassium chloride (KCl)	75 g
Potassium phosphate (dibasic anhydrous) (K_2HPO_4)	60 g
Calcium chloride ($CaCl_2.2H_2O$)	45 g
Magnesium oxide (MgO)	25 g

Table 12. Recommended tube feeding schedule for a 450-kg horse.[133] These allowances should be divided and administered in 3 feedings daily. Maintenance requirements for a 450-kg horse are 13 mcal of digestible energy and 580 g of crude protein.

	Day						
Ingredient	1	2	3	4	5	6	7
Electrolyte mixture (g)[a]	230	230	230	230	230	230	230
Water (L)	21	21	21	21	21	21	21
Dextrose (g)	300	400	500	600	800	800	900
Dehydrated cottage cheese (g)[b]	300	450	600	750	900	900	900
Dehydrated alfalfa meal (g)	2000	2000	2000	2000	2000	2000	2000
Energy (mcal)[c]	7.4	8.4	9.4	10.4	11.8	11.8	12.2

a – Mixture is listed in Table 11.
b – Dehydrated cottage cheese contains 82% crude protein with <2% lactose. Available from Ingredient Specialties, Box 127, Mt. Pleasant, SC 29464, or through a local feed mill.
c – Megacalories of digestible energy.

Monitoring patients receiving partial or total nutritional support is essential. The patient should be weighed and the hydration status (skin turgor, capillary refill time, character and rate of pulse) should be assessed clinically each day. Laboratory evaluation of packed cell volume, total plasma protein level, serum osmolality and serum sodium, potassium, chloride, magnesium and glucose concentrations should be performed intermittently to ensure that the patient is metabolically stable. Serum glucose concentrations should not exceed 200-300 mg/dl.[133] Urine glucose concentrations also should be evaluated. Administration of alimentation solutions should be tailored according to the individual patient's response to nutritional support.

There is little information available regarding nutritional support of horses with gastrointestinal diseases. Acute obstructive diseases usually are resolved surgically or medically within 5 days; therefore, restriction of caloric intake is not often a problem in these cases. After exploratory celiotomy, especially if enterotomy or intestinal resection was performed, a period of restricted oral intake is indicated in the postoperative period. Assuming that gastrointestinal motility returns within 4-8 hours after surgery, a small portion of bran mash may be given within 8 hours after surgery. If bowel was invaded or resected, some surgeons delay the first meal for 24-48 hours after surgery. Hay should be introduced into the diet slowly as intestinal motility, appetite and attitude improve.

Studies of experimental small intestinal resections in ponies have shown that as the length of the small bowel resection increased, weight loss in the postoperative period increased. Resection of more than 60% of the small intestine resulted in significant malabsorption, as indicated by decreased ability to absorb d-xylose.[139] Reduction in small intestinal digestive and absorptive function in patients after resection of shorter segments of small bowel may prove to be clinically significant. Such patients may have decreased ability to digest and absorb nutrients from grain concentrates, and may rely on large bowel digestion and absorption of nutrients from high-quality hay. These issues require clarification.

Horses subjected to experimental transient arterial and/or venous nonstrangulating infarction of the large colon or to resection of 60% of the total length of the large colon had decreased apparent digestion of crude protein 3 weeks after surgery.[140] Horses that had colon resection also had decreased apparent phosphorus and crude fiber digestion 3 weeks after surgery. By 6 months after surgery, all horses had returned to baseline (preoperative) digestive indices. The results of these experiments indicate that diets in the first 3 months after surgery for horses with vascular compromise of the colon, with or without resection, should contain crude protein concentrations in excess of 6-7% and phosphorus in excess of 0.11-0.13% on a dry-matter basis. Feeds containing 15-20% of high-quality protein on a dry-matter basis should be fed during the postoperative period.

Anthelmintic Therapy

Internal parasitism frequently is associated with colic and diarrhea. A regular, effective deworming schedule is an essential part of any herd health program. Prophylactic use of anthelmintics, the problems of anthelmintic drug resistance, and pasture hygiene as a strategy for parasite control have been reviewed.[141-143]

Verminous arteritis associated with migratory phases of larvae of *Strongylus vulgaris* may cause colic that may cause death from secondary ischemia of intestine.[144] This disease is less common these days, presumably because of the accepted use of effective anthelmintic strategies. Diarrhea also has been associated with ulceration of the colon and cecum resulting from *S vulgaris* larval migration.[75] Larvicidal doses of certain anthelmintics are reported to be effective against the migrating larvae of *S vulgaris*. An oral paste of ivermectin (Eqvalan: MSD Agvet) given at 200 μg/kg is 99% effective against adults and arterial larval stages of *S vulgaris*.[145] Killing of susceptible parasites by ivermectin takes several days and resolution of *S vulgaris*-related arteritis may take 5-6 weeks.[145] For this reason, the clinician should allow at least a month after ivermectin treatment before assessing failure or success of therapy.

Other treatment regimens reported to be larvicidal for migrating *S vulgaris* include fenbendazole (Panacur: Hoechst-Roussel) at 50 mg/kg on 3 consecutive days or at 10 mg/kg for 5 consecutive days, and thiabendazole (Equizole: MSD Agvet) at 440 mg/kg (10 times the normal dose) on 2 consecutive days. Thiabendazole therapy may be effective only against the early migratory phases of S vulgaris and may therefore have less effect on larvae in mesenteric arteries. I recommend use of ivermectin for larvicidal therapy.

Small strongyle infection may be associated with colic or diarrhea.[146] Penetration of many small strongyle larvae through the gut wall and presence of larvae in the lumen or encysted in gut wall may be associated with alterations in small intestinal motility or bowel wall inflammation that can cause abdominal pain or diarrhea.[144,146] Diagnosis may be difficult in some cases, as the presence of encysted larvae may not be associated with a patent infection. Oral ivermectin therapy (200 μg/kg) is reported to be 95-100% effective in killing adult, benzimidazole-resistant, and lumen- and mucosal-dwelling small strongyles.[145] A fenbendazole dosage of 60 mg/kg given on 3 consecutive days also is reported to be effective in killing small strongyles in the gut wall.[142] However, results of anthelmintic trials against encysted small strongyles are conflicting and activity against these larvae may not be as complete as desired. Diarrhea associated with immature small strongyles in horses previously treated regularly with ivermectin has been reported.[146]

Infection with the protozoan parasite *Giardia* caused chronic diarrhea in a horse.[147] This horse was successfully treated with metronidazole (Flagyl: Searle) given PO at 10 mg/kg body weight TID for 10 days.

Transfaunation-Transfloration

Imbalance or absence of normal intestinal fauna and flora may predispose to or perpetuate intestinal dysfunction, especially diarrhea. Consequently, reestablishment of a normal enteric environment may speed return to normal function.

Intestinal microfauna may be harvested from a healthy horse. Cecal and colonic contents, obtained at necropsy from a nonparasitized horse with a healthy gastrointestinal system, or via a cecal fistula, are the best sources of viable microfauna. Cecal or colonic ingesta should be strained through cheesecloth and 2-4 L of the filtrate given daily by stomach tube to the recipient as soon as possible after filtering to ensure viability of most microorganisms. The filtrate should be kept warm if it must be stored or transported. Multiple transfaunations may be required before normal feces are passed. Substitutes for fresh ingesta elixir are yogurt and products containing *Lactobacillus* species.

Poor response to transfaunation may indicate that the bowel lumen milieu may be too abnormal to support growth of normal fauna and flora, and that imbalances are the result of rather than the cause of the pathologic process inducing intestinal dysfunction.

Antimicrobial Therapy

Prophylactic Antimicrobials in Surgical Patients: Though use of prophylactic antimicrobials in surgical patients is controversial, use of appropriate antimicrobials is indicated in equine abdominal surgical cases because of the significant risk of bacterial contamination from anastomosis, enterotomy or devitalized bowel.[148] In addition, operative times for these cases are often long, increasing the risk of infection.

Prophylactic antimicrobials should be administered before surgery so that high tissue levels are present when contaminating bacteria arrive via surgical manipulation. Doses appropriate for treating a serious established infection should be used. The antimicrobial agent used depends largely on personal preference. Use of broad-spectrum drugs or drug combinations is recommended. One successful regimen includes procaine penicillin (20,000 IU/kg IM BID) or sodium or potassium penicillin (12,500-100,000 IU/kg IV every 4 hours) and gentamicin (Gentocin: Schering) (2-3 mg/kg IV or IM TID or QID).[149] In the absence of contamination of the abdomen at surgery, use of prophylactic antimicrobials may be discontinued in 72 hours. If significant contamination occurs, antimicrobial therapy should be continued for 5 days or longer, depending on the patient's response. Under these circumstances, metronidazole probably should be given initially PO at 15 mg/kg and then at 7.5 mg/kg QID to combat anaerobic microorganisms.

One complication of antimicrobial therapy in abdominal surgical patients is neuromuscular blockade. Aminoglycosides and other antimicrobials may cause muscular weakness and difficulty getting up in the recovery stall. Calcium salts administered intravenously may reverse the blockade at least partially. This complication may occur especially if paralytic agents are used during anesthesia.[150]

Antimicrobial Agents and Infectious Enterocolitis: Patients with acute enterocolitis, complicated by bacteremia and/or septicemia and characterized by fever, shock, leukopenia and metabolic acidosis, require vigorous antimicrobial therapy. The choice of interim broad-spectrum drugs should be based on identification of the organism most likely to cause enterocolitis in a particular clinical setting or environment. For example, likely causes of acute enterocolitis with fever and septicemia in adult horses in the midwestern United States include *Salmonella* species and *Ehrlichia risticii*. The rationale for use of appropriate antimicrobial agents in animals with acute salmonellosis is to prevent or limit bacteremia/septicemia and dissemination of organisms to other tissues. Antimicrobial agents reportedly do not affect the clinical course of the disease, nor do they limit the duration of diarrhea in horses.[151]

Antimicrobial therapy is not usually recommended for human patients with *Salmonella* gastroenteritis because such therapy may prolong the carrier state, may select for strains with potentially transferable drug resistance and may have no influence on the clinical course of the infection.[152] However, some studies have reported that antimicrobial agents may be useful in treatment of salmonellosis in people, especially when more effective drugs, such as third-generation cephalosporins and quinolones, are used.[152,153] Some authors suggest that antimicrobial therapy is clearly indicated in human patients who are severely ill or bacteremic, or in those with invasive infection by non-*typhimurium* salmonellae.[152-154]

The percentage of horses with acute salmonellosis that are bacteremic/septicemic is unknown; however, one author indicates that extraintestinal distribution of salmonellae occurs most frequently in foals less than 6 months of age and may occur occasionally in adult horses.[151] In a study of human patients infected with *Salmonella typhimurium, S enteritidis, S heidelberg* or *S orangeburg*, the incidence of septicemia was 5.2-13.7%.[155]

An appropriate choice of antimicrobial agents to administer while results of fecal cultures and titers against *Ehrlichia risticii* are pending would be penicillin and gentamicin. If many strains of gentamicin-resistant *Salmonella* are frequently isolated in the geogrpahic area, amikacin (Amiglyde-V: Bristol) given IM or IV at 6.6 mg/kg TID or QID is a good though expensive choice.[149] *In-vitro* susceptibility testing of 7 equine isolates of *Salmonella typhimurium* against trimethoprim-sulfamethoxazole demonstrated that 100% of strains tested had MICs below 0.25 μg/ml. In contrast, MICs for amikacin and gentamicin that inhibited growth of 100% of the strains tested were 2 μg/ml and 1 μg/ml, respectively.[156] These findings and those from other investigations suggest that a potentiated sulfa may be useful for treating acute septicemic/bacteremic salmonellosis.[149,157] Susceptibility patterns for salmonellae may vary geographically, and *in-vitro* susceptibility testing always should be done as a basis for rational selection of antimicrobial agents.

Some clinicians believe that most horses with acute enterocolitis do not require antimicrobial therapy unless fever is extremely high (>105 F) and the horse has a peripheral WBC count <1000 cells/μl. These clinicians base their opinions on published recommendations that people with enteric salmonellosis should not receive antimicrobial agents and the strong clinical impression that withholding antimicrobial therapy has made little difference in the severity or duration of the disease in horses. Unfortunately, there have been no controlled clinical trials to support this contention.

High titers to *E risticii* in a horse with acute enterocolitis, fever and septicemia and from an epizootic area warrant consideration of changing antimicrobial therapy to intravenous oxytetracycline (Liquamycin 100: Pfizer). It should be noted that tetracycline therapy of horses with acute salmonellosis is contraindicated. Every effort should be made to be sure that *E risticii* is the primary problem before therapy with tetracyclines is initiated. However, it often is difficult or impossible to rule out salmonellosis in these cases. Suggested regimens for treating horses with *E risticii* infections are oxytetracycline IV at 6 mg/kg BID or at 10 mg/kg SID for 5 days. An oxytetracycline preparation that does not contain propylene glycol is recommended. Further study of Potomac horse fever under controlled laboratory conditions should soon permit documentation of the best therapeutic approach for this disease.

Proximal enteritis has been associated with both *Salmonella* and *Clostridium perfringens* infections.[158,159] Parenteral antimicrobial therapy for horses with suspected proximal enteritis initially could include penicillin and gentamicin, or penicillin and amikacin. It must be remembered, however, that horses suspected of having this disease have been treated successfully without antimicrobial agents.

In general, most horses with chronic diarrhea do not respond to antimicrobial therapy. Abnormal organisms often proliferate secondary to changes in the intestinal environment and may not be primary pathogens. Antimicrobial therapy may compound the underlying disease. Antimicrobials are not innocuous drugs, especially when used in the clinical setting of Gram-negative enteric disease. Oxytetracycline and ampicillin sodium (Amp-Equine: Beecham) have been reported to potentiate salmonellosis in people and horses.[149,160] These effects may be mediated through a change in normal gut flora. Some normal intestinal flora may produce fatty acids with bacteriostatic or bactericidal activity against salmonellae. Destruction of normal flora by antimicrobial administration allows more resistant pathogens to proliferate. In an outbreak of salmonellosis in a pediatric ward, physicians concluded that transmission of the organism was facilitated by previous use of an antimicrobial to which the organism was resistant.[160] Reestablishment of normal flora may be an important mechanism in clearing the gut of pathogens.[161]

Antimicrobial agents also tend to promote emergence of resistant strains of bacteria. Gram-negative enteric bacteria may develop drug resistance by transfer of a resistance factor from one Gram-negative bacterium to another of the same or a different species. Nonpathogenic bacteria also may transfer resistance to pathogens. The resistance factors may code for resistance to 1 or more antimicrobials, including sulfanilamide, streptomycin, chloramphenicol, tetracycline, neomycin, kanamycin, ampicillin, furazolidone, gentamicin and spectinomycin.[162]

Resistant bacteria proliferate unchallenged when antimicrobials suppress growth of sensitive organisms. Ample opportunity exists for transfer of resistance from one bacterium to another in the gut lumen. For example, data from one study indicated that resistant strains of *Salmonella* may appear after a week of antimicrobial treatment.

Antifungal Therapy

Fungal diseases of the intestinal tract are rare in horses. The most commonly used antifungal drugs have historically been amphotericin B (Fungizone: Squibb) and nystatin (Mycostatin: Squibb). The toxicity of amphotericin B is well known. Nystatin is used only topically. Newer antifungal drugs tend to have a narrow spectrum of action; therefore, accurate diagnosis is essential for selection of an appropriate agent. Recommendations for drug selection and dosage for treating fungal enteritides have been based on drug use in fungal ophthalmic disease.

Antitoxic Therapy

Gastrointestinal diseases caused by heavy-metal poisoning, enterotoxigenic bacteria or endotoxins may require treatment with antitoxic drugs. For example, the specific antidote for inorganic arsenic intoxication, dimercaprol (BAL: Westcott and Dunning), may be beneficial in some cases. Bismuth subsalicylate has antienterotoxic effects in toxigenic *Escherichia coli* infections in people.[163,164] This compound may be useful in treatment of some causes of diarrhea in foals and as empiric therapy in acute diarrhea of adult horses. Salicylate-containing preparations should be used with care in sick, stressed foals and should be withdrawn if clinical signs typical of gastroduodenal ulceration develop. Prostaglandins E and F may be mediators of fluid secretion in some diarrheal diseases, such as secretory diarrheas associated with cholera in people.[165,166] Thus, it has been proposed that cyclo-oxygenase inhibitors, such as flunixin and aspirin, may help control some secretory diarrheal diseases in horses. The mechanism for an antidiarrheal effect of such drugs has yet to be elucidated.

Studies of experimental endotoxemia in horses suggest that systemic absorption of endotoxin from compromised bowel may account for some of the pathophysiologic changes associated with strangulation obstructions and nonstrangulating infarctions. Pretreatment of horses subjected to experimental endotoxemia with flunixin meglumine (1 mg/kg IV) moderated the clinical signs and many of the pathophysiologic effects of endotoxemia.[62] Pretreatment of horses challenged with endotoxin with flunixin meglumine (0.25 mg/kg) attenuated or alleviated signs of colic and reduced endotoxin-mediated lactic acidosis.[167] In the clinical setting, treatment of potentially endotoxic horses with strangulating obstruction, nonstrangulating infarction or toxic enterocolitis using flunixin seems warranted. Use of a low dosage of flunixin (0.25 mg/kg IV BID or TID) is advantageous, especially in dehydrated horses and foals, which are particularly at risk to develop renal papillary necrosis or gut mucosal ulceration secondary to nonsteroidal antiinflammatory drug therapy.

Treatment of endotoxemia in horses has been modified in recent years by the availability of an antiserum preparation (Endoserum: IMMVAC) directed against the endotoxin portion of a mutant *Salmonella*. This antiserum contains antibodies against the core antigen portion of the endotoxin molecule that is similar between various Gram-negative bacteria. Use of the preparation has reduced mortality in horses with clinical evidence of endotoxemia.[168] Using a different preparation with antibodies directed against the J5 mutant of *E coli*, significant improvements in the survival rate and clinical appearance, and shortening of the length of hospitalization have been reported recently.[169] Additional controlled clinical and experimental studies are needed to assess the efficacy of this form of treatment.

Heparin: Heparin (Elkins-Sinn) is thought to facilitate hepatic clearance of endotoxin from the bloodstream. In patients with acute enterocolitis or those recovering from surgery for strangulating obstruction or nonstrangulating infarction, endotoxin may be absorbed from compromised bowel and small doses of heparin may be beneficial. The drug may be given SC at 40 U/kg BID or at higher dosages of 100-150 U/kg to inhibit thrombin.[170]

Immunotherapy

It has been suggested that chronic diarrhea may be associated with immunodeficiency or an inappropriate immune response.[171] Accordingly, intragastric administration of large doses of serum taken from normal horses has been advocated in treatment of horses with chronic diarrhea.[172] The efficacy of this therapy has not been substantiated. Immunosuppressive therapy is recommended as a treatment for chronic granulomatous enteritis and nonspecific chronic diarrhea. Use of dexamethasone (Azium: Schering) or prednisolone acetate has been recommended.[173] Some horses respond to immunosuppressive therapy but may relapse when treatment is stopped. Successful treatment with combinations of ivermectin and dexamethasone in 2 cases of diarrhea caused by immature small strongyles has been reported.[146]

It is difficult to decide when to use immunotherapy, as little is known about the pathogenesis of chronic diarrhea. Immunosuppressive therapy often is used empirically after other treatments have failed. This approach seems justified in selected cases where infectious disease has been ruled out.

Principles of Abdominal Surgery

S.B. Adams

Abdominal surgery often is performed as a diagnostic procedure or for therapy on horses with diseases of the gastrointestinal tract. Abdominal approaches, systematic abdominal exploration, methods of enterotomy, methods of resection and anastomosis, and abdominal closure are common to many of these surgeries. Ventral midline laparotomy has become the standard surgical approach for horses exhibiting colic. This approach provides the best overall exposure to the abdominal contents. Exploratory flank laparotomies are performed less frequently than midline laparotomies. Flank laparotomies are used for evaluation of the abdominal contents in horses with chronic colic, chronic diarrhea, weight loss or abdominal masses. Flank laparotomies provide less exposure to the abdominal contents than the ventral midline approach but can be performed on standing horses following sedation and local anesthesia of the flank. Palpation of most of the intestinal tract, the spleen, kidneys and liver is possible via flank laparotomy. Biopsies may be taken of jejunum, large colon, small colon and cecum.

Indications for Surgery in Horses Exhibiting Colic

Prompt institution of surgery is desirable for horses with colic caused by volvulus, torsions, infarction, strangulation/obstruction, malposition of bowel, intussusceptions, enteroliths, fecaliths and other diseases of the intestine that do not respond to medical therapy alone. Deciding to perform surgery may be difficult. Horses with diseases not requiring surgical therapy may have clinical signs suggesting that surgery is necessary. Medical diseases that cause horses to exhibit signs suggesting surgery is necessary include duodenitis-proximal jejunitis, peritonitis, ileus, primary gastric dilatation and endotoxemia. By comparison, some horses with surgical diseases show few indications that surgery is necessary.

The decision for surgery should be based on information obtained from a complete medical history, a physical examination and laboratory evaluation of blood and abdominal fluid.[7] There is no one pathognomonic sign or criterion that consistently indicates which horses need surgery. However, certain clinical signs and laboratory values strongly suggest that surgery is necessary. When doubt still exists after thorough evaluation as to whether surgery is necessary, laparotomy should be considered as a diagnostic procedure. A veterinarian should err on the side of surgery to avoid allowing horses with surgical diseases to die. This approach occasionally leads to surgery on horses with nonsurgical lesions. These horses usually survive. Prolonged delay in performing surgery on horses with surgical lesions may prove fatal.

Determining whether to perform surgery on horses with colic may be approached from 2 perspectives: the indications for surgery and the contraindications for surgery (Table 13). Interpretation of all available data by experienced clinicians usually results in proper selection of horses requiring surgery. Repeated examinations of horses with unresolved colic may be necessary to determine trends. All data should be recorded for later reference. The reader is cautioned that these are only guidelines; exceptions exist for each listed indication and contraindication for surgery. Following is a brief discussion of indicators that can be used for selection of horses requiring surgery.

Onset and Course of Disease: Sudden onset of colic with severe pain and rapid systemic deterioration suggests a surgical lesion within the abdomen. Horses with normal pulse rates and respiratory rates and good cardiovascular function generally do not have complete bowel obstructions, infarction, strangulation or strangulation-obstruction of bowel.

Rectal Temperature: Most horses with colic requiring surgery have a rectal temperature of ≤ 38.5 C, unless physical activity and high ambient temperature cause hyperthermia. Subnormal rectal temperature has been associated with shock, cardiovascular collapse, and poor perfusion of blood to the skin and extremities. Horses with hypothermia often have cold, sweaty skin and limbs. Rectal temperature >38.5 C, not caused by physical activity or high

Table 13. Guidelines for surgical intervention in horses with colic.

Indications for Surgery

- Persistent pain refractory to analgesics
- Sudden onset
- Rapid deterioration in condition
- Refractory to medical therapy
- Severe abdominal distention
- Absence of intestinal sounds
- Persistent gastric reflux
- Abnormalities detected on rectal examination
- Bloody or serosanguineous abdominal fluid

Contraindications for Surgery

- Rectal temperature >39.5 C
- Loud, frequent intestinal sounds
- Leukopenia (WBC <4000/μl)
- Pain controlled by mild analgesics
- No abnormalities on rectal examination
- Abdominal fluid with WBC count >100,000/μl, normal RBC count and nondegenerate neutrophils

ambient temperature, suggests infectious disease. Surgery is contraindicated.

Pain and Analgesics: Unrelenting pain most often is caused by mesenteric traction, ischemia or strangulation of the bowel. These conditions usually are associated with diseases requiring surgical treatment. Spasmodic colic, flatulent colic, impactions, enteritis and most other causes of colic not requiring surgical intervention usually cause intermittent pain. Though ischemia is painful, once the affected bowel is completely infarcted, pain subsides. Failure of flunixin meglumine or butorphanol to relieve abdominal pain suggests surgery is necessary. Xylazine or detomidine usually is effective for relief of pain caused by torsion, volvulus, strangulation-obstruction and other surgical conditions, but the duration of action may be 30 minutes or less. The need for frequently repeated doses of analgesics suggests surgery is necessary for correction of the disease.

Severe Abdominal Distention: Abdominal distention in adult horses is usually caused by accumulation of gas in the large colon, cecum or abdominal cavity. Gas accumulates within bowel secondary to adynamic ileus, bowel obstruction, strangulation-obstruction or ingestion of highly fermentable feedstuffs. Gas within the abdominal cavity almost always is the result of ruptured bowel. Infrequently, distention of the jejunum causes bloat in mature horses. Distention of the jejunum often causes bloat or abdominal distention in foals because of a thinner abdominal wall and smaller abdominal cavity in relation to the volume of the jejunum. Severe abdominal distention may compromise respiration as well as perfusion to the affected bowel. Severe abdominal distention in the absence of flatus indicates surgical intervention is likely needed. Bloated horses passing gas often recover from colic without surgery.

Intestinal Sounds: Complete absence of borborygmi suggests infarction or other irreversible morphologic damage to the bowel. Adynamic ileus also may cause a lack of borborygmi, though primary ileus causing colic is uncommon. Intestinal sounds should be assessed in horses exhibiting shock and pain after fluids and analgesics have been administered. High sympathetic tone from pain and poor perfusion from shock may suppress intestinal motility in

otherwise healthy bowel. Horses in which borborygmi return after treatment usually are not candidates for surgery. Xylazine and detomidine can suppress intestinal motility and may be a cause of reduced borborygmi when given frequently and in large doses.

Nasogastric Intubation: Reflux of ≥ 4 L of fluid upon intubation of the stomach is abnormal unless the horse has ingested water very recently. Continued reflux suggests obstruction of the stomach or small intestine. Many diseases causing reflux of fluid require surgery. Though continuous gastric reflux is a strong indicator for surgery, this clinical sign should not be used alone to justify surgery. Horses with duodenitis-proximal jejunitis or adynamic ileus often exhibit profuse gastric reflux and may respond to nonsurgical therapy.

Rectal Examination: The rectal examination is extremely useful for determining which horses require surgery. Specific abnormalities that are diagnostic for surgical diseases often are palpable. The decision to perform surgery may be based solely on rectal examination. Abnormalities include left dorsal displacement of the large colon, strangulation-obstruction of the ileum or jejunum in the inguinal canal, enterolithiasis, ileal impactions, intussusceptions, and some large colon displacements. At other times, rectal examination may provide supporting evidence that surgery is required. Abnormalities that support surgery include identification of taut painful mesenteric bands, distended small or large intestine, and nonspecific abdominal masses.

Abdominocentesis: Analysis of abdominal fluid is very useful for determining the necessity of surgery. Abdominal fluid with a serosanguineous or orange color or a total protein concentration >3.5 g/dl is an indication for surgery. Infarction of intestine often causes color changes of abdominal fluid from yellow to pink or red. Green fluid indicates the presence of ingesta; if enterocentesis has not been performed, rupture of bowel likely has occurred. Ruptured bowel also may result in roughened peritoneal surfaces that can be felt on rectal examination.

Abdominal fluid cell counts are useful in determining when surgery is indicated. In a retrospective study, surgery was necessary in 78% of all horses with a red blood cell (RBC) count >20,000 cells/μl.[40] Ischemic, infarcted or strangulated bowel usually elevates the abdominal fluid white blood cell (WBC) count. However, when the WBC count is elevated in the absence of an elevated RBC count, nonsurgical diseases such as peritonitis and enteritis, should be considered. Cytologic examination of abdominal fluid is particularly useful to evaluate the morphology of neutrophils and to determine if bacteria are present. Degenerative changes in neutrophils are caused by toxin-producing microorganisms. Masses of extracellular bacteria of varying morphology are a contraindication for surgery because abdominal cavity contamination is high and survival of the horse is unlikely even if diseased bowel can be resected.

Peripheral Blood Values: The white blood cell count of peripheral blood in horses with colic caused by diseases requiring surgical intervention often is normal or slightly elevated. Nonsurgical diseases, such as enteritis or peritonitis, often cause mild to severe leukopenia. The packed cell volume, anion gap and blood lactate levels differ between groups of horses requiring surgery and those requiring only medical care. However, on an individual basis, these values cannot be used to select surgery or medical care.[174]

Systemic Deterioration: Systemic deterioration in the face of aggressive medical therapy is an indication for surgical intervention. Trends in results of tests that evaluate systemic condition are extremely important. Horses that steadily deteriorate are candidates for exploratory laparotomy when a definitive diagnosis has not been made. However, continued systemic deterioration should not be relied upon as the only indication for surgery. Surgeons who rely on this indication for surgery will find that many horses are too ill to survive the surgical procedure once the decision has been made to perform surgery.

Prognosis for Horses with Colic

Numerous indices can be used individually or in combination to predict survival of horses exhibiting colic before surgery. The ability to predict the outcome has certain advantages to the surgeon and the client. Horses with a very poor probability of survival can be euthanized before expenditure of large amounts of time or money. Practi-cally, however, many owners want to pursue treatment despite a poor prognosis and high costs.

The measurement of serum lactic acid levels was one of the first valuess used to predict survival.[175] This determination seems to be suitable for a prognostic indicator. Blood lactate levels >25 mEq/L indicate a grave prognosis for survival.[176] Other individual values that indicate a poor prognosis are listed in Table 14. Generally, variables that assess cardiovascular function are good prognostic guides.[177] Prediction equations that combine multiple values in an attempt to improve accuracy have been devised. Combined assessment of systolic pressure, hematocrit and blood lactate, and urea nitrogen levels, resulted in a correct prediction of survival in 93% of horses examined.[3] Routine determination of these 4 values is not possible in many practices. However, evaluation of routine clinical values and simple laboratory data comprising the hematocrit, total protein level and color of abdominal fluid also can provide an accurate prognosis for survival.[178] Experienced clinicians often determine an accurate prognosis following physical examination without the use of such formulae.

Observations at the time of surgery may also be used to predict survival. Observation of extensive small intestinal or large intestinal necrosis warrants a poor prognosis. Horses with obstructed or strangulated-obstructed small intestine with mean intraluminal bowel pressures of ≥10 cm of water proximal to the obstruction have a poor prognosis for survival.[53] A poor prognosis also is warranted when histologic examination of bowel proximal and distal to a primary lesion reveals significant mucosal damage.[56]

Table 14. Findings indicating a poor prognosis for survival of horses with colic.

- Marked mental depression
- Capillary refill time >4 seconds
- No palpable facial artery pulse
- Heart rate >100 beats per minute
- Hematocrit >60%
- Venous hemoglobin >13 g/dl
- Systolic blood pressure <70 mm Hg
- Venous blood pH <7.2
- Venous blood lactate >100 mg/dl
- Anion gap >25 mEq/L
- Decreased plasma antithrombin III
- Prolonged thrombin clotting time

Exploratory Laparotomy

Ventral Midline Laparotomy: The ventral midline abdominal incision is the most common approach for abdominal exploration in horses. It provides good exposure to the abdominal contents and facilitates exploration and manipulation of the intestinal tract. Many sections of the gastrointestinal tract can be exteriorized through a ventral midline incision (Fig 14). The ventral midline incision can be made very rapidly because major nerves and vessels are avoided. The incision can extend from the xiphoid to the pubis in nonlactating female horses by splitting the mammary gland on midline. In male horses, the ventral midline can extend from the sheath to the xiphoid. Rarely does a ventral midline incision need to be longer than 40 cm.

Closure of the ventral midline incision is technically easy and can be done rapidly but must be done with proper suture selection and placement. The ventral midline incision must withstand the weight of the viscera in the standing horse and large stresses occurring during movement, defecation and coughing. Postoperative hernias and dehiscence occur with inadequate closure. The most common cause of hernias, however, is postoperative infection.

Exploratory laparotomy via the ventral midline incision is performed with the horse anesthetized and positioned in dorsal recumbency. Following routine surgical skin preparation and draping, a 25-cm incision is made through the skin, subcutaneous tissue and linea alba, starting at the umbilicus and

Figure 14. Sections of the intestinal tract that can be exteriorized through a ventral midline incision (shaded gray).

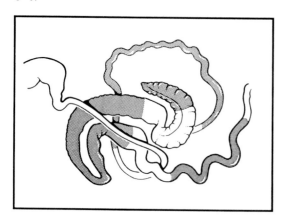

extending cranially, with care taken to stay on midline. The midline can be identified in obese horses at the level of the umbilicus. A finger inserted through the incision to the inside of the body wall then can be used to identify the linea alba. Extreme caution should be observed when entering the abdomen not to perforate greatly distended loops of bowel that may be pushed tightly against the peritoneum. Horses that are bloated present the greatest risk of this complication. Once the linea alba has been incised, the retroperitoneal fat and peritoneum can be perforated with a finger and bluntly separated, or they can be tented up to the incision with thumb forceps and incised with blunt-blunt scissors.

Before abdominal exploration, the incised edges of the body wall can be protected with a plastic barrier drape, and the abdomen should be covered with an impervious drape to prevent soaking through of contaminated fluids. The barrier drape has a ring that expands within the abdomen to hold the drape in place. When the barrier drape is in place, the surgeon can pass contaminated loops of bowel through the incision without contamination of the body wall. The drape reduces the incidence of postoperative incisional infection. No towel clamps or other instruments should be exposed in the operating field once draping is complete so as to avoid damage to exteriorized bowel or misplacement of instruments into the abdominal cavity.

Evaluation of the Abdominal Cavity[179]: Soiling of the abdomen with ingesta noted upon incising the peritoneum indicates a grave prognosis for survival of the horse, and further surgery is unwarranted. Distended jejunum, cecum or large colon often balloons out of the incision. A 12- or 14-ga needle attached to rubber tubing with one end passed out of the surgical field may be used to remove the gas. This facilitates further exploration of the abdomen. Suction on the rubber tubing hastens removal of large quantities of gas (Fig 15). A pursestring suture of 1-0 chromic gut or other absorbable material is placed around the needle and tied after the needle has been withdrawn. The contaminated shaft of the needle should not be touched by the surgeon. The needle should be placed on an isolated area of the surgical table if it is to be used again.

If the needle will not be used again, it is best to discard it. Ideally, a sterile needle is used for each decompression.

The cause of colic may be apparent immediately. If not, exploration deeper in the abdominal cavity is undertaken. The surgeon should wear impervious shoulder length gloves or impervious gown sleeves to prevent from soaking through of contaminating fluids. The abdomen should be explored by gently sweeping the viscera with a hand. Hard masses, turgid loops of intestine, tight mesenteric bands, roughened peritoneal surfaces and fibrous adhesions should be noted. The root of the mesentery and attachments of the cecum and colon should be palpated for volvulus; when present, the direction of any twist is noted. At this point, if the problem has not been identified, a systematic exploration of the intestinal tract is done using the cecum as a reference point (Fig 16). Exteriorized bowel should be kept moist.

Normally the cecum is found slightly to the right of midline and can be exteriorized easily through a ventral midline incision. The cecum often distends with gas from obstruction distal to it. The cecum may be empty when small intestine is obstructed. The cecum should be checked for proper orientation using the cecal bands for reference. The cecocolic fold attaches the cecum to the right ventral colon (Fig 17). This fold should be located on the right side of the cecum. Displacements of the cecum or colon may alter the location of the cecocolic fold.

Figure 15. Removal of gas from the cecum using suction. A 14-ga needle is attached to a rubber tube, which is hooked to the vacuum machine.

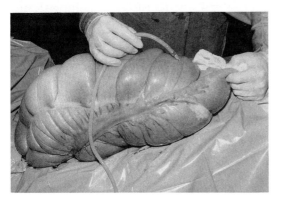

Figure 16. Scheme of abdominal exploration, using the cecum as a reference point.

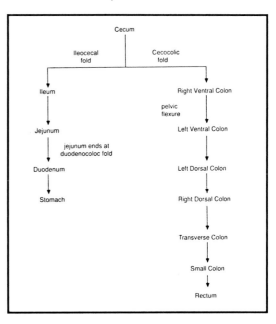

The cecum can be retroverted to expose the dorsal longitudinal band on the lesser curvature. This band extends to the apex of the cecum and has no arteries or veins. The dorsal band is continuous with the ileocecal fold and the antimesenteric ileal fold. The ileocecal junction can be identified by following the dorsal band toward the base of the cecum. In most horses, the ileocecal valve and the most distal part of the ileum cannot be exteriorized through a ventral midline incision. The surgeon should palpate the distal ileum and trace proximally until it can be exteriorized. The ileum is thick and muscular, and has an antimesenteric band and a marginal ileal artery that does not form vascular arches (Fig 18).

The jejunum can be palpated by following the ileum proximally. The jejunum has characteristic vascular arches (Fig 19). Obstructions and other diseases of the jejunum are identified by systematically tracing the jejunum proximally. The jejunum can be exteriorized and palpated to the junction of the duodenum. This junction can be identified by palpating the antimesenteric duodenocolic fold, which is a fibrous band connecting the distal duodenum to the proximal small colon. The surgeon should be able to trace the entire jejunum from ileum to duodenocolic fold without encountering

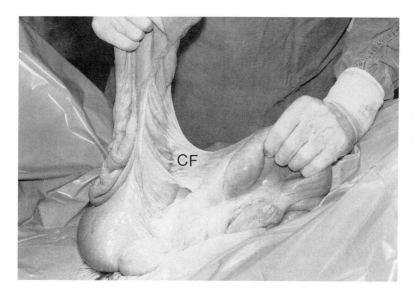

Figure 17. The cecum is exteriorized and retroverted to identify the cecocolic fold (CF). This fold is used to determine the correct position of the cecum and right ventral colon.

fibrous bands, obstructions, rents in mesentery or other anatomic barriers.

Next, the duodenum is traced caudally around the base of the cecum and the root of the mesentery to the right side of the abdomen. The duodenum is the only small intestine that normally is located in the area between the right dorsal colon and body wall as it passes cranially along the liver to the pylorus. The duodenum is traced cranially to the sigmoid flexure and the stomach is palpated for abnormalities. The short mesoduodenum and short attachments of the stomach and pylorus prevent these structures from being exteriorized through

a ventral midline incision. The epiploic foramen lies at the root of the mesoduodenum along the caudate process of the right liver lobe. This foramen is bordered by the hepatoduodenal ligament, caudal vena cava and portal vein. Specific palpation of the epiploic foramen is unnecessary if all bowel is identified and found not to enter the foramen.

The cecum is located again and used as the reference point to examine the large colon. The cecocolic fold is continuous with the lateral band of the cecum and should be located next to the right abdominal wall when properly positioned. The right ventral

Figure 18. The ileum has a marginal artery that runs parallel to the bowel, and an antimesenteric fold (IF). The antimesenteric fold is continuous with the dorsal band of the cecum.

Figure 19. The jejunum has characteristic vascular arcades formed by the anastomosing jejunal arteries.

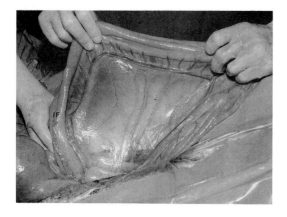

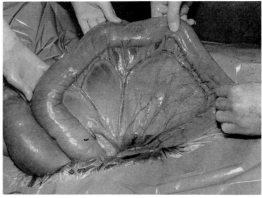

colon, sternal flexure, left ventral colon, pelvic flexure, left dorsal colon, diaphragmatic flexure and right dorsal colon are evaluated in sequence. The large colon is checked for obstructions, torsions and displacements. The left colon often must be exteriorized to reposition twisted or displaced bowel and to perform enterotomies to remove gas and ingesta. The surgeon should place the colon back into the abdominal cavity in the proper position when the examination is complete.

The right dorsal colon becomes much smaller in diameter as it merges with the transverse colon. The transverse colon crosses the dorsal abdomen cranial to the great mesentery and continues caudally as the small colon. The transverse colon is a common site of impactions and obstructions by enteroliths because of its small diameter relative to that of the right dorsal colon. The right dorsal, transverse and proximal small colons cannot be exteriorized but should be evaluated thoroughly by palpation. Finally, the small colon, identified by sacculations and formed fecal balls within the lumen, is examined. Most of the small colon can be exteriorized. The surgeon should palpate the caudal small colon and rectum for abnormalities, as these segments of bowel cannot be exteriorized.

Rapid and complete systematic examination of the intestinal tract can be performed using the cecum as the reference point. However, the cecum may not be in its proper position and the surgeon may not be able to exteriorize the body and apex. Displacement of the cecum most often occurs in association with volvulus or displacement of the large colon. Volvulus of the cecum and large colon close to the mesenteric route is not uncommon and usually occurs in a counterclockwise direction as the surgeon looks upon the ventral midline of the anesthetized horse. The surgeon should identify the left colon and pelvic flexure when the cecum cannot be exteriorized. The left colon should be exteriorized and the direction of the volvulus or displacement determined by following the colons back into the abdomen and to the cecum. After reduction of the colonic displacement, the cecum should return to its normal position. The surgeon should check to be sure the cecocolic ligament, cecum and right ventral colon have the proper orientation. At this point, the systematic examination already described, using the cecum as a reference point, can be initiated.

Correcting Intestinal Diseases Causing Colic

Numerous problems of the gastrointestinal tract can be encountered during colic surgery and must be corrected. Correction of intestinal disease causing colic may require 1 or more of the following procedures: decompression of gas, fluid or ingesta; manual fragmentation of impactions or fecaliths; reposition of displaced bowel; removal of foreign bodies, enteroliths or fecaliths; resection of diseased bowel; and bypass of diseased bowel.

Decompression: Obstruction of the intestines, particularly the large colon, often results in accumulation of gas and/or fluids proximal to the obstruction. Gas and fluid may need to be removed to reposition displaced bowel. Decompression of distended bowel can reduce postoperative complications. Decompression reduces intraluminal pressures that may promote capillary perfusion, removes toxic fluids, can facilitate respiratory ventilation by reducing abdominal pressure and can reduce postoperative ileus.[180-182] Gas evacuation is commonly performed by needle enterocentesis. A rubber tube is attached to the needle to prevent contamination of the surgical field. In many horses with large colon displacements, this is the only procedure necessary before repositioning of the bowel. The gas and fluid in mild to moderately distended jejunum may be massaged or milked into the cecum by digital manipulation. Markedly distended jejunum may require enterotomy for removal of gas and fluids. Enterotomy is necessary for removal of gas and ingesta from the cecum and large colon.

Elimination of Impactions and Fecaliths by Digital Manipulation: Impactions of the stomach, ileum, pelvic flexure, transverse colon and small colon may be fragmented manually without enterotomy in some horses. This procedure requires good judgment by the surgeon. Massage that is too vigorous may result in rupture of the bowel. Large impactions usually do not respond to manual reduction. Fecaliths of the small colon, common in Miniature Horses, may be fragmented with digital pressure and lavaged out of the small colon with a high enema.

Flushing Water Through the Bowel Lumen: Lavaging the small colon with water via a tube or hose passed per rectum can help reduce and eliminate impactions and fecaliths of the small colon. Often this technique is used in combination with digital manipulation. Bowel lavage also can be used to retrograde flush large enteroliths or impacted feed material from the transverse colon back into the right dorsal colon, where enterotomy can be performed for removal of the ingesta or enterolith.[183] Flushing the bowel per rectum requires an assistant to pass a stomach tube or hose into the rectum. The tube should be guided through the small colon by the surgeon to prevent perforation of the bowel. Flow rates of water must be kept low to prevent overdistention of the small colon. A tube for flushing water also may be passed through an enterotomy into the large colon to help remove extensive accumulations of dry ingesta that otherwise would be difficult to massage through the enterotomy site.

Repositioning of Bowel: Large colon displacement, torsions and volvulus are common and are corrected by repositioning the bowel into a normal position. A working knowledge of normal anatomy is necessary to properly reposition bowel.

Enterotomy: Enterotomies are performed to remove foreign bodies, enteroliths, fecaliths, trichobezoars, phytobezoars, gas, fluid and ingesta from the lumen of bowel (Fig 20). Numerous enterotomy techniques have been used. Mastery of a few basic techniques allows the surgeon to perform enterotomies in any section of the bowel. The bowel in which enterotomy is being performed should be exteriorized and isolated from the rest of the abdomen with impervious drapes or sterile towels.

Enterotomies are commonly performed in the jejunum, cecum, large colon and small colon. In the jejunum, enterotomy is performed on the antimesenteric side. Enterotomy commonly is performed on the apex of the cecum, which is positioned to the right side of the horse so ingesta flows away from the surgical site. Enterotomies often are performed at the pelvic flexure of the large colon but also may be performed in the left ventral, left dorsal or right dorsal colon in sections that can be pulled off to

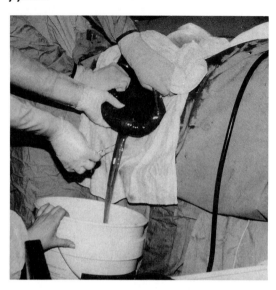

Figure 20. Decompression of fluid from distended jejunum.

one side of the abdomen. A special colon tilt table can be used to hold the left colons for pelvic flexure enterotomy. This table allows the contaminated enterotomy site to be kept away from the abdomen and the incline allows ingesta to flow out of the surgical field (Figs 21, 22). Enterotomies of the large colon should be made on the antimesenteric side over a haustrum. Enterotomies of the small colon should be performed through the antimesenteric band. All enterotomy incisions should be longitudinal in orientation to reduce stricture of the bowel lumen following closure.

Copious lavage of the contaminated edges of incised bowel should be performed before closure. All enterotomies can be closed safely with a 2-layer technique. The first layer of this closure is performed with a simple-continuous suture pattern. The suture bites incorporate the full thickness of the incised edge of the bowel. Copious lavage with sterile fluids is recommended following the first layer of the closure. The second part of the 2-layer closure is performed with a continuous Cushing, Connell or Lembert pattern that inverts the incision (Fig 23). The 2-layer continuous closure pattern is fast and results in minimal stricture of the bowel lumen because only 1 layer is inverted. The advantage to minimal inversion in the cecum or colon is negligible, however, because of the large lumen size. Two-layer closures with inverting patterns

Figure 21. The large colon is placed on a colon table. Enterotomy at the pelvic flexure may be performed away from the abdominal incision and open abdominal cavity.

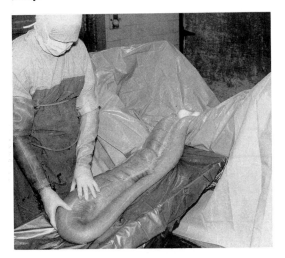

Figure 22. This devitalized large colon is positioned for enterotomy and removal of ingesta. Emptying the colon facilitates correction of certain large colon displacements.

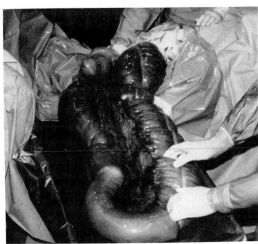

in both suture lines can be used successfully in the cecum and colon. Closure of enterotomies often is done with absorbable suture material, such as polyglycolic acid, polyglactin 910 or polydioxanone. The first layer is closed with 2-0 material and the second layer is closed with 1-0 material. Nonabsorbable suture material, such as 1-0 prolene, can be used for the second layer of the enterotomy closure in the small colon. This section of intestine may be slower to heal due to increased collagenase activity, the high degree of contamination from luminal bacteria and the presence of solid ingesta.

Gastrotomies are uncommon and should be performed only when decompression is absolutely necessary and cannot be performed via a nasogastric tube. In horses, the stomach cannot be exteriorized and must be well isolated with sterile laparotomy drapes before incision. Gastrotomy can be performed midway between the greater and lesser curvature, parallel to the gastric vessels. Closure of gastrotomies is the same as for segments of bowel.

Resection and Anastomosis: The principles for intestinal resection and anastomosis are the same for all segments of the intestinal tract. The anastomotic area should be isolated from the abdominal incision and from other segments of bowel with drapes to reduce contamination. Draping reduces

the incidence of postoperative incisional infections and peritonitis. Contamination and trauma at the site of the anastomosis should be kept to a minimum. The anastomosis should be performed on viable bowel, and the surgeon should use handling and suturing techniques that maintain good blood supply. The most common cause of

Figure 23. Closure of an enterotomy with a 2-layer continuous suture pattern. A full-thickness simple-continuous patter (A) is placed and tied, and a Cushing pattern is used as an oversew (B).

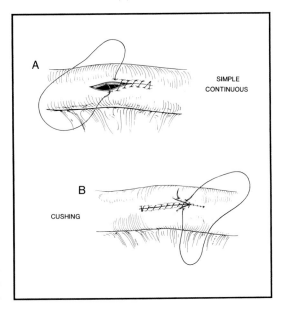

anastomotic failure in people is inadequate blood flow to the resected ends of the bowel. The submucosa should be incorporated in the closure of the anastomosis and the surgeon should avoid placing sutures under tension. Bowel must be carefully apposed on the mesenteric side. Accurate apposition of cut edges of the bowel may be difficult in this area. Mucosa should not evert through the incision with inverting patterns, as leakage of ingesta may occur. All closures should be tight enough to be impervious to water or liquid ingesta immediately after suturing. Mesenteric defects created by resection of bowel should be closed.[182,184]

Bowel that is nonviable or has a high likelihood of becoming nonviable due to ischemia or severe inflammation should be resected. In some horses, clinical assessment of bowel may be satisfactory for determining what areas must be resected. Bowel that is grossly discolored, lacks reflex contraction when pinched, has no pulsation in the mesenteric vessels, has dark hemorrhagic mucosa, or has very friable mesentery should be resected. Not all nonviable bowel has gross changes indicating resection is necessary. The decision to resect may be difficult. A pink color, muscular contractions and perfusion may be evident following correction of strangulating-obstructing lesions in bowel that will become nonviable. This delayed damage may be due to reperfusion injury. Intravenous fluorescein administration, surface oximetry and Doppler flow probes have been used to predict bowel viability. These methods evaluate perfusion at the time of surgery. However, perfusion is not always a good indicator of viability or survivability of bowel. The current approach by many surgeons is to evaluate the bowel grossly for viability and, when in doubt, resect the bowel if technically possible.

Mechanically, it is possible to resect all bowel that can be exteriorized through the abdominal incision (Fig 14). However, there are physiologic limits to the amount of small intestine that can be removed. Ponies with up to 40% of their small intestine resected were able to maintain body weight, whereas those with 60% of the small intestine resected lost weight.[139] Clinical experience with natural disease in horses also indicates that resection of more than 40% of the total length of the small intestine is usu-

ally unsuccessful. Resection of cecum or large colon that can be exteriorized through a ventral midline laparotomy is feasible and does not result in the horse's becoming nutritionally crippled.

Bowel to be resected should be exteriorized and isolated from the rest of the surgical field with moist drapes or towels. Impervious laparotomy sheets prevent soaking through of bacteria from contaminated areas to clean areas. These impervious sheets can be split and used to encircle the section of bowel to be resected. Resection of the jejunum is started by placing intestinal occlusion clamps adjacent to the diseased segment to confine ingesta and toxins to that segment. Ingesta is massaged away from the diseased segments for a distance of 30 cm proximal and distal to the proposed site of resection, and the bowel is clamped with noncrushing intestinal occlusive forceps (Fig 24). Some surgeons prefer to encircle the bowel with a Penrose drain to occlude the lumen of the bowel. The occlusal clamps or Penrose drains prevent gross contamination of the surgery site with ingesta during anastomosis of the cut edges of the bowel. Mesenteric vessels supplying the segment of bowel to be resected are tied off with double ligatures of 2-0 catgut or other suitable material. The vessels should be ligated close to the bowel to leave enough mesentery to close. The resection site should be close to a major mesenteric artery to ensure a good blood supply. At the point of excision, a small defect is made in the

Figure 24. Technique for resection of jejunum. Noncrushing occlusion clamps (OC) are placed next to the diseased segment of bowel and proximal and distal to the resection sites. Intestinal resection clamps (RC) are placed at the site of resection. These clamps are placed at an angle so the antimesenteric side of the incised bowel is shorter than the mesenteric side.

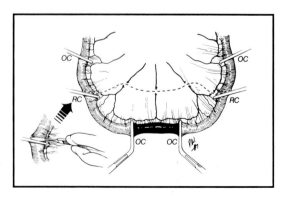

mesentery adjacent to the bowel and crushing clamps are placed at a 60-degree oblique angle to the longitudinal axis of the bowel. This makes the antimesenteric side of the bowel shorter than the mesenteric side. The oblique angle ensures good vascularity on the antimesenteric side and slightly enlarges the lumen of the anastomosis.[182] When all the clamps have been placed and all vessels are ligated, the bowel can be excised so the crushing clamp remains attached to the discarded segment of bowel.

A Parker-Kerr oversew of the ends of the remaining viable bowel may be used to close the stumps in some instances. This procedure is unnecessary if end-to-end anastomosis is anticipated. When the oversew is to be performed, 2 intestinal clamps are placed at each site of resection and the bowel is transected between the clamps. The second pair of clamps should be noncrushing. A continuous Cushing suture pattern is placed over the clamps on the healthy bowel left in the horse. As the clamps are withdrawn, the ends of the suture material are pulled taut to invert the bowel. A continuous Lembert pattern is used as an oversew and is run back to the origin of the Cushing pattern, where the suture strands are tied together (Fig 25). The Parker-Kerr oversew pattern also may be used to close the ileal stump following ileal resection.

The ileum often becomes strangulated/obstructed. Resection of the distal 8-12 inches of the ileum can be difficult with conventional techniques because exteriorization of this section of bowel through a ventral midline incision often is impossible. Two techniques can be used for management of the distal ileum when it is necrotic

Figure 25. Parker-Kerr method of oversewing the end of the jejunum or ileum.

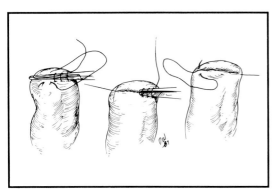

to the ileocecal valve. The ileum can be transected at the level where it is exteriorized and the distal stump oversewn by conventional hand suturing techniques. The stump is then inverted into the cecum and several blind stitches are placed over the ileocecal valve to retain the necrotic stump within the cecum. When the cecum and ileocecal valve are not edematous or thickened, a mechanical stapling device can be placed across the ileum at the junction with the cecum to close the cecum at the ileocecal valve with a double row of staples. The entire ileum is then resected. Anastomosis of jejunum to ileum is rarely performed. Most surgeons prefer jejunocecal anastomoses, even when viable ileal stump is present. The ileum lacks a good collateral blood supply and jejunoileal anastomosis may fail.

The principles for resecting the cecum or large colon are the same as for other segments of bowel, though the lumen of these segments of intestine is much larger. The major vessels in the mesocolon of the small colon or cecal bands of the cecum should be identified and ligated. Large self-retaining intestinal clamps are helpful to minimize contamination of the surgical field. Sections of cecum and large colon that can be exteriorized can be resected.

Numerous surgical techniques and suture materials are satisfactory for intestinal anastomoses. However, mastery of 3 basic techniques allows the surgeon to perform the vast majority of intestinal anastomoses necessary in horses. These techniques are the end-to-end anastomosis, side-to-side anastomosis and end-to-side anastomosis.

The *end-to-end anastomotic technique* is commonly used when bowel segments of equal diameters are being united. Anastomoses of the jejunum or the small colon are usually performed with end-to-end techniques. End-to-end anastomosis also may be performed when small sections of the left dorsal or left ventral colon are removed, making end-to-end anastomosis of nearly equal-sized segments of the remaining bowel possible. A common technique for end-to-end anastomosis is to use simple-interrupted approximating sutures in a single layer. The open ends of the bowel are held together with stay sutures at the mesenteric and antimesenteric sides, with the mesenteric sides slightly offset. The stay sutures are kept under tension to ensure that the 2 open ends have comparable diameters.[185] Sutures are placed 3-5 mm apart and 3-5 mm from the cut edge of the bowel with 2-0 or 3-0 synthetic absorbable suture material (Fig 26).

A 2-layer end-to-end anastomotic technique also may be performed by placing a simple-continuous pattern in the mucosal layer and a continuous Lembert pattern in the serosubmucosal layer. Each layer is interrupted along the circumference of the bowel every 180 degrees (Fig 27) and the first layer is interrupted at 90 degrees around the circumference from the second layer. Synthetic absorbable suture materials are satisfactory for the 2-layer continuous technique. The 2-layer technique results in minimal adhesions and no reduction in the

Figure 26. End-to-end anastomosis using simple-interrupted approximating sutures.

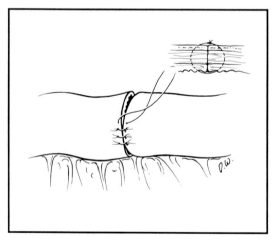

lumen of jejunojejunal anastomoses after healing is complete.[186] The serosubmucosal layer of the 2-layer end-to-end anastomosis in the small colon may be performed with a nonabsorbable monofilament material, such as prolene, which maintains strength for a long period.

Side-to-side anastomoses are used to unite bowel segments with unequal diameters or adjacent segments of the large colon that cannot be positioned end-to-end due to the short mesocolon. Some surgeons routinely use side-to-side techniques for jejunojejunal anastomoses. Side-to-side techniques are commonly used for jejunocecostomy, ileocecostomy, gastrojejunostomy, cecocolostomy and colocolostomy in horses. Side-to-side anastomoses using surgical stapling instruments are now common in horses. Stapling techniques are described in the next section.

A basic 2-layer hand suturing technique can be used for most side-to-side anastomoses. This technique is initiated by apposing the segments of bowel to be anastomosed with stay sutures. Occlusal bowel clamps or Penrose drains are placed proximal and distal to the surgical site whenever possible to prevent spillage of ingesta. The serosubmucosal layers of the 2 segments are joined with a continuous Lembert pattern using 2-0 synthetic absorbable suture material placed parallel to the longitudinal axis of the segments being joined (Fig 28). The length of the continuous Lembert pattern determines the length of the stoma and should be 8-10 cm for jejunocecostomy,

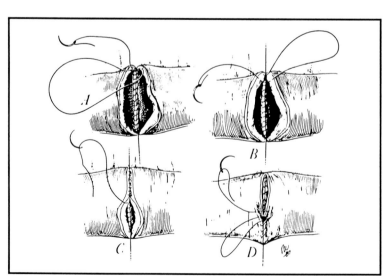

Figure 27. End-to-end anastomosis using 2-layer inverting technique. A simple-continuous pattern (A, B, C) is placed in the mucosa and interrupted one-half way around the circumference of the bowel. A continuous Lembert pattern (D) in the serosubmucosal layer completes the technique.

ileocecostomy or jejunogastrostomy, and 15-20 cm for cecocolostomy and colocolostomy. A linear incision immediately adjacent to the serosubmucosal suture line is made into the lumen of both segments of bowel and a continuous Connell pattern of 2-0 absorbable synthetic suture material is used to join the cut edges of mucosa, thus forming the stoma. Finally, the Lembert pattern in the serosubmucosa is continued around the front of the stoma, back to its origin and tied. All side-to-side anastomoses on blind loops of bowel should be performed near the end of each stump to prevent formation of blind pouches in the proximal segment that may cause postoperative complications.

End-to-side hand-sutured anastomoses may be used for jejunocecostomy in horses. The jejunum is brought into apposition with the cecum and stabilized with stay sutures. A simple-continuous pattern is used to unite the serosubmucosal layer of the jejunum to the serosubmucosal layer of the cecum on the side farthest from the surgeon. An incision into the cecum adjacent to the suture line is made 6-7 cm long. The mucosa of the jejunum and cecum is sutured together around the circumference of the jejunum to form a jejunocecal stoma. Finally, the serosubmucosal layers closest to the surgeon are sutured together to complete the anastomosis. This technique is very similar to the side-to-side technique previously described, except the lumen of the jejunum is open before anastomosis.

The cut edges of the mesentery created by resection of bowel should be sutured to adjacent mesentery or to the serosal surface of adjacent bowel to eliminate all mesenteric defects that may serve as an internal ring for strangulation-obstruction of bowel in the postoperative period. A simple-continuous pattern using small-diameter absorbable suture material is satisfactory. Following jejunocecal anastomosis, the cut edge of the jejunal mesentery is sutured to the serosa of the cecum, the dorsal cecal band, the ileocecal fold of the ileum, over the stump of the ileum and to the ileal mesentery. This technique eliminates any internal mesenteric openings.

Intestinal Stapling: Mechanical stapling instruments for suturing bowel have gained wide acceptance in human and veterinary surgery. Development of mechanical stapling instruments has been pioneered in the US by the United States Surgical Corporation. Instruments have been designed to suture skin, fascia and bowel, and to ligate and divide blood vessels (Fig 29). Mechanical suturing devices have gained popularity because techniques using the staplers are generally quicker than hand-suturing techniques, and stapler use can reduce or minimize contamination during surgical procedures.

The thoracic abdominal staplers form a double row of staples and are used to close enterotomies, close stumps of bowel and perform end-to-end anastomoses. The most popular of the these instruments for equine surgery is the TA90 or the newer TA90 Premium. These instruments form a staple line 90 mm long. The TA90 can be used to tran-

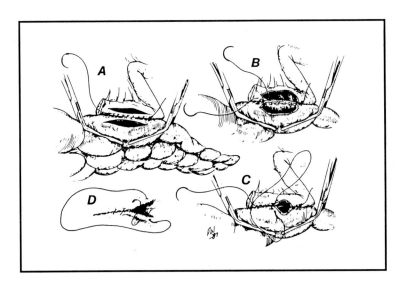

Figure 28. Side-to-side anastomosis using a 2-layer technique. The first layer (A) is a serosubmucosal suture pattern on the far side. After incision into the lumen of both segments of bowel, a continuous Connell pattern is used to form the stoma (B, C). Finally, the Lembert pattern in the seromuscularis (D) is returned to its origin and tied.

sect the ileum close to the ileocecal valve (Fig 30), provided the bowel is not thickened and edematous. Transection is difficult with conventional suturing techniques because of poor exposure of the surgical area. Multiple applications of the TA90 stapler are necessary to close the open lumen of the large colon because of the large diameter. The surgeon must be careful that the thickness of bowel does not exceed the thickness that can be adequately closed with the stapler. All stapling devices were designed for human surgery and not uncommonly the thickness of equine bowel may exceed the limits of the instruments. The TA90 may be used to perform end- to-end anastomoses using a triangulating technique that everts the mucosa. This technique has not gained wide acceptance for jejunojejunal anastomoses in horses because postoperative strictures and adhesions often form.[187] The triangulation technique for end-to-end anastomoses of the small colon using the TA90 has proven satisfactory in experimental models.[188]

The GIA (gastrointestinal stapler) instrument produces 2 double rows of staples 52 mm long and divides the tissues between the double rows of staples. The GIA stapler often is used for side-to-side anastomoses of intestine by equine surgeons. In foals or horses, gastrojejunostomy, jejunocecostomy, ileocecostomy, cecocolostomy and colocolostomy have been performed using the GIA stapler. The most common application of the GIA stapler is for jejunocecostomy in horses following resection of the ileum (Fig. 31). To perform this anastomotic technique, a cecal haustrum between the medial and dorsal cecal bands is occluded with noncrushing intestinal occlusion clamps. The jejunum also is occluded with noncrushing clamps 25-30 cm proximal to the anastomotic site to prevent spillage of ingesta. The jejunum is positioned next to the cecum and stabilized with 3 stay sutures placed about 8 cm apart. A 1-cm stab incision is made into both the jejunum and cecum, and 1 arm of the GIA instrument is inserted into the lumen of each segment of bowel. The instrument is closed and fired to place 2 staple lines and cut between them. The GIA stapler is reloaded with a new cartridge, placed back into the enterotomy with the arms facing the opposite direction and applied again. This double application ensures an ade-

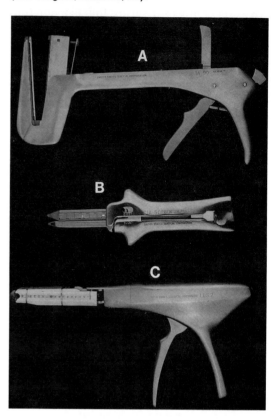

Figure 29. Stapling instruments used for intestinal surgery. A. TA 90 Premium. B. GIA Premium. C. LDS-2 (U.S. Surgical, Stamford, CT).

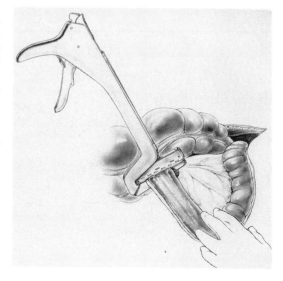

Figure 30. The TA 90 stapler can be used to place a double row of staples across the ileum before transection. (Courtesy of U.S. Surgical)

Figure 31. Side-to-side anastomosis of the jejunum and cecum using the GIA Premium stapler. A. A haustrum on the cecum is occluded with noncrushing clamps. B. Stay sutures are used to stabilize the jejunum and cecum, and a stab incision is made for insertion of the arms of the GIA stapler. C, D. The GIA stapler is used twice to provide a large stoma. The enterotomy site should then be closed perpendicular to the line of staples. E. To form a stoma with the GIA stapler, 2 double rows of staples are placed and the intervening tissue is resected. (Courtesy of U.S. Surgical)

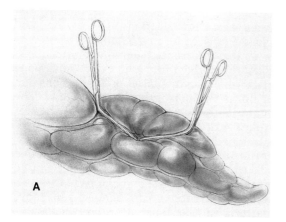

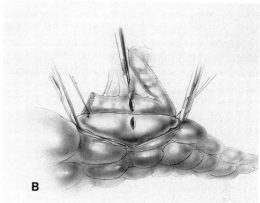

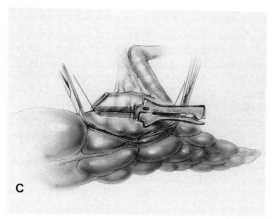

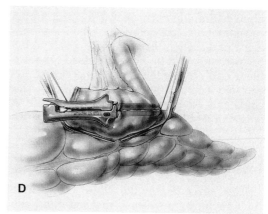

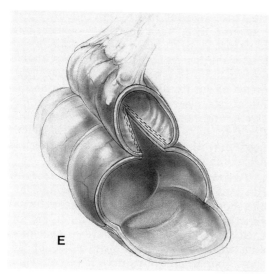

quate stoma. The surgeon should be certain that the staple lines overlap at the point of divergence.

A GIA 90 stapler has been developed that places rows of staples 90 mm long. One application of this instrument should be satisfactory for jejunojejunal or jejunocecal anastomoses. After application of the GIA stapler, the common opening into the cecum and jejunum should be closed with standard suturing methods or by application of the TA90. The common defect should be closed perpendicular to the line of staples forming the anastomosis. The line of staples is supported at each end with a stay suture placed in seromuscular layers of the cecum and jejunum, and the mesenteric defect is closed.

The LDS-2 stapler (ligate-divide stapler) is used to ligate and divide vessels in the mesentery. This instrument forms 2 crescentic staples and divides the tissues between them. Each cartridge holds multiple staples. The LDS-2 can be used for rapid division of mesenteric vessels during resection of jejunum. Reinforcement of the staple with a ligature on the proximal side of the mesentery (side to be left within the abdomen) is recommended to avoid severe hemorrhage if the staple were to slip off the vascular pedicle.

The EEA stapler (end-to-end anastomosis) forms a circular ring of staples and cuts the tissue between the staples. This device is used to perform end-to-end inverting anastomoses. Because the staple ring is small, this instrument is currently limited to jejunojejunal anastomosis in ponies.

Surgeons using mechanical suturing instruments (staplers) should become completely familiar with operating procedures, recommended techniques, indications and contraindications before using the staplers on patients. When properly used, the staplers can reduce surgical time and make possible certain surgical techniques that could not be performed with conventional suturing techniques.

Closure of the Ventral Midline Incision

The surgeon should close the ventral midline incision with a method that adequately apposes the tissues, minimizes wound complications and allows healing to proceed. Adequate wound closure requires knowledge of proper suture techniques, characteristics of suture materials and suture patterns. Numerous methods of closure of the midline celiotomy are satisfactory. The particular method used often is based on training and preference.

Sutures must hold tissues in apposition until healing has created sufficient strength in the wound to withstand stress without mechanical support. The suture material must be at least as strong as the tissues in which it is placed. Extreme stress on the linea alba of the horse requires that strong suture material be used for closure of the linea alba. The physical properties and biologic response of suture materials also are important. Braided synthetic nonabsorbable suture materials harbor microorganisms in their interstices and are associated with a greater incidence of suture sinus formation in infected wounds than absorbable or nonabsorbable monofilament suture materials.

Many equine surgeons use synthetic absorbable suture material for closing the linea alba. Polyglaction 910 can be purchased in sizes up to #3 and can be used in a simple-interrupted or simple-continuous pattern in the linea alba. The continuous pattern is usually placed in 3-4 sections due to limits on the length of suture strand. The material has poor knot security and requires 4 or 5 throws for each knot. Polydioxanone is a monofilament absorbable material with better knot security than braided absorbable materials. This material can be purchased in size #2 and can be placed as a simple-interrupted or simple-continuous pattern in the linea alba. Polydioxanone maintains 70% of its original strength at 14 days after implantation.

Some surgeons prefer to use monofilament synthetic nonabsorbable suture material in the linea alba, particularly in large horses. Generally these materials should not be used in continuous suture patterns due to the difficulty in removing them if an infection develops around the sutures. Number 2 nylon can be placed in a simple-interrupted or far-near-near-far pattern for closure of the linea alba. Degradation products of nylon may be antibacterial. Nylon has been associated with fewer suture sinuses than braided nonabsorbable suture materials. Braided polyester suture materials are exceeded in strength only by stainless steel. They have poor knot security and have lost favor in many clinics to the newer absorbable or monofilament nonabsorbable suture materials because of a higher incidence of suture sinus formation. Monofilament stainless-steel wire is extremely strong and nonreactive but is generally difficult to handle. Stainless steel is seldom used now that synthetic suture materials are available.

Technique for Closure: Before closure of the linea alba, the subcutaneous fat and fascia should be dissected from the external sheath of the rectus muscle for 1 cm on each side. This allows closure of the linea alba without strangulation of adjacent tissues. Abdominal drains may be placed when the abdominal cavity has been grossly contaminated. Linea alba sutures should be placed 1 cm from the wound margins and 1 cm apart for continuous and interrupted patterns (Fig 32). Sutures placed farther laterally from the midline may result in tearing or necrosis of the rectus muscle. Suture knots should be placed to one side of the incised linea so they are not directly on midline. Suggested patterns and materials are given in Table 15 for reference.

Subcutaneous tissues can be closed with a simple-continuous pattern of 1-0 synthetic absorbable material. Tacking the subcutaneous tissues to the rectus fascia every third or fourth bite reduces dead space and postoperative seroma formation. All knots from sutures apposing the linea alba should be carefully covered. The skin may be closed in a number of ways. A simple-continuous pattern is advantageous for speed of application. Following closure of the midline, an adhesive barrier drape should be applied to the ventral abdomen to reduce contamination of the wound during recovery of the horse from anesthesia.

Postoperative Complications

Postoperative complications contribute significantly to deaths of horses following abdominal surgery for colic. Complications may develop during recovery from anesthesia, during the early postoperative period and later following discharge from the hospital.[189] Complications during recovery from anesthesia include postanesthetic rhabdomyolysis, paresis and long bone fracture. During the early postoperative period, incisional infection, ileus, peritonitis, sal-

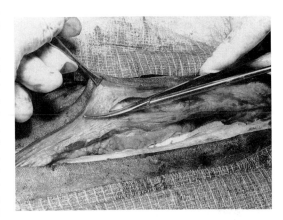

Figure 32. Closure of the ventral midline incision. A. Fat and fascia should be dissected from the linea alba for a distance of 1 cm on each side of the incision. B. A simple-continuous suture pattern is used, with suture bites 1 cm apart and 1 cm from the edge of the incision.

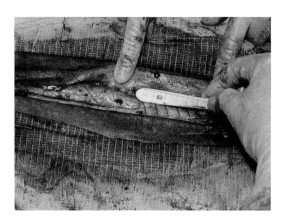

Table 15. Methods of closure for the linea alba after midline celiotomy.

Suture Material	Suture Technique	Comments
#2 Ethilon[a] #2 Novafil[b]	Simple interrupted or far-near-near-far	Far-near-near-far is excellent for very large horses. Simple interrupted for horses <500 kg. Closure is not rapid.
#3 Vicryl[a]	Simple continuous	Material can be doubled for horses >700 kg.
#2 PDS[a]	Simple interrupted, simple continuous or far-near-near-far	Far-near-near-far pattern for horses >700 kg.
#1 Maxon[b]	Simple continuous	Horses <300 kg.

a – Ethicon, Somerville, NJ
b – Davis and Geck, American Cyanamid, Danbury, CT

monellosis, abdominal hemorrhage, laminitis, thrombophlebitis, abortion and shock may occur. In one study, circulatory shock and ileus accounted for 70% of the deaths in the postoperative period.[190] Problems that occur later in the postoperative period, often after discharge of the horse from the hospital, include abdominal adhesions, incisional hernias and malabsorption of nutrients. Long-term problems are not insignificant. The percentage of horses discharged from the hospital, defined as the short-term survival rate, was almost 63% at one veterinary school. Long-term survival rate of this same group of horses was, however, only about 46%.[191]

Postoperative complications should be prevented when possible by adherence to proper surgical techniques, administration of fluids, use of antibiotics, protection of the wound, and attention to the metabolic condition of the horse. Close monitoring of each horse following surgery enables the surgeon to recognize complications early and initiate appropriate therapy. Adhesion formation may be reduced by administration of heparin SC at 40 U/kg every 12 hours in the immediate postoperative period.[192] Laminitis may be prevented by prophylactic use of nonsteroidal antiinflammatory drugs and foot support. The incidence of thrombophlebitis can be reduced by aseptic insertion of catheters and strict adherence to catheter hygiene. In general, the sicker the horse, the more likely that postoperative complications will occur.

DISEASES AFFECTING MULTIPLE SITES
J.E. Sojka and S.B. Adams

Diagnostic and Therapeutic Considerations

Because of the varied nature of diseases of the alimentary system, there is no single set of diagnostic or therapeutic criteria that apply to all diseases. Thorough evaluation of the gastrointestinal tract using clinicopathologic and physical examination findings is indicated for horses with colic, weight loss or anorexia. The reader is referred to the section describing evaluation of the gastrointestinal tract for further discussion.

Congenital and Familial Diseases

Ileocolonic Aganglionosis

White foals born from overo spotted parents are susceptible to a condition known as lethal white syndrome. Except for 1 instance of an affected foal produced from an overo-buckskin cross,[193] all foals have been progeny of overo-overo Paint breedings. There does not appear to be a relationship between the amount of white on the parents and the likelihood of producing an affected foal.[194] Lethal white foals are either completely white or have very little pigmented hair around the muzzle, base of tail or hooves. The irides are blue and the skin is pink.[194] Most foals appear normal at birth, stand and nurse but do not pass meconium. Signs of colic and gastrointestinal distention usually appear within 13 hours after birth, and most affected foals die within 48 hours. If exploratory surgery is performed, areas of the colon may appear stenotic and thin walled.[195]

The syndrome is caused by an absence of myenteric ganglion cells within the intestinal wall. The area of aganglionosis extends from the ileum to the rectum. Often the small colon is contracted and appears atretic. Gaseous dilatation is a common finding in the ileum. The syndrome is thought to be caused by a defect in the embryologic development of the neural crest cells. These cells migrate to the intestinal tract to form the myenteric ganglion cells and also develop into melanocytes in the skin. There may be a defect in development of the intestinal wall itself. This may explain why other tissues derived from neural crest cells are often normal.[196]

Inflammatory, Infectious and Immune Diseases

Anthrax
R.C. Knowles

Anthrax is a bacterial disease, principally of herbivorous animals, characterized by fever and a rapidly fatal course. Anthrax has been reported in areas of Asia, Africa, North America, South America and Europe.

Outbreaks of anthrax in Canada and the United States usually are sporadic.

The most notably affected species are cattle and sheep; however, horses, deer, moose, buffalo and other wild herbivores are highly susceptible. The disease often produces death in people, but people are not as susceptible as herbivorous animals.[197]

Cause: Bacillus anthracis is a large Gram-positive, square-ended bacillus that is regularly encapsulated in tissues. Spores are formed in abundance when the organism is grown in the presence of air. The spores are highly resistant to sunlight, desiccation and gastric juices. Spore-contaminated materials, such as cadavers and animal hides, may serve as a source of infection.[198]

Infection may occur through the alimentary tract, skin and inhalation. It is much easier to infect animals through injured skin and by way of the respiratory tract than by the alimentary tract; nevertheless, it is thought that most natural infections occur through ingestion of contaminated food.[197]

A horse used for pack trips into the Olympic Mountains in the state of Washington died of anthrax.[199] The carcass was fed to large cats on a game farm, resulting in deaths of 42 of a 125 carnivores (*B anthracis* was isolated from 2 cougars and 1 jaguar). The original source of the infection was a pack saddle pad made in New England from coarse goat hair (from Pakistan) and cashmere (from Afghanistan). *Bacillus anthracis* was cultured from both items.

In horses and other equidae, anthrax usually is manifested by severe colic, which might suggest intestinal torsion. The abdominal pain is not accompanied by the accumulation of feces and gas. Typically there is edema of the neck, chest or pharyngeal region. This swelling is distinguished from the swellings of purpura hemorrhagica by its rapid development, painful nature and increased temperature. Hemorrhagic evacuation from the gastrointestinal and urinary tracts is a common sign. Infected animals die within 8-12 hours to 3-8 days.

The gross lesions in fatal cases of disseminated anthrax include edema and hemorrhage throughout the body, particularly in serous membranes. The spleen is greatly enlarged and engorged with dark, unclotted blood. Lymph nodes usually are swollen and edematous.[200]

Diagnosis: A presumptive diagnosis of anthrax can be made from clinical signs; however, it is important to obtain laboratory confirmation, especially when the disease occurs in a previously uninvolved geographic area. The most effective techniques are: microscopic examination of stained blood films for encapsulated bacilli; inoculation of blood or tissue suspensions from anthrax suspects into guinea pigs and demonstration of the anthrax bacillus from the bodies of the guinea pigs; and culture of the bacillus using an inoculum of blood or tissue suspension. Bacteriophage differentiation of anthrax bacilli from nonpathogenic bacilli is employed occasionally.

Control: In most states, anthrax is a reportable disease and laboratory assistance to confirm a diagnosis should be sought from a state diagnostic laboratory. When anthrax is encountered in a herd of horses or other equidae, all members of the herd should be monitored frequently for febrile reactions. Penicillin should be administered to all animals with rectal temperatures 1 degree above normal.

Vaccination of afebrile animals at risk during outbreaks or annually as a precautionary measure in enzootic anthrax areas is recommended. Modified spore vaccines are available in certain countries. A nonencapsulated avirulent spore vaccine (Sterrne Vaccine) is very effective for all species.

In dealing with an outbreak of anthrax, veterinarians should monitor the disposal of animal carcasses. The great resistance of anthrax spores to physical destruction in the environment and the longevity of the spores make carcass disposal critical. Anthrax spores can survive in soil and buffalo bones more than 60 years.

Toxic Diseases

J.E. Sojka and S.B. Adams

Cantharidiasis

(Blister Beetle Poisoning)

Cause: Cantharidin toxicity is caused by ingestion of hay containing blister beetles (*Epicauta* spp). The toxic principle in the blister beetle is cantharidin, which is contained in the hemolymph and other secretions of the beetle. The toxic dosage in horses is as small as 450 μg/kg, which may be contained in as little as 6 mg of dried beetles.[201] There are over 200 species of blister beetle in the United States, but *E lemniscata, vittata, temexa* and *occidentalis* are implicated most often in poisonings.[201,202] Exposure most often occurs by ingestion of dead beetles in baled alfalfa hay. Hay from southern and southwestern states is infested most often. The practice of simultaneous cutting and crimping hay increases the probability of incorporating the beetles into the bales, and thus increases the likelihood of toxicity.[201] Storage does not decrease the toxic principle in the dried beetles.

The pathophysiologic mechanisms of cantharidin toxicosis are not known. It acts as a topical irritant and causes blistering, vesicle formation and severe irritation throughout the gastrointestinal tract. It is excreted in the urine and also causes renal damage.

Clinical Signs: Clinical signs observed after cantharidin ingestion are increased temperature, pulse and respiratory rates.[203] Colic, anorexia and depression are usually noted. Colic may be severe and intestinal strangulation or obstruction may be suspected. Frequent urination may be noted, with hematuria or passage of clotted blood in the urine. Signs of cardiovascular collapse may develop, including increased packed cell volume, congested mucous membranes, prolonged capillary refill time, and forceful cardiac contractions that may be seen through the thoracic wall.

Ulcerative lesions may develop in the mouth and on the tongue, and affected horses often immerse their muzzle in water without drinking. Lack of abdominal sounds is often found, and diarrhea may develop.[201-203] Synchronous diaphragmatic flutter may develop secondary to hypocalcemia.

Clinicopathologic Findings: There are no clinicopathologic findings that are diagnostic of cantharidiasis. The packed cell volume usually is elevated, consistent with the clinical dehydration that develops. Serum sodium, potassium and chloride levels, and acid-base status usually are normal. Hyperglycemia and neutrophilic leukocytosis may develop and indicate a stress response.[201,202] Serum calcium and magnesium levels decrease rapidly after cantharidin ingestion.

Hypocalcemia persists unless treated for prolonged periods.[202,203] Though hematuria is uncommon, urine is usually positive for occult blood. Dilute urine (specific gravity of 1.003-1.006) occurs in the presence of dehydration, indicating renal damage.

Necropsy Findings: Postmortem changes usually are limited to the gastrointestinal and urinary tracts, though myocardial damage has been reported.[202] Gross postmortem lesions consist of fluid-filled intestines, with erosions and ulcerations of the tongue, esophagus, stomach and bladder. Pseudomembranous inflammation may be seen in the small intestine. Histopathologic changes include acute renal tubular necrosis and gastrointestinal tract epithelial acantholysis and sloughing.

Diagnosis: Establishing a definitive diagnosis of cantharidiasis may be difficult. Blister beetles are found in swarms and may be located in only small pockets of hay. If cantharidiasis is suspected, any remaining hay should be examined carefully for additional beetles. Cantharidin can be identified in stomach contents and urine. Samples may be sent to a diagnostic toxicology laboratory with the ability to assay for cantharidin. Hypocalcemia and hypomagnesemia are not commonly associated with other diseases that cause colic and may help differentiate cantharidiasis from other diseases.

Treatment: There is no specific antidote for cantharidin, so treatment is symptomatic. Mineral oil (4 L/450-kg horse) may bind cantharidin and prevent absorption of the toxin. If a poisoning occurs, all potentially exposed horses, even those not showing clinical signs, should be treated with mineral oil. In affected horses, intravenous fluid therapy should be instituted to maintain extracellular fluid volume and establish diuresis. Diuretics may be beneficial early in the course of the disease to help increase the rate of renal excretion. Furosemide at 1 mg/kg may be used, and use of IV 10% DMSO at 1 g/kg has also been advocated.[201] Analgesics often are necessary to control pain. If profound hypocalcemia is present, treatment with calcium- and magnesium-containing solutions is indicated; 500 ml of calcium gluconate may be given slowly to effect. Horses that survive have no long-term residual deficits.

Prevention is by only feeding hay cut in the spring before beetles infest the alfalfa in significant numbers. This is usually before June in the southwestern United States.[201] Fields should be inspected visually before cutting and hay from areas with pockets of beetles should not be baled. Baled hay should be examined before feeding.

Nonsteroidal Antiinflammatory Toxicity

Both the therapeutic and toxicologic effects of nonsteroidal antiinflammatory drugs (NSAIDs) are related to their ability to prevent formation of prostaglandins from arachidonic acid. They act to block the enzyme cyclo-oxygenase that acts to convert arachidonic acid into prostaglandins and thromboxane. Some of the physiologic actions of prostaglandins are to help preserve renal blood flow in volume-depleted states and help maintain the cytoprotective abilities of the gastric mucosa. Not surprisingly, the toxic effects of NSAIDs are related to the loss of the physiologic actions of prostaglandins.

Nonsteroidal antiinflammatory toxicity initially was documented with phenylbutazone, but flunixin meglumine also has been shown to be toxic if sufficient doses are given.[204-207] Formerly, NSAIDs were believed to be very safe drugs, with a wide therapeutic index. It now is apparent that this is not the case, and dosages should not be given in excess of the manufacturer's recommendations. As the effect of different drugs is probably additive, phenylbutazone and flunixin meglumine should be administered concurrently only if the overall NSAID dose is not excessive.

Clinical Signs: The signs of clinical overdose and experimental toxicity are similar. Initial clinical signs are anorexia and depression. As signs progress, colic, diarrhea, peripheral edema and oral ulcers may be observed. Foals appear more susceptible than adult horses. Phenylbutazone acts as a local irritant, and oral ulcers are most common when an oral preparation is given.[205] Gastrointestinal tract lesions are less severe when intravenous forms of the drug are administered.

Clinicopathologic changes include a decreased total plasma protein level, increased blood urea nitrogen level and neutrophilia with a left shift. A low total plasma protein level may be the first detectable change of NSAID toxicity. Labelled albumin studies have documented development of a protein-losing enteropathy.[208] Protein loss occurs before ulcer formation in the gastrointestinal tract. Panhypoproteinemia occurs as both albumin and globulin are lost into the gut. Dependent edema occurs secondary to hypoproteinemia and low plasma oncotic pressure.

Once a significant amount of intestinal mucosa is lost, there is no barrier to prevent endotoxin from entering the systemic circulation, and signs of endotoxemia subsequently develop. Signs include increased heart and respiratory rates, fever, diarrhea, hypotension, dehydration and cardiovascular collapse. If an ulcer perforates and allows ingesta to enter the peritoneal cavity, diffuse peritonitis and death rapidly ensue.

Pathophysiology: The theory that the toxic effects of NSAIDs are due to inhibition of prostaglandin synthesis is supported by the fact that exogenous administration of prostaglandin E_2 prevents many of the signs of phenylbutazone overdose.[209] Prostaglandins help maintain a viable gastric wall by stimulating local blood flow and mucus production. When NSAIDs are given, mucosal atrophy precedes mucosal ulceration.[209] Ulcers usually occur in the glandular portion of the stomach.[205] Colonic and cecal edema also are common and precede cecal ulceration. Renal papillary necrosis has been reported in dehydrated animals but may not occur in animals with adequate hydration.[204-206,210] In volume-depleted states, products of the renin-angiotensin system stimulate local prostaglandin production, which helps preserve renal blood supply.[210] Without maintenance of renal blood flow, ischemic necrosis of the papillae may occur.[210]

Necropsy Findings: Gross postmortem findings of NSAID toxicity include focal, deep ulcers along the gastrointestinal tract. The tongue, hard palate, glandular stomach, cecum and colon are common sites of ulceration. Cecal edema may be present. Linear erosions have been described in the small intestine.

Acute renal necrosis may be observed grossly, with green-yellow cavitation of the papillae and hemorrhage.[210]

Ulcers are sharply demarcated, steep walled and often deep, extending into the submucosa. Small intestine lesions include ulceration, atrophy and protein exudation from intact mucous membranes.

Diagnosis and Treatment: Differential diagnoses of acute NSAID toxicity include infectious enteritis, other causes of colic and Gram-negative septicemia.[211] Signs of chronic or low-grade phenylbutazone toxicity are those of a protein-losing enteropathy and hypoalbuminemia. Differential diagnoses include other causes of protein-losing enteropathy. A history of NSAID administration is critical to diagnosis. A daily phenylbutazone dosage above 8.8 mg/kg for 2 days (4 g/450-kg horse) consistently causes toxicity in foals, ponies and adult horses.[204-206,209] Toxic levels of flunixin meglumine in foals develop after use at 1.1 mg/kg/day for 30 days.[207]

Administration of the NSAID should be stopped immediately when NSAID toxicity is identified. Another class of analgesics should be used if necessary. Opiate agonist-antagonists (butorphanol, pentazocine), sedatives (xylazine) or tranquilizers (acepromazine) may be used as necessary. Fluid therapy should be instituted if the horse is dehydrated, as this minimizes renal necrosis secondary to hypovolemia. Broad-spectrum antibiotics are indicated if severe ulceration is suspected, as the intestinal mucosal barrier is no longer intact and bacteremia and septicemia are likely. Heparin therapy (20-40 IU/kg) has been advocated to prevent laminitis.[211] Histamine-receptor blockers (cimetidine, ranitidine) are indicated if gastric ulceration is suspected. Oral protectants also may be of benefit in foals with gastric ulceration.

Preventing NSAID toxicity is preferable to treating it. Dosage of phenylbutazone should not exceed 8.8 mg/kg/day. It should be decreased from 8.8 mg/kg to 4.4 mg/kg after 2-3 days of treatment. Foals appear to be more sensitive, and phenylbutazone should be carefully administered on a mg/kg basis in young animals. Client education is important to emphasize the narrow therapeutic index and point out wide individual variation in tolerance to larger doses of phenylbutazone. If large doses of phenylbutazone are indicated, IV forms produce less gastrointestinal ulceration, as there are no local irritant effects. If hypoalbuminemia, depression or anorexia develops, therapy should be halted immediately.

Though large doses of phenylbutazone may produce toxicity in a very short time, there is no evidence that small doses produce adverse effects, even if treatment is prolonged.

Neoplasia

The prevalence of gastrointestinal neoplasm is rare.[212] The most common abdominal neoplasms reported are squamous cell carcinoma, lymphosarcoma and lipoma. Common gastrointestinal tumors are described in other sections of the chapter under their specific anatomic location.

Squamous-Cell Carcinoma

Squamous-cell carcinoma is the second most common equine neoplasm, as determined by several tumor surveys.[213-215] It is found most commonly along mucocutaneous junctions of the eye, vulva, penis or prepuce but may be encountered at any location where squamous epithelium exists.[215] Squamous-cell carcinoma of the alimentary tract is found most commonly in the stomach but also has been described in the mouth, pharynx and esophagus.

Squamous-cell carcinoma most often occurs in older horses. Predominant clinical signs are chronic weight loss and exercise intolerance. With the oral or pharyngeal forms, dysphagia and/or dyspnea may also be prominent features. Neither colic nor dysphagia is a common feature of gastric squamous-cell carcinoma, though anorexia is often present.[214] Low-grade fever unresponsive to antibiotic therapy and mild or severe normochromic normocytic anemia is common. There may be indications of liver disease, such as icterus, prolonged sulfobromophthalien dye retention, or increased serum levels of liver enzymes with obstruction of the common bile duct or tumor invasion of the liver (Fig 33). If the horse is dehydrated, prerenal azotemia and electrolyte abnormalities may be identified.

Gastric neoplasia must be differentiated from other causes of chronic weight loss and anorexia in middle-aged or older horses. Metastatic masses often can be palpated on the ventral abdominal wall or within the mesentery via rectal examination.[216] In some instances, exfoliated neoplastic cells may be identified in abdominal fluid. Squamous epithelial cells are not normally found in the abdominal cavity and they suggest squamous-cell carcinoma. Squamous cells are normal constituents of amniotic fluid and care must be taken when interpreting samples collected from pregnant mares. Ultrasonographic examination of the abdominal cavity may reveal splenic, hepatic, diaphragmatic or body wall masses.[23] Tumors in the stomach may be identified by direct viewing if an endoscope of sufficient length is used (3 meters in an adult horse).[14] Neoplastic cells may be recovered from gastric lavage performed with a nasogastric tube, using 0.5 L of saline flushed into and then aspirated from the stomach. Recovered fluid is examined microscopically. If diagnostic samples cannot be obtained any other way, exploratory laparotomy should provide definitive diagnosis.

The prognosis for horses with any form of gastrointestinal squamous-cell carcinoma is grave. By the time clinical signs have appeared, the tumor usually is widely disseminated. Pharyngostomy and/or tracheostomy may provide temporary relief with pharyngeal or oral tumors.

Lymphosarcoma

Lymphosarcoma is an uncommon tumor in horses, accounting for about 1-3% of all tumors surveyed.[214,215] Lymphosarcomas have been classified into 4 groups, according to their origin. These groups are the multicentric, alimentary, thymic and cutaneous forms.[217]

Clinical signs depend upon the location of the tumor, but weight loss and depression are the most common presenting signs. Within the gastrointestinal tract, lymphosarcoma most often is present in the small intestine and mesenteric lymph nodes, though it has also been identified in the soft palate, large intestine and cecum.[212,218] The onset of signs may be chronic or acute, and young animals are often affected. Signs of palatine lymphosarcoma include dysphagia and epistaxis. The tumors are visible via endoscopic examination of the pharynx.[218]

Weight loss and depression are the most consistent clinical findings of intestinal lymphosarcoma. Elevated heart rate, increased temperature, icterus, colic and diarrhea have also been reported.[219]

Anemia is common but atypical lymphocytes in the peripheral blood are rarely found.[219,220] Blood albumin levels often are low secondary to protein-losing enteropathy that develops with extensive intestinal involvement. Blood globulin levels may be increased or normal.

Differential diagnoses include any other cause of chronic weight loss or protein-losing enteropathy. Mesenteric lymphadenopathy or abdominal masses may be present.[219,220] D-xylose or glucose absorption tests document a malabsorptive state and suggest the small intestine as an anatomic site. Ultrasound examination may be useful to identify splenic, hepatic or body wall masses.[23] Diagnosis may be made if atypical lymphocytes are found in peripheral blood, peritoneal fluid or biopsied tissue. Exploratory laparotomy and biopsy of affected areas should provide a definitive diagnosis.

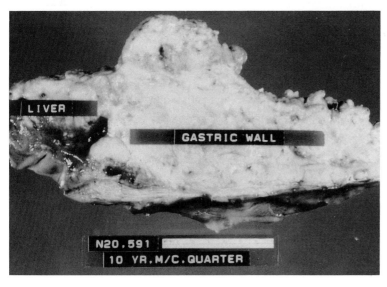

Figure 33. Gastric squamous-cell carcinoma with local invasion from the gastric wall to the liver.

The prognosis is grave. Tumors usually are widely disseminated by the time of diagnosis. Tissue that appears grossly normal when examined often has histologic evidence of tumor invasion. Attempts at tumor resection have been unsuccessful.

Adenocarcinoma

Adenocarcinoma and carcinoma have been reported sporadically involving the intestine and pancreas.[23,212,221,222] Clinical signs include weight loss, anorexia, intermittent colic, pitting edema, exercise intolerance and diarrhea. Hyperglycemia associated with exocrine pancreatic insufficiency has not been described. Clinicopathologic features of pancreatic adenocarcinoma commonly include indications of bile stasis, such as increased gamma glutamyl transferase and alkaline phosphatase activities, increased blood ammonia levels and icterus.[221] Bile stasis presumably occurs due to occlusion of the common bile duct by the neoplasm. Diagnosis may be made via abdominal ultrasonography when metastatic masses can be imaged.[23] Though the prognosis at the time of diagnosis is relatively poor, there has been one report of successful resection of intestinal adenocarcinoma.[222]

Smooth Muscle Tumors

There have been several reports of intestinal leiomyoma and leiomyosarcoma in horses.[212,223-225] These tumors are most common in the small intestine but have been observed at other sites. The most common presenting sign is intermittent or acute colic due to intestinal stasis and distention secondary to lumen obstruction by the tumor. Intussusception associated with the tumor also has been described.[223]

Differential diagnoses include any other cause of intermittent or acute colic. Definitive diagnosis often can be made only during exploratory laparotomy. Resection of the tumor is usually curative, and the long-term prognosis is good.

Mesothelial Tumors

The 2 primary tumors of the mesothelium are the mesothelioma and lipoma. Mesothelioma is an uncommon tumor that may occur in the pleural or peritoneal cavity.[226] Clinical signs may include chronic weight loss, ventral edema and colic. Diagnosis usually can be made by recovery of neoplastic cells from peritoneal or pleural fluid. Reactive mesothelial cells, which may be highly pleomorphic with mitosis, should not be confused with neoplastic cells. The prognosis always is grave due to early dissemination of the tumor throughout the abdominal or pleural cavity.

Lipomas are benign tumors that are extremely common in older horses. An incidence of 3% and 6% of all tumors has been reported in various tumor surveys.[214,215] The tumors do not metastasize and rarely become excessively large. They often develop on long stalks and may cause intestinal strangulation obstruction when the tumor stalk wraps around the small intestine. Acute, severe colic is the usually clinical presentation. Horses with this condition require prompt decompression and resection of the affected intestine and tumor.

Other Neoplasms

Other neoplasms of the gastrointestinal tract have been reported sporadically.[23,212,213] These include hepatic carcinoma, functional pancreatic islet-cell tumor, bony tumors of the teeth and skull, and metastatic ovarian carcinoma or melanoma.[227] In all instances, the prognosis is grave.

Multifactorial Diseases

Nonstrangulating Intestinal Infarction

Nonstrangulating intestinal infarcts may occur in the jejunum, ileum, cecum and large colon. The lesions may be singular and localized, in multiple sites, or diffusely distributed in the bowel. Nonstrangulating intestinal infarction is associated with verminous mesenteric arteritis and thrombotic lesions caused by *Strongylus vulgaris* larval migration.[39,228]

Nonstrangulating intestinal infarction has been commonly termed thromboembolic colic. The term is not accurate, however, because thrombotic disease usually does not cause infarction of the intestines by embolization of the thrombus.[39] Other mechanisms have been proposed to explain the infarction. These mechanisms include: nonocclusive vascular disease associated with low blood flow; vasoconstriction caused by vasoactive substances, such as thromboxane, produced as a product of the coagulation process; complete blockage of the cranial mesenteric artery by thrombotic lesions; hypoxia causing capillary damage; *Strongylus vulgaris* larval damage to small arteries, causing obliterative endarteritis; and diffuse vasoconstriction secondary to blockage of a large vessel supplying the affected segment of intestine.[229,230]

Clinical Signs: Nonstrangulating intestinal infarction causes mild to severe pain, with heart rates ranging from normal to >100 bpm, and reduced or absent borborygmi. Clinical signs are highly variable because of the variable severity of lesions. Depression is common in the later stages of disease. The abdominal fluid may be serosanguineous or orange and may have an elevated white blood cell count and total protein concentration. The red blood cell count in abdominal fluid also may be elevated. The most common findings in horses with nonstrangulating intestinal infarction are mild pain, depression, dehydration and peritonitis.[229]

Treatment: Supportive care with fluids, nonsteroidal antiinflammatory drugs and antibiotics is warranted. Corticosteroids and antithrombotic drugs also may be given. Localized lesions should be resected when surgically accessible. Diffuse and multiple lesions make resection impractical. The prognosis following surgery for localized lesions is poor because the disease is often progressive and new lesions develop. Peritonitis often develops secondary to loss of bowel wall integrity. The sections on surgery, peritonitis and verminous mesenteric arteritis contain more detailed information.

Idiopathic Diseases

Ileus

Ileus is the lack of effective intestinal motility, resulting in failure of intestinal contents to move aborally (distally). This causes a functional obstruction of the intestinal tract.

Cause: Ileus may be caused by exhaustion, colic, peritonitis, enteritis, abdominal surgery, septicemia, and hypoglycemia in foals. Administration of drugs that inhibit intestinal motility, such as atropine, may

also cause ileus.[231] Ileus is most common in horses following colic surgery.[232] Postoperative ileus caused almost 43% of the deaths that occurred following colic surgery in 1 group of horses.[190]

The exact mechanisms by which ileus develops are not understood. Postoperative ileus may in part be due to sympathetic nervous system hyperactivity and parasympathetic hypoactivity. Experimental ileus in ponies was reversed by the dopamine antagonist, metoclopramide.[114] Suppression of excitatory gut peptides and release of inhibitory gut peptides occurs in people with postoperative ileus and may also be a factor in horses.[233] Metabolic derangement, particularly such electrolyte imbalances as hypocalcemia and hypokalemia, also contribute to poor motility.

Postoperative ileus can occur when diseased nonfunctional bowel is present in the abdomen following surgery. This occurs when bowel of questionable viability must be left within the abdomen because resection and anastomosis were not feasible. Peritonitis can cause secondary ileus; a neural inhibitory reflex stimulated by peritoneal irritation and inflammation has been hypothesized to contribute to the ileus. Distention of bowel in one section of the intestinal tract inhibits motility in other sections. Segmental ileus may become diffuse with time.

Persistent ileus results in death via the same mechanisms responsible for death in prolonged mechanical intestinal obstructions. Bowel necrosis, endotoxic shock and circulatory collapse develop.

Clinical Signs: Absence of borborygmi and presence of gastric reflux are hallmark signs of generalized ileus.[231] However, borborygmi may be heard on auscultation when ileus is due to ineffective motility or when ileus is localized to one section of the intestinal tract and sounds are produced in unaffected sections. Gas and fluid accumulation distends the intestine. Fluid from the small intestine refluxes into the stomach and can be removed via nasogastric intubation. Abdominal pain with ileus often is intermittent and, when caused by gastric distention, may be relieved by decompression of gas and fluid from the stomach.

Distention of the cecum and large colons can cause bloat. Rectal examination often reveals distended loops of bowel. Systemic deterioration reflected by an increased pulse rate, respiratory rate, capillary perfusion time and packed cell volume occurs when ileus persists. Abdominocentesis is useful for evaluation of the abdominal cavity and can identify peritonitis and intestinal infarction. Abdominocentesis is particularly helpful in evaluating some horses with postoperative ileus, though the effects of surgical intervention on the abdominal fluid must be taken into account in interpretation of findings.[231]

Treatment: Underlying abdominal diseases that cause ileus, such as peritonitis or intestinal infarction, must be treated before ileus can resolve. Metabolic imbalances should be identified and corrected. Acid-base, electrolyte and fluid disorders can be corrected with appropriate fluid administration.

Decompression of distended bowel is recommended. Distention of bowel contributes to bowel edema, necrosis and perpetuation of ileus. Nasogastric intubation should be performed regularly on the patient to decompress the stomach and reduce the risk of gastric rupture. Rarely, the cecum may need trocarization for removal of gas. Removal of gas and fluid from other segments of the intestinal tract requires laparotomy. A second laparotomy following colic surgery may be necessary when ileus is refractory to medical therapy. Duodenocecostomy may be performed to eliminate profuse gastric reflux caused by duodenitis-proximal jejunitis.[234] This procedure requires resection of the right eighteenth rib to expose the base of the cecum.

Drugs that suppress intestinal motility should be avoided. These include atropine, glycopyrrolate and xylazine.[94] Many drugs singly or in combination have been tried for stimulation of intestinal motility, but none has gained universal acceptance.

D-pantothenic acid has been recommended for horses with ileus. The efficacy is questionable but the drug has few side effects and is inexpensive. Neostigmine may be administered SC at 0.02 mg/kg every hour. This anticholinesterase drug increases propulsive motility of the large colon and segmental motility of the jejunum, but it is less effective after severe intestinal distention has developed and thus may be more valuable as a prophylactic agent than therapeutic. Neostigmine may cause abdominal pain secondary to bowel spasm and should be used with caution when intestinal anastomoses are present. The antidopaminergic drug, metoclopramide, has been used with mixed results to treat postoperative ileus and ileus associated with proximal enteritis. Side effects in adult horses include sweating, abdominal pain, excitement, kicking and nervousness, but undesirable signs are reduced if a dosage of 0.1 mg/kg is given instead of higher dosages.

Sympathetic nervous system blockade with phenothiazines or phentolamine has been used with inconsistent success to treat ileus. Some of the newer prokinetic agents, such as cisapride, provide more promise as effective antiileus agents in horses.[235] Stimulation of intestinal motility with drugs affords poor results if the bowel is severely diseased and underlying conditions are not treated.

Abdominal pain should be controlled with analgesics that do not suppress bowel motility. Pain contributes to increased sympathetic nervous system tone, which inhibits intestinal motility. Management practices that may be beneficial include walking horses every hour and offering intermittent access to small amounts of water when gastric reflux is not present.

Grass Sickness

Grass sickness is a disease of horses limited in its geographic distribution to Scotland, northern England and Sweden. A disease seen in Colombia, South America, is also termed grass sickness, but this condition appears to be caused by *Clostridium perfringens* type A and is not related to the disease of Europe.

Cause: The cause of grass sickness is unknown. Infectious and toxic causes have been proposed, but no causative agent has been identified. Horses 3-6 years of age are usually affected but there is no breed or sex distribution.[2] The disease is most common in pastured horses during the summer months.

Clinical Signs: Clinical signs are colic, depression, dysphagia and drooling. Elevated heart rate and sweating are related to colic episodes. The disease may be acute (1-2 days' duration), subacute (up to 1 week's duration) or chronic (>4 weeks' duration).

Chronically affected horses exhibit marked weight loss and hard, cord-like muscles. Though tenesmus may be observed, feces are not passed and gastrointestinal stasis is the rule. Rectal examination should be performed. In acute cases, gaseous distention of the intestines and impactions are felt. Feces are commonly very hard, firm and covered by mucus. Death often is due to ruptured bowel and subsequent diffuse peritonitis.

The pathologic lesion involves the autonomic nervous system, primarily the sympathetic nervous system. Sites in the central nervous system most often affected include the oculomotor nuclei, facial nuclei, brainstem nuclei, thoracic sympathetic chain ganglia, stellate ganglia, and the intermediolateral nucleus of the spinal cord.[236] Also seen is a loss of myenteric innervation and myenteric plexus neurons. It is thought that neural lesions precede gastrointestinal tract manifestations.[236]

Treatment: There is no known treatment for the disease, though some mildly affected horses may partially recover. Grain supplementation of pastured horses may be preventive.[2]

Regional Nongranulomatous Enteritis

Regional nongranulomatous enteritis and serositis may cause intermittent or continuous colic. Affected horses may exhibit severe abdominal pain, though usually the heart rate does not exceed 60 bpm, and rectal examination findings and abdominal fluid values are normal. Analgesics may result in complete remission of signs, with colic recurring 4-12 hours later. Feces are often passed, and gaseous distention secondary to obstruction does not occur. On exploratory laparotomy, discrete areas of inflamed, hemorrhagic, edematous intestine are identified. Histopathologic examination of biopsied sections reveals edema and acute inflammation. Granulomas are not found. Often the serosa is the most severely affected portion of bowel. No predisposing cause has been identified. A group of 7 horses with similar findings has been described.[237] Parasitism or temporary ischemia were offered as potential etiologies.

Treatment consists of resection of the affected area when possible. If resection is not feasible, use of steroidal or nonsteroidal antiinflammatory agents may be beneficial. In addition to providing analgesia, they also decrease local gut edema and inflammation. The prognosis is excellent if the affected area can be removed. If resection is not possible, affected horses may be subject to repeated bouts of colic that generally respond to symptomatic therapy.

Spasmodic Colic

Cause: Spasmodic colic is caused by spasm and hypermotility of the intestinal tract. This type of colic is probably the most common cause of colic in horses. The disease is characterized clinically by loud gassy intestinal sounds, intermittent abdominal pain, and little or no systemic deterioration of the horse. Pain is caused by bowel spasm. Horses often exhibit spasmodic colic following exercise or excitement. Horses with an excitable temperament may be predisposed to spasmodic colic.[2] An autonomic nervous system imbalance has been hypothesized as the cause.[2] Bowel irritation caused by enteritis, parasitism and moldy feed also may cause spasmodic colic. *Strongylus vulgaris* infection has been associated with altered intestinal motility and spasmodic colic.[144,238] Spasmodic colic rarely is life threatening, and spontaneous resolution is common.

Clinical Signs: Horses with spasmodic colic have mild to severe paroxysmal pain of acute onset and lasting several minutes. Between bouts of pain, the horse may stand quietly. Patchy sweating along the neck may be noted. The pulse rate is often elevated from pain but other metabolic disorders rarely occur. Intestinal hyperactivity is noted as loud rumbling borborygmi that, in some horses, may be heard while standing away from the horse. Auscultation reveals hyperactive bowel and frequent gas sounds. Frequent passage of feces is usual. Any diarrhea suggests onset of enteritis. Rectal examination findings are normal.

Treatment: Many horses recover spontaneously in 10-60 minutes. Treatment of horses that do not recover spontaneously should include analgesic and antispasmodic drug administration. Since pain is caused by spasm, spasmolytic drugs indirectly eliminate pain. Dipyrone may be effective in horses with mild pain. Xylazine suppresses intestinal motility and is a moderately effective analgesic. Other analgesics may be used as deemed necessary by the degree of pain the horse exhibits. Atropine is contraindicated for use as an antispasmodic due to side effects that may lead to adynamic ileus.[120] Many clinicians routinely administer mineral oil via a nasogastric tube. Mineral oil may be beneficial if spasmodic colic is caused by irritation to the bowel.

Intestinal Tympany and Flatulent Colic

Intestinal tympany occurs when gas accumulates in the large colon or cecum, causing distention of the bowel. This gas can be detected by the bloated appearance of the horse, resonance of the affected loops of bowel on percussion, and palpable gas distention of viscera per rectum.

Cause: Primary tympany is caused by microbial digestion of highly fermentable feedstuffs, with increased intestinal gas production. Ingestion of grass from lush pastures, highly fermentable grains or pelleted feeds has been associated with primary tympany. Secondary tympany is caused by obstruction of the colons or cecum. Gas accumulates within the bowel and cannot be passed. Obstruction can be mechanical or functional. Causes of mechanical obstruction include fecaliths or enteroliths in the small colon, large colon torsion, large colon displacement and severe impactions of the large or small colon. Adynamic ileus causes functional obstruction of bowel. The term flatulent colic is used to describe horses with tympany that pass large amounts of gas per rectum. Intestinal obstruction usually is not present; hence, flatulent colic is associated with primary tympany. Primary tympany and flatulent colic have been used synonymously.

Clinical Signs: Horses with primary tympany exhibit moderate to severe pain that is usually intermittent. Bloat, resonance of bowel and flatulence often are noted on physical examination. In the early stages of primary tympany, gas sounds and loud borborygmi may be heard on auscultation. Horses often continue to pass feces. Rectal palpation may reveal distention of the cecum or left colon. Horses show little systemic deterioration in the early stages of primary tympany. Secondary tympany may result in severe distention of the cecum and large colon, respiratory difficulty due to pressure on the diaphragm, severe pain, severe bloat and systemic deterioration. Diseases that cause secondary tympany are discussed in the sections on cecal and colonic diseases.

Treatment: Successful treatment of intestinal tympany depends on differentiation of primary from secondary tympany. Horses with flatulent colic usually recovery following medical therapy. Dipyrone, flunixin meglumine, xylazine or butorphanol may be administered for analgesia. These drugs can be selected based upon the severity of pain. Mineral oil administered via nasogastric tube is indicated, provided gastric distention with gas, fluid or ingesta is not present. Antifermentative and carminative drugs also may be given but have questionable efficacy.[239,240] Walking may promote flatus, though forcing an exhausted horse to walk for long periods serves no purpose.

Trocarization of the cecum to release gas has been advocated when pain from distention is intolerable or the distention causes respiratory difficulty.[239] Trocarization is seldom necessary for horses with primary tympany. These horses often have significant flatus and have no need for trocarization. Trocarization previously has been viewed as a relatively safe procedure. However, intraabdominal hemorrhage, cecal hemorrhage into the bowel lumen or abdominal cavity, localized peritonitis, diffuse peritonitis, and localized abscess formation at the puncture site may occur allowing cecal trocarization.

Horses with secondary tympany from mechanical obstruction usually require surgical intervention. Trocarization may be used to decompress the abdomen before induction of anesthesia to improve respiratory function. However, in absence of a diagnosis, trocarization may delay recognition of a definitive disease and delay the decision to perform surgery. This occurs because horses may improve dramatically after gas is removed. In the absence of correction of the primary problem, this improvement is only temporary. Definitive treatment of horses with secondary tympany is discussed in the sections on colonic and cecal diseases.

DISEASES OF THE LIPS, MOUTH, TONGUE AND OROPHARYNX

P.T. Colahan

Diagnostic and Therapeutic Considerations

Clinical Anatomy

The lips and tongue are composed almost entirely of muscle and are richly supplied with blood vessels and nerves. The blood supply to the lips is via the superior and inferior labial arteries, which are branches of the facial artery. Sensory innervation to the upper lip is provided by the infraorbital branch of the maxillary nerve, while the lower lip is innervated by the mental branch of the mandibular nerve. Both of these nerves are branches of the trigeminal nerve. Motor innervation is by the facial nerve.[241,242]

Blood is supplied to the tongue by the lingual artery, a branch of the linguofacial artery. The sensory nerves supplying the tongue are branches of the trigeminal and facial nerves. Motor function is controlled by the trigeminal, facial, glossopharyngeal and hypoglossal nerves.[241,242] The blood supply to the oral cavity and the oral pharynx is from branches of the external carotid. The trigeminal, facial and glossopharyngeal nerves also control the function of the oral cavity and oropharynx.[241,242]

Examination and Diagnostic Aids

Examination of the lips, mouth and oropharynx can include direct observation, palpation, radiography and endoscopy. Abnormalities involving the lips usually are obvious on inspection, and examination requires only tranquilization and physical restraint. Examination of the rostral mouth and tongue usually is readily accomplished visually and by palpation, requiring only the possible addition of a mouth speculum or dental wedge. Any examination involving use of an oral speculum requires complete control of the horse, generally including both physical restraint and tranquilization or sedation. Oral specula used in equine

practice are dangerous to the horse and the people nearby if the animal becomes excited and swings its head.[243]

Though the caudal oral cavity is visible using a speculum and light source, detailed inspection of the area may require endoscopic examination. Palpation of the deep oral cavity is likewise possible but requires good restraint of the horse and care and experience on the part of the palpator. The oropharynx of a medium-sized to large horse is palpable by examiners with medium-sized to small hands, with the horse under general anesthesia.

In most cases, routine endoscopic examination conducted through the nasal cavity and nasopharynx fails to provide adequate visibility of the oropharynx. In these instances, examination through the mouth is required. Endoscopic examination of the oral cavity and oropharynx through the oral cavity requires general anesthesia to prevent injury to the horse and damage to the endoscope.

Radiographs allow identification of radiodense foreign bodies and fractures of bones surrounding the oral cavity. Radiographic contrast studies may demonstrate dysfunction of the tongue and oropharynx during swallowing.

Surgery

The lips, oral cavity and tongue usually heal readily because they have an extensive blood supply. Though there is nearly constant movement and contamination of the sutured tissues with bacteria, moisture and foreign matter, healing is complete, with minimal scarring.[243-245]

Surgical treatment of the lips is typically limited to suturing wounds or removing tumors. The principles of good surgical technique apply: reduce contamination by debridement and lavage, appose the deep tissues to reduce dead space, provide continuity of the muscular layers, and close the skin carefully using tension sutures on the external surface only (Fig 34).[243]

The same principles also apply to surgical treatment of the tongue. Debridement and lavage of lacerations is very important, as is careful apposition of the muscular layers of the tongue. Attention to these principles helps overcome the causes of wound dehiscence of particular importance for the tongue (contamination, seroma or hematoma formation, motion). Tension sutures are best placed on the dorsum of the tongue, as the tissues in that area provide the greatest strength (Fig 35).[243,245]

Two techniques of partial glossectomy have been used. The first involves amputation of the rostral part of the tongue to remove a nonviable traumatized segment (Fig 36). After removal of the rostral segment, the muscular portion of the tongue is debrided to remove any contaminated tissue and allow apposition of the dorsal and ventral mucous membranes. The muscular layers are sutured with as many layers as necessary to close dead space. Ligation of larger arteries is often necessary. The mucous membranes then are sutured together over the muscular layers to create a smooth margin. For smaller lesions, a V- or wedge-shaped segment of the tongue is removed. The same surgical principles apply, with the added concern that the loss of large segments of tissue on one side of the tongue can cause deviation of the tip of the tongue. For both procedures, healing usually is uncomplicated and occurs with minimal scarring.

A surgical approach to the pharynx through the ventral oral pharynx between the larynx and the basihyoid bone has been described.[246] This pharyngotomy provides limited exposure to the oral pharynx and the approach is more difficult than a laryngotomy. However, for some problems, direct access to the oropharynx rostral to the epiglottis is useful. Some surgeons prefer this approach for resection of the arytenoaryepiglottic fold or pharyngeal cysts.[246]

Congenital and Familial Diseases

Hypoplasia of the Upper Lip

The only congenital condition of the lip reported is hypoplasia of the upper lip. It was noted in conjunction with other congenital abnormalities of the eyes; there was no effective treatment.[247]

Cleft Palate

Cleft palate is an uncommon condition involving either the soft palate or both the hard and soft palates in foals. Though the

Figure 34. Left: Severe, contaminated wound of the buccal commissure and lip, caused by a nail protruding from a stall wall. Right: The wound has been repaired using large tension sutures placed over rubber tubing to reduce stress on the suture line. A Penrose drain has been placed deep in the contaminated fascial layers. Though the suture line later dehisced, it held long enough to allow good second-intention healing.

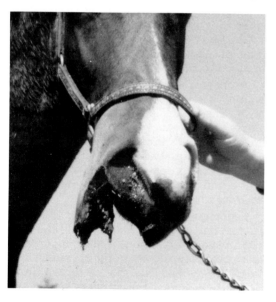
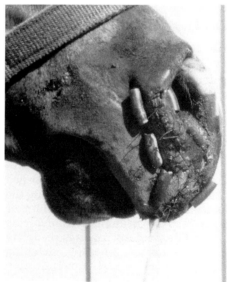

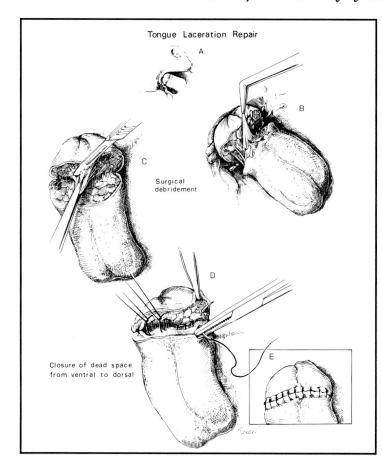

Tongue Laceration Repair

A

B

C

Surgical
debridement

D

Closure of dead space
from ventral to dorsal

E

Figure 35. Repair of lingual lacerations entails careful debridement and closure of dead
space. (Courtesy of Veterinary
Practice Publishing)

condition appears congenitally, the cause is not clear. If possible causes for cleft palate can be extrapolated from other species, the cause could include hereditary, teratogenic, nutritional, infectious, metabolic, intra-uterine mechanical, and ionizing radiation factors may be involved.[243,245]

Clinical Signs: The primary sign of cleft palate is milk dribbling from the nares of a neonatal foal after nursing. Typically, af-fected foals cough, have difficulty nursing, fail to grow normally, may lose weight and are depressed.[243,245] Though some individu-als survive despite these difficulties and the presence of aspiration pneumonia, the out-look for long-term survival without surgical treatment is poor.[248]

Treatment: If treatment of the condition is to be considered, the foal must be muz-zled to reduce the opportunity for aspiration and fed by stomach tube on a scheduled basis until surgical repair is attempted. Serum immunoglobulin levels should be de-termined and, in most cases, supplemented by administration of colostrum if the diag-nosis is made sufficiently early, or by plasma transfusion. Radiographic evalua-tion of the thorax is important to determine the severity of concurrent pneumonia. Broad-spectrum antibiotics are used to con-trol the pneumonia.[243,245]

Surgical access to the palate is difficult and requires mandibular symphysiotomy, division of the mylohyoid muscle and some-times a transhyoid pharyngostomy. The radical nature of the approach is needed to allow careful dissection and suturing. Move-ment of tissues, the moist, contaminated environment and difficulty apposing tissues without excessive tension frequently cause partial or complete dehiscence of the surgi-cal repair. Additionally, the aspiration pneumonia that is almost inevitably pres-ent, the high incidence of osteomyelitis at the symphysiotomy site, the lack of thrift after surgery and the continued discharge of feed material from the nostrils make the prognosis poor even with surgical intervention.[243,245,249,250]

Cysts of the Oropharynx

Retention cysts of the oral cavity originating from mucosal glands or remnants of the thyroglossal ducts can cause difficult swallowing and breathing in young horses. These cysts generally develop slowly and are noticed in animals from a few weeks to 2 years of age. Some retention cysts are evident on endoscopic examination conducted through the nasal cavity, whereas others only are evident on visual examination of the oral cavity or on palpation of the oropharynx. Simple drainage of the contents of the cyst usually results in recurrence. Excision of most of the cyst wall by snaring the cyst through the mouth or resection of the entire cyst through a pharyngotomy or laryngotomy approach is indicated.[243,244]

Diseases With Physical Causes

The most common problems of the lips, tongue and oropharynx have physical causes, including injuries from caustic chemicals, lacerations of the lips, cheeks and tongue, and wounds of the pharynx. Caustic chemicals are no longer as common a cause of oral or lingual injuries as they were when strong counterirritant remedies were commonly used. Red iodide of mercury applied to the limbs was licked by the animal and sometimes caused severe injury to the lips, mouth and tongue. A neck cradle, blanket bib or cross-tying the patient, as well as bandaging the limb, was nearly mandatory when these strong blistering techniques were used.

Injuries to the tongue and lips can be caused by wires, nails, bits, pieces of wood and plant awns (Fig 34). Though the severity and types of these injuries vary tremen-

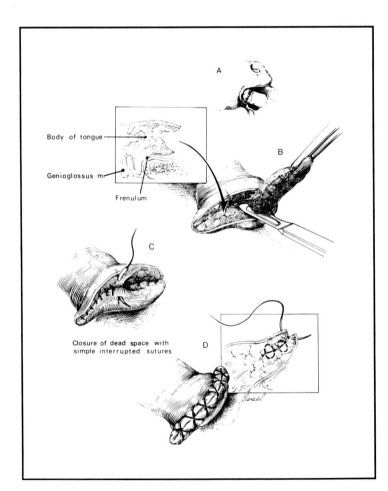

Figure 36. Amputation of the tongue, showing closure of dead space with deep mattress sutures. (Courtesy of Veterinary Practice Publishing)

dously, removal of the foreign bodies or repair of the laceration results in complete return to function.[243,245,251]

Foreign bodies, such as pieces of wire and wood, can be very difficult to locate, particularly if they are lodged in the tongue or deep in the oropharynx. Radiography after infusion of contrast medium into draining tracts can help locate the foreign body.[252] Palpation of the tongue or pharynx, exploration of fistulous tracts, and contrast radiography usually are facilitated by general anesthesia. Nonradiopaque materials, such as wood and plant awns, are the most difficult to find because even the approximate estimation of their location is not provided by plain radiographs. Following removal of foreign bodies, systemic administration of antibiotics is useful to control the cellulitis usually accompanying the foreign body.[252]

Some species of plants produce awns that lodge in the oral mucous membranes and cause chronic granulating wounds. Yellow bristle grass (*Setaria lutescens*) is the most commonly cited plant causing this problem in the United States.[243,253] The wounds usually heal after the awns are removed. Locating and removing all the awns can be difficult, however, and may require repeated efforts.[253]

Lacerations of the lips and tongue heal readily without treatment if they are superficial and small. Large and deep lacerations heal more rapidly and with less scarring if they are sutured using the principles previously described.[243] Repair of some wounds of the lip may require more advanced techniques such as flap transpositions.[254] Suturing lacerations of the tongue always is preferable, both cosmetically and functionally, to partial amputation if the rostral segment is viable; horses can adapt to loss of part of the rostral tongue, however.[243,245]

Injuries of the oropharynx usually are caused iatrogenically by nasogastric tubes, dental floats or balling guns. These injuries usually are located in the dorsal pharyngeal recess, caudal pharyngeal wall, or piriform fossae lateral to the larynx and caudal to the base of the tongue.[243] Caution and training are important in proper use of these instruments. Deep wounds of the pharynx are serious injuries that warrant a guarded prognosis since cellulitis, necrosis, as abcessation frequently complicate these wounds and lead to dysphagia, dyspnea and aspiration pneumonia. Treatment includes cleaning the wound and frequent lavage, if possible, as well as systemic administration of antibiotics.[243,252]

Lacerations of the frenulum of the tongue also occur iatrogenically by unskilled or excessively forceful traction on the tongue during dental procedures or endotracheal intubation. Methods of restraint of horses that incorporate pulling on the tongue are cruel and risk serious injury to the animal.[243,244,252]

Inflammatory, Infectious and Immune Diseases

Stomatitis

Bacterial stomatitis is rare in horses and is presumed to be caused by *Pseudomonas* and *Rhodococcus* spp.[243,245,252] Viral or mycotic causes of stomatitis in horses are discussed elsewhere in this text. These diseases include vesicular stomatitis, horse pox and candidiasis. Generally these conditions are primary oral problems except that candidiasis may occur secondary to prolonged use of broad-spectrum antibiotics in foals.[243]

Horses with stomatitis are treated symptomatically by frequent lavage of the mouth with antiseptic solutions of dilute potassium permanganate or povidone-iodine.[243,252] Severely affected animals may require systemic antibiotic therapy and intravenous fluid administration to prevent dehydration due to reduced fluid intake. Resolution of stomatitis secondary to systemic disease requires successful therapy for the primary disease.[243]

Metabolic and Toxic Diseases

There are several conditions in which stomatitis is one of several signs indicating systemic disease. These include mercury toxicity, uremia, phenylbutazone toxicity and photosensitization. These diseases are discussed elsewhere in this text with other diseases of the skin and kidney.

Lampus

Lampus is a physiologic swelling of the soft tissues of the palate immediately caudal to the incisors. The condition occurs in some horses during eruption of the permanent incisors. Affected horses may be reluctant to eat or may salivate excessively while eating. The condition resolves without therapy; inclusion of less fibrous feeds until the condition resolves may be necessary. Administration of nonsteroidal antiinflammatory drugs, such as phenylbutazone, may help relieve pain and inflammation, and facilitates recovery in severe cases.

Neoplasia

Though tumors of the lips, tongue and oropharynx are rare, several different types of tumors have been identified in this area. Reported neoplasms include squamous-cell carcinoma, fibrosarcoma, malignant melanoma, hemangiosarcoma, rhabdomyoma and lymphosarcoma.[218,243,244,255] Of these, squamous-cell carcinoma and fibrosarcoma are the most common.[243]

Tumors of the lips usually are obvious and easily identified on physical examination. Tumors of the lips and rostral tongue are the most easily and successfully treated because they are noticed sooner by the owner and are accessible to surgical and radiotherapy. Tumors of the palate and pharynx usually are not treated successfully because they generally have become large and may have metastasized to regional lymph nodes before diagnosis.[243]

The most common signs of lingual, oral or oropharyngeal neoplasia are a fetid odor around the horse's mouth and difficulty eating. In some instances, tumors invading the nasal cavity from the oral cavity cause respiratory difficulty as well.

Squamous-cell carcinomas are radiosensitive but tend to recur after resection.[243] Cryosurgery may be useful in treating squamous-cell carcinoma, but a coordinated treatment regimen of radiotherapy, surgical and cryosurgical techniques has not been reported.[243] Laser excision of accessible tumors may increase the success rate, but that also remains to be demonstrated. Fibrosarcomas appear to be less radiosensitive and tend to recur after excision, reducing the prognosis for successful treatment.[243]

Fibrous epulis is a nonmalignant tumor of the gingiva that usually responds to excision.[243]

Some inflammatory problems, such as fungal or parasitic granulomas of the tongue or mouth, bacterial abscesses and problems with physical causes, such as foreign bodies, can cause similar signs, including visible or palpable oral masses.[243,253,256,257]

Diagnosis of the type of tumor and the prognosis associated with tumors of this region depend upon histologic diagnosis from biopsy specimens and information regarding the size and location of the lesion. In some circumstances, such as with small lesions on the lip or tongue, excisional biopsies are possible. For other large or inaccessible masses, only segments of the tumor can be removed with a scalpel or biopsy instrument. In many cases, a uterine biopsy punch and a mouth speculum can be used to obtain biopsies from very deep in the oral cavity of a standing tranquilized horse. A pharyngotomy or laryngotomy incision is necessary to obtain representative samples of some tumors of the oropharynx.

DISEASES OF THE HYOID APPARATUS

P.T. Colahan and B. Watrous

Diagnostic and Therapeutic Considerations

The hyoid apparatus is the bony part of the sling in the intermandibular space that suspends the base of the tongue and the larynx. The hyoid apparatus swings cranially and caudally on its articulation with the temporal bone to facilitate respiration and swallowing. It is pulled cranially by the glossohyoideus and caudally by the sternothyrohyoideus and omohyoideus muscles of the ventral neck.[258]

Primary diseases of the hyoid apparatus are rare and limited to fractures caused by trauma or excessive traction on the tongue.[243,244] Most hyoid problems are associated with inflammatory and/or infectious processes involving adjacent organs, including the guttural pouch, temporal bone and facial and vestibulocochlear nerves (Fig 37).

The obvious sign common to all diseases involving the hyoid apparatus is dysphagia, including flaccidity of the tongue and drooling of saliva (ptyalism). Other signs, such as a drooping lip, deviated muzzle and paralysis of the eyelid, indicate neurologic deficits.[242,259] Involvement of the hyoid apparatus in some inflammatory processes may be occult and only identified radiographically.[260]

Examination and Diagnostic Aids

Definitive diagnosis of abnormalities involving the hyoid apparatus depends primarily upon radiography. Some fractures of the stylohyoid bone are visible on lateral projections of the vertical ramus of the mandible and guttural pouch region. Deformation or fracture of the stylohyoid also may be visible on endoscopic examination of the guttural pouch. Though arthrosis of the temporohyoid articulation and accompanying proliferative bone may be evident on a lateral projection in some cases, most often these lesions are only evident on a dorsoventral view, with the neck extended (Fig 38). The horse must be placed under general anesthesia for this projection.[261] Fractures of the hyoid apparatus that extend through the mucous membrane of the pharynx are visible endoscopically.

Figure 37. Radiograph of a cross-section through the hyoid apparatus and skull at the level of the temporohyoid articulation as viewed from the rear. The left stylohyoid is thickened and the temporohyoid articulation is fused (arrows). The right side is normal. A fibrous nonunion in the petrous temporal bone involving the internal auditory meatus was identified on histologic examination. This 5-year-old mare developed ataxia, head tilt to the left and left facial nerve palsy 10 minutes after being turned out to pasture.

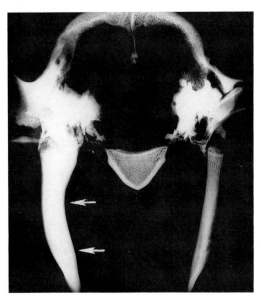

Figure 38. Dorsoventral radiograph of the skull of an 18-year-old stallion showing grand mal seizures. *Actinobacillus equuli* was cultured from the middle ear. Bony proliferation around the right temporohyoid articulation is evident (arrows).

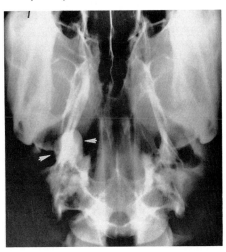

Clinical Anatomy: The hyoid apparatus is composed of paired long stylohyoid bones that articulate with the paired temporal bones at the base of the skull. These bones pass through the guttural pouches and attach to the keratohyoid bones at the level of the oropharynx and tongue. The keratohyoid bones are short and attach to the single basihyoid and the paired thyrohyoid bones in the floor of the oropharynx at the base of the tongue. The muscles that move the hyoid apparatus attach to the basihyoid.[241]

The entire hyoid apparatus is located between the rami of the mandible and hence is relatively protected from external trauma. In the guttural pouches, the stylohyoid is covered only by the mucous membrane lining the pouch. This makes it susceptible to inflammation or infection from the lumen of the eustachian tube. The articulation of the stylohyoid with the temporal bone near the acoustic meatus and middle ear makes it susceptible to extension of otitis media (Figs 37, 38).

Diseases With Physical Causes

Fracture of the Hyoid

Fracture of the hyoid can be caused by trauma, excessive traction on the tongue or can occur secondary to osteomyelitis. External blows cause fracture of the most exposed, ventrally located hyoid bones, the keratohyoid, basihyoid, thyrohyoid and epihyoid. The most frequently fractured bones are the basihyoid or lingual process of the basihyoid and thyrohyoid.[244] Fracture of the stylohyoid by trauma occurs in conjunction with fracture of the ramus of the mandible or with a blow to the poll, as when a horse rears and falls over backward.[262]

Fractures of the hyoid apparatus may be repaired by wiring. This has been especially recommended for traumatic fractures that open into the oropharynx, though the surgical approach was not described.[244] The serious sequelae accompanying these fractures into the oropharynx, most notably cellulitis, dysphagia, aspiration pneumonia and starvation, warrant a poor prognosis for survival. Maintenance of nutrition by alimentation via a nasogastric tube and a tracheostomy to prevent dyspnea due to pharyngeal swelling are useful.[243] Closed unilateral fractures heal in 8 weeks in some horses.[244]

Inflammatory, Infectious and Immune Diseases

The stylohyoid and temporohyoid articulations become involved in inflammatory processes originating in the middle ear and guttural pouch.[260,263] One syndrome describes fractures of the petrous temporal bone caused by chronic otitis media and subsequent inflammation of the tympanic bulla and fusion of the temporohyoid articulation. The action of the hyoideus muscles on the hyoid apparatus causes fracture of the temporal bone and in some cases the stylohyoid bone.[242,259] Inflammation and hemorrhage from the fracture site damage the adjacent vestibulocochlear and facial nerves, and in some cases the glossopharyngeal, vagus and hypoglossal nerves.[242] Affected horses show acute vestibular signs, including a head tilt. Bacterial meningitis can complicate these cases.[259]

Despite treatment, the prognosis for survival was poor in one report.[259] However, other reports indicate that if only the peripheral vestibular system is involved, the prognosis is fair to good in the absence of seizures.[263] Long-term therapy with broad-spectrum antibiotics and nonsteroidal anti-inflammatory drugs is indicated.[261,263,264]

The only prodromal signs that indicate the presence of chronic otitis media is persistent headshaking.[263]

Fistulae may develop in the skin ventral to the parotid salivary gland because of sequestered pieces of hyoid bone.[244] Removal of the sequestered segments is required to eliminate the fistulous tract.[243]

DISEASES OF THE TEETH

G.J. Baker

Diagnostic and Therapeutic Considerations

The Eocene ancestor of the modern horse had simple teeth. As the environment changed and horses changed from browsers to grazers, corresponding modifications in tooth structure occurred. These modifications involved molarization of the cheek teeth (premolar teeth adopting molar form), formation of reserve crowns and continuous eruption with development of crown cementum. The evolution of an efficient food-grinding apparatus and alimentary tract resulted in horses suited to a life of almost continuous grazing. Their lips are selective and prehensile and the incisor teeth form an efficient cutting apparatus. The cheek teeth function as a serrated arcade and the temporomandibular joint accommodates the side-to-side movements of the mandible that grind food.

Tooth Eruption

The deciduous (milk) teeth are represented by the dental formula 303/303 (Table 16). Within a week of birth, the first incisors erupt, and within 2 weeks, all 3 premolars erupt. The second incisors usually appear at 1 month and the third at 6-9 months of age. The deciduous incisors are shell shaped as compared with the rectangular permanent incisors and are much smaller. A 2-year-old horse should not be confused with a 5-year-old on dental appearance (Fig 39).

The first molar (fourth cheek tooth) erupts at 9-12 months of age and the first permanent incisors at 2 1/2 years of age. By 5 years of age, all deciduous teeth have been shed and the horse has its complete perma-

Table 16. Times of deciduous and permanent tooth eruption. (From Sisson and Grossman's *Anatomy of the Domestic Animals*)

Tooth	Eruption
Deciduous Teeth	
1st incisor	(Di 1) birth or 1st week
2nd incisor	(Di 2) 4-6 weeks
3rd incisor	(Di 3) 6-9 months
Canine	(Dc)
1st premolar	(Dp 2)
2nd premolar	(Dp 3) birth or 1st 2 weeks
3rd premolar	(Dp 4)
Permanent Teeth	
1st incisor	(I1) 2 1/2 years
2nd incisor	(I2) 3 1/2 years
3rd incisor	(I3) 4 1/2 years
Canine	(C) 4-5 years
1st premolar (wolf tooth)	(P1) 5-6 months
2nd premolar	(P2) 2 1/2 years
3rd premolar	(P3) 3 years
4th premolar	(P4) 4 years
1st molar	(M1) 9-12 months
2nd molar	(M2) 2 years
3rd molar	(M3) 3 1/2-4 years

The periods given for P3 and P4 refer to the upper teeth; lower ones may erupt about 6 months earlier.

nent arcade represented by the dental formula:

$$\frac{3}{3} \quad \frac{1}{1} \quad \frac{3 \text{ (or 4)}}{3} \quad \frac{4}{3}$$

Types of Teeth

The first permanent premolar may be absent or rudimentary and is popularly termed "wolf tooth." In horses, the term molar may be applied to any maxillary or mandibular tooth, irrespective of the true definition of the term; that is, a molar is a tooth not represented in the deciduous dentition. In this discussion, the teeth are described as cheek teeth, upper or lower, and numbered 1 to 6.

Canine teeth usually are absent or rudimentary in the mare. Like wolf teeth, canine teeth have a simple crown, long embedded root and very little crown cementum. Incisors and cheek teeth differ in that they have considerable reserve crowns that erupt as the exposed crown is worn away by mastication.

Incisor teeth have a deep enamel invagination partly filled with cementum. As the teeth wear, the occlusal surface has a central ring of enamel surrounding the infundibulum and a peripheral enamel ring. The infundibulum darkens due to food deposits

Figure 39. Skull of a 2-year-old colt dissected to show embedded teeth. The upper first premolar (wolf tooth) is present but not visible; the lower one is indicated by an arrow. Temporary premolars are numbered 1, 2, 3; permanent premolars and molars are designated by Roman numerals. Dc is the upper temporary canine, C is a lower permanent canine not ready to erupt, Di2 and Di3 are the 2nd and 3rd temporary incisors and I1 is the first permanent incisor not ready to erupt. (From Sisson and Grossman's *Anatomy of the Domestic Animals*)

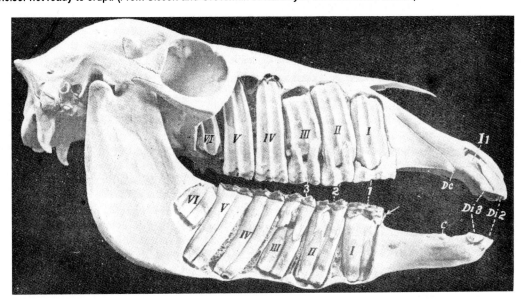

Figure 40. Occlusal surfaces of maxillary (left) and mandibular (right) cheek teeth.

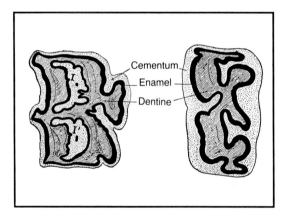

As the complex enamel folds are worn away, the dental arcades take on a slight wave-like formation so that 10 transverse ridges are formed, (2 for each tooth except the first and last). Corresponding valleys and ridges form on the opposing arcade.

Tooth Anatomy

Each tooth is composed of pulp, dentine, enamel and cementum. The pulp is a soft, gelatinous tissue that occupies the central part of the tooth, the pulp cavity. In the upper teeth, the pulp cavity has 5 main divisions within the folds of enamel and 2 main divisions in the lower teeth. Dentine forms the bulk of the tooth and progressively encroaches on the pulp cavity with age. It is hard and yellow-white, whereas enamel is very hard and blue-white. Cementum is the peripheral tooth substance. Progressive cementation of peripheral enamel irregularities levels up the surface. Cementum is very similar to bone in structure. The embedded part of the tooth is united to the alveolus by a vascular layer of connective tissue, the alveolar periosteum.

and is lost as the crown is worn away (see Determination of Age below).

There is intimate contact between adjacent cheek teeth to maintain a continuous row of tooth substance. Upper cheek teeth differ from lower teeth in that the enamel is formed from an enamel organ folded vertically across the tooth, as well as longitudinally. As these folds erupt and are worn away, an upper tooth is produced with its distinctive enamel lakes filled with cementum and a central canal, the infundibulum (Fig 40).

In all horses, the distance between the left and right mandible, measured at any tooth, is 30% narrower than the space between the maxillary arcades (anisognathism). Consequently, the teeth in the lower arcades erode more on the buccal aspect and those of the upper arcades on the lingual aspect, and sharp enamel edges form.

The position of the embedded crowns and roots of the last 4 upper cheek teeth varies at different ages and in different types of horses. All of these teeth develop in the caudal part of the maxilla and are related to the maxillary sinuses. The third and fourth teeth commonly project dorsad into the rostral maxillary sinus, and the fifth and sixth into the caudal maxillary sinus. This relationship is important clinically in that periapical infection of these 4 teeth may lead to maxillary sinus empyema.

Table 17. Timing of changes in the occlusal surfaces of the lower incisors.

Stage	1st Incisor	2nd Incisor	3rd Incisor	Canine
Deciduous	1 week	1 month	6 months	
Permanent	2 1/2 years	3 1/2 years	4 1/2 years	4 1/2-5 years
Loss of enamel cup	6 years	7 years	8 years	
Appearance of dental star	8 years	9 years	10 years	
Change from oval to triangular shape	11 years	12 years	14 years	
Loss of enamel star	12 years	13 years	15 years	

Determination of Age

The age of horses up to 8 years is determined by examination of the state of eruption and the amount of wear of the incisors. An estimate of later age is gained by examination of incisor occlusal surface shape and changes in the angle of the incisor profile.[265-268]

Table 17 summarizes the changes that occur up to 15 years of age on the occlusal surfaces of the lower incisors. Variations in occlusal surface wear occur in cribbers, sand-eaters and horses with malocclusion.

Cementogenesis within the base of the enamel invagination ceases when the incisor erupts. Consequently, the depth of the enamel cup (infundibulum) within the invagination and its subsequent erosion depend on the rate of erosion and on the amount of cementum that persists up to 12, 13 and 15 years, respectively, until the enamel star is lost (Fig 41).

Dental Examination and Diagnostic Techniques

Dental Examination: A complete history should be obtained and inquiry made of eating habits, quidding, biting and riding problems, headshaking, shyness, loss of condition or halitosis. The quality and quantity of the normal diet should be noted. By correlating the history with the animal's age and clinical signs, a presumptive diagnosis often can be made (Table 18).

It is impossible to examine a nervous, frightened or stubborn horse satisfactorily. Therefore, one must take every precaution not to increase the animal's natural suspicion and distrust of strangers. It is uncommon for a horse to permit dental examination without suitable preliminaries to convince it that the examiner intends no harm. This may be impossible without sedation or even general anesthesia for examination of some painful disorders.

The incisors should be examined first by rolling back the horse's lips. The angle of the bite and any external abnormalities should be noted. The deciduous incisors should be checked for looseness if evidence indicates they are about to be shed. The mouth is opened by reaching into the interdental space and withdrawing the tongue or by applying opposing pressure on the upper and lower lips. The animal's age should be determined because it can be an important clue to disorders encountered in further examination of the mouth and dental arcades.

The buccal edges of the first 3 cheek teeth can be assessed for sharpness by external palpation through the cheeks. Examination of cheek teeth without a speculum is not difficult once the technique is mastered. Such an examination is simpler, neater, less objectionable to the patient, and more impressive to the owner. Two methods may be employed. In one method, both hands are used and in the other, only one hand is used. Each method has its advantages and disadvantages and should be carefully eval-

Figure 41. Changes in the occlusal surface of the first incisor as a horse ages. (Modified from Sisson and Grossman's *Anatomy of the Domestic Animals*)

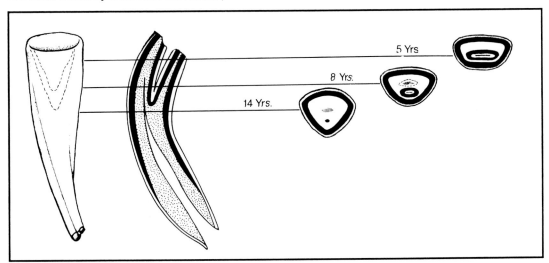

uated by the individual practitioner before being employed.

In the 2-handed method, the right side of the dental arcade is palpated by approaching the horse from the left. The left labial commissure is parted with the right hand, and the tongue is grasped through the left interdental space and withdrawn through the left side of the mouth. A light cotton glove on the right hand facilitates this manipulation and keeps the tongue from slipping. At this time, the horse opens its mouth and tends to pull back, which provides a good chance to observe the table surfaces of the upper incisors and right upper cheek teeth. A flashlight held by the clinician or an assistant facilitates this examination.

With the horse's tongue held in the left labial commissure, the left hand is passed between the right dental arcade and the cheek, with the knuckles toward the cheek and palm toward the teeth. The upper and lower cheek teeth are palpated with the fingertips. As long as the tongue is held in the labial commissure, the horse (ordinarily) will not close its mouth and there is little chance of finger injury.

Do not conduct the examination in a leisurely fashion because it annoys a horse to have its tongue clutched for long periods while each tiny ridge or cavity of cheek teeth is being examined. When the right side has been examined, repeat the process on the left, using the opposite hand and labial commissure. Examiners with large hands may find this unsatisfactory.

For experienced operators, the 1-handed technique is more suitable. It also is applicable to otherwise manageable horses who dislike specula or tongue-holding. The horse is approached from the front and the right side of the mouth is palpated by inserting the right hand into the right interdental space with the palm facing laterad (Fig 42). The hand should be slightly dorsiflexed (overextended) and should lie between the lingual surface of the cheek teeth and the tongue. This forces the tongue between the left rows of cheek teeth and keeps the horse from closing its mouth completely.

The hand is advanced into the oral cavity, and the thumb and forefinger are used to palpate the buccal, lingual and table surfaces of the teeth (Fig 43). During this examination, one also should palpate the buc-

Table 18. Dentistry procedures at various ages.

Age	Examine For Necessary Dentistry	Dental Procedure
2-3 years	1. 1st premolar vestige (wolf teeth)	1. Remove wolf teeth if present
	2. 1st deciduous premolar (upper and lower)	2. Remove deciduous teeth if ready. If not, file off corners and points of premolars
	3. Hard swelling on ventral surface of mandible beneath 1st premolar.	3. Make radiographs. Extract retained temporary premolar if present.
	4. Cuts or abrasions on inside of cheek in region of the 2nd premolars and molars.	4. Lightly float or dress all molars and premolars if necessary.
	5. Sharp protuberances on all premolars and molars.	5. Rasp protuberances down to level of other teeth in the aracde.
3-4 years	1. 1, 2, 4 and 5 above.	1. 1, 2, 4 and 5 above.
	2. 2nd deciduous premolar (upper and lower)	2. Remove if present and ready.
4-5 years	1. 1, 4 and 5 above.	1, 4 and 5 above.
	2. 3rd deciduous premolar.	2. Remove if present and ready.
5 years and older	1. 1, 4 and 5 above.	1. 1, 4 and 5 above.
	2. Uneven growth and "wavy" arcade.	2. 1, 4 and 5 above.
	3. Unusually long molars and premolars.	3. Unusually long molars and premolars may have to be cut if they cannot be filed down.

cal mucosa, gingiva and right side of the tongue. The left side of the mouth is examined in the same manner using the left hand. There is danger of being bitten when using this technique, particularly if one is careless. The operator's hands may be scratched by sharp edges of the upper cheek teeth. This ordinarily results from failure to palpate the outside of the cheeks before inserting the hand into the horse's mouth.

The cheek region around the labial commissures is readily palpated by placing the thumb in the commissure with the ball toward the buccal mucosa. Wolf teeth can be felt by inserting the thumb or forefinger into the interdental space and palpating the first upper and lower cheek teeth on the close side. Do not attempt to palpate the premolars on the side of the jaw opposite the one in which your finger is inserted. Wolf teeth feel much smaller than the adjacent rostral premolar. Because wolf teeth may occur in the maxilla or mandible, both upper and lower arcades should be examined. At the same time the arcades are examined for wolf teeth, the first definitive premolars should be palpated for protuberances and sharp edges. It is in this area that the bit draws the cheek or tongue against the teeth and sharp edges of the

Figure 42. Hand position to enter the mouth in the 1-handed technique for dental examination.

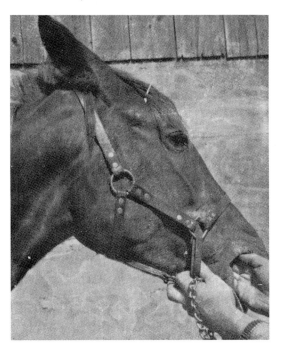

Figure 43. Palpating the upper fourth cheek tooth using the 1-handed method.

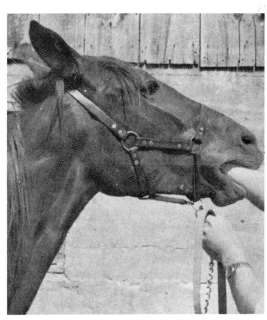

first premolars can cause painful lacerations.

Great care should be exercised if a mouth speculum (gag) is used to examine an untranquilized horse. Such specula are designed to forcibly hold the mouth open and usually are constructed of heavy metal. The device can be hazardous when attached to the swinging head of an excited horse.

General anesthesia enables detailed inspection of molar arcades and gingival pockets, biopsy and cauterization of buccal ulcers and lesions, and probing of dental tissues. For complete investigation of tooth root infections, radiographs are invaluable in revealing the extent of maxillary or mandibular bone disease.

Radiography: Satisfactory radiographs can be produced with standard veterinary equipment at exposures equivalent to 60-70 kVp at 40 mAs. Lateral and oblique films are made using stationary grids, fast film and screens. The mouth is held open with the anesthetized horse in lateral recumbency and the diseased side next to the cassette. In most cases, root and reserve crown detail, rather than exposed crown detail, is desirable on radiographs. This detail is achieved by using a 30- to 45-degree oblique beam to project the image of the normal arcade away from the diseased area.[269]

Greater detail of individual maxillary roots can be obtained from intraoral (occlusal) dental films wedged 45 degrees to the hard palate, the x-ray tube head correspondingly angled, and the affected side up. A mandibular arcade occlusal film is placed between Perspex sheets to prevent ensalivation, and is wedged vertically between the tongue and mandibular arcade.

Floating: Floating teeth usually is performed without anesthesia and with minimum restraint. It must be emphasized that the objective of routine regular dental prophylaxis is to maintain normal dental occlusion. In this way, many of the problems of irregular wear and periodontal disease may be prevented. During the eruption phase of teeth, horses in training and older horses should have biannual dental examinations and prophylactic work. Annual examination and flotation should be done in all other domestic horses.

When viewed from the front, the table surfaces of the lower cheek teeth are angled dorsad and mediad, and the table surfaces of the upper cheek teeth are angled ventrad and laterad. Sharp edges may be found on the buccal borders of the upper arcade and the lingual borders of the lower. Table surfaces must be rough to be efficient but must be even and complementary to opposing teeth. A speculum may be used or the tongue grasped and withdrawn to make the horse open its mouth. Often this is not necessary, as passage of the float (rasp) itself causes the horse to open its mouth enough for removal of the sharp edges. When more severe floating is necessary, as when grinding down a protruding tooth, a speculum should be used and the horse tranquilized, sedated, restrained or given general anesthesia as warranted.

There is a tendency to overtreat rather than undertreat dental lesions. The only floating usually necessary is to remove sharp projections that can abrade or cut the tongue or cheeks and to level any projections of the table surface that are incompatible with opposing teeth. These projections usually are removed by 5-6 strokes with a sharp float over the arcade, depending on how much pressure is used and the consistency of the teeth. The float should not be placed flat on the arcade but should be held at an angle of slightly less than 90 degrees to the lingual surface of the lower

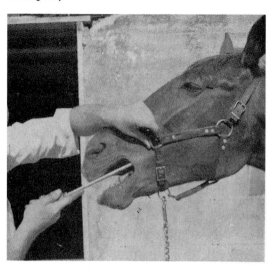

Figure 44. Floating the upper dental arcade. The halter is pulled away from the horse's cheek so that it does not compress the underlying buccal mucosa against the moving rasp.

arcade and to the buccal surface of the upper. A slightly angled float is used on the lower arcade and a straight rasp is used on the upper (Figs 44, 45). When floating the upper arcade, the assistant's arm or the noseband of the halter or speculum should not press against the horse's cheek, as that causes the back of the rasp to injure the buccal mucosa. If the horse shakes its head or moves it up or down quickly, it is important to move with the horse so the rasp does not injure the mouth. The assistant should

Figure 45. Floating the lower dental arcade.

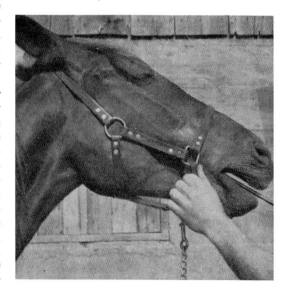

hold the head firmly and steadily but should not hold the soft part of the nose too firmly, as that may hinder air passage through the nostrils.

If the horse is ridden, driven or in training, the rostral premolars should be floated to remove sharp projections or edges that may cut or abrade the cheeks or tongue from bit action. This is best accomplished with a 45-degree float, using a file blade rather than a float. Most of the procedure can be accomplished with relative ease if the instrument is held close to the blade. Lingual and buccal edges of the rostral premolars are rounded to prevent injury to adjacent soft tissues. In yearlings, it sometimes is necessary to remove enough of the tooth surface to prevent teeth from contacting one another at all because some snaffle bits force a portion of the buccal mucosal between these teeth. Pieces subsequently may be bitten out, resulting in mouth injury and excessive objection to the bit or any attempt at manipulation. This is of great importance in young Saddle Horses in training for the rack and slow gaits that requires much bit manipulation. In many of these cases, corrective dentistry must be performed before training is resumed.

Removal of Wolf Teeth and Dental Caps: There is no single satisfactory method for removal of wolf teeth; the method used often is dictated by the size of the tooth, angle of growth and position of the tooth in relation to the second premolar. A dental elevator is used to loosen the tooth before extraction.

Deciduous teeth often are so firmly lodged that the underlying permanent tooth becomes impacted. When an upper permanent premolar with its root immediately beneath the floor of the maxillary sinus is involved, there is swelling over the sinus wall and evidence of pain when the area is percussed. This apparently reflects an exaggerated physiologic reaction that accompanies the teething process. Removal of the cap provides almost immediate relief to the horse. Removal of the impediment to normal eruption results in gradual reduction of pain and swelling over the sinus. Sinusitis that requires surgical drainage or medical therapy rarely develops. Retained caps commonly occur in pairs. Therefore, the corresponding tooth on the opposite arcade

should be examined and removed after removal of the affected cap.

One method of cap removal involves use of a rongeur or bone cutter, particularly one that is double-faced and offset; however, an ordinary bone cutter is satisfactory. The tooth is palpated with the thumb or forefinger and the bone cutter applied caudal to the finger between the first and second premolar with the flat face toward the second premolar. It is guided into place while the thumb or forefinger palpates the tooth. The instrument is placed high enough so the points close, to 1/2 inch above the gingiva. As the forceps is closed, it is given a rotating twist or prying motion by moving the handles caudad. If properly done, the tooth is loosened with minimal pain to the horse and minimal effort by the operator. The tooth is then removed with fingers or forceps.

A canine root elevator also works well for this operation and is used in the same manner as bone cutters. A root elevator must be quite strong, however, and it is difficult to obtain one that can withstand the pressure. An ordinary screwdriver also may be used in the same manner but does not fit the tooth as well as a root elevator and must be employed carefully to prevent injury to the roof of the mouth. The area around the first premolar may be locally anesthetized in horses that resist manipulation of the mouth. This is accomplished by injecting local anesthesia solution into the gingival area through a fine-gauge needle. If one is working on a group of horses, an anesthetic dental ointment containing butyl sulfate or some other topical anesthetic may be massaged into the gum around the tooth every 10 minutes until the area is sufficiently anesthetized to permit painless tooth removal.

Extensive oral manipulation, extraction and dental radiography are most satisfactorily done with the horse in lateral recumbency and under general anesthesia. A range of dental equipment should be available.

Tooth Cutting: Cutting forceps with hardened jaws have been designed to remove projecting portions of molars. Forceps with a compound fulcrum apply sufficient force to the cutting edge to sever the tooth cleanly, though an operator with strong arms can use simple forceps satisfactorily.

A speculum should be used in this operation. The tooth is engaged in the jaws of the cutter and severed in much the same way that steel bolts are severed with a bolt cutter. Undesirable sequelae include loosening or splitting of the tooth. Teeth of old animals tend to be fragile and should be cut with caution.

The tooth should be floated after cutting to remove loose fragments or sharp corners. If special cutters are not available, large hooks and irregularities can be removed by careful striking with a heavy hammer and a sharpened heavy cold chisel.

Tooth Extraction: Extraction should be performed with the horse under general anesthesia, with a speculum in place and the airway intubated.

One must determine the firmness of the tooth's attachment in the alveolus. In cases of alveolar periostitis, the molar may be loose enough to be extracted with forceps. If extraction can be accomplished this way, the forceps are placed on the affected tooth close to the gingival line and rotated in a gradually increasing arc as the tooth loosens. Progress can be determined by the change in character of a sucking sound around the alveolus and by palpation.

When the tooth has been thoroughly loosened, an object used as a fulcrum may then be placed on the table surface of the teeth rostral to the affected one and the forceps used to pull the tooth from the alveolus. As the tooth is raised from the alveolus, the forceps should be moved down the root to facilitate removal. If the tooth is too long to be removed without coming into contact with the table surfaces of the opposing teeth, it sometimes can be moved mediad and extracted. If this is not possible, the top of the tooth must be cut off with molar cutters to allow room for removal. After the tooth is removed, the alveolar cavity should be carefully searched to be sure all loose pieces of the tooth and its roots have been removed. The cavity is then flushed with a mild antiseptic solution and packed with gauze or cotton soaked with suitable antiseptic. Gelfoam or dental wax may be use to prevent feed from contaminating the alveolar space. The horse should be fed mash or ground feed, and hay should be withheld for 2-3 days until granulation tissue forms.

Tooth Repulsion: Repulsion of teeth is preferred when oral extraction is difficult.

The operation should be performed with the horse under general anesthesia and a speculum in place.

Repulsion involves trephining to gain access to the base of the tooth and using a dental punch and mallet to drive the tooth from its socket. The principal difficulties are gaining access to the base of the tooth without producing excessive damage to the supporting bone and driving the tooth from its socket without fracturing the jaw, splintering the tooth or causing excessive damage to the alveoli or adjacent teeth. The surgeon should elevate the gingiva and attempt to loosen the tooth by rotating it with extraction forceps before repelling the tooth. Use of these techniques minimizes the risks of alveolar bone complications.

Repelling is confined to the upper and lower cheek teeth. Postoperative care may be required for a few days to several weeks, depending on how soon the infection is overcome, involvement of adjacent tissue, and how rapidly healthy granulation tissue fills the vacated alveolus. The owner should be warned that removal of the tooth results in elongation of the opposing tooth and that the horse will need yearly dental care.

With repulsion of the upper cheek teeth, it is essential to position the trephine opening properly to avoid damage to the nasolacrimal duct and the lacrimal canal, both of which run from the medial canthus of the eye rostroventrad to the floor of the nasal cavity near the external nares. A baseline constructed from the medial canthus of the eye through the infraorbital foramen and extending rostrad to the nares marks the location of the nasolacrimal duct. Trephine openings should be made below this line. Due to the length of the teeth in young horses, the trephine opening must be kept as close to the line as possible. In older animals, it may be made some distance ventral to the line to compensate for shortening of tooth length and sharpening of facial contours.

Each tooth requires a differently located trephine opening. For the first and second cheek teeth, a line is drawn vertically through the center of the tooth and the opening is made along this line and just ventral to the baseline. For the third through fifth cheek teeth, the opening is made ventral to the baseline along a line passing dorsad, parallel to the caudal border of the tooth. It is fortunate that this tooth seldom needs to be repelled because it is not easily accessible, particularly in young animals in which the base of the tooth lies ventral to the floor of the orbit. As a horse becomes older, the teeth become progressively easier to reach via trephine openings, as gradual eruption of the teeth leaves more space between the baseline and the trephined opening.

After surgical preparation of the area and application of a speculum to the horse's mouth, an X-shaped or circular incision is made over the site where the trephine will be placed. The center of the incision should mark the center of the opening. The skin flaps are reflected and held back from the surgical field with stay sutures or Backhaus forceps. Subcutaneous tissues are dissected until the periosteum is reached. The periosteum is incised with an X-shaped incision and carefully elevated from the bone and pushed back under the soft tissues, leaving enough bone exposed to accommodate the trephine. The center punch of the trephine is set in the center of the field and, with firm pressure on the handle, the instrument is rotated back and forth in an arc until the blades cut through the exposed bone. The instrument should not be tipped as it is being rotated so as to avoid breaking the cutting drum. The disc of bone usually remains in the trephine when the instrument is removed, but in some cases the disc must be freed from the underlying attachments with forceps and a bone chisel.

After the trephine opening has been made, the base of the affected tooth is located carefully by palpation of the exposed portion of the tooth inside the mouth and projection the direction of the tooth into the bone. The punch then is placed on the base of the tooth and an assistant strikes the end of the punch with a mallet. The first few blows should be only sufficiently hard to seat the punch against the base of the tooth. If there is insufficient room to do this, the opening should be enlarged with rongeurs or a bone chisel. The accuracy of the punch setting is determined by palpation of the impact area with fingers on the affected tooth (and on adjacent teeth). If the punch is properly placed, mallet blows subsequent to seating have a characteristic ring and rebound not observed when the punch is penetrating soft tissue. The tooth then should

be loosened by blows heavy enough to loosen but not heavy enough to splinter the base. When the tooth has been loosened, subsequent blows can be lighter as the tooth is repelled from its alveolus.[270]

After the tooth is repelled, its base must be examined carefully to determine if it is complete. Any dental fragments remaining in the alveolus should be removed with splinter forceps. Great care must be taken to remove all fragments of the tooth and nodules of cementum from the alveolar cavity. Thorough curettage and postoperative radiographs to check the alveolus are essential. After the socket has been cleaned, it should be packed with antiseptic gauze or dental wax. The periosteum and skin flaps should be apposed over the incision. If the packing is tied, a small central portion of the skin flap should be removed to allow the tie to pass through. An alternative procedure is to remove the skin over the trephine opening and let it heal by second intention.

When repelling the fourth, fifth and sixth cheek teeth, it may be necessary to cut the tooth off with a molar cutter when it is partially repelled because of insufficient space between the table surfaces to allow total repulsion. Movement mediad may not be possible without causing undue injury to the alveolus.

The trephine openings for repulsion of the lower cheek teeth are made on the lateroventral border of the mandible, using similar surgical techniques for placing the trephine as employed in the maxilla. The opening for repelling the first lower cheek tooth should be made directly ventral to the table surface of the tooth. For the second through the fifth lower cheek teeth of horses <9 years old, the opening is made ventral to the caudal border of the tooth. In horses >9 years old, the opening is aligned more closely with the center of the table surface until the animals is 12 years old. In horses 12 years of age and older, the opening should be ventral to the center of table surface.

The trephined opening for the fourth and fifth lower cheek teeth may be near the external maxillary artery and vein and the parotid duct. These should be carefully exposed, freed and retracted from the surgical field.

Removal of the sixth lower cheek tooth presents several special problems. The tooth root ends about midway between the table surface of the tooth and the greatest curvature of the ramus of the mandible. This necessitates trephining on the lateral side of the mandible rather than on the lateroventral surface. The trephine point underlies the thick and expansive masseter muscle, creating considerable difficulty in exposing the operative site properly. Finally, the curvature of this tooth is greater than that of any other and requires careful attention during repulsion, as the line of force established by the mallet and punch must be at an angle rather than a straight line.

A 3- to 4-inch incision is made through the skin, parallel to the fibers of the masseter muscle. The center of this incision should lie midway between the table surface of the tooth and the greatest curvature of the mandible. The muscle fibers are then bluntly separated until the bone is reached. A retractor is inserted at this time to separate the musculature and provide exposure of the site. The most ventral part of the tooth bed is located by finding the bulging bony prominence of the root, and the trephine opening is made at this point.

Rarely can the entire tooth be repelled into the mouth in one piece, as the upper sixth tooth is so close. Therefore, the lower tooth must be cut once or twice with a suitable instrument during removal. Care should be taken to avoid injury to major branches of the facial nerve and the masseteric artery, which are found 1-2 inches dorsal to the ventral border of the mandibular ramus.

As in the maxilla, the punch should be placed as nearly as possible in alignment with the long axis of the tooth. The technique of repulsion is the same. A method of identifying the root of the tooth when excessive enlargement of the mandible is present is to apply forceps to the tooth and rotate it slightly while palpating through the trephine opening with the finger of the dental punch.

Postoperative radiographs can reveal any alveolar fragments remaining after the alveolar socket has been searched.[269,271] The alveolar socket is irrigated with warm saline solution and packed to prevent contamination with food. Dental wax is the most satisfactory product for the purpose, though gauze rolls, gutta percha or soft acrylic may be used.

Truwax Dentsply baseplate wax has a melting point of 37.8 C (100 F), which is above the temperature of the mouth, and remains solidified when placed in the oral cavity. After the tooth has been removed and the alveolus cleansed of fragments, 2 sheets of the wax, measuring 3 x 6 x 1/8 inches each, are submerged in hot water (95-100 C). Within a few seconds, the wax becomes soft and pliable and can be molded in roughly the shape of the tooth just extracted. This should be done hurriedly so that the molded shape may be inserted into the alveolus before the wax has "set." As the soft wax plug is inserted into the alveolus, it conforms to the shape of the cavity; the little irregularities therein stabilize the plug and prevent its dislodgement during mastication.

The entire plug should be about half the length of the root of the removed tooth to allow room for development of granulation tissue in the root socket. The plug should extend only slightly above the top of the gingiva so that it is not involved in chewing. After the wax is in place, its surface is molded carefully with a finger to build a slight flange over the gingival line to seal the alveolus (Fig 46).

Removal of the plug postoperatively for drainage of a sinus, medication or inspection is done by inserting a hemostat through the trephine opening and dislodging the wax. A new plug may be inserted without anesthesia, as its application is attended by little or no discomfort. Each re-

Figure 46. The wax plug should extend about half way down into the alveolar cavity and extend slightly above the gum line.

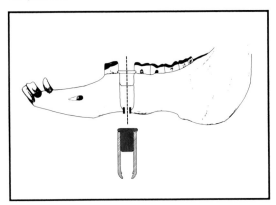

placement of the plug requires less wax because of rapidly developing granulation tissue. After the need for treatment has ended, a final plug of appropriate size is inserted. Granulation tissue filling the alveolus gradually pushes the wax plug into the oral cavity until it is finally expelled. During convalescence, a gauze dressing is used over the exterior trephine wound.

In some cases, the dental sinus may persist postoperatively because remaining dental fragments act as a necrotic focus. In such cases, secondary alveolar curettage, drainage and irrigation may be necessary.

Congenital and Familial Diseases

Maxillary and Mandibular Deformities

The most common congenital and developmental oral deformity is a maxilla that is relatively longer than the mandible, the so-called "parrot mouth" (Fig 47). The condition is called "sow mouth" or "monkey mouth" when the mandible is longer than the maxilla. These conditions also are referred to as maxillary and mandibular prognathism, respectively. Perhaps these terms are confusing because so-called maxillary prognathism actually is mandibular brachygnathia (short mandible). Conversely, mandibular prognathism is caused by maxillary shortening, ie, maxillary brachygnathia.[271] For these reasons, it is convenient to use the colloquial terms of parrot mouth, sow mouth or monkey mouth.

Both conditions are thought to be inherited. Some correction of incisor malocclusion occurs up to 5 years of age.[271] The following definitions have been adopted for use in North America and the United Kingdom. In North America, normal occlusion is complete contact of the occlusal (table) surface of the incisor teeth. Partial maxillary prognathism (overshot) or partial mandibular prognathism (undershot) results in 10-90% contact of the table surface of the incisors. In total maxillary prognathism (parrot mouth) or total mandibular prognathism (monkey mouth), there is gross malalignment of any incisors and/or no contact of the table surface of the incisors.

In the United Kingdom, parrot mouth in horses should be determined at 2 years of age and is defined as that condition in which there is no occlusal contact between the upper and lower central incisors, with the lower teeth caudal to the upper teeth. Horses should be examined in a halter. The horse's mouth should be closed and the chin elevated as the lips are rolled away from the incisors to assess the amount of occlusal contact.

Parrot Mouth: This deformity is congenital and may be heritable; affected horses are considered unsound (Fig 47). Abnormal incisor apposition results in abnormal wear and overgrowth. The central incisors develop a rabbit-toothed appearance and a characteristic parrot beak overhang of the upper incisors. There may be abnormal molar wear in grossly affected animals, with formation of hooks on the first maxillary and sixth mandibular teeth and, in some cases, shear mouth formation.[272]

Treatment usually is only palliative and involves regular rasping or sawing of the incisor arcade and chiseling of molar hooks. It is possible to arrest growth of the incisive area by circumferential wiring and anchoring to the first cheek tooth. Caution must be exercised before using orthodontic procedures in show animals because of the implication of unethical action.

Sow Mouth: This defect is not as common as parrot mouth but occurs frequently in some pony lines. As in parrot mouth, malocclusion leads to secondary infections and digestive disorders. The lesion is regarded as an unsoundness and treatment is palliative.

Figure 47. Parrot mouth resulting from mandibular brachygnathia in a Thoroughbred.

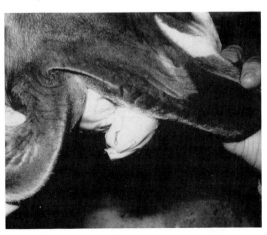

Shear Mouth: Shear mouth arises from an excessive difference in width between the maxilla and mandible. In normal horses, the upper arcade always is wider than the lower. A slight excess of this inequality results in excessive angulation of the table surfaces of the cheek teeth and development of long, extremely sharp edges. This condition may occur in horses of any age but is more common in old animals with irregularities in wear and age changes involving mandibular shape. From 1-2 cheek teeth to all premolars and molars may be involved. It may be unilateral or bilateral. The signs and lesions are similar to those associated with sharp enamel points but are more severe. Treatment usually is unsatisfactory and involves cutting and rasping to improve alignment. Giving the horse hard feed may postpone recurrence, but it seldom does.

Supernumerary Teeth

A wolf tooth should not be regarded as a supernumerary tooth, as it is part of the normal permanent dentition. By definition, supernumerary teeth are those found in addition to the normal number (polyodontia).

Extra incisors occur most frequently and may arise as a result of division of the permanent tooth germ. In some horses, there may be a complete double row but, more often, only 1 or 2 extra teeth (Fig 48). Treatment depends upon how the teeth develop. Those that wear more or less evenly and cause no apparent trouble should be left alone. However, if the extra teeth become elongated, they should be cut off or extracted to prevent damage to the mouth.

The type of operation depends upon the location of the teeth and judgment of the veterinarian. Owners frequently want supernumerary incisors removed for cosmetic reasons and it may be necessary to accede to such a request when there are no other reasons for extraction.

An extra cheek tooth may be present at the caudal end of the arcade or, less frequently, may appear displaced to the lingual or buccal aspect of the normal arcade. Extra cheek teeth should be extracted to prevent malocclusion.

Dentigerous Cysts

Dentigerous cysts are abnormal tooth developments of epithelial origin from Hertwig's sheath or its precursor, the enamel organ.[273] Such cysts frequently contain tooth fragments and may distort the surrounding maxilla or mandible.[274]

Dentigerous cysts arising from misplaced tooth germs of the branchial arch appear as temporal cysts and may drain into the ear.[275] The cysts are lined by stratified squamous epithelium and may contain one or more teeth (Figs 49, 50). Temporal teratoma or heterotopic polyodontia are terms used to describe such lesions. Clinical signs depend upon the affected site. In rare cases, cysts may form inside the cranial vault, but they more commonly occur as temporal cysts with aural fistulae and as maxillary or paranasal sinus cysts.[272] Treatment consists of careful dissection and removal of the cyst, followed by obliteration of the dead space and fistula or draining and packing the area with sterile rolled gauze.

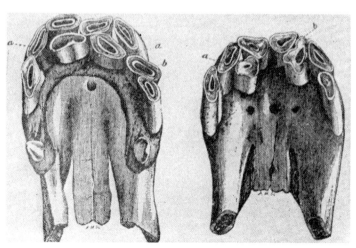

Figure 48. Supernumerary incisors. (From *The Viscera of the Domestic Mammals*, courtesy of Verlag Paul Parey)

The reader also is referred to the discussion of Heterotopic Polyodontia in the chapter on Diseases of the Skin.

Cystic Sinuses

This condition is also referred to as mucoid degeneration of the nasal turbinates, multiple mandibular cysts or osteodystrophia fibrosa cystica. It is seen typically in newborn or young horses. Affected animals may have facial and/or mandibular distortion, nasal occlusion, dyspnea and nasal discharge from contact ulcers on the turbinates (Fig 51). Differentiating between multiple mandibular cysts and dentigerous cysts may be difficult in mild cases. The lesions in this condition are similar to those of classic hyperparathyroidism with osteopenia due to excessive resorption of bone and fibrous tissue replacement.[275,276] However, there is no evidence that this condition is influenced by dietary factors, such as abnormal Ca:P ratios, and it is more likely that genetic defects are involved.

Though severely affected animals do not respond to treatment, they can survive satisfactorily for several years. Surgical drainage may benefit mildly affected animals.[274,277]

Abnormal Tooth Eruption

Tooth eruption is a complex phenomenon involving interplay between dental morphogenesis and the vascular forces responsible for creation of the eruption pathway. Table 16 lists the normal eruption times of the deciduous and permanent teeth. It should be noted that the third cheek tooth (fourth premolar) is the last permanent tooth to erupt and is most frequently impacted, rotated or medially misplaced.

Figure 49. Dentigerous cyst and aural fistula in an 8-month-old Thoroughbred colt.

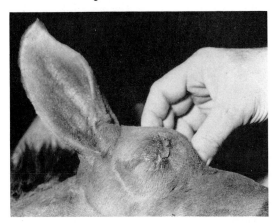

Figure 50. Dentigerous cyst opened to show enclosed tooth.

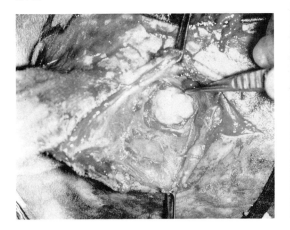

Figure 51. Ventrodorsal radiograph showing maxillary distortion from a multiloculated cyst in a 1-day-old Thoroughbred.

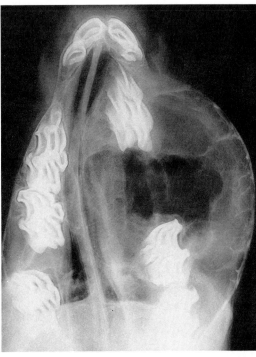

Mandibular, maxillary or incisive bone fractures may severely damage, displace, rotate or even destroy the permanent tooth germ and may result in a deficiency in permanent dentition, dental impaction or maleruption.

Delayed Eruption: Wolf teeth may be displaced in a labial and rostral direction or delayed in eruption. Such abnormalities result in contact ulcers at the area of bit contact. Such teeth are extracted easily in sedated horses.

Occasionally there may be marked variations in canine tooth eruption in males and 1 may be impacted. The gingiva should then be split allowing the crown to emerge.

Overcrowding and Displacement: If there is relative shortening of the maxilla or mandible, the third cheek tooth is unable to fit into the arcade. The upper third cheek tooth may be displaced medially into the palate, or there may be diffuse alveolar periostitis and facial swelling. It is normal for erupting permanent teeth to cause symmetric, nonpainful swelling along the ramus of the mandible, as well as dorsal and rostral to the facial crest. Such swellings result from periapical hyperemia and alveolar bone resorption and usually resolve spontaneously (Fig 52). In an overcrowded mouth, there is abnormal resistance to the erupting tooth.[278] This may exacerbate alveolar bone changes so that swelling becomes painful and may progress to sinus formation and periapical infections.

Early removal of deciduous caps and filing the mesial edges of adjacent teeth may facilitate normal eruption of impacted

Figure 52. Lateral radiograph showing an eruption pseudocyst around the apex of a premolar in a 3-year-old pony.

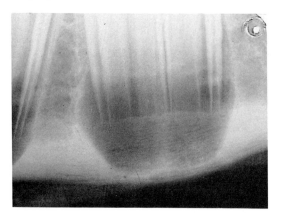

teeth; however, extraction is the only effective treatment in the presence of dental sinus formation and periapical infection.

Absence of Teeth (Oligodontia): Failure of teeth to develop is more common than polyodontia. Canines may be absent in some stallions and always are rudimentary in mares. There may be fewer than normal numbers of teeth in the arcades of any horse. Pseudo-oligodontia may result from loss of individual teeth or from total impaction (Fig 53).

Mandibular fractures in young horses may severely damage or even destroy the permanent tooth germ to result in deficiency in permanent dentition.

Unless there is interference with normal occlusion, no treatment is indicated for oligodontia. Malocclusion should be surgically corrected, as with acquired overgrowth from loss of the opposing tooth.

Figure 53. Lateral radiograph at necropsy showing impaction of the third cheek tooth within the mandible.

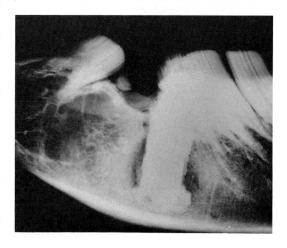

Wolf Teeth

These represent the vestiges of the first premolar tooth. Over 20% of aborted Thoroughbred fetuses examined contained wolf teeth. Over 90% of Plains Zebra had wolf teeth in the upper arcade and 60% in the lower arcade.[271] In the latter case, the teeth were large and, in some cases, occlusal contact was made.

In domestic horses, the mandibular wolf tooth is rarely present. The maxillary wolf tooth normally is in contact with the rostral margin of the first maxillary cheek tooth (Fig 54).

It is commonly believed by horse owners and trainers that all wolf teeth interfere with the bit and thus handicap the horse in training. This is true if the tooth is displaced or delayed in eruption, but there is no solid evidence to support the common procedure of routine wolf tooth extraction.

Diseases With Physical Causes

Abnormal Dental Wear

Sharp Enamel Points: Normal grinding action of dental arcades leads to formation of complex transverse ridges across the occlusal surface of teeth. Full lateral movement of the mandible results in incomplete wear of buccal surfaces of the upper arcade and lingual surfaces of the lower arcade so that small, sharp enamel points form along the edges. At the same time, there is slight caudal retraction of the mandible so the first maxillary and last mandibular teeth tend to develop small hooks (Fig 55). Such points and hooks can cause buccal or lingual ulcerations and may result in poor bit contact and bit-shy horses. Sharp enamel points are corrected by regular floating.

Wave Mouth: Abnormal mastication results in changes in the shape and position of the normal transverse ridges across the occlusal surfaces. Some ridges and valleys are enhanced, and the arcades attain a wave form. In severe cases, the teeth in one arcade may be worn to the gingival margin,

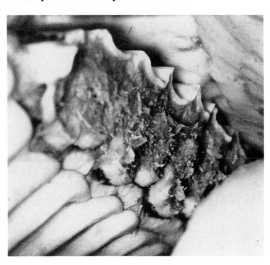

Figure 55. Labial enamel points and rostral hook on the maxillary arcade of a 6-year-old Hunter.

permitting the opposing molar to lacerate the gingiva.

If the history and clinical examination suggest minimal malocclusion and the arcades are relatively complementary, only floating is necessary. If mastication is grossly impaired or if there is much salivation and quidding, an attempt should be made to level the arcades with a dental rasp, chisels and compound molar cutters. In most cases, this is best accomplished under general anesthesia with the horse in lateral recumbency and a speculum applied. In mild cases, the procedure can be accom-

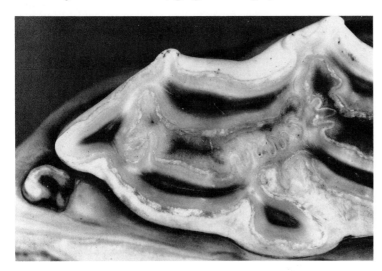

Figure 54. Wolf tooth (left) in its normal position at the rostral margin of the first cheek tooth (right).

plished with the horse standing in stocks or a stall. Treatment of severe cases seldom is satisfactory despite adequate removal of the projecting portions of the wave.

Step Mouth: Step mouth is characterized by marked variation in the height of individual premolars and molars. This may be due to unequal wear of opposing teeth in the dental arcade or a sequel to surgical removal of teeth. Signs of this condition are similar to those of other dental disorders, but malnutrition and emaciation usually are more evident because a step-mouthed animal cannot chew food properly. Treatment involves leveling projecting teeth at regular (usually semiannual) intervals.

Smooth Mouth: In extreme old age, the teeth may become completely smooth or lost entirely. Smooth mouth usually is found in old horses but may be encountered in young animals. The table surfaces of the teeth become smooth through complete erosion of the crowns and through defects in the lamellar arrangement of enamel, cementum and dentine. Individual teeth of the entire arcade may be affected, though an animal ordinarily is not called smooth-mouthed until most of the teeth are involved. Because the smooth table surfaces of the teeth prohibit proper grinding of feed, associated signs include colic and poor condition. Smooth table surfaces are detected readily by palpation. In young animals, smooth mouth occasionally may be caused by improper floating, during which the table surfaces of cheek teeth are filed smooth.

Treatment of smooth mouth in old and young animals with defective teeth is useless. Feeding mashed and chopped feed to young animals that have been mishandled gives the teeth an opportunity to reestablish their normal rough table surfaces.

Retention of Deciduous Teeth

Dental caps are deciduous cheek teeth that remain attached to the permanent teeth after the permanent ones have erupted. Deciduous teeth sometimes are movable on palpation; however, even if they are not loose, the caps should be removed once it has been definitely determined that the permanent tooth has grown beyond the gingival line. It is best not to attempt to remove caps if it requires a great deal of effort to loosen them. Age and pain generally

dictate removal of offending caps. Sometimes the cap partially detaches and rotates laterally, causing buccal laceration and facial deformity.

To remove a cap in the lower arcade, medium-sized forceps should be applied and the cap rocked loose and removed. Caps on the upper arcade are best removed by inserting a dental elevator or screwdriver blade into the junction between the cap and permanent tooth and prying the cap loose. The extracted tooth should be examined to make sure that a portion has not broken off and remains in the maxilla or mandible, as that may hinder eating, cause the permanent tooth to grow unevenly, cause local gingivitis and predispose to infection.

Dental caps should be removed before the teeth are floated because sharp edges or points sometimes are present on underlying permanent teeth. Removal of deciduous teeth at the proper time allows the permanent teeth to grow normally and results in less chance of training interruption due to mastication difficulties or interference with the bit.

Retained temporary incisors are similar to dental caps except that they may remain embedded more or less firmly in the gingiva and the permanent incisors erupt caudal to them rather than displacing them. Ordinarily these teeth are loose and easily removed with a pair of dental forceps; however, occasionally they must be loosened with a bone gouge or dental elevator. The cavity should be searched with a probe or splinter forceps to make sure all tooth fragments are removed. Occasionally the gingiva must be incised under local anesthesia and dental fragments removed. The surgical wound ordinarily heals without suturing, though 1 or 2 sutures of nonabsorbable material may be placed in the gum to appose the divided tissues; these sutures should be removed within 10 days. Most horses do not object much to this procedure and removal can be accomplished with minimal restraint.

Inflammatory, Infectious Immune Diseases

Paranasal Sinus Cyst

This topic is discussed in the chapter on Diseases of the Respiratory System.

Periodontal Disease

Periodontal disease in horses is inflammatory and dystrophic in nature, and may cause malnutrition, halitosis, maxillary and mandibular osteitis (quidding), paranasal sinusitis, nasal discharge, colic and death in severely affected animals. It has been described as the dental scourge of horses and is the most common dental disease of horses (Fig 56).[279,280]

The initial lesion is marginal gingivitis, with hyperemia and edema (Fig 57). The lateral gingival sulcus becomes eroded and a triangular pocket is formed, usually on the buccal aspect. This cavity harbors food materials and a cycle of irritation, inflammation and erosion destroys gingival tissue to the lingual aspect and deeper into the periodontium (Fig 58). Ultimately, gross alveolar sepsis develops and the tooth is lost. Transient gingivitis may be caused by the first instars of the bot fly.[281]

In all species, the shearing forces produced by normal mastication are essential for maintenance of healthy periodontium.[282] Gingivitis, which may lead to periodontitis, occurs in any situation in which there is abnormal occlusion and alteration in shearing forces.[283] The most severe form of periodontal disease, with gross pocketing, periodontal suppuration and loosening of

Figure 56. Incidence of periodontal disease in horses at various ages.

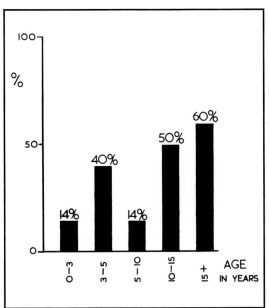

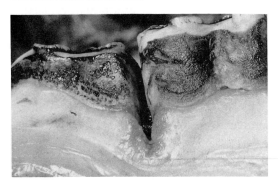

Figure 57. Marginal gingivitis between the first and second mandibular cheek teeth.

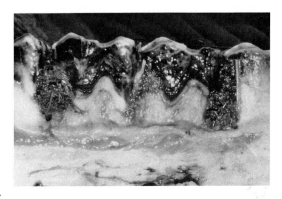

Figure 58. Severe periodontitis with debris-filled pockets.

teeth, is associated with extreme abnormalities of wear, such as irregular arcades, hooks, loss of teeth with corresponding overgrowth of the occluding arcade, misplaced or split teeth, and mandibular fractures.

The disease affects all teeth during eruption of permanent dentition, but lesions heal once the normal grinding pattern is established. In severe cases, gross alveolar sepsis, unthriftiness and halitosis may necessitate the horse's destruction.

The importance of this disease should be understood. Regular dental examination and prophylaxis to maintain normal teeth and grinding action can help prevent its onset.

Alveolar Periostitis

(Chronic Ossifying Periostitis)

These terms have been used to describe the diffuse bone changes seen in association with periodontal disease in young horses. In particular, they refer to the changes seen at eruption of the permanent cheek teeth.[278-280] However, there are inflammatory periosteal changes in all horses at this stage, and the differentiation between normal and pathologic changes is by no means clear. Progression of inflammation of rhinitis, paranasal sinusitis and apical infection of teeth causes corresponding clinical signs.

Dental Decay

Some question has been expressed as to the use of the term caries as applied to horses.[269,284] By definition, caries is a disease of the calcified tissues of teeth resulting from the action of microorganisms on carbohydrates and characterized by decalcification of the inorganic portion of the tooth. This is accompanied or followed by disintegration of the organic portion.

Horses commonly have an expanding, debris-filled cavity within the cementum of enamel invagination of maxillary teeth. Formation of cementum within the enamel lakes is incomplete at eruption and blood supply through the infundibulum is lost. Consequently, the lake cementum in all erupted maxillary teeth is dead tissue. As the tooth surface is worn away, areas of hypoplastic cementum are exposed and appear as necrotic cavities.[271,285] Secondary to hypoplasia, there may be fermentation of impacted food in the infundibulum and acid dissolution of the surrounding cementum, enamel and dentine. Such lesions are then true caries of cementum (Fig 59).[271,272,286]

The lesion is benign in many teeth. Though there may be local extension within an individual cementum lake, formation of secondary dentine protects the pulp from infection. Pulpitis and even splitting of the tooth result when the lesion spreads (Fig 60). This may lead to alveolar sepsis, sinus empyema and nasal discharge.

The primary lesion, hypoplasia of cementum, rarely is detected in life, and only after alveolar sepsis or sinus infection has developed do signs of disease appear. Tooth extraction or repulsion, alveolar or sinus curettage and irrigation then should be performed. Similar lesions exist in the teeth of wild equidae. Though it can be argued that some management and feeding regimens influence development of primary periodontal disease, it is not the case that caries of

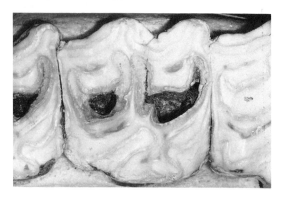

Figure 59. Caries of cementum of the fourth cheek tooth in an 8-year-old Hunter.

cementum is a disease of domestication, as has been suggested.[287]

Caries of cementum is not the only route of infection into the pulp cavity. Pulpitis may arise from tooth fracture, periodontal disease or, as seen more commonly in the mandible, as a result of maleruption and lysis of alveolar bone. Figure 61 is a schematic representation of the possible sequelae of apical infections and pulpitis in horses. Table 19 demonstrates that second and third upper and lower teeth are affected most frequently and emphasizes the etiologic significance of dental impactions.

Apical infections cause maxillary and mandibular swelling, and usually are of only minor discomfort to the horse. Clinical signs may include dental sinus formation, paranasal sinusitis and nasal discharge (Fig 62). Oblique radiographs are useful in eval-

Figure 60. Fusion of rostral and caudal caries.

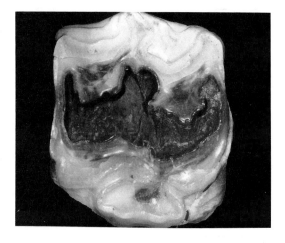

Figure 61. Sequelae of pulpitis.

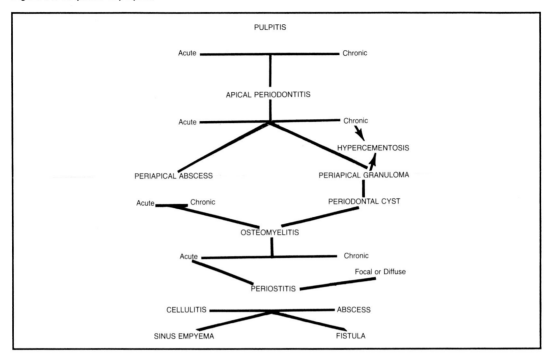

uating the lesion. There may be cystic osteitis of alveolar bone and production of new bone and cementum from the irritated periodontal ligament (Fig 63).[283]

Apical infections can be treated only by extraction of the affected tooth or teeth, followed by thorough curettage of the osteitic bone, and irrigation and cleansing of sinus tracts and paranasal sinus empyema as indicated.

Neoplasia

Dental tumors are classified, according to their origin, as epithelial or mesenchymal. Odontoma describes any tumor of odontogenic origin and refers to a tumor in which both the epithelial and mesenchymal cells produce functional ameloblasts and odontoblasts (and, therefore, enamel and dentine within the tumor).

Table 19. Comparative prevalence of apical infections at various cheek teeth.

							Cheek Tooth						Number
	1		2		3		4		5		6		
	R*	C*	R	C	R	C	R	C	R	C	R	C	Affected
Maxillary	2	7	9	9	10	11	7	8	0	0	0	0	
Total		9		18		21		15		0		0	63
Mandibular	0	4	18	22	13	10	5	3	3	1	0	0	
Total		4		40		23		8		4		0	79
													142

*R = rostral root, C = caudal root

Most dental tumors occur in young horses and, if originating from a deciduous tooth germ or the first true molar tooth germ, are congenital.[288,289] They usually are benign but defy treatment because of their size and degree of facial or mandibular distortion created. However, affected animals may survive for several months or years before euthanasia is necessary.

The most common dental tumors are ameloblastic odontomas of the maxilla, which are mixed tumors of epithelial and mesenchymal origin. Clinical signs may include facial swelling, nasal obstruction, dyspnea, dysphagia, quidding and unthriftiness.

Multifactorial Diseases

Dental Calculus

With normal dental occlusion, the frictional forces generated by the grinding action of mastication prevent accumulation of plaque and dental calculus in horses. Calculus commonly accumulates on the canine teeth of all male horses because their teeth do not make occlusal contact. Similarly, dental irregularities, loss of teeth, oral ul-

Figure 62. Facial swelling and nasal discharge caused by apical infection of the third right maxillary cheek tooth in an 8-year-old pony.

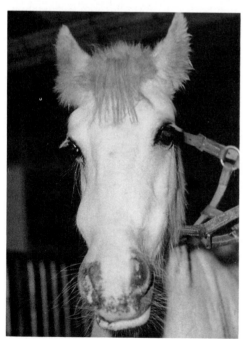

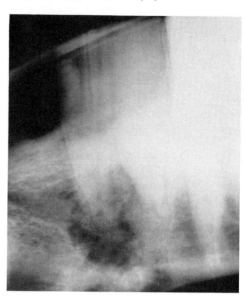

Figure 63. Lateral radiograph showing mandibular osteitis and a dental sinus caused by apical root infection.

cers and jaw injuries change the pattern of mastication and hence allow calculus accumulation (see Floating). Systemic disease, septicemia, toxemia and renal disease may all cause gingival edema, ulceration, and plaque and calculus formation.

DISEASES OF THE SALIVARY GLANDS

J.N. Moore

Diagnostic and Therapeutic Considerations

The salivary glands of horses provide the large volume of saliva required for softening roughage during mastication and for initial digestion of feedstuffs. As evidence of the importance of this function in an animal that normally consumes roughage, salivary flows approaching 50 ml/minute have been measured during mastication in ponies.[290] The parotid gland is the largest of the salivary glands in horses. Of the salivary glands, the parotid secretes an electrolyte-rich fluid, the composition of which is directly influenced by the rate of flow.[291] Presumably the submaxillary glands of horses secrete an electrolyte-poor fluid. Based on studies using a saliva-collecting bit in pony mares, it has been determined that there is considerable variation in the electrolyte composition of whole saliva.[292] Fortunately, diseases affecting the salivary glands are rare and the need to collect samples of saliva or determine its constituents arises uncommonly.

Congenital Diseases

Parotid Duct Atresia

There has been a report in the literature of atresia of the parotid duct in a foal. Rather than penetrating the oral mucosa, the affected duct ended in a cul-de-sac.[293]

Diseases With Physical Causes

Trauma to the Salivary Gland and Ducts

Of the conditions affecting the salivary glands, trauma to the parotid duct occurs most often. Generally the duct is traumatized by kicks to the mandible, lacerations or surgery performed in the area of the guttural pouch. Damage to the parotid duct usually occurs where the duct passes around the mandibular border and often results in a salivary fistula; the flow of saliva is most noticeable when the horse eats.

Fortunately, most wounds to the salivary gland itself are self-limiting and heal by second intention without need for intervention. Similarly, many wounds involving the parotid duct result in leakage of saliva for a short time and then heal by second intention. In other instances, the flow of saliva may be sufficient to prevent healing of the wound and a salivary fistula develops. If the defect in the skin heals or if the parotid duct ruptures, saliva may collect in a subcutaneous space. This salivary mucocele can be distinguished from a seroma by aspiration of the fluid and determination of the electrolyte content. Saliva has higher concentrations of potassium and calcium than plasma.

If the parotid salivary gland is traumatized, the area should be cleansed, devitalized tissue debrided, and the skin sutured. It is probably appropriate to feed the horse through a nasogastric tube for several days to avoid any potential problems due to stimulation of salivation by eating. Generally, these wounds heal satisfactorily. If a salivary fistula occurs secondary to trauma to the glandular tissue, treatment should be conservative, as these fistulae usually heal spontaneously. If, however, the fistula involves the duct and persists for several weeks, surgery is needed to reestablish continuity of the duct or to destroy the salivary gland.

If the aim of the surgery is to reconstruct the duct, an incision is made over the fistula and the dissection is continued down to isolate the duct. Medical-grade polyethylene tubing is then passed caudad through the duct toward the gland and rostrad through the parotid papilla. The duct is then sutured end-to-end with interrupted sutures of 5-0 material and the tubing is secured to the cheek. This tubing should remain in place for 2-3 weeks.[294] Alternatively, a tunnel may be created into the oral cavity and a silk suture placed in the oral mucosa is passed from the oral cavity to the rostral end of the duct. This suture then serves as a scaffold for development of a fistula into the mouth.

Though the above procedures are designed to reestablish the patency of the parotid duct, a simpler solution to the problem is to ligate the proximal end of the duct. This procedure induces atrophy of the glandular tissue. It has been suggested that heavy suture or umbilical tape be used for this ligation and that the suture not be tied too tightly. Otherwise, the suture may cut through the duct before the gland atrophies. As an alternative approach, the lining of the duct may be curetted and iodine solution injected locally to cause scarring of the walls of the fistula.

Trauma to the sublingual salivary gland most often results in formation of a mucocele on the floor of the mouth, lateral to the frenulum. These mucoceles respond to marsupialization into the mouth by creating a permanent fistula. An opening is created into the mucocele and tubing is used to connect the mucocele with the oral cavity.

Salivary Calculi

Though uncommon, salivary calculi occasionally form and become lodged at the orifice of the parotid duct. Clinical findings may include swelling along the duct or acute inflammation of the gland secondary to complete obstruction. The calcium carbonate calculus forms around a nidus of desquamated cells and exudate, and may enlarge to several centimeters in size. Treatment involves excision of the calculus through an incision made directly over the swelling and suturing of the edges of the duct with fine sutures. Generally it is advisable to restrict access to feed for several days postoperatively to reduce parotid salivation.

Inflammatory, Infectious and Immune Diseases

Sialoadenitis

As with other abnormalities involving the salivary glands, inflammation of the glands is uncommon. The most common causes of sialoadenitis are trauma to the gland and obstruction of the salivary duct. Trauma-induced sialoadenitis generally responds favorably to symptomatic therapy and antibiotics if there is evidence of infection. Obstruction of the salivary duct by plant material may induce secondary inflammation of the gland due to accumulation of exudate, mucus and desquamated cells. Treatment includes removal of the obstruction and appropriate antimicrobial therapy.

Neoplasia

Neoplasms rarely affect the salivary glands of horses. Adenocarcinomas, acinar-cell tumors, melanomas and mixed tumors involving the salivary glands have been reported in horses.[295] Though rare, these tumors most often involve the parotid salivary gland. Affected horses are usually aged, and clinical signs include pain over the gland, edema and a palpable enlargement of the area. Examination of histologic sections permits determination of the tumor type and the prognosis.

Generally, benign mixed tumors and acinar-cell tumors are locally invasive and tend to recur; wide excision is required. Adenocarcinomas generally have metastasized to the regional lymph nodes by the time the mass is evident. Consequently, treatment is often unsuccessful. Malignant melanomas generally fail to respond adequately to excision.

DISEASES OF THE ESOPHAGUS

J.A. Stick

Diagnostic and Therapeutic Considerations

The clinical signs, diagnosis and therapy of esophageal disease are specific and unlike those of the rest of the alimentary system. Clinical evaluation of the equine patient with esophageal disease includes physical, radiographic and endoscopic examinations. Early and definitive diagnosis is paramount when dealing with esophageal injury, especially when signs of disease recur following initial treatment. Therapy of esophageal disorders is centered around conservative medical and manipulative management, with dietary alterations being a primary component of therapy. However, surgical management of esophageal disease in the equine patient has become more commonplace in recent years and necessitates discussion of surgical anatomy, approaches and complications.[280,296,297]

Clinical Manifestations

The obstructive disease of "choke" may be manifested by ptyalism, dysphagia, coughing, and regurgitation of food, water and saliva from the mouth and nostrils. Attempts at ingestion often are followed by odynophagia (painful swallowing), repeated extension of the head and neck, and other signs of distress or agitation. The time interval from swallowing until these signs are shown by the patient depends upon the location of the lesion within the esophagus. With obstruction of the distal esophagus, odynophagia and retching may occur 10-12 seconds after swallowing. With proximal esophageal obstruction, the signs may be evident immediately. This occurs because the propagation speed of the equine esophagus is about 9.4 cm/second in the proximal two-thirds but only 4.6 cm/second in the distal one-third. Therefore, over an average length of 116 cm, a bolus of food would take about 16 seconds to traverse the body of the esophagus.[298,299] Intermittent signs of choke, followed by periods of relief, may indicate a disease other than simple feed impaction, and further diagnostic procedures are warranted. Anorexia, electrolyte imbalances and dehydration accompany cases of long duration (see Complications of Surgery below). Aspiration pneumonia frequently follows esophageal obstruction, and the clinical signs may be present as early as 1 day after the onset of choke.

Physical Examination

A thorough oral examination should be performed to rule out an oral foreign body, dental disease, cleft palate or oropharyngeal neoplasms. Observation and palpation of the neck in the area of the jugular furrows may reveal enlargement of the cervical esophagus. Simple food impaction of the cervical esophagus may be localized in this manner. Crepitation of a diffuse, firm enlargement may indicate loss of integrity of the esophageal wall. Passage of the nasogastric tube often confirms luminal obstruction and localizes the site of involvement. Gentle lavage of warm water through the tube may permit material to be flushed free of the obstruction if feed or consumption of bedding is the cause of the problem. At this time, sedation of the animal with xylazine (Rompun: Haver) IV at 1.1 mg per kg lowers the horse's head and prevents further aspiration. Lavage may be continued until the obstruction is relieved, and further diagnostic studies may be unnecessary. However, reobstruction indicates that other esophageal disease may be present and the diagnosis should be pursued.

With any esophageal disease, auscultation and radiography of the thorax are indicated to monitor development of aspiration pneumonia. This complication is common when an esophageal problem is encountered.

Radiographic Evaluation

Esophagography in horses is diagnostic in most instances and should be considered as part of the complete esophageal examination in problems other than simple obstruction. A survey film is necessary to establish radiographic technique and the presence or absence of disease without contrast material (*eg,* feed impaction or foreign body) (Fig 64). Barium paste (85% w/v with water, 120 ml) given by mouth outlines the longitudinal mucosal folds of the esophagus with the lumen undistended and localizes the obstruction or any disruption of the lumen (Fig 65). A feed impaction becomes coated with the barium, a complete obstruction halts barium flow at the site of the lesion (Fig 66), and rupture of the esophagus permits barium to escape into surrounding soft tissues. If possible, sedation of the patient should be avoided during this procedure because it suppresses the swallowing reflex and causes barium to be held in the mouth, reducing the amount available to coat the esophagus.

Liquid barium (72% w/v with water, 480 ml) may be administered under pressure by a dose syringe through a cuffed nasogastric tube to prevent reflux into the pharynx (Fig 67). This technique demonstrates strictures and associated prestenotic dilatation of the esophagus. Liquid barium (480 ml) followed by air (480 ml), delivered by dose syringe under pressure, provides a double-contrast study (Fig 68), permitting examination of mucosal folds with the esophagus distended. This latter technique gives the best definition of mucosal lesions, such as circumferential mucosal ulcers following feed impaction. Though a diagnosis often can be made

Figure 64. Lateral cervical radiograph of a 9-year-old gelding with anorexia and odynophagia. A metallic foreign body (fishing lure) is lodged in the cranial esophageal sphincter (arrow).

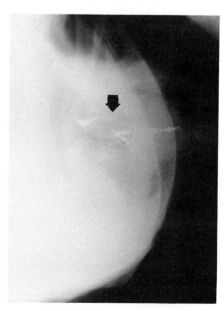

without using all 3 techniques, each technique demonstrates lesions not seen with the other 2.

In the cranial cervical area, where the esophagus lies dorsal to the trachea, lesions that restrict distention of the esophageal lumen can be demonstrated with negative-contrast radiography. A flexible endoscope can be used to localize the lesion and to permit insufflation of the esophagus during radiography. Alternatively, air (480 ml) can be delivered by dose syringe under pressure through a cuffed nasogastric tube to achieve the same results. However, negative-contrast radiography alone does not yield much information about the caudal cervical and thoracic portions of the esophagus because of superimposition of the air density of the trachea and lungs.

Swallowing during contrast studies, when the lumen is being distended, produces false signs of esophageal stricture (Fig 69). Xylazine, given IV at 1.1 mg/kg 5 minutes before the barium-under-pressure, double-contrast or negative-contrast esophagogram, helps eliminate this swallow artifact by decreasing the reflex "secondary swallows" that follow luminal distention.

Figure 65. Barium paste (120 ml) given by mouth outlines the normal longitudinal folds of the mucosa in the undistended lumen of the esophagus.

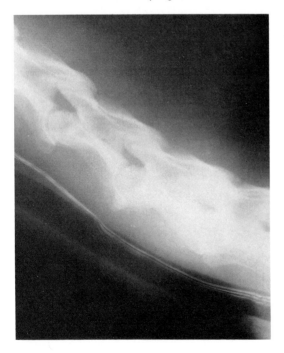

Figure 66. Complete obstruction of the esophagus is localized on esophagography following barium paste swallow. This adult horse had an esophageal stricture. Note the prestenotic dilatation.

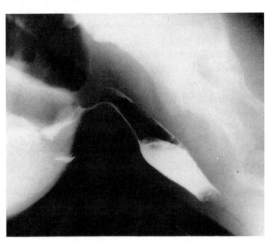

Endoscopic Evaluation

Esophagoscopy may better define the severity and extent of esophageal lesions diagnosed on radiography and can be used as an ancillary diagnostic aid. However, endoscopic examination always should be performed when radiographic findings are not diagnostic. If the endoscope is 150 cm or longer, the entire esophagus may be examined and esophageal lesions in the thorax of the adult horse undetected on radiographic examination can be diagnosed. A flexible endoscope that allows irrigation and insufflation is necessary to provide good observation of mucosal disease and changes in luminal size.

Endoscopic examination may be performed safely on the restrained standing animal in most instances. Diagnostic observations are best made by starting with the endoscopy fully inserted and the esophageal lumen insufflated; then one slowly withdraws the endoscope tip toward the horse's head. After each swallow, the endoscope should be cleared by irrigation and the esophagus dilated before further withdrawal. Several passes should be made over any area of suspected disease.

Longitudinal mucosal folds in the esophagus normally are seen when the endoscope tip is moved proximad and the esophagus is in the relaxed position (Fig 70). Insufflation flattens these folds and permits observation of luminal size. Inability to insufflate the esophagus and flatten the longitudinal mucosal folds usually indicates disease. This is noted cranial and caudal to a stricture. Transverse folds can be produced iatrogenically by moving the endoscope tip toward the stomach (Fig 71). When the cervical esophagus in insufflated, the outline of the trachea often can be seen through the esophageal wall (Fig 72). Swallowing produces changes in the lumen that give the appearance of diverticula or strictures to the untrained observer (Fig 73). The normal mucosa is white to light pink; reddened discolorations are evidence of mucosal disease.

The cranial aspect of the cervical esophageal sphincter is difficult to examine because of repeated stimulation of the swallowing reflex and the larynx's directing the endoscope tip dorsally. Radiographic assessment of this area may be more diagnostic. Additionally, the longitudinal mucosal folds found along the rest of the esophagus are absent in this area.

Frequently endoscopic appearance of an esophageal obstruction is obscured by saliva mixed with ingesta that collects proximal to the obstruction. This should be removed by suction through a nasogastric tube and the

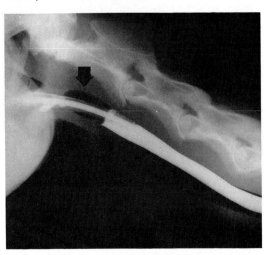

Figure 67. Positive-contrast esophagogram using liquid barium administered under pressure through a nasogastric tube fitted with an inflatable cuff (arrow) shows the distended lumen of the normal esophagus. The inflatable cuff prevents reflux of barium into the pharynx and aspiration into the trachea.

endoscope should be reinserted immediately to observe the area of obstruction.

Manometric Evaluation

Esophageal dysfunction in people is routinely evaluated using intraluminal pressure manometry. Manometric techniques have been developed and reference esoph-

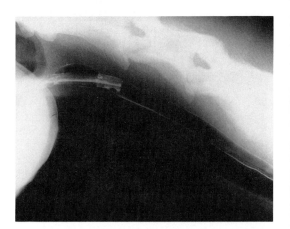

Figure 68. Double-contrast esophagogram using liquid barium, followed by a bolus of air shows the normal esophagus with the lumen distended. This technique can outline any abnormal transverse mucosal folds.

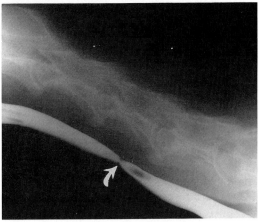

Figure 69. Barium esophagogram shows false signs of a stricture (arrow) when barium is administered under pressure and the radiograph is made during swallowing. This swallow artifact can be avoided if xylazine is administered 5 minutes before the study is attempted.

Figure 70. Appearance of the normal longitudinal mucosal folds of the undistended esophagus when the endoscope is pulled craniad (toward the head).

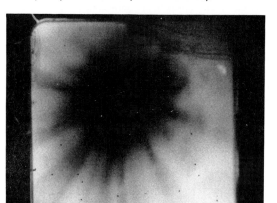

Figure 72. The tracheal rings (arrow) are seen through the wall of the normal distended esophagus during endoscopy.

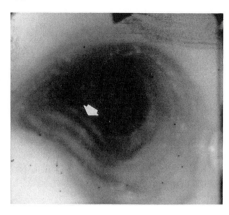

Figure 71. Endoscopic photograph shows transverse folding of esophageal mucosa occurring when the scope is passed towardthe stomach. These folds are not considered pathologic unless they are seen when the esophagus is insufflated and the scope is pulled craniad.

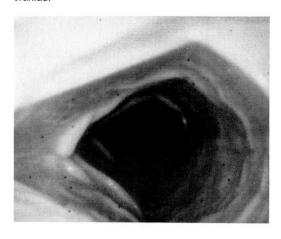

Figure 73. Endoscopic photographs show the transient changes of the esophageal lumen after swallowing, mimicking a diverticulum (top) or stricture (bottom).

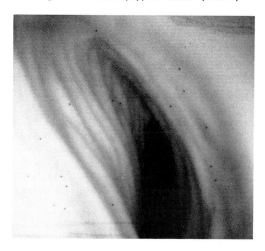

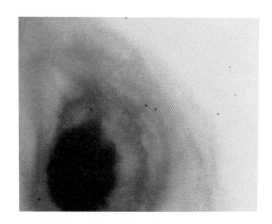

ageal pressure profiles have been established in healthy horses.[298,299] Four functionally distinct regions of the esophagus were demonstrated: cranial esophageal sphincter, caudal esophageal sphincter and "fast" (cranial two-thirds) and "slow" (caudal one-third) regions in the body of the esophagus (Fig 74). In some physiologic disorders of the equine esophagus, manometry may better define problems in which more conventional methods have not yielded a diagnosis. Manometry has yielded new information on clinical manifestations of esophageal obstruction. However, the availability and technical difficulty of manometry have limited its use as a diagnostic tool in equine practice.

Figure 75 outlines a systematic scheme of examination using physical, radiographic and endoscopic findings to diagnose esophageal disorders. Alternate pathways may be used, depending on the disease, clinical signs, available diagnostic aids and experience of the clinician. Physical examination, including passage of a nasogastric tube and esophageal lavage, and radiography yield a diagnosis for most common esophageal problems. Endoscopy allows definitive diagnosis of some anatomic disorders not observed with radiography. Manometry, cine-

Figure 74. Manometric recording (in mm of Hg) of a swallow as it passes through the 4 functionally distinct regions of the esophagus. UESG = cranial (or upper) esophageal sphincter region; FER = fast esophageal region; SER = slow esophageal region; LESR = caudal (or lower) esophageal sphincter region.

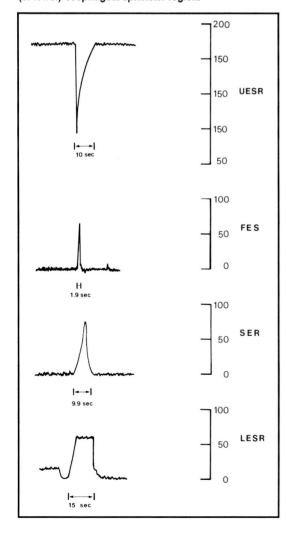

Figure 75. Scheme of examination of esophageal disorders. Arrows outline pathways that usually are diagnostic for the conditions shown at the right.

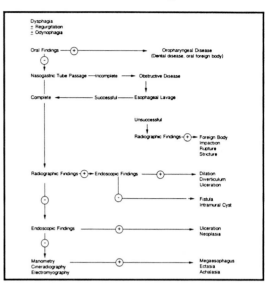

radiography and electromyography seldom are necessary and have not been used commonly in diagnosis of esophageal diseases.

Surgical Anatomy

The esophagus of adult horses varies in length from 125 to 150 cm, depending on the size of the animal, and consists of cervical, thoracic and abdominal parts. As it courses caudally, it deviates from a position dorsal to the trachea in the cranial one-third of the neck, to the left side of the medial plane in the middle one-third of the neck, and comes to lie ventral to the trachea at the thoracic inlet.[300] The cervical part of the equine esophagus is most accessible to surgery and comprises over 50% of the total length of the esophagus.

The wall of the esophagus is comprised of 4 layers: a fibrous layer (tunica adventitia); muscular layers (tunica muscularis); a submucosal layer (tela submucosa) and a mucous membrane (tunica mucosa). The muscular layers are striated from the pharynx to the base of the heart, where they gradually blend into smooth muscle. As the esophagus courses caudally, its muscular layers increase in thickness while the lumen diminishes. Except at the upper esophageal sphincter, the 2 muscular layers are arranged spirally and elliptically.[301] On surgical incision, the esophageal wall separates easily into 2 distinct layers. The elastic inner layer, composed of mucosa and submucosa, is freely movable within the relatively inelastic outer muscular layer and adventitia (Fig 76). The mucosa, which provides the greatest tensile strength upon closure of an esophageal incision, is covered with stratified squamous epithelium and lies in longitudinal folds that obliterate the lumen except during deglutition.

The arterial supply to the cervical part of the esophagus originates from the carotid arteries. The thoracic and relatively short (2-3 cm) abdominal esophagus is supplied by the bronchoesophageal and gastric arteries. The vascular pattern is arcuate but segmental without generous collateral circulation, necessitating careful preservation of vessels during surgery.

Innervation of the esophagus is derived from the ninth and tenth cranial nerves and the sympathetic trunk, as well as mesenteric ganglion cells within the muscle layers.

Surgical Approaches

Three surgical approaches to the equine esophagus can be used. Each approach is dictated by anatomic location of the lesion and purpose of the surgery. The ventral cervical approach is best used for esophagostomy, esophagomyotomy and resections involving the proximal three-quarters of the

Figure 76. Traction on the incised esophagus, with a nasogastric tube in place, shows the elastic properties of the mucosa and submucosa (inner layer).

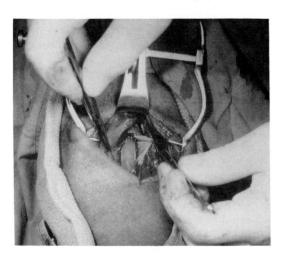

cervical esophagus. A ventrolateral approach is recommended for placing a feeding tube in the mid-cervical esophagus or for approaching the distal one-fourth of the cervical esophagus, especially near the thoracic inlet.[296] Thoracotomy is necessary to approach the distal half of the esophagus; the choice of intercostal space is dictated by the aim of the surgery and location of the lesion.

If the surgeon expects to invade the esophageal lumen, broad-spectrum antibiotics are indicated, based on sound surgical principles, expected complications and recognized bacterial colonization of this organ.[280,301,302] Before induction of anesthesia, a nasogastric tube should be passed as far into the esophagus as the surgical site (or beyond if possible) to facilitate identification of the esophagus at surgery. It also is necessary to avoid damage to the recurrent laryngeal nerve and vagosympathetic trunk, which are easily traumatized when retracting the carotid artery away from the esophagus.

Ventral Approach: Surgical procedures are conducted with the animal under general anesthesia and placed in dorsal recumbency. A 10-cm skin incision permits exposure of about 6 cm of the esophagus. The skin and subcutaneous fascia are divided sharply using a scalpel. The paired muscles of the sternothyroid, sternohyoid and omohyoid are separated along the midline to expose the trachea (Fig 77). Blunt separation of fascia along the left side of the trachea permits identification of the esophagus containing the nasogastric tube. Retraction of the trachea to the right of the median plain and gentle sharp dissection of overlying loose adventitia expose the ventral wall of the esophagus.

Ventrolateral Approach: Placement of a feeding tube using this approach facilitates firm anchorage of the tube to the skin and permits it to lie in a comfortable position on the patient's neck while avoiding impingement of the feeding tube on the trachea (Fig 77). This approach also affords better access to the distal cervical esophagus where the ventral cervical musculature becomes more heavily developed, making the ventral approach less desirable. This surgical approach may be made with the horse standing, using local anesthesia, or with the horse in dorsal or right lateral recumbency, under general anesthesia.[303]

A 5-cm skin incision (for feeding tube placement) is made just ventral to the jugular vein. The sternocephalicus and brachiocephalicus muscles are separated and the deep cervical fascia is incised to expose the esophagus. It may be necessary to incise the cutaneous colli muscle in the distal cervical area.

Approach to the Thoracic Esophagus: This approach can be used for vascular ring anomalies (2 patients in my experience in which the left fourth or right fifth interspace was used) or when the suspected lesion can be resolved surgically without entering the esophageal lumen. A 5-month-old foal was successfully treated for an intrathoracic esophageal stricture with esophagomyotomy through the eighth intercostal space.[304]

The patient is placed in right lateral recumbency under general anesthesia and positive-pressure ventilation is used. The skin, subcutaneous tissue, cutaneous trunci, serratus ventralis and latissimus dorsi are sharply divided. A subperiosteal rib resec-

Figure 77. Placement of a feeding tube ventral to the jugular vein permits it to lie in a comfortable position on the neck. Note the "butterfly" tape bandage sutured to the skin to firmly anchor the tube (black arrow), and saliva loss around the tube (white arrow).

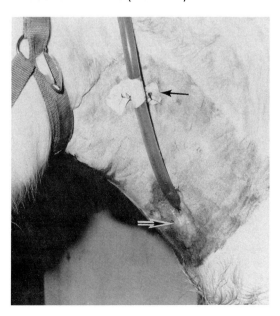

tion has been described.[304] However, in my experience, this is not necessary in foals, as rib retractors provide adequate exposure.

Complications of Esophageal Surgery

The surgeon has 3 clinical objectives: to obtain leakproof healing of a primary anastomosis or incision; to dilate a restricted aperture; and to return the enlarged or disrupted esophagus to near normal size and function. Despite meticulous technique, complications can occur. If managed properly, however, they can be resolved with a favorable outcome for the patient.

Dehiscence and Stricture: The key to handling breakdown of a sutured esophageal incision is early recognition and treatment. For this reason, a suction drain placed next to the esophagus at the time of surgery serves a second function in addition to drainage of serum and blood from the surgical site: it provides a method to detect salivary leakage. Not all incisions that leak saliva dehisce, especially if the saliva is removed from periesophageal tissues. However, if extreme amounts of saliva are leaking through the incision or complete dehiscence occurs, the original approach incision should be completely opened and lavaged daily to remove any ingesta or saliva. Dissection planes ventrally along the trachea should be drained to the outside to prevent eventual mediastinitis or pleuritis. Dissecting infections can occur following esophagostomy as well, and inadvertent placement of a dislodged feeding tube into a dissection plane or the thorax obviously would have an unfavorable outcome.[302]

The patient may be permitted to drink which, in many cases, lavages the wound. Nutritional requirements may be met by oral feeding or placement of a feeding tube into the esophagus at the point of dehiscence or distally through a separate esophagostomy. The outcome of this complication from this point depends on management of water and electrolyte balance. The most common complication following treatment of an annular lesion is stricture (Fig 78). This complication is the bane of the esophageal surgeon and its successful treatment is limited to case reports.

Acid-Base and Electrolyte Alterations: In the face of adequate nutrition, daily losses of large amounts of saliva results in hyponatremia, hypochloremia (Fig 79) and transient metabolic acidosis followed by progressive metabolic alkalosis (Fig 80).[305] The alkalosis probably results from renal compensation for electrolyte imbalances. Oral administration of sodium chloride daily reverses the electrolyte imbalance (potassium requirements are adequately met in feed); alkalosis is corrected through renal mechanisms.

Laryngeal Hemiplegia: Manipulative procedures and/or disease of the esophagus in the cervical area can easily result in laryngeal hemiplegia because of the close proximity of the recurrent laryngeal and vagus nerves. The surgeon should be aware that apparently minor manipulations of these nerves can have deleterious effects on their function.

Congenital and Familial Diseases

Intramural Cyst

Esophageal cysts are uncommon in all species, and only 2 equine cases have been documented.[306,307] I have seen 2 additional horses with esophageal cysts, a 3-year-old Morgan mare, in which the cyst lining had radiographic signs of calcification, and a yearling Quarter Horse colt admitted for dysphagia. In all 4 horses, an epithelial inclusion cyst (lined by stratified squamous epithelium and filled with keratinaceous de-

Figure 78. Positive-contrast esophagogram using liquid barium administered under pressure through a cuffed nasogastric tube shows stricture (arrow) with prestenotic dilatation. The stenosis was subsequently resolved by esophagomyotomy.

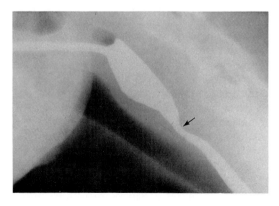

Figure 79. Influence of salivary depletion on serum electrolyte levels (Na, K, Cl) before (day 0) and after esophageal fistulation. Bars indicate ±1 SE (n=6). Stars indicate days on which serum electrolyte levels were significantly different from baseline values (0 day).[302]

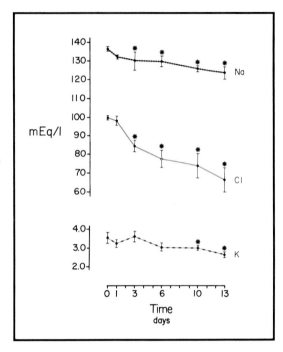

Figure 80. Effect of salivary depletion and serum electrolyte alterations on acid-base values [pH, P_{CO2} (mm of Hg), T_{CO_2} = total CO_2 (mEq/L), HCO_3^- (mEq/L), and BE (mEq/L)] before (day 0) and after esophageal fistulation. Bars indicate ±1 SE (n=6). Stars indicate days on which each value was significantly different from baseline values (0 day).

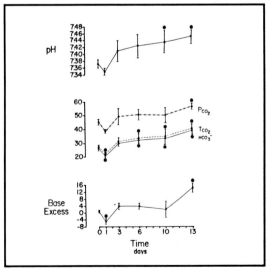

bris) was found in the esophageal wall. Mural cysts probably are a developmental anomaly.

Clinical findings include dysphagia, regurgitation, a palpable soft tissue mass in the neck, and resistance to passage of a nasogastric tube at the site of the cyst. The diagnosis is confirmed on contrast radiography by the classic appearance of a filling defect caused by a mural lesion (Fig 81). Endoscopically, the esophageal lumen may appear partially occluded, but significant gross changes usually are not observed because the mucosa appears normal.

Intramural esophageal cysts may be removed through enucleation with inversion or resection of redundant mucosa. The esophagus is exposed and the cyst is identified by manipulation of a nasogastric tube within the esophageal lumen. A longitudinal incision is made through the muscularis over the cyst. By careful dissection, the cyst is separated from its position between the mucosa-submucosa and muscularis. The cyst can be mistaken for an abscess if inadvertently incised by the inexperienced surgeon (Fig 82). Positioning the nasogastric tube caudal to the cyst helps prevent inadvertent perforation of the mucosa. The cyst is removed intact, leaving an area of redundant mucosa or a sac, which may be treated as a pulsion diverticulum, *ie*, by inversion preferably, or by diverticulectomy. The muscularis is closed with simple-inter-

Figure 81. Barium esophagogram shows the classic appearance of an intramural lesion of the esophagus, in this case, an epithelial inclusion cyst. The esophageal lumen is narrowed caudally and is dilated but not filled with barium cranially because the mural mass produces a filling defect.

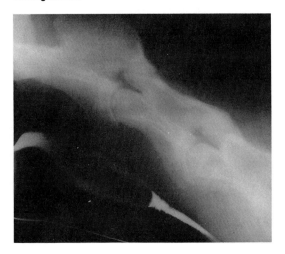

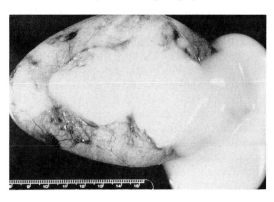

Figure 82. An excised intramural inclusion cyst following puncture. The epithelial-cell contents could be mistaken for an abscess if ruptured during surgery.

rupted 3-0 sutures of polydioxanone or polypropylene at the surgeon's preference.

Megaesophagus

Megaesophagus is dilatation and muscular hypertrophy of the esophagus oral (proximal) to a constricted distal segment. This term, as used here, includes congenital ectasia (dilatation of unknown origin), achalasia (failure of the distal esophagus to relax because of neural dysfunction, resulting in proximal dilatation), and megaesophagus secondary to vascular ring anomalies. One case of vascular ring anomaly causing megaesophagus in a foal has been reported.[308] The anomalous defect was a result of a persistent right aortic arch and was suspected on radiographic examination and confirmed on necropsy.

Though hypomotility of the esophagus has been documented in 1 foal and neural defects of the esophagus were found in another, achalasia as defined in dogs and people has not been reported.[309,310] Treatment of these horses was not successful, even with a modified Heller's myotomy in 1 foal.[309] I have treated congenital ectasia conservatively with good results. A 5-month-old foal was admitted because of recurrent choke that began at the time of weaning. Esophageal lavage produced 8 L of feed regurgitated through the nasogastric tube. On radiography and endoscopy, generalized ectasia was found from the midcervical to the midthoracic esophagus (Fig 83), with an annular ring noted at the point where the esophagus passed through the thoracic inlet (Fig 84). The foal was fed a mash diet (pellets mixed with warm water) for 6 months, with the feed trough elevated above the animal's withers. The mash diet was changed to complete pelleted feed for an additional 6 months before the horse was fed normal feed. Though fluid did not pool in the lumen of the esophagus after 6 months of the mash diet and the size of the dilated esophagus did not change over the next 24 months during several radiographic examinations, the horse could eat normally and is being used for show and pleasure riding. Conservative management of this problem should be considered if the owners are willing to provide the extensive nursing care (no access to roughage, including bedding in the stall and total confinement with exercise in-hand only) and are willing to face the possibility of several episodes of "choke" requiring treatment.

Reduplication

It is not clear if reduplication of the esophagus is a congenital or acquired condition, but it is included here for the sake of completeness. A single case of this condition has been reported.[311] Clinical signs were similar to those of other forms of esophageal obstruction. Diagnosis may be difficult and the problem does not appear to be amenable to surgery. This condition closely resembles one of the complications of esophagostomy tube feeding, wherein a dissecting tract develops parallel to the esoph-

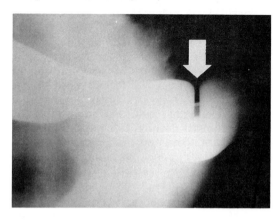

Figure 84. Barium pressure esophagogram shows megaesophagus in the same foal as Figure 83. Note the narrowing of the esophageal lumen as it passes through the thoracic inlet (arrow).

ageal wall or within it, causing signs of obstruction.[302]

Diseases With Physical Causes

Diverticulum

In horses, diverticula of the esophagus only occasionally cause esophageal dysfunction. Usually they are acquired lesions that result from contraction of periesophageal fibrous scar tissue, causing outward traction and tenting of all layers of the esophageal wall (traction or true diverticulum), or from protrusion of mucosa and submucosa through a defect in the esophageal muscularis (pulsion or false diverticulum).

A traction diverticulum commonly develops at the site of a healed esophagostomy, a postsurgical or posttraumatic wound of the esophagus that is allowed to heal by second intention as a fistula, or following penetration of the esophageal lumen (traumatic or surgical) where leakage of saliva has caused inflammation or abscess.[302,312] Pulsion diverticula are caused by fluctuations in esophageal intraluminal pressure and overstretch damage to esophageal muscle fibers by impacted feedstuffs. A more probable cause is external trauma to the cervical area.[313,314]

Diverticula in the cervical esophagus should be considered when an enlargement in the neck results in dysphagia and yet a nasogastric tube can be passed. On barium

Figure 83. Double-contrast esophagogram shows megaesophagus at the mid-thorax level. The foal was managed with a mash diet and recovered esophageal function over a 1-year period.

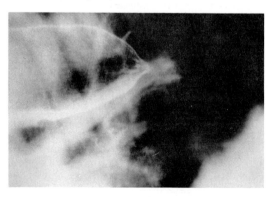

swallow esophagograms, traction diverticula are spherical and have a wide neck (Fig 85), whereas pulsion diverticula are flasklike in configuration with a narrow neck. Differentiation of these 2 types of diverticula can be aided by additional contrast techniques that distend the esophageal lumen and outline the opening into the evagination. Esophagoscopy also defines the relative size and configuration of the opening of a diverticulum (Fig 86).

A traction diverticulum, even when quite large, produces few clinical signs and seldom requires treatment. A pulsion diverticulum, however, has a tendency to enlarge progressively so that risk of obstruction and rupture increases with time. Surgical repair is indicated.

A pulsion diverticulum can be repaired by diverticulectomy with resection of the mucosal-submucosal sac, followed by reconstruction of the mucosa-submucosa and muscularis, or by inversion of the mucosa-submucosal sac with reconstruction of the muscular layer. Diverticulectomy should be used when the mucosal sac is very large and the neck of the diverticulum very narrow. There is a single report of repair of an apparent congenital esophageal diverticulum using this technique.[315] However, mucosal inversion is the preferred technique because it decreases the chance of postoperative leakage, infection or fistula formation, and

Figure 85. Barium swallow in a horse with an esophagotomy that healed by second intention shows a traction diverticulum (arrows). Note the wide neck of the diverticulum. A fistula remains from an esophagostomy distally.

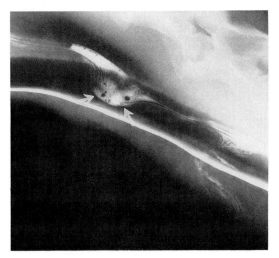

Figure 86. Endoscopic appearance of an opening into an esophageal diverticulum.

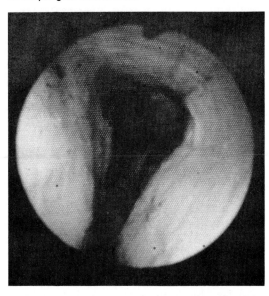

does not appear to predispose to postoperative obstruction complications.[313,314]

The esophagus is exposed and the diverticulum and defect in the muscularis are identified by careful dissection. Inadvertent perforation of the mucosa-submucosa should be repaired immediately. The edges of the muscular defect should be debrided back to healthy-appearing tissue. The sac is inverted and the edges of the muscularis are apposed with simple-interrupted sutures of 3-0 polypropylene in a manner to avoid undue tension on the closure and prevent stenosis of the esophageal diameter. Postoperatively, feeding should consist of soft foods for 4-6 weeks.

Impaction

The most common type of obstructive esophageal disease is impaction with ingesta or bedding. It can occur in the normal esophagus of a gluttonous animal and has a typical radiographic appearance (Fig 87). Nasogastric tube passage and gentle warm water lavage usually are successful in relieving the obstruction. Xylazine sedation to lower the patient's head during this procedure greatly reduces the hazard of aspiration of ingesta that is flushed free and passes up the esophagus into the nasopharynx.[316]

Several alternative techniques may be necessary if gentle lavage meets with failure. A cuffed nasogastric tube may be placed, the animal sedated, and water lavaged under pressure with a dose syringe or stomach pump. The tube helps prevent reflux or ingesta into the pharynx while permitting pressure of the water to push the obstruction distally. External massage and to-and-fro movement of the water resolve most impactions. If this technique is not successful, the animal should be muzzled to prevent food and water intake, left alone for 8-12 hours, and the treatment repeated. Frequently the initial treatment softens the impaction and it becomes dislodged by swallowing or is easily relieved by a second treatment. Some clinicians claim that atropinization (0.02 mg/kg) of a horse with esophageal impaction aids dissolution of the impaction by promoting esophageal relaxation and reduces salivary secretions that might otherwise be inhaled.

Refractory cases or intractable horses may benefit from general anesthesia and water lavage under pressure. This method has the advantages of providing some relaxation of the esophageal musculature, reducing the chances of aspiration because the horse's head is lowered and decreasing the risk of esophageal perforation with the tube in an intractable horse. Gentle manipulation is mandatory with this technique to avoid rupture of the esophagus.

Impactions that do not respond to conservative therapy should be definitively identified by radiographic and endoscopic examination and, if amenable, relieved by longitudinal esophagotomy (see Foreign

Figure 87. Lateral cervical radiograph shows typical appearance of impaction of ingesta in the cranial cervical esophagus.

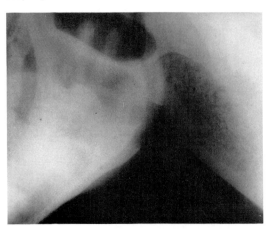

Figure 88. Lateral cervical radiograph of a horse after impaction of the esophagus has been relieved shows fluid line (arrow) in an area of dilatation that extends from the distal point of obstruction proximally to the upper esophageal sphincter. The fluid line is produced by saliva that has collected in the dilatation.

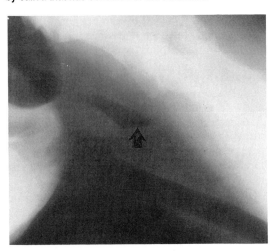

Body below). Surgery is preferable to repeated trauma of the esophagus through attempts to relieve the obstruction with a nasogastric tube. Use of the nasogastric tube as a probang is not recommended. Cervical esophagotomy can be performed with the horse standing or under general anesthesia, and obstructions can be lavaged through the incision if necessary.

One aftermath of simple impaction is fusiform dilatation of the esophagus that predisposes to reobstruction (Fig 88). This condition resolves in 24-48 hours, provided the dilatation is kept free of ingesta. Food should be withheld or only small quantities of a soft diet fed for 2 days after an episode of choke to permit the lumen to resume its normal diameter. Glucose-electrolyte solutions for drinking should be provided in addition to fresh water so the electrolyte abnormalities secondary to salivary loss may be compensated.

Broad-spectrum antimicrobial therapy is indicated for 5-7 days because the risk of aspiration pneumonia is high after choke. If pneumonia is not the major limiting factor in this disease, simple obstruction has a favorable prognosis.

When an obstruction has been present for several days or is refractory to initial treatment, examination using radiography and/or endoscopy is warranted after the obstruction has been relieved. Circumferential mucosal ulceration is not uncommon in these cases and usually results in esophageal stricture.

Dilatation

Dilation of the esophagus or acquired megaesophagus, other than that following impaction, usually is the result of a distal constricting lesion of the esophagus. Differential diagnoses should include vascular ring anomalies in foals and stricture.[317] Once the primary lesion has been identified and corrected, this form of esophageal dilatation should not remain as a permanent problem, providing it is not of long duration.

Foreign Body

Small pieces of wood, wire, fishing tackle and medication boluses can become esophageal foreign bodies in horses.[318,319] They often perforate the esophageal wall resulting in phlegmon or abscessation (Fig 89). The swelling that accompanies these conditions usually obstructs the esophageal lumen and results in impaction. Diagnosis is made by radiography and/or esophagoscopy.

Retrieval of small sharp foreign bodies under endoscopic guidance is possible but difficult; general anesthesia is recommended to prevent the swallowing movements during manipulation that may produce pain and further esophageal trauma. It is necessary to relieve the impaction before attempting this method of treatment. Blunt or round foreign bodies may be treated similar to feed impactions. Though the nasogastric tube may be used as a probe to push the object into the stomach, the risk of perforation is great. Gentle manipulation is mandatory to avoid rupture. Additionally, this technique has the risk of moving the foreign body from the cervical region only to have it lodge in the thorax, a more inaccessible site. Longitudinal esophagotomy with primary closure results in minimal complications when performed in a region of normal esophagus and has become the accepted method of removing many foreign bodies.[280,312,319,320]

Surgery is preferred to manipulations that induce further esophageal trauma. Passage of a nasogastric tube as far as the foreign body (or beyond, if possible) facilitates identification of the esophagus during surgery. General anesthesia is preferred if closure is to be attempted. The patient is placed in dorsal recumbency and the skin of the ventral surface of the neck is prepared and draped for aseptic surgery. A 10-cm skin incision is made. Care should be taken to preserve the small vessels that supply the esophagus. Elevation of the esophagus from its bed of adventitia should be avoided. The left carotid sheath, containing the carotid artery and vagus and recurrent laryngeal nerves, should be retracted laterally. Pediatric-size Balfour abdominal retractors aid exposure to the esophagus, which then can be sharply incised through the muscle, submucosa and mucosa cranial to, caudal to or directly over the foreign body (Fig 90). Where the incision is made into the esophagus depends upon the mobility of the foreign body within the lumen and the amount of swelling in the esophageal wall.

After removal of the foreign body, if the esophagus has a normal appearance in the area of the incision, closure should be completed using a simple-continuous suture of 3-0 polypropylene suture material with the knots tied in the lumen (Fig 91). Esophageal musculature may be apposed with simple-interrupted sutures of 3-0 monofilament nonabsorbable suture material or polydioxanone, at the surgeon's preference. Muscular layers, subcutaneous tissue and

Figure 89. Lateral cervical radiograph of a 5-year-old Quarter Horse gelding with cervical swelling, dysphagia and odynophagia. A metallic foreign body (fishhook) is lodged in the ventral wall of the cranial esophagus. A nasogastric tube passed easily despite the abscess (arrow) that has developed secondary to perforation of the esophagus.

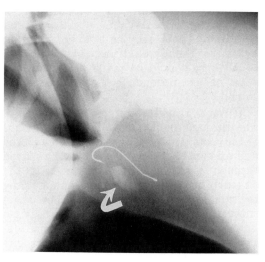

Figure 90. In the longitudinal esophagotomy technique, a scalpel is used to incise both the outer layer (muscularis and adventitia) (left) and inner layer (mucosa and submucosa) (right). A nasogastric tube or the foreign body is used to stabilize the esophagus during incision.

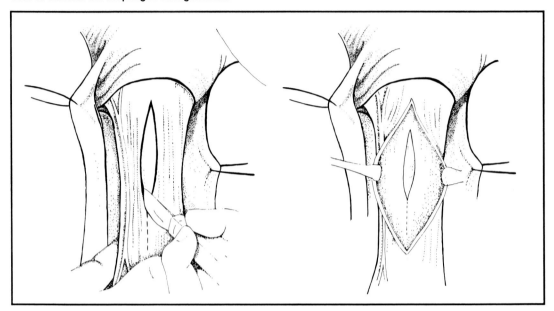

skin may be apposed with 2-0 monofilament nonabsorbable suture material in a simple-interrupted pattern. A polyethylene drain with an outer diameter of 0.25 inch (0.63 cm) is placed beside the esophagus and exits ventral to the skin incision through a small stab wound. This drain is maintained under constant suction for 48 hours to remove serum and blood from the surgical site and to provide early detection of salivary leakage should dehiscence occur.

Postoperatively, feed should be withheld for 48 hours. Parenteral administration of electrolyte solution, the composition of which depends on the horse's acid-base and hydration status, may be used to maintain hydration. Small quantities of pelleted feed in a slurry should be fed over the next 8 days before normal feeding can be resumed.[320]

If removal of the foreign body is necessary through an obviously diseased segment of the esophagus, the incision may be closed and an esophagostomy tube may be placed through a separate incision closer to the stomach or directly into the esophagotomy incision. Feeding of a complete pelleted diet through the esophagostomy tube can begin immediately after surgery. Particular attention to the patient's water and electrolyte

balance is necessary when closure of the esophagus is not possible.[305,312]

Figure 91. Technique used to close an esophagotomy showing simple-continuous sutures in the inner layer (mucosa and submucosa) and simple-interrupted sutures in the outer layer (muscularis and adventitia).

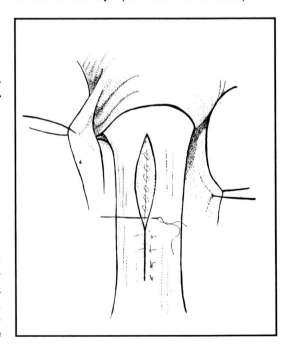

Inflammatory or Infectious Diseases

Ulceration and Esophagitis

Mucosal ulceration and esophagitis commonly occur secondary to long-standing impactions. Longitudinal mucosal ulcers can be produced from impactions; more frequently, circumferential ulcerations occur. Other causes of esophageal ulceration in foals include phenylbutazone toxicity, in which generalized gastrointestinal mucosal disease is a feature, and severe gastroduodenal ulcer disease that produces secondary reflux esophagitis. Diagnosis of esophageal ulceration is best made by endoscopy (Fig 92), though contrast radiography frequently defines the margins of the ulcer (Fig 93).

Conservative management should be instituted to minimize trauma to the mucosa, reduce inflammation and control infection. A low-bulk, minimally abrasive diet (mash), nonsteroidal antiinflammatory drugs (only if they are not implicated as causative agents) and broad-spectrum antimicrobial therapy are indicated. Because this diet results in hunger, and the patient should be muzzled between feedings or all bedding should be removed from the stall to avoid ingestion of straw or wood chips. Re-

Figure 92. Endoscopic appearance of esophagitis with circumferential ulceration 24 hours after feed impaction. A stricture subsequently formed but responded to medical management (see Figures 93 and 98).

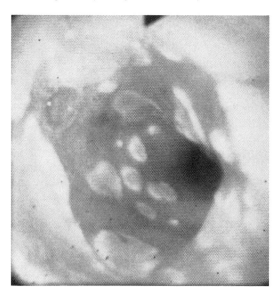

Figure 93. Double-contrast esophagogram shows the length of the circumferential esophageal ulcer 24 hours after relief of feed impaction.

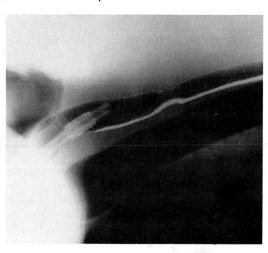

examination is recommended every 10-14 days. Stricture (see below) may occur within 30 days of the original insult when the circumferential ulcer is >2.5 cm long.[321] Longitudinal mucosal ulcers (especially if they are not extensive and are localized to one area of the esophagus) and circumferential ulcers <2 cm long usually heal without stricture.

Rupture

Rupture of the esophagus can occur secondary to long-standing obturation, from repeated or aggressive nasogastric tube passage, foreign body perforation, external trauma to the cervical area (usually a kick), or extension of infection from surrounding strictures.[322-326] Cervical swelling usually prevents successful passage of a nasogastric tube, even after irrigation of the esophagus with water. Swallowed air escapes from the rupture and causes subcutaneous emphysema; this can be recognized on radiographs (Fig 94). Positive-contrast techniques demonstrate escape of barium into surrounding tissues (Fig 95).

Perforations and Lacerations

Ruptures that cannot drain to the outside result in leakage of saliva and ingesta into tissues of the neck, where severe infection and phlegmon develop. Ruptures or perforation that allow escape of saliva and ingesta through the skin are less likely to cause systemic illness and extension of infection into the thorax. As discussed above, early establishment of drainage, preferably on the ventral midline, is necessary with all ruptures of the esophagus to avoid mediastinitis, pleuritis and even septicemia.

Perforation or lacerations of the esophagus accompanied by minimal escape of saliva and ingesta can be repaired using the technique described for esophagotomy.[324] Drainage and the feeding regimen used following esophagotomy should be employed. Secure closure of a ruptured or perforated defect usually is possible only in patients operated on shortly after the perforation has occurred (within 12 hours). In early cases in which esophageal tissues are too damaged to hold sutures or when infection and/or contamination with ingesta has already occured, some means of draining the esophageal contents to the outside must be provided. The patient should receive systemic antibiotics and water; electrolyte and nutritional requirements should be met by tube feeding. In some cases, the feeding tube can be placed through the site of rupture into the stomach. An alternative method of feeding that allows spontaneous healing of the rupture, or successful repair of the rupture when edema and infection have been controlled, is an esophagostomy performed distal to the rupture (closer to the stomach).

Figure 94. Barium swallow in a horse with a penetrating foreign body (arrow) showed swallowed air that has escaped into the periesophageal tissue.

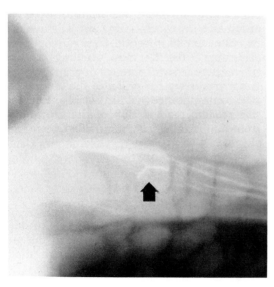

Figure 95. Barium liquid under pressure shows a rupture in the esophageal wall (arrow). Barium is seen in the periesophageal tissue.

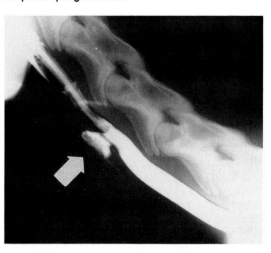

Cervical esophagostomy is an excellent method of extraoral alimentation that avoids the discomfort and irritation of the indwelling nasogastric tube.[303] An additional advantage is avoidance of deleterious influences on healing of an esophageal wound by an intraluminal tube located in the immediate region.[326,327] To use this advantage, obviously the esophagostomy should be placed distal to the area of esophageal injury. The surgery can be performed with the horse in lateral recumbency under general anesthesia or standing under mild tranquilization and local anesthesia.[303] Passage of a nasogastric tube facilitates identification of the esophagus at surgery. Though the same approach can be used as for esophagotomy, a more lateral incision may provide better access to the esophagus while avoiding impingement of the tube against the trachea.

The skin over the left jugular furrow is prepared for surgery in the desired area. The esophagus occasionally is located on the right side of the trachea and should be approached over the right jugular furrow in those horses. A 5-cm skin incision is made. The esophagus is sharply incised longitudinally for 3 cm down to the indwelling nasogastric tube. The nasogastric tube is removed and a polyethylene nasogastric tube (14-24 mm outer diameter) is placed into the stomach through the esophagostomy. Failure to place the tube into the stomach allows easy dislodgement. Care should be taken to ensure that the end of the tube is placed into both the elastic inner layer and inelastic outer muscle layer of the esophagus. Difficulty in tube placement usually is an indication that the incision in the muscle layer is inadequate to accommodate the diameter of the tube. Sutures can be placed in the mucosa to form a seal around the tube but probably are unnecessary because they do not prevent leakage of saliva. The tube should be secured firmly, first with butterfly tape bandages sutured to the skin (Fig 77), then with elastic tape bandages (Fig 96). Tubes of large diameter are preferred to avoid plugging with ingesta during feeding. They should be capped between feedings and flushed with water at the end of each feeding to maintain patency.

Esophagostomy tubes should remain in place for a minimum of 7-10 days to permit granulation tissue to form a true stoma. A longer period is necessary if the tube is placed in the area of a rupture or perforation. When the tube is removed, normal feeding may be resumed. A large portion of swallowed feed may be lost through the stoma when the patient is fed from the ground. When feed is placed at the height of the withers, however, less of the bolus is lost through the stoma with each swallow. The stoma heals spontaneously after the tube is removed and fistula formation is rare.[302,303]

However, complications of this form of alimentation are well documented and can

Figure 96. Esophagostomy tube is firmly secured with elastic tape bandages to prevent dislodgement.

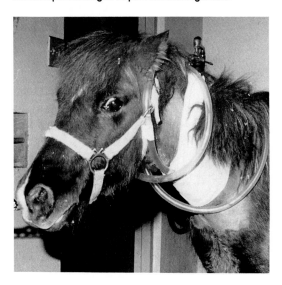

result in death.[302,327] Early detection and ventral drainage of infections that dissect along the trachea and esophagus are vital for a successful outcome. Patients should be maintained on antimicrobial therapy until a mature stoma develops (7-10 days).

Resection of the esophagus following rupture is warranted if the muscular layer is obviously necrotic and does not act as a tube along which the mucosa may regenerate, and if the proximal and distal segments of the esophagus can be anastomosed without undue tension (see Partial Resection and Complete Resection and Anastomosis below). Few ruptures of the esophagus requiring resection occur without necrotizing cellulitis. Usually a delay in repair is necessary to permit acute inflammation to subside before surgery. During this period, the patient may be accommodated with a change in diet.

Stricture

Narrowing of the esophageal lumen because of stricture formation usually is an annular lesion and can be classified into 3 types, depending on the anatomic location of induration and fibrosis: mural lesions that involve only the adventitia and muscularis; esophageal rings or webs that involve only the mucosa-submucosa; and annular stenosis that involves all layers of the esophageal wall. Stenosis of the esophagus may be acquired as a result of external or internal trauma to the esophageal walls (especially following impactions that produce circumferential ulceration), leakage of saliva or dehiscence after surgery, or external compression by or attachment to adjacent structures. In most instances, strictures are less likely to occur when traumatic insults involve only a portion of the circumference of the esophagus. For this reason, mobilization of the esophagus from its fascial attachments during surgery should be avoided when possible.

Strictures usually impede complete passage of the nasogastric tube and are best demonstrated by positive-pressure contrast esophagograms (Fig 97). Conservative management of a stricture is aimed at dilatation of the stenotic segment. Bougienage or pneumatic or hydrostatic dilators have limited practical value in horses because of the inaccessibility of special equipment and chronicity of the problem. Early lesions, such as postsurgical strictures or those following circumferential ulceration, can be dilated with the frequent feeding of small quantities of soft food over a period of several months. In 7 horses that developed stricture following esophageal impaction, observation over 2 months revealed that the esophageal lumen was maximally reduced (strictured) 30 days after circumferential ulceration was observed (Fig 98), after which lumen diameter increased to normal by 60 days.[321] This also has been documented following experimental resection and anastomosis.[327] Therefore, a low-bulk diet and antiinflammatory and antimicrobial therapy should be used and surgical intervention be delayed for 60 days after the original insult. It is important to impress upon horse owners that several episodes of "choke" may occur up to 40 days following the original obstruction.

Strictures more than 60 days old usually have matured to the point where the cicatrix is too firm to yield to dilatation by this method and, therefore, may be classified as chronic. Chronic strictures of the esophagus may be corrected by esophagomyotomy, partial or complete resection and anastomosis, or patch grafting. Any of these surgical treatments are met with complications and the surgeon should take care to pick the most conservative therapy that will meet the aim of treatment. Leakage of luminal contents and reformation of the stricture requiring prolonged medical management are to be expected following resection and patch grafting.

Strictures that are mural in origin respond to myotomy and have the best prognosis for recovery without restricture. Three successful reports appear in the literature; I have had similar experience with 2 other horses.[304,328,329] The surgery should be performed with the horse under general anesthesia, with a nasogastric tube passed to the level of the stricture to permit easy identification of the involved area. The approach for esophagotomy or esophagostomy is at the surgeon's discretion.

The esophagus is incised longitudinally to the level of the mucosa, through the stricture, and 1 cm distal and proximal to it (Fig 99). The nasogastric tube may be passed through the stenotic area at this point. From this single incision, the muscularis is

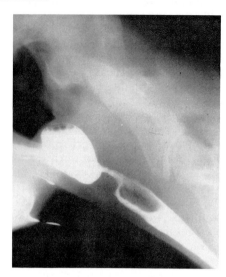

Figure 97. Positive-pressure esophagogram showing a stricture in a foal. Note the pre- and poststenotic dilatations. The lesion was resolved by partial resection and anastomosis.

separated by sharp dissection from the mucosa around the entire circumference of the esophagus (Fig 100). When the mucosa is freed in this manner, it makes removal of a portion of the muscularis or multiple myotomy incisions seldom necessary. The myotomy is not sutured and the approach incision is closed and drained in a routine manner. If the mucosa is opened inadvertently, it should be closed immediately with

Figure 98. Endoscopic appearance of a stricture 30 days after circumferential ulceration (see Figures 92 and 93).

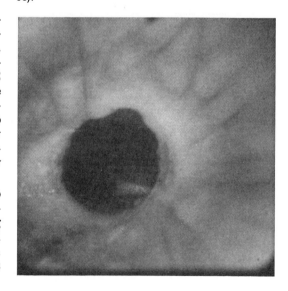

3-0 polypropylene sutures in a simple-interrupted pattern.

Postoperatively, feeding small but frequent quantities of soft feed may be necessary if a prestenotic dilatation is present before surgery. When this dilatation is no longer evident radiographically, normal feeding may be resumed.

Recurrence of postsurgical cicatricial stricture is slow to develop, with clinical signs occurring weeks or months after the operation. Conservative treatment (a change from hay to complete pelleted diet) may be all that is necessary to resolve recurrent obstructions. A postsurgical stricture seen long after the original operation usually is due to mature nonresilient cicatrix and may not respond to dilatation. If surgery is necessary, the surgeon should not hesitate to perform a second esophagomyotomy; however, performing another surgery in a stenotic area of the esophagus before allowing the acute inflammation of the previous surgery to subside greatly increases the propensity for restricture. If such is the case, a more hazardous procedure may have to be selected eventually to correct the problem.

Longitudinal esophagomyotomy combined with mucosal resection provides relief of stricture caused by esophageal rings or webs or annular stenosis of all muscle layers.[330,331] Performed under general anesthesia, the procedure is indicated when the cicatrix involves the mucosa and prevents

Figure 99. Longitudinal incision of the outer layer of the esophageal wall in esophagomyotomy.

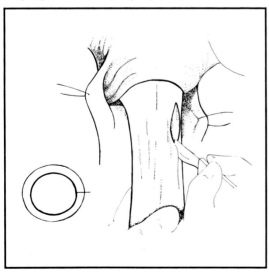

Figure 100. Technique used to elevate and separate the outer (muscularis and adventitia) and inner (mucosa and submucosa) layers of the esophageal wall to complete esophagomyotomy.

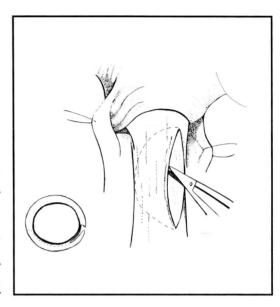

passage of a nasogastric tube following myotomy.

The esophagus is exposed and incised as described previously for esophagomyotomy. A longitudinal incision is made through the mucosa long enough to permit identification of the diseased segment. The mucosal scar is separated by sharp dissection from normal or diseased muscle layer. Circumferential incisions are made at the proximal and distal edges of the mucosal cicatrix and it is removed, leaving the muscular tube intact.

If cut edges of the mucosa can be brought into apposition without undue tension, they are apposed by 3 equally-spaced 3-0 polypropylene simple-continuous sutures with the knots tied in the lumen (Fig 101). When mucosal rings or webs are the cause of stenosis, the normal esophageal muscle should be apposed over the mucosal anastomosis but, in the case of an annular stenosis that involves the entire esophageal wall, the muscularis should not be sutured. A drain is placed next to the esophagus and the approach incision is closed. If space permits, tube feeding through an esophagostomy placed through a separate incision distal to the stricture is ideal. When this is not possible, frequent feeding of small quantities of soft food may begin 48 hours after surgery and should be continued for 10 days before normal roughage is offered to the patient.

When the stricture is extensive and the mucosa cannot be sutured, regeneration within the muscle tube occurs readily.[327] The muscularis may be sutured if it is healthy or left open if only scar tissue remains. Spontaneous healing is aided if esophagostomy tube feeding (located closer to the stomach than the operative site) is used.[327,330,331] When the stricture is located too close to the thoracic inlet to permit placement of a separate esophagostomy incision, the tube may be inserted directly through the stricture site. Recurrence of stricture following this procedure may be an indication for esophagomyotomy or an esophagostomy tube placed through the stricture.[331]

Complete resection and anastomosis should be reserved for rupture of the esophagus in which the muscularis is not viable. The esophagus is exposed as described previously. The area to be resected and several centimeters of normal esophagus distal and proximal to it are mobilized. Umbilical tape or rubber drain tubing (0.25 inch, 0.63 cm) is placed around the esophagus and held in place with hemostatic forceps to occlude the lumen a convenient distance from the area to be resected. Crushing clamps of any type should not be used on the esophagus. A point is selected proximal to the diseased segment where the esophagus is sharply

Figure 101. Technique for partial resection and anastomosis. Following longitudinal incision of the outer layer, the inner layer is resected and, when possible, closed using several simple-continuous sutures.

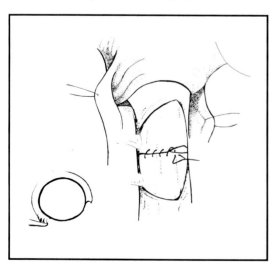

transected, leaving healthy tissue for closure. This procedure is repeated distally and the diseased portion is removed. The mucosal-submucosal layer is apposed with 3-0 simple-interrupted monofilament nonabsorbable polypropylene sutures placed about 3 mm from the cut edge, 2-3 mm apart, with the knots tied in the lumen. Tension of the sutures is adequate to form a tight seal without interference of blood supply.

The esophageal muscle is apposed with interrupted horizontal mattress sutures of 2-0 polydioxanone or monofilament nonabsorbable suture material. The muscle layer has limited elasticity and, if necessary, a relief incision in the form of a circular myotomy 4-5 cm proximal or distal to the anastomosis can decrease tension on the repair. The approach incision is closed as described previously.

Alternative successful methods of closure have been described, but postoperative management is a major determinant of the outcome of this procedure, regardless of closure technique.[332,333] Prevention of undue tension on the anastomosis by use of a standing martingale and special feeding regimen is necessary. If oral alimentation is elected, soft foods should be given only after 48 hours and until endoscopic or radiographic evaluation of the surgery shows primary healing has occurred. Esophagostomy is the preferred method of feeding, if possible.

An extensive cervical esophageal stricture produced by annular stenosis of the entire wall may preclude successful repair by techniques described previously. The diameter of the equine esophageal lumen can be increased by using a patch graft of the sternocephalicus muscle.[334]

Antibiotics should be given preoperatively and maintained for 6-10 days after surgery. With the horse under general anesthesia, a ventral midline or lateral approach to the esophagus is made and, depending on location of the defect and the approach used, the brachiocephalicus and sternocephalicus muscle serve as donors for the graft. With a nasogastric tube passed to the level of the stenosis, a longitudinal incision is made through the muscularis from a point 3 cm distal to and extending 3 cm proximal to the stricture. The mucosa-submucosa is sharply incised as the nasogastric tube is passed into the stomach. A caudal portion of the muscle belly of the brachiocephalicus or sternocephalicus is mobilized by blind separation of muscle fibers. The strip of muscle should maintain its proximal and distal attachments, and should be freely movable so as not to exert tension on the closure when the patient's head and neck are moved. The graft should be wide enough to appreciably increase the lumen of the esophagus.

The edges of the mucosa-submucosa are sutured to the muscle graft using 3-0 interrupted through-and-through polypropylene mattress sutures, and the edges of the muscularis are sutured to the graft with 3-0 simple-interrupted sutures of monofilament polypropylene. Preplacement of mattress sutures and closure of both layers on one side of the esophageal defect at a time facilitate repair. The nasogastric tube should be removed before the second edge is closed. Suction drains are placed next to the esophagus and the approach incision is closed.

Postoperatively, extraoral alimentation is preferred for 10 days (by esophagostomy, if space allows, or intravenous feeding), but soft foods may be given per os as early as 48 hours if salivary leaking has not occurred. An indwelling nasogastric tube provides a stimulus for salivation and increases the incidence of fistula formation.[327,334]

Fistula

Fistulae of the esophagus result from causes previously described for ruptures

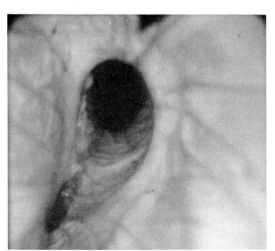

Figure 102. Endoscopic appearance of a large esophageal fistula. Smaller fistulae often are difficult to locate endoscopically.

and may be treated similarly. However, small fistulae may be a diagnostic challenge. Occasionally they may be observed endoscopically (Fig 102). More frequently, findings of endoscopic examinations and barium swallow esophagograms are normal. When cervical swelling, fever and dysphagia are present, a nasogastric tube can be passed to the stomach and endoscopic findings are normal, esophageal fistulae should be included in the differential diagnosis. Contrast radiography, using liquid barium administered under pressure, best demonstrates the lesion (Fig 103).

When ventral drainage has been established, fistulae almost always heal spontaneously. If healing does not occur, resection of the sinus tract and closure of the esophageal stoma may be necessary.[302,303]

Neoplasia

Squamous-Cell Carcinoma

Neoplasms causing signs of esophageal obstruction are very rare.[213] Squamous-cell carcinoma is the most common neoplasm and has been reported in detail in 3 cases. One was an extension of gastric carcinoma, one was located in the tracheal bifurcation, and one was located in the distal cervical esophagus.[335-337] Biopsy and cytologic examination of brush samples obtained through the endoscope may provide an early diagnosis before stenosis of the esophagus develops, but advanced cases may be detected on radiography.[337] The value of resection is questionable.

DISEASES OF THE STOMACH

M. Campbell-Thompson

Diagnostic and Therapeutic Considerations

Gastric Anatomy

The equine stomach accounts for about 4% of the entire gastrointestinal tract capacity and is positioned mainly to the left of midline up against the diaphragm.[300,338] The stomach is separated from the esophagus and duodenum by distinct sphincters, the cardia and pylorus, respectively. The esophagus joins the stomach at the cardia at

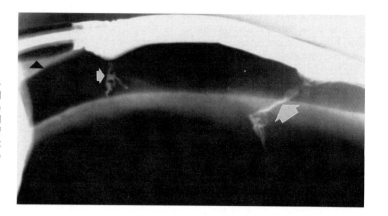

Figure 103. Positive-contrast esophagogram shows a sinus tract (small white arrow) and a fistula (large white arrow) remaining after removal of the esophagotomy tube. The cuff on the nasogastric tube (black arrow) prevents reflux of barium into the pharynx.

such an acute angle that passage of a nasogastric tube may be difficult if the stomach is distended. The left portion of the stomach dorsal to the cardia is termed the saccus cecus. The pylorus lies just to the right of midline only about 4 inches ventral to the cardia.

The stomach has 2 curvatures, known as the lesser and greater curvatures, and 2 surfaces, parietal and visceral.[300,338] The lesser curvature is very short and extends from the cardia to pylorus, while the greater curvature is much longer and is in contact with the spleen and large colon as it courses from the cardia to pylorus. The 2 curvatures are important surgically because of their relation to the major vascular arcades.[338] The arterial supply along the lesser curvature originates from the left gastric artery, which is derived from the celiac artery. The left gastric artery connects with the right gastric artery, a branch of the hepatic artery. Along the greater curvature, the right gastroepiploic artery, a branch of the gastroduodenal artery, connects with the left gastroepiploic artery, a branch of the splenic artery. The parietal surface of the stomach lies against the diaphragm and liver. The visceral surface faces caudoventrally and is in contact with the greater omentum, pancreas, small intestine, and portions of the large colon.

Several ligaments attach to the stomach.[300,338] The gastrophrenic ligament connects the greater curvature from the cardia to saccus cecus with the left crus of the diaphragm. The gastrosplenic ligament connects the greater curvature at the saccus cecus to the hilus of the spleen. The gastropancreatic fold attaches from the left dorsal aspect of the cardia to the duodenum and connects ventrally to the pancreas. The lesser omentum extends from the lesser curvature and proximal duodenum to the liver. The greater omentum extends from the ventral part of the greater curvature to the transverse and small colons. The greater omentum is very thin and usually is folded up between the visceral surface of the stomach and the intestines.

The equine gastric mucosa is composed of about one-third stratified squamous and two-thirds glandular epithelium, demarcated by a thickened fold of squamous mucosa known as the margo plicatus.[300,338] The stratified squamous mucosa is devoid of glands but has a thick layer of keratinized epithelium. Though the glandular region is classically divided into 3 regions, based on primary glandular architect use, these regions are less distinct in horses than in other species. The cardiac region forms a narrow band along the margo plicatus and contains branched tubular glands lined with mucous and endocrine cells.[339] The pyloric region extends from the margo plicatus to the pylorus and contains branched tubular glands with mucous, serous and endocrine cell types. The cardiac and pyloric gland regions are partially commingled. The G and D cells are found in the pyloric gland region and are the sources for gastrin and somatostatin, respectively (Figs 104, 105). The fundic zone comprises roughly half of the entire glandular region and is the site of acid and pepsinogen production by parietal and chief cells, respectively. Mucous and endocrine cells are also located in this region.

Gastric Function-Secretion

The stomach receives masticated food mixed with bicarbonate-rich saliva. As the stomach fills, muscular contractions mix the ingesta. Large food particles are retained in stratified layers while liquids and small particles are rapidly passed through the pylorus.

Stimulation of gastric secretion has been described in terms of 3 phases.[340] The first is the cephalic phase, which involves vagal reflexes following the sight, smell or taste of food. One early report suggests that teasing with food does not stimulate gastric secretion in horses.[341] The gastric phase involves reflexes initiated by food within the lumen of the stomach. Complex neural, hormonal and paracrine stimuli regulate secretion. Mechanical and chemical stimuli activate sensory receptors in the gastric mucosa, which then activate motor neurons within the submucosal (Meissner's) and myenteric (Auerbach's) plexuses. These neurons activate secretory cells directly or through intermediate cell types, such as mast and endocrine cells. Gastrin is released from pyloric G cells in response to vagal reflexes and luminal products, such as calcium, polypeptides and certain amino acids. Fasting gastrin concentrations generally are low in foals and adult horses, with only moderate increases after feeding.[342-344] Finally, the intestinal phase of gastric secretion is initiated by the presence of digestion products in the duodenal lumen and involves neural and hormonal mediators.

Inhibition of gastric secretion is also highly regulated by neural and hormonal mediators. Acid in the gastric lumen producing a pH of less than 3 inhibits gastrin release. Entry of acid into the duodenum triggers inhibitory mechanisms via the release of such hormones as secretin. Hypertonicity and fat within the duodenum decrease both secretion and gastric emptying.

The equine stomach continually secretes gastric acid and pepsin, even during fasting. This also occurs in several other species, such as people, monkeys, ruminants, pigs and rodents.[340] In weaning horses, gastric fluid with a pH of 2.0 is produced at about 1 L/hour. As in other species, stimulation of maximum acid secretion can be achieved with intravenous administration of pentagastrin, a synthetic analog of the hormone gastrin. In addition to acid, intrinsic factor is produced by parietal cells in other species, but this has not yet been characterized in horses. Pepsin, a proteolytic enzyme, is secreted by chief cells as an inactive precursor, pepsinogen. The pepsinogen content in equine gastric fluid is relatively low in comparison to that in other species, particularly carnivores.[340] Several isoenzymes are found in equine gastric fluid with different pH optima.[345] A small amount of pepsinogen also exists in serum and urine. Equine gastric fluid contains sodium, potassium and chloride ions in addition to hydrogen ions. Stud-

Figure 104. Three gastrin cells (G cell) in the pyloric mucosa of an adult horse. (Immunoperoxidase, 400X)

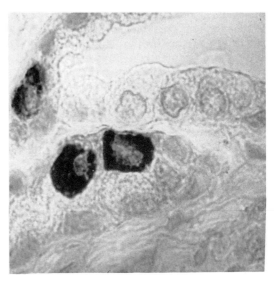

Figure 105. A somatostatin-containing cell (D cell) in the pyloric mucosa has a typical process extending to adjacent cells. (Immunoperoxidase, 400X)

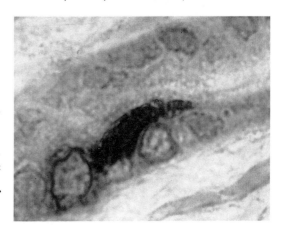

ies in horses indicate that acid concentrations never reach the maximum levels reported for other species, while sodium secretion always is very high, decreasing only slightly during maximal acid stimulation.[340] Lactate and the volatile fatty acids acetate, propionate and butyrate are also produced by intragastric bacteria.[44,346]

The gastric mucosa has developed several defense mechanisms to protect itself from acid and pepsin.[347] A thin layer of mucus that is constantly formed spreads out to protect the mucosa. Mucus is secreted as very-high-molecular-weight glycoproteins that form a thin adherent layer on the mucosa and lubricate the luminal contents. Surface epithelial cells secrete bicarbonate ions that are trapped beneath the mucous layer. This bicarbonate creates a neutral pH at the luminal aspect of the epithelium and neutralizes any acid that diffuses through the mucous layer. Epithelial cells are constantly shed every 2-4 days so that damaged cells are replaced quickly. Epithelial cells also are capable of rapid migration over areas of denuded epithelium. Prostaglandins may play a role in stimulation of these protective and repair mechanisms, including an increase in mucosal blood flow. As a result, acid and pepsinogen can be secreted in various amounts without causing significant mucosal damage.

Motility

The stomach differs from other areas of the digestive tract in having 3 muscle layers composed of an external longitudinal, a middle circular and an internal oblique layer.[338] The circular layer is thickest at the pylorus, where it forms the pyloric sphincter. Gastric volume can fluctuate considerably and the stomach is moderately full under normal conditions. During feeding, relaxation of the fundus allows the stomach to accommodate large increases in volume without change in intragastric pressure.[348] Even though there is food in the stomach, fluid and ingesta usually do extend proximally beyond the margo plicatus. This is evident during endoscopic or radiographic examination of the stomach. Studies on gastric emptying in ponies indicate that liquid material is rapidly moved through the pylorus, while particulate markers remain in the stomach for several hours.[349]

Myoelectrical activity can be recorded as continuous slow-wave potentials (basal electrical rhythm) or with superimposed action potentials.[348,350] Slow-wave potentials have been recorded at a frequency of 2-5/minute from the antrum in ponies and horses.[350,351,352] Action potentials combine to form migrating myoelectrical complexes consisting of: a period of intense repetitive spike activity (phase 3); a period of no spiking activity that follows phase 3 (phase 1); and a period of intermittent spiking activity comprised of both propagated and non-propagated spike events (phase 2).[348] Phase-3 activity has not been observed in the antrum of horses; phase-2 and phase-1 activity are timed with a duodenal migrating myoelectrical complex.[350] *Ad libitum* feeding does not disrupt the interval between these complexes, as occurs in dogs.[350]

Clinical Signs and Clinicopathologic Findings

Horses of all ages are susceptible to gastric disease. Horses with gastric disease may have a nonspecific history of depression, anorexia and abdominal pain. Gastric diseases must be differentiated from intestinal disorders or liver failure.[353] Yawning or teeth grinding also can be observed. Weight loss, weakness and fever may be present in chronic conditions. Abnormalities of mastication or refusal to feed may be caused by dental problems. The horse may drool saliva or make retching movements. If gastric contents are fluid, retching may result in expulsion of fluid through the nares (rather than the mouth) because the soft palate is positioned ventral to the epiglottis except during swallowing. A dilated stomach may exert considerable pressure on the diaphragm and, to ease this pressure, some horses assume a "dog-sitting" position.[354]

On physical examination, the horse with gastric disease may be acutely painful, with fluid at the nares. In chronic conditions, the animal may show depression, weight loss and fever. A nasogastric tube should be passed in all cases. Rectal examination may not be rewarding in primary gastric conditions, though it is very helpful to rule out other abdominal disorders. Laboratory analyses consisting of a complete blood count and serum chemistry analyses, with glucose, creatinine, electrolyte concentrations, and liver function tests are required to evaluate the metabolic status and to rule out other diseases. Loss of gastric fluid by repeated aspiration through the nasogastric tube may cause hypochloremic hypokalemic alkalosis though, in horses, renal failure also can result in a similar acid-base abnormality. This abnormality results from combined loss of hydrogen, chloride and potassium ions. The resulting chloride depletion may enhance renal tubular resorption of bicarbonate, leading to the characteristic finding of aciduria associated with alkalosis.

Abdominocentesis is performed and the fluid is analyzed for cell type, white blood cell numbers and total protein level. For instance, gastric squamous-cell carcinoma has been diagnosed by cytologic examination of peritoneal fluid. The clinician may elect not to perform an abdominocentesis if there is gross abdominal distention that would increase the likelihood of entering the bowel. Impaired gastric emptying may be diagnosed by delayed peak absorption or low plasma levels of d-xylose, though impaired intestinal absorption also must be considered in the differential diagnosis.

Gastroscopy

Gastroscopy is extremely valuable in diagnosis of gastric disease, as it makes direct observation and biopsy possible.[14,355,356] Gastric fluid pH and cytologic examination also may be helpful diagnostic procedures. Gastroscopy is performed with fiberoptic equipment or the newer videoendoscopes with greater lengths (up to 3 m) for adults and smaller diameters (10 mm) for foals. Foals usually are fasted for at least 6 hours, while adults are fasted 10-48 hours.[356,357] Complete gastric emptying usually is not achieved, as horses continuously secrete gastric fluid. Even in fed animals, food does not occupy much more than the region of the glandular mucosa. The procedure is tolerated quite well in animals of all ages with restraint or sedation. General anesthesia occasionally may be required.

The esophagus is inspected for mucosal defects, such as erosions or ulceration, before the stomach is entered. Gastric fluid can be seen refluxing into the distal esophagus in foals and adult horses with gastric emptying problems. The squamous mucosa appears as a white, glistening, fairly smooth surface. The entire squamous mucosa and margo plicatus can be inspected by advancing the endoscope dorsally along the greater curvature in foals and ventrally in adults to view the lesser curvature. The musculature of the lesser curvature forms a shelf at the margo plicatus, beyond which the pylorus may be observed. The glandular mucosa contains folds or rugae, and is pinkish-red with a thin mucous coating. Sheets of desquamated epithelium are commonly observed dorsal to the margo plicatus in foals <1 month old.[355,357] Crater-like ulcerations may be seen in the squamous mucosa where *Gasterophilus* larvae have been attached.

Radiographic Examination

The radiographic anatomy of the normal equine stomach has been characterized in foals and adult horses.[358-360] Contrast studies with 30-50% barium sulfate solutions (3-5 ml/kg) and/or air insufflation are useful. After fasting as for gastroscopy, right-to-left standing films are acquired. The stomach is inclined in a dorsocaudal to ventrocranial direction just caudal to the left crus of the diaphragm. Gastric dimensions and the amount of air in the stomach vary, depending on the amount of fluid and ingesta; however, the width of the stomach is generally one-half of the vertical length.[359] Air within the duodenal bulb can be seen superimposed over the caudal aspect of the gastric shadow. Plain radiographs may document failure of gastric emptying despite prolonged fasting.

Despite technical problems of variable air distention and barium coating and retained ingesta that obscures detail, contrast studies have been used to diagnose gastroduodenal ulcer disease and pyloric and duodenal stenosis in foals, and gastric tumors and stenosis in adult horses.[360-366]

Medical Therapy

Medical therapy is initially directed at primary correction of the disease and any fluid or electrolyte deficits, especially acid-base, calcium and potassium imbalances. Dilation must be relieved as quickly as possible due to the risk of gastric rupture. If resistance to passage of the nasogastric tube is encountered at the cardia, administration of 5-10 ml lidocaine may relax the cardia enough to allow passage.[367] With gastric impactions, lavage with large-bore tubes may be attempted if the contents are fluid enough. Administration of mineral oil generally is contraindicated, as it only adds to distention and, therefore, increases pain. In many cases, gastric contents can be removed only by suction and frequent siphoning. Gastric siphoning should be continued even after fluid and gas are removed, as coarse material may not siphon out readily. Reflux volume can be measured and the fluid checked for digested or occult blood, pH, sand and seeds. The nasogastric tube generally is left in place by taping it to the halter.

Administration of drugs to stimulate gastric motility has not been uniformly successful and the resultant increase in muscle tone may predispose to rupture. Neostigmine, an anticholinesterase drug, delays gastric emptying in normal horses.[116] Metoclopramide, an antidopaminergic agent, has been reported to enhance gastroduodenal coordination in ponies with experimental postoperative ileus.[114]

Medical management of primary gastritis or gastric ulceration is directed at reducing total acid output or improving in local mucosal defense.[368] Three endogenous substances that stimulate parietal-cell acid secretion are gastrin, histamine and acetylcholine. Several drugs can reduce the rate of acid secretion by interacting with receptors for these substances or their intracellular pathways.[369] The histamine H_2-receptor antagonists, cimetidine and ranitidine, are used for treatment of equine peptic ulceration.[370,371] Substituted benzimidazoles, such as omeprazole, block hydrogen ion transport at the parietal cell membrane and are being evaluated.[372] Acid output not only is reduced by inhibiting its secretion rate, but also by neutralization with basic antacids.[373] Oral antacids often are used in adult horses, primarily for monetary reasons, despite the fact that these agents require frequent administration.

Sucralfate, an aluminum hydroxide salt of sucrose, is widely used for improving the gastric mucosal defense system.[369] At a pH of less than 4, sucralfate becomes a sticky, yellow-white gel that adheres to ulcer craters, preventing exudation of protein, and adsorbing pepsin, bile acids and trypsin. Sucralfate also may stimulate local production of prostaglandins that are thought to play a crucial role in mucosal defense.[369] Prostaglandin analogues expedite ulcer healing by inhibiting acid secretion, stimulating mucosal bicarbonate secretion, and increasing gastric blood flow.[369,374]

Surgical Therapy

Gastric surgery in horses is directed at 2 major problems: perforation (rupture) and obstruction. Gastric ulcer hemorrhage, which is primarily a complication of peptic ulceration in people, occurs rarely in foals, and surgical correction has not been attempted.[375]

Preoperative evaluation should include a complete blood count, serum biochemical profile, liver function tests, blood gas determination and abdominocentesis. Thoracic and abdominal survey radiography help detect aspiration pneumonia and assess gastric distention. Medical therapy should involve gastric decompression via nasogastric tube (partially to avoid gastric rupture during casting) and correction of fluid and electrolyte deficits. Parenteral administration of H_2 antagonists (cimetidine, ranitidine) and nutritional supplementation also should be considered. Antibiotics are required when enterotomies are performed and are administered parenterally immediately before surgery to achieve adequate levels in tissues.

Gastrotomy is performed within the abdomen and is therefore technically difficult, especially in adult horses. A ventral midline incision is made extending to the xiphoid cartilage and retractors inserted. The cecum and large intestine may need to be exteriorized. The stomach is isolated with towels from other organs and toweling is packed beneath the stomach to raise it toward the incision. The caudal (visceral) surface of the stomach is then stabilized between 2 stay sutures. A stab incision is made into the lumen and gastric contents are aspirated with a suction tip. Suction and lavage also can be attempted for treatment of gastric impaction. The stab incision is closed with a pursestring or linear pattern to invert the incised edges. After close inspection of the repair site, the abdominal cavity is lavaged copiously and all fluid aspirated. The most common complication is sepsis from intraoperative contamination or partial dehiscence of the incision.

Repair of gastric perforations and rupture would be attempted early in the course of the disease when contamination is minimal. Retractors are inserted and any free fluid aspirated after collecting a sample for culture. Fluid may be bile stained. All surfaces of the stomach are explored. The site of gastric perforation may be sealed by omentum or only the seromuscular layer may be torn in a gastric rupture. The stomach is isolated and stabilized as for a gastrotomy incision. An inverting closure is performed and omentum or jejunum may be sutured over the repair site for additional reinforcement.

Various procedures are available for surgical treatment of gastric obstruction, depending on whether the stomach or proximal duodenum is involved. Partial gastrectomy has been reported in foals and an adult horse with proximal obstructions.[362,366] More commonly, pyloroplasty has been used for pyloric obstructions. The pylorus is isolated and stay sutures placed at the edges of intended incisions. A Heinecke-Mikulicz pyloroplasty is performed by making a vertical incision centered over the pyloric ring and closing it transversely with a 2-layer closure.[376] A Finney pyloroplasty involves a curvilinear incision from the antrum, across the pylorus to the duodenum. This procedure increases the size of the stoma; however, care must be taken to ensure that the distal duodenum is not kinked in the process.

A Jaboulay pyloroplasty is a side-to-side gastroduodenostomy.[376] The descending duodenum is joined to the distal stomach with a running seromuscular stitch. The duodenum and pylorus are incised close to each side of the running stitch. Fluid is aspirated carefully and the bowel interior checked for lesions. The adjacent duodenal and pyloric walls are joined with a continuous stitch, carrying this layer onto the caudal walls to encircle the anastomosis. The running seromuscular stitch is continued around to bury the first layer of sutures, completing a 2-layer anastomosis. The anastomosis also can be accomplished using the GIA stapler (Auto Suture: US Surgical, Norwalk, CT). The duodenum and pylorus are brought together with a running seromuscular stitch. Stab incisions are made into the duodenum and pylorus at the distal aspect of the intended anastomosis.

The separated limbs of the stapler are placed into the incisions with the points toward the pylorus. The limbs are locked together so they lie above the running seromuscular stitch with no intervening tissue. The stapler is activated and inserts 4 parallel rows of staples and cuts between the middle rows. The stapler is removed and the anastomosis inspected. The stab incisions can be closed by suture or with a TA-55 stapler (Auto Suture: US Surgical, Norwalk, CT) by drawing the defect into an everted slit. If desired, the running seromuscular suture can be continued from the cranial wall to the caudal wall to bury the stapled line.

Gastrojejunostomy has been performed in foals and weanlings with not only pyloric obstruction but also duodenal stricture or duodenitis.[361,362,377] The technique generally is without complication if the disease has been recognized early. Exposure of the stomach is accomplished as for gastrotomy. Proximal jejunum is selected and without tension, is positioned going right to left (isoperistaltic) on the visceral surface of the stomach near the pylorus. The anastomosis is stapled or hand sewn depending upon the surgeon's preference, similar to a gastroduodenostomy. I have not seen complications from stoma closure after a stapled anastomosis if 2 applications of the instrument and a transverse closure of the enterostomy are used.[361] A side-to-side jejunojejunostomy is added by some surgeons to allow duodenal contents to bypass the stomach; however, others believe the duodenal contents continue to follow the normal path of ingesta flow. Long-term complications from stagnant loop syndrome (local stasis and bacterial over growth) and stomal ulceration have been encountered in human patients but not in foals.[374]

Congenital and Familial Diseases

Pyloric Stenosis

Pyloric stenosis is a functional resistance to gastric emptying at the pylorus. It may be congenital, as with hypertrophic pyloric stenosis or acquired due to peptic ulceration or carcinoma.[273,378,379] Hypertrophic pyloric stenosis is produced by thickening of the pyloric musculature. The condition has been reported in foals and a yearling.[380-382]

Clinical signs associated with pyloric stenosis include abdominal pain, salivation, teeth grinding, retching, gastric reflux, and relief of pain after removal of gastric contents.[379] Clinical signs may appear when the foal begins to consume solid feed. The diagnosis is confirmed by endoscopy; gastric reflux is seen entering the distal esophagus, and distal esophagitis and gastric ulceration are present. Radiography shows gastric dilatation on plain or contrast studies, with megaesophagus and aspiration pneumonia in severe cases. Exploratory laparotomy reveals gastric distention, a thickened, small pyloric orifice, and an empty intestinal tract.

Medical therapy consists of fluid, electrolyte and nutritional support, plasma transfusions if necessary, and antiulcer medication for the gastric and esophageal lesions. Definitive therapy entails surgical correction by pyloroplasty or gastroenterostomy.

Diseases With Physical Causes

Gastric Dilatation

Gastric dilatation has been classified as primary, in which only the stomach is affected, or secondary, resulting from a more distal obstruction to the flow of gastric contents. Primary gastric dilatation occurs from grain engorgement, consumption of excessive grass or hay, rapid intake of water (especially after exercise), excessive swallowing of air (cribbing) or parasitism.[251,383,384] Secondary gastric dilation occurs more frequently and can occur with primary intestinal ileus or obstruction leading to stasis of intestinal contents that later reflux into the stomach. The more proximal the obstruction, the sooner the stomach fills. For instance, duodenal obstruction produces gastric reflux within 4 hours.[385,386] Gastric dilatation also can be seen with large intestinal obstruction.

Historical findings associated with gastric dilatation may include ingestion of large quantities of feed or water. The primary clinical sign is acute onset of moderate to severe, continuous pain.[251] To relieve abdominal pressure and assist diaphragmatic movement, the horse may lean back or assume a "dog-sitting" position. Ingesta may be seen at the nares.

Retching and vomiting can occur but are rare in horses and may indicate a terminal event. Most horses with gastric dilation have hemoconcentration, hypokalemia and hypochloremia.[251,379] A nasogastric tube always should be passed and gastric fluid siphoned out continually to reduce the chance of rupture. Rectal palpation is performed routinely to rule out distal intestinal obstruction.

Medical therapy is supportive for fluid losses, pain and secondary complications of aspiration pneumonia and laminitis.

Gastric Impaction

Gastric impaction results from gastric atony (adynamic ileus, peritonitis, enteritis, trauma, chronic distention), ingestion of feed that tends to swell if improperly masticated (wheat, barley, persimmon seeds), or accumulation of dry ingesta or foreign substances (hairballs, rubber fencing).[251,354,379] Insufficient water, poor dentition resulting in poor mastication, and rapid eating may predispose to impaction.

Clinical signs include acute or chronic abdominal pain, retching, salivation, and ingesta at the nares. Endoscopic and radiographic examinations are used to confirm the diagnosis and determine the type and consistency of the impacted material. Treatment consists of nasogastric lavage, if possible, or exploratory laparotomy with infusion of fluid and massage to soften the impacted mass.[387] Gastrotomy has successfully relieved such impactions.[388] Attempts at stimulating gastric motility are contraindicated due to the risk of rupture.

Gastric Rupture

Generally, gastric rupture is a rare complication of gastric impaction or dilatation because these problems usually are recognized early by clinicians.[5,389,390] In 2 retrospective studies of equine colic cases, the incidences of gastric rupture were 5 and 8%.[191,391] In a necropsy survey, gastric rupture was found in 3% of 1659 horses.[5] Primary (or idiopathic) gastric rupture results from gastric dilatation or impaction, whereas secondary gastric rupture can result from obstructive, peritoneal and enteric etiologies.[5] Results of one study suggest that geldings, and horses on a diet of grass hay or grass/alfalfa hay only, are at an increased risk of gastric rupture.[390]

Historical findings are of acute or chronic gastric dilatation, with clinical signs lasting from hours to days.[354,384] Affected horses may have markedly elevated heart rates, hypochloremia, septic peritoneal effusion and concurrent intestinal disease. The presence or absence of gastric reflux may not be a reliable indicator of gastric rupture and, unfortunately, rupture may occur even if a nasogastric tube has been in place. Abdominal radiography may reveal free air near the diaphragm and surrounding the kidneys, while abdominal ultrasonograms may show excessive fluid. When the stomach ruptures, a horse that has been previously exhibiting abdominal pain suddenly appears calm. Signs of shock soon appear, along with a cold sweat and muscle fasciculations. Food particles may be recovered by abdominocentesis unless the rupture is small or occurs into the omental bursa. Rectal palpation may permit detection of gritty ingesta free in abdominal cavity and on serosal surfaces. Most ruptures occur along the greater curvature, and the margins show evidence of antemortem hemorrhage (Fig 106).[273]

Surgical closure of the rupture has been described in horses.[392,393] Generally, the seromuscularis tears first along the greater curvature before the mucosal layer.[273] Inaccessibility of the stomach and excessive contamination of the peritoneal cavity limit attempts to repair these lesions.

Inflammatory, Infectious and Immune Diseases

Gastric Parasitism

Parasites of the equine stomach include *Gasterophilus* spp, *Habronema* spp, *Draschia megastoma* and *Trichostrongylus axei*.[394] Infection by these parasites is common but rarely results in clinical signs. The eggs or larvae of *Habronema* and *Draschia* are not usually recovered by conventional fecal flotation methods, while *T axei* eggs can be mistaken for those of other strongylid worms.[395] Endoscopy may reveal *Gasterophilus* larvae or mural abscesses caused by *Draschia megastoma*. The anthelmintic, ivermectin, appears effective against all gastric parasites.[396]

The most frequent cause of chronic gastritis is infection with *Gasterophilus* larvae.[397,398] The larvae, commonly known as bots, are red, 1- to 2-cm long maggots that attach to the squamous gastric mucosa or first ampulla of the duodenum. They may also be seen in feces. Adult flies are active in warm months and lay their white eggs on the legs of horses. The eggs either hatch spontaneously or when stimulated by the horse while grooming and migrate via the mouth to the stomach. The larvae survive for 10-12 months before being passed out to pupate in feces. *Gasterophilus intestinalis* larvae attach in clusters to the squamous gastric mucosa at the margo plicatus along the parietal surface and in the dorsal aspect of the saccus cecus (Fig 107).[398] *Gastero-*

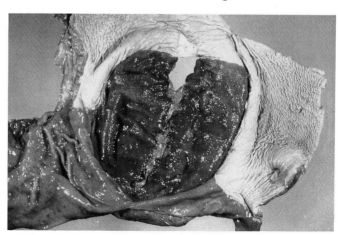

Figure 106. Gastric rupture in an adult horse as viewed from the mucosal surface. The rupture is along the greater curvature. Severe mucosal infarction is present. (Courtesy of Dr. L. Roth)

philus nasalis larvae attach to the dorsal aspect of the first ampulla of the duodenum.[398] Despite ulcerative lesions in the stomach, horses can carry a large number of *Gasterophilus* larvae without ill effects. Gastric rupture, perforating ulcers, abscesses and peritonitis have been attributed to damage caused by the larvae.[399]

Habronema larvae are 1-2.5 cm long and live in the mucous layer over the glandular mucosa. They may cause a subclinical catarrhal gastritis with excess mucus production (Fig 108).[394] The major clinical significance of *Habronema* is in contamination of skin wounds, known as "summer sore" lesions. Conjunctivitis or pulmonary abscessation also can be produced by *Habronema* or *Draschia*. *Draschia megastoma* infection is very similar to *Habronema* infection except it is more damaging and frequently causes abscessation and granulomatous lesions in the glandular wall where the worms live in colonies (Fig 109).

Trichostrongylus axei are hair-like, 0.5-cm long worms.[400] *Trichostrongylus axei* is a common abomasal parasite of ruminants and is found in horses grazing on common pastures.[401] Clinical signs are not remarkable and infected horses may exhibit only weight loss and an irregular appetite. Worm burdens tend to be low, but in heavy infections, proliferative circumscribed lesions with nodules, ulcers, plaques and polyps are found in the glandular epithelium.[402,403]

Acquired Pyloric Stenosis

Fibrous masses may result in acquired pyloric stenosis.[404,405] Diagnosis is based on clinical signs of gastric obstruction, such laboratory data as an abnormal d-xylose absorption test, and endoscopic and radiographic examinations.

Toxic Diseases

Nonsteroidal Antiinflammatory Drug Toxicity

Nonsteroidal antiinflammatory drugs (NSAIDs), such as phenylbutazone and flunixin meglumine, can produce oral, squamous and glandular gastric, and intestinal ulceration when given in large doses.[205,209,406,407] Gastric ulcers are localized primarily to the glandular region (Fig 110). Ulceration results from absorption of the drug across the surface epithelium, direct cyto-

Figure 108. *Habronema* larvae in the mucous layer of the cardiac gland region in an adult horse. (Courtesy of Dr. M. Riggs)

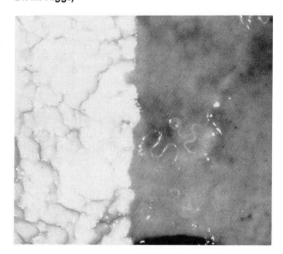

Figure 107. *Gasterophilus intestinalis* larvae in the squamous mucosa on the parietal surface, while *Gasterophilus nasalis* larvae are attached to the dorsal aspect of the duodenal bulb. Despite the heavy infection, clinical signs were not present. (Courtesy of Dr. L. Roth)

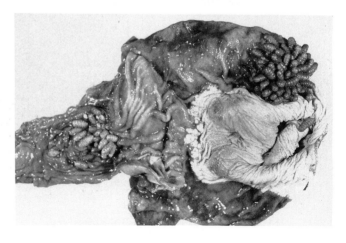

toxic action of the drug and from impairment of mucosal protective mechanisms due to inhibition of endogenous prostaglandin synthesis.[373] Prostaglandins inhibit histamine-stimulated acid secretion, stimulate mucus and bicarbonate secretion, and increase gastric blood flow. Additionally, prostaglandins have protective properties for epithelial cells and damaged epithelium that are independent of their antisecretory properties.

Clinical signs associated with NSAID toxicity include diarrhea, oral ulceration, excessive salivation and depression.[407] Ulcer perforation may occur. Serum protein and albumin concentrations decrease if intestinal ulceration is severe. Therapy includes removal of NSAID therapy and administration of antisecretory agents (cimetidine, ranitidine, antacids) and surface protectants (sucralfate). Synthetic prostaglandins have been approved for use in people with NSAID-associated gastric ulceration, but the cost of these agents is prohibitive for use in horses. Daily feeding of corn oil, which is high in linoleic acid, at 2-3 ml/kg may be a practical approach to inducing endogenous gastric prostaglandin production.[408]

Neoplasia

Squamous-Cell Carcinoma

The incidence of primary gastrointestinal neoplasia is <1% of necropsied horses, while squamous-cell carcinoma is one of the most common tumors of this system.[273,409] Other tumors reported include adenocarcinoma, leiomyoma and lymphosarcoma.[213]

Figure 109. *Draschia* brood nodule in the fundic mucosa. (Courtesy of Dr. L. Roth)

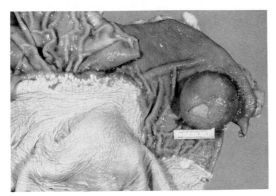

Figure 110. Glandular ulcers at the pylorus in an adult horse treated with a nonsteroidal antiinflammatory drug. (Courtesy of Dr. L. Roth)

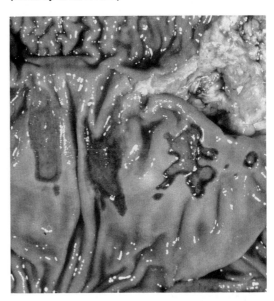

Squamous-cell carcinoma occurs only in the squamous mucosa and generally in horses over 6 years of age.[410] In younger horses, exuberant granulation tissue and fibrous masses have been reported.[404,411] Clinical signs are nonspecific and usually consist of anorexia, progressive weight loss and colic (especially after ingesting a meal) for several weeks.[23,216,335,412-416] Other signs may include anemia, dysphagia, pleural effusion and salivation.

The diagnosis is supported by anemia and neutrophilia on a complete blood count. A fecal parasite examination may rule out other causes for chronic weight loss. Cytologic examination of abdominal fluid may reveal an increased number of nucleated cells and protein but rarely reveals malignant cells.[417] Survey and contrast radiographs have been used to demonstrate the tumor.[360,417] Finally, endoscopy or exploratory laparotomy with biopsy can confirm the clinical diagnosis. Histologic examination reveals typical whorls of cells that form cyst-like structures lined by keratinized cells (epithelial pearls). At the time of diagnosis, the mass usually is large and often cauliflower-like, with necrotic areas, and metastasis has already occurred to the liver, spleen and visceral peritoneum (Fig 111). Invariably, the prognosis is grave.

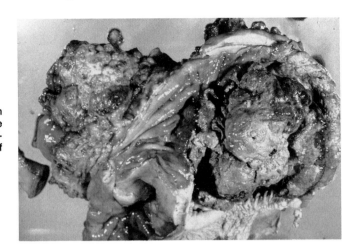

Figure 111. Squamous-cell carcinoma in the squamous mucosa of an aged horse with infiltration through the serosal surface toward the duodenum. (Courtesy of Dr. L. Roth)

Multifactorial Diseases

Gastritis

The squamous portion of the gastric mucosa frequently is involved in erosive and ulcerative conditions. An erosion is a mucosal defect that does not penetrate the muscularis mucosa, whereas an ulcer extends beyond this layer.[370] Gastritis can be divided into acute and chronic stages. During the acute stage, mild thinning of surface epithelium with a raised border develops. Extensive inflammation and bacterial colonization lead to frank hemorrhage as submucosal vessels are eroded. In chronic stages, hypertrophy of the squamous mucosa occurs. The most common site of erosion or ulceration is along the margo plicatus in the squamous mucosa, usually at the lesser curvature or extending from the junction of the pyloric and fundic glandular regions (Fig 112).[418] Others have reported that squamous ulceration is more prevalent at the greater curvature.[419]

In a study of necropsy findings in foals in the United States and Europe, about 25% of foals had ulceration, primarily in the gastric squamous mucosa.[370] The overall prevalence of gastric ulceration in adult horses undergoing routine necropsy in Hong Kong was 66%,; those that had been in training recently had a higher prevalence.[418] The antemortem prevalence of gastritis in foals and adult horses was not fully appreciated until the introduction of endoscopic equipment with sufficient length and resolution.

Horses with gastritis may be asymptomatic, with lesions found only as incidental findings at endoscopy or necropsy.[420] Symptomatic foals show anorexia, mild depression and colic, salivation, teeth grinding (bruxism), gastric reflux or regurgitation and diarrhea.[421,422] Adult horses may have mild colic, poor condition, anorexia or poor exercise tolerance.[356] On nasogastric intubation, ulcer hemorrhage may produce a serosanguineous fluid or "coffee grounds" due to the action of acid on hemoglobin.

Gastric ulceration in the squamous mucosa can be diagnosed by direct endoscopic inspection and, only rarely, by contrast radiography. Multiple erosions or confluent ulceration are commonly observed on endoscopy. Within an ulcer, islands of residual squamous epithelium often can be found. Hyperkeratosis in chronic stages of gastritis appears as thickened, yellow areas raised from the normal white glistening squamous mucosa. These lesions perforate only rarely. In radiographic studies, an ulcer crater can be seen as a barium-filled defect or as a persistent fleck of barium on multiple exposures.

Medical therapy most often includes administration of H_2 antagonists (cimetidine, ranitidine).[373] The effect of cimetidine on gastric acid secretion has been studied in horses following intravenous and oral administration.[126,127,423] One pharmacokinetic study revealed poor bioavailability following oral administration, and dosages of 11 mg/kg/day IV and 48 mg/kg/day PO were needed to achieve blood levels similar to therapeutic levels in people.[424] Ranitidine (0.5 mg/kg IV) apparently is more effective than cimetidine when given PO or IV.[128,370,423] Ranitidine given PO at 2.2 mg/kg BID was not effective in prevention of phenylbutazone-induced gastric ulceration in suckling foals but was effective when given IV at 2 mg/kg BID in weaned foals.[425,426] In adult horses, ranitidine dosages of 5 mg/kg/day IV and 15 mg/kg/day PO are required to achieve serum levels found in people.[427]

These studies suggest that the dosages of cimetidine and ranitidine commonly used in the field have minimal impact on reducing gastric acid production in horses and that dosages that produce a desired effect are almost prohibitively expensive. One study in horses indicated successful therapy with H2 antagonists; however, a control group was not included.[371] Other clinicians use antacids and sucralfate for therapy.[370] Rest and hay diets are also recommended for adult horses with gastritis.

Gastroduodenal Ulcer Disease

Gastroduodenal ulcers are most commonly seen in 2- to 6-month-old foals and can occur as a herd outbreak.[361,362] Diarrhea frequently precedes other clinical signs, which include bruxism (teeth grinding), excessive salivation, depression, anorexia and colic (especially postprandial). Delayed gastric emptying (with or without a physical stricture) usually results in squamous gastritis and reflux esophagitis. Foals with chronic gastric outflow obstruction from pyloric or duodenal ulceration may appear cachectic, and have a rough haircoat, oral candidiasis and gastric reflux. Unfortunately, gastroduodenal ulcers may perforate and result in rapid, life-threatening deterioration within 48 hours of the first clinical signs of ulcer disease.[428]

Endoscopy is the primary diagnostic tool. Linear, hemorrhagic lesions usually are found in areas of reflux esophagitis that extend from the cardia to the thoracic inlet in severe cases. Gastritis frequently is present; the glandular and duodenal mucosa may only be inspected if sufficient fluid is removed. Glandular ulcers in the pyloric region and on the antimesenteric surface of the duodenal bulb are the most common sites. Radiographic findings may include aspiration pneumonia, megaesophagus with fluid, and gastric distention. Air and/or contrast material may be seen within the hepatic duct and the first duodenal ampulla if the duodenal stricture is distal to the hepatopancreatic ampulla (see the section on liver diseases).[361,377] Ultrasonic examination may reveal excessive peritoneal fluid if perforation is suspected; otherwise, abdominal free air can be seen surrounding the diaphragm and kidneys on plain radiographs.[363,364] Free air may be a misleading finding if abdominocentesis has been performed before radiography.

Medical therapy is the same as for gastritis. Surgery in foals is directed at relieving gastric outflow obstruction.[429] Foals can be positioned on a small animal table in dorsal recumbency, which improves the view of and accessibility to the duodenum and stomach. Ulcer perforation is a frequent

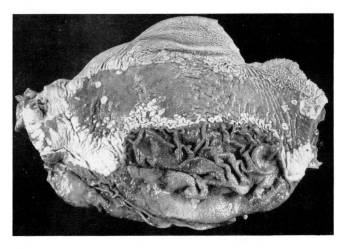

Figure 112. Extensive gastritis involving most of the squamous mucosa, extending toward the greater curvature in an adult horse. (Courtesy of Dr. M. Riggs)

complication of duodenal ulceration and, less frequently, gastric ulceration. Gastric ulcer perforation has been treated successfully by simple closure of the site and peritoneal lavage.[430] Following gastric decompression, a pursestring pattern or 2-layered series of Lembert sutures can be placed over a gastric ulcer or a wedge resection attempted with an omental patch. Perforating lesions of the duodenum can be inverted using a 2-layer continuous pattern, with proximal jejunum used as a serosal patch.[361] Pyloric stenosis has been treated by pyloromyotomy, pyloroplasty and gastrojejunostomy.[380,381,429]

Following surgery, the foal should be returned to the mare and but should remain muzzled for at least 24 hours, after which limited nursing is allowed if signs of abdominal pain are not observed. Nasogastric decompression can be attempted during any painful episode, which usually is associated with ileus or ulcer perforation. Parenteral nutrition can extend the duration of fasting; this may hasten healing of the anastomotic site or help prevent ulcer perforation. Replacement fluids and parenteral nutrition may be provided according to the foal's needs. Teeth grinding and salivation diminish gradually over several days as reflux esophagitis resolves.

H_2-receptor antagonists (cimetidine, ranitidine) should be given parenterally until the foal resumes a normal diet; then oral formulations and sucralfate are given for at least 1 month. Use of NSAIDs for analgesia should be avoided in these foals because these drugs can produce glandular gastric ulcers.

Postoperative abdominal contrast radiographs should be used to evaluate gastric emptying or if abdominal pain recurs. In normal foals, the contrast material ascends through the duodenum but, following gastrojejunostomy, contrast material initially follows a ventral course. Liver function tests and thoracic radiographs should be used to monitor biliary stasis and aspiration pneumonia, respectively. Though reflux esophagitis resolves, a mild degree of esophageal stricture may persist for several months after surgery.

Glandular Gastric Ulcer

Primary glandular ulcers are rare and usually are found in severely ill or traumatized neonates and older horses, or following administration of NSAIDs.[370,422,431] Glandular ulcers located near the margo plicatus or in the pyloric region can result in pyloric stenosis. Unfortunately, in very ill neonates, ulcer perforation may occur insidiously and is only recognized at necropsy. Diagnosis is based on clinical signs of teeth grinding or retching, blood in the gastric fluid, and endoscopic verification.

DISEASES OF THE SMALL INTESTINE

Diagnostic and Therapeutic Considerations

J.T. Robertson

Small Intestinal Obstruction

A horse with small intestinal obstruction usually has colic and thus is evaluated by physical and rectal examinations, passage of a nasogastric tube, complete blood count, serum electrolyte determinations and abdominocentesis. A foal's abdomen can be further evaluated by ultrasonographic and radiographic examinations. The history taking should emphasize prior administration of medication, as certain drugs, such as flunixin meglumine, initially may mask the severity of clinical signs.

Small intestinal obstruction must be further categorized as to whether it is complete or incomplete, high (proximal) or low (distal), simple or strangulating. This must be done because in each of these instances the clinical findings and potential outcome of the disease are different.

Complete obstruction refers to total occlusion of the bowel lumen and thus a greater degree of nasogastric reflux and more rapid deterioration than an incomplete obstruction, in which the bowel lumen is not completely obstructed. A functional obstruction may occur when no physical obstruction is present but an imbalance in intestinal motility causes signs consistent with complete obstruction.

The level where the lesion occurs, whether proximal or distal in the small intestine, affects the type of electrolyte imbalances and metabolic abnormalities observed. A high (proximal) obstruction at the level of the duodenum may cause a metabolic alkalosis, whereas one more distal in the small intestine usually produces metabolic acidosis.

The terms simple or strangulating refer to whether or not the lesion compromises the blood supply to the bowel. A simple obstruction is not the life-threatening emergency that a strangulating lesion represents. Signs associated with a strangulating obstruction include: moderate to severe, unrelenting abdominal pain; rapid deterioration of cardiovascular status as evidenced by elevated heart rate, prolonged capillary refill time, and injected or purple mucous membranes; decreased or absent intestinal sounds; and sanguineous or serosanguineous peritoneal fluid, indicating bowel wall necrosis. These cases represent surgical emergencies.

Malassimilation Syndromes

J.E. Sojka

Many diseases of various causes can interfere with absorption and metabolism of nutrients from the small intestine. These diseases often are described as causing malabsorption syndrome, though true malabsorption may not be present; the term malassimilation syndrome is more correct.[432] Malassimilation may be caused by inability to digest nutrients into the simple products that can be absorbed across the gut wall and used to meet metabolic needs, or by inability of the gut to absorb properly digested nutrients.

Malassimilation syndromes are characterized by a negative energy balance, weight loss and low serum protein concentrations. Diarrhea may be present but is not a consistent feature. In adult horses, diarrhea indicates large intestinal disease. Extensive small intestinal disease may exist before diarrhea is not present because the colons can compensate and absorb the increased fluid load. Malassimilation syndromes are less common in horses than in people or small animals.[432] This may be due to the horse's ability to partially compensate by volatile fatty acid production in the colon.

Maldigestion

Though there are many potential mechanisms of maldigestion, most have not been described in horses and their clinical significance is unknown.[432] A small intestinal brush border enzyme defect has been described in foals.[433] The equine pancreas normally secretes low concentrations of digestive enzymes.[434] Exocrine pancreatic deficiency as a cause of maldigestion has not been identified in horses.

Malabsorption

Malabsorption of nutrients may result from an insufficient absorptive surface area or an intrinsic defect in the intestinal wall. Insufficient surface area may be caused by loss of villi, as seen in viral enteritis or by resection of the small intestine. Inability of the intestinal wall to absorb nutrients may be caused by local infiltrative or inflammatory disease or by gut edema or lymph obstruction secondary to local or systemic causes.[432] This discussion is limited to small intestinal diseases. Causes of malabsorption are discussed in their appropriate sections.

If an ischemic insult to the small intestine results in necrosis, intestinal resection is a necessary, life-saving technique. If too much of the intestine is resected, however, malabsorption results. In instances of small intestinal necrosis, the surgeon is obligated to remove all devitalized bowel. If more than 60% of the small intestine is devitalized and removed, the long-term prognosis is poor. A horse with extensive small intestine resection benefits from a high plane of nutrition. High-quality fiber, which can be metabolized in the cecum and colons to volatile fatty acids, may partially compensate for small intestinal loss. Feeding increased amounts of all feedstuffs is also beneficial.

Mucosal Absorptive Defects

The most well-described mucosal absorptive defect in horses is granulomatous enteritis. Many other diseases present a similar clinical picture. Often definitive diagnoses can be made only via biopsy taken during exploratory laparotomy or at necropsy. Diseases that cause mucosal absorptive defects include granulomatous enteritis, infectious granulomatous diseases, chronic postinfarctive inflammation, eosinophilic gastroenteritis, basophilic enteritis and alimentary lymphosarcoma.

A common feature of these diseases is a negative energy balance due to malabsorption of nutrients and protein-losing enteropathy. Both the malabsorption and enteric protein loss contribute to the catabolic state. Protein-losing enteropathy can occur due to several mechanisms. With severe inflammatory infiltrative disease of the gut wall, all of these mechanisms may be acting at once. Protein may diffuse into the gut lumen through cell junctional pores, which are increased in size due to inflammation.[435] Protein may passively exude through ulcerations in the mucosa or be secreted actively by mucosal cells.[435] Normal protein loss due to sloughing of villus tip cells may be accelerated if there is an increased rate of villus cell turnover.[435]

Protein-losing enteropathy reduces serum albumin through decreased hepatic formation, albumin loss into the gut lumen, and catabolism of albumin to meet protein and energy requirements. All 3 of these mechanisms may occur concurrently. Though all classes of proteins may be lost into the gut lumen in protein-losing enteropathy, the blood albumin is generally decreased in relation to serum globulin levels. This may be due to an increased rate of globulin production in response to inflammation. The total plasma protein level in the blood is variable and may be in the normal range. Thus, serum albumin and globulin determinations, rather than simply a total protein measurement, are important when evaluating a horse with suspected protein-losing enteropathy.

Clinical signs associated with protein-losing enteropathy include lethargy or exercise intolerance, weight loss and dependent edema. Edema is secondary to low plasma oncotic pressure caused by hypoalbuminemia and usually is most prominent in the pectoral region, ventral abdomen and prepuce. Diarrhea may not be present. Definitive diagnosis is by administering [51]CR-labelled albumin parenterally and then documenting increased fecal protein loss. If this technique is not feasible, protein-losing enteropathy can be diagnosed presumptively by ruling out other causes of protein loss, such as renal disease, and by excluding the possibility of decreased albumin production as in liver disease. Oral absorption of glucose or d-xylose may be decreased if the small intestine is involved but may be normal if other sections of the intestinal tract are the primary site of disease.

Diseases that cause dilated lymph vessels or gastrointestinal edema may result in protein-losing enteropathy even though they affect areas other than the small intestine. These diseases include verminous arteritis from large strongyle migration, acute salmonellosis or other forms of infectious enteritis, congestive heart failure, mesenteric abscess due to *Rhodococcus equi, Streptococcus equi* or other bacteria, gastric or large intestinal ulceration or peritoneal adhesions.[173,432]

Congenital and Familial Diseases

J.T. Robertson

Meckel's Diverticulum

The omphalomesenteric duct serves as a communication between the gut of the young embryo and its temporary source of nutrition, the yolk sac. This duct is obliterated early in gestation as placental nutrition becomes established. Persistence of the proximal portion of the duct produces a tubular, finger-like projection from the antimesenteric surface of the ileum known as Meckel's diverticulum.[436,778] The lumen of this diverticulum may be continuous with that of the ileum. Impaction or empyema of the diverticulum can cause chronic colic, and rupture of the diverticulum can result in fatal peritonitis.[273,436]

A complete, persistent duct that attaches to the umbilicus is known as a vitelloumbilical band. A vitelloumbilical band may predispose to volvulus of the jejunum and ileum. Affected horses show signs of an acute strangulating obstruction. Definitive diagnosis is by exploratory celiotomy. The fibrous band must be ruptured or cut to correct the volvulus. Because there may be a communication between the lumen of the ileum and the proximal portion of the duct, the band should be ligated before it is severed. The necrotic bowel is resected and an anastomosis is performed.

Mesodiverticular Band

A persistent vitelline artery may form an anomalous mesodiverticular band.[438] This band, located in the jejunum, is continuous with the jejunal mesentery; its attachment extends to the antimesenteric side of the small intestine (Fig 113). In 4 reported cases, there were no associated Meckel's diverticula.[438]

The mesodiverticular band and adjacent mesentery and jejunum form a potential internal hernia sac. Small bowel may enter the sac and become incarcerated. Pressure from this distended, incarcerated bowel may lead to rupture of the jejunal mesentery. Intestine passes through the mesenteric rent, leading to strangulation and predisposing to volvulus of the jejunum and ileum.

Clinical signs are consistent with those of an acute strangulating obstruction. Diagnosis is by exploratory celiotomy. Surgical repair involves correction of the volvulus and strangulation. The necrotic jejunum and ileum are resected and jejunocecal anastomosis is performed.

Diseases With Physical Causes

Malabsorption Due to Extensive Resection

Resection of more than 60% of the small intestine in experimental ponies resulted in serious malabsorption and weight loss.[139] Some ponies also developed diarrhea and liver dysfunction. In all of these ponies, a portion of the ileum was resected and the ileocecal valve was bypassed by jejunocecal anastomosis. Evidence of a true malabsorption syndrome was a flattened d-xylose absorption curve and progressive weight loss. An unexpected finding in control ponies was reduced d-xylose absorption. Because these ponies had only a short segment of small intestine removed but did have an ileocecal bypass, it is possible that ileal bypass procedures may have more adverse effects than previously recognized.

A number of factors probably contributed to development of the malabsorption syndrome in these experimental studies.[139] Extensive resection of intestine significantly reduces the absorptive surface area of the small bowel. Ileal resection and bypass of the ileocecal valve may contribute to decreased small intestinal transit time and reflux of cecal or colonic contents into the small intestine.[139,223] Bacterial contamination of the small intestine with colonic contents can contribute to malabsorption,

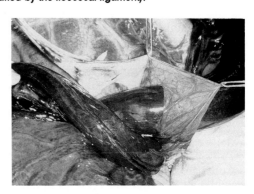

Figure 113. An anomalous mesodiverticular band in the jejunum predisposed to strangulation of the ileum (identified by the ileocecal ligament).

which may have been the cause of xylose malabsorption in control animals. Chronic changes in the colonic environment secondary to small intestinal malabsorption may have caused diarrhea in some ponies. Hepatic dysfunction and inadequate feed intake also may have contributed to malabsorption and weight loss. These ponies were fed only maintenance diets.

These findings should be given clinical consideration if more than 30 feet of small intestine must be removed. If possible, the ileum should be preserved.[223] The client should be forewarned of the possibility of malabsorption syndrome and the need for dietary management.

Postoperative Adhesions

One of the most serious and undesirable complications of equine abdominal surgery is formation of peritoneal adhesions.[191] Though adhesions may form and never interfere with intestinal function, they frequently cause kinking and distortion of the normal anatomy or result in stricture that produces obstruction. Fibrous adhesions also may form a potential internal hernial orifice or predispose to volvulus. Horses subjected to intestinal resection and anastomosis or an enterotomy are at high risk for developing adhesions. It was reported in one study that adhesions were responsible for producing obstruction in 22% of horses having small intestinal surgery. The overall occurrence of adhesion formation following all types of colic surgery is likely much higher.[437] Repeat celiotomies increase the likelihood of intraabdominal adhesion formation.[437]

Peritoneal adhesions form in response to tissue anoxia or hypoxia, infection and the presence of foreign material.[326,439] Factors that contribute to adhesion formation include intestinal ischemia or necrosis, peritoneal contamination, tissue dehydration, hemorrhage, rough tissue handling, and inappropriate suture material and technique.[439] The duration of the strangulating or obstructive lesion before surgery and the ileus following surgery are also important factors.[437] Following surgery, adhesions may be well formed by 5-7 days and produce signs of obstruction as early as 10-14 days. Most obstructions associated with postoperative adhesion formation become apparent within 2 months of surgery.[437] Adhesions also may form as a result of peritonitis caused by verminous arteritis, parasite larval migration, bacterial infection, and internal abdominal abscess formation.

Peritoneal adhesions should be suspected as a cause of small intestinal obstruction in horses with recurrent colic and a history of peritonitis or abdominal surgery. The severity of clinical signs depends on the degree of obstruction. A partial obstruction of the small intestine is likely to produce intermittent episodes of mild to moderate pain. On rectal examination during an episode of colic, the obstructed bowel feels distended and may be thickened proximal to the chronic obstruction. If the adhered bowel is within reach, the adhesion may also be palpable. Fever, peripheral leukocytosis and alterations in the peritoneal fluid indicate active peritonitis.

Internal abdominal abscesses can produce intestinal structure secondary to adhesive peritonitis. Recurrent, prolonged colic and/or chronic weight loss are consistent features of internal abdominal abscessation.[440] Some horses have anorexia and a fever, and increased heart and respiratory rates. Associated clinicopathologic features include neutrophilia, anemia, hypergammaglobulinemia and hypoalbuminemia. Peritoneal fluid analysis often reveals elevated protein content (2.5 g/dl) and a high WBC count (10,000/μl). Free bacteria are rarely seen and bacterial culture of peritoneal fluid almost always is negative for aerobic and anaerobic growth.[440] The abscess may be palpable per rectum.

The occurrence of postoperative adhesions can be reduced by practicing good surgical technique and minimizing peritoneal injury. Horses with peritonitis should be treated with appropriate antibiotics, anti-inflammatory agents and peritoneal lavage, if necessary. Irritating peritoneal lavage solutions should be avoided. One study showed that small doses of heparin, administered parenterally at surgery and continued for 2 days, decreased formation of adhesions in ponies with experimentally induced intestinal ischemia.[192]

When adhesions produce intestinal obstruction, the type of surgical repair is dependent on their location and severity. If an adhesion forms in a very localized area severing the adhesion may be adequate to restore luminal patency. More extensive adhesions necessitate intestinal resection and anastomosis or a bypass procedure if the intestine is adhered to an inaccessible area or incorporated into an abdominal abscess. Even after surgical repair of adhesions, there is a great likelihood for recurrence. Horses with widespread adhesions usually are euthanized.

Intestinal Stricture

Stricture of the small intestine occurs as a result of peritonitis and fibrous adhesion formation around the intestine, or as a sequel to fibrosis associated with severe mucosal ulceration. Strictures often occur at the site of an intestinal anastomosis if there has been excessive fibrosis or inversion of the bowel. Occasionally secondary strictures develop at the site of an anastomosis performed with a stapling device. Duodenal stricture is seen in foals 1-16 weeks of age that have severe gastroduodenal ulceration.[361,362]

Clinical signs associated with strictures depend on the location and severity of the obstruction. Foals with duodenal stricture show weakness, depression and anorexia. These foals usually grind their teeth, salivate excessively, protrude their tongues, and regurgitate after nursing.[362] Distention of the stomach with fluid produces abdominal pain, and reflux of gastric fluid into the esophagus produces esophagitis and ulceration. Frequently there is megaesophagus, and some of these foals demonstrate metabolic alkalosis.[361]

A diagnosis of duodenal obstruction is confirmed by contrast abdominal radiography. After draining the stomach, barium is administered by stomach tube and sequential standing lateral abdominal radiographs are made at 10, 20, 30 and 60 minutes.[361,362] If the duodenum is obstructed, barium remains in the stomach after 60 minutes.

Strictures associated with peritonitis or an intestinal anastomosis usually involve the jejunum or ileum and frequently produce recurrent episodes of mild colic that often respond to analgesics. When the obstruction becomes complete, clinical signs become more acute and pain may be unrelenting. The stricture can be resected, surgically dilated or effectively bypassed, and the horse should have a good prognosis. The prognosis for surgical correction of duodenal stricture following gastroduodenal ulceration is guarded. Foals with concurrent cholangitis and pancreatitis have a poor prognosis.[361]

Epiploic Foramen Hernia

Epiploic foramen herniation is an example of an internal hernia and displacement of bowel through an opening within the abdominal cavity without formation of a hernial sac. The epiploic foramen (foramen of Winslow) is located dorsal to the portal fissure on the visceral surface of the liver. It is bound dorsally by the caudate process of the liver and the caudal vena cava, and ventrally by the pancreas, hepaticoduodenal ligament and portal vein.[441] Strangulating epiploic foramen hernias occur more frequently in horses older than 6 or 7 years of age due to hepatic atrophy and enlargement of this potential hernial opening.[442,443] A loop of small intestine may pass through the epiploic foramen in a right-to-left fashion into the omental bursa. Less frequently, the intestine passes through the foramen from the left, pushing the omentum before it or causing it to rupture.[436,444] The walls of the foramen form a tight constrictive ring around the loop of strangulated intestine.

Clinical signs associated with this condition are not always typical of small intestinal strangulation.[444] Signs of shock frequently are less severe than would be expected. Pain may be only slight and often there is no gastric reflux or distention of intestine on rectal examination. Grasping the ventral band of the cecum and pulling it

during the rectal examination may elicit a painful response in horses in which the ileum is taut as a result of incarceration.[445] Peritoneal fluid analysis appears to be the most useful determinant for surgical intervention (Table 2).[444] Serosanguineous fluid is found in most cases and the WBC count in peritoneal fluid increases as the disease progresses.

Decompression of the strangulated intestine and manual dilation of the hernial opening facilitate reduction. Manipulations around the foramen must be performed cautiously to prevent fatal rupture of either the caudal vena cava or portal vein. Intestinal resection and anastomosis are necessary in almost all cases. Frequently the ileum is involved, necessitating jejunocecal anastomosis. Closure of the epiploic foramen is not attempted due to its inaccessibility and the potential for damage to surrounding structures. The prognosis for incarcerations through the epiploic foramen is poor.

Mesenteric Hernia

Mesenteric defects, whether congenital or acquired, also predispose to formation of internal hernias. Such defects occur more commonly in the small intestinal mesentery than in mesentery of the large and small colons (Fig 114).[436,446] Acquired defects or tears may result from trauma, such as a blow to the abdomen, or rough handling of the mesentery during surgery.[436] It has been postulated that a hyperperistaltic segment of bowel striking a taut or fixed segment of mesentery may also produce a

Figure 114. Mesenteric defect of the jejunum. A loop of proximal jejunum passed through the defect and became strangulated.

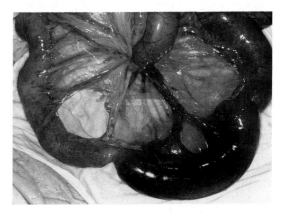

tear.[447] Persistence of an anomalous meso-diverticular band also may predispose to rupture of the adjacent jejunal mesentery.[438] A loop of small intestine enters the mesenteric defect, and incarceration and strangulation of the herniated loop may follow. The herniated bowel subsequently may twist to produce a volvulus.

Clinical signs and findings of physical and laboratory examinations depend on the location and size of the hernial opening and the length of small intestine incarcerated or strangulated. In most cases, mesenteric herniation ultimately results in a strangulating obstruction.

Repair of a strangulated mesenteric hernia usually requires enlargement of the hernial opening to allow reduction and resection of the strangulated section of small intestine. Anastomosis and repair of the mesenteric defect are then performed. If the tear extends toward the root of the mesentery, exposure and repair are difficult and care must be taken to avoid damaging jejunal vessels. Tears in the mesentery that are produced while handling the intestine at surgery should always be repaired. The prognosis associated with strangulated mesenteric hernias is guarded.

Other Forms of Internal Hernia

Small intestinal herniation also can occur through tears or defects of the omentum and various abdominal ligaments and through the rings formed by fibrous bands and adhesions.[436,442,448] These forms of internal herniation are relatively rare. Incarceration of small bowel through a ligamentous defect frequently produces clinical signs and strangulation consistent with that type of obstruction. Small intestine can become incarcerated in the renosplenic space, though it is far more common for the large colon to displace and become entrapped over the renosplenic ligament.

Inguinal Hernia

Inguinal or scrotal hernia in stallions almost always produces acute intestinal obstruction. Acquired inguinal hernias usually are unilateral and most are indirect, with the intestine passing through the vaginal ring into the cavity of the tunica vaginalis.[449] As the bowel invades the inguinal canal and scrotum, it lies next to the sper-matic cord, epididymis and testis. Herniation may be spontaneous or caused by recent breeding, trauma, strenuous exercise or abnormally large inguinal canal openings.[450] Inguinal herniation and evisceration also occur as complications of castration. There appears to be a high incidence of scrotal herniation in Standardbred stallions.[443,451] It is possible, though rare, for an inguinal hernia to occur in a gelding, even though the inguinal canal is narrowed or closed in most castrated horses.[436]

Incarceration of the intestine within the inguinal canal usually produces intense, persistent abdominal pain. Only in rare cases in which the vaginal ring, internal inguinal ring and vaginal cavity are exceptionally large is there an absence of colic or small intestinal obstruction.

The affected testis is usually swollen, cool and firm when palpated. There may be no scrotal swelling, however, if the bowel is within the inguinal canal and not in the scrotum (Fig 115). A rectal examination always should be performed on stallions showing signs of abdominal pain. A definitive diagnosis can be made if the small intestine can be palpated as it enters the inguinal canal. Reduction of the hernia per rectum should be attempted only in the very early stages of the disease before the bowel becomes strangulated.

Incarceration for longer than 6-8 hours produces strangulation of the herniated bowel and signs of shock. Rapid surgical

Figure 115. Scrotal swelling associated with an inguinal hernia.

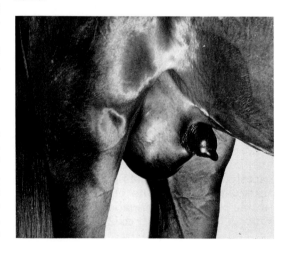

correction is imperative. Inguinal celiotomy is indicated in cases of inguinal herniorrhaphy.[452] A second incision (ventral midline or paramedian) may be necessary for hernia reduction or resection and anastomosis. Both the inguinal and abdominal incision sites must be surgically prepared.

Reducible inguinal hernias may be corrected without opening the tunica vaginal communis.[450,453] Unilateral castration is optional. If the bowel is incarcerated, the tunic should be incised carefully along its longitudinal axis and the affected bowel exteriorized. The internal ring can be enlarged digitally, or carefully with scissors, to allow mobilization of the intestine. The degree of vascular compromise varies from mild venous congestion and edema, to strangulation and ischemic necrosis. Resection of jejunum may be performed via the inguinal approach. A ventral abdominal or paramedian incision is necessary if the ileum is strangulated, necessitating ileal resection and jejunocecal anastomosis.

If the testis is salvageable, the diameter of the vaginal canal should be decreased by placing an imbricating pursestring suture through the tunical vaginalis communis as close to the vaginal ring as possible. Care should be taken not to incorporate any bowel or part of the spermatic cord into this suture. If castration is indicated, the vaginal tunic and spermatic cord are transfixed to the vaginal ring and the cord is emasculated distal to the ligature. The edges of the external inguinal ring should be apposed with interrupted sutures. A ventral scrotal skin incision is made for drainage, the inguinal skin incision is closed, and the space between the external inguinal ring and the ventral incision is packed with gauze. Providing the repair can be accomplished within a few hours of herniation, the prognosis for life is good. The longer the duration of the condition, the poorer the prognosis.[451]

Strangulating Umbilical Hernia

Most umbilical hernias are reducible; rarely do their contents become incarcerated. Incarceration is more likely to occur if the hernial ring is small. Should a previously reducible herniated segment or loop of small bowel become filled with ingesta, gas or fluid, outflow may become obstructed due to kinking and compression of the bowel at the hernial ring.[436] Congestion and edema of the bowel wall follow. Externally, the umbilical area appears diffusely swollen and the hernia becomes irreducible. The hernia and surrounding tissues are edematous and very sensitive to palpation. Incarceration of only a portion of the bowel wall circumference is known as Richter's hernia. This type of hernia is rarely encountered and usually involves the ileum.[774]

Acute, severe abdominal pain is associated with umbilical incarceration. Clinical findings, other than the obvious herniation, are typical for acute small intestinal obstruction. If the peritoneal sac ruptures, herniated bowel can migrate subcutaneously.

It is often difficult to surgically reduce the hernia without enlarging the hernial ring. This is accomplished by extending the ventral midline incision through the ring. Care must be taken to avoid lacerating the intestine. The incarcerated bowel is examined for viability and resected if necessary. Herniorrhaphy is then performed.

Intussusception

Intussusception is a result of abnormal intestinal peristalsis. A segment of intestine (intussusceptum) and its mesentery invaginates into the lumen of a segment of bowel immediately distal to it (intussuscipiens) (Fig 116). Predisposing factors include sudden dietary changes, enteritis, heavy ascarid infection, mesenteric arteritis, bowel surgery and intestinal neoplasia.[447,455,456] Other factors include obstruction secondary to foreign bodies or intraluminal polyps, anthelmintic administration and tapeworm infection (*Anoplocephala perfoliata*).[457] Though it has been suggested that intussusception occurs more frequently in horses <3 years of age, it also occurs in older horses and ponies.[442,443,458]

Clinical signs associated with jejunal and ileocecal intussusceptions usually are acute in onset and characterized by persistent, moderate to severe abdominal pain. The body temperature may be normal or slightly elevated, and heart and respiratory rates are increased. Defecation ceases, the obstructed bowel fills with fluid, and gas and fluid accumulate in the stomach. The abdomen of affected foals may be distended. The bowel usually is hypomotile on auscultation.

The rectum may contain a scant amount of mucus-covered feces or dry, tenacious mucus. Distended loops of small intestine are palpable per rectum and, in cases of ileocecal intussusception, the animal may be very sensitive to manipulation around the ileocecal region. In the neonate, ultrasonographic examination of the ventral abdomen may demonstrate a small intestinal intussusception.[454] The peritoneal fluid has an increased cell count, and ranges from amber yellow and slightly turbid in early cases, to serosanguineous in advanced cases. Peritoneal fluid changes associated with a strangulating ileocecal intussusception may not reflect the degree of ileal necrosis because the invaginated ileum is contained within the cecum and essentially "walled off" from the peritoneal cavity.[353]

Ileal intussusception may produce an initial episode of moderate to severe pain, followed by intermittent subacute colic that persists for weeks or months, terminated by an acute episode when the bowel becomes completely obstructed.[458,459] A subacute form of intussusception also been reported as a sequel to diarrhea in young foals.[380] Clinical signs include anorexia, depression, intermittent episodes of moderate colic, unthriftiness and teeth grinding. Chronic small intestinal intussusception has been reported to cause partial obstruction and repeated episodes of colic for as long as a year.[458,460] A chronic form of ileocecal intussusception has been reported to cause signs of chronic, intermittent, mild to moderate abdominal pain for as long as 40 days. Other, nonspecific findings included chronic

Figure 116. Jejunal intussusception found at necropsy. The intussusceptum can be seen invaginating into the intussuscepiens (arrow).

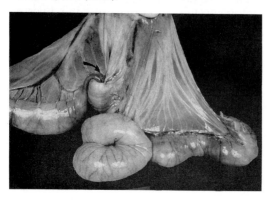

low-grade fever, poor appetite, weight loss, and colic within 2 hours after eating.[775]

Treatment of intussusception involves surgical intervention through a ventral midline or paramedian celiotomy. Initially, attempts should be made to reduce the intussusception. Some are irreducible due to their length, swelling of the invaginated bowel or fibrous adhesions between the serosal surfaces. Even if the intussusception is reducible, resection and anastomosis or an ileocecal or jejunal bypass should be considered to increase the chance of survival. Though the intestine may appear viable, there may be mucosal necrosis.[461] Simple reduction, without resection, increases the risk of acute and chronic postoperative obstruction, and formation of adhesions.

A jejunal intussusception is resected and end-to-end anastomosis performed. An ileal-ileal intussusception can be corrected with resection and jejunocecal anastomosis. In one report, a chronic ileal-ileal intussusception in the distal ileum was left intact and successfully bypassed with a side-to-side ileocecal anastomosis.[460] In most cases of ileocecal intussusception, the intussusception is reduced, the terminal ileum is blind-stumped, the remaining ileum is resected, and a jejunocecal anastomosis is performed. If the distal ileal stump appears necrotic, attempts should be made to invert it into the cecum.[462] With an irreducible ileocecal intussusception, the options are to either amputate the ileum near the cecum and perform a jejunocecal anastomosis, or create a side-to-side jejunocecal bypass of the intussusception.

With early diagnosis and prompt surgical treatment, the prognosis for successful repair of an intussusception is good. The prognosis is poor in horses with an advanced intussusception that has become necrotic and irreducible, and for those that have developed ileus and/or peritonitis.

Volvulus

Volvulus of the small intestine is produced when a loop of jejunum and/or ileum twists ($\geq$180 degrees) about the long axis of its mesentery.[273] Many affected animals have obvious predisposing lesions, such as small intestinal incarceration, intestinal infarction, severe ascarid infection, Meckel's diverticulum or a mesodiverticular band.[438,447] In animals without obvious causative lesions, such factors as verminous arteritis and rapid dietary changes should be considered.[447]

One author postulates that abnormal intestinal motility, whether hyperperistalsis, segmental atony or both, can produce rotation of the bowel.[447] A certain degree of rotation may be normal.[273,436] However, when this rotated loop of intestine becomes fixed, it may provide an axis for further rotation. Active peristalsis in the intestine proximal to this fixed, rotated portion causes further mesenteric rotation and twisting. The length of small intestine involved is variable, but the distal limit is often the terminal ileum. Another author describes a "knotting process that produces volvulus and suggests an anatomic predilection for the terminal ileum due to its fixed nature."[380] In severe cases involving most of the small intestine, the twist is located at the root of the mesentery.

The onset of colic is acute, and pain is severe and unrelenting. The rate of systemic deterioration varies with the length of bowel involved and the degree of strangulation. As the disease progresses, the heart rate increases, mucous membranes become injected, and hemoconcentration is evidenced by progressive increases in the PCV and total plasma protein values. Rectal examination reveals multiple distended loops of small intestine. The wall of the intestine incorporated in the volvulus may be palpably thickened and edematous. Passage of a stomach tube is essential to relieve fluid distention of the stomach and reduce the risk of gastric rupture.

Peritoneal fluid is amber yellow and lightly turbid in early cases, and serosanguineous and turbid in more advanced cases.[463] Cytologic examination of this fluid shows marked neutrophilic leukocytosis, red blood cells, and an elevated protein concentration. In advanced cases of strangulation, bacteria may be seen on Gram stain.

At surgery, the distended, edematous loops of small bowel are located and their mesentery palpated to determine the direction and degree of the twist. There may be a predisposing lesion, such as incarceration of small intestine through the epiploic fora-

men or through a rent in the mesentery.[447] If the volvulus is proximal or distal to an incarceration, the primary lesion should be corrected before attempts are made to correct the volvulus. In some cases, the volvulus may involve the incarcerated bowel. Affected loops of bowel are exteriorized and the volvulus corrected by rotating this bowel *en masse* (Fig 117). Gentle manipulation is essential to prevent rupture of the friable bowel and mesentery, particularly in foals.

The bowel should be evaluated for viability after correction. In most cases, the diseased bowel is resected and end-to-end anastomosis performed. Involvement of the terminal ileum requires jejunocecal anastomosis.[464] The prognosis for successful surgical correction of small intestinal volvulus is poor.

Figure 117. Small intestinal volvulus. Affected loops of bowel were exteriorized for decompression and correction.

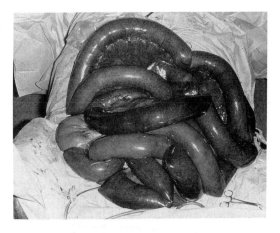

Pedunculated Lipoma

A common cause of small intestinal strangulation in horses over 8 years of age is the pedunculated lipoma.[442,443] Pedunculated lipomas, usually multiple, are suspended on mesenteric pedicles that may reach 20-30 cm in length and are often incidental findings during exploratory celiotomy or necropsy.[465] The lipomatous mass and pedicle have the potential to wrap around a loop of intestine, form a "knot" and produce strangulation (Fig 118). Occasionally the lipoma passes through a rent in

Figure 118. This lipoma (L), suspended on a relatively short stalk (arrow) from the jejunal mesentery, wrapped around an adjacent segment of jejunum (J) and produced an acute obstruction. During manipulation, the lipoma pulled free of the stalk, releasing the bowel.

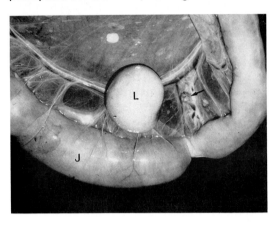

the mesentery. Though pedunculated lipomas may wrap around intestine at any point from the pylorus to the rectum, most often the small intestine is strangulated.[465]

Lipomatous strangulation of the small intestine produces obstruction characterized by acute, persistent abdominal pain, ileus and hemoconcentration. Multiple distended loops of small intestine are palpable per rectum, and fluid accumulates in the stomach. Increases in both the count and protein concentration in the peritoneal fluid reflect the degree of necrosis.

Surgical correction of strangulation is accomplished by severing the avascular pedicle and lipoma, and resecting the devitalized section of intestine. Ileocecal or jejunocecal anastomosis is indicated if the terminal ileum is strangulated. The prognosis is favorable, provided there are early diagnosis and prompt treatment of the disease. If the condition is advanced or the strangulated bowel cannot safely be resected, the prognosis is poor.

Inflammatory, Infectious and Immune Diseases

J.E. Sojka

Strongyloides westeri Infection

Strongyloides westeri (thread worm) has a worldwide distribution. A large percentage of all foals are infected, and it is the first species of parasite to establish a patent infection in young foals. Eggs have been detected in the feces of 2-week-old foals. Older horses appear to be resistant, and infection is a problem only in foals <6 months of age.

The ability of *S westeri* to cause naturally occurring disease is controversial.[466] It does not appear to be an important cause of naturally occurring foal diarrheal diseases.[129] Clinical signs in foals that received boluses of 4.5-13 million *S westeri* larvae included diarrhea, fever and death.[466] This is an infective number far above natural levels, however.

In clinical settings, a presumptive diagnosis of *S westeri* infection has been made in cases of foal diarrhea that responded to thiabendazole therapy. Heavy enteric infections have been demonstrated in foals without diarrhea or other clinical disease.[466] Extremely severe transdermal infestations may result in dermatitis or allow for the penetration of pathogenic bacteria.[2]

Life Cycle: Foals ingest the infective larvae in mare's milk. Larvae migrate into the mammary gland at the time of parturition and may be detected in the milk 4 days after onset of lactation. Alternatively, foals also may ingest infective larvae or eggs from their environment, or infective larvae may penetrate the skin directly. The eggs and free-living forms are quite susceptible to cold temperatures and drying, and ingestion via the milk is thought to be the major mode of infection. Larvae that penetrate the skin travel via the capillaries to the lungs, where they penetrate into the alveoli, travel to the pharynx and are swallowed. Parthenogenetic females develop and reside in the small intestine and pass shelled, embryonated eggs.

Diagnosis: Diagnosis can be made from identification of eggs by fecal flotation. The eggs are smaller than strongyle eggs and contain a vermiform embryo. Fresh feces should be examined, as strongyle eggs that are embryonated may be difficult to distinguish from eggs of *Strongyloides*.

Treatment: Adult parasites can be eliminated from infected foals by a wide range of anthelmintics at recommended dosages. Prevention of infection by treating mares with anthelmintics shortly after foaling has been attempted. Treatment of mares with ivermectin (Eqvalan: Merck) 200 μg/kg at parturition decreases but does not eliminate fecal egg numbers in their foals.[467] Keeping the environment clean and dry helps decrease the numbers of free-living forms of the parasite and helps prevent intradermal penetration.

Ascariasis

Clinical disease due to *Parascaris equorum* is found predominantly in weanling foals between 3 and 12 months of age. The primary presenting complaint varies, depending on the stage of the parasite life cycle, age and condition of the horse, and the worm burden.

Respiratory disease has been associated with migration of larvae through the lungs. Gastrointestinal manifestations of infection with the adult worms include stunting, poor growth, weight loss, CNS signs, rough haircoat, colic, intestinal perforation and death.

Parascaris equorum has a worldwide distribution and may become a severe problem in areas where a high concentration of foals leads to accumulation of many eggs in the environment.

Life Cycle: Eggs are produced by mature females and passed in the feces. Females are extremely prolific and infected foals may pass millions of eggs daily. The infective larvae develop in the environment within 1-2 weeks. The larvae remain in their shells, and thus are extremely resistant to environmental conditions. Eggs remain infective for up to 5 years. The eggs are sticky and may be found in manure, on stable surfaces or on the mare's udder. Ingested eggs hatch and larvae migrate through the gut wall, through the liver, to the lungs, and are then brought up in respiratory secretions and swallowed. The average time between ingestion of eggs and appearance of immature adults in the gastrointestinal tract is 2-4 weeks. The complete prepatent period is 72-110 days. These parasites preferentially reside in the duodenum and proximal jejunum but may occupy the entire small intestinal tract in heavy infections (Fig 119).[468]

The size of the adult parasite depends on the number present. The larger the infective dose, the smaller the individual worms.[468] Generally the worms are quite long, averaging 2.5-14 cm in length.

Foals >6 months of age are less susceptible, and acquired resistance and self-cure

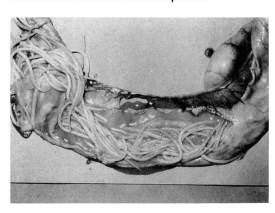

Figure 119. Necropsy specimen of jejunum in which a massive ascarid burden caused impaction.

are common. It is rare for a horse >2 years of age to develop a patent infection with shedding of eggs. If infective larvae are given to older animals, a pronounced inflammatory reaction may be seen in the liver or lungs, but no adults develop in the intestinal tract. Adult animals with *P equorum* infection may be immunosuppressed.[469] Foals usually are infected by ingesting eggs produced by the previous year's foals, not from adult horses with patent infections.

Clinical Signs and Diagnosis: The predominant initial clinical signs of *P equorum* infection are referable to the respiratory tract. Coughing and a mucopurulent nasal exudate may be noted 3-4 weeks after infection. Diagnosis at this point is based primarily on the history and elimination of other respiratory tract diseases. A frothy white material may be seen in the trachea on endoscopic examination, but the larvae are microscopic and cannot be seen endoscopically. Signs associated with the intestinal forms of infection are ill thrift, poor haircoat, poor growth and anorexia. Plasma protein levels may be low and total body water is increased, indicating poor body composition.[468] Serum albumin levels are lower than in unaffected foals.

More severe manifestations include diarrhea, colic, and ultimately an ascarid impaction that may result in bowel rupture, peritonitis and death. Clinical signs of ill thrift and stunting associated with *P equorum* infection are caused by the mature worms in

617

the intestine, not by pulmonary or hepatic larvae migration. With the exception of cough and mucopurulent discharge, infection by the larval stages is largely asymptomatic.

The clinical picture classically associated with a heavily parasitized foal is a small individual with poor muscle mass and a pendulous abdomen. Depression, poor appetite, and frequent episodes of colic and diarrhea are common.

The likelihood of intestinal rupture is not correlated directly to worm numbers. Administration of an anthelmintic that paralyzes rather than kills the worms seems to predispose to impaction and rupture. Diagnosis of the patent infection is by identifying the characteristic eggs on fecal examination. The number of eggs per gram of feces is not a reliable estimate of the worm burden, as 1 female may lay thousands of eggs per day and eggs are not produced by immature worms.

Treatment: Adult ascarids are susceptible to a wide variety of anthelmintics, but no formulation is completely effective against the migrating larvae. Foals in contaminated areas should be dewormed at 6-week intervals until 6 months of age. Ivermectin at 2 µg/kg is highly effective against immature adults in the intestinal tract. Treatment prevents immature worms in the intestinal tract from developing into fertile adults. If a foal is to be treated for the first time when a heavy infection is suspected, using a benzimidazole product initially may decrease the likelihood of an ascarid impaction. concurrent administration of mineral oil also may be beneficial. If the medical approach to relieving the obstruction is unsuccessful, surgical intervention is necessary. Multiple incisions in the small intestine may be needed to remove the worms. In those cases, the prognosis is guarded.

Tapeworm Infection

Paranoplocephala mamillana, Anoplocephala magna and *Anoplocephala perfoliata* are the 3 species of tapeworm found in horses. Of these, *A perfoliata* is most common and has been reported in approximately 50% of horses examined at necropsy in Kentucky.[470] *Paranoplocephala mamillana* is found primarily in the duodenum and proximal jejunum, *A magna* is found in the

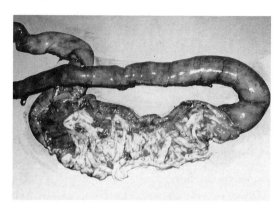

Figure 120. Heavy *Anoplocephala magna* infection of the small intestine.

distal small intestine (Fig 120), and *A perfoliata* is found from the distal jejunum to the colons. *Anoplocephala perfoliata* appears to have a predilection for sphincters and orifices, and large numbers of tapeworms often are found clustered around the ileocecal junction. Cestodes (tapeworms) are seen most often in younger horses, though all ages may be affected.

It is not clear that cestodes cause clinical disease; horses experimentally infected do not exhibit signs. Enteritis, mucosal erosions and ulcers, perforation, peritonitis and intussusceptions have been attributed to tapeworm infection.[432,471]

Life Cycle and Treatment: The life cycle of all tapeworm species is indirect. Proglottids or eggs are passed in the feces of infected horses and are consumed by free-living orbatid mites. The life cycle is complete when the infected mites are consumed by horses eating forage. Diagnosis is by fecal examination. The proglottids are generally passed singly and are about the size of a grain of rice. The typical angular eggs may be found on fecal flotation. Pyrantel pamoate, at 13.2 mg/kg, is effective against mature cestodes. Niclosamide at 100 mg/kg is also effective.

Protozoal Infections

As with tapeworms, intestinal protozoans have not clearly been identified as pathogens in horses. Because of their predilection for the small intestine, *Eimeria leukarti* and *Cryptosporidium* are discussed here.

Diagnosis: A 59% prevalence of *Eimeria leukarti* infection was found in one study.[472] Because of the difficulty in identifying oocysts, the actual prevalence may be higher than is usually thought. Though the brown, thick-walled oocyst is quite distinctive, it is not easily concentrated using standard hypertonic solutions. It is best to use a saturated sodium nitrate solution.[473] The exact life cycle is not yet known, but the prepatent period is 16-35 days.[473] Various intestinal diseases have been ascribed to *E leukarti* infection, including diarrhea, intestinal hemorrhage and jejunitis.[473] Disease has not been produced experimentally by *E leukarti* administration, and this protozoan is generally believed to be nonpathogenic.

Cryptosporidium spp are parasites of a broad range of mammalian species, including people. Infection rates in horses, as judged by serum antibody titers, may be as high as 91%. The parasite develops within the limiting membrane but outside the cytoplasmic space of the enterocytes of the distal small intestine. They are extremely small (2-6 μm) and difficult to identify by light microscopy. Diagnosis is by examination of histopathologic sections or identifying the oocytes in feces. Oocysts take up acid-fast stain and may be identified on acid-fast or acridine orange-stained fecal smears. Infective oocytes are ingested and develop within the intestinal tract. Sporozoites develop within the oocysts while they are within enterocytes. Thus, infective oocysts may develop within the intestinal lumen and self-infection without repeated ingestion may be possible. Fecal identification is best done by a laboratory with experience in identifying the oocysts.[473]

Clinical Signs and Treatment: The primary clinical sign associated with cryptosporidiosis is severe, persistent diarrhea. Infection is most persistent in foals with combined immunodeficiency and was found in 5 of 6 affected foals examined.[474] To what extent *Cryptosporidium* causes disease in immunocompetent horses is unknown. Experimentally, the presence of oocysts in feces was correlated with periods of diarrhea in helminth-free foals. Diarrhea lasted 1-3 weeks. No viral or bacterial pathogens could be found to explain the clinical signs.[475] There is no effective therapeutic agent available against *Cryptosporidium* infection.

Viral Enteritis

Viral agents produce malabsorption by destruction of absorptive enterocytes at the tips of the intestinal villi. This leads to loss of brush border enzymes and subsequent maldigestion, as well as clubbing or loss of villi with ensuing decrease in the absorptive surface area and subsequent malabsorption. The net result is an increased osmotic load within the gut lumen. The increased amount of osmotically active material draws fluid into the gut lumen, resulting in diarrhea. In addition, immature crypt enterocytes hypertrophy and migrate distally on the villi at an increased rate. Crypt enterocytes have mainly secretory abilities and may contribute to a secretory diarrhea.

Cause: In foals, rotavirus is the most common viral agent, though coronavirus, adenovirus and parvovirus also are implicated as pathogens.[84,129,476,477] Adenovirus has been isolated from foals with combined immunodeficiency but does not appear to be pathogenic in immunocompetent foals.[129,476]

The role of rotavirus in foal diarrhea is still not clear. It has been isolated on farms with epizootics of foal enteritis, but did not produce disease when administered experimentally to colostrum-deficient foals.[84,477,479] Rotavirus generally is believed to be a true pathogen when a large infective dose is ingested or when present in combination with other pathogens, such as *Salmonella*.[129,476,480]

Rotavirus is ubiquitous and it is probable that most foals come in contact with this agent, though in most instances the infections are subclinical. Nearly all adult horses have serum antibody titers against rotavirus.[476] Clinical infection and disease are present when high rotavirus concentrations are found in the environment. A large infective dose overwhelms a foal's enteric defense mechanisms and the protective effect of colostral antirotavirus antibody.[481] Rotavirus is quite stable; thus, virus particles may accumulate in the environment if poor sanitation and overcrowded conditions are present.

Clinical Signs: Affected foals are usually < 1 month old and clinical disease rarely occurs in animals >2 months of age. Initial clinical signs are depression and anorexia. Profuse watery diarrhea follows in 12-24 hours. Fever and leukopenia are variable findings and, when present, may be due to concurrent bacterial infection.[129] Weight loss and stunting may occur after prolonged diarrhea. The disease may occur as epizootics, with most foals on a farm affected.

Diagnosis: Diagnosis is by detection of virus particles in feces or gut sections via electron microscopy, or by use of a commercial ELISA kit. All rotavirus species contain a common group-specific antigen; thus, the ELISA need not be species specific and reacts with all equine rotavirus particles. However, a foal with diarrhea due to another factor may be positive for rotavirus and, conversely, a foal with rotavirus diarrhea may not be shedding enough virus particles when it is tested to be positive.[129] A supportive history and environmental conditions also are important for diagnosis.

Treatment: Therapy should be aimed at preserving adequate hydration and electrolyte balance. Antibiotics are indicated in the debilitated foal or if a bacterial septicemia is also present. In most foals, the diarrhea resolves in 7-14 days, though in some instances it may continue for prolonged periods. Additional support with parenteral nutrition may be necessary in severely debilitated foals. Lactase deficiency due to loss of brush border disaccharides may develop and should be suspected in cases of prolonged diarrhea.

Prevention should be attempted by changing the environment. Good hygiene and low population densities of foals are essential. Adequate passive transfer of antibody should be ensured in all foals. Rotavirus is quite hardy and may survive in the environment for up to 9 months.[129] Disinfection and drying of foaling stalls between use help prevent accumulation of virus particles in the environment. Rotavirus vaccines developed for food animal species are not protective in foals.[129,476]

Infectious Granulomatous Diseases

Several infectious agents cause granulomatous small intestinal disease. Clinically they may be impossible to distinguish from other causes of granulomatous enteritis. Histopathologic examination and gut or fecal cultures may be required for specific identification.

Mycobacterium tuberculosis (avium) and *Mycobacterium paratuberculosis* have been isolated from horses with chronic gastrointestinal disease.[81,482,483] Histopathologically, acid-fast bacteria can often be found within the gut wall or lymph nodes.[81,482] Despite histopathologic evidence of acid fast bacteria, culture results may be negative.[482] Horses experimentally infected with *M paratuberculosis* developed signs of disease, including weight loss and rough haircoat. *Mycobacterium paratuberculosis* was reisolated from the infected horses and from fecal cultures, and infected horses could transmit the disease. Infected horses did not react to intravenous or intradermal *M paratuberculosis* antigen tests.[483] Skin testing is of little or no value in diagnosis of mycobacterial infection.

Antemortem diagnosis is by identification of acid-fast bacteria on intestinal biopsy sections or via intestinal tissue or fecal cultures. There are no reports of attempts to treat affected horses, but isoniazid at 3-20 mg/kg/day or rifampin at 10 mg/kg BID may be of some benefit. Histoplasmosis has been isolated from horses with diarrhea, low serum protein level and weight loss.[484,485] No attempt at treatment was reported.

Rhodococcus equi was isolated from 2 foals with weight loss and diarrhea.[486] Pathologic findings included inflamed, ulcerated Peyer's patches, mucosal ulcerations, enlarged mesenteric lymph nodes, villus atrophy in the jejunum and ileum, and PAS-positive macrophages filled with Gram-positive pleomorphic rods. *Rhodococcus equi* was cultured from all tissues and pulmonary disease was present in 1 foal. Treatment of foals infected with *Rhodococcus equi* involves use of rifampin at 10 mg/kg BID and erythromycin estolate at 25 mg/kg QID. There are no reports of treating foals with the granulomatous enteric form of the disease, however.

Clostridial Enteritis

Clostridium perfringens and *Clostridium welchii* types B and C have been described as causes of peracute hemorrhagic enteritis and death in foals.[129,487-489] Foals may be found dead or moribund, and most die within 24 hours of the onset of signs. Colic has been described as an initial presenting sign.[489] Bloody diarrhea may be present if the foal does not die peracutely. Successful treatment has not been described. Fluid therapy, high levels of penicillin, and non-steroidal antiinflammatory agents should be used if an attempt to save the foal is made. Necropsy findings include blood- and gas-filled small intestine, with a fibrous diphtheritic membrane on the mucosal surface (Fig 121). Histopathologically, hemorrhagic enteritis with necrosis of the villi and superficial mucosal layer is found. The deeper mucosa often is unaffected. Large, Gram-positive bacteria may be seen lining the small intestinal villi.

Definitive diagnosis is by identifying the type C toxin in the intestinal contents by mouse inoculation tests. *Clostridium perfringens* is normally a resident in the intestinal tract and soil; thus, isolation of the organism but not the toxin is not diagnostic. Extremely high numbers of *Cl perfringens* organisms in the small intestine suggest the diagnosis, however.

The principal toxin elaborated by *Cl perfringens* type C, beta toxin, is trypsin labile. Because older animals produce sufficient trypsin to destroy the toxin, the problem is limited to neonates. Occurrence usually is sporadic, though herd outbreaks have been reported.[467,488] In instances of yearly outbreaks in young foals, vaccination of pregnant mares with *Cl perfringens* toxoid types C and D may prevent recurrent annual problems.[488]

Ascarid Impaction

Foals, weanlings and yearlings with a very heavy infection of *Parascaris equorum* are susceptible to ascarid impaction of the small intestine. It occurs most commonly in weanlings and usually follows administration of an effective anthelmintic, such as ivermectin, piperazine or an organophosphate. These drugs paralyze the ascarids, and masses of roundworms subsequently accumulate and partially or completely obstruct the small intestinal lumen.[776] Perforation and rupture of the small intestine can occur as a sequel to massive accumulation of ascarids in weanlings.

Clinical signs include mild to severe abdominal pain, gastric reflux, often containing ascarids if the obstruction is complete,

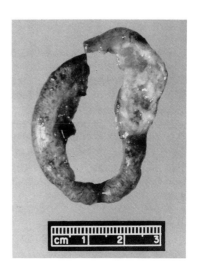

Figure 121. Cross-section of small intestine affected with clostridial enteritis. Note the gas bubbles within the gut wall.

and debilitation consistent with chronic ascariasis. Complete small intestinal obstruction with ascardids can produce shock, which is compounded by the apparent toxic or allergenic effects of the dead ascarids. Diagnosis is based on evidence of a heavy ascarid burden and a history of a recent deworming.

Foals with a suspected heavy ascarid burden should be treated with low-efficacy drugs, such as thiabendazole or fenbendazole, to reduce the risk of impaction. A second treatment, with a high-efficacy wormer, can then follow.[777] Treatment of ascarid impaction includes administration of mineral oil PO as an intestinal lubricant in cases of incomplete obstruction, and parenteral analgesics. If the medical approach to relieving the obstruction is unsuccessful, surgical intervention is necessary. Multiple incisions in the small intestine may be necessary to remove the bulk of the obstructing ascarids. In those cases, the prognosis is guarded.

Neoplasia

Alimentary Lymphosarcoma

Alimentary lymphosarcoma may cause protein-losing enteropathy and malabsorption syndrome. Historical findings may include weight loss, mild colic, diarrhea, fever, edema and icterus.[219,490] In a study of 9 horses with alimentary lymphoma, 7 had anemia but only 2 showed atypical mononuclear cells on peripheral blood smears.[219]

Lymphoma tends to be a disease of young horses, with a typical age ranging from 2-11 years. Malabsorption has been confirmed via oral glucose tolerance tests.[490] Diagnosis is by finding atypical lymphocytes present in the blood or peritoneal fluid, or by intestinal or mesenteric lymph node biopsy. Often the gut wall is grossly normal, though patchy or diffuse thickening may be present.

There are reports of attempted tumor resection, but usually the disease is widely disseminated at the time of diagnosis and the prognosis is grave.

Other Intestinal Neoplasms

J.T. Robertson

Other types of abdominal neoplasia that may cause gastrointestinal disturbances are mesothelioma, carcinoma, malignant melanoma and vascular tumors.[273,463,465,491] Any of these tumors may metastasize. A leiomyoma, a benign neoplasm of smooth muscle origin, can produce discrete, focal obstruction of the small intestine.[224]

Clinical signs depend on the type, location and size of the tumor, and the degree of metastasis and intestinal infiltration. Signs may include anorexia, depression, progressive weight loss, exercise intolerance, diarrhea, abdominal distention, ascites and colic.[465] Though cytologic examination of peritoneal fluid from affected horses does not usually reveal malignant cells, other abnormalities may be noted.[463] Melanin granules were observed in the macrophages of a horse with malignant melanoma; a horse with generalized carcinoma had blood peritoneal fluid with an increased nucleated cell count.[463] The author of that report also suggested vascular tumors have the potential to produce bloody peritoneal fluid.

A tentative diagnosis of neoplasia of the abdominal viscera can be based on the age of the horse, history, clinical signs and findings of physical examination. Rectal examination may reveal enlarged mesenteric lymph nodes, thickened bowel or abdominal masses. Ultrasonographic examination of the abdomen may reveal intraabdominal tumor masses. The horse should be examined carefully for evidence of metastasis to other organs, especially the lungs. Definitive diagnosis is by histologic examination of a biopsy specimen from a tumor mass. Such a specimen may be obtained by an ultrasound-guided needle biopsy or may be obtained at the time of exploratory celiotomy. Resection of metastatic neoplastic lesions is useless. If the tumor is solitary and in an accessible area, resection can be contemplated.

Multifactorial Diseases

J.E. Sojka

Lactase Deficiency

Though a primary, congenital lactase deficiency has been described in people, in domestic animals lactase deficiency has been described only as a sequel to an underlying primary enteric disorder.[28] Lactase is found in 2 forms within the equine small intestine: a digestive enzyme, neutral beta-galactosidase, and a lysosomal enzyme, acid beta-galactosidase.[492] The digestive enzyme is found in the brush border cells of enterocytes of the small intestine. Enzyme activity is highest at birth and declines to nearly undetectable levels after 3 years of age.[492]

As lactose is the primary energy source for the nursing foal, a deficiency of the lactase enzyme may be devastating. Undigested lactose is osmotically active in the gastrointestinal tract or it may be broken down by colonic bacteria producing additional osmotically active agents.[433] This causes influx of water and electrolytes into the intestinal tract that results in diarrhea. The original disease may be any that results in loss of mature enterocytes from villi tips. Viral enteritis most often is implicated as the cause. In severe cases, other disaccharidases may be lost as well, resulting in more severe maldigestion.[433]

The primary clinical sign of lactose intolerance is severe diarrhea, with dehydration, acidosis and loss of electrolytes in an unweaned foal. These signs can be identical to those produced by the original causative agent. Lactose intolerance should be considered in any foal with prolonged diarrhea. Hypoglycemia may be present due to a lack of a glucose substrate precursor.[433]

Diagnosis is by an oral lactose tolerance test.[28,433] Following a 4-hour fast, a 20% solution of lactose is given at 1 g/kg by naso-gastric tube.[28] Blood glucose levels should be determined for a baseline blood sample and 30, 60 and 90 minutes after lactose administration. Foals should remain muzzled throughout the test. An increase in blood glucose levels of at least 35 mg/dl is normal; often the level in the 90-minute sample is 2 times the control value.[28] A lactase-deficient foal shows no increase in blood glucose levels following lactose administration. A foal with partial lactose intolerance shows a rise in glucose intermediate between baseline and normal control values.

Treatment consists of temporarily or permanently removing lactose from the diet. If the foal is of sufficient age, weaning is indicated. For a younger animal, muzzling the foal prevents nursing the mare. Oral rehydration formulas available for calves or foals may be used for electrolyte and fluid supplementation. Glucose or dextrose may be used as a carbohydrate source. If a foal requires extended lactose restriction, a soy-based lactose-free milk replacer may be used, or milk to which a lactase enzyme preparation has been added (Lactaid, Sugarlo) may be given.[433]

Chronic Postinfarctive Inflammation

Chronic postinfarctive inflammation has been described as a cause of small intestinal granulomatous disease.[482] Clinical signs were anorexia, weight loss and colic. Hypoproteinemia was present. Gross postmortem changes included thrombosis of the cranial mesenteric artery, enlarged mesenteric lymph nodes, thickened small intestine and vascular granulomatous patches on the jejunal and ileal serosa.[482] Histologically, there was evidence of recent thrombosis and ischemic and granulomatous changes. The mucous membrane was replaced with granulation tissue that in places extended to the subserosal surface of the bowel.

Idiopathic Diseases

Ileal Impaction

J.T. Robertson

Impaction in the small intestine occurs most frequently in the ileum. The pathophysiology of this condition is unclear; however, mesenteric vascular disease and feed-ing hay with a high fiber content may be contributing factors.[493,494] Horses in Florida and other southern coastal states fed Bermuda grass hay appear to be at greater risk.[493] Presumably, as feed material accumulates in the ileum, the ileum contracts spasmodically, extruding water and causing the impaction to become firmer.[494]

In the initial stages of the disease, clinical findings are consistent with those of a simple obstruction. There is acute onset of mild to severe abdominal pain, the heart rate is elevated, intestinal sounds are decreased and the impacted ileum may be felt on rectal examination.[494] As the disease progresses, there is persistent abdominal pain and cardiovascular deterioration. Distended small intestine is palpable per rectum and there is nasogastric reflux. The peritoneal fluid, which was normal earlier in the course of the disease, shows elevations in the WBC count and total protein content.

Medical treatment with analgesics, intravenous fluids and mineral oil PO may be effective early in the course of the disease before small intestinal distention develops. Surgery is indicated if medical therapy fails to soften the impaction and progressive signs of complete obstruction develop. These clinical findings include the presence of distended loops of small intestine on rectal examination, nasogastric reflux, and elevations in the peritoneal fluid protein content (>2.6 g/dl).

At surgery, attempts should be made to massage the impaction and move the contents of the ileum into the cecum. If necessary, a very firm and dry mass can be softened by injecting saline into the impaction. If the impaction cannot be softened and reduced, it must be removed through a distal jejunostomy.[493] Following reduction of the impaction, the ileum should be examined and the ileocecal valve palpated. If there is ileal thickening, ileocecal valve swelling or evidence of vascular damage to the ileum, an ileal resection or ileocecal bypass procedure should be performed to prevent recurrence of the impaction.[495]

Muscular Hypertrophy of the Ileum

Muscular hypertrophy of the distal ileum produces luminal narrowing and partial obstruction.[496-499] Primary or idiopathic hypertrophy of the muscularis externa and muscularis mucosa may be the result of an autonomic imbalance that produces uncontrollable peristalsis or in response to neurogenic stenosis of the ileocecal valve. Secondary muscular hypertrophy may occur as a result of mucosal damage or strongyle larval migration.[436,497] Both the circular and longitudinal layers of the muscularis layer are thickened and the transition from normal to abnormal bowel is gradual.[497] Signs of partial obstruction include intermittent subacute episodes of colic and vague signs of lethargy and weight loss.[498,499] As the hypertrophy increases and the lumen narrows, the transient, recurrent episodes of colic become more severe and there is small intestinal distention.

The options for surgical correction include ileal myotomy or ileocecal bypass. The prognosis is good, provided there has been no chronic distention of the small intestine.

Granulomatous Enteritis

J.E. Sojka

Granulomatous enteritis was first described in horses in 1974.[80] It is most common in young-adult horses 2-5 years old, but it has been identified in yearlings and aged horses.[80,81,482] There is no sex predilection. Standardbreds are the breed most commonly affected with granulomatous enteritis, and a familial incidence has been reported.[500]

Cause: An etiologic agent or initiating pathophysiologic mechanism has not been identified. The disease appears similar in some respects to Crohn's disease of people.[80,81] Suggested causes include an un-identified bacterium, perhaps a cell wall-defective mycobacterium, hypersensitivity reactions to a common antigen, or immune dysfunction. One theory combines these possibilities and suggests that the disease is due to an aberrant host immunologic response to a microbial or environmental agent. Decreased phagocytic function of peritoneal macrophages has been described in horses with granulomatous enteritis, indicating a possible immunologic defect.[81] This has been an inconsistent finding, however.

The most common presenting sign is chronic weight loss. Appetite may be increased, normal, decreased or variable, though generally it is increased initially. Weight loss is usually insidious, and the clinical course may last many months. Diarrhea is not often present; if it is, large intestinal and rectal involvement should be suspected. Decreased exercise tolerance may precede onset of other signs. Generally, horses are bright and alert initially but become increasingly depressed as they become debilitated and cachectic. Roughened haircoat, alopecia, dry flaky skin and pruritus may be present, particularly with the eosinophilic form of the disease.[501] If the animal becomes hypoproteinemic, dependent edema may develop. Enlarged mesenteric lymph nodes may be palpated on rectal examination.

Diagnosis: Complete blood counts are often normal or may show neutrophilia with a mild left shift.[501] Hypoalbuminemia is the most consistent laboratory finding. Total plasma protein concentration can be low or normal, depending on the globulin levels, but it rarely if ever is high. Monosaccharide absorption tests, using glucose or d-xylose, reveal decreased small intestinal absorption if the small intestine is involved significantly. Peritoneal fluid findings usually are normal, though macrophages may exhibit decreased phagocytic ability.[81] Rectal biopsy may provide a diagnosis if the rectum is involved. Definitive diagnosis is by intestinal biopsies taken via exploratory laparotomy, though a debilitated, hypoproteinemic patient is a poor surgical candidate. Duodenal biopsy taken via endoscopic examination may become a valuable diagnostic aid in.

Pathologic Changes: Histopathologic findings include villus atrophy and clubbing. The gut wall contains a diffuse mononuclear infiltrate in the lamina propria and submucosa. The variety of cell types and severity of lesions varies from horse to horse and between anatomic sites within the same horse. The ileum usually is the first site affected and bears the most severe changes. The entire length of the intestinal tract, pancreas, liver and lung may be involved in severe cases. Common cell types involved in the granulomatous reactions include lymphocytes, macrophages and epithelioid cells, with plasma cells and multinucleated giant cells identified less frequently.[80] Lymph nodes commonly exhibit diffuse lymphoid hyperplasia.[80] Portal fibrosis is common in the liver.

In severe cases, the gut wall is thickened with a "cobblestone" appearance, and linear or patchy ulcerations may be seen during necropsy. The lymph nodes are enlarged and edematous (Fig 122). The carcass is emaciated with minimal body fat. The gut may have adhesions to the abdominal wall and the serosal surface of the intestines may be nodular or contain plaques.[501] Acid-fast bacteria, fungi, parasites or other pathogens cannot be identified by culture or by histologic examination.

Treatment: Treatment generally is unrewarding. Feeding a high-quality ration free choice is a necessity. Therapy has been aimed at modulating the host's immune response with immunosuppressive drugs. Treatment with parenteral prednisolone at 2.2 mg/kg SID has been described, and some horses may improve initially. Parenteral nutrition or hyperalimentation may be indicated in an extremely valuable individual. Resection is not indicated as, in most instances, areas of gut that are grossly normal have histologic evidence of disease. The long-term prognosis is grave.

Eosinophilic Gastroenteritis

The presenting complaints of eosinophilic gastroenteritis are chronic weight loss, poor condition, protein-losing enteropathy, dermatitis and variable diarrhea.[82,482,502,503] A wide range of organs may be affected, including the skin, intestinal tract, pancreas, salivary gland, mesenteric lymph nodes and lungs, though not all organ systems are affected in every horse. A common histopathologic finding in all organs affected is eosinophilic aggregates and granulomas. Clinicopathologic abnormalities include hypoalbuminemia and hypoproteinemia consistent with protein-losing enteropathy and occasionally eosinophilia in the peripheral blood and peritoneal fluid.

Diagnosis is based on biopsy of affected sites. Skin, rectal mucosa or the oral cavity are easily accessible areas.[502,503] Biopsies taken during exploratory laparotomy or at necropsy would provide a definitive diagnosis in other instances. Gross postmortem changes typically consist of a fibrotic, enlarged pancreas, biliary fibrosis, enlarged lymph nodes, ileitis and colitis.[502] Histologic changes primarily consist of lymphocytic

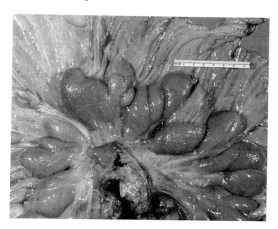

Figure 122. Mesenteric lymphadenopathy in a horse with granulomatous enteritis. These enlarged lymph nodes may be palpated rectally around the mesenteric root and may develop along the mesenteric attachments to the large colon.

and eosinophilic infiltrative granulomas and fibrous tissue deposition.

The cause of this condition is unknown. Eosinophils are implicated in hypersensitivity reactions, and the most widely held theory is that there is an unrecognized allergen responsible for the condition. Ingested, inhaled or parasitic antigens are potential sensitizing agents. Degenerative nematode remnants have been identified among the eosinophilic granulomas; thus, parasites may be involved in the pathogenesis of the disease.[482]

Unlike other granulomatous diseases, successful therapy has been reported with eosinophilic enteritis.[503] An initial loading dosage of dexamethasone at 0.2 mg/kg daily for 5 days is followed by decreasing doses of oral prednisolone, starting at an initial dosage of 0.55 mg/kg BID. The dose should be decreased to the smallest amount necessary to control clinical signs.[503] Affected horses may need life-long corticosteroid therapy.

Basophilic Enterocolitis

Horses with basophilic enterocolitis show signs characteristic of protein-losing enteropathy, with peripheral basophilia. The postmortem findings of basophilic enterocolitis are distinct from those of eosinophilic enteritis. An allergen has not been identified, though a immediate hypersensitivity reaction may be involved.

Duodenitis – Proximal Enteritis

Acute colic has been associated with a syndrome that primarily involves the duodenum and jejunum.[505] It has been referred to as proximal enteritis, duodenitis-proximal jejunitis, anterior enteritis, gastroduodenojejunitis and hemorrhagic fibrinonecrotic duodenitis-proximal jejunitis. Most cases occur in adult horses, with a mean age of 9 years.[158] The syndrome is most common in the southern United States, but it has been recognized in other areas of the US and Europe. An etiologic agent has not been identified. Clostridial or *Salmonella* infection has been proposed, but the disease has not been produced experimentally with either agent.[505-507]

Clinical Signs: This syndrome is characterized by an initial fever and acute onset of colic, followed by depression. Initially the colic may be extremely severe and the horse may traumatize itself by rolling. Signs of dehydration and endotoxic shock, such as increased heart rate, "toxic" cyanotic mucous membranes and delayed capillary refill times, may be present.[158,159,506] Borborygmi may be absent, and gastric reflux, often in voluminous amounts, can be obtained via nasogastric intubation. Rectal examination findings are variable, ranging from no significant changes to distended small intestine that is full of fluid or gas.[158,159] Once the stomach has been decompressed, colic signs usually abate and depression is the most prominent finding.

Diagnosis: Clinical laboratory findings are variable. Often, the gastric reflux is orange-brown or blood tinged, fetid and alkaline. Usually blood gas determinations reveal a normal acid-base status, though alkalosis may be present in the early stages of the disease, and acidosis may be present if severe hypovolemic shock has developed. Peripheral white blood cell counts may reveal leukocytosis with band neutrophils and toxic changes.[159] Increased packed cell volume, increased serum alkaline phosphate activity and azotemia are often found as well. Peritoneal fluid usually is yellow although it may be serosanguineous. Protein concentrations in peritoneal fluid usually are >3 g/dl and total cell numbers are near the normal range (<6000 WBC/dl).[158,506]

All clinical examination and laboratory findings should be evaluated together when trying to differentiate proximal enteritis from small intestinal strangulating obstruction lesions that require prompt surgical correction. It is important to remember that abdominal fluid with elevated protein levels and normal cell counts is not pathognomonic for proximal enteritis and cannot be used solely to differentiate it from surgical diseases.[158] If rectal examination does not reveal a condition that requires surgery, the peritoneal fluid has a normal cellularity, and the colic dissipates after gastric decompression, a diagnosis of proximal enteritis is likely and surgery should not be performed until repeat evaluation demonstrates clear surgical indicators.[507]

Gross pathologic changes found at necropsy or surgery are limited to the stomach, duodenum and proximal jejunum. Gross findings include in distention and discoloration with serosal petechial and ecchymotic hemorrhages (Fig 123).[159] The intestinal mucosa is bright red with focal ulceration and necrosis; often red or red-brown fluid is found in the intestinal lumen.[159] Microscopic lesions may be found in the stomach and entire small intestine, though they are most severe in the duodenum and jejunum. Lesions vary from edema of the mucosa and submucosa, to extensive loss of surface mucosa, villus atrophy, neutrophilic infiltrate and hemorrhage.[159]

Treatment: Treatment is primarily supportive. The first priority is to prevent gastric rupture by removing accumulated gastric contents with a nasogastric tube. Initially, extremely large volumes of reflux may be recovered (up to 8 L/hour), and it is most expedient to leave the nasogastric tube in place. The nasogastric tube should be siphoned if necessary to initiate the flow of reflux. Intravenous fluid therapy with a balanced electrolyte solution should be instituted to maintain adequate fluid balance in the face of intestinal fluid losses and homeostatic needs. Bicarbonate should not be given unless a blood gas analysis indicates acidosis. Gastric reflux may be present for several days, thus nasogastric intubation and intravenous fluid therapy may be required for prolonged periods. Serum electro-

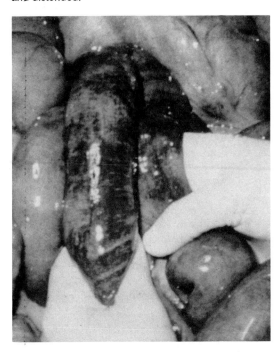

Figure 123. Proximal enteritis seen during exploratory laparotomy. The affected small intestine is hemorrhagic and distended.

lyte concentrations should be determined and any imbalances corrected. Broad-spectrum antibiotics should be administered as septicemia may develop.[506] Flunixin meglumine at 1 mg/kg may be given to protect against the effects of circulating endotoxin and for relief of pain. One should first ensure adequate gastric decompression before administering an analgesic if a horse with proximal enteritis demonstrates colic.

Heparin administration has been advocated if bacterial or endotoxin absorption is suspected.[506] In cases with severe, prolonged gastric reflux, such bypass procedures as duodenocecostomy or duodenojejunostomy may be of benefit. Once the bypass has been performed, gastric reflux decreases dramatically.

Mortality for horses with proximal enteritis varies significantly among institutions.[158,159] With prompt, vigorous medical therapy, the prognosis for life is good.[158] Long-term survival may be less than during the short term due to development of life-threatening complications including laminitis, pleuropneumonia, hepatitis, renal disease and peritoneal adhesions.[159] Early diagnosis and treatment afford the best chances of survival.

DISEASES OF THE CECUM

M.W. Ross

Diagnostic and Therapeutic Considerations

The cecum is 1 meter long, has a capacity of 16-68 L and occupies the right caudal abdominal quadrant.[300] The cecum is comma-shaped and comprised of a base and body. The cecal base is functionally divided into cranial and caudal parts by a dorsally directed fold arising from the ventral floor during contractions.[508] The cecal body has 4 distinct taeniae (bands): the dorsal, medial, ventral and lateral bands. The ventral band joins the medial band near the cecal apex. The medial and lateral cecal arteries, branches of the cecal artery from the ileocolic artery, and cecal veins course in a loose mesenteric attachment along the medial and lateral cecal bands, respectively.[509] The cecum is attached to the dorsal body wall by a dense mesenteric attachment. Additional attachments include the cecocolic ligament, running from the lateral cecal band to the right ventral colon, and the ileocecal fold, coursing from the antimesenteric band of the ileum to the dorsal cecal band. These attachments render the cecum immobile without movement of the right ventral colon or ileum.

The major functions of the cecum include retention of particulate digesta for microbial fermentation and water absorption. Liquid markers are rapidly moved through the cecum, but particulate markers are retained for 12-24 hours. The ventral and dorsal colons are much more important sites for retention of digesta. The cecum is the most important site for net water absorption in the equine large intestine. Partial or complete typhlectomy increases fecal water content and decreases fiber digestibility.[510,511]

The motor events of the cecum are complex and have yet to be understood completely. An important progressive motility pattern has been identified; it starts in the cecal body and is propagated aborally (distally) to the cecal base and into the right ventral colon.[512] This pattern is thought to propel digesta from the cecum to the right ventral colon, occurs about once each 3 minutes, and is associated with a loud "rush" of digesta that can be heard easily with a stethoscope. A pacemaker area in the cecal body is thought to initiate this progressive motility pattern.[508,512,772] Interruption of progressive motility from the cecum by damage to the cecal pacemaker could lead to accumulation of feed material or abnormal motility.

Physical examination of horses with cecal diseases should include visual inspection, transabdominal auscultation and rectal examination. Because the cecum is located in the right flank region, distention with gas causes right abdominal distention. Normal cecal sounds heard by auscultation include tinkling and gurgling sounds associated with mixing movements. About once every 3 minutes, the loud rush of digesta is associated with progressive motility. Therefore, auscultation of the cecum should be performed for a minimum of 5 minutes. Failure to hear progressive motility could indicate outflow dysfunction. A high-pitched sound or "ping" can be heard on simultaneous auscultation and percussion in horses with cecal tympany.

Rectal examination is most important in evaluation of the equine cecum. The caudal aspect of the cecal base and ventral aspect of the cecal body can be palpated in normal horses. The ventral band is readily identified as a flaccid narrow band, without covering by mesocolon or associated vessels. When abnormal conditions exist, the examiner must differentiate the cecum from such structures as the right dorsal colon or portions of the ventral colon in abnormal positions. Because of the dorsal mesenteric attachment, the examiner's hand cannot pass dorsal to the cecum. However, even with cecal distention, it often is possible to pass the hand to the right side of the cecum. Therefore, if a distended organ is felt in the right caudal abdominal quadrant, has a distinct tenia without vessels or mesocolon, and is attached to the dorsal body wall, it is most likely the cecum.

Congenital and Familial Diseases

Congenital abnormalities of the cecum are rare. I have observed a single horse with absence of the dorsal mesenteric attachment of the cecum that appeared to contribute to chronic large colon and cecal displacement. At exploratory surgery, the entire cecum, including the base and ileocecal junction, could be exteriorized easily through a ventral midline incision.

Diseases With Physical Causes

Cecal Torsion

As a primary disease entity, cecal torsion is rare and may occur only under the unusual situations of adhesions or entrapment. Cecal torsion developed in a weanling filly with hypoplasia of the cecocolic ligament.[773] As mentioned above, the cecum is relatively immobile and cannot move freely without movement of the right ventral colon and ileum. It often is displaced or twisted in horses with associated large colon volvulus (torsion). Occasionally the axis of the volvulus involves the dorsal mesenteric attachment of the cecum. Surgical correction of the torsion is the only viable treatment. Large colon torsions involving the cecum usually are severe, and the prognosis depends on the amount of edema and necrosis of the bowel wall. If a true cecal torsion is present, a partial or complete typhlectomy may be necessary.

Adhesion

Adhesion of the cecum to adjacent structures is unusual except following exploratory celiotomy. The cecum often becomes adherent to the ventral body wall in association with a previous abdominal incision. There are anecdotal accounts of horses with intermittent mild pain after exploratory surgery as a result of chronic cecal adhesions. Rectal examination may reveal chronic malposition or an inappropriate amount of tension on the ventral cecal band in horses with such adhesions.

Fistula

A cecal-cutaneous fistula has been reported after application of an umbilical hernia clamp.[513] Therefore, incarceration and strangulation of the cecal apex in an umbilical hernia is possible, but incarceration of the small intestine is much more likely.

Infectious, Inflammatory and Immune Diseases

Typhlitis

Typhlitis, or inflammation of the cecum, occurs with enteric salmonellosis. Severe mucosal ulceration, mural edema and serosal discoloration may be present. Typhlitis generally is not a primary disease entity without concomitant involvement of the large colon.

Tapeworm Infection

Tapeworm infection, most commonly with *Anoplocephala perfoliata* and less often with *Anoplocephala magna*, usually is associated with generalized parasitism. Clinical signs include weight loss, unthriftiness and poor haircoat. A possible specific sign of tapeworm infection of the cecum is flank biting. Tapeworms have been implicated as causative factors in horses with cecal perforation or cecocolic intussusception, but these conditions occur more commonly without the presence of tapeworms. Tapeworms may cause superficial mucosal ulceration, particularly around the ileocecal junction. Pyrantel pamoate at twice the recommended dosage (13.2 mg/kg body weight) has been reported to be effective.

Multifactorial Diseases

Cecal Impaction

Cecal impaction is the most important and common disease of the cecum but represents only about 5% of all intestinal impactions.[442,514,515]

Cause: Sand impaction of the cecum can occur, but the most common cause is fibrous feed material. Classic descriptions of the disease attributed the cause of cecal impaction to old age, poor feedstuffs and poor dentition. However, recently there seems to be a relative increase in the number of younger horses affected, particularly those being treated for unrelated conditions, such as musculoskeletal disorders or other gastrointestinal problems.[515] The disease can also occur in foals but is rare in that age group.

The cause of cecal impaction is not known but it appears that no outflow obstruction exists. Parasite-induced damage or altered blood flow to the cecal body may alter the cecal pacemaker and interrupt or slow progressive motility. Abrupt dietary changes, treatment for other unrelated diseases or general anesthesia may alter cecal motility as well. Transit of small volumes of digesta occurs, as the horse continues to pass a low volume of feces. The colon continues to empty and becomes quite small. The digesta retained in the cecum becomes drier than normal due to increased water absorption. Horses treated with analgesics and allowed to continue to eat are at risk, as the cecum continues to enlarge and perforation eventually occurs. Recurrence of cecal impaction is common, suggesting that the cause is a persistent motility derangement rather than a simple accumulation of dry digesta.

Clinical Signs: Horses with cecal impaction typically show signs of mild abdominal pain, including pawing, lying down and occasionally rolling. These signs may be evident for 2-7 days. Appetite is reduced and often the horse is depressed. There is a decrease in fecal production and feces may range from dry to "cow flop" in nature. Gastrointestinal sounds are depressed, especially on the right side, and cecal progressive motility is not heard. Vital signs are generally normal except during painful episodes.

Careful rectal examination is diagnostic, but the clinician must differentiate cecal impaction from other diseases, including left colon impaction, right dorsal colon impaction, right dorsal displacement of the colon and cecal-colic intussusception. In horses with cecal impaction, a firm to hard digesta-filled viscus is felt with a distinct ventral band. The examiner may be able to pass a hand to the right of but not dorsal to the viscus. Typically, the cecal base fills before the body and little or no gas distention occurs. Another characteristic of horses with cecal impaction is inability of the clinician to identify the pelvic flexure on rectal examination, as the cecum is large and the colon is relatively empty (Fig 124). Early in the disease, it may not be possible to detect the abnormal cecum on rectal examination, and serial examinations may be necessary.

Laboratory data, including the hemogram, serum electrolytes and acid-base values, usually are normal. The PCV and total plasma protein values may be mildly elevated, reflecting mild dehydration. Peritoneal fluid analysis usually is normal.

Treatment: Treatment of horses with cecal impaction is controversial; both medical and surgical management have been advocated. Because affected horses show only low-grade abdominal pain and little or no change in vital signs, the severity of the problem must be based on rectal examination findings and the known duration. If the abnormal cecum is small to moderate in size and the digesta is relatively easily identifiable, medical treatment is recommended. Successful medical treatment includes liberal intravenous and oral fluid therapy, and withholding oral food until the cecum is completely normal, based upon rectal examination. As a general recommendation, a balanced polyionic electrolyte solution should be given IV at 1-2 L/hour. After ensuring that no gastric fluid or gas distention is present, 8 L of warm water can be given by nasogastric tube 3 times daily. Xylazine is quite effective in controlling abdominal pain but abolishes cecal motility for up to 40 minutes and should be avoided if possible.[93]

Intestinal stimulants have been used previously with varied success. In preliminary studies, the cholinesterase inhibitor neostigmine sulfate increased cecal progressive motility in normal ponies.[516] Neostigmine given at 0.0125-0.025 mg/kg (5-10 mg/450 kg) SC, IM or slowly IV causes mild colic, increased intestinal sounds, apparently increased intestinal wall tone as judged by rectal examination findings, and defecation. However, one should be extremely careful using neostigmine in horses with large, tense cecal impaction, as cecal perforation could occur. Neostigmine use should be reserved for horses with mild impaction or recurrent cecal dysfunction, or for cases in which economic concerns prevent surgical intervention.

Once the cecum returns to normal, based on rectal examination findings, the horse should be reintroduced to its normal diet gradually. Initial addition of laxative feedstuffs, such as bran mash or grass, may help. A low-residue diet consisting of pelleted feed has been tried with varied success.[516,517] Pelleted feed may increase fecal water content and decrease intestinal transit time.

Surgical management should be considered if the cecum is large and the digesta is very firm, or if the impaction is refractory to medical treatment. Good results have been reported with infusion and massage, and with enterotomy (typhlotomy) and manual evacuation of ingesta, but I have not shared the same success.[518,519] Neither of these methods addresses the likely cause of a motility disturbance and the potential for recurrence. Typhlotomy is performed midway between the lateral and ventral cecal teniae near the apex; manual evacuation of the contents is necessary. Because only the cecal apex can be exteriorized, much fecal contamination occurs and careful cleaning of the bowel is necessary. The enterotomy incision is closed with a double inverting pattern with 0 absorbable suture material. Evacuation of the cecum, combined with strict dietary management and close postoperative monitoring, may result in a successful outcome.

Two procedures have been described for surgical management of cecal impaction. Cecocolic anastomosis with or without typhlotomy resulted in a successful outcome in 12 of 14 horses, but 4 had mild colic caused by gas accumulation after surgery.[517] Cecocolic anastomosis resulting in an alternative route for digesta transit after surgery prevented recurrence of cecal impaction. Anastomosis is done by creating a 15- to 20-cm stoma midway between the dorsal and lateral cecal bands and between the lateral free band and lateral mesocolic

Figure 124. Postmortem view of a severely impacted cecum. The emptiness of the left ventral colon makes rectal palpation of this part of the large intestine difficult with long-standing cecal impaction.

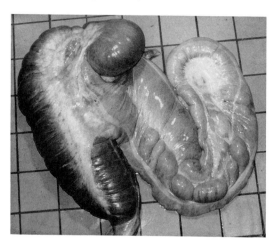

band of the right ventral colon. The technique is best done with a combination of hand-sewn and autosuturing techniques. Back and front seromuscular layer closures with 2-0 absorbable suture material, combined with 4 applications of the GIA surgical stapling instrument, provide a good anastomosis with minimal contamination.

Jejunocolic (or ileocolic) anastomosis to bypass the cecum and reroute intestinal contents into the right ventral colon may be superior to cecocolic anastomosis.[516,520] Complete jejunocolic anastomosis prevents digesta or gas from entering the cecum after surgery.[520] This can be combined with a typhlotomy to empty the cecum. To perform this technique, the ileum is oversewn in 2 inverting layers to create a blind stump. An end-to-side anastomosis is performed between the distal jejunum and right ventral colon between the medial free band and medial mesocolic band. Alternatively, a side-to-side anastomosis can be created using the GIA surgical stapling instrument after oversewing the end of the jejunum to create a blind stump.

Complete typhlectomy and ileocolic anastomosis have been described for surgical management of horses with cecal impaction.[521] The horse is placed in left lateral recumbency and the surgical approach to the cecum is made by eighteenth rib resection. Complete typhlectomy is an extremely difficult procedure but remains a viable alternative.

The prognosis for horses with cecal impaction is guarded due to the possible sequelae of perforation and recurrence. Client education concerning the differences between impaction of the cecum and impaction of the large colon is important to avoid communication problems should these serious complications arise.

Cecal Perforation

Cause: Cecal perforation in horses is a relatively recently recognized syndrome. The pathogenesis of cecal perforation may involve 2 pathways: a primary entity in broodmares at the time of parturition without evidence of a previous cecal outflow dysfunction; and a secondary disease in horses with cecal outflow dysfunction, leading to cecal filling and later perforation. In 11 mares, cecal perforation and death occurred within 24 hours after foaling.[522-526] In 1 mare, cecal perforation occurred during late pregnancy.[527] None of these mares had any evidence of cecal disease before death. In 1 mare, the cecum and colon were of normal size and no outflow obstruction or impaction was present.[522] It is possible that cecal motility is altered in late pregnancy or during parturition, and gas distention with subsequent perforation occurs due to increases in intraabdominal pressure. Though the exact cause is unknown, cecal perforation in mares appears to be similar to perforation in people with intestinal pseudo-obstruction or Ogilvie's syndrome. Women undergoing obstetric procedures or who have other unrelated gastrointestinal or systemic disorders may develop cecal perforation. Cecal perforation should be suspected in any broodmare dying unexpectedly.

Cecal perforation is more common as a sequel to interrupted outflow or impaction. In a study of 22 horses with this form of cecal perforation, ages ranged from 6 weeks to 13 years, and there was no breed or sex predilection. Thirteen horses were hospitalized and 16 were administered nonsteroidal antiinflammatory agents. All horses died unexpectedly. Necropsy revealed a large digesta-filled cecum, empty colon and a single site of perforation. The size of the cecum relative to the colon was remarkably similar to that seen in horses with cecal impaction. In this series of horses, the signs of cecal disease were either missed or masked by administration of analgesics.

Horses that are hospitalized or being treated for other disorders appear to be at risk of developing cecal impaction and later perforation. The clinician should investigate even the most subtle clinical signs, such as reduced appetite, mild depression or a subtle change in fecal quality from normal to soft feces, in any hospitalized horse. This should include careful auscultation and rectal examination.

Clinical Signs: Clinical signs after perforation are characteristic of endotoxin shock or Gram-negative sepsis, with subsequent rapid cardiovascular deterioration and death. Changes in clinical and laboratory values reflect the length of time after perforation. There is no treatment alternative, though complete typhlectomy remains a theoretical consideration because gross fecal contamination of the abdomen results in certain death.

Cecal Tympany

Gas distention of the cecum occurs most frequently secondary to abnormal conditions of the large colon and only rarely as a primary disease. Cecal tympany is a common finding on clinical and rectal examination in horses with nonstrangulating colonic displacements or volvulus of the colon.

Moderate to severe abdominal pain may accompany cecal tympany but may be related to the other primary disease process. Right-sided abdominal distention is often present and a cecal ping is heard on simultaneous auscultation and percussion. Rectal examination is diagnostic, and the clinician usually can differentiate gaseous distention from digesta accumulation. Generally there is a moderate to extreme amount of tension on the ventral cecal band.

If the condition is mild and associated with spasmodic colic, successful treatment can be achieved with analgesics, antifermentives, oral fluids and fasting. In horses with cecal tympany secondary to colonic displacement or volvulus, surgical correction of the primary problem is necessary. In severe cases, trocarization of the cecal base to remove accumulated gas may provide relief from pain. Trocarization should only be performed after careful clinical and rectal examinations confirm the presence of a gas-distended cecum.

Following aseptic preparation of the right paralumbar fossa, a 14-ga, 5-inch needle or intravenous catheter can be inserted through the body wall into the cecal base. An extension set or rubber tubing can be connected to a suction device or submerged in water to ensure gas outflow with no inflow. One must consider the possible risks associated with the procedure including leakage of digesta with localized peritonitis, or contamination of the flank area with attendant cellulitis.

Idiopathic Diseases

Cecocecal, Cecocolic Intussusception

Intussusception of the body of the cecum into the base or a continuation of the invagination process into the right ventral colon occurs uncommonly.[528-532] There appear to be 3 distinct clinical syndromes associated with the disease, based on severity of abdominal pain. These syndromes include acute, subacute and chronic wasting forms. It is unlikely that the disease is breed or sex specific; it occurs in all ages of horses.

Cause: The cause of cecocecal or cecocolic intussusception has not been established, but various authors have suggested the involvement of the tapeworm, *Anoplocephala perfoliata*. Tapeworms were present in only 3 of 10 horses in a retrospective study of horses with cecal intussusception.[532] Abnormal motility, induced by tapeworms or following organophosphate administration, has been proposed as a possible cause.[530,533] An intramural abscess or other damage to the cecal wall remain possible causes as well.

Diagnosis: The history, clinical examination and laboratory findings depend on the form of the disease. The presentation may also depend on when the veterinarian is first called. An important point is that intussusception of the cecum may mimic other causes for various grades of abdominal pain. In general, changes in vital signs and laboratory values, including elevated peritoneal fluid protein concentration and WBC and RBC counts, are more pronounced with the acute form. Presumably the increased pain reflects greater compromise to the invaginated bowel and damage to the nervous and vascular supply of the cecum. In the subacute form, horses may be depressed, have intermittent abdominal pain and show reduced fecal production. In the chronic form, horses have weight loss, fever and intermittent mild abdominal pain. Eventually, when the invaginated portion of the cecum becomes devitalized, the horse begins to show signs of increased abdominal pain and cardiovascular deterioration, with typical changes in laboratory values indicating dehydration and acidosis. Peritoneal fluid becomes serosanguineous.

Rectal examination is most helpful in establishing the diagnosis. In one report, 4 of 8 horses had an enlarged viscus felt on rectal examination;[532] In some horses, however, the cecum may not be palpable. Exploratory celiotomy often is necessary to establish the definitive diagnosis.

Treatment: Surgical management is necessary for a successful outcome. Typically the cecal apex is absent on exploration of the abdomen and a firm mass is present in the cecal base and/or right ventral colon. Manual reduction of cecocecal intussusception is usually possible and is followed by resection of the diseased portion. The cecum is closed with a double inverting closure. The surgeon must remember that the medial and lateral cecal vessels must be double ligated.

Manual reduction is often impossible with cecocolic intussusception. Enterotomy in the right ventral colon between the lateral and medial free bands is necessary and reveals the darkened, often necrotic mucosal surface of the cecum. The cecum often can be manually reduced. This procedure os then followed by enterotomy closure and partial typhlectomy. Partial resection of the cecum can be performed from within the right ventral colon and is followed by reduction of the cecum. The enterotomy incision is closed in a double inverting pattern with absorbable suture material. After thorough cleansing of the right ventral colon and a change of gowns and drapes, the enterotomy site should be oversewn.

The prognosis is good with surgical management if all of the diseased cecum can be removed. If tapeworms are present, the horse should be given pyrantel pamoate (13.6 mg/kg) at about 30 days after surgery.[534]

Infarction

Because both the medial and lateral cecal arteries arise from the single cecal artery, the equine cecum is particularly susceptible to thromboembolism secondary to verminous arteritis. Additionally, the cecal arteries are located 180 degrees apart and lack the extensive communications present between the colonic vessels. Fortunately, the disease is rare.

Cecal infarction can occur at any age, but I have seen it most frequently in foals <1 year of age. Clinical signs vary from acute, severe abdominal pain and cardiovascular collapse requiring surgical intervention, to low-grade abdominal pain, diarrhea and evidence of peritonitis. Changes in peritoneal fluid reflect ischemic necrosis of the cecum, including pronounced elevations in protein concentrations and WBC and RBC counts.

Surgical therapy, consisting of partial typhlectomy, may be successful if only a portion of the cecal body is affected. However, the condition may be progressive, and more dorsal portions may become necrotic following resection.[518] If the entire cecum is necrotic, complete typhlectomy is possible, but severe peritonitis may warrant a grave prognosis.

DISEASES OF THE LARGE COLON

K.E. Sullins

Diagnostic and Therapeutic Considerations

Disease of the large colon is responsible for about half of colic cases. The severity of disease varies from mild to fatal. As a group, diseases of the colon respond more favorably to surgical treatment than those of the small bowel. With the possible exception of volvulus of the large colon/cecum, postoperative complications are comparatively few. The colon is not subject to peritoneal adhesions to the degree of the small intestine.

Some conditions (impactions, flatulence, nonstrangulating displacements) may respond to intense medical therapy. However, because severe gas distention and pain may be a feature of any large colon disease, including large colon volvulus, surgeons may elect early exploratory laparotomy to rule out the latter condition.

Thus, when presented with a horse with large bowel distention and severe pain, it may not be possible to distinguish between "simple" flatulence and volvulus of the large colon. The difference lies in the fact that horses with less severe obstructive diseases may respond to trocarization and supportive therapy, whereas volvulus is a surgical disease in which time is of the essence. If it is not possible to make the distinction, and surgical intervention is an option, laparotomy is recommended. If the pain was caused by distention or displacement, these conditions are corrected. If volvulus is present, the best care has been given to the horse. If a horse does not have the option of surgery, trocarization is performed and supportive therapy is provided. If signs resolve, the horse is saved. If signs return, euthanasia is the eventual outcome.

Congenital and Familial Diseases

G.M. Shires

Atresia Coli

Any portion of the large colon may be atretic (Fig 125). Evidence suggests that this condition is heritable in foals.[535] One widely accepted hypothesis of the pathogenesis of atresia coli is an ischemic vascular accident with resultant necrosis during the fetal stage.

Three basic types of atresia are recognized: Type 1 is membrane atresia due to a diaphragm of membranous tissue obstructing the intestinal lumen. Type 2 is cord atresia characterized by a fibrous or muscular cord-like remnant of gut connecting blind ends. Type 3 is blind-end atresia caused by the absence of a segment of intestine, disconnected blind ends and a gap in the mesentery.

Atresia coli may be the animal's only problem or it may occur in conjunction with other anomalies. For this reason, affected animals should be completely evaluated. This condition usually mimics intestinal obstruction from meconium or other conditions causing abdominal pain and is noticed early, usually within 24-72 hours after birth. Clinical signs include discomfort and pain, tenesmus, abdominal splinting, abdominal distention and lack of meconium. Differential diagnoses include atresia ani, impacted meconium, intestinal obstruction (intussusception and volvulus), ruptured bladder and diaphragmatic hernias.

The initial examination should easily rule out atresia ani and impacted meconium. For definitive diagnosis of atresia coli, radiographs may be obtained after a carefully controlled barium enema. Great care must be taken to avoid rupturing the rectum and colon with large quantities of barium under pressure.

Once the diagnosis has been established, it may be possible to connect the 2 blind ends of the atretic colon by end-to-end or side-to-side anastomosis. This is greatly facilitated with automatic suturing instruments. If most of the proximal colon is present, it may be possible to perform a "pull-through" operation, though the mesentery and its blood vessels may prevent this. If there is a large defect, it is possible to create a permanent colostomy via the left flank. It is probably not practical, however, to create a permanent colostomy in a foal. In foals intended for breeding purposes, one should always be concerned about the genetic implications of this type of anomaly when called upon to repair them.

Diseases With Physical Causes

K.E. Sullins

Colonic Impaction

Though feed material usually forms the bulk of the physical obstruction, the impaction may be promoted by reduced water intake, coarse roughage, poor dentition, extraneous material in the feed, or alterations in colonic motility.

Water consumption is reduced if the source of water freezes. Alternatively, the horse may voluntarily diminish drinking during cold weather. Horses on pasture during winter may consume a higher percentage of coarse roughage; this coupled with reduced water intake, can cause impaction.

Such material as sand or gravel, when consumed with feed, can progressively col-

Figure 125. Atresia of the large colon, starting at the pelvic flexure, in a neonatal foal Note the distention of the left ventral colon with impacted contents. (Courtesy of Dr. A. Koterba)

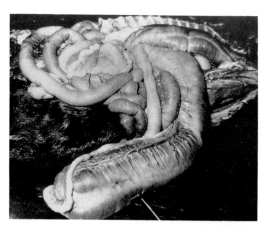

lect in the colon until an obstruction is formed. Horses with insufficient pasture grass available or too little roughage in their diets are prone to consume sand while attempting to gather feed from the ground. The composition of the soil has a bearing on the incidence of sand impaction. Access to other material, such as rubber fencing or feeders with nylon cord, or inadvertent inclusion of foreign material in hay bales predisposes to obstruction.

The horse may have a recent history of intermittent colic that gradually worsens. Subtle signs of colic include rolling of the lip, playing in water, looking at the abdomen, stamping the feet and backing up. As complete obstruction develops or pressure necrosis of bowel develops around the impaction, the signs worsen. Mucous membrane color, capillary refill and pulse rate generally are normal or mildly altered until the horse's condition deteriorates.

Clinicopathologic values reflect physical findings. An increase in the peritoneal fluid total protein concentration may indicate bowel wall deterioration before changes in metabolic signs occur. Systemic signs of toxemia appear after degeneration or perforation of the bowel. Intestinal sounds may be normal or decreased, depending upon the amount of pain, intestinal distention or bowel ischemia. A mass in the pelvic flexure or ventral colon may be present upon rectal examination. Impaction of the transverse colon may cause gas distention or accumulation of ingesta in the oral (proximal) portions of the colons and cecum. It is not possible to palpate the transverse colon by rectal examination (Fig 3).

Later in the course of the disease (which may take days), conditions can worsen. Complete obstruction of the colon allows gas to accumulate, leading to obstructive shock and respiratory compromise. Continuing mural pressure from the impaction results in necrosis and eventual perforation of the bowel. Accumulation of heavy feed material, coupled with rolling, can tear the colonic wall. In horses with severe impaction, metabolic deterioration and compromise of the bowel make medical therapy impossible and complicate surgical therapy.

The prognosis depends on the cause. Simple feed impactions often respond to medical therapy consisting of laxatives, fluids and pain control. Gut motility is aided by controlling pain, allowing access to small amounts of hay, and administration of warm water and/or mineral oil via nasogastric tube. Continued accumulation of large amounts of feed oral (proximal) to the impaction should be prevented. If sand is detected in the feces, repeated treatments of mineral oil or Metamucil can be given in an attempt to purge the colon, providing the bowel is patent. Though the signs of colic may subside, thorough removal of the material is never actually confirmed.

Passage of mineral oil is an encouraging sign because complete obstruction of the colon is unlikely. However, mineral oil can pass through or around some obstructions caused by sand, gravel or foreign bodies. The appearance of large amounts of feces, sand in the feces, or other material is more likely to signify that the problem has been relieved.

In severe cases, large volumes of intravenous fluids (20-50 L/24 hours) maintain fluid and electrolyte balance, improve intestinal motility and appear to hydrate the fecal mass. Medical therapy resolves many cases of impaction colic. If the horse's pain can be controlled and the metabolic status stabilized, conservative therapy should be pursued. With lack of improvement or worsening of signs, surgical intervention is indicated. If surgery is not an option, several days may be spent with fluid therapy, pain control and use of laxatives before improvement is seen. Changes that can occur in the bowel during prolonged impaction can complicate surgical therapy.

Enteroliths, Fecaliths, Bezoars

Enteroliths are mineral concretions that form in the colon over a long period. A nidus, which is considered to be the inciting cause of phosphate salt precipitation, usually is in the center of the stone (Fig 126).[536,537]

There is a geographic predisposition to enterolithiasis, as more cases are seen in California and the southern region of the United States. Though less common elsewhere, the condition should be considered in any horse with signs of large colon obstruction. In a series of 30 cases, no affected horses were <4 years of age.[536]

Clinical signs are similar to those of impaction, with the exception that they may be intermittent over a long period. Radiography may confirm enteroliths if the proper equipment is available.[17] With rectal or radiographic confirmation of an enterolith, surgery is indicated. Without confirmation of an enterolith, surgery is indicated if there is evidence of complete colonic obstruction; however, a high probability of an enterolith should cause the surgeon to be more aggressive than with most impactions. The prognosis depends upon the location, condition of the bowel around the enterolith, and metabolic status of the horse. The location of the stone(s) depends upon its size. Enteroliths usually are located in the transverse colon, small colon or, less often, pelvic flexure.

If the bowel segment containing the stone can be exteriorized, a colotomy may be performed over the stone or in healthy bowel adjacent to the stone. When the stone

Figure 126. Top: Enteroliths from 2 horses. Bottom: Radiograph of an enterolith showing a nidus in the center.

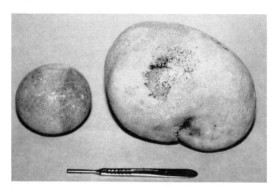

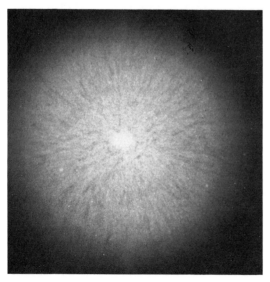

Figure 127. Normal orientation of the large colon and cecum. (Courtesy of Veterinary Practice Publishing)

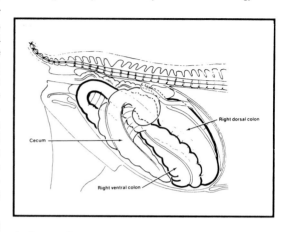

is located in the transverse colon and cannot be manipulated to a portion of right dorsal colon outside the celiotomy incision, a colotomy must be performed in the left dorsal colon and an arm passed intraluminally to the stone. Manipulation should be gentle because the surrounding bowel can be adherent or necrotic. This makes retrograde flushing via the small colon a delicate procedure. Following removal of the enterolith, bowel should be thoroughly explored to identify other enteroliths. Removal of enteroliths with shapes other than spherical should alert the surgeon to the possibility of other stones.

Figure 128. 360-degree volvulus of the large colon at the cecocolic junction (drawn). (Courtesy of J.B. Lippincott.)

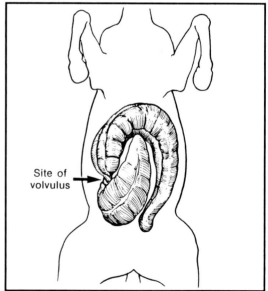

Site of volvulus

Colonic Volvulus

One of the most common and most dangerous colic conditions in horses is volvulus of the large colon. This displacement consists of rotation of the double loop of dorsal and ventral colons about their long axis. The point of attachment of these structures is the root of the mesentery, the most common location for the twist (Figs 127, 128). Rarely the twist may be found in the middle of the colons. Viewing the horse in dorsal recumbency, the colon usually twists counterclockwise with respect to the root of the mesentery. The cecum may or may not be involved in the twist. In any instance, normal repositioning of the colon and cecum is confirmed when the cecocolic ligament lies lateral to the ileocecal ligament with the apex of the cecum pointed craniad and the entire colon can be traced.

The large colon and cecum also can rotate together around the vertical axis of the mesentery. They can come to lie in a seemingly normal position with the mesenteric root strangulated. This condition is just as life threatening.

Cause: As with other colonic displacements, the exact cause is unknown. One may hypothesize that hypomotility due to pain or electrolyte abnormalities results in gas distention of the colon and movement of the larger ventral colon over the smaller dorsal colon.

Clinical Signs: The most commonly affected type of horse is the periparturient broodmare, most often after foaling. While horses of all types are affected, immature horses are affected far less often.

The onset of signs is sudden and severe, with pain that is often difficult or impossible to control. Xylazine (0.6 mg/kg IV) or detomidine (20-40 μg/kg IV) offers relief, but this may be of short duration. Butorphanol (0.01-.02 mg/kg) can provide additional pain control. The tachycardia from pain and anxiety is sustained by obstructive shock. The mucous membranes may be normal or pale due to vasoconstriction and decreased venous return. As gaseous distention progresses, respiration becomes compromised and respiratory acidosis may occur. Further metabolic deterioration may not be observed unless the horse receives treatment. An increased total protein concentration in the peritoneal fluid

is associated with a poor prognosis. Hemoconcentration occurs but is masked somewhat by intramural sequestration of whole blood in the colonic wall and eventually in the lumen. When such changes are present, the prognosis is grave.

On rectal examination there is extreme distention of the large colon with mural and mesenteric thickening. If the twist exposes the mesocolon, the edema is easier to palpate. The colon may be oriented transversely across the pelvic inlet due to elongation of the colon by distention or rotation of the colon and cecum on the mesenteric axis.

Treatment: Successful therapy depends upon expedient surgical correction. The intraoperative appearance of the typically affected bowel is cyanotic to blue-black. The tissue seems to retain a dry appearance despite repeated moistening. To prevent absorption of the toxic material, a pelvic flexure colotomy is performed and the contents are lavaged from the bowel before the volvulus is corrected. Removal of the heavy bowel contents also allows safer and easier reduction of the volvulus. Following correction of the volvulus, the viability of the tissue must be evaluated. Thickness of the bowel, the amount of mucosal hemorrhage, return of color following correction, and evaluation of circulation with fluorescein dye or oximetry are all considered in making the decision.[538,539]

Bowel with a reddened mucosa that is not bleeding into the lumen has a better prognosis than one that is blackened and hemorrhagic. Horses with colons of marginal viability can be recovered from anesthesia and supported with intensive fluid, antibiotic and antiendotoxic therapy. If sufficient viable cells remain in the mucosal crypts, the epithelium regenerates in about 48 hours. In the interim, the horse usually remains endotoxemic and passes dark hemorrhagic diarrhea. Provided other complications of stress and toxemia have not occurred, a good result can be expected. Some horses lose the absorptive function of the colon and continue to have diarrhea and protein loss. This may resolve over several weeks or remain permanently. Should this occur, elective resection of the affected colon should be considered.

If the affected colon is nonviable, colonic resection or euthanasia are the only options. The surgical procedure consists of creating a side-to-side anastomosis of the viable lateral (juxtaparietal) aspects of the dorsal and ventral colons, and amputating the nonviable dorsal and ventral colons leaving blind stumps. The side-to-side anastomosis should be accomplished first so the entire colon is available for stabilization of the tissue. Once the left colons are amputated, the remaining stumps retract into the abdomen.

To perform the resection, there must be enough integrity of the right colons to hold sutures. Stapling equipment expedites the surgery and minimizes contamination of the field. For these reasons, I recommend use of the linear stapler to create the dorsal and ventral colon stumps even when the tissue is thickened. Double-sutured inversion of the staple rows is necessary under these circumstances. The anastomosis instruments do not work as well in thickened tissue, and a completely hand-sutured side-to-side anastomosis may be necessary.

The anastomosis of the dorsal and ventral colons should be 10-15 cm long. Such limits should be identified with stay sutures. Whether staples or sutures are to be used, a Connell suture is placed between the stay sutures to ensure appropriate apposition of the colons and to secure the inner surface of the anastomosis, which will become inaccessible. For sutured anastomoses, the suture and needle can be clamped and laid aside. If staples are to be used, the suture can be trimmed. For stapled anastomoses, stab incisions for the anastomosis instrument (GIA: U.S. Surgical, Norwalk, CT, and Proximate: Ethicon, Somerville, NJ) entry portals are placed adjacent to the suture line. The staple instrument is applied parallel to the suture line in each direction and can be repeated in one direction if a 15-cm stoma is desired (Fig 129a, 129b). After the staple rows and their intersections are inspected, the instrument portal is closed using a double-inverting suture (Fig 129c). Sutures are placed to reinforce the ends of the staple rows. If any difficulty was experienced when firing the instrument, the staple rows are oversewn with a Cushing pattern.

For hand-sutured anastomoses, dorsal and ventral colonic incisions are made parallel to the initial suture line. The apposed inner edges of the bowel are sutured with a continuous horizontal mattress pattern of

Figure 129A. Stapled resection of the large colon. A. One limb of the anastomosis instrument has been inserted into a stab incision. The second instrument portal can be seen in the ventral colon (solid arrow), and the Cushing suture line lies between (open arrows).

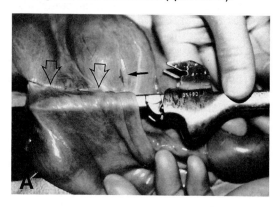

Figure 129B. The staple instrument has been closed parallel to (but excluding) the suture line (arrow).

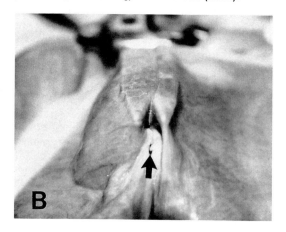

Figure 129C. Final doubly inverted instrument portal (between forceps). The anastomosis is indicated by arrows.

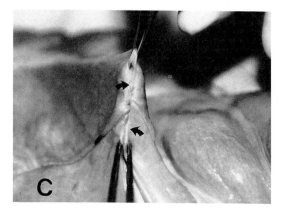

absorbable suture. When the end of the incision is reached, the suture is tied and continued along the outer (near) tissue margins as a Connell pattern. Once the seal is complete, the tagged suture from the first Cushing suture is retrieved for completion of the double-inverting pattern.

To amputate nonviable colon, a site is selected within 1-2 cm of the distal limit of the anastomosis adjacent to a large vessel entering the viable colonic wall (Fig 129d). Clamps are placed across the colon in tissue to be resected. If the tissue is thickened, sutures placed around the instrument help prevent slippage. This procedure requires dissection between the dorsal and ventral colonic walls and the mesentery, excluding the mesentery and colonic vessels. Angled slightly toward the viable bowel, the TA-90 stapling instrument is placed just distal to the selected vessel (Fig 129e). As the instrument closes, the tissue should be spread as flatly as possible manually, and the pin should be observed to seat properly in the opposing jaw of the staple cartridge. The instrument is fired and about 8 cm of tissue are transected using the cartridge as a guide (Fig 129f). The instrument is reloaded and placed across the first staple line, and the procedure is repeated until the entire width of colon is amputated. I prefer to amputate the larger ventral colon first. The colonic vessels and mesentery are clamped flatly with large Oschner forceps. The dorsal and ventral colonic vessels are separately double ligated and transected. An identical procedure is performed on the dorsal colon.

Inspection of the tissue margins for integrity of the staples and sutures must be accomplished while stabilizing the stumps, which retract into the abdomen when released (Fig 129G). If the tissue is thickened, the staples should be doubly inverted with sutures. The staples reduce contamination even with severely abnormal tissue.

Irreversible ischemic damage seemingly occurs before clinical signs are evident in some cases. One study reports a 36% survival rate.[540] Success depends upon the speed of referral and surgical correction. A higher survival rate can be achieved if surgery is performed early. The fact that survival was not related to duration of signs indicates that the actual twist sometimes

Figure 129E. The stapler and colon clamp in place on the ventral colon. Care has been taken to seat the pin correctly in the staple cartridge through the bowel wall. Note the suture (arrow) around the colon clamp to prevent slippage.

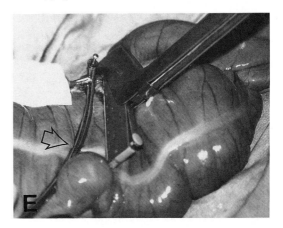

Figure 129D. A curved hemostat is placed adjacent to the bowel wall of the ventral colon. The blunt dissection exits adjacent to the bowel wall on the visceral surface, excluding the mesentery and vessels.

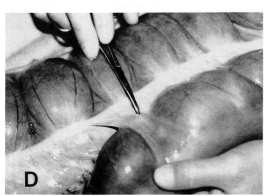

Figure 129F. Transection of the first 8 cm of the stapled tissue, leaving 1 cm of secure (nonleaking) anastomosis (arrow) for reapplication of the staple instrument.

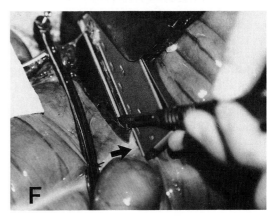

Figure 129G. Completed parietal view showing the anastomosis (solid arrows) and colonic stumps (open arrows).

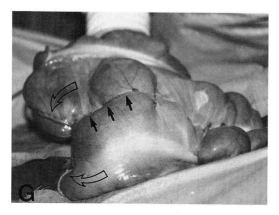

Figure 130. Right dorsal displacement of the large colon in the most common presentation. (Courtesy of Veterinary Practice Publishing)

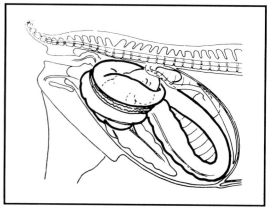

occurs later in the course of a simpler colic.[540]

One study reported recurrence in 2 of 9 survivors of surgery to correct colonic volvulus.[540] Limited experience indicates that suture fixation of the ventral colon to the ventral abdominal wall (colopexy) is feasible, and no recurrences have been observed following the procedure.[541,542] Partial colonic resection is another prophylactic procedure that would reduce the tissue mass presumably required to accomplish the twist. Though elective removal of the colon in an asymptomatic horse may cause the surgeon to hesitate, some mares have suffered the condition often enough to justify the procedure.

Right Dorsal Displacement of the Colon

This condition involves displacement of the left colons to the right of the cecum (between the cecum and the right body wall). Most commonly, the pelvic flexure travels to the right, cranial to the base of the cecum, transversely across the pelvic inlet, and comes to lie at the sternum. The right colons are oriented transversely across the pelvic inlet (Fig 130).[11,543] Less commonly, the left colons travel directly caudad from their normal position to the right around the base of the cecum and come to lie to the right of the cecum (Fig 131). The pelvic flexure still comes to rest at the sternum, but the direction of displacement is opposite to the first instance. This is right dorsal displacement with medial flexion.[11] A variable amount of volvulus is possible with either displacement. As with any colonic displacement, the exact cause is unknown. Horses that are large for their breed have been reported to have a higher incidence of this condition.[11]

The signs vary from insidious pain to violent uncontrollable colic. The amount of pain seems related to the amount of gaseous distention and tension on the mesentery. Metabolic indicators also vary from normal to those of obstructive shock. Severe toxemia is not a common finding, and clinicopathologic values generally are near normal despite the severe pain that may be observed. With significant distention, respiratory acidosis may exist.

On rectal examination, the right colons commonly are oriented transversely across the pelvic inlet, and edema from partial ve-

Figure 131. Right dorsal displacement of the less common medial flexion presentation. (Courtesy of Veterinary Practice Publishing)

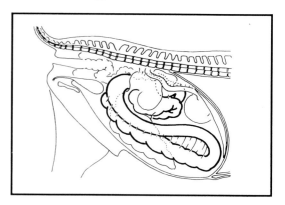

nous obstruction may be palpable in the colonic wall. The dorsal and ventral colons may be felt to disappear into the right flank caudal to the cecum, and the left colons may extend beyond reach into the cranial abdomen to the left of the cecum. Early cases have been described in which the pelvic flexure can be palpated before it extends out of reach toward the sternum. In the case of right dorsal displacement with medial flexion, the mesocolon is not palpable if no volvulus exists because it has merely extended from its normal position.

Right dorsal displacement requires surgical correction. The prognosis is good in uncomplicated cases. Edema of the colon may be present but is of no concern if the tissue is not strangulated.

Left Dorsal Displacement of the Colon

Left dorsal displacement results from displacement of the left colons dorsal to the renosplenic ligament, such that the colon adjacent to the pelvic flexure hangs over the ligament.[12,544] It is not known whether the colon achieves this position by passing through the renosplenic space from cranial to caudal or if the colon swings lateral to the spleen and over the top.

Clinical Signs: The typical clinical course resembles that of colonic impaction in that signs are mild to moderate, intermittent, but slowly worsening. Because the obstruction is only the "kink" of the colon hanging over the renosplenic ligament, the bowel may remain patent for some time. Eventually either ingesta accumulates in the region of the pelvic flexure or ileus causes gaseous distention, and the signs become acute and unrelenting. The amount of pain also seems related to the tension on the renosplenic ligament, and the horse may resent rectal palpation of this area.

The horse's metabolic status and clinicopathologic findings depend upon the duration and severity of the condition. Abdominocentesis often produces blood because the spleen is displaced ventrally and toward the midline. Rectal findings may be incriminating in that it may be possible to trace the colon over the renosplenic ligament. Usually the spleen is rotated caudally away from the left abdominal wall because of ventral tension on its suspensory ligament.

Treatment: Exploratory laparotomy reveals the mid-left colons located dorsal to the spleen, with the pelvic flexure approximating its normal position or lying flexed to the right or cranially. The entire colon should be located before attempting to exteriorize the pelvic flexure because the displacement is tightened by pulling on the pelvic flexure. Correction is achieved by lifting (ventrad) and rotation of the spleen and, with the same arm, reversing the hand under the colon dorsal to the spleen. After reduction, the colon should be exteriorized to confirm its normal position and to determine whether the contents must be emptied to facilitate return to function. In most cases, the ingesta accumulated in the pelvic flexure can be manually redistributed, and colotomy is not required. Strangulation of the entrapped portion of colon occurs rarely. In these rare cases, it is necessary to resect the devitalized colon.

In a few patients, the colon displaces from the renosplenic space during induction of anesthesia and positioning of the horse in dorsal recumbency. Displacement usually occurs in a cranial direction, and the left colon gathers in the left craniodorsal abdomen cranial to the spleen. When the bowel is exteriorized, the characteristic bruise is observed where the colon was hanging over the ligament. This observation has led some to suggest that most cases can be corrected by rolling the horse or elevating the hindquarters. Though strong evidence exists for correction of the displacement by rolling of the horse, it must be remembered that the diagnosis has never been definitively observed in cases that seemingly self-correct. I prefer to correct the condition surgically so the exact final position and condition of the colon are known. Results of conservative therapy have been unrewarding. In one study, 3 of 5 horses died after treatment with supportive therapy alone.[545]

In 122 cases, there was a 92% survival rate.[545] Complications directly attributable to the condition included rupture of the bowel during reduction of the displacement (4), recurrence of the displacement (3), and strangulation of the left colons (1). Another study reported significant complications in 4 of 9 cases.[546] These consisted of recurrence (twice in 1 horse), focal necrosis of the colon, omental adhesions presumably a result of ischemia during a previous episode of the condition, and significant incisional problems in 2 horses.

A surgical procedure to prevent recurrence of left dorsal displacement has been described.[545] The approach is made via the left flank, and the last rib is resected. The renosplenic space is obliterated by suturing the renosplenic ligament to the dorsomedial surface of the spleen. Of 8 reported cases, none experienced recurrences. I have had no experience with the procedure but believe it should follow complete midline exploratory and correction of the displacement. A subjective difference has been noticed in the depth of the renosplenic space among individual horses. An alternative would be elective performance of the preventive procedure in horses that had the condition more than once.

Displacement of the Pelvic Flexure and/or Left Colons

Because the large colon is quite mobile, it is possible for the left colons and pelvic flexure to become displaced. The most common situation is cranial flexion of the left colons that causes the pelvic flexure to lie toward the sternum.[543] Usually this is a nonstrangulating displacement but can result in obstructed flow of ingesta.

Entrapment of the pelvic flexure in a rent in the intraabdominal mesoductus deferens also has been reported in horses.[547] Displacement of the left colons through a rent in the gastrosplenic ligament into the omental space or, similarly, through a rent in the diaphragm has been observed.[518]

The clinical presentation is as variable as for right and left dorsal displacements. The severity of pain and the metabolic status depend upon the duration and amount of gaseous distention. Rectal examination usually cannot locate the pelvic flexure. If strangulation occurs, the signs increase in severity accordingly.

As with other nonstrangulating colonic displacements, the prognosis for survival is good. It is not known whether such a displacement occurs and self-corrects with pain control and supportive therapy.

Rents in inaccessible areas must be left with the hope that displacement will not recur. Diaphragmatic defects should be repaired because recurrence is almost certain.

Some diaphragmatic defects have been repaired, but many affected horses must be euthanized.

Intussusception of the Large Colon

Intussusception of the left ventral colon, pelvic flexure and left dorsal colon has been reported in horses.[542,548,549] The exact cause of intussusception is unknown; however, hypermotility of the bowel has been speculated to play a role. In other areas of bowel, a solid mass in or on the bowel wall forms the leading edge of the intussusceptum. Such intramural colonic masses occur. Intussusception is classically a disease of young animals. Of 3 reported colonic cases, 2 were in yearlings and 1 in a 3-year-old.

The course of the disease is that of mild recurrent pain with continued passage of soft feces. More severe signs of colic develop when obstruction leads to gaseous distention. Mild tachycardia persists with variable depression of intestinal sounds. A mild temperature elevation may be present. Leukocytosis in the peripheral blood and peritoneal fluid has been a feature. The peritoneal fluid protein concentration was marginally increased in 1 horse and 1 horse had a plasma fibrinogen level of 1000 mg/dl. Rectal findings included a mass in the left colons in only 1 of 3 cases; gaseous distention was present in the other 2 cases.

Treatment consists of surgical exploration, identification of the condition, and reduction or resection of the affected segment. Of 3 reported cases, 2 were reduced manually and experienced no recurrence or other postoperative complication. The remaining lesion could not be reduced and was resected successfully. The prognosis appears to be good with timely recognition and correction of the problem.

Inflammation, Infectious and Immune Disease

Intramural Lesions of the Colon

Plaques of variable size occur in parts of the colon and produce functional obstruction to the flow of ingesta. Eventually an impaction results; however, the impaction recurs if the lesion is not removed. Examples of such plaques include eosinophilic granulomas, hematomas and fibrotic plaques that presumably were hematomas earlier.

The exact cause of intramural lesions is rarely known. Ischemia, local inflammation or trauma must be considered. The lesions produce functional obstruction that causes accumulation of ingesta. The clinical signs are similar to those described for impaction.

Surgery is the eventual course of treatment because the "impaction" does not resolve. Lesion may not be evident until the impaction has been reduced or the colon has been lavaged via colotomy at the pelvic flexure, and the colonic wall can be palpated well. The prognosis is good if resection is possible. The site of occurrence is anywhere from the pelvic flexure to the transverse colon, making consideration of resection an individual matter.

Salmonellosis

J.E. Palmer and R.H. Whitlock

Salmonellosis refers to any disease caused by *Salmonella* spp. Though the term usually denotes acute enterocolitis, numerous clinical syndromes may occur. These include peracute enterocolitis with sudden death, bacteremia, enteritis without diarrhea, and mild enteritis resulting in colic.[550] The following discussion centers around salmonellosis associated with acute enterocolitis and diarrhea.

Cause: Any age, breed or type of horse may develop salmonellosis. In adult horses, the groups most frequently affected are broodmares, young racehorses, performance horses and horses that have undergone recent surgery under general anesthesia or that have other serious illnesses. In a study of a nosocomial outbreak of salmonellosis at a university hospital, horses receiving parenteral antibiotics, horses intubated with nasogastric tubes, and horses with colic were at greatest risk of developing the disease.[551]

There is a complex group of interacting factors that determine whether or not a horse develops salmonellosis. These include exposure to a contaminated environment, the dose received in relation to that required for infection, the level of stress on the horse, virulence of the bacteria, and immune status of the horse. The relative importance of these factors is poorly understood.[552] The ultimate source of the

Salmonella bacteria is the environment. The horse's local environment is most intimately shared by other horses and they are the most likely source of contamination.[129,175] Thus, most horses develop the disease secondary to shedding of the organism by other horses. This may be especially true in foals. The most likely source of contamination of the foal's environment is the mare. In most cases of salmonellosis in foals, the mare is shedding the organism. Whether the mare is the source of the organism for the foal or the foal is the source for the mare is not clear. Other possible sources include rodents, birds, insects, dogs, cats, goats and other animals.

Once an environment is contaminated, *Salmonella* can survive within it for prolonged periods. The organism can be recovered from soil for more than 300 days, from dried feces for more than 30 months, and in the water for more than 9 months.[465] *Salmonella* survives freezing. However, it usually does not multiply outside the host unless the contaminated area is warm, moist and dark, and contains abundant organic substrate. Drying and exposure to sunlight kill the organism.

The exposed horse must ingest the infective dose during a finite period. Ingestion of small numbers of bacteria over a prolonged period may increase resistance of the host rather than result in infection. The size of the infective dose may be quite different from situation to situation. Generally it is believed that large doses are required (10^6-10^{12} bacteria), but as few as 100-1000 bacteria may result in infection in people.[553]

Stress plays an important role in determining whether the animal shows signs of infection. The most commonly involved stressful situations include exhaustion, changes in diet, weaning, pregnancy, adverse weather conditions, transport over long distances, changes in environment, such as moving from one farm to another, general anesthesia, surgery and antibiotic therapy. Changes in the horse's normal intestinal flora probably play a major role in increasing its susceptibility to salmonellosis. The normal bacterial flora of the large intestine of horses is hostile to *Salmonella*.[554] When the normal floral balance is disrupted, the dose of organisms required for infection is reduced drastically. Stress may produce rapid changes in intestinal flora or changes in intestinal motility. If the ingested bacteria are retained in the lumen because of decreased progressive motility, bacterial invasion of the mucosa is more likely. Much is yet to be learned about stress as a factor favoring development of acute salmonellosis. Horses shedding *Salmonella* while experiencing the stresses of colic and exploratory celiotomy may not develop acute disease.[552] Unstressed horses may also develop salmonellosis.

There are well over 1800 serotypes of *Salmonella*. None of these is host specific or host adapted for horses. The most common isolate is *Salmonella typhimurium*, though numerous others may be found.[555-557] Multiple serotypes may be isolated from a singe patient.[555,556] This, in combination with the frequent isolation of *Salmonella typhimurium*, makes epizootiologic conclusions based on serotypes difficult. A more useful epizootiologic tool is plasmid analysis of isolates.[558-560] The plasmid profile of *Salmonella* isolates from a common source is usually identical, giving the investigator a means of following the *Salmonella* from horse to horse. Groups of bacteria isolated during an epizootic can be shown, based on plasmid analysis, to be closely related, distinguishing them from community isolates, even if they represent different serotypes or species of bacteria.[558-560] This simple yet powerful tool has proven to be valuable in investigating equine *Salmonella* outbreaks just as it has in epidemics in people.[558]

Finding the same serotype in a number of horses does not necessarily imply cross-contamination. This was demonstrated when an outbreak of *Salmonella senftenburg* enteritis occurred in a group of horses from one region of the United States.[175,556] This was a rare equine isolate, yet appeared to occur in a number of geographically separate animals at one time. This implies a common source rather than horse-to-horse spread of the disease.

Clinical Signs: The history of horses with salmonellosis is similar to that of horses with other acute enteritis syndromes. Though occasionally there is a lack of prodromal signs, most horses that are observed closely initially become depressed, febrile and anorectic. This may be followed within 24-48 hours by varying degrees of abdominal pain. The pain may be manifested by prolonged periods of recumbency, restlessness, looking at the flanks, pawing, playing in water, stretching out or rolling.

Diarrhea is usually delayed 24-48 hours after the onset of these initial signs, though it may appear within a few hours or may be delayed as long as 7 days. During the early phase of the disease while the horse experiences abdominal pain, there may be a noticeable absence of feces. The diarrhea can begin as "cow-flop" manure that gradually becomes watery, or there may be an apparent sudden onset of watery and projectile diarrhea. The feces are often dark and have a characteristic foul "septic tank" odor. The presence of gross blood is very rare.

Abdominal distention develops early in the course of the enteritis. Once the diarrhea has been present for a time there is a gaunt, tucked-up appearance. The diarrhea most frequently is profuse and dehydrating. Initially, fibrous material is passed; however, as the contents of the colon are emptied, less and less fibrous material may appear and the dry-matter content of the diarrhea decreases. There may be evidence of diarrhea in the perineal region or on the tail. Some horses have diarrhea devoid of particulate matter that soaks through straw, resulting in what appears to be urine stains. Thus, close examination of the stall or paddock environment may be needed to confirm the frequency and consistency of the diarrhea. Manifestations of abdominal pain usually subside as the diarrhea begins; however, some animals may show signs of discomfort each time feces are passed. The horse's appetite and degree of depression may be variable and independent of the fluidity of the feces. The horse's attitude usually improves after initiation of diarrhea. Horses that remain alert and continue to eat have a much better prognosis than those that become depressed and completely anorectic.

Affected horses are depressed and have a moderately elevated heart rate. The mucous membranes often have an injected appearance, with a blue "toxic ring" on the gums at the gingival margin. Capillary refill time may be prolonged secondary to dehydration or may be more rapid than normal as a result of venous pooling secondary to endotoxemia. The diarrhea itself may be variable in frequency and consistency; however, watery material is most commonly seen. It may vary in color from green to black.

Though loud isolated gas sounds may be heard on auscultation of the abdomen, borborygmi generally are decreased. Simultaneous auscultation and percussion of the right side frequently reveals a large hyperresonant area in the dorsal paralumbar fossa that corresponds to the cecal base. There may be a hyperresonant area on the left side as well. Ballottement of the abdomen usually results in splashing noises, indicating a gas-fluid interface in the colon.

Rectal examination usually is unrewarding. The examiner is often met by fluid manure in the rectum. The rectal mucosa may be edematous and, on rare occasions, ingesta adheres to the mucosal surface. Rectal palpation causes extreme straining and evidence of discomfort. The colon feels heavy and full of very fluid ingesta. Though there may be gas in the colon and cecum, the walls of the intestine are not taut. Occasionally the wall of the large colon or cecum is edematous. Rectal examination may result in tenesmus.

Diagnosis: Diagnosis of salmonellosis is established by isolation of *Salmonella* from feces or tissues. The feces of all horses with acute diarrhea should be cultured for *Salmonella* because salmonellosis can closely mimic diarrhea syndromes caused by any other agent. Multiple cultures are necessary because of intermittent shedding during the disease.[175] Fecal cultures may be negative until the manure becomes formed. *Salmonella* is shed most consistently before the onset of diarrhea;[561] thus, it may be best to obtain samples for culture at the onset of depression and fever. We suggest a minimum of 5 cultures taken no more frequently than daily, using 10-30 g of feces cultured by an enrichment technique. The most useful enrichment media are tetrathionate brilliant green broth and selenite broth. The latter may inhibit some *Salmonella* spp, whereas the former may be less effective in isolating others. Isolation of *Salmonella* is a routine bacteriologic procedure, though the success is directly proportional to the experience and enthusiasm of the bacteriology technician.

If there is a high index of suspicion but the initial fecal cultures are negative, a rectal mucosa culture should be obtained using small basket uterine biopsy forceps.[562] The tissue should be placed in enrichment medium and cultured in a routine manner. The rectal mucosa appears to concentrate *Salmonella*. Histologic examination of the biopsy usually shows proctitis, but this is not specific for salmonellosis.

If the horse does not survive, culture samples should be taken at necropsy. The most rewarding sites for culture are the cecal wall, large colon wall, ileum, and cecal or colonic lymph nodes. Obviously, the most likely site to culture *Salmonella* is from or near a lesion. Despite extensive efforts to culture tissues, only 64% of horses with antemortem *Salmonella* isolation have positive postmortem cultures.[563]

Other clinical laboratory findings follow a typical pattern during various phases of the disease but are not specific for salmonellosis. Early in the disease, often there is leukopenia with neutropenia and often lymphopenia. This type of leukogram may occur in any disease associated with endotoxemia. Hyponatremia, hypochloremia and hypokalemia are typical, as is acidemia and azotemia. Protein-losing enteropathy is frequently noted by a decline in plasma protein concentration. Proving that the site of protein loss is the gastrointestinal tract can be accomplished only by using research techniques. Showing that there is no other likely site of loss usually is sufficient. Laboratory evidence of disseminated intravascular coagulation also may be found.

Leukocytes may be shed in the feces of horses with salmonellosis.[564] Of affected horses, 50% have >10 WBC/20 high-power fields; 20-30% of horses with diarrhea not associated with *Salmonella* also have the same number. Thus, the finding of fecal leukocytes is not specific for salmonellosis but rather indicates invasive colitis. *Salmonella* spp are the most common invasive pathogens that affect horses.

Treatment: Therapy usually is symptomatic. The most important aspect of therapy is fluid replacement, with attention to electrolyte deficiencies and acid-base status. The fluids should be tailored to the imbalances found in the patient, as discussed elsewhere in this book.

Some controversy exists over use of antimicrobials in acute salmonellosis in adult horses. It is fairly clear that appropriate antimicrobials do not shorten the course of diarrhea. Inappropriate antimicrobials, however, may kill the normal microflora and may enhance the ability of *Salmonella* to grow within the lumen of the intestine. This may be the reason why hospitalized horses given oral and parenteral antimicrobials had 40 times greater risk of developing clinical salmonellosis than those not given such therapy.[551] Some clinicians believe antimicrobials are indicated to prevent seeding of other tissues because all horses may become bacteremic during their clinical course. Though bacteria may be found periodically in the blood, seeding of other tissues with *Salmonella* is rarely the cause of serious complications in adult horses. Thus, we believe that it is not necessary to treat adult horses with salmonellosis with parenteral antimicrobials. However, horses treated with large volumes of intravenous fluids through an indwelling intravenous catheter occasionally develop septic thrombophlebitis. Parenteral antimicrobials may decrease the sepsis, though they do not decrease the incidence of thrombosis of major vessels. The thrombosis may be due to the attendant endotoxemia in concert with irritation caused by infusion of medications through the catheter or bacterial colonization of the catheter tip.[565]

A better case for antimicrobial therapy can be made in treatment of foals. Foals are more likely to develop serious infections at other locations, such as the physes, kidneys, lungs and meninges secondary to bacteremia. These infections may be prevented by appropriate antimicrobial therapy; however, seeding of these tissues often occurs so early in the disease that prevention is not possible. If infection is established, antimicrobials may be beneficial therapeutically.

If the clinician decides to use antimicrobials, several things should be kept in mind. *Salmonella* is primarily an intracellular parasite. Maintaining adequate blood levels above the MIC of the organism may not be sufficient if the drug does not readily enter cells. Thus, an aminoglycosides is not the drug of choice. The sensitivity patterns of the isolate cannot be predicted without susceptibility testing. *Salmonella* spp are notorious for their resistance patterns.[1] Resistance factors are carried on plasmids that are readily transferred between *Salmonella* spp and between *Salmonella* and other members of Enterobacteriaceae.[566,567] Drugs commonly used on the farm or in the area are likely to be ineffective because of the prevalence of plasmids in resistent microflora carrying resistance factors to these drugs.[568] Antimicrobials that have been used to treat *Salmonella* infections include chloramphenicol, aminoglycosides, trimethoprim-sulfa and ampicillin. Antimicrobials to avoid include tetracycline, neomycin, streptomycin, lincomycin, tylosin and poorly absorbed oral antimicrobials. Resistance to chloramphenicol and gentamicin is not uncommon, though most isolates are sensitive to amikacin.[1]

Antidiarrheal drugs, such as bismuth subsalicylate or activated charcoal, may be helpful. If the course of the diarrhea does not change within 48-72 hours, these medications are ineffective and their use should be discontinued. Small doses of nonsteroidal antiinflammatory drugs, especially flunixin meglumine (0.25 mg/kg TID), may be helpful for their antiendotoxic action.[569] Large doses of these drugs are contraindicated because of the intestinal toxicity that can result. Plasma transfusions may be helpful.

Many problems can complicate a case of salmonellosis. Probably the most common yet least disruptive is dependent edema. This is seen frequently in horses that receive large volumes of intravenous fluids. It appears to be independent of the hypoproteinemia that often occurs concurrently. The edema may be a result of total body sodium overload, which may occur when large volumes of intravenous fluids are given.

Another frequent problem is hypoproteinemia secondary to the protein-losing enteropathy. The total plasma protein concentration may decline to <3 g/dl and on rare occasions <2 g/dl. Horses appear to adapt to these levels and very few complications occur, with the possible exception of an increased thrombotic tendency associated with low antithrombin III levels. Horses with such low plasma protein levels often become cachectic and may have a prolonged recovery period before the protein level rises. It is not unusual to have hypoproteinemia (4-6 g/dl) persist for months.

Coagulation disorders are a more serious problem. Disseminated intravascular coagulation is a frequent finding. Injection sites occasionally bleed or venous thrombosis occurs at a dramatic rate. These signs are accompanied by the expected clinical laboratory results diagnostic of disseminated intravascular coagulation. Venous thrombosis may occur with or without sepsis and is associated with long-term indwelling catheters. The high prevalence of this complication may be associated with low antithrombin III levels secondary to protein-losing enteropathy.

Azotemia is a frequent complication of salmonellosis. Usually it is prerenal in origin and associated with hypovolemia and endotoxemia. Infarcts secondary to disseminated intravascular coagulation, tubular necrosis secondary to hypovolemia, drug toxicity (vitamin K3, aminoglycosides, nonsteroidal antiinflammatory drugs) or, more rarely, septic emboli may result in renal failure. In such situations, the prognosis is grave. At times, horses with acute enteritis develop fungal pneumonia late in the course of infection. This is associated with severe necrosis of the intestinal tract. Though signs of pneumonia may be observed before death, this condition is diagnosed most often at necropsy.

The most devastating complication of acute salmonellosis is laminitis. Its occurrence and course are unpredictable. It is severe and progresses as long as the enteritis persists. It may continue to progress after recovery of the animal and be the reason for euthanasia. Occasionally it is not seen until after complete recovery from the enteritis.

The prognosis for horses with acute salmonellosis is as variable as the clinical syndrome. Patients that are not peracutely infected, that receive aggressive fluid therapy, that continue to eat and that do not develop complications have a fair prognosis. Peracute infection, dehydration and electrolyte changes that cannot be corrected, plummeting total plasma protein levels and devastating complications warrant a grave prognosis. It is not uncommon for the diarrhea to last 3-4 weeks. On occasion the diarrhea does not resolve for 6-18 months. A prolonged convalescent period frequently is required because of dramatic loss of body condition.

Control: After recovery from the disease, the affected horse should be considered a threat to other horses as long as *Salmonella* continues to be shed in the feces. The active shedder should be distinguished from the latent carrier.[175] An active shedder continues to shed the organism in the feces and thus contaminates the environment. A latent carrier does not shed the bacterium in the feces and thus is no risk to the environment; however, such a horse may begin to shed and contaminate the environment sometime in the future. Latent carriers cannot be detected short of necropsy.

Active shedders are a threat to the herd. The active shedding state does not persist indefinitely. If 5 serial fecal cultures taken at weekly intervals are negative, it is unlikely that future cultures will be positive.[175] This can be used as a definition of the end of the active shedding state. Based on this criterion, most horses do not remain an active shedder more than 8 weeks after recovery from the disease, though about 10% may actively shed for a year or more.[175]

The most important factor in controlling and preventing salmonellosis is good management. Enzootic premises usually include racetracks, large training farms and large breeding farms. Salmonellosis occurs in these facilities during the warm months when many transient animals are brought to an area with high-density housing and are then placed under a variety of stresses. The management challenge is to decrease the amount of stress, decrease commingling of transient horses and use low-density housing, yet still meet the primary function of the facility.

Transient animals should not be commingled with permanent residents. There should be minimal movement of people and equipment between the 2 population groups. Factors that can be manipulated, such as changes in diet, vaccination schedules, anthelmintic therapy, training schedule and breeding schedule, should be coordinated so that the stress is minimized. Adequate time to acclimate should be allowed before horses are placed into heavy work. Routine vaccination and anthelmintic care should be performed before, not after, shipping the animal and placing it in a new environment. Careful attention to environmental hygiene also is important. Once an outbreak occurs, cleaning and disinfecting protocols should be reviewed, strengthened and strictly enforced. Movement of people and equipment should be regulated carefully to minimize the spread of the contagion.

Intestinal Clostridiosis

Intestinal clostridiosis in adult horses is a proposed disease characterized by abnormal colony counts of *Clostridium perfringens* type A in feces or intestinal contents at necropsy of horses with typical clinical signs.[570-573] Horses with this disease may have histories and clinical signs very similar to those of colitis X. In fact, some of these horses probably have colitis X. Two major differences from colitis X are the reported survival rate and the longer clinical course of some patients. There is a rapid onset of severe illness, with an associated foul-smelling diarrhea and 40% mortality.[571]

Cause: Dietary factors have been associated with increased colony counts of *Cl perfringens* in horse feces.[571] When protein supplements containing the amino acids lysine and methionine are fed, fecal colony counts of *Cl perfringens* type A increase. This is especially true in comparatively young racehorses in hard training. However, these increases have not been associated with development of disease.[571] Use of antibiotics, specifically tetracycline, also may be associated with increased fecal clostridial counts and diarrhea.[574] The intestinal tract of horses normally is quite resistant to colonization by *Cl perfringens*.[571] In the presence of stress, antibiotics or feed changes that may disturb the normal flora, the organism may be capable of establishing itself in great numbers.

Experimental production of intestinal clostridiosis is possible through oral administration of broth cultures; however, only one-third of challenged horses develop signs. Induced intestinal clostridiosis is much milder than the clinical form, with horses developing loose feces only occasionally despite administration of ≥ 2 L of broth culture with 10^9 to 10^{12} *Clostridium* organisms.[571] Intravenous administration of *Cl perfringens* type-A enterotoxin causes severe abdominal pain and hemorrhagic gastroenterocecocolitis.[572]

Clinical Signs: Naturally occurring cases are noted for their acute onset. Rarely are there prodromal signs; however, a few hours before onset of the major manifestations of the disease, there may be some apparent depression and a decrease in appetite. This is followed rapidly by severe diarrhea.[571]

All physical findings typical of severe acute toxic enterocolitis syndrome frequently are found in clostridiosis. Colic, if present, usually is mild. There may or may not be sweating associated with abdominal pain. Rectal temperature may vary from normal to 40 C. The heart rate is elevated in proportion to the severity of the syndrome. Diarrhea may be variable. Usually it is severe, watery, dark and foul smelling. Occasionally the feces may be normal but decreased in volume. Some horses may have a mild prolonged course, with primary signs of listlessness and fetid, semisolid manure. Dehydration is proportional to the severity of the diarrhea. Rectal findings are not contributory to a diagnosis.[571]

The course of the disease is variable but usually short. Death usually occurs within 14 hours and rarely more than 48 hours after development of the disease. The horse may survive for a prolonged time with intensive therapy. Recovery, if it occurs, usually is dramatic and occurs within 24-48 hours after initiation of therapy.

Clinicopathologic Findings: Clinical laboratory findings are not unique to the disease. Early in the disease there may be leukopenia, and leukocytosis may occur later. An increase in packed cell volume and plasma total protein concentration is associated with dehydration, though there may be hypoproteinemia. Serum concentration of liver enzymes and total bilirubin may be elevated. Prerenal azotemia may be associated with severe dehydration. Disseminated intravascular coagulation also may be present.

The major postmortem finding is typhlocolitis. The severity varies from catarrhal to hemorrhagic to necrotizing. There often is acute catarrhal or hemorrhagic enteritis, though this is not a consistent finding. Lesions also occur in the liver, kidneys and heart of severely affected horses.

Diagnosis: Diagnosis of intestinal clostridiosis is by finding higher than normal clostridial counts in the feces or intestinal luminal contents.[571,573] Most horses have <5 colony-forming units per gram of feces.[571] Counts above 10^3 colony-forming units per gram are highly unusual. Though there is a clear association with higher than normal clostridial counts and disease, the association has not been proved to be causal. Isolation of the organism in the presence of enteritis does not prove its role. It is possible that the high clostridial counts are secondary to the enteritis, rather than the cause. The change of flora that occurs during enteritis and the presence of intraluminal protein secondary to protein-losing enteropathy may produce an intraluminal environment favoring clostridial multiplication. Thus, proliferation of clostridial organisms actually may be secondary to a primary underlying etiologic agent rather than the cause of the enteritis.

Ideally, to prove that *Clostridium* is causing disease, clostridial toxins should be demonstrated in the intestinal lumen. This is a difficult task and generally is not available as a diagnostic aid. Postmortem findings associated with the disease are not unique. Thus, the only practical means of diagnosing intestinal clostridiosis at this time is by demonstrating increased clostridial colony counts associated with typical signs of enteritis in the absence of other pathogens.

Treatment: Therapeutic considerations for the most part are identical to those in colitis X. Aggressive fluid therapy and supportive therapy are warranted. One adjunctive therapy that has been reported anecdotally is use of cultured "sour milk," which is derived from strains of *Streptococcus* that metabolize lactic acid. Unfortunately, this product generally is not available in the United States. When 4-6 L of this solution are given via stomach tube every 6 hours, a dramatic improvement is claimed. *In-vitro* studies have demonstrated that this solution has a strong antibacterial effect against *Cl perfringens* but not against other bacteria.[575]

Early in the disease, the prognosis is grave because of high mortality. However, if the horse survives the first 48 hours of the disease, the prognosis is fair. Barring any complications, recovery is complete and the horse can return to its former level of work.

Granulomatous Colitis

Granulomatous colitis usually is part of the granulomatous enteritis syndrome, particularly if tuberculosis is the cause. For details, see the description of this problem in the section on Diseases of the Small Intestine. It should be stressed here that if the colonic disease is sufficiently diffuse, rectal biopsy may be diagnostic.

Parasitic Diarrhea

Diarrhea in horses may be caused by *Strongylus* spp or *Cyathostoma*.[75,76,146,576-578] These helminths may cause enteritis during their mucosal phase of development. *Strongylus vulgaris*, *S edentatus* and *S equinus* also may cause peritonitis during their migration that may result in diarrhea. *Strongylus vulgaris* may disturb the blood flow to the intestine, which may also be associated with colonic dysfunction.[75]

The history commonly includes poor parasite management, especially with regard to pasture management and total farm management, allowing for exposure to a highly contaminated environment. Though frequently the animal in question receives anthelmintic therapy, the pastures may be overstocked or some animals on pasture are not dewormed as frequently as the patient. Occasionally there is a history of recent anthelmintic therapy in an individual that is heavily parasitized. However, by removing the adult parasites from the lumen, the dormant immature forms are stimulated to develop, resulting in mass exodus of larvae from the mucosa. This causes widespread tissue damage. Thus, the onset of diarrhea may be associated with deworming.

Strongylus vulgaris: Diarrhea caused by *S vulgaris* may vary in severity from mild chronic, intermittent diarrhea to acute, watery, profuse diarrhea. Fulminant colitis with marked endotoxemia, severe colic and watery low-volume diarrhea may occur when colonic infarcts are associated with the disease. Historically, the horse may have had febrile episodes, colic or weight loss. The animal may be unthrifty and have a poor haircoat with mild dermatosis. Often, however, the horse is normal and there may have been no indication of parasitism before onset of disease. Physical findings often are not helpful in distinguishing this disease from that with other causes. Rectal examination may detect fremitus in the ileocecocolic (cranial mesenteric) artery; however, active disease is often present without positive rectal findings.

Because of its long prepatent period, *S vulgaris* seldom is considered as a potential cause of foal diarrhea. However, the larvae penetrate the mucosa by day 3 postingestion and can be found in the ileocecocolic artery by 14-21 days. Thus, if a foal is exposed to a heavily contaminated environment early in life, it may show signs of the intestinal phase of migration as early as the first 2 weeks of life and signs of the arterial phase within the first month of life.

During the early intestinal phase, the larvae penetrate and molt to the fourth stage in the mucosa. Associated with this stage of infection is generalized arteritis in the bowel submucosa and serosa, resulting in marked inflammation. The intestinal phase is associated with fever, anorexia, dullness, abdominal pain and diarrhea.[433,481,579,580] Because this period probably does not last more than a week, diarrhea from a single massive exposure should be short lived.[433]

The arterial phase begins about 3 weeks after infection and is associated with thrombosis, intimal thickening, and narrowing of the lumen of the ileocecocolic artery. This period may also be associated with fever, anorexia, depression, colic and diarrhea or constipation.[581] If conditions are appropriate, the diarrhea may become chronic. We have observed foals that developed diarrhea within the first 2 weeks of life, continued with chronic watery diarrhea for 2-3 months, and had severe verminous lesions of the ileocecocolic artery and its branches. Such foals are refractory to symptomatic therapy and have no other detectable underlying causes at necropsy.

Diagnosis of *S vulgaris*-associated diarrhea may be difficult. A presumptive diagnosis may be made from the signs and history of poor antiparasitic management. The neutrophilia, eosinophilia and increase in plasma beta globulin levels associated with experimental infections in foals may be seen in foals with massive exposure to the parasite early in life.[579] However, because most foals and older horses have repeated exposures, these changes usually are not evident. Peritoneal fluid occasionally contains excessive numbers of eosinophils. A therapeutic trial with thiabendazole (440 mg/kg on 2 consecutive days), fenbendazole (10 mg/kg on 5 consecutive days) or ivermectin may be rewarding in suspected cases. Repeated larvicidal therapy occasionally is helpful. Though most of the damage heals, leaving only fibrosis, the repair process may

take 1-2 months.[579] We believe that therapy should not be delayed in suspected cases for fear of exacerbating the disease. If colic or diarrhea is caused by parasites, they must be removed. Waiting may further jeopardize the patient.

Cyathostoma: The role of small strongyles in producing colitis has been underestimated in the past. Coincident with the increased occurrence of anthelmintic-resistant cyathostomes, there have been a number of reports of cyathostome-induced colitis.[76,578] In some cases there may be a history of fever, colic or weight loss, and the animal may be unthrifty and have a poor haircoat.[76,578] However, the onset of signs is often sudden and without warning.[146,577] Occasionally the severity of the diarrhea varies and periods of apparent remission are followed by severe diarrhea.[76,576] Horses heavily infected with *Cyathostoma* spp may have severe weight loss and diarrhea beginning in the late winter or early spring, associated with development of larvae that have wintered in the gastrointestinal mucosa.[76,146,576]

There may be a history of frequent anthelmintic therapy without effect. Apparently, encysted forms may be resistant to otherwise effective drugs that achieve adequate tissue levels, such as ivermectin or high levels of fenbendazole.[146] The anthelmintic therapy may, in fact, exacerbate the condition by killing mature luminal forms. This stimulates *en-masse* maturation of encysted larvae. If the parasite load is high enough, colitis results. Thus, the history may indicate therapy shortly before the onset of disease. The owner also may say that the animal consistently passed adult parasites for months despite frequent anthelmintic therapy.

Physical findings depend on the severity of the underlying disease. Some horses have mild, intermittent diarrhea and few other signs, whereas others have severe diarrhea with all the signs of acute toxic colitis. Large numbers of small strongyles occasionally are found in the feces or on the examiner's rectal sleeve early in the disease.

No diagnostic tests are specific for cyathostomiasis. Though occasionally there is peripheral or peritoneal eosinophilia, this is not a consistent finding. Changes in the plasma protein profile, such as increases in beta globulins, are also inconsistent. Fecal egg counts are variable and eggs may be absent.[76,146,577,578] Rectal biopsies or biopsies taken during exploratory surgery may reveal encysted larvae.[146] Usually, however, the diagnosis is made tentatively on clinical grounds and is not proven unless a necropsy is performed.

Once the diagnosis is strongly suspected, larvicidal therapy should be administered without delay to avoid further damage. Thiabendazole at 440 mg/kg on 2 consecutive days or fenbendazole at 10 mg/kg on 5 consecutive days may be used. Oxifendazole at 10 mg/kg for 1 or 2 days has also been effective.[76] Though ivermectin is larvicidal, our clinical experience indicates that it is not as consistently effective in correcting the clinical signs as fenbendazole. Often, especially in cases of cyathostomiasis, the therapy must be repeated several times because encysted larvae are resistant. It is important to correct management factors that led to the problem, or recurrence is likely.

Potomac Horse Fever

(Ehrlichial Colitis)

Potomac horse fever is an acute enterotyphlocolitis caused by *Ehrlichia risticii*. It also has been referred to as acute equine diarrheal syndrome, equine monocytic ehrlichiosis and equine ehrlichial colitis.[582-587] Though clinical signs result from enterocolitis, a wide range of severity may be seen.[584,588-590]

Epizootiology: Potomac horse fever should be on the differential diagnosis list in any case of enterocolitis that occurs in a previously identified enzootic area. Enzootic areas have been noted along major rivers in Virginia, Maryland, Pennsylvania, New York, Connecticut and Ohio.[584] Outbreaks have been identified in 33 states.[583,584,591] In all likelihood, such enzootic areas will be found throughout the country in the near future.

The disease appears to be seasonal, with the first cases occurring in the late spring and the last cases occurring in the fall. Most cases occur in July, August and September.[584,589,592] The disease is sporadic within the enzootic areas, both temporally and geographically. A large number of cases on any one farm is unusual unless the farm has a large population.[584] The usual pattern consists of 1-2 cases per farm. Thus, a large number of farms is affected in enzootic areas. On large farms where 5 or more horses are affected, the pattern continues to be sporadic, with horses on all parts of the farm affected rather than a concentration of disease in one location.[584] Horses seemingly develop the disease at random.

A notable exception occurs in areas with unusually high prevalence.[585] Some farms in these areas have a high prevalence, with up to 80% of horses on the farm affected clinically and 100% with positive titers. This may reflect a high density of infected vectors in the area, making challenge likely. Alternatively, the possibility of oral infection has been proposed.[583] Contact with recovered or currently ill animals, in most cases, is not associated with development of disease. There is no apparent age-related resistance, and horses under all management and housing conditions seem to be affected.[582] It is not unusual for an aged retired horse that has been isolated from other horses and housed at pasture for many years to develop the disease.[584,585]

Though the mode of transmission is unproven, the disease is not transmitted by direct contact. Because of the ehrlichial etiology and the ability to experimentally transmit the disease with whole blood, an arthropod vector has been sought. Initial studies trying to implicate ticks as a vector have not been productive;[593,594] however, an arthropod should be considered the vector until proven otherwise.[594-596] Some evidence indicates that oral transmission may be possible.[597]

The reservoir for the causative agent is not known. It is common for the disease to occur on successive years in the same area.[584,585] Thus, a mechanism for overwintering must exist. Horses are only one possible source and may be dead-end hosts. If transovarial and transstadial passage occurs in an arthropod vector, the vector itself may be the reservoir. Also, specific antibodies to the agent have been detected in pigs, goats, dogs, field mice, foxes and a rabbit within enzootic areas.[594,596,598,599] The possibility of a reservoir in wild mammals or birds should be investigated as well. Potomac horse fever may be a zoonotic disease, as the organism can cause mild clinical signs in primates.[600]

In some ehrlichial diseases, such as *E canis* infection in dogs, a long-term carrier state occurs for years after initial infection. In others, such as *E equi* infection in horses, the infection is cleared soon after acute signs subside. The chronic carrier state in Potomac horse fever has been studied using 2 different approaches. First, there is no chronic ehrlichemia in most cases. Using a mouse concentration technique, *Ehrlichia* could not be detected in ponies tested 6-20 months after initial infection. Second, culture of tissues from ponies 4-36 months after infection have failed to isolate the agent, with one exception. Fetal tissues from one pony grew *E risticii*.[591] The importance of this finding in terms of fetal infection or production of a compliant infection resulting in carrier offspring is unclear and deserves further study. Also, inability to culture intestinal mucosa, the most likely site of chronic infections, leaves these studies incomplete.

Clinical Signs: Historical complaints usually include anorexia and depression. A transient fever as high as 105 F (40.6 C) may be noted with few other signs, followed in 2-7 days by a second febrile episode accompanied by depression, anorexia and ileus. Affected horses typically develop other signs of gastrointestinal disease, such as abdominal pain or diarrhea. Laminitis may be part of the initial complaint on rare occasions.

At the time of initial examination, the horse usually is mildly depressed. If diarrhea has not begun, there may be moderate abdominal distention. Mucous membrane injection is not as dramatic as in other acute toxic enteritis syndromes; however, a prominent "toxic ring" may be seen as a blue rim around the gingival margin. Mild tachypnea and tachycardia may be noted. Rectal temperature can be variable but usually is 102-106 F (38.9-41.1 C). Auscultation of the intestinal tract reveals a dramatic decrease in the frequency and volume of borborygmi. The gastrointestinal tract is quiet, with only occasional loud gaseous-type sounds. Simultaneous ballottement and auscultation of both flanks usually elicits increased splashing sounds. Simultaneous auscultation and percussion of the abdomen frequently reveals a large hyperresonant area in the right paralumbar fossa corresponding to the area of the cecal base.

Findings of rectal examination are not remarkable, with the occasional exception of mild gaseous distention and fluid within the large colon. Diarrhea, if present, may be of "cow-flop" consistency to watery and profuse. If no diarrhea has been passed and there is marked abdominal distention, there usually is extreme tachycardia, profoundly injected mucous membranes and signs of abdominal pain. Indications of dehydration are present, such as decreased skin turgor, decreased moisture of mucous membranes and prolonged capillary refill time.

There is a wide range of clinical syndromes as a result of the variable host response to the agent.[585,590] About 40% of affected horses do not have diarrhea, and about 50% develop some signs of abdominal pain. Some horses suddenly stop passing feces after a period of profuse diarrhea; they become distended, painful and depressed, and die within 24 hours despite aggressive therapy. Some horses show mild signs of anorexia, depression and fever. Once Potomac horse fever has been shown to exist in the area, any horse showing these signs should be considered infected until proven otherwise.[584,585,588,589,601]

Clinicopathologic Findings: Clinical laboratory changes resemble those of other acute toxic enteritis syndromes.[585,588] Hyponatremia, hypokalemic and hypochloremic acidosis should be expected. The degree of azotemia is directly proportional to dehydration and is usually prerenal. Initially there may be mild to extreme leukopenia with neutropenia and lymphopenia. This may be followed by dramatic leukocytosis. However, the blood picture is so variable that it is not diagnostic. Some individuals have total WBC below 2000/μl, followed in a few days by counts above 25,000/μl. Others may maintain WBC counts between 6000/μl and 10,000/μl throughout the disease.[602]

Diagnosis: Though the cause of Potomac horse fever is unique, the clinical signs are no different from those seen in other diseases resulting in acute toxic colitis and are not diagnostic.[584,585,588,589,601] The most accurate method of diagnosing Potomac horse fever is isolation of the causative *Ehrlichia* species.[587] A less difficult and thus more useful diagnostic test is measurement of serum antibody titers. An indirect fluorescent antibody assay has been modelled after similar tests used for other *Ehrlichia* (eg, *Ehrlichia canis* and *Ehrlichia equi*).[583] Preliminary studies indicate that this is a relatively specific test, though its sensitivity has not yet been proved.[583,586]

Detection of any antibody titer is not sufficient for a diagnosis, as titers may persist at high levels for more than a year.[586] Antibody titers during the acute phase of disease may be quite high (up to 1:5120) and then drop rapidly or may follow the more expected pattern of a rapid rise. Thus, a dramatic decrease or increase may be sufficient for diagnosis of current disease. Unfortunately, both experimental and field experience have shown that acute and convalescent antibody titers determined at appropriate times often are within one dilution of each other despite recent infections. Thus, though the indirect fluorescent antibody test is a very useful tool epidemiologically, this is not the ideal test for individual cases.[585,586]

Several other diagnostic tests have been developed but none is more useful than the indirect fluorescent antibody test. A plate latex agglutination test has been produced.[586] Lack of sensitivity and specificity of this test (false negatives and false positives) indicates that this is not a reliable acute-phase diagnostic test.[586] Though ELISA determination of antibody level is possible, it is no more useful than indirect fluorescent antibody tests.[603] At present, there is no completely satisfactory test for diagnosing individual cases of Potomac horse fever.[585,586] Introduction of a vaccine has further decreased the utility of diagnostic tests based on serologic reactions.

Treatment: As with other acute enterocolitis syndromes, the primary and most important therapeutic aim is to maintain fluid and electrolyte balance. Recommendations regarding therapy currently are based on the experience of a few disease outbreaks and several experimental trials. Uncontrolled anecdotal experience from one outbreak indicated that trimethoprim-potentiated sulfa drugs, moderate doses of flunixin meglumine and small doses of sodium heparin (20 units/lb SC, BID or TID) may have improved the survival rate. Though chloramphenicol is rickettsiostatic, field experience with this drug indicates that it does not change the course of the disease. Use of oxytetracycline during the incubation period was ineffective in preventing the disease, but it prolonged the incubation period. This is the expected response of a rickett-

siostatic drug used during the incubation period.[604] Limited field experience indicates that oxytetracycline may shorten the period of clinical signs and decrease the severity of the disease when used therapeutically.

Experimental trials support these observations.[585] Oxytetracycline given IV at 6.6 mg/kg once a day beginning 24 hours after development of a fever results in rapid recovery and dramatic decrease in mortality.[585] The oral combination of erythromycin (30 mg/kg BID) and rifampin (10 mg/kg BID) shows similar results.[585] However, the practitioner must face the dilemma of trying to definitively diagnose the disease during the acute phase, when therapeutic modalities will be useful. At present, there is no rapid diagnostic test and the clinical signs of Potomac horse fever so closely mimic those of other enteric diseases, such as acute salmonellosis and antibiotic-associated enteritis, that use of oxytetracycline in undiagnosed cases could be questioned. Nevertheless, it has proven to be very effective, especially when used early in field cases of Potomac horse fever. It should be noted that Potomac horse fever and salmonellosis may occur concurrently, so that diagnosis of one disease should not preclude investigations of the other.

Vaccination: A formalin-killed vaccine was introduced in the spring of 1987. In one experimental study, after 2 inoculations at 3-week intervals, 78% of the challenged ponies developed transient fevers of 102 F (38.9 C) or greater and 22% developed sufficient signs to be considered by investigators to be unprotected.[604] No controlled field trial of the vaccine has been undertaken. Though there are anecdotal reports of lack of protection, the level of protection of the vaccine in the field is unknown. Experimentally infected ponies are resistant to reinfection for up to 20 months. The duration of protection after vaccination is much shorter, with only 50% of vaccinated horses protected at 6 months. This has led to the suggestion that horses in areas with a high prevalence of Potomac horse fever should be vaccinated every 4 months.[771]

Colitis X

In the past, the definition of this disease has been confusing. The term "colitis X" originally was coined to describe an acute to peracute, highly fatal, sporadic diarrheal disease.[570,605,606] In typical cases, death occurs within 3-24 hours of onset of signs.[607,608] On rare occasions, horses may recover with intensive treatment; however, most die. The diagnosis in survivors is open to debate, as the only diagnostic method available is necropsy.[605] More recently, some authors have used the term to describe cases of undiagnosed enteritis of longer duration before death or that are not fatal.[570,571,609] Synonyms used in the past for this disease include acute colitis syndrome, hemorrhagic edematous colitis syndrome, poststress diarrhea syndrome and equine anaphylaxis.

Horses of all ages may be affected with colitis X. There is no breed or sex predilection. The disease may occur any time during the year.[605-608] This disease in infrequent and sporadic except on racetracks, where it may become epizootic.[606-608]

Cause: The cause of colitis X is not known. A number of agents and factors probably cause similar clinical syndromes and postmortem findings. None of the proposed theories explains all occurrences of the disease. Endotoxic shock has been proposed as a possible cause.[605-608,610] Studies on the effects of this toxin in horses make a causal role unlikely, though certainly it occurs secondarily. Anaphylaxis may mimic colitis.[605,611] The phenomenon of exhaustive shock has also been proposed as a possible cause.[605,608,610] According to this theory, prolonged stress exhausts the animal's resistance. This stress may be in the form of training, respiratory disease or other diseases. A secondary insult, such as a change in diet or a change in weather, causes complete collapse of the horse's resistance, resulting in shock. However, some authors have stated that many cases occur in seemingly unstressed horses.[605,609]

There has been interest in the possibility that colitis X is a *Cl perfringens* type-A enterotoxemia.[570,572,573] This hypothesis is based on finding unusually large numbers of the bacterium ($>10^3$ colony-forming units/g) in the feces or intestinal contents of horses with typical signs. Of course, mere isolation of *Clostridium* from the lumen does not prove a role in disease. Indeed, because of the expected disturbance of microflora secondary to enteritis, such findings may be secondary to a primary under-lying problem. Isolation of toxin from the intestinal contents would be the ideal way of implicating clostridia. Nevertheless, the association is present and may be causal. Peracute salmonellosis also may mimic this disease.

Clinical Signs: A history of "stress" 10-14 days before onset of clinical signs is common. This may include shipping, respiratory disease or heavy training, though the disease may occur without these historical events.[605-607,609] A sudden change in diet or a diet rich in protein and low in cellulose also have been associated with the disease.[570]

Horses with colitis X have a sudden onset of severe disease with no premonitory signs. Affected horses may be febrile with a temperature as high as 106 F, but more commonly they are hypothermic secondary to severe shock. Profound depression and complete anorexia are seen. If diarrhea has not developed, significant abdominal distention may be present. Colic may be mild to severe.

The oral and vaginal mucous membranes are red-purple, dry and tacky, with a capillary refill time approaching 4-5 seconds. Scleral vessels are significantly congested. A weak, rapid pulse with poor filling of the jugular veins is present. Tachypnea may be present. If diarrhea is present, it is watery, profuse and foul smelling but not bloody. Rectal examination is difficult because of straining. If one is performed, it reveals fluid-filled bowel. Edema of the colonic and cecal walls and mesenteric lymph nodes may be detected. The rectal mucosa may be normal or edematous and friable.

Clinical signs are a result of the combination of severe hypovolemic and toxic shock. Hypovolemia is secondary to massive loss of fluid into the intestinal lumen and edematous large intestinal wall. Toxemia is a result of absorption of endotoxin or other bacterial toxins (eg, clostridial exotoxins) through the compromised intestinal wall. There may be marked leukopenia (<3000 cells/μl).[605,607] Signs progress rapidly and a fatal outcome is expected within 24 hours of onset. On rare occasions, an affected horse survives.

Diagnosis: The diagnosis of colitis X should be based on observing the typical clinical course and finding the usual lesions at necropsy. The most dramatic changes occur in the cecum and large colon. A large amount of odoriferous ingesta is found in the cecum and colon. The mucosa may be hyperemic with petechial hemorrhages, or green-black and intensely hemorrhagic with necrosis but no ulceration. There may be dramatic edema and occasional hemorrhage in the submucosa. On rare occasions there is free blood in the gastrointestinal tract. Lesions are most severe in the cecum and ventral colon, though they may extend to the rectum and rarely to the ileum. There are no changes in the stomach, duodenum or jejunum.[605-608] Edema, hyperemia and emphysema may be seen in the lungs.[605,608] Evidence of disseminated coagulopathy may be present.

Treatment: Aggressive fluid therapy is of prime importance in treating horses with colitis X. These animals are extremely hypovolemic, even before the onset of diarrhea and, therefore, need large volumes of replacement fluids delivered rapidly. Initially this may require simultaneous catheterization of both jugular veins for administration of fluids. The disease progresses too rapidly to wait for laboratory values to direct fluid and electrolyte replacement. These horses can be assumed to be acidotic, hyponatremic, hypochloremic and hypokalemic. Intravenous fluids should be given as rapidly as possible.

Use of corticosteroids have been advocated in treatment of colitis X.[570,605,609,610] Though large doses of corticosteroids may decrease apparent injection of the mucous membranes, any beneficial effect induced by them, in our opinion, is transient and not dramatic. Pain relief may be afforded with judicious use of nonsteroidal antiinflammatory drugs. These drugs also may lessen the severity of endotoxic shock.

The prognosis is grave in this disease, and up to 90% of affected horses die despite therapy. However, if the animal survives more than 2 days, the prognosis for full recovery is fair.

Toxic Diseases

Cantharidin Toxicosis

(Blister Beetle Toxicosis)

Cause: Cantharidin toxicosis, also known as blister beetle poisoning or striped beetle poisoning, is a syndrome caused by inges-

tion of beetles of the genus *Epicauta* (blister beetles). Though there are several thousand beetles in this genus, the ones associated with toxicosis in horses are *E occidentalis, E lemniscatta, E vittota, E temexa* and the black blister beetle, *E pennsylvanica.* Adult blister beetles are leaf and flower feeders. They tend to move in swarms in hay fields and are particularly attracted to alfalfa leaves and blooms. With the advent of modern hay-harvesting machinery, which cuts and crimps forage simultaneously, groups of beetles may be killed at the time of harvest and be concentrated in a section of a bale of alfalfa hay.

Cantharidin is a bicyclic terpenoid found in the hemolymph, genitalia and possibly other tissues of these beetles. The toxin is extremely irritating and causes acantholysis and epidermal vesiculation on contact with the skin. It usually is absorbed through the gastrointestinal tract and excreted in the urine; however, it causes irritation with topical application and may be absorbed topically.[202,203,612] The minimum lethal dose is thought to be <1 mg/kg.[612,613]

Clinical Signs: Cantharidin toxicosis is a sporadic disease that may be seen in a single animal or in a group that shares the same pasture or area of the barn. Because the beetles usually are found in only one bale or even a part of a bale of hay, one horse or a small group fed from the same bale can be the only horses affected.

The severity of the disease varies with the dose of toxin ingested. Signs become apparent within a few hours of beetle ingestion. Some horses have profuse salivation initially and place their nose in water and splash continually.[612] Others may become anorectic and depressed, though any oral lesions do not necessarily discourage eating.[203] Oral erosions are not consistent findings. When they are present, they may found on the gingival mucosa or oral mucosa, especially the tongue.[202,614] Affected horses may exhibit a short-strided gait that resembles that of myositis.[203] Synchronous diaphragmatic flutter also may occur.

Varying degrees of abdominal pain, ranging from very mild to quite severe, can be seen. Small amounts of urine may be voided frequently.[202,614] Though hematuria with gross blood clots can occur, the urine usually appears normal. The skin may be irritated where urine has contacted it. Diarrhea may develop and range from watery feces to a mucoid, bloody discharge.[615] Diarrhea is not a consistent sign and usually is mild. Though initially showing signs of colic, some animals may exhibit mild depression followed by sudden death. When fever is present, the temperature may be as high as 41 C (105.8 F). Usually tachycardia, tachypnea, congested mucous membranes and prolonged capillary refill time are noted.

Clinicopathologic Findings: The packed cell volume is elevated and may be as high as 60%. Though the toal plasma protein level is initially elevated due to dehydration, there may be some protein loss into the tissues and intestinal tract, resulting in a decrease in total plasma protein concentration.[202,614] The leukocyte count is variable but usually high.[202,203,614,615] Most serum electrolyte levels are normal to slightly decreased. If acute tubular necrosis occurs, serum creatinine and urea nitrogen levels are elevated.

Striking abnormalities consistently found during the clinical laboratory investigation are hypocalcemia and hypomagnesemia, which probably cause synchronous diaphragmatic flutter. In field cases, the serum calcium level may be as low as 5.9 mg/dl and experimentally as low as 4.1 mg/dl.[202,614] The low serum calcium level persists for at least 48 hours and is relatively refractory to therapy. Serum CPK activity also may be elevated; this is not dramatic, however.

Diagnosis: Tentative diagnosis is by finding blister beetles in uneaten hay or around the manger. However, for definitive diagnosis, detection of the toxin in stomach contents or urine is required. Analytic methods for cantharidin detection using high-pressure liquid chromatography and gas chromatography-mass spectrometry are useful diagnostically.[613] Urine appears to be a reliable sample for toxin detection and may retain toxin longer than stomach contents. When sampling stomach contents, a large, well-mixed sample is required because the amount in stomach fluid may be small, especially if it has been several days since exposure.[613]

Postmortem lesions are not diagnostic but may be helpful. Even when no lesions are found in the oral cavity, there usually are erosions of the esophagus and stomach. Sheets of epithelium may be lifted off the surface, with normal epithelium in between lesions. In the small intestine, changes range from a normal intestine filled with mucoid contents to pseudomembranous enteritis. The large intestine frequently has watery contents and occasionally may be ulcerated. The walls of the small and large intestine may be edematous. Hemorrhagic ulcerative cystitis and mild acute renal tubular necrosis can occur. Lesions generally are very mild in the upper urinary tract and most severe in the lower urinary tract. Ulcerative lesions in the bladder can be dramatic despite a lack of gross hematuria during life. Ventricular myocardial necrosis also can occur.[202,614]

Treatment: Therapy is largely symptomatic and supportive. Maintaining the hydration status is very important, both to minimize associated hypovolemic shock and to maintain adequate hydration to encourage diuresis. Particular attention should be paid to the acid-base status and serum calcium and magnesium concentrations. Use of mineral oil has been advocated to prevent absorption of the intraluminal toxin because cantharidin is soluble in organic solvents.[615] However, therapeutic trials have not been performed and there is at least a possibility that mineral oil may, in fact, increase toxin absorption.[202] Analgesics may be required but nonsteroidal antiinflammatory drugs should be used with care, as they can exacerbate renal and gastrointestinal lesions.

Mortality can be as high as 60%. However, if the horse does not die during the initial 72 hours, it is likely to survive. There are no long-term followup studies to determine if long-lasting sequelae develop. The potential for cardiac arrhythmias secondary to myocardial necrosis is present, as well as renal disease secondary to tubular necrosis.

Control: Prevention of toxicosis may be difficult. All suspect hay should be removed and the new hay replacing it should be examined very carefully. Animals that may have been exposed but are not showing signs of illness should be observed closely and allowed adequate access to water.

Multifactorial Diseases

Antimicrobial-Associated Diarrhea

Therapy with certain antimicrobials is associated occasionally with diarrhea in horses.[574,616-619] The antimicrobials involved most commonly are tetracyclines and trimethoprim-potentiated sulfa drugs. Other drugs associated more rarely with diarrhea include erythromycin, high levels of penicillin, lincomycin, metronidazole and cephalosporins.

Cause: Antimicrobials probably cause diarrhea secondary to a disturbance of the intestinal flora. During antimicrobial administration, sensitive organisms may be decreased or eliminated from the gastrointestinal flora. Consequently, resistant bacteria may proliferate.[574,620,621] Trimethoprim-potentiated sulfa combinations have a marked effect on Enterobacteriaceae of the gastrointestinal tract in people. There usually is a marked decrease in these organisms and there may also be a decrease in enterococci and clostridia. The effect of this drug on anaerobic organisms, such as *Bacteroides* and anaerobic lactobacteria, is irregular and dependent on the individual.[620] There may be a marked decrease in *E coli* numbers during therapy unless the *E coli* strain is resistant to the drug, in which case they maintain their population in the gastrointestinal tract. After cessation of drug use, reconstitution of the gastrointestinal flora may include new bacterial serotypes.[620] Thus, there not only is a possibility of diarrhea associated with the onset of antimicrobial therapy, but also at the time of cessation of therapy.

In our experience, trimethoprim-potentiated sulfa-associated diarrhea may occur 24-48 hours after cessation of therapy, as well as 24-48 hours after initiation of therapy. Experience with the antimicrobial has been variable. In some parts of the country, anecdotal experience has convinced equine clinicians that the association of trimethoprim-potentiated sulfa drugs and diarrhea is real. In other parts of the country, no problem has been noted. In our opinion, though the association between the 2 exists, the complication is not so frequent that it should preclude use of this drug when indicated.

Similar floral changes have been observed in horses after administration of oxytetracycline. Suppression of certain anaerobic bacteria (*Veillonella* spp) and proliferation of *Cl perfringens* type A, coliforms, *Streptococcus* and *Bacteroides* have been found.[574,621] These types of floral changes certainly may lead to diarrhea, especially considering the possible role of *Cl perfringens* type A in acute enteritis. Though oral therapy probably produces more profound floral changes, large doses of intravenous preparations also may be associated with problems because oxytetracycline is excreted in the bile.

Clinical Signs: Typically the horse has a history of antimicrobial therapy for a problem unrelated to the gastrointestinal tract. Diarrhea develops suddenly a few days after initiation of therapy or a few days after cessation of therapy. All degrees of severity may be experienced, from mild "cow-flop" diarrhea to full-blown toxic enteritis with depression, high fever, anorexia, injected mucous membranes and profuse dehydrating diarrhea.

Diagnosis: It is impossible to make anything but a tentative diagnosis of this condition. The association of antimicrobial therapy with the onset of diarrhea is an absolute requirement. Clearly, implicating the antimicrobial almost always is impossible. Though a causative relationship is difficult to prove, when there is a historical association of initiation or cessation of antimicrobial therapy and the onset of an otherwise unexplained diarrhea, a tentative diagnosis of antimicrobial-associated diarrhea can be made.

Treatment: The most important step in therapy is removing the offending antimicrobial. Ideally, the horse should not be given any antimicrobials. If antimicrobials are required for treatment of other problems, they should be parenteral and preferably those that do not achieve high levels in the intestinal lumen or that have a minimal effect on gut flora.

As with other diarrheal diseases, symptomatic and supportive therapy are required. If the normal flora has only been suppressed and not completely eliminated, discontinuing antimicrobial use may be followed rapidly by complete recovery. However, if the flora is severely disturbed and pathogens become established, diarrhea may be protracted and quite severe, requiring intensive therapy. If diarrhea becomes chronic, transfaunation using fecal fluid, cecal/colonic fluid or *Lactobacillus* preparations may be of value.

Nonstrangulating Infarction of the Colon

K.E. Sullins

Spontaneous ischemia of the colon results in necrosis of the affected segment. The most popular etiologic theory in the past has been that ischemia results from damage and stenosis and/or embolism due to verminous arteritis of the cranial mesenteric artery or its immediate branches. However, most horses with nonstrangulating infarction lack evidence of physical vascular occlusion when examined at necropsy.[39] Consequently, it has been proposed that vasospasm may occur in the affected region. This hypothesis is based on the fact that the collateral capability of the colonic circulation should compensate for most emboli unless an extensive thrombus ensues. The absence of thickening of the infarcted bowel at some sites supports the possibility of complete local functional arterial occlusion.

Though the cause for the proposed vasospasm has not been identified, human patients with reduced blood flow due to arteriosclerosis experience vasospasm capable of producing clinical ischemia.[622,623] Both species have potential sources for partial mesenteric arterial occlusion (arteriosclerosis and verminous arteritis, respectively), yet a comparative few individuals suffer bowel ischemia. Both clinical syndromes are potentially reversible but have high mortality when severe.

No predisposition to nonstrangulating infarction has been identified, though most affected horses had verminous lesions in the mesenteric arteries.[39] Aside from circumstantial evidence, however, a connection between the 2 conditions has not been proven.

Clinical Signs: The severity of the clinical picture is quite variable and not related to the presence of irreversible ischemia in the bowel. Because no physical obstruction exists in most cases, bowel distention is not a consistent feature. Peritoneal fluid changes may be present (increased protein level or WBC numbers, darker color); however, normal peritoneal fluid does not rule out lethal intestinal disease. The amount of pain observed also is not necessarily correlated to the severity of the infarction. Signs of toxemia depend upon the progression of infarction.

Some cases resolve with medical therapy consisting of pain relief and fluid therapy. This is a reasonable therapy as long as the horse's condition is stable or improving. With deterioration, surgery is indicated. Use of flunixin meglumine should be evaluated carefully where this disease is concerned. Without severe pain from intestinal obstruction, alterations in the peritoneal fluid and the severity of toxemia may be the only indicator of the status of the horse. If the degree of toxemia is masked pharmacologically, deterioration of the horse's status and indications for surgery can be missed.

In surgical cases, resection of the affected bowel may be curative if the process is not too extensive. The outcome can be complicated by postoperative continuation of the problem in additional segments, making the prognosis somewhat unpredictable.

Idiopathic Diseases

Tympany

Rapid fermentation of feed may result in accumulation of large amounts of gas or may cause functional obstruction of the colon. Either condition results in flatulence and clinical signs of colic.

Changes in feed that allow rapid changes in gas-producing intestinal flora represent the most common cause of colonic tympany. This may occur after excessive carbohydrate intake, such as with grain overload or following ingestion of roughage with increased surface area, such as mown grass.

Signs depend upon duration and severity of tympany. Horses with flatulent colic mimic horses with other nonstrangulating disorders, such as impaction. As gas accumulates and the bowel becomes distended, the bowel wall is stretched and the horse feels pain. This is one of the most difficult types of pain to control. The horse may develop visible distention of the flanks or distention may be palpable per rectum. The horse's metabolic status and clinicopathologic findings depend upon the severity of the condition. However, once distention begins to increase, obstructive shock and respiratory compromise progress rapidly.

Horses with mild to moderate tympany frequently respond to analgesics and fluid therapy. Resolution of signs in early stages of the condition depends upon maintaining colonic motility so the gas can be expelled. This is accomplished by controlling pain to minimize sympathetic inhibition of motility. Oral administrations of mineral oil helps minimize absorption and aids excretion of any offending material. As distention becomes excessive, trocarization may be required to slow the course of events until the process subsides. This should be performed via the right and/or left flank, depending upon the location of the distention.

DISEASES OF THE SMALL COLON

G. M. Shires

Diagnostic and Therapeutic Considerations

The blood supply to the small colon is via the cranial mesenteric, caudal mesenteric, and internal pudendal arteries, and the veins flow to the portal and internal pudendal veins. Lymphatic drainage is to the colic lymph nodes and then the cisterna chyli. The nerve supply is derived from the mesenteric and pelvic plexuses of the sympathetic system. The small colon is where fecal balls are formed through final desiccation of the ingesta.

Local blood flow is one of the most important factors contributing to the healing process. While submucosal blood flow is maintained better in the colon than in the small intestine, the incidence of anastomotic leakage in other species is higher in the colon. This apparent paradox appears to be caused by alterations in blood flow caused by differences in tensile loads due to intraluminal pressure. Intraluminal pressure in dogs, and possibly horses, is higher in the colon than in the small intestine. The different sensitivity of the local microcirculatory systems of the intestinal segments to

tension thus may be one of the factors adversely affecting healing in the small colon.[624] This reinforces the practice of maintaining soft feces following enterotomy and may be most important with enterotomy of the small colon.

Survival rates for horses with colic have been significantly higher for small colon problems than for small intestine and large colon problems.[10] Problems with the small colon in adult horses are easier to recognize via rectal palpation than most other conditions involving the large bowel. The broad and prominent antimesenteric band on the small colon makes this area of the bowel easily identifiable. In some cases, such as impactions or volvulus of the small colon, rectal examination is limited, as the arm cannot be advanced deep into the rectum. In these cases, the caudal mesenteric root may be palpable as it is under tension.

Studies have shown that an everting staple closure of the small colon enterotomy had a greater incidence of adhesion formation, smaller lumen diameter and poor healing as compared to a simple-interrupted pattern.[625] Comparison of suture patterns indicates a 2-layer appositional pattern was mechanically and clinically better than single-layer appositional and 2-layer inverting patterns.[626]

Following segmental colectomy in dogs, animals pretreated with methylprednisolone had a significant overall increase in motility on the first postoperative day. Though this positive effect of corticosteroids may exist in some species, the potential for corticosteroid-induced laminitis always should be considered in horses.

When treating colic in horses, possible effects of drugs upon gut motility always should be kept in mind. Of the commonly employed analgesics, flunixin meglumine (Banamine: Schering) has no effect on colonic motility in normal ponies. General anesthesia, however, reduces intestinal motility and may cause postanesthesia colic in normal horses.

Diseases With Physical Causes

Meconium Impaction

If a foal 48-72 hours of age begins to show signs of mild abdominal discomfort, indicated by intermittent uneasiness, kicking and looking at the abdomen and/or stretching into a "sawhorse" stance, meconium impaction should be suspected. This suspicion would, of course, be enhanced by the history that no one had seen the foal defecate since birth. These early signs sometimes can progress quite rapidly to the point where the foal is continually and markedly painful, and prefers to remain in dorsal recumbency.

Short of an accurate history, clinical differentiation of meconium impaction from other causes of intestinal obstruction in foals can be difficult, especially if the animal is extremely painful. The aboral (distal) end of the meconium mass may be palpated digitally per rectum in some cases, but this is hardly reliable. Because of its position, meconium impaction causes more gaseous obstruction, but this does not eliminate the possibility of colonic torsion or atresia coli. In general, the foal's cardiovascular status (membrane color, capillary refill time, extremity temperature) is better than in many of the other more catastrophic intestinal problems that can beset a neonatal foal. One of the most useful diagnostic procedures is radiography if appropriate equipment is available; the impacting mass and gas-distended viscera proximal to the impaction may be identifiable.

The most direct therapeutic approach to meconium impaction is the enema. Though many enema formulations exist, simple soap and water probably is as effective as any. The important thing to remember is that too-vigorous infusion of the enema could result in serious electrolyte imbalance or a ruptured rectum. If gentle infusion of fluid does not achieve the desired results after 30-45 minutes of effort, surgical intervention can, in the long run, result in much less stress on the foal. Cholinomimetics or other drugs that putatively promote colonic motility are definitely contraindicated.

The surgical approach should be a caudal midline laparotomy. Gentle massage of the impactus, perhaps combined with transmural infusion of 0.9% NaCl mixed with some dioctyl sodium sulfosuccinate (DSS) via a small hypodermic needle, often loosens the mass so that it may be flushed out per rectum. If any enterotomy must be performed to relieve the obstruction, intraoperative

and postoperative broad-spectrum antibiotic therapy is indicated.

Ingesta Impaction

Clinical signs of small colon impaction vary from mild discomfort and straining to defecate, to shock and dehydration accompanied by pressure necrosis of the small colon. Rupture of the colon may occur in protracted cases. Rectal examination reveals enlargement of the small colon, with distention of the large colon and occasionally the cecum. In rare cases, an obstructing enterolith or bezoar may be palpable rectally.

If findings do not warrant surgical intervention, these obstructions can be managed adequately with medical therapy. Rehydration of the patient, accompanied by strict attention to the electrolyte and acid-base status, should be initiated as early as possible and followed by oral administration of emollients (mineral oil) and warm water if no reflux is present on placement of the nasogastric tube.

Fecal softeners, such as dioctyl sodium sulfosuccinate (DSS), may be administered orally via a tube but may affect the action of emollients; these agents preferably should not be administered simultaneously. The oral dose of DSS is 120-180 ml of a 5% solution for a 500-kg adult horse. This can be repeated after 24 hours but should not be administered too frequently. Use of hygroscopic cathartics, such as magnesium sulfate, should be limited to animals in which dehydration is not a problem. Other fecal softeners, such as 1-8-dihydroxyanthraquinone (Danthron: Sigma) can be given PO at 10-20 g every 36-48 hours to maintain soft feces once the impaction has loosened. Because such complications as diarrhea may follow an episode of obstruction, care should be taken to monitor the hydration and metabolic status of the patient during treatment, as well as for 24-48 hours following resolution of the problem. The eager surgeon must exercise patience and not turn to the scalpel blade without adequate indications. With vigorous and proper medical treatment, most simple obstructions of the small colon resolve.

Pain associated with simple impaction of the small colon usually is controlled adequately with the common analgesics used for colic. If dehydration is present, use of the phenothiazine tranquilizers should be avoided due to their potentially hypotensive effect.

Simple obstruction is routinely resolved medically, but some horses may require surgical intervention, and the clinician should be alert to this and carefully evaluate every alteration in clinical signs and blood values. Should surgery be indicated, exposure via ventral midline celiotomy should reveal the impacted small colon and distended large bowel. It may be possible to massage the impacted ingesta and break it down into smaller pieces. This may be aided by injection of sterile saline into the lumen of the small colon and gentle kneading of the mass. If not possible, an enterotomy must be performed to remove the obstruction. If an area of bowel over the obstruction is compromised, the enterotomy should be made adjacent to this tissue and the obstruction moved to the healthy area for removal. If pressure necrosis is present, it may be necessary to resect the compromised bowel and anastomose the 2 healthy segments. As with any enterotomy, great care must be taken to prevent contamination of the abdomen and viscera. As such, antibiotics should be administered during surgery and postoperatively for at least 5 days.

If the abdomen has been contaminated and peritonitis is likely, postoperative peritoneal lavage with 6-8 L of warm sterile saline via a Foley catheter placed ventrally may be performed several times. This lavage may be sufficient to lower the intensity of the peritonitis and reduce ileus. Once the saline has been introduced via the catheter into the abdominal cavity in the standing horse, the catheter is pinched to prevent leakage and covered to retain sterility. The patient is then walked around vigorously for several minutes, after which the catheter is opened and the fluid drained. Samples from the first and last fluid flow can be examined for cell counts. This procedure can be repeated several times until the clinician is satisfied that lavage has been successful in reducing contamination. With a suitable level of properly selected antibiotics being administered parenterally, there is no need for antibiotics or antiseptics to be included in the sterile saline lavage.

Enterolith, Fecalith or Bezoar Obstruction

Blockage of the small colon due to solid matter that has passed from the transverse colon or has formed in the small colon itself is well recognized. Some foreign objects such as pantyhose, which are used frequently on Walking Horses, have been the cause of small colon obstruction. Obstruction of the lumen by this type of obstacle may be palpated rectally, making definitive diagnosis simple. Abdominal radiographs may be diagnostic in small horses (Fig 132). Clinical signs usually are not too acute and may delay the decision to perform surgery. In instances where the object is very large in comparison to the lumen of the small colon, any delay adversely affects the prog-

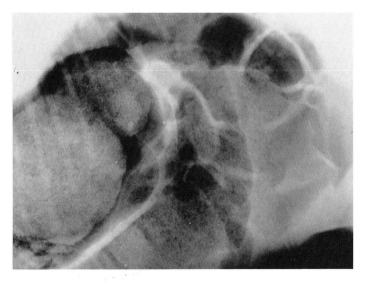

Figure 132. Radiographic demonstration of a 5-cm-diameter enterolith (top center) lodged in the small colon of a 5-month-old Miniature Horse with acute onset of colic and subsequent abdominal distention. Note the marked distention of the right dorsal colon with gas and gut contents. (Courtesy of Dr. A.M. Merritt)

nosis, as the bowel wall may become ischemic when stretched over the object, and necrosis develops quickly.

In early cases, the offending enterolith can be easily located through a ventral midline celiotomy and, if possible, moved via gentle massage to an uncompromised area of bowel. Enterotomy can then be performed and the enterolith removed. Very often the enterolith is in a section of bowel that cannot be exteriorized for enterotomy; this type should be moved along the bowel to a more suitable area, if possible. Retrograde flushing via the rectum or injection of saline around the blockage may help dislodge the obstruction. Great care must be exercised to avoid rupturing the small colon while the enterolith is being moved. In more severe cases, the bowel surrounding the object has become necrotic and must be resected.

Enteroliths usually form slowly over a lengthy period, during which no signs of colic are displayed, or there may be a history of recurrent colic that responds to medical therapy. Smaller enteroliths may pass from the large colon without causing any problems. In some cases of incomplete obstruction, mineral oil, soft feces and gas may bypass an enterolith and thereby confuse the diagnosis. If it is known that a horse has previously passed an enterolith, care should be taken to ensure that other enteroliths are not still present. The prognosis for survival is excellent, provided the bowel is not compromised.

Colonic Adhesions

Blockage of the small colon may occur due to adhesions caused from peritonitis due to a multitude of causes. Adhesions in this area are most likely to follow inflammation or injury to the distal bowel following meconium impaction in foals or as a result of complications following rectal trauma in adults.

Adhesions are rarely limited to the small colon and usually involve the rectum in horses with rectal tears and/or abscesses. Alternatively, the adhesions may be spread widely over the viscera in cases of diffuse peritonitis. In isolated instances following surgical intervention in the small colon, localized adhesions may restrict movement of the small colon and cause obstruction.

As with most intraabdominal adhesions, treatment is difficult and unrewarding, and may include a variety of drugs, most of which have very little effect on mature adhesions. Surgical intervention may resolve the problem if local adhesions can be located and broken down, but often the adhesions recur following surgery. The most successful treatment for adhesions is prevention by minimizing the inciting causes or aggressively treating conditions likely to have peritonitis as a sequel.

Colonic Volvulus

Volvulus is not a common condition of the small colon as compared to volvulus involving other intestinal segments. With the long mesentery, one would expect a higher incidence of both volvulus and intussusception; perhaps the small colon does not move as much as other sections of bowel. In instances of small colon volvulus, surgery is indicated and the prognosis depends on the extent of vascular compromise, bowel necrosis and location of the lesion.

Colonic Incarceration

Due to its anatomic position, the small colon has little opportunity to become incarcerated. Any rents or openings in the mesocolon are potential areas through which the small colon can become incarcerated. Other potential opportunities include rents in the broad ligament or related ovarian ligaments. Treatment for incarceration is via surgical exploration and correction. Most often this includes resection and anastomosis due to severe compromise to the affected areas. The prognosis is directly related to the condition of the affected portions of bowel and necessity for resection.

Obstruction by Pedunculated Lipoma

The cord-like pedicle of intraabdominal lipomas may encircle and strangulate the small colon as with other areas of the intestines. Affected horses usually require surgery and recover if treated early by celiotomy and resection of the strangulating cord. In more advanced cases, there may be pressure necrosis and rupture of the bowel wall. Surgical intervention may include resection and anastomosis of a portion of the small colon, and the surgeon should be prepared for this eventuality. Pedunculated lipomas are most likely to be found in mature to aged horses.

Inflammatory, Infectious and Immune Diseases

Abscessation

Abscessation following generalized septicemia may result in strictures or adhesions that obstruct the small colon. Though a specific diagnosis can usually be made only via exploratory celiotomy, rectal examination may be very helpful, as with other problems in the small colon.

If the abscess is in an area accessible to the surgeon, attempts can be made to break down the adhesions and/or drain and flush the abscess. If contamination is from injuries to the rectum, an approach via the rectum may allow the abscess to be drained and flushed. In most cases, however, some stricture results. This is discussed more completely in the section on Rectal Tears.

Idiopathic Diseases

Intramural Lesions

Intramural hematoma and submucosal edema of the small colon have been treated successfully with surgery.[627] Bruising of the small colon during parturition may initiate colic due to ileus of the small colon. In most cases, this condition can be treated successfully by medical therapy with fecal softeners and emollients, as well as analgesics and dietary control.

Intussusception

Intussusception of the small colon occurs rarely in foals. Presenting signs are acute colic with significant abdominal distention and rapidly deteriorating condition. Very often the colic episode is preceded by diarrhea. Radiography may help distinguish this problem from severe colitis. Surgical intervention is the only choice, and early diagnosis and exploration are imperative.

The prognosis is poor because a fairly large section of the small colon must be resected, unless the condition is identified early enough that the intussuscepting section can be reduced via gentle traction and massage. Unfortunately, this is not often the case, and resection and anastomosis of a significant section of the small colon usually are required. Early and proper treatment of parasites and diarrhea to limit small colon inflammation and straining may help prevent this condition.

Veno-occlusive Disease

This problem is very difficult to diagnose before surgery but is characterized by bouts of severe, barely controllable abdominal pain and sometimes straining to the point where the rectum begins to prolapse. Early in the course of the problem, rectal examination may not reveal anything definitive enough to warrant immediate surgery. Later in the course of the disease, very diffusely edematous small colon may be appreciated by rectal examination, but the horse may strongly resist this procedure because of the pain it causes. Even as the problem progresses, however, the animal's metabolic status remains relatively normal, as does the peritoneal fluid. The unrelenting pain usually provokes surgical exploration.

Segmental Ischemic Necrosis

Ischemic necrosis of the small colon occurs rarely in postparturient mares.[628] Affected mares generally are pluriparous, exhibit signs of colic within 12 after parturition, and have increased numbers of leukocytes in the peritoneal fluid. Necrosis of a segment of small colon occurs due to tearing of the small colon mesentery and disruption of the blood supply. If possible, treatment of the condition involves resection of the devitalized small colon and anastomosis. The condition must be distinguished from cecal rupture and hemorrhage from the middle uterine artery.

DISEASES OF THE RECTUM

G.M. Shires

The rectum is the terminal portion of the gastrointestinal tract extending for about 25-30 cm from the pelvic inlet to the anus. Only the most proximal section is covered with peritoneum; this is an important fact in relation to rupture of the rectal wall.

Congenital and Familial Diseases

Atresia Ani and Atresia Recti

Atresia ani and/or recti is the most common of the rare atretic anomalies in horses. In some cases, lack of a tail and vagina has been seen together with atresia ani. Because other defects, such as atresia coli, may occur with this condition, affected foals should be evaluated carefully for other problems. Even the unobservant horse owner is alerted because of the lack of passed meconium. Routine postfoaling physical examination should identify this condition immediately after the foal has risen.

The difficulty lies in deciding if the atresia is limited to a persistent membrane blocking the anus or if a sections of the rectum or colon are missing. Obviously, the prognosis depends on these findings. In simple cases, anal tone is present and the membrane over the opening to the rectum is thin and bulging outward due to pressure of the rectal contents. In such cases, a simple incision without damaging the sphincter solves the problem. In more severe cases, a rectal "pull-through" procedure under local anesthesia or via laparotomy may be required. Because the metabolic status of the foal may deteriorate rapidly, early diagnosis and treatment improve the prognosis. Care must be taken to inform the owner of the potential heritability of this problem, as well as the possibility of other anomalies that are not as easily identifiable.

Diseases With Physical Causes

Rectal Tear

Cause: Rupture of one or all layers of the rectal wall due to trauma is a relatively common problem. It most often is associated with rectal palpation for reproductive evaluation in the mare, or during rectal examination as a diagnostic procedure. The prognosis following rectal tears is guarded, and insurance claims for this problem are not uncommon.

Though the risk of rectal tears may be related to the examiner's inexperience, it is not necessarily restricted to inexperienced palpators. A disparity in size between the palpator's arm and the horse's rectal lumen increases the risk of trauma to the rectal structures. Restlessness and straining of the horse during examination or extreme debility of the animal also increase the risk of tears.

Other causes of tears can include accidental damage during breeding, or injury following parturition in mares. In foals, rectal trauma may be caused by attempts to remove impacted meconium. Various other causes have been reported.[629,630]

In most cases, tears occur 20-25 cm cranial to the anus on the dorsal wall of the rectum. The prognosis depends on several factors, not the least of which are the extent of the tear and number of tissue layers torn. Commonly, only the mucosal layer is penetrated. The only indication to the palpator may be a sensation of "give" in the wall of the rectum and blood on the glove when the arm is withdrawn. Classification of rectal tears varies from tearing of only the mucosa (Grade 1) to rupture of all layers and the sudden ability to easily palpate the organs in the abdominal cavity (Grade 4).

Tears of the muscularis only, with intact mucosa and serosa (Grade 2), are seldom diagnosed primarily. The palpator might feel a sensation of something "giving," but after carefully feeling the mucosa and inspecting the glove for blood is unable to detect any blood or any tear in the mucosa. These Grade-2 tears can lead to herniation of the mucosa and possible rupture.

Initial Management: Initial discovery of trauma to the rectum should be followed by a series of actions aimed at evaluation of the problem and communication with the owner. A database of information should be obtained and used to monitor the animal's progress. The horse should be treated to reduce tenesmus and for peritonitis. The owner should be fully informed of the problem and prognosis. The patient must be treated aggressively or referred elsewhere if treatment cannot be undertaken.

Initial evaluation of the extent of the tear must be done with great care to prevent further damage to the rectal wall. Straining can be reduced by giving an epidural anesthetic, a sedative and/or probanthine IV at 25-30 mg/450 kg. In some cases, rectal infusion of lidocaine (15-20 ml of 2% solution in 30-40 ml water) may aid examination.

A complete physical examination should be done and the findings recorded so that any changes can be evaluated. This initial database should include abdominoparacentesis so that development of peritonitis can be assessed (Table 2). Medical therapy should include a tetanus booster and broad-spectrum antimicrobials, such as trimethoprim-sulfas, a combination of penicillin and gentamicin sulfate, or the newer-generation antibiotics.

Surgical Management: Surgical choices include attempts at suturing mucosal (Grade-1) tears via the anus; however, most tears are beyond reach with routine surgical instruments, making this procedure very difficult and not very successful. One report describes use of new instrumentation developed to facilitate direct visual examination and repair of some rectal tears per rectum.[631,632] It must be remembered that unless the wound and its surroundings can be properly cleaned and lavaged, closure of the mucosa over any debris may lead to formation of an abscess and subsequent stricture.

If the tear is close to the anus and easily visible, cleaning and repair may be performed simply in the standing animal under epidural anesthesia. Most tears, however, are at least 20-25 cm cranial to the anus and, therefore, are beyond reasonable access in the standing animal.

With perforation of the mucosa, submucosa and muscularis but not the serosa (Grade 3), or perforation of all 4 layers (Grade 4), several options are available. If the decision is made to treat the horse, vigorous antimicrobial and supportive therapy are required. Very careful, thorough communication with the owner is essential from the outset to fully explain the prognosis and treatment regimen. Initially, baseline data should be recorded, including evaluation of abdominal fluid, to begin carefully monitoring of the animal's progress and any complications that may arise.

If repair per rectum is not an option, then ventral midline laparotomy may be needed to repair the tear. In most cases, however, visual examination of the lesion through a ventral midline incision is as difficult as it would be per rectum due to the location of the wound and immobility of the organ.

Attempts at prolapsing the rectum and associated structures and suturing the lesion while the mucosa is everted have rarely been successful in my experience. To prolapse enough rectum to exteriorize the lesion, considerable tissue must be forced into the pelvic canal. Thrombosis of the vessels in this tissue causes serious problems once the procedure has been completed.

Diversion of the fecal mass through a colostomy also has been described as a temporary means of allowing the rectal tear to heal. This colostomy can be performed in the standing animal and should be positioned in the left flank area. Two methods are described.[629,634] In one technique, the small colon is severed, the distal end oversewn, and the proximal end sutured to the skin. Once the rectal tear has healed, the 2 ends of the small colon are anastomosed via a ventral laparotomy incision.[633] The second technique involves making an incision through the antimesenteric band of a section of small colon that has been exteriorized and sutured to an incision in the left flank. This technique has been termed a "loop colostomy." Once the tear has healed, this enterotomy is closed, the small colon is replaced and the wound closed. Both procedures are done with the animal standing.

The principle of a colostomy is diversion of fecal material from the tear in the rectum or small colon to permit healing without impaction and additional contamination. Aggressive support against infection, peritonitis and expected complications must accompany any surgical attempts if success is to be expected. Initially, careful and gentle gravitational retrograde flushing of the distal small colon and rectum with sterile isotonic fluid via the anus is performed to remove any remaining fecal material and to keep the distal bowel functional.

The colostomy site lends itself to abuse by the patient, accidentally or purposefully, and may prolapse even when located correctly. Careful attention to correct location of the incision and section of small colon used as well as to dietary and medical aftercare can make the temporary colostomy a successful procedure. If such complications as strictures or stenoses make the rectal tube nonfunctional, a semipermanent colostomy may be very practical. In one unreported case, a valuable broodmare was salvaged for the latter period of her pregnancy and early lactation by a loop colostomy following severe complications subsequent to a rectal tear. A permanent colostomy probably is not desirable in most cases.

Use of a temporary rectal liner has been proposed as another means of protecting the tear from fecal contamination. With this method, an indwelling liner, made from a rectal prolapse ring, and a plastic sleeve is sutured in the lumen via a ventral midline or a standing flank incision. The plastic sleeve then serves as a protective cover for the tear until it heals.[635] This procedure appears to be successful provided the tear has not progressed to a Grade-4 lesion.

An intelligent choice of corrective measures, coupled with suitable medical therapy, helps improve the prognosis for rectal tears. No matter what the choice, it is still a very serious lesion demanding immediate diagnosis and therapy if any success is to be achieved. Full and candid communication with the client should be initiated early and maintained throughout the course of treatment. In many cases, euthanasia may be an early or eventual choice, and this should be explained at the outset to avoid unrealistically optimistic expectations.

Stenosis and Stricture

Narrowing of the rectal lumen, to the extent that normal passage of fecal material is impaired, causes impaction and colic. Very often this obstruction is a sequel to a rectal tear and is located in the retroperitoneal section of the rectum. Simple abscessation may be resolved via drainage and flushing per rectum; however, great care must be taken to avoid further contamination of the peritoneal cavity. In some cases, these perirectal abscesses have been opened, drained and flushed per vagina with success. Frequently, however, these resolved abscesses constrict and form a restrictive band around the rectum, resulting in blockage.

Treatment of rectal strictures is unrewarding and may call for diversion of the feces via a colostomy. In less severe cases, careful and continuous attention to diet may enable the feces to be kept sufficiently soft that impactions do not occur often. The regularity of the horse's bowel movements must be constantly monitored to identify these impactions early.

Strangulation

The stalk a pedunculated lipoma may completely strangulate the rectum. Other space-occupying lesions, such as a neo-plasm, or even excessive fat depots, may fill the pelvic canal sufficiently to cause stricture or strangulation of the rectum. Treatment involves surgical intervention and the prognosis hinges on early recognition of the condition.

Infectious, Inflammatory and Immune Diseases

Pruritus Ani

The most common cause of persistent irritation to the anus and tailhead is infection with pinworms (*Oxyuris equi*). Alternatively, constant rubbing of the area may be a vice or due to hypersensitivity to *Culicoides*. In these instances, irritation is not limited to the tailhead. Irritation following a food allergy or persistent enteritis and diarrhea may also produce pruritus ani.

Multifactorial Diseases

Prolapse

Rectal prolapse may be partial, involving only the mucosa, or complete, in which case the full thickness of the rectal wall is prolapsed (Fig 133). Great care must be taken to differentiate a rectal prolapse in mares from other conditions, such as prolapse of the bladder via a rectovaginal tear. Any increase in abdominal pressure or excessive

Figure 133. Complete rectal prolapse. The prolapsed portion of the rectum was congested and edematous. (Courtesy of Dr. L. Bramlage)

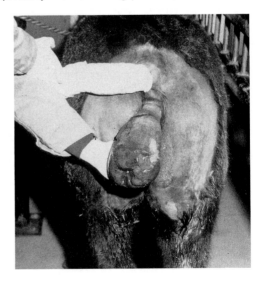

straining from inflammation of the bowel or urogenital organs may initiate prolapse of the rectal wall.

Depending on the condition of the tissue, treatment may be medical and/or surgical. In very early cases in which the prolapsed tissue is not severely traumatized and the initiating cause is resolved to eliminate tenesmus, the prolapsed tissue may simply be reduced. Careful manipulation and use of lubricants may suffice to replace the tissue. Permanent resolution of the prolapse depends upon removal of the inciting cause.

In some cases, an early and small prolapse may be resolved by a simple alteration in feed and feeding practices. More often, however, the prolapsed portion of rectum is traumatized and contaminated, and has been exteriorized for some time. Frequently the blood supply to the prolapsed tissue has been interrupted, and edema and necrosis are present. If possible, after cleaning and lubricating, the exteriorized section should be replaced and retained with a pursestring suture. Epidural and local anesthesia are required, and tenesmus must be controlled. If, however, tissue damage is severe and replacement of the prolapse is impossible, surgical intervention, including submucosal resection or even amputation of the prolapsed portion, must be performed. Complications following either of these procedures are common due to stenosis and impaction of the distal rectum.

Rectovaginal Tear and Fistula

This lesion consists of a connecting passage between the rectum and the vagina. It can range from a small perforation that is difficult to identify, to a complete communication between the distal rectum and caudal vagina. The perineum may be completely torn. Suffice it to say that rectovaginal tears are very seldom life threatening, and repair is usually best postponed until edema has abated and local tissue architecture has become discernable. Because this lesion usually is a complication of dystocia, it is discussed in detail in the chapter on Diseases of the Reproductive System: The Mare.

If the foal responsible for the tear is alive and suckling, surgical repair is best postponed until after weaning. Successful surgical repair hinges upon reduction of the

mare's fecal output as well as maintenance of very soft feces before and after surgery. To accomplish this, dietary changes must be made and maintained which usually adversely affect lactation and, therefore, the foal.

DISEASES OF THE PERITONEUM AND MESENTERY
S.D. Semrad

Diseases With Physical Causes

Intraabdominal Hemorrhage
(Hemoperitoneum)

Cause: Bleeding or effusion of blood into the peritoneal cavity (hemoperitoneum) with no visible blood loss is rare in horses.[636] Blunt trauma, vascular accidents, surgical complications, tumor necrosis with vascular encroachment, intestinal accidents and coagulopathies have been associated with intraabdominal bleeding. Blunt abdominal trauma may cause rupture of the spleen, liver or blood vessels, with massive blood loss and rapid death. Contusion of the spleen or liver, with bleeding beneath the capsular surface and hematoma formation, results in less obvious blood loss until capsular rupture occurs. Laceration of the liver, spleen or major blood vessels following penetration of the abdomen with a foreign body results in either rapid blood loss and death or blood loss slow enough to allow for presentation of the animal for treatment.

Traumatic rupture of the diaphragm also may result in hemoperitoneum. Pressure necrosis of the portal vein, vascular rupture and acute death have been reported following long-standing incarceration of bowel in the epiploic foramen. Intramural hematomas of the intestine may cause considerable blood loss into the abdomen. Minor to moderate hemorrhage with hematoma formation occurs following tears in the mesentery. Postoperatively, hemoperitoneum occurs due to faulty hemostasis or mesenteric vessel ligature failure.

Massive hemorrhage and rapid death following rupture of an aneurysm of the abdominal aorta or cranial mesenteric artery occur occasionally in racehorses during exercise. Blood loss is less acute if the hemorrhage originates from an aneurysm or thrombus of the more distal mesenteric blood supply. Rupture of the utero-ovarian, middle uterine or large intraabdominal blood vessels during late pregnancy, parturition or correction of an uterine torsion often leads to rapid demise. Postpartum hemorrhage is not always fatal if the bleeding remains contained within the peritoneal layers of the broad ligament. Older (>8 years of age) multiparous mares are prime candidates for peripartum hemorrhage.[637] Bleeding into the abdomen after castration is most commonly seen after the procedure has been done with the horse standing.

Clinical Signs: Signs of intraabdominal hemorrhage depend on the primary injury and the rapidity and amount of blood loss. Acute, severe blood loss following rupture of a major vessel or parenchymal organ progresses rapidly to hemorrhagic shock and death. Clinical manifestations include colic, rapidly progressive weakness, tachycardia, tachypnea, dyspnea, sweating, pale or blanched mucous membranes, cold extremities, agitation or severe depression and prostration. When bleeding occurs less rapidly, signs may be more subtle. Mild depression, intermittent or mild colic, partial anorexia, lethargy, reluctance to move, pale or icteric mucous membranes, dehydration, and mild increases in heart rate, respiratory rate and body temperature may be seen. Signs of hemorrhage during parturition are difficult to distinguish from the second and third stages of labor. Findings on rectal examination usually are normal unless secondary ileus and bowel distention occur. A hematoma may be palpated rectally if hemorrhage occurred into the broad ligament or mesentery.

Diagnosis: Intraabdominal hemorrhage should be suspected from the history (blunt trauma, penetrating wound, recent abdominal surgery, castration, late pregnancy, recent parturition) and clinical manifestations. Abrasions, bruises and lacerations suggest trauma and possible internal injury and bleeding. The hematocrit, hemoglobin level and erythrocyte count do not decrease for 8-10 hours or more following significant blood loss and are of little aid when assessing conditions with severe acute hemorrhage. The hematocrit may be normal or elevated due to splenic contraction during the

early response to blood loss. Total plasma protein concentrations decrease gradually. Baseline values for hematocrit and total plasma protein should be obtained so that blood loss may be estimated and progression monitored. Neutrophilic leukocytosis reflecting stress may be present.

Hemoperitoneum usually is diagnosed by abdominocentesis. Care must be taken to differentiate hemoperitoneum from contamination by puncture of the spleen or subcutaneous vessels. Unless the horse is severely dehydrated, splenic blood has a higher hematocrit than does peripheral blood. Consequently, the hematocrit of the peritoneal fluid and of the peripheral blood should be compared. Following splenic puncture, bleeding into the peritoneal cavity continues. A second abdominocentesis at another site may appear bloody but should not yield a large volume of fluid following splenic puncture. When true hemoperitoneum is present, erythrophagocytosis is observed on direct blood smear, and a large volume of bloody fluid usually can be obtained from multiple sites by abdominocentesis. The protein content of abdominal fluid usually is elevated. A hematoma in the broad ligament or mesentery may be identified by rectal palpation or ultrasonographic examination.

Treatment: Management of intraabdominal hemorrhage is difficult, as the underlying cause often is not known. Assessment of the rapidity and amount of blood loss may help determine the appropriate therapeutic approach. Rupture of a major vessel (aorta, main uterine artery, cranial mesenteric artery) or parenchymal organ usually results in death before therapy is possible. If this is suspected, supportive measures, including treatment for shock and hypovolemia, are begun and surgery undertaken to stop the hemorrhage. If splenic rupture is suspected, resection of the seventeenth rib on the left side is the preferred surgical approach. Occlusion of a bleeding uterine artery may be attempted through a vaginal approach. If fatal hemorrhage occurs during delivery of a foal, the foal should be extracted per vagina if possible.[637] If vaginal delivery is not possible, an emergency cesarean section should be performed.

When bleeding is less severe or hemorrhage following uterine vessel rupture is confined within the broad ligament, conservative measures should be undertaken initially. Conservative therapy includes support of the cardiovascular system (IV fluids, or plasma or blood transfusions if indicated), pain relief, and maintenance of a positive energy balance. The horse should be housed in a quiet environment; exercise should be severely restricted, and stress or agitation minimized. Tranquilizers should be used judiciously, as most agents lower the blood pressure and may contribute to cardiovascular compromise. Intravenous administration of hypertonic saline solutions is of short-term benefit in treatment of hemorrhagic shock.[638] Use of corticosteroids and antibiotics is controversial. Parenteral administration of oxytocin to encourage uterine contraction and thus vascular contraction has been recommended when rupture of a uterine vessel is suspected. If hemorrhage cannot be arrested within 12 hours, laparotomy should be considered.

Prognosis: The prognosis is grave following rupture of the spleen, liver or major blood vessels. Recovery from less severe intraabdominal hemorrhage may be complicated by peritonitis, intraabdominal hematoma or abscess, or laminitis. In cases of postpartum hemorrhage, blood transfusions, plasma expanders and fluid therapy do not seem to affect the outcome. In any case of intraabdominal hemorrhage, a guarded to poor prognosis should be given.

Penetrating Abdominal Wounds

Penetrating abdominal wounds are serious, require immediate attention and often are difficult to treat. The spectrum of injuries occurring with penetrating wounds of the abdomen ranges from minor injury to the abdominal wall, with no involvement of the internal organs, to intestinal and vascular perforation, with subsequent septic and hemorrhagic shock.

Cause: The abdominal cavity may be entered through wounds in the abdominal wall, rectum, vaginal vault or uterus. Penetration of the abdominal wall may occur accidentally (hunting accidents, impalement on a fencepost, jump, sharp branches, racetrack rail or driving shafts), result from malice (gunshot wounds, stab wounds) or iatrogenically (liver biopsy, cecal trocarization, abdominocentesis). Rupture of the rectum results from mechanical trauma during rectal palpation, from sadistic acts or, less

commonly, it occurs spontaneously. Penetration of the vaginal vault most commonly results from trauma during breeding. Uterine perforation may occur during endometrial biopsy, artificial insemination, parturition, or correction of uterine torsion. "The external appearance of the penetration site often does not reflect the extent of internal injuries."[639] "Low-velocity penetrating injuries caused by sticks, knives, shotgun pellets, pistols and air guns may produce minimal damage to nearby tissues, whereas rifle bullets fired at high velocity often result in extensive, widespread tissue damage."[639,640]

Clinical Signs: Penetrating wounds of the abdomen may have serious complications, the most common of which are hemorrhage, peritonitis, intestinal herniation and organ dysfunction.[640] Acute severe abdominal bleeding results in abdominal pain, hypovolemia, shock and death. Injury to the liver, spleen, kidneys or large intraabdominal vessels can produce extensive bleeding. Intestinal perforation with gross contamination of the abdomen leads to overwhelming toxemia, septic shock and death. Minor injury to the bowel wall may be contained within the omentum and/or seal spontaneously. In such cases, manifestations of peritonitis are slower to develop and are less severe.

Traumatic disruption of the blood supply to the intestine or other organs may cause severe maceration and devitalization of tissue. The full extent of such injuries may not be evident for several days. Laceration or perforation of the liver, pancreas or bladder results in release of chemical irritants that predispose to secondary bacterial peritonitis.[639] Intestinal herniation may induce severe pain and profound shock. Additional damage to the bowel occurs upon contact with objects in the environment or as the horse steps on the herniated abdominal contents. Damage to the nerve supply of the intestine and other internal organs may follow intestinal herniation or penetrating wounds to the abdomen.

Diagnosis: Diagnosis is based on the history and physical examination. Observation of blood in the urine or manure, bleeding from body orifices, inability to micturate, and deterioration in clinical status may help determine the severity of the injury. The animal must be carefully examined to identify entrance and exit wounds. Alterations in the hemogram and blood chemistry depend on the duration of the wound and degree of abdominal contamination and toxemia. Abdominocentesis may help differentiate types of abdominal injury and help assess the degree of contamination of the peritoneal cavity.

The usefulness of abdominal radiography depends on the size of the animal and facilities available. Free gas, free fluid or alterations in size or position of major abdominal organs may be observed on abdominal radiographs in foals or small horses. Generalized loss of abdominal contrast suggests fluid in the abdomen (hemorrhage, urine, exudate). Free gas in the abdomen results from intestinal rupture, infection with gas-producing organisms or penetration of the abdominal wall.[639] Contrast radiography may be used to determine the integrity of the bladder. Though physical examination and supportive data may suggest severe intraabdominal injury, definitive diagnosis and treatment often require surgical intervention.

Immediate therapy is aimed at controlling life-threatening shock and hemorrhage and protecting any exposed viscera. When appropriate, intravenous fluids are administered to reestablish circulating volume. Sedation may be necessary, depending on the mental status of the animal. When the animal is uncontrollable by physical or chemical restraint, general anesthesia may be necessary to proceed with emergency care. Care must be taken not to further compromise the cardiovascular status to induce severe hypotension. After stabilization of the animal, exploratory laparotomy may be indicated to determine the source of intestinal contamination and bleeding, or to correct bowel damage following intestinal herniation. Depending on the degree of injury, exposed abdominal viscera are cleansed and returned to the abdomen, or intestinal resection and anastomosis are performed.

Until proven otherwise, perforation of the intestinal tract should be assumed following a penetrating abdominal wound, and broad-spectrum antimicrobial therapy should be initiated. The optimal antimicrobial agent(s) for penetrating abdominal injuries remains undetermined.[641] If severe peritonitis develops, placement of a peritoneal drain may be warranted. Paralytic ileus frequently results from trauma to the peritoneal cavity and often is difficult to manage. Wounds involving the abdominal wall and inguinal region can act as one-way valves and thus can trap air, promoting subcutaneous emphysema and poor wound healing. Placement of an abdominal wrap or closure of the wound with sterile packing may help prevent air trapping.

The prognosis depends on the site and extent of internal injury, as well as the degree of contamination of the peritoneal cavity. If the wound is accompanied by perforation of abdominal viscera, laceration of major blood vessels or tearing of the mesentery and enclosed vessels, a grave prognosis is warranted.

Inflammatory, Infectious and Immune Diseases

Peritonitis

The peritoneal cavity, which includes the abdominal cavity, pelvic cavity and extraabdominal extensions or vaginal processes, is the largest extravascular space in the body.[642] It is a closed sac in the male but is opened to the exterior at the oviduct in the female. A single layer of mesothelial squamous cells, overlying loose areolar connective tissue and adipose tissue, lines the peritoneal cavity and covers the intraabdominal viscera.[642,643] The surface of this mesothelial lining is covered with microvilli.

The peritoneum secretes a serous fluid that lubricates the abdominal cavity, minimizes intraabdominal adhesion formation, and has minimal antibacterial properties. It also acts as a bidirectional semipermeable barrier to diffusion of water and low-molecular-weight solutes between the blood and abdominal cavity.[642,643] Defects in the peritoneal surface normally heal rapidly by connective tissue deposition and transformation of fibroblasts and other cell types into mesothelial cells.[642,643] Inflammation of the mesothelial lining of the peritoneal cavity is termed peritonitis.

Cause: Peritonitis is characterized by marked exudation of serum, fibrin and protein into the peritoneal cavity. It may be classified according to origin (primary or secondary), onset (peracute, acute, chronic), region affected (diffuse, localized), and presence of bacteria (septic, nonseptic).

Though rare in animals, primary peritonitis may result from hematogenous spread and may be associated with impaired host defenses.[642] In horses, peritonitis is usually acute, diffuse and secondary to traumatic or chemical insults or infectious processes (bacterial, viral, mycotic, parasitic). Any agent or disease that causes irritation of the peritoneum or inflammation in abdominal viscera, or compromises the wall of hollow abdominal organs may foster development of peritonitis.

Peritonitis most commonly occurs secondary to contamination of the peritoneal cavity by bacteria from the intestinal tract. The infectious organisms that cause strangles, influenza, viral arteritis and African horse sickness have an affinity for serosal surfaces, predisposing to peritonitis.[643] Chemical peritonitis resulting from exposure to irritants or foreign fluids (urine, bile) often progresses to septic peritonitis. Localized peritonitis in horses most frequently is associated with abdominal abscesses.[643] Chyloabdomen has also been associated with an intraabdominal abscess in a foal.[644]

Pathogenesis: Contamination of the abdomen and injury to the mesothelial cells initiates an inflammatory response and a cascade of events that results in: release of catecholamines and vasoactive substances from peritoneal mast cells; vasodilatation and hyperemia; an increase in peritoneal and vascular permeability; influx of protein-rich fluid, macrophages, polymorphonuclear cells, humoral opsonins, natural antibodies and serum complement into the peritoneal cavity; chemotaxis and phagocytosis; depression of peritoneal fibrinolytic activity; fibrin deposition on the peritoneal surface; and reflex ileus.[642,643,645-648] Though initially of benefit by confining the contamination and infection, these processes become deleterious, resulting in: hypovolemia; hypoproteinemia; dilution of opsonin concentrations; reduction of peritoneal oxygen tension; ileus with bowel distention, ischemia of bowel wall and absorption of bacteria and toxins; and adhesion formation.[642,645-648] The cardiovascular compromise, renal insufficiency and endocrine and metabolic alterations observed reflect the degree of hypovolemia and endotoxic shock present.

The severity of peritonitis is related to the primary underlying disease process, nature of the infective agent, natural host defenses, type and number of organ systems involved and site of intestinal leakage. A mixed population of bacteria is present in the intestinal tract, but the quantity of bacteria and prevalence of anaerobic species increase in the distal segments.[642,645] High mortality is associated with contamination from the distal bowel.[645]

Clinical signs of peritonitis depend on the primary disease, infectious agent involved and stage of disease when the animal is first examined. The spectrum of pathologic changes ranges from peracute or acute generalized peritonitis with overwhelming toxemia and shock, to chronic low-grade localized infection with minimal clinical signs. Common presenting signs in 30 horses (aged 2 months to 16 years) with peritonitis were colic, ileus, fever, anorexia, weight loss and diarrhea.[649] Horses with peracute peritonitis, as might be observed after rupture of the intestine, show profound toxemia, weakness, depression, elevated heart and respiratory rates, circulatory failure and rapid deterioration. Death may occur within 4-24 hours. Fever and abdominal pain may or may not be evident, depending on the stage of shock and mental status of the animal.

Signs associated with acute diffuse peritonitis include abdominal pain, sweating, pawing, muscle fasciculations, elevated heart and respiratory rates, "thready" peripheral pulses, red to purple mucous membranes, prolonged capillary refill time, dehydration, depression and anorexia. The body temperature may be high, low or normal.

Abdominal pain is most evident in the early stages of the disease. The abdominal discomfort associated with peritonitis results from a combination of visceral and parietal pain; parietal pain predominates in most cases. Parietal pain is characterized by immobilization, reluctance to move, splinting of the abdominal wall, and sensitivity to external abdominal pressure.[643,649] The horse may groan and have an increased heart rate and rapid shallow breathing pattern when forced to move.

Gastrointestinal motility and fecal output may be transiently increased early in the disease. Ileus, however, is seen more frequently, and the resultant stasis may lead to intestinal distention, gastric reflux and abdominal discomfort. Reluctance to perform an abdominal press due to pain and dehydration causes decreased fecal output, constipation or impaction. Findings on rectal examination are inconsistent. Abnormalities reported include a "gritty" feeling to the serosal and parietal surfaces of the peritoneum due to fibrin deposition, a dull "dry" texture to the peritoneum, decreased fecal or dry fecal material in the intestine, pain on palpation of fibrous adhesions, mesenteric band or inflamed surfaces of the peritoneum, intestinal impaction or distention secondary to ileus, and an abdominal mass (abscess or neoplasia).[636,643,649] In many cases, no abnormalities can be detected on rectal examination.

Horses with localized, subacute or chronic peritonitis show chronic or intermittent colic, depression, anorexia, weight loss, intermittent fever, ventral edema, exercise intolerance, decreased or absent intestinal sounds and mild dehydration. The heart and respiratory rates may be normal. Fecal output may be normal; however, chronic diarrhea and weight loss have been reported. Alternatively, mild chronic or localized peritonitis may be characterized by loss of body condition, depression and partial anorexia without a history or evidence of abdominal discomfort. Infrequently, pleurisy, polyuria and polydipsia have been associated with chronic peritonitis. Rectal examination may reveal no abnormalities, or may reveal evidence of inflammation, adhesions or an abdominal mass.

Diagnosis: Peritonitis should be suspected in a horse with a history of predisposing factors, suggestive clinical signs and compatible laboratory data. Alterations in the peripheral blood depend on the stage of disease and primary underlying disease process. In peracute or acute peritonitis with overwhelming toxemia or contamination, severe leukopenia with absolute neutropenia and a degenerative left shift are present due to margination of neutrophils and accumulation of neutrophils in the peritoneal cavity. Protein sequestration and fluid exudation into the peritoneal cavity lead to hypoproteinemia and dehydration. An elevated packed cell volume with a proportionate increase in total plasma protein concentration may be present early in the disease, reflecting the degree of dehydra-tion. As protein loss into the abdomen continues, the packed cell volume may be elevated while a normal or disproportionally low plasma protein level exists. Serum fibrinogen concentrations are elevated if the process has been present for ≥ 48 hours.

In cases of acute peritonitis of longer duration and in localized or chronic peritonitis, the changes in the complete cell count may not be as dramatic. White blood cell counts may be normal or neutrophilic leukocytosis may be present. A small number of immature neutrophils, lymphopenia, lymphocytosis or monocytosis may be present. No correlation between peripheral WBC count and prognosis was noted in a study of 30 cases of peritonitis.[649] Hyperproteinemia due to hypergammaglobulinemia in association with hypoalbuminemia and decreased albumin:globulin ratio is frequently seen. Normocytic normochromic anemia reflective of chronic disease may be observed.

Alterations in blood chemistry values depend on the underlying cause of the peritonitis, organ compromise induced by toxemia, and hydration status of the animal. In peracute and acute peritonitis, metabolic acidosis and electrolyte (sodium, potassium, chloride) losses may be significant. Such alterations are uncommon in chronic peritonitis.

Abdominocentesis confirms peritonitis but may not identify the cause of the primary pathologic process. Peritoneal fluid may vary in quantity and color (serosanguineous, turbid, flocculent, purulent). Early in the disease, the elevation in peritoneal fluid WBC count is due primarily to an increase in polymorphonuclear cells (degenerative or nondegenerative). In more chronic cases, mononuclear-cell and macrophage numbers increase in relation to polymorphonuclear-cell numbers. Mesothelial cells may become hyperplastic and mimic neoplastic cells in chronic cases. Reportedly, WBC counts in the peritoneal fluid of horses with acute peritonitis (100,000/μl) are higher than those with chronic peritonitis (20,000-60,000/μl); however, this is not always the case.[649,650] White blood cell counts reflect the degree of peritoneal effusion and hydration status of the animal. No correlation between peripheral and peritoneal WBC counts has been noted.[649] Peritoneal protein levels are increased.

Bacteria may be seen free or phago-cytized by peritoneal leukocytes. Failure to identify bacteria on cytologic examination does not rule out septic peritonitis. Samples for Gram stain and aerobic and anaerobic cultures of the peritoneal fluid should be submitted in an attempt to identify the of-fending organism. Frequently, bacterial cul-tures may be negative when cytologic evalu-ation and Gram stain have indicated the presence of bacteria. Gram stain may be es-pecially helpful in horses that have already received antibiotic therapy or in which an anaerobic infection is present. Special transport media must be used correctly if anaerobic organisms are to be isolated.

Diagnosis of peritonitis following surgery is more difficult, as manipulation of the bowel causes an increase in the WBC count and total protein concentration in the peri-toneal cavity. Infection is suspected if the WBC appear degenerative and bacteria are present. Examination of the peritoneal fluid for plant fibers, fecal material, foreign sub-stances, bile, blood and chyle may give some indication of the disease that initiated the peritonitis.

Treatment: Early, aggressive therapy is required if treatment of peritonitis is to be successful. Treatment is based on 3 princi-ples: stabilization of the animal's condition; treatment of any infection; and isolation and correction of the primary insult or un-derlying disease process.[651] In the acute phase, primary consideration must be given to arrest of endotoxic and/or hypovolemic shock, correction of metabolic and electro-lyte abnormalities, dehydration and hypo-proteinemia, and management of pain.[646-648,651-653] An alkaline fluid is recommended for correction of metabolic acidosis. Specific electrolyte abnormalities, commonly hypo-kalemia and hypocalcemia, must be identi-fied and corrected to help reestablish ho-meostasis and gastrointestinal motility. In the absence of blood gas and electrolyte de-terminations, adequate volumes of a bal-anced electrolyte solution are recommended to correct dehydration and support the car-diovascular system. If the animal is hypo-proteinemic (total plasma protein level of <4 g/dl) and dehydrated, administration of plasma should be considered before large volumes of fluid are infused because of the risk of inducing pulmonary edema and fur-ther fluid loss into extravascular spaces.

Specific guidelines for fluid therapy and treatment of endotoxic shock are discussed elsewhere in this text. Surgical exploration after stabilization of the animal's condition may be necessary to correct the primary problem, decrease peritoneal contamina-tion, or remove a foreign body.[651]

Analgesics to relieve abdominal discom-fort and promote return to voluntary water and food consumption are recommended. Nonsteroidal antiinflammatory agents should be used cautiously in hypovolemic, hypoproteinemic, compromised horses, as toxicity may result. If gastric reflux is pres-ent, decompression through a nasogastric tube may aid in relief of pain and correction of ileus.

The mainstays of therapy in peritonitis are broad-spectrum antimicrobials and cor-rection of the underlying disease.[651-653] An-timicrobial therapy should be initiated as soon as peritonitis is diagnosed and after a sample of peritoneal fluid is obtained for culture and sensitivity testing. Delay in ini-tiation of therapy until laboratory results are returned (24-48 hours after sampling) may decrease the likelihood of a successful outcome. Antimicrobial therapy can be al-tered, if necessary, when culture and sensi-tivity results are obtained. Intravenous ad-ministration of antimicrobials is preferred in shock because of unreliable perfusion of tissues and resultant delay in uptake and distribution with other routes of admini-stration.[651-653] Infections are typically multimicrobial, involving both aerobes (*E coli, Streptococcus equi, Streptococcus zoo-epidemicus, Rhodococcus equi*) and anaer-obes (*Bacteroides, Peptostreptococcus, Clos-tridium, Fusobacterium*).[251,645,651]

In people, synergistic bacterial activity is important in the pathogenesis of peritonitis, and different organisms account for differ-ent stages or types of the disease.[251] Coli-forms (*E coli, Proteus*) may account for early death in acute bacterial peritonitis, while later intraabdominal abscess forma-tion is associated with aerobic infection.[251, 654] As peritonitis progresses, predominantly Gram-negative aerobes (primarily *E coli*) and Gram-positive anaerobes (*B fragilis*) are isolated.[655]

Antimicrobial combinations are com-monly used and decrease mortality and ab-scess formation in rat peritonitis models.[652] The peritoneal fluid level of most antimicrobials exceeds 50% of the serum level after systemic administration.[652,653] Bactericidal antibiotics are generally preferred, as the immune response and phagocyte activity may be decreased by the disease.[656,657] Aminoglycosides are effective against the majority of Gram-negative aerobes but are ineffective against anaerobes.[656,657] These drugs must be used cautiously in hypovolemic animals and animals with evidence of renal dysfunction. Though most Gram-positive aerobes and anaerobes are sensitive to penicillin, *Bacteroides fragilis* commonly is resistant to penicillin and cephalothin.[656,657] Metronidazole may be effective against anaerobes resistant to penicillin but is not effective against aerobes. In a study of 30 cases of peritonitis, 70% were treated successfully with antimicrobials and supportive therapy excluding peritoneal lavage.[649]

Intermittent drainage of abdominal fluid through a catheter or indwelling drain may be of benefit. Abdominal drainage is advocated to: remove of offending bacteria, toxic bacterial byproducts, lysosomal enzymes from degenerate neutrophils, cellular debris, blood and bacterial growth factors, and foreign matter; decrease adhesion formation and pain; increase antimicrobial contact with the peritoneal surface; and foster return of intestinal motility.[646,651,652] Complications associated with use of abdominal drains or repeated peritoneal penetration to drain fluid include retrograde infection, local irritation, pneumoperitoneum, subcutaneous seepage and cellulitis around the drain, and protein, electrolyte and fluid volume loss. If the animal is hypovolemic and hypoproteinemic, volume replacement and administration of plasma should be considered before large quantities of fluid are removed from the abdomen.

Peritoneal lavage is controversial, especially in horses with localized or chronic peritonitis in which there is the possibility of spreading infection. Lavage may be more beneficial in horses with generalized peritonitis in which little response has been seen to therapy with antimicrobials and fluid drainage. It should not, however, be used as the sole therapy. Two approaches to peritoneal lavage are commonly described: retrograde irrigation through a ventrally placed ingress-egress drain (Foley catheter); and placement of ingress catheters in both paralumbar fossae for infusion of fluids,

with placement of a drain along the ventral abdominal midline for removal of infused fluid and peritoneal exudate.[643,658] Due to the anatomy and massive amount of intestinal contents and mesentery, effective abdominal lavage is difficult in horses and the efficacy of both methods has been questioned. Greater success may be attained by peritoneal lavage at the time of surgical exploration to identify and correct the underlying cause of peritonitis. In certain instances (uroperitoneum, renal failure) in which blood chemistry derangements are severe, peritoneal dialysis has been attempted.[659]

Therapy with heparin (intravenous, subcutaneous or in peritoneal lavage fluid) has been recommended to prevent adhesion formation and to render bacteria more susceptible to cellular and noncellular clearing mechanisms. Studies on the effectiveness of heparin in preventing abdominal adhesions in other species have had inconsistent results. An experimental study in ponies with ischemic small intestine indicated that IV administration of heparin (40 U/kg) at surgery and then BID for 48 hours reduced formation of adhesions.[192]

Larvicidal doses of anthelmintics should be administered after the horse's condition is stabilized if peritonitis secondary to parasite migration or verminous arteritis is suspected.

The prognosis depends on the severity and duration of the peritonitis, primary etiologic insult and occurrence of such complications as abdominal adhesions, abdominal abscesses, laminitis and organ failure. With early, aggressive therapy and rapid correction of the primary lesion, the prognosis generally is fair to good in localized and mild acute diffuse peritonitis. In cases with severe abdominal contamination, intestinal penetration and coincident diarrhea or in chronic cases, the prognosis is poor.

Abdominal Abscesses

Cause: "Though bacteria usually are present in abscesses, neutrophils alone can cause abscess formation and are essential for their development."[642] A mixed population of bacteria, similar to the spectrum seen in diffuse peritonitis, may be associated with abscess formation in the abdominal cavity.[642] The organisms most commonly isolated from abdominal abscesses in horses include *Streptococcus equi, Streptococcus zooepidemicus, Corynebacterium pseudotuberculosis* and *Salmonella* spp.

Abdominal abscesses commonly occur as a sequel to respiratory infections and/or septicemia. The infectious agents localize in abdominal or mesenteric lymph nodes and subsequently lead to abscess formation in a variety of abdominal organs (spleen, liver, kidney, uterus). Most abscesses, however, are located in or around the mesentery. Abscesses have also been associated with umbilical infections, foreign body penetration of the small intestine, ascarid infection in foals, verminous arteritis, peritonitis, gastric granulomas and parturition accidents.[353,440,660,661] Abdominal abscesses may occur in any animal but are seen most commonly in horses less <5 years old. One study reports a higher incidence in mares than in geldings or stallions.[443]

The pathogenesis of internal abscess formation has not been delineated. It has been proposed that internal infections with *Streptococcus equi* ("bastard strangles") develop due to individual variations in the immune response to infection rather than because of any innate difference in the bacteria.[662,663] Inadequate antimicrobial levels at the site of infection and treatment before abscess maturation also have been proposed to contribute to metastatic abscess formation. Research, however, has shown that delaying treatment to allow abscess maturation does not prevent septicemia or spread of infection. Therefore, it has been suggested that penicillin may affect the streptococcal organism in a manner that results in an inadequate host immune response.[662,663] Alternatively, abscess formation may result from failure of antimicrobial therapy to control an organism already disseminated throughout the host.[662,663]

Clinical Signs: Three clinical presentations associated with abdominal abscesses have been reported. In the first syndrome, intermittent or prolonged colic may not be responsive to medical therapy. Chronic pain without intestinal obstruction may result from intestinal adhesions, stricture or compression of the bowel, or tension on the mesentery in association with the abscess. Intermittent leakage of bacteria or debris from the abscess may result in low-grade, chronic or recurrent peritonitis. Depression and anorexia are consistent findings, whereas the effects on intestinal motility are variable.[251,636] The horse may continue to defecate, but total fecal output and intestinal sounds may be depressed. Elevations in heart and respiratory rates, persistent or intermittent fever, and dehydration usually are noted.

In the second syndrome, chronic weight loss may be seen, ranging from severe emaciation to thinness with an inability to gain weight. Depression and anorexia are seen frequently. Alterations in temperature, heart rate and respiratory rate are inconsistent. Urination, defecation and intestinal sounds usually are normal, though profuse diarrhea may be present. Clinical signs reflecting specific organ involvement may occur.

In the third syndrome, acute intractable abdominal pain may occur in horses in good body flesh or with evidence of weight loss. Tension on the mesentery due to the weight of the abscess, abscess rupture or acute intestinal obstruction causes acute discomfort and deterioration in physical status, and may progress to shock. The horse may lie on its back in an attempt to relieve the pressure on the mesentery. Acute colic in foals with streptococcal abscesses of the umbilical cord and mesentery has been reported.[459] With all 3 presentations, rectal examination may reveal no abnormalities or may reveal an abdominal mass palpable within the mesentery. Adhesions or tight mesenteric bands may be felt in association with the mass.

Diagnosis: Abdominal abscess always should be considered in horses with a suggestive medical or clinical history. Previous illness due to septicemia or respiratory disease or close association with horses with *Streptococcus equi* infections should increase the level of suspicion. Horses with a history of recurrent or vague abdominal pain, weight loss and intermittent or continuous fever are prime candidates. The maintenance of good body condition and attitude, however, does not rule out an abdominal abscess.

Clinicopathologic alterations vary with the stage of abscess formation, location of the abscess and effectiveness with which the abscess is "walled off." The complete blood count may be normal, but, more often, neutrophilic leukocytosis, hyperfibrinogenemia and mild normocytic normochromic anemia are evident. A mild left shift, lymphopenia or absolute monocytosis may be seen. Neutropenia with a degenerative left shift and toxic changes in WBC may occur following leakage of toxic products from the abscess. Plasma protein and gamma globulin levels are increased, while the plasma albumin level is normal or decreased, resulting in a decreased albumin:globulin ratio.

In most affected horses, a normal or mildly elevated WBC count and protein concentration are present in the peritoneal fluid. The WBC are primarily nondegenerative neutrophils when the abscess is "walled off." Free and phagocytized bacteria may be seen if the abscess is penetrated, leaking or ruptured. The abscess may be penetrated during abdominocentesis when it is close to or attached to the ventral abdominal wall. Fluid obtained on penetration of the abscess has a marked elevation in WBC numbers and protein level. Fluid obtained by abdominocentesis or abscess aspiration should be submitted for cytologic examination, Gram stain, culture and sensitivity tests. Though intracellular and/or free bacteria may be recognized on cytologic examination, aerobic and anaerobic cultures of the peritoneal fluid may be negative.

In young foals and smaller horses, abdominal radiographs may offer some diagnostic aid. Technical limitations make abdominal radiography less diagnostic in adult horses. Ultrasonographic detection of abdominal abscesses transabdominally or may be especially helpful in foals and smaller horses. Laparoscopy or laparotomy may be necessary for definitive diagnosis (Fig 134).

Long-term antimicrobial therapy (for $\geq$ 2-6 months) with appropriate agents and adequate drug levels is the mainstay of medical therapy for an abdominal abscess. Ideally, drug selection is based on culture and sensitivity testing of abscess contents, or of peritoneal fluid if the former is not available. Major pathogens commonly associated with abdominal abscesses are sensitive to penicillin or ampicillin. When Gram-negative organisms (*E coli*, *Salmonella*) are involved, antimicrobials with an appropriate spectrum of activity (trimethoprim-sulfadiazine, gentamicin, amikacin) are included in the therapeutic regimen.

Aminoglycosides or erythromycin provide adequate coverage for abscesses secondary to *Rhodococcus equi* infection. Rifampin, because of its broad-spectrum activity, ability to penetrate and to foster penetration of other antimicrobials into abscesses, and ease of administration, frequently is included in the therapeutic regimen. Metronidazole is effective with anaerobic infections, especially those due to *Bacteroides fragilis*. After initiation of antimicrobial therapy, marked improvement in clinical status is often noted. Recurrence of clinical signs is seen frequently if antimicrobial therapy is withdrawn prematurely.

Penetration of the abscess during diagnostic abdominocentesis may allow for therapeutic drainage of the abscess. Care must be taken not to contaminate the surrounding body cavity and tissues, as peritonitis and/or cellulitis may ensue. Supportive measures include maintenance of hydration and electrolyte balance through oral or intravenous supplementation, analgesics for pain relief, and maintenance of a positive energy balance. Response to medical therapy may be evaluated by monitoring clinical signs, clinicopathologic data, peritoneal fluid cell count and protein concentration, and assessing abscess size by rectal palpation or ultrasonographic examination.

In cases of bowel obstruction, intractable pain or lack of response to medical therapy, abdominal exploration with excision or drainage of the abscess is recommended. If

Figure 134. Large abscess on the base of the cecum of a foal with abdominal discomfort and anorexia. (Courtesy of Dr. L. Hovda)

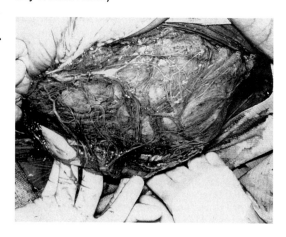

a segment of intestine or its blood supply is compromised or incorporated in the abscess, bypass of the affected area in combination with medical therapy may be attempted. Marsupialization of the abscess to the outside may help reduce the abscess without contaminating the peritoneal cavity. The abscess must be manipulated carefully, as abscess rupture with contamination of the abdomen is possible.

The prognosis depends on the size, location and causative organism of the abscess, and secondary involvement of visceral organs. Complications, including abdominal adhesions, peritonitis and laminitis, may interfere with recovery. Streptococcal abscesses often respond well to antimicrobial therapy if abdominal viscera are not extensively involved.

Abdominal Adhesions

Cause: Adhesions are bands of fibrinous material on the surface of a serous membrane and connected to an apposing surface. During the first 3 days after a peritoneal insult, fibrinous adhesions form. Infiltration of phagocytes and fibrinolytic enzymes may lead to resolution of these adhesions in 4-6 days. Alternatively, infiltration of capillaries and fibroblasts with collagen deposition leads to formation of fibrous adhesions in as few as 7-10 days.[664,665] Beneficial effects of adhesions include stabilization of mobile viscera, localization of infectious processes, prevention of visceral leakage, and structural support for neovascularization of ischemic or compromised vascular segments.[664,665] Intestinal obstruction, interference with nonintestinal organs, pain and discomfort are some deleterious side effects of adhesions that lead to clinical problems.

Adhesions commonly occur secondary to infectious, ischemic, inflammatory or traumatic insults to the bowel, peritoneum or other abdominal organs. Conditions predisposing to adhesion formation include gastrointestinal or abdominal surgery, peritonitis, abdominal abscess or tumor, penetrating abdominal wound, ischemic or devitalizing bowel disease, abdominal foreign body, dystocia, metritis, uterine rupture, castration, cryptorchid surgery, cystitis, pelvic inflammatory disease, and strongyle infection and migration.[251,665] Uncommonly, fibrous bands occur in association with embryonic anomalies (Meckel's diverticulum, mesodiverticular bands). Mesenteric herniation through or intestinal volvulus around these bands may occur.

Peritoneal adhesions frequently occur as part of the healing process following abdominal disease or surgery and remain asymptomatic. Once adhesion formation interferes with intestinal or organ function, clinical manifestations become apparent. Adhesions may lead to compression, malpositioning or stricture of the bowel, internal herniation, or interference with intestinal motility. Intestinal impaction or diarrhea may result from disruption of normal intestinal motility. Adhesions involving the large or small colon may be associated with recurrent impaction.

Clinical Signs: Clinical signs are related to the degree, location and duration of intestinal obstruction. Peritoneal adhesions result in a spectrum of syndromes ranging from acute intestinal obstruction to chronic weight loss and poor performance. Partial obstruction or alteration in intestinal motility may cause mild intermittent abdominal discomfort of up to a week or more. Painful episodes after eating, mild elevations in heart and respiratory rates, and altered intestinal sounds may be observed. Fecal output usually is decreased. Between painful episodes, the animal may appear normal. Alternatively, chronic partial obstruction may result in recurrent or chronic colic, weight loss, anorexia and/or diarrhea. On rectal examination, intermittent or chronic distention of the same bowel segment may be noted. Until complete obstruction occurs, the repeated bouts of colic appear responsive to medical therapy. Signs (decreased intestinal sounds and fecal output, pain, elevated heart and respiratory rates, intestinal distention, ileus, gastric reflux) become more severe and persistent as the obstruction progresses from incomplete to complete. Active peritonitis may be present.

Adhesions involving the reproductive organs may cause difficulty at breeding, affect conception rate or interfere with pregnancy or parturition. Urine pooling occurs if adhesions pull the uterus cranioventrad and interfere with normal outflow of urine. Chronic cystitis results from adhesions that prevent complete bladder emptying. Adhesions affecting the urogenital tract often are palpable on rectal examination.

Diagnosis: A history of previous peritoneal disease or abdominal surgery with signs of colic and/or weight loss suggests abdominal adhesions and/or abscess. After abdominal surgery, adhesions begin to form within a few hours. Rectal examination may reveal no abnormalities or may reveal evidence of bowel distention, impaction or inflammatory bowel disease. Depending upon their location, the adhesions may be palpable rectally. The significance of adhesion formation often is not confirmed until laparotomy, laparoscopy or necropsy is performed.

Clinicopathologic alterations vary with the state of adhesion formation and underlying disease. The white blood cell count and total plasma protein and fibrinogen concentrations may be normal or increased. Postoperatively, inflammatory changes in the peritoneal fluid are common and neither confirm nor rule out the possibility of adhesions. In chronic cases not associated with surgery, peritoneal fluid may be normal or may only show a mild to moderate increase in protein concentration.

Treatment: The therapeutic approach depends on the stage of maturation, location and number of adhesions, and also on involvement of adjacent viscera. Mild or chronic colic due to adhesions is clinically responsive to analgesics and medical management. Medical management using fibrinolytic agents is not effective in resolving adhesions. Heparin may be of some value as a preventive or therapeutic agent in management of adhesions.[192]

Manual separation of adhesions per rectum has been attempted in the early stage of adhesion formation. This approach is limited to the area of the abdominal cavity that is palpable rectally, by the danger of rectal perforation, and by reccurrence of adhesions. Surgical intervention to reestablish intestinal patency is required when adhesions are more than 7 days old or multiple, or when they involve adjacent viscera.[666] A single or localized adhesion may be managed successfully by separation and excision, intestinal resection and anastomosis, or intestinal bypass. Recurrence of adhesions is discouraged by oversewing all severed or roughened areas resulting from adhesion "breakdown."[251,665]

When multiple adhesions are present, the involved area is bypassed and the original adhesions are left undisturbed. Extensive adhesions involving large or multiple bowel segments and/or adjacent viscera are usually not amenable to surgical correction, and euthanasia is recommended. The prognosis always is guarded due to the progressive nature of the disease and frequency of adhesion reccurrence after surgical intervention.

Prevention of abdominal adhesions, rather than therapy, is preferred. Measures to minimize the initial insult and inflammatory response, and to control fibrinous adhesion formation and organization should be initiated when abdominal disease is suspected or abdominal surgery is performed. Minimizing tissue trauma and peritoneal contamination by blood, bacteria or foreign bodies discourages adhesion formation. Antiinflammatory agents must be used judiciously so as not to interfere with normal healing.

Uroperitoneum

Uroperitoneum, or urine within the peritoneal cavity, occurs following rupture of the bladder, urachus, ureter or kidney. Usually it is seen in neonatal foals due to traumatic rupture of the bladder or urachus during parturition. Though congenital weaknesses may make a bladder more susceptible to rupture during parturition or following urachal closure, this is not the primary cause of uroperitoneum. The reported frequency of bladder rupture in foals ranges from 0.2% to 2.5%; most cases occur in males.[667] Bladder rupture is not common in adults. In any aged horse, rupture may occur secondary to urethral obstruction with calculi or blunt trauma, or during urinary catheterization. In mares, bladder rupture may result from trauma during parturition. Rupture of the ureter and kidney is uncommon and usually is traumatic in origin.

Uroperitoneum causes chemical peritonitis. Clinical signs are often nonspecific, making early diagnosis difficult. Depression, anorexia, mild abdominal discomfort, straining, and passage of small amounts of urine may be observed within 24-36 hours of bladder rupture in foals.[667] In adult horses with induced bladder rupture, physical responses were absent until 50 hours after rupture, when elevation in heart and respiratory rates, mild colic, anorexia and abdominal distention were noted.[668] Clinical signs of uroperitoneum, including abdominal distention, generally are less striking in adult horses than in foals. Ballottement of the abdomen to detect a fluid wave is more rewarding in foals. Rupture of the urachus is clinically indistinguishable from rupture of the bladder. Clinical signs may develop more slowly following perforation or rupture of one ureter.

Uroperitoneum causes few changes in the hemogram. Elevations in PCV and total plasma protein concentration occur as the animal becomes dehydrated. A stress leukogram often is noted. If chemical peritonitis progresses to septic peritonitis, neutropenia with a left shift may be seen. Serum electrolyte changes become striking as uroperitoneum progresses. Hyponatremia, hyperkalemia and hypochloremia are observed consistently.[667,668] Decreased serum osmolality and increased serum creatinine and urea nitrogen levels also occur.[667,668] Metabolic acidosis may be present. The severity of these changes is related to the duration of uroperitoneum and the initiating cause. Changes are less striking following ureter or kidney rupture, as compensation by the remaining healthy ureter or kidney may mask some of the electrolyte and biochemical disturbances.

Varying quantities of a clear to turbid yellow fluid are obtained on abdominocentesis. Inconsistently, an ammonia odor to the fluid may be observed. Heating the fluid may accentuate the ammonia odor. Hematologic and cytologic examinations of fluid show an inflammatory response. Elevated potassium, inorganic phosphorus and creatinine levels are observed in the peritoneal fluid.[667,668] An elevated blood urea nitrogen level is seen less consistently. The ratio of peritoneal fluid creatinine to serum creatinine levels is the most useful antemortem laboratory diagnostic aid.[668]

A ruptured bladder, urachus or ureter may be delineated by contrast radiography in foals. Recovery of the dye in the peritoneal fluid after instillation of dye into the bladder suggests rupture of the bladder or urachus. Rupture of the kidney is often not diagnosed until exploratory laparotomy or necropsy. Measures to correct serum electrolyte and acid-base abnormalities usually are undertaken before surgical correction of the primary cause of urine leakage. Perito-

neal dialysis has been used successfully to correct electrolyte derangements before surgery in foals.[659]

Verminous Mesenteric Arteritis

Cause: Mesenteric thromboarteritis associated with migration of *Strongylus vulgaris* larvae can be found in most horses. Though several clinical entities have been associated with larval migration, most infections are asymptomatic. Development of clinical signs depends on the number of larvae involved, period over which larvae are acquired, number and size of arteries affected, and age and immune status of the host.[229,669,670]

The cranial mesenteric artery and its ileocecocolic branch are the vessels most commonly and severely affected by migration of the strongyle larvae.[353] Larval migration within the cranial mesenteric artery and its major branches and the body's reaction to this insult have been termed "verminous arteritis."[670] Infarction of gut segments (nonstrangulating infarction, thromboembolic colic), mesenteric hemorrhage, infected verminous aneurysm and abdominal abscess formation, and impaired nervous innervation to the intestine all have been associated with verminous mesenteric arteritis.[229,669,670]

Common lesions associated with larval migration are edema, hemorrhage and cellular infiltration in the wall of the intestine, and inflammation, thrombus formation and marked thickening of the branches of the cranial mesenteric artery.[669,670] Thickening of the arterial wall results from leukocyte infiltration, edema and connective tissue replacement of elastic and muscle fibers of the media. Mineralization of the arterial wall may occur. Ischemia and necrosis of the intestinal wall secondary to alterations in intestinal blood supply contribute to nonstrangulating infarction (thromboembolic colic) of the intestine.

Clinical Signs: Clinical signs most commonly associated with larval migration are recurrent or intermittent abdominal discomfort (colic), chronic weight loss or chronic diarrhea. During the prepatent period, heavy larval burdens may produce acute illness in horses of any age, but suckling and weanling foals appear most susceptible.[671] Diarrhea, fever, depression, anorexia, colic and occasionally death may result. Yearlings are more prone to emaciating disease.[671] Chronic diarrhea has been associated with cecal and colonic ulceration as a result of migration of larvae back into the intestine.

Though migrating larvae have been incriminated as a frequent cause of colic in horses, evidence for and definition of the role that migrating larvae play is lacking.[670] Suggested mechanisms by which larvae may induce colic include: penetration of the wall of the ileum by ingested larvae with hemorrhage into the intestinal wall; migration against arterial blood flow, causing arterial irritation, thrombus formation, and altered intestinal blood flow; reduced blood flow and altered intestinal motility due to a thrombus, aneurysm or abscess in the cranial mesenteric artery and its major branches, with a predisposition to intestinal displacement, impaction or necrosis; chronic lesions with arterial wall thickening, dilatation or narrowing of the arterial lumen, and alterations in blood flow; occlusion and erosion of small arteries as the larvae leave the mesenteric arterial branches to return to the cecum and large colon; and impaired innervation of the intestine by pressure on or stretching of the nerves as a result of the arterial lesion, release of toxins by degenerating larvae, or hypersensitivity or allergic response to *S vulgaris*.[229,669,670]

Diagnosis: The diagnosis of verminous arteritis is often based on a history of a poor deworming program, compatible clinical signs, elimination of other causes of diarrhea, colic and weight loss, and response to therapy. On rectal examination, a mass in the cranial mesenteric artery or its proximal branches may be palpated. Fremitus may or may not be felt in the artery. The significance of these rectal findings in relation to presenting clinical signs is questionable. With a heavy parasite burden, adult strongyles may be observed in the feces or on the rectal sleeve after rectal palpation. Peripheral eosinophilia, anemia, hyperproteinemia and hyperbetaglobulinemia (especially IgG [T]) suggest parasite infection but do not confirm verminous arteritis.[229,672] Turbid to hemorrhagic peritoneal fluid with elevated protein levels and neutrophil, eosinophil and red blood cell counts

may be seen. Verminous arteritis and nonstrangulating infarction often are not confirmed until exploratory laparotomy or necropsy. Other causes of colic, chronic weight loss or chronic diarrhea must be carefully ruled out before verminous mesenteric arteritis can be diagnosed with any certainty.

Treatment: The therapeutic approach depends on the history, clinical signs and degree of systemic involvement. When verminous mesenteric arteritis is the suspected cause of weight loss, or for chronic or intermittent colic in horses without evidence of bowel infarction, anthelmintic therapy at larvicidal doses is indicated. Anthelmintics considered effective include thiabendazole PO at 440 mg/kg on 2 successive days, fenbendazole PO at 50 mg/kg on 3 successive days or at 10-15 mg/kg on 5 successive days, or ivermectin at 0.2 mg/kg as a single dose repeated every 4-8 weeks for a total of 3 doses. Horses should be carefully observed for signs of colic or laminitis following deworming. Nonsteroidal antiinflammatory agents are often administered concurrently to decrease this risk and to alleviate any adverse inflammatory response following killing of the parasites. The prognosis for horses with verminous arteritis without intestinal infarction is fair to good.

Horses with intestinal infarction are usually hypovolemic and endotoxemic, and have significant metabolic and electrolyte derangements. Extensive fluid therapy for cardiovascular support and correction of metabolic derangements is often necessary. Nonsteroidal antiinflammatory agents and anti-endotoxin antiserum (Endoserum: Imvac, Columbia, MO) may be helpful in controlling endotoxemia. After the patient is stabilized, intestinal resection and anastomosis are indicated if infarcted intestine is present. Surgical correction is only possible if the lesion is focal and damage not extensive. Nonstrangulating infarction is a progressive disease, and further infarction may occur in bowel that appeared healthy at surgery. Thus, the prognosis remains guarded. Horses that recover following intestinal resection should be treated with larvicidal doses of anthelmintics when their condition is considered stable. The prognosis is guarded due to the possibility of progression of the disease.

Neoplasia

Neoplasms of the Peritoneum and Abdominal Cavity

Neoplasia of the abdominal cavity is rare in horses. Malignant tumors are found in only 0.5-0.8% of all necropsies.[636] Primary gastrointestinal neoplasia is rare, with an estimated incidence of <0.1% at necropsy.[212] Squamous-cell carcinoma of the stomach and alimentary form of lymphosarcoma are the most common primary neoplasms, but lipoma of the mesentery, adenocarcinoma, leiomyoma and ameloblastic odontoma have also been reported.[23,212,673,674] Malignant melanoma, transitional-cell carcinoma, multicentric lymphosarcoma, adenocarcinoma, reticulosarcoma, teratoma and others may metastasize to the intestinal tract and the abdominal cavity.[212,636,637] Primary neoplasia of the equine peritoneum has not been reported. Several tumor types (squamous-cell carcinoma, hemangiosarcoma, lymphosarcoma, mesothelioma, malignant melanoma) can spread throughout the abdominal cavity and may involve the peritoneal surface.[23,212,636,637,673-680]

Most abdominal neoplasms occur in middle-aged to older horses, though they may be observed at any age. Alimentary lymphosarcoma is not uncommonly observed in younger horses, and lymphosarcoma has been reported in foals.[219,680]

Clinical Signs: Clinical signs depend on location, size and extent of metastasis of the tumor, and degree of secondary intestinal or lymphatic obstruction. Neoplasms causing intestinal obstruction may induce an acute abdominal crisis characterized by violent colic and rapid deterioration of the animal. Lymphosarcoma, mesothelioma and pedunculated lipoma also have been associated with acute colic.[212,637,676]

More commonly, onset of neoplastic disease is insidious, with nonspecific clinical signs. Chronic weight loss, anorexia, depression, exercise intolerance, icterus and intermittent or chronic colic are common. Diarrhea, ascites and edema of the limbs, prepuce or ventral abdomen are noted less consistently. If peritoneal effusion is prominent, pleural effusion may also be present.

An abdominal mass or mesenteric lymphadenopathy may be identified on rectal examination. Rapid deterioration of the horse's condition may be seen later.

Diagnosis: Neoplasia may be suspected from the history, clinical signs, rectal palpation and clinicopathologic alterations. Though hematologic findings may be normal, alterations suggesting chronic disease or inflammation often accompany neoplasia. Anemia, neutrophilic leukocytosis, hyperproteinemia, hypoalbuminemia and hyperfibrinogenemia are frequently present. Abnormal circulating lymphocytes, elevated serum alkaline phosphatase. glucose/xylose malabsorption, lactic dehydrogenase or sorbitol dehydrogenase activities and immunologic dysfunction may be seen with lymphosarcoma.[219,677-681] Hypercalcemia has been seen with lymphosarcoma, squamous-cell carcinoma and malignant mesenchymoma.[682]

Neoplasms do not usually exfoliate in the peritoneal fluid, with the exception of lymphosarcoma. Often it is difficult to differentiate inflammatory changes in the peritoneal fluid secondary to neoplasia from similar changes caused by infectious peritonitis. Melanin granules in macrophages may suggest malignant melanoma. Bloody peritoneal fluid with increased RBC and WBC cell counts (predominantly mononuclear cells) may occur with carcinoma, hemangiosarcoma and other necrotizing neoplasms.[650] A mass may be detected by radiographic or ultrasonographic examination of the abdomen, depending on its size and location, size of the animal and equipment available.

Diagnosis of abdominal neoplasia usually is not confirmed until biopsies obtained at laparotomy or necropsy are examined. Histologic examination of neoplastic tissue is necessary to identify origin of the neoplasm.

Treatment: Response to medical and surgical therapy is generally poor. A temporary improvement in condition may be noted with antimicrobial or corticosteroid therapy. Discrete, localized neoplasms (*eg*, lipoma) may be successfully resected. Attempts to resect solitary lymphosarcoma lesions in the intestine have met with little success.[683]

Multifactorial Diseases

Ascites

Ascites is a sign of disease rather than a disease in itself. It is defined as a collection of serous fluid within the peritoneal cavity. The accumulated fluid may be adipose (fatty), biliary, chylous, exudative, hemorrhagic, hydremic, pseudochylous or transudative.

Cause: Ascites results from transudation or exudation of fluid from the surface of the liver or from the surfaces of the gut and mesentery.[684] Uroperitoneum is a special type of ascites. The mechanism by which ascites occurs is complex and incompletely understood. Factors implicated in formation of ascites include portal hypertension, hypoalbuminemia and renal retention of sodium and water.[639] In liver disease, decreased serum osmotic pressure due to hypoalbuminemia and portal hypertension result in movement of fluid into the peritoneal cavity and other extravascular spaces. According to the "traditional" theory of ascites, renal sodium retention in response to a decreased effective circulating plasma volume occurs secondary to ascites.[639] More recently, the "overflow" theory suggested that a primary inability of the kidneys to excrete sodium and water results in water and sodium retention.[639]

A *transudate* is colorless with a low cell count ($<9000/\mu l$), low protein level (<3 g/dl) and specific gravity of <1.015. It usually occurs due to congestion in the area of the portal vein or vena cava. Subacute or chronic hepatic disease, renal disease, congestive heart failure and tumors of the mediastinum may be accompanied by a fluid transudate.[636] Hypoproteinemia secondary to parasitism and protein-losing renal disease may also induce ascites.

An *exudate* is white, yellow or pink, with a high cell count ($>5000/\mu l$), high protein level (3 g/dl) and specific gravity of >1.015. Neoplastic and inflammatory lesions of the abdominal cavity and gastrointestinal tract often produce an exudate.[636] A bloody exudate that is high in RBC and WBC but of low volume occurs with intestinal necrosis. Neoplasia of the abdominal cavity and organs may be associated with large volumes

of a turbid or hemorrhagic exudate.[650] Chyloabdomen, due to impaired lymphatic drainage or erosion of the lymphatics, has been reported in a foal with an abdominal abscess.[644] Rupture of the bladder, ureter or kidney in adult horses and newborn foals results in uroperitoneum.

Clinical Signs: Clinical signs reflect the underlying disease process. In horses, ascites often is not visibly evident until massive fluid accumulation is present. Nonspecific abdominal distention with dyspnea suggests ascites. Ascites usually occurs secondary to a chronic debilitating disease; anorexia, weight loss, weakness, lethargy and dependent edema are observed frequently. Rectal examination may reveal no abnormalities, or the intestine may appear to "float" in the abdomen when massive fluid accumulation is present.[636] Fibrin deposits and/or adhesions may be palpable when the underlying cause is an inflammatory process, abdominal tumor, abscess or hematoma.[636] Occasionally an abdominal mass may be palpable rectally.

Diagnosis: The history, clinical signs and clinicopathologic data reflect the primary disease. In foals and small horses, a fluid wave may be appreciated on ballottement of the abdomen. In larger horses, due to their size and tightness of the abdominal musculature, ballottement of the abdomen is less productive. Ascites is diagnosed definitively by abdominocentesis. The character of the fluid is determined by the underlying disease. Radiographic examination of the abdomen may be helpful in foals or small horses. A loss of contrast or a hazy, opaque, "ground glass" appearance to the abdominal cavity suggests fluid accumulation. Due to technical limitations, this may be difficult to appreciate. Ultrasonographic examination also may help identify excessive fluid in the peritoneal cavity. Ascites must be differentiated from other causes of abdominal distention, such as pregnancy, hydroallantois, intestinal tympany and dilatation or torsion of the large colon.

Treatment: Therapy and prognosis are determined by the underlying disease. Except for uroperitoneum following bladder, urachal or ureter rupture, ascites usually warrants a guarded to grave prognosis. Therapy usually is not attempted.

DISEASES OF THE ABDOMINAL WALL

E.P. Tulleners

Congenital and Familial Diseases

Umbilical Hernia

Cause: Umbilical hernias occur in an estimated 0.5-2% of foals. Proposed causes include manually breaking the umbilical cord, excessive straining, umbilical cord ligation, umbilical cord trauma and umbilical cord infection.[685] In foals, most umbilical hernias are small (<5 cm) and uncomplicated by underlying organic diseases. As such, they represent a cosmetic defect and potential site of bowel incarceration.[686]

Treatment: Rarely, evisceration occurs immediately postpartum as a result of trauma to the umbilical cord. This condition necessitates emergency surgical reconstruction of the abdominal wall. Preoperative administration of broad-spectrum antibiotics, appropriate intravenous fluid therapy, and colostrum should be provided before or in conjunction with administration of general anesthesia. The exposed bowel must be cleansed meticulously with copious volumes of sterile balanced polyionic electrolyte solution or isotonic saline before being replaced in the abdominal cavity. After transfixation ligation and excision of remaining umbilical cord remnants, abdominal wall closure may be performed with a synthetic absorbable suture material such as #1 polyglactin 910. Closure of the subcutaneous tissue and skin is done with small-diameter synthetic absorbable suture material placed in a simple-continuous pattern.

Routine small umbilical hernias are non-painful and completely reducible. A watch-and-wait attitude may be adopted with daily reduction performed by owners. Because of the more sloping contour of the foal's abdomen and relatively caudal position of the umbilicus, abdominal bandaging is not as effective as in calves. Usually the cotton and elastic tape bandage slips caudally, producing a "bucking strap effect" and causing considerable annoyance to the foal.

If the hernia is not resolved by 4-6 months of age, intervention is necessary. Hernia clamps may be custom made by bisecting a length of dowel rod and drilling transverse holes at either end, to which a screw and wingnut can be attached. Alternatively, commercially available clamps may be used. The hernia to be clamped should be less than 5 cm in diameter and completely reducible. The foal should undergo a complete physical examination and should not be fed for 24 hours before induction of general anesthesia with a short-acting agent. Ideally, the foal is placed in dorsal recumbency and the umbilical area is clipped and aseptically prepared. Viscera are massaged into the abdominal cavity and traction is placed on the overlying skin and peritoneum of the hernial sac with 3 thyroid traction or Babcock forceps placed at equal intervals. The hernia clamps then are applied gently and extreme caution is exercised to be certain no abdominal viscera are interposed between the clamp edges. Then the clamps are positioned against the body wall and the wingnut is tightened. The clamp and wingnuts may be padded to prevent abrasions.

Hernia clamps work by producing ischemic necrosis in the exposed hernial sac. Inflammation on the abdominal wall induces fibroblast infiltration and healing by collagen deposition (fibrosis). The clamp and hernial sac usually slough in 10-12 days and the skin defect subsequently heals in 7-10 days by second intention through contraction and epithelialization.[686]

If surgical closure of the hernia is contemplated, it should be done when the animal is about 6 months of age. The animal should be placed under general anesthesia and positioned in dorsal recumbency, and aseptic techniques used. The open technique of excising the hernial sac containing skin and peritoneum is preferred. A gently curving elliptic incision is made around either side of the hernial defect. The dissection is extended down to the white fascia of the hernial ring, paying particular attention not to stray too far laterally.

In completely reducible, uncomplicated hernias, the hernial sac is tented up and a small incision is made with Metzenbaum scissors in an area devoid of any palpable contents. The surgeon's finger is introduced into the hernial sac and the hernial ring palpated circumferentially for any viscera. The hernial sac incision is extended to the hernial ring and the sac is excised circumferentially at the body wall. Closure of defects less than 5 cm long is completed with a simple-interrupted pattern using #2 polyglactin 910 or other synthetic absorbable suture material. Alternatively, 25-ga stainless-steel wire or monofilament nonabsorbable suture material may be used.

Other appropriate suture patterns include cruciate or near-far-far-near patterns. The imbricating Mayo mattress ("vest over pants") pattern does not have any advantages over a simple appositional technique closure in people.[686] In rabbits, the bursting strength of the wounds closed with imbricating techniques decreases almost proportionally to the extent of the overlapping.[686] Subcutaneous tissue is closed with 0 or 2-0 synthetic absorbable material in a simple continuous pattern and the skin with 0 or 2-0 synthetic nonabsorbable or monofilament absorbable material, such as polydioxanone.

Incarceration of intestine in an umbilical hernia occurs in 2-10% of cases, usually in foals 6 months or older with large hernias.[685] Foals with strangulated umbilical hernias have swelling, warmth and firmness of the hernial sac. The umbilical mass may be partially reducible or not reducible. Abdominal pain or enterocutaneous fistulae occasionally may be seen.

Correction of intestinal incarceration is by open reduction, with the foal under general anesthesia as previously described for excision of umbilical cord remnants. If an enterocutaneous fistula is present, this should be temporarily closed by inverting the skin edges over the defect with a continuous Lembert suture of #2 nylon. If the mass cannot be reduced, a 10- to 15-cm celiotomy is made just cranial to the hernial ring. Bowel and/or omentum can then be freed. If an enterocutaneous fistula is present, the mass can be removed *en bloc*. This is accomplished by elliptically excising around the viscera, guided by a hand placed in the abdomen. After tending to the specific visceral problem by reduction of healthy bowel or resection and anastomosis if devitalized bowel is encountered, the abdominal wall defect is closed with simple-in-

terrupted sutures of #2 polyglactin 910. Alternatively, #2 nylon or stainless-steel wire can be used if the surgical site has not been contaminated. If contamination is severe or the defect is fairly large, reconstruction with full-thickness body wall closure should be considered strongly.

Large (>5-10 cm) umbilical hernias are seen occasionally in older foals or secondary to disruption of previous herniorrhaphy attempts. In the absence of infection, prosthetic reconstruction with synthetic mesh should be performed.[687]

Inguinal Hernia

Nonstrangulating congenital inguinal hernias are occasionally encountered in young colts, but these hernias usually resolve without surgery during the first few months of life. If the hernia appears relatively small, the colt can be confined to a box stall and observed, or the owner can be instructed to manually reduce the hernia several times daily to encourage closure. Larger hernias may benefit from support provided by a figure-eight inguinal bandage constructed from roll cotton, gauze and 4-inch elastic bandage material passed between the colt's legs and over the opposite side of the tail head. Initial reduction and bandaging may require heavy sedation with xylazine. Alternatively, it may be necessary to cast the animal into lateral recumbency or even administer a short-acting intravenous anesthetic. Care must be exercised to avoid incorporating the colt's penis into the bandage because of the risk of urine contamination. The foal should be restricted to a box stall and carefully observed for abdominal discomfort, mobility, freedom to urinate and defecate, and general attitude. The bandage should be checked for looseness daily and changed every 2-3 days to avoid soiling and rub sores.

Congenital inguinal hernias occasionally persist beyond 6 months of age or an excessive amount of bowel herniates through the defect, causing abdominal discomfort or inappetence. In these instances, manual reduction and conservative bandaging management techniques may be impossible. In most foals, the bowel remains within the common vaginal tunic. Occasionally, however, the tunic is disrupted, allowing dissection of small intestine into subcutaneous planes on the medial aspect of the foal's thighs. If not corrected, the hernia may approach 20 cm in diameter, resulting in excoriation of overlying skin.

Bilateral suture closure of the external inguinal rings is performed using aseptic technique with the foal under general inhalation anesthesia and positioned in dorsal recumbency. Reduction usually occurs spontaneously when the foal is rolled onto its back but may be facilitated by elevating the animal's hindquarters slightly. A 10- to 15-cm incision is made parallel and just medial to the affected inguinal ring. After incising the subcutaneous fascia, the external ring is exposed manually by blunt dissection. The testis is isolated by disrupting the scrotal ligament and stripping off any peritunical soft tissue attachments. Reduction of the hernia usually can be maintained by placing mild traction on the testis and twisting the common vaginal tunic on its longitudinal axis. The testis and cord can be removed by routine emasculation, followed by oversewing the transected tunic or placement of a transfixation ligature. The external inguinal ring(s) are closed with simple-interrupted sutures of synthetic absorbable material. The subcutaneous fascia and skin are closed separately with 2-0 polydioxanone in a simple-continuous pattern.

Two techniques are available if the testis must be preserved. Through an inguinal approach, the common vaginal tunic and the external inguinal ring are isolated. The hernia is reduced and confirmed distally, if necessary, through a small vertical incision into the common vaginal tunic adjacent to the external inguinal ring. The common vaginal tunic is imbricated to within a few millimeters of the spermatic cord with a series of interrupted or continuous mattress sutures using 0 or 2-0 synthetic absorbable suture. The external inguinal ring is closed from cranial to caudal with simple-interrupted absorbable suture, size 1 or 2 depending on the foal's age, allowing about 25-30 mm (width of 1-2 fingers) for the common vaginal tunic and cord structures. The remainder of the closure is routine. The success rate with this technique is estimated to be 50%; the remaining incisions dehisce and require revision.

The second technique involves partial closure of the vaginal ring. This may be used initially or if the previously described techniques fail. Though this technique is more difficult to perform in older foals or yearlings, it may provide a more secure closure. In young foals with bilateral hernias, the vaginal rings may be approached through a caudal midline incision. In older foals and yearlings, the affected ring is approached through a caudal (prepubic) paramedian incision made large enough to admit one hand. The hernia is reduced, and the vaginal ring palpated internally and the cord externally to be certain that only structures associated with the spermatic cord pass through the vaginal ring. Exposure is facilitated by large hand-held or self-retaining retractors and by using moistened laparotomy sponges to isolate the intestines.

Partial closure of the vaginal ring is achieved from cranial to caudal with simple-interrupted sutures of synthetic absorbable material size 0, 1 or 2. The sutures are preplaced to allow about 15-20 mm for the cord structures to exit. The fascia of the internal and external rectus muscles are closed in 2 layers with simple-interrupted, synthetic absorbable sutures. Subcutaneous tissue and skin are closed routinely. The animal should be restricted to a box stall for 30 days during the early phases of wound healing. Mild abdominal discomfort and scrotal edema may be treated with judicious use of small doses of phenylbutazone of flunixin meglumine.

Diseases With Physical Causes

Incisional Hernias With Acute Total Dehiscence

Acute dehiscence of properly sutured ventral midline incisions is rare in horses. Because of its ventral position, however, total disruption of the incision leads to evisceration, which may be catastrophic. Abdominal distention, incisional trauma from excessive struggling during recovery from general anesthesia or postoperatively from rolling associated with uncontrolled pain, and severe postoperative debility due to diarrheal disease or peritonitis may be factors in breakdown of the incision. Of these, the 2 most common factors involved are excessive postoperative incisional trauma and wound infection.

Disruption of the incision usually occurs in the first 3-8 days postoperatively and is preceded by a brown serosanguineous discharge from the wound 24 hours before dehiscence. Early recognition of dehiscence may be facilitated by observing excessive peritoneal fluid leaking from the incision and by palpating gaps in the sutured abdominal wall.[688] Support of the wound may be provided by an elastic bandage that encircles the abdomen and by sterile compresses. Bandaging cannot prevent evisceration, however.

Once incisional disruption is recognized, emergency reconstructive surgery is necessary with the horse positioned in dorsal recumbency under general inhalation anesthesia.[688] After aseptic preparation of the wound, all sutures are removed. All infected and devitalized tissue along the wound edge is sharply excised, until the wound margins appear healthy and are bleeding. Samples of appropriate tissues are submitted for aerobic and anaerobic bacterial cultures. Protecting the abdominal viscera with saline-moistened laparotomy sponges, the incision is copiously lavaged with sterile physiologic saline containing 10% povidone-iodine, 0.5% chlorhexidine or another appropriate antimicrobial solution. Excessive fluid is removed by suction.

Monofilament stainless-steel wire (22-ga) is used to close the abdominal wound. Interrupted vertical mattress sutures are placed through all layers of the body wall (Fig 135). The sutures are spaced 2-3 cm apart and are passed through skin, fascia and rectus abdominis muscle about 5 cm from the wound edge. The wire then is passed through a 2.5-cm length of hard rubber tubing before placing the close bites of the ver-

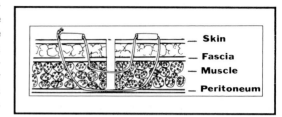

Figure 135. Diagrammatic cross-section of a ventral abdominal wound, showing placement of a vertical mattress retention suture. (Courtesy of *JAVMA*)

tical mattress pattern. These bites are taken about 2.5 cm from the wound edge and only through the skin and fascia, thus minimizing eversion of tissue. After completing the near bite, a second piece of hard rubber tubing is placed over the needle to reduce the tendency of the wire to cut the skin and underlying tissue. All sutures are preplaced and the wound is closed by putting tension on all sutures simultaneously. The ends of the wire sutures are then twisted together with a wire twister or Vice-Grips. The ends beyond the twists are cut and the twisted wire is bent back into the lumen of the rubber tubing. If the tissues are infected, the skin edges are left unsutured to facilitate drainage (Fig 136).

After the horse recovers from general anesthesia, the incision is protected with 55 x 55-cm sterile abdominal compresses secured with 15-cm-wide roll gauze and elastic adhesive bandage material. This initial compress is changed within 24 hours to remove effluent from the wound and thereafter as needed every 48-72 hours. Abdominal bandaging is continued until the incisions have healed (about 30 days). The horse is restricted to a box stall for 60 days, with handwalking permitted after 30 days. Alter-

Figure 136. Ventral abdomen of a Thoroughbred mare after abdominal reconstruction with stainless-steel wire and retention sutures.

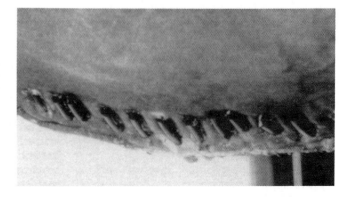

nate wire sutures and rubber tubing are removed beginning on the fourteenth day after surgery, and all remaining sutures are removed by the twenty-first day. Any evidence of local infection due to pressure necrosis is treated with povidone-iodine or chlorhexidine scrub and by flushing draining tracts with 10% povidone-iodine or 0.5% chlorhexidine in physiologic saline solution. Broad-spectrum parenteral antibiotics (penicillin and gentamicin) are administered perioperatively with adjustments in coverage determined by culture results and progression of wound healing. Prolonged administration of antibiotics usually is not necessary.

Traumatic Hernia

Traumatic hernias occur primarily from blunt trauma, such as kicks or injuries involving fence posts or farm machinery. Large penetrating abdominal wounds may require immediate debridement and reconstruction to treat or prevent evisceration. If the surrounding tissue has been traumatized extensively, stainless-steel wire retention sutures placed in a vertical mattress pattern over hard rubber tubing through the full thickness of the body wall may be necessary.[688]

More commonly, traumatic wounds are not penetrating and the horse can be treated with debridement, local therapy and, if necessary, abdominal bandaging. After inflammation has subsided and soft tissue healing has occurred in 30-60 days, residual defects in the body wall are treated by primary suture apposition or, if very large, by prosthetic reconstruction with synthetic mesh.[687]

Inflammatory, Infectious and Immune Disease

Umbilical Cord Remnant Infection

Umbilical cord remnant infections are an infrequent but potentially serious problem that may be caused by poor umbilical hygiene and a dirty environment at the time of birth.[689] Most affected foals are less than 3 weeks old and show heat, swelling, pain on palpation and discharge of urine or purulent material from the umbilicus. Though one or more umbilical structures may be af-

fected, patent urachus is seen most commonly. Ultrasonography may be useful in delineating which structures are involved and the extent of involvement. Bacterial septicemia with dissemination to other organs, particularly bone, joint and lung, is a common serious sequela; hence, surgical extirpation is recommended.

Surgical correction begins as described for uncomplicated umbilical hernias. Strict adherence to aseptic technique, meticulous hemostasis, and careful soft tissue handling is essential to reduce the incidence of subsequent intestinal obstruction due to adhesions. After exposing the hernial ring, the abdomen is entered on the midline just cranial to the umbilical remnants through a 10- to 15-cm celiotomy. The umbilical vein, which runs cranially to the liver, is isolated and divided between transfixation ligatures. The remaining umbilical mass can be defined and avoided by placing one hand in the abdominal cavity and continuing the sharp dissection elliptically around the perimeter.

The umbilical arteries and urachus are isolated as the entire mass is reflected caudally. The umbilical arteries are divided between transfixation ligatures at an appropriate level proximal to sites of infection and adjacent to the bladder. The bladder may be drained by catheterization but, preferably, may be emptied through a needle and rubber tubing using suction decompression, thus avoiding gross contamination of the abdomen with urine. After isolating the bladder and urachal remnant from the remaining abdominal viscera with saline-moistened laparotomy sponges, the bladder is stabilized and suspended by Babcock forceps placed 1-2 cm from either end of the proposed site for cystectomy.

The urachal remnant then is excised by partial fundic cystectomy. The bladder is closed with 2 inverting layers using a Lembert followed by a Cushing pattern with 3-0 polyglactin 910 suture material on a tapered needle. Abdominal wall closure is as described previously. If there is concern about hypoproteinemia or abdominal wall contamination, 22- to 25-ga stainless-steel wire or #1 or #2 synthetic nonabsorbable suture may be used to provide prolonged suture tensile strength with minimal reactivity.

Broad-spectrum antibiotics are administered intravenously after removal of the mass. Tissue or fluid obtained during surgery should be submitted for appropriate aerobic and anaerobic cultures to help determine the necessity and extent of postoperative antimicrobial therapy. Enteric Gram-negative and streptococcal organisms are commonly isolated from these structures.

If extensive involvement of the umbilical vein precludes safe transection of the umbilical remnant, the condition may be treated by marsupialization of the vein adjacent to the liver through a separate stab incision to the right of the abdominal incision. After securing the vein to the external fascia of the rectus abdominis muscle and the skin, the primary abdominal incision should be closed. The umbilical vein is then opened, drained and flushed after the foal recovers from general anesthesia.

Multifactorial Diseases

Incisional Hernias

Cause: Large defects in the abdominal wall requiring prosthetic reconstruction with synthetic mesh are uncommon in horses. These defects most commonly arise from partial incisional dehiscence after ventral midline celiotomy or following failed umbilical herniorrhaphy. Careful soft tissue handling and aseptic technique, attention to proper suture selection in terms of size and material, and proper suture placement allow for first-intention healing in a high percentage of cases. One study indicated that incisional edema, drainage, and a history of a previous ventral midline incision were associated with an increased risk of herniation.[690] In that study of 210 horses undergoing midline celiotomy, the incidence of incisional hernias was 16%, and all hernias were evident within 4 months of surgery.

The same factors responsible for acute total wound disruption may, in less severe cases, result in partial dehiscence and eventual hernia formation. Incisional infection precedes hernia formation in most cases. Incisional trauma from excessive struggling during recovery from general anesthesia or during uncontrolled bouts of postoperative pain may weaken the closure or predispose to bacterial infection. In some horses, chronic debility from low-grade peritonitis or protein-losing enteritis, as in salmonellosis, may result in partial wound breakdown.

Treatment: In most horses, primary wound healing proceeds unimpeded without the need for abdominal bandaging. If a serious wound infection develops or if gaps in the abdominal wall are palpable, chronic abdominal support with a snug elastic bandage is strongly recommended. The wound should be cultured for aerobic and anaerobic bacterial growth and, when economically feasible, the animal should be treated with an appropriate antimicrobial agent based on the sensitivity of the organism. Several skin sutures should be removed to facilitate drainage, and as much exudate as possible should be expressed frequently using aseptic technique. Initially, sterile abdominal compresses may need to be changed once or twice daily if the exudate is copious. If the infection is localized, flushing is not recommended due to the likelihood of disseminating the infection. Generalized incisional infections may be flushed once or twice daily with 10% povidone-iodine or 0.5% chlorhexidine solution in 1 L of physiologic saline using sterile tubing and aseptic technique.

Chronic abdominal bandaging for 1 or 2 months during treatment of wound infections usually limits the overall size of the subsequent hernia. Some small body-wall defects may not require reconstruction due to fibroplasia adjacent to the defect and in subcutaneous tissue.

Ideally, all infection should be eradicated before prosthetic reconstruction of the defect with knit polypropylene mesh (Marlex: Davol, Cranston, RI) or woven plastic mesh (Proxplast: Goshen Labs, Goshen, NY). Both types of mesh are strong, elastic and inert, have high melting points and resist infection. Granulation tissue and capillaries can grow through the interstices of both types of mesh. Woven plastic mesh is less elastic than polypropylene mesh, but the woven edges tend to unravel when cut. Though woven plastic mesh can be autoclaved repeatedly, it sustains about 10% shrinkage with each sterilization. Plastic mesh is easy to handle, and unraveling has not been a problem. Because plastic is about 40 times less expensive than polypropylene mesh and has less sag, it may be preferable in spanning large defects in horses, particularly when only supportive hernial sac fascia is lacking and only subcutaneous tissue and skin will cover the mesh.

Surgery is done with the horse in dorsal recumbency under general inhalation anesthesia, with strict adherence to aseptic technique. A straight or elliptic skin incision is made adjacent to the defect. The wound is widened by sharp dissection vertically to the hernial ring. The fascia and fibrous tissue overlying the hernial ring are incised for 180 degrees at the margin of the hernial ring (Fig 137). A double layer of mesh is cut to correspond to the size and contour of the defect. When possible, a retroperitoneal dissection is created and the peritoneum is left intact. Ideally, the mesh is placed retroperitoneally and subfascially. In some horses, only intraperitoneal and subfascial placement is possible. If the defect is very large, only intraperitoneal placement is possible and the mesh is covered by skin and subcutaneous tissue.

In either case, horizontal mattress sutures are preplaced about 2.5 cm from the cut edge of the mesh, 1.5-2.5 cm wide and 1.5-2.5 cm apart. Either #2 Mersilene or #2 monofilament nylon swaged on double-armed needles is used. When properly placed, the mesh should fit flat and snugly under moderate tension beneath (deep to) the hernial ring. Excessive gaping or pucker between sutures should be avoided, as this may allow incarceration of the small intestine. If available, the onlay hernial flap is trimmed and the free edge sutured to the hernial ring for reinforcement with simple-interrupted synthetic absorbable sutures (Fig 137). Subcutaneous tissues and skin are closed in a routine fashion.

After the horse recovers from general anesthesia, the incision is supported with sterile compresses and an abdominal bandage to help prevent seroma formation and excessive edema. The initial bandage is changed after 1 day and then every 2-3 days as needed for 2-4 weeks. Broad-spectrum parenteral antibiotics (penicillin and gentamicin) are given before surgery and discontinued on the second or third day if the horse's vital signs are normal and the incision is dry and well apposed. Horses are confined to a stall for 60 days, with hand-walking exercise only. The prognosis for recovery and future use is excellent in about 80% of affected horses.

Diaphragmatic Hernia

Diaphragmatic hernias are rare in horses, with only 35 cases recorded in the literature before 1986.[691] Congenital defects can result from failed fusion of any of the 4 embryonic components of the diaphragm or from rupture *in utero* or during dystocia. Affected adult horses may have a history of

Figure 137. Top: The onlay fascial flap is reflected back and the peritoneum is separated from the hernial ring margins. Two layers of mesh are cut to the appropriate size, and horizontal mattress sutures are preplaced around the perimeter of the mesh 1.5-2.5 cm from the cut edge, 1.5-2.5 cm wide and 1.5-2.5 cm apart. The mesh is placed retroperitoneally and subfascially, and the sutures are tied. Bottom: The onlay fascial flap is trimmed and sutured to the free edge of the hernial ring. Subcutaneous tissue and skin are closed in routine fashion. (Courtesy of *JAVMA*)

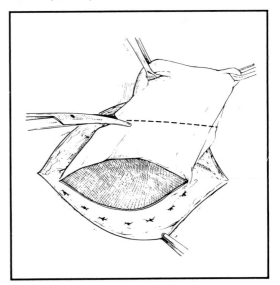

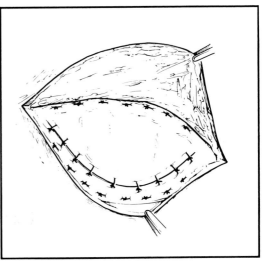

trauma. Though diaphragmatic hernias may result in low-grade, chronic, recurrent abdominal pain and may even be found incidentally at necropsy, most horses are presented in distress with a serious abdominal crisis and the lesion is found during ventral midline exploratory celiotomy. Once the defect is discovered and the viscera returned to the abdominal cavity, ventilatory assistance is necessary if it has not already been instituted.

Small defects, particularly those ventrally positioned, are accessible and may be closed by primary apposition using monofilament nonabsorbable or synthetic absorbable suture material. Large defects, estimated to be larger than 10 cm in diameter, require prosthetic reconstruction with synthetic mesh (Marlex: Davol, Cranston, RI or Proxplast: Goshen Labs, Goshen, NY). Two layers of mesh are cut to the appropriate size and contour, approximately 2 cm larger than the defect under medium tension. The mesh is secured to the perimeter of the defect with simple-interrupted horizontal mattress sutures with appropriately sized synthetic nonabsorbable material. These sutures are preplaced about 1-2 cm from the edge of the hernial ring, 2-3 cm from the edge of the mesh, and about 3 cm apart. The sutures are tied in succession after drawing the mesh up snugly to the hernia ring. Tension should be maintained and sutures alternately tied on opposite sides. In some instances, the defect may be repaired with a flap of adjacent peritoneum and transversus abdominis muscle.[691]

Some very large defects and/or dorsally positioned defects may be inaccessible, precluding safe closure. It may be necessary to extend the midline incision to the xiphoid. Large, self-retaining rib retractors (Burford Retractors: Lawton, Moonachie, NJ) are used, and the large colon is exteriorized. The remaining viscera are isolated with laparotomy sponges, and the surgery table tilted so the horse's head is elevated to permit access to the defect. Thoracotomy may be required if access is still poor.

Before complete closure of the defect, the lungs should be expanded maximally to help evacuate air from the pleural cavity. If pneumothorax is present postoperatively, thoracentesis should be performed to remove as much air as possible.

Abdominal Wall Hernias and Prepubic Tendon Ruptures in Pregnant Mares

Cause: Abdominal wall hernias in pregnant mares resemble rupture of the prepubic tendon; it may be difficult initially to differentiate the 2 clinically.[692] These hernias are associated with hydrallantois, twins, trauma, and excessive edema of the ventral portion of the abdomen. Though the problem is seen more commonly in older draft mares, it has been encountered in other breeds.[687,692]

Clinical Signs: In the acute phase, mares with abdominal wall hernias and prepubic tendon ruptures show mild to moderate abdominal discomfort and progressive ventral abdominal enlargement with extensive pitting edema. Mares with prepubic tendon rupture have a stiff gait, are reluctant to move, and prefer not to lie down. They may assume a sawhorse stance, with lordosis and elevation of the tailhead and tuber ischii. Tipping of the pelvis is due to loss of cranial pelvic support. Conversely, mares with abdominal wall defects prefer to lie down and do not strongly resist walking. Elevation of the tail head or tuber ischii is not present.[692]

Because of the amount of edema, it may be impossible to delineate the exact site and

Figure 138. Abdominal wall hernia in an aged Standardbred broodmare. Abdominal bandaging has resolved ventral edema. The hernial margins are clearly palpable and the hernia is completely reducible.

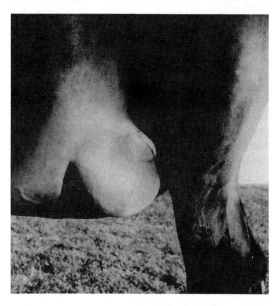

extent of the defect by external palpation. The caudal abdominal floor should be palpated per rectum to determine if it is intact and if herniation is present.

Treatment: A worsening of vital signs and abdominal pain not responsive to aggressive intravenous fluid and analgesic therapy may indicate intestinal incarceration in mares with abdominal wall hernias. If the economic value of the mare is sufficient, emergency ventral midline celiotomy may be necessary to relieve the incarceration and assess the size and location of the defect. Terminating pregnancy by cesarean section should be strongly considered to help avoid irreversible damage to the body wall. Herniation appears to be fairly common through a rent of an aponeurosis of the internus abdominis muscle and the transverse abdominis muscle, or of the externus abdominis muscle and the transversus abdominis muscle just ventral to the flank fold (Fig 138). Unilateral or bilateral defects may occur.

If edema and tissue disruption are severe, closure of the defect with synthetic mesh should be postponed for several weeks until inflammation has subsided and the hernial ring is well defined. After the horse has recovered from general anesthesia, the defect should be supported with a snug abdominal bandage for several weeks.

In heavily gravid mares not showing signs of incarceration, parturition should be induced to reduce the weight on the abdominal defect. After delivery of the foal, the hernia is reduced and the defect supported with abdominal bandaging. Parturition in mares with rupture of the prepubic tendon should likewise be induced with a veterinarian in attendance. Abdominal bandaging is required for several weeks. In both instances, the prognosis for survival of the dam is guarded to poor, depending on the extent of the defect and whether intestine becomes incarcerated.

Ideally, prosthetic reconstruction of the defect with synthetic mesh should be delayed until 1-2 months after parturition, when all inflammation has subsided and the hernial ring is thick, contains mature fibrous tissue and is well delineated. The principles of mesh placement and pre- and postoperative management have been described earlier in this section.[687] The hernial ring usually is well developed and there is an abundant onlay fascial flap to cover the mesh. For unilateral hernias, the approach is through a curvilinear incision made adjacent to the hernial ring (Fig 137). Bilateral defects in the prepubic area may have a narrow strip of intact fascia on the ventral midline under the mammary gland. Ideally, these defects are approached by 2 teams of surgeons positioned on either side of the surgery table.

Bilateral semicircular incisions are made around the lateral aspect of each hernia. The dissection plane is continued to the hernial ring and the flaps are reflected toward the midline. One large double-layered piece of mesh is cut to fit the size and oval shape of the entire defect. The mesh is placed intraabdominally and pulled underneath (deep to) the intact strip of tissue. Beginning medially on the midline and working circumferentially, sutures are then preplaced around the perimeter by both surgeons. Because of the size and location of the defect, the mesh must be stretched flat and taut without excessive wrinkling or bunching. Horizontal mattress sutures must be placed carefully at least 2.5 cm from the edges of both the mesh and the hernial ring. The sutures should be spaced close enough to avoid incarcerating a segment of small intestine under the mesh edge between sutures. The fascia of the hernial sac is trimmed and sutured with synthetic absorbable material. Subcutaneous layers and skin are closed routinely and deadspace is obliterated. Drains are not used routinely.

After the horse has recovered from general anesthesia, the caudal abdomen is kept bandaged for 2-4 weeks or longer, if necessary. Use of perioperative broad-spectrum antibiotics (penicillin and gentamicin) is discontinued in 2-3 days, provided the wound edges are dry and well-apposed, and the horse's vital signs are normal. Because of the dependent location of the wound and extensive tissue dissection, seroma may form. If it does not resolve with bandaging, time and hot-packing, then needle aspiration using strict aseptic techniques may be necessary in addition to bandaging. Aspirated fluids should be submitted for cytologic examination, Gram stain and bacteriologic cultures. Antibiotic therapy may need to be reinstituted depending on results of these examinations.

The prognosis for complete recovery after mesh reconstruction of abdominal wall hernias in mares is fair to good. However, serious and even fatal complications have occurred, including implant disruption with and without infection, adhesion of intestine to the mesh, intestinal incarceration under the mesh, and fatal peritonitis from full-thickness small bowel defects created by intestine apparently rubbing on the mesh.

DISEASES OF THE LIVER

J.K. Johnston

Diagnostic and Therapeutic Considerations

The liver plays a central role in maintaining normal homeostasis through its numerous metabolic functions. Adequate production and excretion of bile are essential for absorption of dietary fat and fat-soluble vitamins. Hepatic glycogen storage and gluconeogenesis are important for maintenance of normal blood glucose concentrations. The liver also is responsible for production of clotting factors, albumin, fibrinogen and many nonessential amino acids. With venous drainage from the gastrointestinal tract serving as its primary blood supply, the liver is a center for detoxification and elimination of a variety of toxic substances.

Because of its diverse involvement in many metabolic processes, the liver is subjected to injury by numerous infectious, metabolic and toxic processes. Fortunately, the liver has great reserve capacities and can continue to function in the presence of significant damage; liver failure and its associated clinical signs do not become apparent until 50-75% of the hepatocellular mass is destroyed.[693] Clinical signs and clinicopathologic findings associated with failure are referable to the liver's inability to perform its many essential functions. Regardless of the cause and duration of liver disease, clinical signs of failure often develop suddenly, making it difficult to establish a relationship with a potential cause.[694]

Treatment of liver disease often is difficult due to the extensive damage that usually occurs before the onset of clinical signs.

While the prognosis for horses with liver failure generally is unfavorable, those suffering from acute failure may recover if appropriate supportive therapy is administered while hepatocellular regeneration is occurring. Conversely, the prognosis for failure resulting from chronic disease usually is poor because of disruption of the normal hepatocellular architecture and replacement with fibrosis. Therefore, when contemplating therapy and offering the client a prognosis, it is important to determine whether the degree of liver failure and associated clinical signs are the result of acute or chronic disease.[695]

Clinical Signs of Liver Disease

Icterus (jaundice) occurs as the result of accumulation of bilirubin in the plasma and other tissues. Bilirubin is produced when heme from senescent red blood cells is broken down by the reticuloendothelial system. Initially the insoluble unconjugated bilirubin is bound to albumin and transferred to the liver, where it is conjugated by hepatocytes. In horses, more than 50% of the bilirubin in bile is conjugated with glucose.[696] Conjugated bilirubin then is actively excreted into the bile ducts. If the energy metabolism of the hepatocyte is disturbed or the biliary system is obstructed, the liver's excretory capacity is overwhelmed. Subsequently, the excretion of conjugated bilirubin into bile is limited and plasma concentrations of bilirubin increase.

Icterus of the mucous membranes and sclera usually is evident when serum concentrations of bilirubin exceed 3 mg/dl and is marked when concentrations are greater than 12 mg/dl.[697] Increased bilirubin concentrations usually precede clinically detectable icterus. Because conjugated bilirubin has a greater affinity for connective tissue than does the unconjugated form, the degree of icterus reflects levels of the conjugated bilirubin fraction. Thus, pronounced icterus should be expected with cholestatic liver disease.[693,698]

While most normal horses do not appear icteric, 10-15% may have mild yellow discoloration of the mucous membranes and sclera.[699] Critical evaluation of the mucous membranes and sclera is best performed in direct sunlight so as to minimize the variations that can occur with artificial lighting.

It is easiest to detect subtle icterus by evaluating nonpigmented sclera. The normal pink color of the mucous membranes makes them difficult to evaluate; by applying temporary pressure to the gingival mucosa, one can reduce blood flow to the area, enhancing inspection of the underlying tissues.

Horses have a higher serum unconjugated bilirubin concentration than most other species; therefore, equine plasma normally has a higher icterus index, limiting the value of the index in evaluation of clinically significant icterus.[693] Any condition that causes decreased food intake in a horse results in a more rapid increase in plasma unconjugated bilirubin concentration.[700] Hemolytic anemia, anorexia, intestinal obstruction and enteritis can cause icterus and should be ruled out before primary liver disease is diagnosed. Marked icterus is a relatively consistent finding in acute liver failure, but it is more variable in chronic failure.[699]

Hepatic encephalopathy can occur in any form of liver failure, but it is probably most severe in horses with an acute fulminant process.[693] Multiple factors are involved in the pathogenesis of hepatic encephalopathy and are only partially understood.[701] Ammonia is produced primarily in the gastrointestinal tract by the action of colonic bacteria and mucosal enzymes on protein. The ammonia is then transported via the portal circulation to the liver for conversion to urea. If ammonia is not metabolized completely, it enters the systemic circulation. The mechanism of ammonia neurotoxicity still is not understood totally, but the reaction and distribution of free ammonia (NH_3), the more toxic moiety, depend upon blood pH and the potassium concentration (*ie*, the higher the pH, the more NH_3 there is and the less NH_4^+ there is). Though increased blood ammonia levels occur frequently in horses with liver failure, the severity of clinical signs is not always correlated with blood ammonia concentrations.[702]

High blood ammonia levels stimulate glucagon production in people with liver failure. This results in increased hepatic gluconeogenesis from amino acids.[701] To maintain normal blood glucose concentrations, insulin secretion is initiated; this stimulates uptake and metabolism of branched-chain amino acids by muscle.[701,702] Decrease in the ratio of branched-chain to aromatic amino acids in the plasma from a normal value of ≤ 1.5-4:1 may cause severe neurologic dysfunction.[703] Aromatic amino acids not readily metabolized by a diseased liver accumulate and interfere with normal neurotransmission.[701,703]

Because of the importance of normal liver function in maintaining adequate blood glucose concentrations, liver failure can result in profound hypoglycemia that may contribute to hepatic encephalopathy; blood glucose concentrations of ≤ 20 mg/dl have been reported.[699] Neurologic dysfunction can vary from mild behavioral changes and depression, to fulminant, maniacal activity. Clinical signs include depression, somnolence, muscle tremors, ataxia, compulsive circling and aimless walking. Dementia, head pressing and violent thrashing may become severe, posing a threat to handlers. Occasionally these signs can be mistaken for those of colic.

Both acute and chronic liver failure can cause photosensitization that may result in photodermatitis. Phylloerythrin, a porphyrin derivative of chlorophyll, is produced by intestinal bacteria and excreted primarily in the feces. Normally the portion of phylloerythrin that is absorbed by the portal circulation is effectively removed by the liver and excreted in the bile. In liver failure, phylloerythrin passes into the systemic circulation and accumulates in the skin where, it absorbs radiant energy from the sun. This process results in free radical formation, ultimately causing inflammation and necrosis of unpigmented skin. The most common site of photodermatitis is the muzzle, which has minimal protective hair and often is unpigmented, though any area with unpigmented skin may be affected.

Depression and anorexia are commonly observed in liver failure. Abdominal pain also may occur due to a rapid increase in liver size. Cholelithiasis can cause recurrent, mild abdominal pain due to intermittent, partial or complete biliary obstruction. Clotting abnormalities, as evidenced by petechial and ecchymotic hemorrhage, excessive bleeding from venipuncture sites and frank hemorrhage, also can occur. Ascites and edema are not common in horses with liver failure.

Clinicopathologic Abnormalities

Numerous clinicopathologic abnormalities occur in response to liver damage, and no single diagnostic test provides a complete measure of the liver's status. An accurate assessment of the condition of the liver is best achieved by serial determination of a battery of tests that provide reliable diagnostic and prognostic information. By providing an estimate of the degree of damage and progression of the disease process, these tests also may serve as valuable prognostic indicators.[704] Serum hepatic enzyme activity provides a measure of active or ongoing hepatocellular damage. Measuring circulating levels of products normally produced and excreted by the liver and timing hepatic clearance of specific dyes provide valuable information regarding changes in functional capacity.

Increased serum enzyme activity can result from enzyme leakage due to active hepatocellular damage, altered hepatocellular membrane permeability, biliary obstruction, severe anemia, heart failure, general anesthesia, endotoxemia and systemic infectious diseases that do not result in primary hepatocellular damage. The active disease frequently has passed before clinical evidence appears, so transient increases in serum enzyme activity may not be detected. Enzyme release in chronic liver disease is variable and, in some cases, serum activities are normal.[703] Therefore, it is important to evaluate the serum enzyme activity in conjunction with the progression of clinical signs and other diagnostic information.

Sorbitol dehydrogenase (SDH) is a sensitive indicator of hepatocellular necrosis in horses.[704] The enzyme's short half-life makes serial increases in serum activity a useful indicator of ongoing liver necrosis. In acute processes, serum sorbitol dehydrogenase activity should return to normal 4-5 days after the initial insult.[705] Unfortunately, the instability of this enzyme makes it difficult to assay in the practice setting.

Lactate dehydrogenase is not liver specific, and increases in plasma activities of this enzyme can occur with a variety of diseases.[704] However, isoenzyme 5 of lactate dehydrogenase (LDH-5) is a useful indicator of hepatocellular disease in horses.[706] In response to hepatocellular damage, serum LDH-5 levels increases rapidly. It has a short half-life and is stable at room temperature for 48 hours. Because its automated assay (ACA: DuPont) is less complicated and more readily available than assays for SDH, LDH-5 may be more useful in assessing the degree of ongoing hepatocellular necrosis.[706]

Aspartate aminotransferase (AST) activity is found in many tissues, particularly heart, muscle and liver. It has a longer half-life than SDH; thus, increased serum concentrations persist longer after hepatic injury. Increases in serum AST activity can be diagnostic of liver disease once nonhepatic causes have been ruled out.[704] Alkaline phosphatase activity is not specific for liver disease. However, persistent increases in serum activity of this enzyme occur most commonly in chronic liver diseases that involve biliary obstruction.[699,703,704]

Serum activity of gamma glutamyl transferase (GGT) is increased in a variety of liver disorders. This may be the enzyme of choice for detection of hepatic disease in horses; GGT is located primarily in the kidneys, pancreas and liver.[707] Racehorses tend to have higher normal ranges of GGT activity than other types of horses. Though serum GGT activity is not increased significantly in very early hepatic necrosis, persistent increases are quite common in chronic liver disease.[703,704,708] Because GGT originates in the biliary tract, increased enzyme concentrations consistently occur with cholestasis.

As mentioned previously, horses have higher normal serum bilirubin concentrations than do other domestic species. Usually the total bilirubin concentration is 0.3-2.0 mg/dl, but higher concentrations have been observed in otherwise normal individuals.[693,697,703] The largest proportion of the total bilirubin value is normally unconjugated, with less than 25% conjugated.[704] Unconjugated hyperbilirubinemia occurs as a result of overproduction, as in hemolytic anemia, or when hepatic uptake or conjugation is depressed. Fasting results in decreased hepatic transport of bilirubin into bile, which probably is responsible for the hyperbilirubinemia (up to 10 mg/dl) observed in horses with reduced feed intake due to nonhepatic causes.[693,709] Vitamin K and certain drugs also can impair bilirubin conjugation.[710]

Conjugated bilirubin often represents a smaller proportion of the total bilirubin concentration in the horse than in other species with liver failure. Though concentrations of conjugated bilirubin greater than 25% of total bilirubin indicate cholestasis, even with complete biliary obstruction the conjugated fraction usually does not exceed 50% of the total.[711,712]

Hyperbilirubinemia associated with acute liver failure typically has bilirubin concentrations >10 mg/dl.[711] Proportionately greater increases in unconjugated bilirubin are expected, but concentrations of the conjugated form may increase due to intrahepatic obstruction. Total bilirubin concentrations are increased with acute liver failure because of decreased bilirubin uptake, conjugation and excretion, and increased heme production due to increased erythrocyte destruction.[699] Horses with chronic liver failure usually have elevated total bilirubin concentrations; however, the increases are variable and often less than those observed with acute disease. Even if there is no increase in total bilirubin concentration with chronic disease, the ratio of conjugated to total bilirubin levels usually is noticeably increased and diagnostically important.[699]

Bile acids are synthesized by the liver, conjugated with glycine or taurine, and excreted in the bile. The detergent properties of bile acids are important for small intestinal absorption of fat. Because bile acids are absorbed efficiently and recirculated through the liver about 38 times a day, they are sensitive indicators of liver disease in horses.[7,13] Normal bile acid concentration in horses is less than 15 μmol/L; concentrations exceeding that may indicate liver disease.[713] Bile acids appear most useful in diagnosis of chronic disease, as enough functional tissue may remain for reexcretion of the acids during early disease states.[713]

Ammonia is produced by bacterial degradation of protein in the intestinal tract and is carried by the portal circulation to the liver for amino acid production via the urea cycle.[708] Though ammonia is of pathologic significance in development of hepatic encephalopathy, ammonia is difficult to assay; sample handling is crucial and normal concentrations vary widely. For these reasons, serum ammonia levels are not measured routinely in horses. Ammonia tolerance tests are used in other species for assessment of liver function, but use of this test in equine practice is limited and requires further investigation.[714] Urea is a product of the liver's metabolism of ammonia. Consequently, when ammonia metabolism is impaired, blood urea nitrogen concentration may be decreased.[708] Liver diseases should be suspected in the presence of a blood urea nitrogen level below 10 mg/dl, though this alone is not diagnostic. If residual liver function is sufficient, the blood urea nitrogen level often remains normal.

Most horses with liver disease have normal blood glucose concentrations. However, if liver function is sufficiently impaired, profound hypoglycemia can result. Blood glucose concentrations as low as 20 mg/dl often are accompanied by signs of encephalopathy that often abate after intravenous administration of 50-100 g of glucose.[699]

Though the liver is responsible for protein production, hypoproteinemia is not a consistent finding in equine liver disease. Hypoalbuminemia may occur in the later stages, though this decrease usually is offset by increases in beta and/or gamma globulins, maintaining normal plasma protein concentration. Thus, it is extremely important to know how much of each of these components makes up the total protein concentration.

Prothrombin, a vitamin K-dependent clotting factor, is produced by the liver.[715] Its concentration may be reduced with extensive hepatic necrosis or when insufficient bile reaches the small intestine to permit intestinal absorption of vitamin K.[708] The serum fibrinogen level is normal in many horses with liver disease. However, with severe hepatocellular damage, serum fibrinogen concentrations may be as low as 100 mg/dl.[699] Because primary cholestatic disease may be accompanied by a relative sparing of hepatocellular function, serum fibrinogen concentrations may be normal or increased in cholelithiasis.[716]

Sulfobromophthalein (BSP) dye excretion has proven useful in assessment of liver function in horses, especially when occult liver disease is suspected and the results of other liver function tests are equivocal. Normal BSP clearance times range from 2.0 to 3.7 minutes; times longer than 5 minutes are abnormal. Invariably, BSP clearance is prolonged in markedly icteric individuals. Therefore, this test seldom is used in horses with serum bilirubin concentrations exceeding 6 mg/dl. Because the initial slope of the clearance curve is independent of the dose, a standard 1-g dose is administered intravenously to adult horses (450 kg). Heparinized blood samples are taken from another vein before administration of the dye and then every 3-4 minutes for 15 minutes after dye injection. Plasma concentrations of these are plotted against time on semilog paper and the half-life determined from the graph.

Aberrant BSP clearance can occur because of failure to record proper time of blood sampling, contamination of blood collection equipment from BSP on hands, or unintentional perivascular injection of the dye. Fasting hyperbilirubinemia can prolong BSP clearance time, but it does not appear to alter interpretation of results. Though its availability is limited, BSP is the most commonly used dye for evaluation of hepatic functions. Indocyanine green clearance has been studied in fed and fasted horses, but clinical use of the dye for diagnosis of liver failure has not been reported.[717] Normal values of selected liver tests are presented in Table 20.

Liver Biopsy, Ultrasonography and Radiography

Percutaneous liver biopsy is a useful method for obtaining information regarding the liver that otherwise is unavailable except by exploratory laparotomy or necropsy. Prognostic and diagnostic information can be obtained regarding hepatocyte loss, fibrosis, altered architecture, regeneration and repair. In horses, diffuse hepatic involvement occurs most often in liver disease. Therefore, lesions seen on liver biopsy usually correlate well with lesions throughout the organ. Focal hepatic lesions occur occasionally; in these cases, diagnostic ultrasonography can be useful in detection and guided biopsy of such lesions. The biopsy specimen can be obtained with a variety of instruments. Disposable 6-inch biopsy needles (Tru-Cut: Travenol) work very well. The approach is through the right eleventh to fourteenth intercostal space, just ventral to a line drawn from the point of the hip to the point of the shoulder. The more cranial site usually gives the best result. Several

Table 20. Normal values for clinicopathologic assays used to detect liver disease. (From the Clinical Laboratory, University of Pennsylvania, Kennett Square)

Constituent		Range
Sorbitol dehydrogenase (SDH)		206 IU/L
Lactate dehydrogenase (LDH)		251-548 IU/L
Lactate dehydrogenase-5 (LDH-5)		0-20 IU/L
Aspartate aminotransferase (AST)		199-441 IU/L
Gamma glutamyltransferase (GGT)		2-18 IU/L
Alkaline phosphatase		118-487 IU/L
Bilirubin	Total	0.7-2.8 mg/dl
	Direct	0.1-0.4 mg/dl
Blood urea nitrogen		11.1-21.5 mg/dl
Ammonia		13-108 mg/dl
Glucose		51-95 mg/dl
Fibrinogen		75-210 mg/dl

techniques have been described.[718-720] Samples should be submitted not only in formalin for histopathologic diagnosis, but also in appropriate culture media for bacteriologic culture when suppurative cholangitis is suspected.

If available, diagnostic ultrasonography is indicated in horses with suspected liver disease. Sector scanners of 3.3-3.5 MHz are most useful. On the right side of the animal, the liver is adjacent to the diaphragm, ventral to the lung margin and caudal to the level of the right kidney. The size of the liver varies between individuals but is considered of normal size if a moderate wedge with a sharp border is visible. On the left side, the spleen usually rests medial to the liver. The hepatic and portal veins usually are outlined in the normal liver, while the biliary system with its bright echogenic walls is not.

Obstructive biliary disease results in hepatomegaly with a larger than normal amount of liver visible on ultrasound examination. Dilated bile ducts are present. Occasionally a highly reflective focal hyperechoic region, indicative of cholelithiasis, is seen within the distended ducts.

When hepatomegaly and alterations in the texture of the liver are observed ultrasonographically, hepatic neoplasia should be considered. Fibrosis can result in hepatomegaly or atrophy. If focal lesions are observed, ultrasound-guided biopsies of the lesions are indicated.[721]

The most useful application of radiography for assessment of liver damage is for the gastroduodenal ulcer disease syndrome. It is common to identify markedly dilated bile ducts in young horses with the chronic form of this disease in which there is duodenal fibrosis and stricture. In fact, this radiographic finding provides further evidence of the syndrome and is a strong indication that surgical intervention may be needed.[361]

Treatment of Liver Failure

Treatment of horses with liver failure is largely supportive and should be directed toward alleviation of clinical signs. Horses with acute liver failure have a reasonable prognosis for survival and should be treated aggressively until signs of recovery are evident or the disease has progressed to a point where management is impossible. Management of hepatic encephalopathy should be undertaken with caution. Horses with severe neurologic dysfunction and those that are in danger of injuring themselves or people should be sedated. Sedatives that are metabolized by the liver should be used judiciously, as adverse reactions and prolonged half-lives may occur because of liver failure. Though the phenothiazine tranquilizers are useful, most horses with liver failure can be sedated successfully with xylazine.[703,722] Oral or intravenous administration of glucose can result in a dramatic reversal of neurologic dysfunction in some individuals. A continuous infusion of 5% dextrose at 1 L/hour provides 50 g of glucose/hour and maintains blood glucose concentrations at about 100-160 mg/dl.[703] Though this infusion rate does not provide the total caloric requirements of an adult horse, it usually is beneficial and does not cause significant glucosuria.[703] Blood and urine glucose concentrations can be monitored to guide the rate of glucose administration. If prolonged intravenous glucose therapy is indicated, a balanced electrolyte solution should be added to the treatment regimen.

To reduce production of ammonia and other potential neurotoxins by the intestinal bacteria, oral administration of neomycin sulfate (50-100 mg/kg) has been recommended.[693,723] However, prolonged use should be avoided as it may predispose to salmonellosis.[703] In people, lactulose (150-200 mg) given PO every 6 hours acidifies the colonic contents and promotes conversion of free ammonia to ammonium ion, which is absorbed poorly. This reduces the ammonia load delivered to the liver.[693,723] This technique has not been evaluated in horses but would be very expensive. Cathartics and mild enemas also may be beneficial in preventing absorption of toxins and ammonia. Acidosis should be corrected slowly and alkalosis treated vigorously, as a sudden increase in blood pH can promote conversion of the ammonium ion to ammonia, which can easily cross the blood-brain barrier by nonionic diffusion.

An increase in the ratio of aromatic to branched-chain amino acids appears to be important in development of hepatic encephalopathy. Therefore, oral administration of branched-chain amino acids (isoleucine, leucine, valine) may help prevent this problem.[724] Sorghum and beet pulp have high concentrations of branched-chain amino acids and are palatable if mixed with molasses.

Nutritional support of affected horses is essential. If the animal is not eating or drinking, administration of electrolyte solutions and glucose via a nasogastric tube may be indicated. If a hypertonic glucose solution is administered PO, it is important to ensure adequate hydration, as fluids are drawn into the gastrointestinal tract, potentially decreasing intravascular and extravascular fluid volumes. Feeds containing a low level of high-quality proteins are recommended. The diet should be highly digestible and made as palatable as possible because many horses in liver failure have a poor appetite. A good-quality grass hay and grain diet is appropriate, especially as the patient's appetite improves. Alfalfa hay should be avoided due to its high protein content. Intolerance of dietary protein, with progression of clinical signs and neurologic dysfunction despite attempts to optimize the diet, is considered a poor prognostic sign.[693] Parenteral administration of B-complex vitamins is indicated to decrease the demands on the liver for production, as well as to ensure an adequate supply for energy metabolism. Administration of the fat-soluble vitamins A, D and E may be beneficial but usually is not required. Vitamin K supplementation may be important if coagulopathy is evident.[723] It must be remembered, however, that vitamin K_3 is nephrotoxic in horses.

697

Use of corticosteroids in treatment of liver failure remains controversial. Corticosteroids are gluconeogenic and stimulate protein breakdown, thus indirectly increasing the workload of the liver. No studies support their therapeutic efficacy, as corticosteroids do not inhibit development of liver fibrosis and may potentiate ascites.[693]

Antimicrobials are indicated if an infectious process is suspected. Horses with suppurative cholangitis or cholelithiasis should be treated with a broad-spectrum antimicrobial combination, such as penicillin with an aminoglycoside or trimethoprim with sulfamethoxasole. If culture and sensitivity results of a biopsy are available, antimicrobial therapy should be directed accordingly. If treated appropriately, horses with acute liver failure have a reasonable chance for survival.

If hepatoencephalopathy, coagulopathy and secondary complications persist despite therapy, the prognosis is less favorable. However, horses with only slight to moderate alterations in plasma activities of hepatic enzymes and liver function test results have a better prognosis. Serial monitoring of laboratory values can provide prognostic information and index the progression of the disease state.

Treatment of horses with chronic liver disease should not be considered hopeless, though the prognosis is less favorable than for acute liver disease. Close monitoring of disease progression or regression is indicated so that clients can make informed decisions regarding continuation of treatment. Treatment can be complex and prolonged; but if clinical signs are alleviated within a reasonable time, the horse can recover if further insults to the liver are minimized.[723]

Congenital and Familial Diseases

Biliary Atresia

Biliary atresia, an uncommon anomaly in animals, has been described in a foal.[725] The foal was normal at birth but its condition soon deteriorated. The foal showed mild abdominal pain, icterus and lethargy.

It failed to gain weight over the next several weeks. Laboratory values were consistent with obstructive biliary disease and the foal was euthanized. Necropsy findings revealed an enlarged, firm, pale liver. The entrance to the bile duct and the main bile duct to the liver and duodenum were absent. The cause and pathogenesis remain unknown.

Inflammatory, Infectious and Immune Diseases

Tyzzer's Disease

Tyzzer's disease is an acute multifocal hepatic necrosis and hepatitis caused by *Bacillus piliformis*.[726-735] Natural infection with *Bacillus piliformis* is thought to occur by ingestion. The disease can be reproduced experimentally with bacteria recovered from foals that died from multifocal hepatic necrosis.[736] Experimentally, the disease appears highly contagious, but natural infections are sporadic. Predisposing factors in the natural disease of foals are not well understood. In experimental models with other species, corticosteroid administration, poor sanitation, overcrowding and environmental contamination have been associated with the disease.[737] It may be that adult horses or rodents serve as a reservoir for environmental contamination of foals.

This disease is highly fatal in foals, most often but not exclusively at 7-42 days of age. Affected foals usually are in excellent health before the onset of clinical signs, which include depression and rapid progression to a comatose state. Fevers as high as 105 F (40.6 C) have been reported, though subnormal temperatures may be associated with shock. Icterus may or may not be present. In many cases, sudden death is the only clinical sign. Serum hepatocellular-specific enzymes and bilirubin concentrations and BSP clearance may be increased.

Multifocal, pale pinpoint areas in the liver capsule and parenchyma consistent with necrotizing hepatitis are observed and hepatomegaly is common in Tyzzer's disease. Icterus, petechiation and focal necrosis of other organs usually are present. Histologic evaluation of the liver typically reveals filamentous bacilli arranged in parallel or haphazard fashion in the hepatocytes at the periphery of necrotic foci. These foci more frequently are seen in the periportal areas. Silver stains are required to identify the organisms best.[729,733] Unfortunately, the disease is rapidly progressive and highly fatal; treatment has not been uniformly successful. Broad-spectrum antibiotics and fluid therapy with supportive care may be attempted, though the prognosis is extremely poor.

Toxic Diseases

Hepatoxicosis

A toxic hepatopathy in newborn foals 2-5 days of age that received a microorganism culture product (Primipaste SL) PO after birth, and most likely before gut closure, has been described.[738,739] Clinical signs include icterus, depression and neurologic dysfunction. Laboratory findings, in conjunction with clinical signs, supported the diagnosis of liver failure. The disease was uniformly fatal.

Pathologic findings included a small rubbery liver with massive hepatocellular necrosis, marked bile duct proliferation and occasional fibrosis on histopathologic examination. These changes suggested of a subacute to chronic disease process. The product responsible for the disease contained live organisms, fermentation products, vitamins and ferrous fumarate. The last ingredient was most likely responsible for hepatoxicosis.[740] The product no longer is available.

Pyrrolizidine Alkaloid Toxicity

In certain geographic locations, pyrrolizidine alkaloid intoxication is the most common cause of liver failure in horses.[699] *Amsinckia intermedia, Crotolaria* spp, *Heliotropium europium, Echium lycopsis* and *Senecio* spp are the plants incriminated most commonly. Usually these plants are unpalatable, and ingestion with subsequent toxicity occurs only if other feeds are limited. Most cases occur after ingestion of contaminated hay, grain or processed feeds. The toxic moiety appears to be concentrated in the seeds, which may contaminate the pasture or hay fields. Consequently, hay and pastures should be evaluated thoroughly for hepatotoxic plants. If cubed hay or pellets are the suspected source, chemical analysis of the feed may be necessary.[703]

Acute intoxication may occur, with clinical signs developing within several weeks of exposure.[741] However, chronic progressive hepatopathy is more common and usually occurs subsequent to prolonged low level exposure. Clinical signs typically do not develop for several months, often making it difficult to identify the source of the toxin. In those cases, the diagnosis must be based on the characteristic histopathologic changes associated with pyrrolizidine alkaloid toxicity.

Though the disease usually is chronic, the onset of clinical signs often is abrupt. Variable degrees of hepatic encephalopathy may be present and include periodic somnolence, head pressing, belligerence, blindness, aimless walking and seizures. The degree of icterus is variable, and photosensitization occurs in about 25% of the cases. Many horses are unthrifty and presented for chronic weight loss. Other clinical signs referable to the gastrointestinal tract include anorexia, decreased borborygmi, intermittent diarrhea and, very infrequently, ascites. Abdominal pain may be present in rare cases. Defective clotting, as evidenced by petechiation, excessive bleeding from venipuncture sites and internal hemorrhage, is seen occasionally. Hypoalbuminemia as a result of decreased hepatic synthesis occurs rarely and only in late hepatic failure.

While clinical signs, laboratory findings and history of exposure to the toxin may suspect pyrrolizidine alkaloid intoxication, a liver biopsy is essential for accurate diagnosis. Classical histopathologic lesions include fibrosis, megalocytosis and bile duct proliferation (Fig 139).[742] Consumption of large amounts of the toxin can result in acute liver failure and zonal or centrilobular necrosis that later may progress to the characteristic histopathologic changes.[703]

The progressive hepatocyte loss, fibrosis and destruction of the normal hepatic architecture often result in terminal liver failure or necessitate euthanasia. Treatment generally is unrewarding. Therefore, management of horses exposed to the toxin but not yet showing clinical signs is more important. Those horses should be denied further

Figure 139. Microscopic section of liver from a horse intoxicated with pyrrolizidine. Note the prominent megalocyte (arrow) within the section. These are characteristic of the histopathologic changes induced by this toxin. (100X) (Courtesy of Dr. L. Roth)

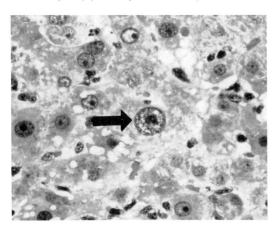

access to any of the contaminated feed or hay and offered supplemental grain. Care should be taken to avoid feeding alfalfa hay due to its high protein content.

Mycotoxicosis

Corn contaminated with the molds *Penicillium rubrum* or *Aspergillus flavus* or *A parasiticus* may contain rubritoxin or aflatoxin, respectively, and can be extremely hepatotoxic. Clinical signs after consump-

Figure 140. Lateral radiographic view of the caudal thorax and cranial abdomen of a 3-month-old foal with duodenal stricture, a serious complication of the gastroduodenal ulcer disease syndrome. The arrow points to the dilated bile ducts that are a common finding with this disease. (Courtesy of Dr. A.M. Merritt)

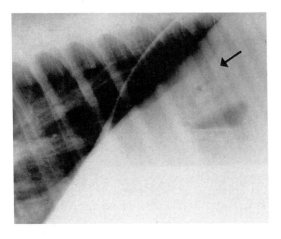

tion of such corn are similar to those seen with Theiler's disease and some cases of pyrrolizidine toxicity. Definitive diagnosis is based upon finding the toxin in hepatic tissue from the affected animal.

Multifactorial Diseases

Obstructive Cholangitis

Cholangitis with marked bile duct dilatation occasionally is evident in foals with advanced gastroduodenal ulcer disease and duodenal stricture (Fig 140). When present, this finding indicates the need for surgical intervention to bypass the duodenal stricture. Though this condition may occur secondary to stricture involving the opening of the common bile duct, similar findings have been seen with minimal involvement of the duct opening. Primary cholangitis resulting from bile stasis or reflux of ingesta into the bile duct may occur if the stricture is located distal to the opening of the bile duct.[743]

Idiopathic Diseases

Acute Hepatitis

(Theiler's Disease)

Theiler's disease, a diffuse hepatitis, is one of the most common causes of acute liver failure in horses.[694] This disease occurs only in adult horses and often develops 4-10 weeks after administration of an equine-origin biologic.[703,744] However, many horses develop a similar acute hepatitis with no history of equine antiserum administration.[694] Multiple-horse involvement on some farms and seasonal occurrence suggest a blood-borne infectious agent, yet no etiologic agent ever has been identified. There is speculation that the disease may be similar to human viral hepatitis B, but serologic testing of affected horses has been negative. Experimental transmission of the disease using tissue or blood from affected individuals has been unsuccessful, suggesting that dietary and/or other environmental toxins may play a role in the pathogenesis.[694,745]

Most affected horses first show neurologic dysfunction. Clinical signs include depression, excessive yawning, ataxia and circling, but often there is a rapid progression to head pressing, nondirected charging and belligerence that may terminate in coma. Marked icterus is common but is not always present at the onset of neurologic signs. Photosensitization and excessive hemorrhage occur less commonly. Hemoglobinuria occasionally accompanies this acute hepatic failure syndrome; when present, it indicates a grave prognosis.

Diagnosis of Theiler's disease is based upon the history, clinical signs and laboratory findings consistent with hepatic failure. Because the liver often is smaller than normal, biopsy may be difficult without ultrasonographic guidance. Histopathologic evaluation of the liver usually reveals severe, widespread hepatocellular necrosis, primarily of the centrilobular to mid-zonal areas. Bile duct and fibroblastic proliferation usually are present.[746] Some horses that respond quickly to therapy and continue to eat eventually recover. If the prothrombin time, serum bilirubin concentration and liver enzyme activity return toward normal values, a more favorable prognosis can be offered.

Chronic Active Hepatitis

Many of the above causes of hepatopathy can result in chronic active hepatitis. The most common sign is progressive weight loss. The animal may not be icteric unless there is attendant anorexia, but the conjugated portion of the serum bilirubin concentration usually exceeds 25% of the total bilirubin concentration. Serum activities of hepatic enzymes may be elevated to varying degrees, depending upon current activity of the inflammatory process and amount of intrahepatic cholestasis. Definitive diagnosis of the problem is based upon histopathologic examination of a biopsy specimen.

Cholelithiasis

The frequency of reports of cholelithiasis in horses has increased recently.[22,747-752] Cholelithiasis appears primarily to be a disease of horses older than 9 years of age, though horses as young as 5 years of age have had the disease.[694,717]

Cause: The cause of cholelith formation remains unknown. In one study, the composition of choleliths from 6 horses was predominantly calcium bilirubinate, similar to that of brown-pigmented stones in people.[716,754] Infection is closely associated with

brown-pigment stone formation, and enteric organisms can be cultured from the choleliths and biliary tree at necropsy. Because horses have no gallbladder and are thought to continually secrete bile, ascending infection causing biliary stasis before cholelith development seems a reasonable sequence of events. However, this theory remains speculative.

Clinical Signs: Clinical signs of obstructive biliary disease and cholelithiasis include recurrent abdominal pain, icterus and fever. Intermittence of the signs is common and most likely represents partial or complete biliary obstruction. The duration of signs is variable, from acute onset to a chronic problem of several months' duration accompanied by progressive weight loss.

Because obstructive biliary disease results in primarily conjugated hyperbilirubinemia, icterus is common. Hepatic encephalopathy occurs less frequently, probably due to sparing of hepatocellular functions. Photosensitization also may be observed.

Diagnosis: Serum GGT activity usually is markedly increased in horses with cholelithiasis. Serum activities of hepatocellular enzymes also may be increased, but usually to a lesser extent than GGT. These findings are consistent with primary cholestatic disease and secondary hepatocellular changes. Leukocytosis, hyperproteinemia and hyperfibrinogenemia often are observed.

Ultrasonography is invaluable in diagnosis.[753] The liver often appears larger than normal, with increased echogenicity compatible with hepatomegaly and fibrosis. Dilated bile ducts often are present and appear as thin-walled anechoic vessel-like structures. Multiple choleliths are common and appear as hyperechoic regions, either within distended ducts or the hepatic parenchyma, and they often cast an acoustic shadow (Fig 141). It is important to scan the right ventral abdomen, as choleliths commonly are seen in the sixth through eighth intercostal spaces.[716] A liver biopsy is indicated to assess the degree of structural alteration. Variable degrees of periportal fibrosis and bile duct proliferation usually are observed and, in most cases, are representative of diffuse liver involvement.

Treament: Unfortunately, due to the chronic diffuse nature of the disease, the extent of hepatic fibrosis by the time of diagnosis and the multiplicity of choleliths,

Figure 141. Left: Two choleliths are visible (arrows), with one showing weak acoustic imaging. Right: Image of the liver showing the parallel channel sign associated with dilitation of the biliary tree adjacent to the portal vein.(Courtesy of Dr. V. Reef)

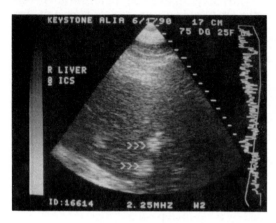
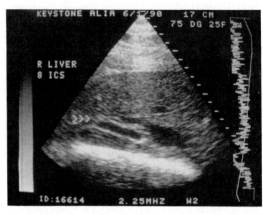

treatment options are limited. If a cholelith is obstructing the common bile duct and the horse has minimal parenchymal changes on liver biopsy, choledolithotripsy may be accomplished via exploratory laparotomy. Most choleliths are easily crushed within the duct and can be flushed into the duodenum. This method is preferred over removal via a choledocotomy because of the difficult exposure and associated complications of bile-induced peritonitis. Multiple stones often are scattered throughout the biliary system and cannot be retrieved, making it difficult to recommend surgical intervention. Medical management, which includes supportive care and broad-spectrum antibiotics, should be attempted in view of the theoretical pathogenesis of the stones. Unfortunately, this therapy proves unrewarding due to the extent of liver damage by the time the condition is diagnosed.

DISEASES OF THE PANCREAS

J.K. Johnston

Diagnostic and Therapeutic Considerations

Though the pancreas of horses serves important metabolic and digestive functions, it has received little investigative attention. As an exocrine gland, the pancreas provides sodium bicarbonate and digestive enzymes necessary for intestinal assimilation of food. Its endocrine function includes secretion of insulin and glucagon from the islet cells of Langerhans. These products are essential to regulation of carbohydrate, lipid and protein metabolism.

At rest, pancreatic secretion in horses is profuse and continuous, yet it can be increased greatly with neural and hormonal stimulation. However, the enzyme concentration and thus the proteolytic activity of equine pancreatic juice is much lower than that in many other species.[290] Vagal stimulation of the pancreas increases the amylase concentration to only 2-4 U/ml in horses versus 50-80 U/ml in pigs and dogs, implying that equine pancreatic juice has less digestive importance than in other monogastric species.[290,755]

Unlike that of other species, chloride rather than bicarbonate is the primary inorganic anionic component of equine pancreatic juice. Bicarbonate concentration is low and never exceeds that of chloride at any rate of secretion.[290] In some species, including horses, bicarbonate is excreted into the terminal ileum in exchange for chloride.[66,756] Thus, the pancreatic juice provides a medium rich in chloride for such anionic exchange in the ileum, making sufficient bicarbonate available to buffer the products of fermentation of the cecum.

Diagnosis of Pancreatic Disease

Clinical pancreatic diseases rarely are diagnosed in horses. Clinical and laboratory confirmation of the disease is not achieved easily and is not attempted routinely. The pancreas is difficult to see with most routine surgical approaches to the abdomen and often is overlooked at necropsy. Only lethal cases of pancreatitis usually are confirmed in horses; thus, little information is available regarding the clinical and pathologic changes that occur in less severe forms of disease.

Serum amylase and lipase activity, peritoneal fluid amylase activity and fractional excretion of amylase can be useful in diagnosis of pancreatic disease in horses.[757] Because methodologies differ, normal values for the above must be established for each laboratory. Amylase is a small molecule (MW 50,000) and is stable when refrigerated. Serum samples should be used, as amylase activity requires the presence of calcium, which is chelated in plasma samples.[758] Serum amylase activity in normal horses is 15-20 IU/L. Values less than 50 IU/L are considered normal.[757] Amylase activity in peritoneal fluid of normal horses usually has slightly lower activity than that in serum.[757]

Fractional excretion of amylase can be calculated by the following equation:

$$\text{Fractional excretion of amylase} = \frac{\text{urine amylase}}{\text{serum amylase}} \times \frac{\text{serum creatinine}}{\text{urine creatinine}} \times 100$$

Normally the fractional excretion of amylase in horses is less than 1%. Renal function should be assessed before interpretation of serum amylase activity or the fractional excretion because abnormal renal function may result in decreased urinary excretion of amylase and increased serum activity.[758] Serum amylase activity is best determined early in the disease. At one time, despite the complex methodologies required, serum lipase was the diagnostic test of choice in diagnosis of pancreatic disease. Currently, greater diagnostic accuracy is achieved if both amylase and lipase are evaluated simultaneously in dogs.[758] Lipase activity remains elevated longer and does not appear to be affected by renal dysfunction as readily as amylase activity.[758] Normal serum lipase activity in horses is less than 0.2 Sigma-Tietz U/L.[757]

Though increased pancreatic enzyme activity in serum and peritoneal fluid suggests pancreatic disease, damage to other intra-abdominal organs may cause the enzyme to leak the enzyme into the peritoneal cavity.

Clinically significant pancreatic disease often results in serum amylase activity exceeding 700 U/L and lipase activity greater than 3.5 Sigma-Tietz U/L. Less marked increases may be present with other gastrointestinal lesions.

As mentioned earlier, hypocalcemia is a rather common finding associated with acute and subacute pancreatitis in horses. The pathogenesis is not well understood. Interrelationships between glucagon and thyrocalcitonin could explain some if not all of the phenomenon, however.[759-761]

Neoplasia

Adenocarcinoma

Like many chronic intraabdominal diseases, pancreatic adenocarcinoma initally causes progressive weight loss with vague signs of gastrointestinal disturbance, including intermittent mild colic. Clinical signs may falsely indicate hepatic rather than pancreatic disease, though icterus rarely is seen. Serum chemistry results also may appear compatible with liver disease especially because there is marked elevation of liver-specific enzyme activity.[221,762] This may be due primarily to obstruction of biliary outflow by the tumor, but there is a large amount of gamma glutamyl transferase (GGT) in equine pancreatic tissue as well.[763] Definitive diagnosis depends upon exploratory laparotomy or necropsy.

Idiopathic Diseases

Acute Pancreatitis

Acute pancreatitis in horses is characterized by acute, intractable abdominal pain, progressive gastric distention and hypovolemic shock, often culminating in death.[757,764] The cause of acute pancreatitis in horses remains unknown. In other species, furosemide and corticosteroid administration, pancreatic duct obstruction, vitamin A and vitamin E/selenium deficiency, and vitamin D intoxication have been implicated. Parasitic migration may be a cause, as *Strongylus equinus* larvae pass through the pancreas as part of their normal developmental cycle, and *S vulgaris* and *S edentatus* larvae may reach the pancreas during aberrant migration.

Gastric distention, contributing to the abdominal pain and cardiovascular compromise, is relieved by nasogastric intubation. Large volumes of fluid are lost in this manner. This fluid loss, combined with release of vasoactive substances from the pancreas, contributes to progressive dehydration and shock. Tachycardia, poor peripheral perfusion, mucous membrane congestion and other signs consistent with shock denote the severity of the condition. Auscultable borborygmi vary in intensity, and rectal examination findings are usually unremarkable. Abdominocentesis usually yields peritoneal fluid containing an increased number of neutrophils indicative of inflammation. Frank hemorrhage into the fluid also may be observed.

Treatment is symptomatic and includes repeated gastric decompression via nasogastric intubation to prevent gastric rupture. Analgesic administration to control abdominal pain is important, especially if the horse's violent signs pose a threat to itself or people. Large volumes of intravenous balanced electrolyte solutions are required to combat progressive dehydration and shock. Plasma electrolyte concentrations should be monitored closely and supplemented as indicated. If hypocalcemia occurs, 22% calcium borogluconate (10 g of available Ca/500 ml) should be added to the balanced electrolyte solution. If primary or secondary bacterial infection is suspected, broad-spectrum antibiotics are indicated.

Most cases are diagnosed at necropsy; therefore, the expected prognosis for horses with acute pancreatitis is poor. However, further investigation may show that pancreatitis plays a role in some medically responsive colics.

Chronic Pancreatitis

Subacute and chronic pancreatitis are rare antemortem diagnoses in horses and usually are recognized only when endocrine dysfunction is evident.[765] The cause is uncertain, but parasitic migration has been strongly implicated.[766-768] Clinical signs include chronic weight loss, intermittent abdominal pain, icterus and fever. Some animals have recurrent bouts of hypocalcemic tetany. Because the biliary and pancreatic ducts share a common duodenal papilla, mild hepatitis and cholangitis usually occur with pancreatitis. Steatorrhea and voluminous stool, common signs of exocrine pancreatic insufficiency in other species, are not seen in affected horses.[765] This may indicate that pancreatic enzyme activity in horses is less important to digestion than in most other animals because there is little fat in the equine diet.[765] If the disease is severe, destruction and fibrosis of the islets of Langerhans occur, with resultant hypoinsulinism and diabetes mellitus.[766,769]

Chronic interstitial pancreatitis is commonly observed in horses at necropsy.[742] It is thought to arise as an inflammatory process beginning in the ducts and spreading to the interstitial tissue. Ascending infections by gastrointestinal bacteria, as well as parasitic migration, may be responsible for this damage. In horses with chronic interstitial pancreatitis, the pancreas often is enlarged as normal parenchyma is replaced by scar tissue.[765] Pancreatic necrosis, occlusion of the ampulla and proximal duodenitis also have been documented.[770]

Exocrine pancreatic disease is often diagnosed by excluding other differential diagnoses for weight loss and abdominal pain. Evaluation of serum pancreatic enzyme activity in conjunction with hypocalcemia in cases of medically responsive abdominal diseases may identify less severe cases. Unfortunately, in many patients, necropsy may be necessary to diagnose this condition definitively.

References

1. Kelly WR: *Veterinary Clinical Diagnosis.* 3rd ed. Bailliere Tindall, London, 1984. pp 192-195.

2. Blood DC *et al: Veterinary Medicine.* 6th ed. Bailliere Tindall, London, 1983. pp 1240-1241, 185-186, 911-912.

3. Parry BW *et al:* Prognosis in equine colic: a comparative study of variables used to assess individual cases. *Equine Vet J* 15:211-215, 1983.

4. Alexander F: Certain aspects of the physiology and pharmacology of the horses digestive tract. *Equine Vet J* 4:166-169, 1972.

5. Todhunter RJ *et al:* Gastric rupture in horses: a review of 54 cases. *Equine Vet J* 18:288-293, 1986.

6. Barclay WP *et al:* Primary gastric impaction in the horse. *JAVMA* 181:682-683, 1982.

7. Colahan PT: Evaluation of horses with colic and the selection of surgical treatment. *Compend Cont Ed Pract Vet* 7:S141-S150, 1985.

8. Greatorex JC: Rectal exploration as an aid to the diagnosis of some medical conditions in the horse. *Equine Vet J* 1:26-30, 1968.

9. Kopf N, in Robinson NE: *Current Therapy in Equine Medicine 2.* Saunders, Philadelphia, 1987. pp 23-27.

10. Adams SB and McIlwraith CW: Abdominal crisis in the horse: a comparison of presurgical evaluation with surgical findings and results. *Vet Surg* 7:63-69, 1978.

11. Huskamp B and Kopf N: Right dorsal displacement of the large colon in the horse. *Equine Pract* 5(2):20-29, 1983.

12. Milne DW et al: Left dorsal displacement of the colon in the horse. *J Equine Med Surg* 1:47-52, 1977.

13. Becht JL et al: Colic caused by verminous arteritis: laboratory and clinical diagnosis. *Proc Equine Colic Res Symp*, 1983. pp 35-39.

14. Brown CM et al: Fiberoptic gastroduodenoscopy in the horse. *JAVMA* 186:965-968, 1985.

15. Traub-Dargatz JL: Endoscopy of the digestive tract of the horse. *Proc 5th Ann ACVIM Forum*, 1987. pp 742-744.

16. Reid CF: Radiography of the alimentary canal of the horse. *J So Afr Vet Assn* 46:69-72, 1975.

17. Rose JA et al: Radiography in the diagnosis of equine enterolithiasis. *Proc 26th Ann Conv AAEP*, 1980. pp 211-220.

18. Evans DR et al: Diagnosis and treatment of enterolithiasis in equidae. *Compend Cont Ed Pract Vet* 3:S383-S390, 1981.

19. Powis CL: Ultrasound science for the veterinarian. *Vet Clin No Am* (Equine Pract) 2:3-28, 1986.

20. Rantanen NW: General considerations for ultrasound examinations. *Vet Clin No Am* (Equine Pract) 2:29-32, 1986.

21. Rantanen NW: Diseases of the abdomen. *Vet Clin No Am* (Equine Pract) 2:67-88, 1986.

22. Traub JL et al: Surgical removal of choleliths in the horse. *JAVMA* 182:714-716, 1983.

23. Traub JL et al: Intraabdominal neoplasia as a cause of chronic weight loss in the horse. *Compend Cont Ed Pract Vet* 5:S526-S534, 1983.

24. Schalm OW et al: *Veterinary Hematology.* 3rd ed. Lea & Febiger, Philadelphia, 1975.

25. Moore WE, in Anderson NV: *Veterinary Gastroenterology.* Lea & Febiger, Philadelphia, 1980. pp 44-58.

26. Becht JL: Interpretation of erythrocyte and leukocyte responses, dynamics of plasma proteins and assessment of fibrinogen. *Proc 32nd Ann Conv AAEP*, 1986. pp 605-612.

27. Divers TJ et al: Interpretation of electrolyte abnormalities in clinical disease in the horse. *Proc 32nd Ann Mtg AAEP*, 1986. pp 69-80.

28. Martens RJ et al: Oral lactose tolerance test in foals: Technique and normal values. *Am J Vet Res* 46:2163-2165, 1985.

29. Merritt T et al: D-xylose absorption in growing foals. *Equine Vet J* 18:298-300, 1986.

30. Jacobs KA et al: Effect of diet on the oral D-xylose absorption test in the horse. *Am J Vet Res* 43:1856-1858, 1982.

31. Jacobs KA and Bolton JR: Effect of diet on the oral glucose tolerance test in the horse. *JAVMA* 180:884-886, 1982.

32. Bolton JR et al: Normal and abnormal xylose absorption in the horse. *Cornell Vet* 66:183-197, 1976.

33. Tulleners EP: Complications of abdominocentesis in the horse. *JAVMA* 182:232-234, 1983.

34. Schumacher J et al: Effects of enterocentesis on peritoneal fluid constituents in the horse. *JAVMA* 186:1301-1303, 1985.

35. Blackford JT et al: Equine peritoneal fluid analysis following celiotomy. *Proc 2nd Symp Equine Colic Res*, 1985. pp 130-133.

36. Brownlow MA: Polymorphonuclear neutrophil leukocytes of peritoneal fluid. *Equine Vet J* 15:22-24, 1983.

37. Nelson AW: Analysis of equine peritoneal fluid. *Vet Clin No Am* 1:267-274, 1979.

38. Swanwick RA and Wilkinson JS: A clinical evaluation of abdominal paracentesis in the horse. *Aust Vet J* 52:109-117, 1976.

39. White NA: Intestinal infarction associated with mesenteric vascular thrombotic disease in the horse. *JAVMA* 178:259-262, 1981.

40. Hunt E et al: Interpretation of peritoneal fluid erythrocyte counts in horses with abdominal diseases. *Proc 2nd Equine Colic Res Symp*, 1986. pp 168-174.

41. Adams SB et al: Cytologic interpretation of peritoneal fluid in the evaluation of equine abdominal crises. *Cornell Vet* 70:232-245, 1980.

42. Fischer AT et al: Diagnostic laparoscopy in the horse. *JAVMA* 3:289-292, 1986.

43. Witherspoon DM et al, in Harrison RM and Wildt DE: *Animal Laparoscopy.* Williams & Wilkins, Baltimore, 1980. pp 157-167.

44. Argenzio RA, in Anderson NV: *Veterinary Gastroenterology.* Lea & Febiger, Philadelphia, 1980. pp. 172-198.

45. Argenzio RA: Functions of the equine large intestine and their interrelationship in disease. *Cornell Vet* 65:303-330, 1975.

46. Aryenzio RA, in White NA: *The Equine Acute Abdomen.* Lea & Febiger, Philadelphia, 1990. pp 33-34.

47. Adams SB: Equine intestinal motility: An overview of normal activity, changes in disease, and effects of drug administration. *Proc 33rd Ann Mtg AAEP*, 1987. pp 539-556.

48. Sellars AF et al: Retropulsion-propulsion in equine large colon. *Am J Vet Res* 43:390-396, 1982.

49. Lowe JE et al: Equine pelvic flexure impaction: A model used to evaluate motor events and compare drug responses. *Cornell Vet* 70:401-412, 1980.

50. Ruckebusch Y: Motor functions of the intestine. *Adv Vet Sci Comp Med* 25:345-369, 1981.

51. Moore JN et al: Particular fecal markers in the diagnosis of large intestinal obstruction. *J Equine Med Surg* 2:541-544, 1978.

52. Granger DN et al: Effect of luminal distention in intestinal transcapillary fluid exchange. *Am J Physiol* 239:G516-G523, 1980.

53. Allen D et al: Factors for prognostic use in equine obstructive small intestinal disease. *JAVMA* 189:777-780, 1986.

54. Sullins KE et al: Pathologic changes associated with induced small intestinal strangulation, obstruction and non-strangulating infarction in horses. *Am J Vet Res* 46:913-916, 1985.

55. White NA et al: Mucosal alterations in experimentally induced small intestinal strangulation obstruction in ponnies. *Am J Vet Res* 41:193-198, 1980.

56. Meschter CL et al: Histologic findings in the gastrointestinal tract of horses with colic. *Am J Vet Res* 47:598-605, 1986.

57. Roy RS and McCord JM, in Greenwald RA and Cohen G: *Oxy Radicals and Their Scavenger Systems.* Vol II. Elseiver Science Publishers, New York, 1983. pp 145-150.

58. Parks DA and Granger DN, in Greenwald RA and Cohen G: *Oxy Radicals and Their Scavenger Systems.* Vol II. Elseiver Science Publishers, New York, 1983. pp 134-144.

59. Moore JN *et al:* Equine endotoxemia: an insight into cause and treatment. *JAVMA* 179:473-477, 1981.

60. Moore JN *et al:* Prevention of endotoxin-induced arterial hypoxemia and lactic acidosis with flunixin meglumine in ponies. *Equine Vet J* 13:95- 98, 1981.

61. Bottoms GD *et al:* Thromboxane prostaglandin I2 and the hemodynamic changes in equine endotoxin shock. *Am J Vet Res* 43:999-1002, 1983.

62. Moore JN *et al:* Modulation of arachidonic acid metabolism in endotoxic horses: Comparison of flunixin meglumine, phenylbutazone, and a selective thromboxane synthetase inhibitor. *Am J Vet Res* 47:110-113, 1986.

63. White NA *et al:* Scanning electron microscopic study of *Strongylus vulgaris* larva-induced arteritis in the pony. *Equine Vet J* 15:349-353, 1983.

64. Argenzio RA *et al:* Colonic compensation in transmissible gastroenteritis of swine. *Gastroenterology* 86:1501-1509, 1984.

65. Argenzio RA and Stevens CE: Sites of organic acid production and absorption in the equine gastrointestinal tract. *Am J Physiol* 226:1043-1050, 1974.

66. Argenzio RA *et al:* Interrelationship of Na, HCO3 and volatile fatty acid transport by equine large intestine. *Am J Physiol* 233:E469-E478, 1977.

67. Bertone AL *et al:* Digestion, fecal, and blood variables associated with extensive large colon resection in the horse. *Am J Vet Res* 50:253-258, 1989.

68. Ooms L and Degryse A: Pathogenesis and pharmacology of diarrhea. *Vet Res Comm* 10:355-398, 1986.

69. Cheney CP *et al:* Species specificity of *in vitro Escherichia coli* adherence to host intestinal cell membranes and its correlation with in vivo colonization and infectivity. *Infect Immun* 28:1019-1027, 1980.

70. Holtand RE *et al:* Isolation of enterotoxigenic *Escherichia coli* from a foal with diarrhea. *JAVMA* 194:389-391, 1989.

71. Argenzio RA and Whipp SC: Effect of *Escherichia coli* heat stable enterotoxin and theophylline on ion transport in porcine colon. *J Physiol* 320:469-487, 1981.

72. Smith BP: *Salmonella* infections in horses. *Compend Cont Ed Pract Vet* 3:S4-S16, 1981.

73. Murray MJ: Enterotoxin activity of a *Salmonella typhimurium* of equine origin *in vivo* in rabbits and the effect of *Salmonella* culture lysates and cholera toxin on equine colonic mucosa *in vitro*. *Am J Vet Res* 86:769-773, 1986.

74. Drudge JH and Lyons ET: The chemotherapy of migrating strongyle larvae. *Proc 2nd Intl Conf Equine Infect Dis*, 1970. pp 310-322.

75. Greatorex JC: Diarrhoea in horses associated with ulceration of the colon and caecum resulting in *S vulgaris* larval migration. *Vet Record* 97:221- 225, 1975.

76. Chiejina SN and Mason JA: Immature stages of *Trichonema* spp as a cause of diarrhoea in adult horses in spring. *Vet Record* 100:360-361, 1977.

77. Klei TR *et al:* Morphologic and clinicopathologic changes following *Strongylus vulgaris* infections of immune and nonimmune ponies. *Am J Vet Res* 43:1300-1307, 1982.

78. Sims LD *et al:* Hemorrhagic necrotising enteritis in foals associated with *Clostridium perfringens.* *Aust Vet J* 62:194-196, 1985.

79. Bertone JJ *et al:* Diarrhea associated with sand in the gastrointestinal tract of horses. *JAVMA* 193:1409-1411, 1988.

80. Cimprich RE: Equine granulomatous enteritis. *Vet Pathol* 11:535-547, 1974.

81. Merritt AM *et al:* Granulomatous enteritis in nine horses. *JAVMA* 169:603-609, 1976.

82. Pass DA and Bolton JR: Chronic eosinophilic gastroenteritis in the horse. *Vet Pathol* 19:486-496, 1982.

83. Lindberg R: Pathology of equine granulomatous enteritis. *J Comp Pathol* 41:1699-1703, 1984.

84. Conner ME and Darlington RW: Rotavirus infection in foals. *Am J Vet Res* 41:1699-1703, 1980.

85. Tzipori S: The relative importance of enteric pathogens affecting neonates of domestic animals. *Adv Vet Sci Comp Med* 29:103-206, 1985.

86. Masri MD *et al:* Faecal composition in foal heat diarrhea. *Equine Vet J* 18:301-306, 1986.

87. Kazunori I *et al:* Establishment of intestinal ciliates in new-born horses. *Jpn J Vet Sci* 47:39-43, 1985.

88. Lowe JE: Xylazine, pentazocine, meperidine, and dipyrone for relief of ballon induced equine colic. A double blind comparative evaluation. *J Equine Med Surg* 2:286-291, 1978.

89. Pippi NL and Lumb WV: Objective tests of analgesic drugs in ponies. *Am J Vet Res* 40:1082-1086, 1979.

90. Kohn CW and Muir WW: Selected aspects of the clinical pharmacology of visceral analgesics and gut motility modifying drugs in the horse. *J Vet Int Med* 2:85-91, 1988.

91. Kalpravidh M *et al:* Effects of butorphanol, flunixin, levorphanol, morphine, and xylazine in ponies. *Am J Vet Res* 45:217-223, 1984.

92. Muir WW and Robertson JT: Visceral analgesia: Effects of xylazine, butorphanol, meperidine, and pentazocine in horses. *Am J Vet Res* 46:2081-2084, 1985.

93. Ross MW *et al:* Normal and altered cecocolic motility patterns in ponies. *Vet Surg* 14:1, 1985.

94. Adams SB *et al:* Motility of the distal portion of the jejunum and pelvic flexure in ponies: effects of six drugs. *Am J Vet Res* 45:795-799, 1984.

95. Adams SB *et al:* Effects of selected drugs on intestinal motility in the horse. *Proc 2nd Symp Equine Colic Res*, 1986. pp 85-88.

96. Clark ES *et al:* Effects of xylazine on cecal mechanical activity and cecal blood flow in healthy horses. *Am J Vet Res* 49:720-723, 1988.

97. Muir WW *et al:* Evaluation of xylazine, guaifenesin and ketamine hydrochloride for restraint in horses. *Am J Vet Res* 39:1274-1278, 1978.

98. Knight AP: Xylazine. *JAVMA* 176:454-455, 1980.

99. Lowe JE and Hilfiger J: Analgesic and sedative effects of detomidine compared to xylazine in a colic model using IV and IM routes of administration. *Acta Vet Scand* 82(Suppl):85-95, 1986.

100. Hamm D and Jochle W: Sedation and analgesia in horses treated with various doses of domosedan: Blind studies on efficacy and the duration of effects. *Proc 30th Ann Mtg AAEP*, 1984. pp 235-242.

101. Jochle W and Hamm D: Sedation and analgesia with Domosedan (detomidine hydrochloride) in horses: Dose response studies of efficacy and its duration. *Acta Vet Scand* 82 (Suppl):69-94, 1986.

102. Short CE et al: Cardiovascular and pulmonary function studies of a new sedative/analgesic (Detomidine) for use in horses. *Proc 30th Ann Mtg AAEP*, 1984. pp 243-250.

103. Clarke KW and Taylor PM: Detomidine: A new sedative. *Equine Vet J* 18:366-370, 1986.

104. Jochle W et al: Comparison of detomidine, butorphanol, flunixin meglumine, and xylazine in clinical cases of equine colic. *Equine Vet J* Suppl 7:111-116, 1989.

105. Davis LE, in Anderson NV: *Veterinary Gastroenterology*. Lea & Febiger, Philadelphia, 1980. pp 263-292.

106. Roberts MC and Argenzio A: Effects of amitraz, several opiate derivatives and anticholinergic agents on intestinal transit in ponies. *Equine Vet J* 18:256-260, 1986.

107. Roger TH et al: Colonic motor responses in the pony: Relevance of colonic stimulation by opiate antagonists. *Am J Vet Res* 46:31-35, 1985.

108. Stout RC and Priest GT: Clinical experience using butorphanol tartrate for relief of abdominal pain in the horse. *Proc 2nd Ann Symp Equine Colic Res*, 1986. pp 68-70.

109. Sojka J et al: The effect of 2 opiate agonist-antagonists on intestinal motility in the pony. *Proc 2nd Ann Symp Equine Colic Res*, 1986. pp 102-104.

110. Combie J et al: Pharmacology of narcotic analgesics in the horse: Selective blockade of narcotic-induced locomotor activity. *Am J Vet Res* 42:716-721, 1981.

111. Muir WW et al: Hemodynamic and respiratory effects of a xylazine-acetylpromazine drug combination in horses. *Am J Vet Res* 40:1518-1522, 1979.

112. Watney GCG et al: Effects of a demand valve on pulmonary ventilation in spontaneously breathing, anaesthetised horses. *Vet Record* 117:358-362, 1985.

113. Vernimb GD and Hennessey PW: Clinical studies on flunixin meglumine in the treatment of equine colic. *J Equine Med Surg* 1:111-116, 1977.

114. Gerring EL and Hunt JM: Pathophysiology of equine postoperative ileus: effect of adrenergic blockade, parasympathetic stimulation and metoclopramide in an experimental model. *Equine Vet J* 18:249-255, 1986.

115. Gerring EL and King JN: Cisapride in the prophylaxis of equine post-operative ileus. *Equine Vet J* Suppl 7:52-56, 1989.

116. Adams SB and MacHarg M: Neostigmine methylsulfate delays gastric emptying of particulate markers in horses. *Am J Vet Res* 46:2498-2499, 1985.

117. Pinder RM et al: Metoclopramide: A review of its pharmacological properties and clinical usage. *Drugs* 12:81-131, 1976.

118. Burrows CF: Metoclopramide. *JAVMA* 183:1321-1343, 1983.

119. Hunt JM and Gerring EL: A preliminary study on the effects of metoclopramide on equine gut activity. *J Vet Pharmacol Therap* 9:109-112, 1986.

120. Ducharme NG and Fubini SL: Gastrointestinal complication associated with the use of atropine in horses. *JAVMA* 82:229-231, 1983.

121. Davis LE and Knight AP: Review of the clinical pharmacology of the equine digestive tract. *J Equine Med Surg* 1:27, 1977.

122. Haynes RC and Murad R, in Gilman AG et al: *Goodman and Gilman's The Pharmacological Basis of Therapeutics*. 7th ed. MacMillan, New York, 1985. pp 1517-1543.

123. Hood DM et al: Phenoxybenzamine for the treatment of severe nonresponsive diarrhea in the horse. *JAVMA* 180:758-762, 1982.

124. Zelders JN et al: Ranitidine: A new H2-receptor antagonist. *N Eng J Med* 309:1368-1373, 1983.

125. Douglas WW, in Gilman AG et al: *Goodman and Gilman's Pharmacological Basis of Therapeutics*. 7th ed. MacMillan, New York, 1985. pp 624-627.

126. MacAllister CG et al: The effects of cimetidine and ranitidine on the gastric pH of fasted horses. *Proc 2nd Ann Symp Equine Colic Res*, 1986. pp 123-125.

127. Campbell-Thompson ML and Merritt AM: Gastric cannulation in the young horse: A new technique for studying gastric fluid secretion. *Proc 2nd Ann Symp Equine Colic Res*, 1986. pp 120-122.

128. Campbell-Thompson ML and Merritt AM: Effect of ranitidine on gastric acid secretion in young male horses. *Am J Vet Res* 48:1511-1515, 1987.

129. Palmer JE: Gastrointestinal diseases of foals. *Vet Clin No Am* (Equine Pract) 1:151-168, 1985.

130. Clark ES and Becht JL: Clinical pharmacology of the gastrointestinal tract. *Vet Clin No Am* (Equine Pract) 3:101-122, 1987.

131. Murray MJ: Equine gastric ulcer syndrome. *Equine Vet Data* 6:309-367, 1985.

132. Harvey SC, in Gilman AG et al: *Goodman and Gilman's Pharmacological Basis of Therapeutics*. 7th ed. MacMillan, New York, 1985. p 988.

133. Naylor JM et al: Alimentation of hypophagic horses. *Compend Cont Ed Pract Vet* 6:S93-S100, 1984.

134. Naylor JM and Freeman DE, in Robinson NE: *Current Therapy in Equine Medicine 2*. Saunders, Philadelphia, 1987. pp 421-426.

135. Della Ferra MA: Benzodiazepines stimulate feeding in clinically debilitated animals. *Fed Proc* 307:401, 1978.

136. Baile CA: Endotoxin-elicited fever and anorexia and elfazepam-stimulated feeding in sheep. *Physiol Behavior* 27:271, 1981.

137. Hansen TO et al: Total parenteral nutrition in four healthy adult horses. *Proc 2nd Ann Symp Equine Colic Res*, 1986. p 204.

138. Sweeney R, Univ Pennsylvania: Personal communication, 1990.

139. Tate LP et al: Effects of extensive resection of the small intestine in the pony. *Am J Vet Res* 44:1187-1191, 1983.

140. Ralston SL et al: Digestion in horses after resection or ischemic insult of the large colon. *Am J Vet Res* 47:2290-2293, 1986.

141. Herd RP, in Robinson NE: *Current Therapy in Equine Medicine 2*. Saunders, Philadelphia, 1987. pp 328-331.

142. Herd RP, in Robinson NE: *Current Therapy in Equine Medicine 2*. Saunders, Philadelphia, 1987. pp 331-332.

143. Herd RP, in Robinson NE: *Current Therapy in Equine Medicine 2*. Saunders, Philadelphia, 1987. pp 334-336.

144. Berry CR *et al:* Evaluation of the myoelectrical activity of the equine ileum infected with *Strongylus vulgaris* larvae. *Am J Vet Res* 47:27-30, 1986.

145. Bennett DG: Clinical pharmacology of ivermectin. *JAVMA* 189:100-104, 1986.

146. Church S *et al:* Diagnosis and successful treatment of diarrhoea in horses caused by immature strongyles apparently insusceptible to anthelmintics. *Equine Vet J* 18:401-403, 1986.

147. Kirkpatrick CE and Skand DL: Giardiasis in a horse. *JAVMA* 187:163-164, 1985.

148. Holmberg DL: Prophylactic use of antibiotics in surgery. *Vet Clin No Am* 8:219, 1978.

149. Brumbaugh GW: Rational selection of antimicrobial drugs for treatment of infections in horses. *Vet Clin No Am* (Equine Pract) 3:191-220, 1987.

150. Pittinger C and Adamson R: Antibiotic blockade of neuromuscular function. *Ann Rev Pharm* 12:169, 1972.

151. Palmer JE, in Robinson NE: *Current Therapy in Equine Medicine 2*. Saunders, Philadelphia, 1987. pp 88-92.

152. Jewes LA: Antimicrobial therapy of non-*typhi* *Salmonella* and *Shigella* infections. *J Antimicrob Chemotherap* 19:557-600, 1987.

153. Bryna JP *et al:* Problems in salmonellosis: Rationale for clinical trials with newer B-lactam agents and quinolones. *Rev Infect Dis* 8:189-207, 1986.

154. Gorbach SL: Bacterial diarrhea and its treatment. *Lancet* 2:1378-1382, 1987.

155. Cherubin CE *et al:* Septicemia with non-typhoid *Salmonella*. *Medicine* 53:365-376, 1974.

156. Hirsh DC and Jang SS: Antimicrobial susceptibility of bacterial pathogens from horses. *Vet Clin No Am* (Equine Pract) 3:181-190, 1987.

157. Whitlock RH: Therapeutic strategies involving antimicrobial treatment of the gastro-intestinal tract in large animals. *JAVMA* 185:1210-1213, 1984.

158. Johnston JK and Morris DD: Comparison of duodenitis/proximal jejunitis and small intestinal obstruction in horses: 68 cases (1977-1985). *JAVMA* 191:849-854, 1987.

159. White NA *et al:* Hemorrhagic fibrinonecrotic duodenitis-proximal jejunitis in horses: 20 cases (1977-1984). *JAVMA* 190:311-315, 1987.

160. Rosenthal SL: Exacerbation of Salmonella enteritis due to ampicillin. *N Eng J Med* 280:147, 1969.

161. Dixon JMS: Effect of antibiotic treatment on duration of excretion of *Salmonella typhimurium* in children. *Brit Med J* 2:1343, 1965.

162. Watanabe J: Infectious drug resistance. *Sci Am* 217:19, 1967.

163. Ericsson CD: Bismuth subsalicylate inhibits activity of crude toxins of *Escherichia coli* and *Vibrio cholerae*. *J Infect Dis* 136:693, 1977.

164. Dupont HL: Symptomatic treatment of diarrhea with bismuth subsalicylate among students attending a Mexican university. *Gastroenterology* 73:715, 1977.

165. Tothill A: Prostaglandin E2: A factor in the pathogenesis of cholera. *Prostaglandins* 11:925-933, 1976.

166. Waller SL: Prostaglandins and the gastrointestinal tract. *Gut* 14:402-417, 1973.

167. Semrad SD *et al:* Low dose flunixin meglumine: Effects on eisosanoid production and clinical signs induced by experimental endotoxaemia in horses. *Equine Vet J* 19:201-206, 1987.

168. Garner HE *et al:* Active and passive immunization for blockade of endotoxemia. *Proc 31st Ann Mtg AAEP*, 1985. pp 525-532.

169. Spier SJ *et al:* Protection against clinical endotoxemia in horses using plasma containing antibody to an Rc mutant *E. coli* (J5). *Circ Shock* 28:235-248, 1989.

170. Gerhards H and Eberhardt C: Plasma heparin values and hemostasis in equids after subcutaneous administration of low-dose calcium heparin. *Am J Vet Res* 49:13-18, 1988.

171. Targowski SP: Serum immunoglobulin, dermal response, and lymphocyte transformation studies in horses with chronic diarrhea. *Infect Immunol* 12:48, 1975.

172. Targowski SP: Treatment of horses with chronic diarrhea: Immunologic status. *Am J Vet Res* 37:29, 1978.

173. Meuten DJ *et al:* Chronic enteritis associated with malabsorption and protein-losing enteropathy in the horse. *JAVMA* 172:326-333, 1978.

174. Parry BW *et al:* Assessment of the necessity for surgical intervention in cases of colic: a retrospective study. *Equine Vet J* 15:216- 221, 1983.

175. Donawick WJ *et al:* The diagnostic and prognostic value of lactate determinations in horses with acute abdominal crises. *J So Afr Vet Assn* 48:127, 1975.

176. Bristol DG: The anion gap as a prognostic indicator in horses with abdominal pain. *JAVMA* 181:63-65, 1982.

177. Parry BW *et al:* Prognosis in equine colic: A study of individual variables used in case assessment. *Equine Vet J* 15:337-344, 1983.

178. Pascoe PJ *et al:* Accuracy of clinical examination in the prognosis of abdominal pain in the horse. *Proc 2nd Equine Colic Res*, 1986. pp 149-152.

179. Adams SB: Surgical approaches to and exploration of the equine abdomen. *Vet Clin No Am* 4:89-104, 1982.

180. Miller LD *et al:* The pathophysiology and management of intestinal obstruction. *Surg Clin No Am* 42:1285-1309, 1965.

181. Singleton AO and Montalbo P: Effects of decompression during removal of intestinal obstruction. *Am J Surg* 167:909-911, 1968.

182. Stashak TS: Techniques for enterotomy, decompression and intestinal resection/anastomosis. *Vet Clin No Am* 4:147-165, 1982.

183. Taylor TS *et al:* Retrograde flushing for relief of obstructions of the transverse colon in the horse. *Equine Pract* 5(6):22-28, 1979.

184. Richardson DC: Intestinal surgery: A review. *Compend Cont Ed Pract Vet* 3:259-270, 1981.

185. Edwards GB: Resection and anastomosis of small intestine: Current methods applicable to the horse. *Equine Vet J* 18:322-330, 1986.

186. Dean PW and Robertson JT: Comparison of three suture techniques for anastomosis of the small intestine in the horse. *Am J Vet Res* 46:1282- 1286, 1985.

187. Sullins KE *et al:* Evaluation of intestinal staples for end-to-end anastomosis of the small intestine in the horse. *Vet Surg* 14:87-92, 1985.

188. Hansen RR and Nixon AJ: Small colon anastomoses: A comparison of stapled and sutured techniques. *Vet Surg* 16:91, 1987.

189. Robertson-Smith RG and Adams SB: Management of postoperative complications following equine abdominal surgery. *Compend Cont Ed Pract Vet* 8:844-849, 1986.

190. Hunt JM et al: Incidence, diagnosis and treatment of postoperative complications in colic cases. *Equine Vet J* 18:264-270, 1986.

191. Ducharme NG et al: Surgical treatment of colic-Results of 181 horses. *Vet Surg* 12:206-209, 1983.

192. Parker JE et al: The use of heparin in preventing intra-abdominal adhesions secondary to experimentally induced peritonitis in the horse. *Vet Surg* 16:459-462, 1987.

193. Schneider JE and Leipold HW: Recessive lethal white in foals. *J Equine Med Surg* 2:479-482, 1978.

194. Hultgren BD: Ileocolonic aganglionosis in white progeny of overo spotted horses. *JAVMA* 180:289-292, 1982.

195. Jones WE: The Overo white foal syndrome. *J Equine Med Surg* 3:54-56, 1979.

196. Loeven K: Overo crosses and aganglionosis. *J Equine Vet Sci* 7:249-250, 1987.

197. Bruner DW and Gillespie JH: *Hagan's Infectious Diseases of Domestic Animals.* 6th ed. Cornell Univ Press, Ithaca, 1973.

198. Horsch F, in Dietz O and Wiesner E: *Diseases of the Horse.* Vol Part II. Karger, New York, 1984. pp 293-296.

199. US Dept HEW: *Veterinary Public Health Notes.* Washington, DC, 1974.

200. Smith HA et al, in Smith HA et al: *Veterinary Pathology.* 4th ed. Lea & Febiger, Philadelphia, 1972. pp 570-572.

201. Schmitz DG and Reagor JC, in Robinson NE: *Current Therapy in Equine Medicine 2.* Saunders, Philadelphia, 1987. pp 120-122.

202. Schoeb TR and Panciera RJ: Blister beetle poisoning in horses. *JAVMA* 173:75-77, 1978.

203. Shawley RV and Rolf LL: Experimental cantharidiasis in the horse. *Am J Vet Res* 45:2261-2266, 1984.

204. MacKay RJ et al: Effects of large doses of phenylbutazone administration to horses. *Am J Vet Res* 44:774-780, 1983.

205. Traub JL et al: Phenylbutazone toxicosis in the foal. *Am J Vet Res* 44:1410-1418, 1983.

206. Collins LG and Tyler DE: Phenylbutazone toxicosis in the horse: A clinical study. *JAVMA* 184:699-703, 1984.

207. Traub-Dargatz JL: Potential atoxicity of nonsteroidal anti-inflammatory drug therapy in the foal. *Proc 5th Ann ACVIM Forum*, 1987. pp 5:451-452.

208. Snow DH et al: Phenylbutazone toxicosis in equidae: A biochemical and pathophysiological study. *Am J Vet Res* 42:1754-1759, 1981.

209. Collins LG and Tyler DE: Experimentally induced phenylbutazone toxicosis in ponies. Description of the syndrome and its prevention with synthetic prostaglandin E2. *Am J Vet Res* 46:1605-1615, 1985.

210. Gunson DE and Soma LR: Renal papillary necrosis in horses after phenylbutazone and water deprivation. *Vet Pathol* 70:603-610, 1983.

211. Murray JJ: Phenylbutazone toxicity in a horse. *Compend Cont Ed Pract Vet* 7:S389-S394, 1985.

212. Boulton CH, in Robinson NE: *Current Equine Therapy 2.* Saunders, Philadelphia, 1987. pp 107-109.

213. Cotchin EA: A general survey of tumors in the horse. *Equine Vet J* 9:16-21, 1977.

214. Sendberg JP et al: Neoplasms of equidae. *JAVMA* 170:150-152, 1977.

215. Kerr KM and Alden CL: Equine neoplasia: A ten-year survey. *Proc 17th Ann Mtg Am Assn Vet Lab Diagnost*, 1974. p 183.

216. Meagher DM et al: Squamous cell carcinoma of the equine stomach. *JAVMA* 164:81-84, 1974.

217. Van den Hover R and Franken P: Clinical aspects of lymphosarcoma in the horse: A clinical report of 16 cases. *Equine Vet J* 15:49-53, 1983.

218. Lane PC: Palatine lymphosarcoma in two horses. *Equine Vet J* 17:465-467, 1985.

219. Platt H: Alimentary lymphomas in the horse. *J Comp Pathol* 97:1-10, 1987.

220. Rebhun WC and Bertone AL: Equine lymphosarcoma. *JAVMA* 184:720-721, 1984.

221. Church S et al: Two cases of pancreatic adenocarcinoma in horses. *Equine Vet J* 19:77-79, 1987.

222. Honnas CM et al: Small intestinal adenocarcinoma in a horse. *JAVMA* 191:845-846, 1987.

223. Collier MA and Trent AM: Jejunal intussusception associated with leiomyoma in an aged horse. *JAVMA* 182:810-821, 1982.

224. Hanes GE and Robertson JT: Leiomyoma of the small intestine in a horse. *JAVMA* 182:1398, 1983.

225. Livesay MA et al: Colic in two horses associated with smooth muscle intestinal tumors. *Equine Vet J* 18:334-337, 1986.

226. Wallace SS et al: Mesothelioma in a horse. *Compend Cont Ed Pract Vet* 9:210-216, 1987.

227. Ross MW et al: Hypoglycemic seizures in a Shetland pony. *Cornell Vet* 73:151-169, 1983.

228. Wright AI: Verminous arteritis as a cause of colic in the horse. *Equine Vet J* 4:169-174, 1972.

229. White NA: Thromboembolic colic in horses. *Compend Cont Ed Pract Vet* 7:S156-S173, 1985.

230. Davies JV and Gerring EL: Effect of experimental vascular occlusion on small intestinal motility in ponies. *Equine Vet J* 17:219-224, 1985.

231. Adams SB: The recognition and management of ileus. *Vet Clin No Am* 4:91-104, 1988.

232. Becht JL and Richardson DW: Ileus in the horse: Clinical significance and management. *Proc 27th Ann Mtg AAEP*, 1981. pp 291-297.

233. Rennie JA et al: Neural and humoral factors in postoperative ileus. *Brit J Surg* 67:694-698, 1980.

234. Huskamp B: Diagnosis of gastroduodenojejunitis and its surgical treatment by a temporary duodenocecostomy. *Equine Vet J* 17:314-316, 1985.

235. King JN and Gerring EL: Actions of the novel gastrointestinal prokinetic agent cisapride on equine bowel motility. *J Vet Pharmacol Therap* 11:314-321, 1988.

236. Gilmour JS: Observations on neuronal changes in grass sickness of horses. *Res Vet Sci* 15:197-200, 1973.

237. Barclay WP et al: Chronic nongranulomatous arteritis in seven horses. *JAVMA* 190:684-686, 1987.

238. Bueno L *et al:* Disturbances of digestive motility in horses associated with strongyle infection. *Vet Parasitol* 5:254-260, 1979.

239. Robertson JT, in Mansmann RA and McAllister ES: *Equine Medicine and Surgery.* 3rd ed. Vol 1. American Veterinary Publications, Goleta, CA, 1982. pp 559-579.

240. Byars TD, in Robinson NE: *Current Therapy in Equine Medicine.* Saunders, Philadelphia, 1983. pp 236-238.

241. Dyce CM *et al: Textbook of Veterinary Anatomy.* Saunders, Philadelphia, 1987. pp 462-485, 511-513.

242. Geiser DR *et al:* Tympanic bulla, petrous temporal bone and hyoid apparatus diseases in horses. *Compend Cont Ed Pract Vet* 10:740-755, 1988.

243. Koch DB, in Mansmann RA and McAllister ES: *Equine Medicine and Surgery.* 3rd ed. American Veterinary Publications, Goleta, CA, 1982. pp 458-476.

244. Schleiter H, in Dietz O and Wiesner E: *Diseases of the Horse.* Vol Part I. Karger, New York, 1984. pp 124-139.

245. Scott EA: Surgery of the oral cavity. *Vet Clin No Am* (Large Anim Pract) 4:3-31, 1982.

246. Haynes PF, in Jennings PB: *The Practice of Large Animal Surgery.* Saunders, Philadelphia, 1984. pp 388-487.

247. Saperstein G: Hypoplasia of the upper lip in a foal. *VM/ SAC* 78:869, 1983.

248. Haynes PF and Qualls JCW: Cleft soft palate, nasal septal deviation, and epiglottic entrapment in a Thoroughbred filly. *JAVMA* 179:910-913, 1981.

249. Bowman KF *et al:* Complications of cleft palate repair in large animals. *JAVMA* 180:652-657, 1982.

250. Bowman KF, in Robinson NE: *Current Therapy in Equine Medicine 2.* Saunders, Philadelphia, 1987. pp 1-3.

251. McIlwraith CW, in Jennings PB: *The Practice of Large Animal Surgery.* Saunders, Philadelphia, 1984. pp 554-663.

252. Dietz O, in Dietz O and Wiesner E: *Diseases of the Horse.* Part I. Karger, New York, 1984. pp 149-155.

253. Linnabary RD *et al:* Oral ulceration in a horse caused by grass awns. *J Equine Vet Sci* 6:20-22, 1986.

254. Smyth GB *et al:* Delayed repair of an extensive lip laceration in a colt using an Estlander flap. *Vet Surg* 17:350- 352, 1988.

255. Terechow PF, in Dietz O and Wiesner E: *Diseases of the Horse.* Part I. Karger, New York, 1984. pp 441-462.

256. Cho DY *et al: Micronema* granuloma in the gingiva of a horse. *JAVMA* 187:505-507, 1985.

257. Verstraete FJM and Ligthelm AJ: Excessive granulation tissue of periodontal origin in a horse. *Equine Vet J* 20:380-382, 1988.

258. Sisson S, in Getty R: *Sisson and Grossman's The Anatomy of Domestic Animals.* 5th ed. Saunders, Philadelphia, 1975. pp 376-453.

259. Blythe LL *et al:* Vestibular syndrome associated with temperohyoid fusion and temporal bone fractures in three horses. *JAVMA* 185:775-781, 1984.

260. Cook WR, in Brunsell CSG: *The Veterinary Annual.* John Wright and Sons, Bristol, 1971. pp 12-43.

261. Power HT *et al:* Facial and vestibulocochlear nerve disease in six horses. *JAVMA* 183:1076-1080, 1983.

262. Cook WR: Skeletal radiology of the equine head. *Vet Radiol* 11:35-55, 1970.

263. Watrous BJ: Head tilt in horses. *Vet Clin No Am* (Equine Pract) 3:353-370, 1987.

264. Spurlock SL *et al:* Keratoconjunctivitis sicca associated with fracture of the stylohyoid in a horse. *JAVMA* 194:258-259, 1989.

265. Goubaux A and Barrier G: *The Exterior of the Horse.* 2nd ed. Lippincott, Philadelphia, 1892.

266. Huidekoper RS: *Age of the Domestic Animals.* 2nd ed. Eger, Chicago, 1903.

267. Galvayne S: *Horse Dentition.* 2nd ed. Thomas Murray, Glasgow, 1919.

268. *Official Guide for Determining the Age of the Horse.* American Association of Equine Practitioners, Lexington, KY, 1966.

269. Baker GJ: Some aspects of equine dental radiology. *Equine Vet J* 3:46-51, 1971.

270. Baker GJ: Dental disease in the horse. *Vet Record* Suppl 1:19-26, 1979.

271. Baker GJ: *A study of dental disease in the horse.* PhD thesis, University of Glasgow, 1979.

272. Becker E: *Handbuch der Speziellen Pathologischen Anatomie der Haustiere.* Paul Parey, Berlin, 1962.

273. Jubb KVF and Kennedy PC: *Pathology of Domestic Animals.* Vol 2. 2nd ed. Academic Press, New York, 1970. pp 65-190.

274. Cannon JH *et al:* Diagnosis and surgical treatment of cystlike lesions of the equine paranasal sinuses. *JAVMA* 169:610- 613, 1976.

275. Espersen G: *Multiple Kaebecyster Hos Hesten.* Mortensen, Copenhagen, 1962.

276. Rubarth S and Krook L: Etiology and pathogenesis of so-called mucoid degeneration of nasal conchae in the horse. *Acta Vet Scand* 9:253-267, 1968.

277. Lane JG *et al:* Equine paranasal sinus cysts: A report of 15 cases. *Equine Vet J* 19:537-544, 1987.

278. Eisenmenger F: Surgical treatment of alveolar periostitis in young horses. *Wien Tierrztl Mschr* 46:51-70, 1959.

279. Hofmeyr CFB: Comparative dental pathology (with particular reference to caries and paradontal disease in the horse and dog). *J So Afr Vet Assn* 29:471-480, 1960.

280. McIlwraith CW and Turner AS: *Equine Surgery - Advanced Techniques.* Lea & Febiger, Philadelphia, 1987. pp 12-19, 264-267.

281. Tolliver SL *et al:* Observations on the specific location of *Gasterophilus* spp larvae in the mouth of the horse. *J Parasitol* 60:891-892, 1974.

282. King JD: Experimental investigations of paradontal disease. *Brit Dent J* 82:61-69, 1947.

283. Baker GJ: Dental disorders in the horse. *Compend Cont Ed Pract Vet* 4:S507-S515, 1982.

284. Merillat LA: *Veterinary Surgery.* Eger, Chicago, 1921.

285. Baker GJ: Some aspects of equine dental decay. *Equine Vet J* 6:127-130, 1974.

286. Honma K *et al:* Statistical study on the occurrence of dental caries in domestic animals. I. Horse. *Jpn J Vet Res* 10:31- 36, 1962.

287. Colyer F: *Abnormal Conditions of the Teeth of Animals and Their Relationship to Similar Conditions in Man*. Dental Board of the United Kingdom, London, 1931.

288. Peter CP et al: Ameloblastic odontoma in a pony. *Am J Vet Res* 29:1495-1498, 1968.

289. Lingard DR and Crawford TB: Congenital ameloblastic odontoma in a foal. *Am J Vet Res* 31:801-804, 1970.

290. Alexander F and Hickson JCD, in Phillipson AT: *Physiology of Digestion and Metabolism in the Ruminant*. Oriel Press, Newcastle-on-Tyne, England, 1970. pp 375-389.

291. Alexander F: A study of parotid salivation in the horse. *J Physiol* 184:646-656, 1966.

292. Eckersall PD et al: Equine whole saliva: Variability of some major constituents. *Equine Vet J* 17:391-393, 1985.

293. Fowler ME: Congenital atresia of the parotid duct in a horse. *JAVMA* 146:1403-1404, 1965.

294. Hofmeyr CFB, in Oehme FW and Prior JE: *Textbook of Large Animal Surgery*. Williams & Wilkins, Baltimore, 1974. pp 391-392.

295. Bowman KF, in Robinson NE: *Current Therapy in Equine Medicine 2*. Saunders, Philadelphia, 1987. pp 3-6.

296. Stick JA: Surgery of the esophagus. *Vet Clin No Am* (Large Anim Pract) 4:33-59, 1982.

297. Stick JA, in Robinson NE: *Current Therapy in Equine Medicine 2*. Saunders, Philadelphia, 1987. pp 12-15.

298. Stick JA et al: Equine esophageal pressure profile. *Am J Vet Res* 44:272-275, 1983.

299. Clark ES et al: Esophageal manometry in horses, cows, and sheep during deglutition. *Am J Vet Res* 48:547-551, 1987.

300. Nickel R et al: *The Viscera of the Domestic Animals*. 2nd ed. Springer-Verlag, New York, 1973. pp 99-101, 180-199.

301. Slocombe RF et al: Quantitative ultrastructural anatomy of esophagus in different regions of the horse: Effects on alternate methods of tissue processing. *Am J Vet Res* 43:1137-1142, 1982.

302. Stick JA et al: Equine cervical esophagostomy: Complications associated with durations and location of feeding tubes. *Am J Vet Res* 42:727-732, 1981.

303. Freeman DE and Naylor JM: Cervical esophagostomy to permit extraoral feeding of the horse. *JAVMA* 172:314-320, 1978.

304. Nixon AJ et al: Esophagomyotomy for relief of an intrathoracic esophageal stricture in a horse. *JAVMA* 183:794-796, 1983.

305. Stick JA et al: Acid-base and electrolyte alterations associated with salivary loss in the pony. *Am J Vet Res* 42:733- 737, 1981.

306. Scott EA et al: Intramural esophageal cyst in a horse. *JAVMA* 171:652-654, 1977.

307. Stick JA et al: Esophageal intramural cyst in a horse. *JAVMA* 171:1133, 1977.

308. Bartels JE and Vaughan JT: Persistent right aortic arch in the horse. *JAVMA* 154:406-409, 1969.

309. Bowman KF et al: Megaesophagus in a colt. *JAVMA* 172:334- 337, 1978.

310. Rohrback BW and Rooney JR: Congenital esophageal ectasia in a Thoroughbred foal. *JAVMA* 177:65-67, 1980.

311. Swanstrom OG and Dade AA: Reduplication of the esophageal lumen in a Quarter Horse filly. *VM/SAC* 74:75-76, 1979.

312. Stick JA et al: Esophageal healing in the pony: A comparison of sutured vs non-sutured esophagotomy. *Am J Vet Res* 42:1506-1513, 1981.

313. Aanes WA: The diagnosis and surgical repair of diverticulum of the esophagus. *Proc 21st Ann Mtg AAEP*, 1975. pp 211-221.

314. Hackett RP et al: Surgical correction of esophageal diverticulum in a horse. *JAVMA* 173:998-1000, 1978.

315. Haasjes C: Esophageal diverticulum. *JAVMA* 109:2789, 1946.

316. Kerz PD: A technique for relieving esophageal obstruction in the horse. *VM/SAC* 71:216, 1976.

317. Honnas CM et al: What is your diagnosis? *JAVMA* 190:699-700, 1987.

318. Lundvall RL and Kingrey BW: Choke in Shetland ponies, caused by boluses. *JAVMA* 133:75-76, 1958.

319. DeBowes RM et al: Esophageal obstruction by antibiotic boluses in a Thoroughbred filly: A case report. *J Equine Vet Sci* 2:23-26, 1982.

320. Stick JA et al: Esophagotomy in the pony: Comparison of surgical techniques and form of feed. *Am J Vet Res* 44:2123-2132, 1983.

321. Todhunter RJ et al: Medical management of esophageal stricture in seven horses. *JAVMA* 185:784-787, 1984.

322. Raker CW and Sayers A: Esophageal rupture in a Standardbred mare. *JAVMA* 133:371-373, 1958.

323. DeMoor A et al: Surgical treatment of a traumatic oesophageal rupture in a foal. *Equine Vet J* 11:265-266, 1979.

324. Wingfield-Digby NJ and Burguez PN: Traumatic oesophageal rupture in the horse. *Equine Vet J* 14:169-170, 1982.

325. Lunn DP and Peel JE: Successful treatment of traumatic oesophageal rupture with severe cellulitis in a mare. *Vet Record* 116:544-545, 1985.

326. Peacock EE: *Wound Repair*. 3rd ed. Saunders, Philadelphia, 1984. pp 451-455, 483-484.

327. Todhunter RJ et al: Comparison of three feeding techniques after esophageal mucosal resection and anastomosis in the horse. *Cornell Vet* 76:16-29, 1986.

328. Wagner PC and Rantanen NW: Myotomy as a treatment for esophageal stricture in a horse. *Equine Pract* 2(3):40-45, 1980.

329. Steward KA and Reinertson EL: Congenital esophageal stricture in a pony foal. *MVP* 64:753-754, 1983.

330. Derksen FJ and Stick JA: Resection and anastomosis of esophageal stricture in a foal. *Equine Pract* 5(4):17-20, 1983.

331. Craig D and Todhunter RJ: Surgical repair of an esophageal stricture in a horse. *Vet Surg* 16:251-254, 1987.

332. Lowe JE: Esophageal anastomosis in the horse. *Cornell Vet* 54:636-641, 1964.

333. Suann CJ: Oesophageal resection and anastomosis as a treatment for oesophageal stricture in the horse. *Equine Vet J* 14:163- 164, 1982.

334. Hoffer RE et al: Esophageal patch grafting as a treatment for esophageal stricture in a horse. *JAVMA* 171:350-354, 1977.

335. Moore JN and Kintner LD: Recurrent esophageal obstruction due to squamous cell carcinoma in a horse. *Cornell Vet* 66:589-596, 1976.

336. Pommer A: Carcinomstenose des oesophagus beim pferd. *Wein Tierrztl Monatsh* 34:193-197, 1947.

337. Roberts MC and Kelly WR: Squamous cell carcinoma of the lower cervical oesophagus in a pony. *Equine Vet J* 11:199-201, 1979.

338. Sisson S, in Getty R: *Sisson and Grossman's The Anatomy of Domestic Animals*. 5th ed. Saunders, Philadelphia, 1986. pp 447-482.

339. Kitamura N *et al:* Immunochemical distribution of endocrine cells in the gastrointestinal tract of the horse. *Equine Vet J* 16:103-107, 1984.

340. Campbell-Thompson ML *et al:* Basal and pentagastrin-stimulated gastric secretion in young horses. *Am J Physiol* 259:R1259-R1266, 1990.

341. Troitskii A: The undulating character of the gastric secretion in the horse. *Veterinariya* (Moscow) 2:117-126, 1940.

342. Brown CM *et al:* Serum immunoreactive gastric activity in horses: basal and postprandial values. *Vet Res Comm* 11:497-501, 1987.

343. Young DW and Smyth GB: Validation of a radioimmunoassay for measurement of gastrin in equine serum. *Am J Vet Res* 49:1179- 1183, 1988.

344. Smyth GB *et al:* Postprandial serum gastrin concentrations in normal foals. *Equine Vet J* 21:285-287, 1989.

345. Gonchar MV *et al:* Multiple forms of equine pepsin. *Biochem* 49:882-891, 1984.

346. Alexander F and Davies ME: Production and fermentation of lactate by bacteria in the alimentary tract of the horse. *J Comp Pathol* 73:1-8, 1963.

347. Silen W, in Johnson LR *et al: Physiology of the Gastrointestinal Tract.* Raven Press, New York, 1987. pp 1055-1070.

348. Meyer JH, in Johnson LR *et al: Physiology of the Gastrointestinal Tract.* Raven Press, New York, 1987. pp 613-630.

349. Argenzio RA *et al:* Digesta passage and water exchange in the equine large intestine. *Am J Physiol* 226:1035-1042, 1974.

350. Merritt AM *et al:* Effect of xylazine treatment of equine proximal gastrointestinal tract myoelectrical activity. *Am J Vet Res* 50:945-949, 1989.

351. Phaneuf LP *et al:* Electromyenterography during normal gastrointestinal activity, painful or nonpainful colic and morphine analgesia in the horse. *Can J Comp Med* 36:128-134, 1972.

352. Hunt JM and Gerring EL: The effect of prostaglandin E1 on motility of the equine gut. *J Vet Pharmacol Therap* 8:165-173, 1985.

353. Robertson JT: Conditions of the stomach and small intestine: Differential diagnosis and surgical management. *Vet Clin No Am* 4:105-127, 1982.

354. Jaksch W, in Wintzer HJ: *Equine Diseases.* Springer Verlag, New York, 1986. pp 110-112.

355. Murray MJ *et al:* The prevalence of gastric lesions in foals without signs of gastric disease: An endoscopic survey. *Equine Vet J* 22:6-8, 1990.

356. Murray MJ *et al:* Gastric ulcers in horses, a comparison of endoscopic findings in horses with and without clinical signs. *Equine Vet J* Suppl 7:68-72, 1989.

357. Wilson JH: Serial gastric endoscopy of foals in a research herd. *Equine Vet J* Suppl 7:138, 1989.

358. Bargai U: *The radiological examination of the digestive system of the horse.* Thesis, Pretoria, South Africa, 1971.

359. Campbell ML *et al:* Radiographic anatomy of the foal gastrointestinal tract. *Vet Radiol* 25:194, 1984.

360. Dik KJ and Kalsbeek HC: Radiography of the equine stomach. *Vet Radiol* 26:48-51, 1985.

361. Campbell-Thompson ML *et al:* Gastroenterostomy for treatment of gastroduodenal ulcer disease in 14 foals. *JAVMA* 188:840-844, 1986.

362. Orsini JA and Donawick WJ: Surgical treatment of gastroduodenal obstruction in foals. *Vet Surg* 15:205-213, 1986.

363. Cudd TA *et al:* The use of clinical findings, abdominocentesis and abdominal radiographs to assess surgical versus non-surgical abdominal disease in the foal. *Proc 33rd Ann Mtg AAEP*, 1987. pp 41-53.

364. Fischer AT *et al:* Radiographic diagnosis of gastrointestinal disorders in the foal. *Vet Radiol* 28:42-47, 1987.

365. Fischer AT: Diagnostic and prognostic procedures for equine colic surgery. *Vet Clin No Am* (Equine Pract) 5:335-350, 1989.

366. Peterson FB *et al:* Gastric stenosis in a horse. *JAVMA* 160:328-332, 1972.

367. Whitlock RH, in Anderson NV: *Veterinary Gastroenterology.* Lea & Febiger, Philadelphia, 1980. pp 392-395.

368. Bass NM *et al*, in Andreoli TE *et al: Cecil's Essentials of Medicine.* Saunders, Philadelphia, 1986. pp 293-300.

369. Roberts A,in Johnson LR *et al: Physiology of the Gastrointestinal Tract.* Raven Press, New York, 1987. pp 1071-1088.

370. Campbell-Thompson ML and Merritt AM: Diagnosis and treatment of gastric and duodenal ulceration and gastric outflow obstruction in foals and adults. *Proc 35th Ann Mtg AAEP*, 1989.

371. Furr MO and Murray MJ: Treatment of gastric ulcers in horses with H2 receptor antagonists. *Equine Vet J* Suppl 7:77-79, 1989.

372. Campbell-Thompson ML *et al:* Efficacy of omeprazole versus ranitidine in inhibiting equine gastric acid secretion. *Proc 3rd Equine Colic Res Symp*, 1988. p 16.

373. Geor RJ and Papich MG: Medical therapy for gastrointestinal ulcers in foals. *Compend Cont Ed Pract Vet* 12:403-412, 1990.

374. McGuigan JE in Braunwald E *et al: Harrison's Physiology of Internal Medicine.* McGraw-Hill, New York, 1987. pp 1239-1250.

375. Traub-Dargatz J *et al:* Exsanguination due to gastric ulceration in a foal. *JAVMA* 186:280-281, 1985.

376. Kirk RM, in Kirk RM and Williamson RCN: *General Surgical Operations.* 2nd ed. Churchill Livingstone, New York, 1987. pp 69-81.

377. Orsini JA and Donawick: Hepaticojejunostomy for treatment of common hepatic duct obstructions associated with duodenal stenosis in two foals. *Vet Surg* 18:34-38, 1989.

378. Crow MW and Swerczek TW: Equine congenital defects. *Am J Vet Res* 46:353-357, 1985.

379. Freeman DE, in Mansmann RA and McAllister ES: *Equine Medicine and Surgery.* 3rd ed. American Veterinary Publicationns, Goleta, CA, 1982. pp 509-516.

380. Crowhurst RC *et al:* Intestinal surgery in the foal. *J So Afr Vet Assn* 46:59-67, 1975.

381. Barth AD *et al:* Pyloric stenosis in a foal. *Can Vet J* 21:234-236, 1980.

382. Munroe GA: Pyloric stenosis in a yearling with an incidental findings of *Capillaria hepatica* in the liver. *Equine Vet J* 16:221-222, 1984.

383. Huskamp B: The diagnosis and treatment of acute abdominal conditions in the horse: The various types and frequency as seen at the animal hospital in Hochmoor. *Proc Equine Colic Res Symp*, 1982. pp 261-272.

384. Huskamp B, in Dietz O and Wiesner E: *Diseases of the Horse.* Part I. Karger, New York, 1984. pp 164-167.

385. Datt SC and Usenik EA: Intestinal obstruction in the horse: physical signs and blood chemistry. *Cornell Vet* 65:152-172, 1975.

386. Puotunen-Reinert A and Huskamp B: Experimental duodenal obstruction in the horse. *Vet Surg* 15:420-428, 1986.

387. Honnas CM and Schumacher J: Primary gastric impaction in a pony. *JAVMA* 187:501-502, 1985.

388. Clayton-Jones DG *et al:* Gastric impaction in a pony: relief via laparotomy. *Equine Vet J* 4:98-99, 1972.

389. Becht J, in Robinson NE: *Current Veterinary Therapy in Equine Medicine.* Saunders, Philadelphia, 1983. pp 196-200.

390. Kiper ML *et al:* Gastric rupture in horses: 50 cases (1979-1987). *JAVMA* 196:333-336, 1990.

391. Pascoe PJ *et al:* Mortality rates and associated factors in equine colic operations - a retrospective study of 341 operations. *Can Vet J* 24:76-85, 1983.

392. Von Boening KJ and Plocki vKA: Über die chirurgische versorgung einer partiellen, zirkularen magenruptur biem pferd. *Prakt Tierarzt* 7:608-612, 1982.

393. Steenhaut M *et al:* Surgical repair of a partial gastric rupture in a horse. *Equine Vet J* 18:331-332, 1986.

394. Jacobs DE: *A Colour Atlas of Equine Parasites.* Bailliere Tindall, London, 1986. pp 4.4-4.16.

395. Urquhart GM *et al:* *Veterinary Parasitology.* Churchill Livingstone, New York, 1987. pp 78-80.

396. Torbet BJ *et al:* Efficacy of injectable and oral paste formulations of ivermectin against gastrointestinal parasites in ponies. *Vet Res Comm* 43:1451-1453, 1982.

397. Drudge JH and Lyons ET, in Robinson NE: *Current Therapy in Equine Medicine.* Saunders, Philadelphia, 1983. pp 283-286.

398. Price RE and Stromberg PC: Seasonal occurence and distribution of the *Gasterophilus intestinalis* and *Gasterophilus nasalis* in the stomachs of equids in Texas. *Am J Vet Res* 48:1225-1232, 1987.

399. Rainey JW: Equine mortality due to *Gasterophilus* larvae (stomach bots). *Aust Vet J* 38:12-13, 1948.

400. Herd RP: Epidemiology and control of equine strongylosis at Newmarket. *Equine Vet J* 18:447-452, 1986.

401. Esker M *et al:* Alternate grazing of horses and sheep as control for gastrointestinal helminthiasis in horses. *Vet Parasitol* 13:273-280, 1983.

402. Leland SE *et al:* Studies on *Trichostrongylus axei* VII. Some quantitative and pathologic aspects of natural and experimental infections in the horse. *Am J Vet Res* 22:128-138, 1961.

403. Herd RP: Serum pepsinogen concentrations of ponies naturally infected with *Trichostrongylus axei.* *Equine Vet J* 18:490-491, 1986.

404. McGill CA and Bolton JR: Gastric retention associated with a pyloric mass in two horses. *Aust Vet J* 61:190-195, 1984.

405. Church S *et al:* Gastric retention associated with acquired pyloric stenosis in a gelding. *Equine Vet J* 18(4):332-334, 1986.

406. Traub-Dargatz JL *et al:* Chronic flunixin meglumine therapy in foals. *Am J Vet Res* 49:7-12, 1988.

407. Carrick JB *et al:* Clinical and pathologic effects of flunixin meglumine administration to neonatal foals. *Can J Vet Res* 53:195-201, 1989.

408. Cargile J and Merritt A, Univ Florida: Personal communication.

409. Moulton JE: *Tumors in Domestic Animals.* 2nd ed. Univ California Press, Berkeley, 1978. pp 259-262.

410. Tennant B *et al:* Six cases of squamous cell carcinoma of the stomach of the horse. *Equine Vet J* 14:238-243, 1982.

411. MacKay RJ *et al:* Exuberant granulation tissue in the stomach of a horse. *Equine Vet J* 13:119-122, 1981.

412. Titus RS *et al:* Gastric carcinoma in a mare. *JAVMA* 161:270-273, 1972.

413. Meuten DJ *et al:* Gastric carcinoma with pseudohyperparathyroidism in a horse. *Cornell Vet* 68:179-195, 1978.

414. Wrigley RH *et al:* Pleural effusion associated with squamous cell carcinoma of the stomach of the horse. *Equine Vet J* 13:99-102, 1981.

415. Keirn DR *et al:* Endoscopic diagnosis of squamous cell carcinoma of the equine stomach. *JAVMA* 180:940-942, 1982.

416. Schmitz DG: Diagnosis of gastric squamous cell carcinoma. *Equine Pract* 9:18-21, 1987.

417. Zicker SC *et al:* Differentiation between intra-abdominal neoplasms and abscesses in horses, using clinical and laboratory data: 40 cases (1973-1988). *JAVMA* 196:1130-1134, 1990.

418. Hammond CJ *et al:* Gastric ulceration in mature Thoroughbred horses. *Equine Vet J* 18:284-287, 1986.

419. Murray MJ: Endoscopic appearance of gastric lesions in foals: 94 foals (1987-1988). *JAVMA* 195:1135-1141, 1989.

420. Rooney JR: Gastric ulceration in foals. *Vet Pathol* 1:497-503, 1964.

421. Rebhun WC et al: Gastric ulcers in foals. *JAVMA* 180:404-407, 1982.

422. Becht JL and Byars TD: Gastroduodenal ulceration in foals. *Equine Vet J* 18:307-312, 1986.

423. Sangiah S *et al:* Effects of cimetidine and ranitidine on basal gastric pH, free and total acid contents in horses. *Res Vet Sci* 45:291-295, 1988.

424. Smyth GB *et al:* Pharmocokinetic studies of cimetidine hydrochloride in adult horses. *Equine Vet J* 22:48-50, 1990.

425. Smith JM *et al:* Efficacy of oral ranitidine in the reduction of gastric acid output and the prevention of phenylbutazone-induced gastric ulceration in nursing foals. *Proc 33rd Ann Mtg AAEP,* 1987. pp 113-127.

426. Geor RJ *et al:* The protective effect of sucralfate and ranitidine in foals experimentally intoxicated with phenylbutazone. *Can J Vet Res* 53:231-238, 1989.

427. Duran SH *et al:* Pharmokinetics of intravenous ranitidine in adult horses. *J Vet Int Med* 3:136, 1989.

428. Acland HM *et al:* Ulcerative duodenitis in foals. *Vet Pathol* 20:653-661, 1983.

429. Campbell-Thompson ML: Upper gastrointestinal surgery in the foal. *Vet Clin No Am* (Equine Pract) 5:351-362, 1989.

430. Probst CW *et al:* Surgical repair of a perforated gastric ulcer in a foal. *Vet Surg* 12:93-95, 1983.

431. Furr MO and Murray MJ: Effects of stress on gastric ulceration and serum T3, T4 and cortisol in neonatal foals. *J Vet Int Med* 3:114, 1989.

432. Roberts MC: Malabsorption syndrome in the horse. *Compend Cont Ed Pract Vet* 7:S637-S646, 1985.

433. Martens RJ and Scrutchfield WL: Foal diarrhea: Pathogenesis, etiology and therapy. *Compend Cont Ed Pract Vet* 4:S175-S187, 1982.

434. Merritt AM, in Anderson NV: *Veterinary Gastroenterology.* Lea & Febiger, Philadelphia, 1980. pp 463-522.

435. Roberts MC: Protein-losing enteropathy in the horse. *Compend Cont Ed Pract Vet* 5:S550-S558, 1983.

436. Neiberle K and Cohrs P: *Textbook of Special Pathological Anatomy of Domestic Animals.* Pergamon Press, Oxford, 1967. pp 289-566.

437. Baxter GM *et al:* Abdominal adhesions after small intestinal surgery in the horse. *Vet Surg* 18:409-414, 1989.

438. Freeman DE *et al:* Mesodiverticular bands as a cause of small intestinal strangulation and volvulus in the horse. *JAVMA* 175:1089-1094, 1979.

439. Henderson RA: Controlling peritoneal adhesions. *Vet Surg* 11:30-33, 1982.

440. Rumbaugh GE *et al:* Internal abdominal abscesses in the horse: A study of 25 cases. *JAVMA* 172:304-309, 1978.

441. Getty R, in Getty R: *Sisson and Grossman's The Anatomy of Domestic Animals.* 5th ed. Saunders, Philadelphia, 1975. pp 454-497.

442. Tennant BC *et al:* Observations on the causes and incidence of acute intestinal obstruction in the horse. *Proc 18th Ann Mtg AAEP,* 1972. pp 251-257.

443. Sembrat RF: The acute abdomen in the horse: epidemiologic considerations. *Arch Am Coll Vet Surg* 4:34-38, 1975.

444. Turner TA *et al:* Small intestine incarceration through the epiploic foramen of the horse. *JAVMA* 184:731-734, 1984.

445. Kopf N: Rectal findings in horses with intestinal obstruction. *Proc Symp Equine Colic Res,* 1982. pp 236-260.

446. Meagher DM: Intestinal strangulations in the horse. *Arch Am Coll Vet Surg* 4:59-64, 1975.

447. Rooney JR: Volvulus, strangulation and intussusception in the horse. *Cornell Vet* 55:644-653, 1965.

448. Yovich JV *et al:* Incarceration of small intestine through rents in the gastrosplenic ligament in the horse. *Vet Surg* 14:303-306, 1985.

449. Ashdown RR: The anatomy of the inguinal canal in the domesticated mammals. *Vet Record* 75:1345-1351, 1963.

450. Moore JN *et al:* A case report of inguinal herniorrhaphy in a stallion. *J Equine Med Surg* 1:391-394, 1977.

451. Schneider RK *et al:* Acquired inguinal hernia in the horse: a review of 27 cases. *JAVMA* 180:317-320, 1982.

452. Vaughan JT: Surgical management of abdominal crisis in the horse. *JAVMA* 161:1199-1212, 1972.

453. Heinze CD *et al*, in Catcott EJ and Smithcors JF: *Equine Medicine and Surgery.* 2nd ed. American Veterinary Publications, Goleta, CA, 1972. pp 157-179.

454. Bernard WV *et al:* Ultrasonographic diagnosis of small intestinal intussusception in three foals. *JAVMA* 194:395-397, 1989.

455. Pearson H *et al:* The indications for equine laparotomy - an analysis of 140 cases. *Equine Vet J* 7:131-136, 1975.

456. Lowe JE: Intussusception in three ponies following experimental enterotomy. *Cornell Vet* 58:288-292, 1968.

457. Barclay WP *et al:* Intussusception associated with *Anoplocephala perfoliata* infection in five horses. *JAVMA* 180:752-753, 1982.

458. Edwards GB: Surgical management of intussusception in the horse. *Equine Vet J* 18:313-321, 1986.

459. Mason TA *et al:* Laparotomy in equine colic: A report of thirteen cases. *Aust Vet J* 46:349-355, 1970.

460. Scott EA and Todhunter RJ: Chronic intestinal intussusception in two horses. *JAVMA* 186:383-385, 1985.

461. Owen R ap R *et al:* Jejuno- or ileocecal anastomosis performed in seven horses exhibiting colic. *Can Vet J* 16:164-169, 1975.

462. Vasey JR and Julian JR: Elective inversion of the distal ileal stump into the caecum of the horse. *Equine Vet J* 19:223-225, 1987.

463. Bach LG and Ricketts SW: Paracentesis as an aid to the diagnosis of abdominal disease in the horse. *Equine Vet J* 6:116-121, 1974.

464. Donawick WJ *et al:* Resection of diseased ileum in the horse. *JAVMA* 159:1146-1149, 1971.

465. Blood DC *et al:* *Veterinary Medicine.* 5th ed. Lea & Febiger, Philadelphia, 1979. pp 99-155, 476.

466. Drudge JH and Lyons ET, in Robinson NE: *Current Therapy in Equine Medicine.* Saunders, Philadelphia, 1983. pp 281-283.

467. Ludwig KG *et al:* Efficacy of ivermectin in controlling *Strongyloides westeri* infections in foals. *Am J Vet Res* 44:314-316, 1983.

468. Clayton HM: Ascarids, recent advances. *Vet Clin No Am* (Equine Pract) 2:313-327, 1986.

469. Herd RP, in Robinson NE: *Current Therapy in Equine Medicine 2.* Saunders, Philadelphia, 1987. pp 323-327.

470. Lyons ET *et al:* Prevalence of *Anoplecephala perfoliata* and lesions of *Draschia megastoma* in Thoroughbreds in Kentucky at necropsy. *Am J Vet Res* 45:996-999, 1984.

471. Drudge JH and Lyons ET, in Robinson NE: *Current Therapy in Equine Medicine.* Saunders, Philadelphia, 1983. p 287.

472. McQueary CA *et al:* Observations on the life cycle and prevalence of *Eimeria leuckarti* in horses in Montana. *Am J Vet Res* 38:1673-1674, 1977.

473. Mayhew IG and Griener EC: Protozoal diseases. *Vet Clin No Am* (Equine Pract) 2:439-459, 1986.

474. Snyder SP *et al:* Cryptosporidiosis in immunodeficient Arabian foals. *Vet Pathol* 15:12-17, 1978.

475. Klei TR: Other parasites: Recent advances. *Vet Clin No Am* (Equine Pract) 2:329-336, 1986.

476. Becht JL and Semrad SD: Gastrointestinal diseases of foals. *Compend Cont Ed Pract Vet* 8:S367-S375, 1986.

477. Kanitz CL: Identification of an equine rotavirus as a cause of neonatal foal diarrhea. *Proc 22nd Ann Mtg AAEP*, 1977. pp 155-165.

478. Baker JC and Ames TR: Total parenteral nutritional therapy of a foal with diarrhea from which parovirus-like particles were identified. *Equine Vet J* 19:342-344, 1987.

479. Tzipori S *et al:* Enteritis in foals induced by rotavirus and enterotoxigenic Escherichia coli. *Aust Vet J* 58:20-23, 1982.

480. Eugster AK and Whitford HW: Concurrent rotavirus and *Salmonella* infections in foals. *JAVMA* 173:857-858, 1978.

481. Woode GN and Crouch CF: Naturally occuring and experimentally induced rotaviral infections of domestic and laboratory animals. *JAVMA* 173:522-526, 1978.

482. Platt H: Chronic inflammatory and lymphoproliferative lesions of the equine small intestine. *J Comp Pathol* 96:671-684, 1986.

483. Larsen AB *et al:* Susceptibility of horses to *Mycobacterium paratuberculosis. Am J Vet Res* 33:2185-2189, 1972.

484. Dade AW *et al:* Granulomatous colitis in a horse with histoplasmosis. *VM/SAC* 69:279-281, 1973.

485. Goetz TE and Coffman JR: Ulcerative colitis and protein losing enteropathy associated with intestinal salmonellosis and histoplasmosis in a horse. *Equine Vet J* 16:439-441, 1984.

486. Cimprich RE and Rooney JR: Corynebacterium equi enteritis in foals. *Vet Pathol* 14:95-102, 1977.

487. Dickie CW *et al:* Enterotoxemia in two foals. *JAVMA* 173:306-307, 1978.

488. Pearson EG *et al:* Hemorrhagic enteritis caused by *Clostridium perfringens* type C in a foal. *JAVMA* 188:1309-1310, 1986.

489. Howard-Martin M *et al: Clostridium perfringens* type C enterotoxemia in a newborn foal. *JAVMA* 189:564-565, 1986.

490. Roberts MC and Pinsent PJN: Malabsorption in the horse associated with alimentary lymphosarcoma. *Equine Vet J* 7:166-172, 1975.

491. Ricketts SW and Peace CK: A case of peritoneal mesothelioma in a Thoroughbred mare. *Equine Vet J* 8:78-80, 1976.

492. Roberts MC *et al:* Small intestinal beta-galactosidase activity in the horse. *Gut* 14:535-540, 1973.

493. Embertson RM *et al:* Ileal impaction in the horse. *JAVMA* 186:570-572, 1985.

494. Allen D Jr, in Robinson NE: *Current Therapy in Equine Medicine 2.* Saunders, Philadelphia, 1987. pp 51-53.

495. Doran RE *et al:* Clinical aspects of ileal impaction in the horse. *Proc 2nd Equine Colic Res Symp*, 1986. pp 182-185.

496. Horney FD and Funk KA: Ileal myotomy in the horse. *MVP* 52:49-50, 1971.

497. Rooney JR and Jeffcott LB: Muscular hypertrophy of the ileum in a horse. *Vet Record* 83:217-219, 1968.

498. Lindsay WA *et al:* Ileal smooth muscle hypertrophy and rupture in a horse. *Equine Vet J* 13:66-67, 1981.

499. Schneider JE *et al:* Muscular hypertrophy of the small intestine in a horse. *J Equine Med Surg* 3:226-228, 1977.

500. Sweeney RW *et al:* Chronic granulomatous bowel disease in three sibling horses. *JAVMA* 188:1192-1194, 1986.

501. Cimprich RE: Granulomatous enteritis of horses: Clinical and postmortem findings. *Compend Cont Ed Pract Vet* 3:S437-S440, 1981.

502. Nimmo Wilkie JS *et al:* Chronic eosinophilic dermatitis: A manifestation of a multisystemic, eosinophilic, epitheliotropic disease in five horses. *Vet Pathol* 22:297-305, 1985.

503. Gibson KT and Alders RC: Eosinophlic enterocolitis and dermatitis in two horses. *Equine Vet J* 19:247-252, 1987.

504. Pass DA *et al:* Basophilic enterocolitis in a horse. *Vet Pathol* 21:362-364, 1984.

505. Blackwell RB and White NA: Duodenitis-proximal jejunitis in the horse. *Proc 1st Equine Colic Res Symp*, 1982. p 106.

506. Blackwell RB, in Robinson NE: *Current Therapy in Equine Medicine 2.* Saunders, Philadelphia, 1987. pp 44-45.

507. Merritt AM *et al:* Is *Salmonella* infection a cause of the acute gastric dilatation/ileus syndrome in horses? *Proc 1st Equine Colic Res Symp*, 1982. pp 119-124.

508. Sellers AF *et al:* The reservoir function of the equine cecum and ventral large colon: its relation to chronic non-obstructive disease with colic. *Cornell Vet* 72:233-241, 1982.

509. Sack WO and Habel RE: *Rooney's Guide to the Dissection of the Horse.* Veterinary Textbooks, Ithaca, NY, 1977. p 54.

510. Meyer H *et al:* Untersuch-ungen uber die verdaulich-keit und vertraglichkeit verschiedener Futtermittel bei typhlotomierten Ponys. *Dtsch Tierrztl Wochenschr* 86:384-390, 1979.

511. Sauer WS *et al:* Effective cecectomy on digestibility coefficiences and nitrogen balance in ponies. *Can J Anim Sci* 59:141-151, 1979.

512. Ross MW *et al:* Normal motility of the cecum and right ventral colon in ponies. *Am J Vet Res* 47:1756-1762, 1986.

513. Brown MP and Meagher DM: Repair of an equine cecal fistula caused by application of a hernia clamp. *VM/SAC* 73:1403-1407, 1978.

514. Boles C: Surgical techniques in equine colic. *J So Afr Vet Assn* 46:115-119, 1975.

515. Ross MW *et al:* Cecal impaction and idiopathic cecal perforation in the horse. *Vet Surg* 13:57, 1984.

516. Ross MW *et al:* Jejunocolic anastomosis for the surgical management of recurrent cecal impaction in a horse. *Vet Surg* 16:265-268, 1987.

517. Ross MW et al: Cecocolic anastomosis for the surgical management of cecal impaction in horses. Vet Surg 15:85-92, 1986.

518. Foerner JJ: Diseases of the large intestine. Differential diagnosis and surgical management. Vet Clin No Am (Large Anim Pract) 4:129-146, 1982.

519. Campbell ML et al: Cecal impaction in the horse. JAVMA 184:950-952, 1984.

520. Craig DR et al: Ileocolostomy: A technique for surgical management of equine cecal impaction. Vet Surg 16:451-455, 1987.

521. Huskamp B and Kopf N: Typhlectomy in the horse-experimental and clinical experiences. Dtsch Tierrztl Wochenschr 85(1):1-7, 1978.

522. Ross MW et al: Cecal perforation in the horse. JAVMA 187:249-253, 1985.

523. Littlejohn A and Ritchie JDS: Rupture of the caecum at parturition. J So Afr Vet Assn 46:87-98, 1975.

524. Voss JL: Rupture of the cecum and ventral colon of mares during parturition. JAVMA 155:745-747, 1969.

525. Platt H: Caecal rupture in parturient mares. J Comp Pathol 93:343-346, 1983.

526. Donelan E and Sloss V: Two cases of rupture of the large intestine in the mare associated with unassisted parturition. Aust Vet J 48:413-414, 1972.

527. Platt H: Sudden and unexpected deaths in horses: a review of 69 cases. Brit Vet J 138:425, 1982.

528. Allison CJ: Invagination of the caecum into the colon in a Welsh pony. Equine Vet J 9:84-86, 1977.

529. Robertson JT and Johnson FM: Surgical correction of cecocolic intussusception in a horse. JAVMA 176:223-224, 1980.

530. Cowles RR et al: Cecal inversion in a horse. VM/SAC 72:1346-1348, 1977.

531. Semrad SD and Moore JN: Invagination of the caecal apex in a foal. Equine Vet J 15:62-63, 1983.

532. Martin BB et al: Unpublished data, 1988.

533. Beroza GA et al: Cecal perforation and peritonitis associated with Anophlocephala perfoliata infection in 3 horses. JAVMA 183:804-806, 1983.

534. Bello TR, in Mansmann RA and McAllister ES: Equine Medicine and Surgery. 3rd ed. American Veterinary Publications, Goleta, CA, 1982. p 73.

535. Huston R et al: Congenital defects in foals. J Equine Med Surg 1:146-161, 1977.

536. Blue MG: Enteroliths in horses: a retrospective study of 30 cases. Equine Vet J 11:76-84, 1979.

537. Blue MG and Wittkopp RW: Clinical and structural features of equine enteroliths. JAVMA 179:79-82, 1981.

538. Sullins KE et al: Intravenous fluorescein dye as an indicator of equine large and small intestinal viability. Proc 2nd Colic Res Symp, 1985. pp 280-289.

539. Snyder JR et al: Surface oximetry for determination of intestinal perfusion and viability in the horse. Proc 2nd Colic Res Symp, 1985. pp 289-290.

540. Barclay WP et al: Volvulus of the large colon in the horse. JAVMA 177:629-630, 1980.

541. Markel MD: Personal communication, 1986.

542. Dyson S and Orsini J: Intussusception of the large colon in a horse. JAVMA 182:720-721, 1983.

543. Hackett RP: Nonstrangulated colonic displacement in horses. JAVMA 182:235-240, 1983.

544. Speirs VC et al: Dorsal displacement of the left ventral and dorsal colon in two horses. Aust Vet J 55:542-544, 1979.

545. Huskamp B and Kopf N: Die verlagerung des colon ascendens in den milznierenraum beim pferd (2). Tierrztl Prax 8:495-506, 1980.

546. Markel MD et al: Complications associated with left dorsal displacement of the large colon in the horse. JAVMA 187:1379-1380, 1985.

547. Yovich JV et al: Colic resulting from an internal pelvic hernia in a horse. Compend Cont Ed Pract Vet 6:S343-S344, 1984.

548. Wilson DG et al: Intussusception of the left dorsal colon in a horse. JAVMA 183:464-465, 1983.

549. Meagher EM and Stirk AJ: Intussusception of the colon in a filly. MVP 7:951-952, 1974.

550. Palmer JE: Acute diarrheal disease of the adult horse. Proc 2nd Ann ACVIM Forum, 1984. pp 247.

551. Hird DW et al: Case-control study of risk factors associated with isolation of Salmonella saintpaul in hospitalized horses. Am J Epidem 120:852, 1984.

552. Palmer JE et al: Subclinical salmonellosis in horses with colic. Proc 2nd Equine Colic Res Symp, 1982. pp 180-186.

553. D'Aoust JY and Pivnik H: Small infectious doses of Salmonella. Lancet 1:866, 1976.

554. Meynell GG and Subbaiah TV: Antibacterial mechanisms of the mouse gut. I. Kinetics of infection by Salmonella typhimurium in normal and streptomycin-treated mice studied with abortive transductants. Brit J Exp Pathol 44:197, 1963.

555. Morse EV et al: Salmonellosis in equidae: A study of 23 cases. Cornell Vet 66:198, 1976.

556. Palmer JE et al: Salmonella shed by horses with colic. JAVMA 187:256-257, 1985.

557. Carter JD et al: Salmonellosis in hospitalized horses: Seasonality and case fatality rates. JAVMA 188:163-167, 1986.

558. Farrar WE: Molecular analysis of plasmids in epidemiologic investigations. J Infect Dis 148:1-6, 1983.

559. Brunner F et al: The plasmid pattern as an epidemiologic tool for Salmonella typhimurium epidemics: Comparison with the lysotype. J Infect Dis 148:7-11, 1983.

560. Taylor DN et al: Salmonellosis associated with marijuana: A multistate outbreak traced by plasmid fingerprinting. N Eng J Med 306:1249-1253, 1982.

561. Owen R ap R et al: Studies on experimental enteric salmonellosis in ponies. Can J Comp Med 43:247-254, 1979.

562. Palmer JE et al: Comparison of rectal mucosal cultures and fecal cultures in detecting Salmonella infection in horses and cattle. Am J Vet Res 46:697-698, 1985.

563. Palmer JE, Univ Pennsylvania: Unpublished data, 1985.

564. Morris DD et al: Fecal leukocytes and epithelial cells in horses with diarrhea. Cornell Vet 73:265-274, 1983.

565. Ettlinger JT et al: Unpublished data, 1988.

566. Marsik FJ et al: Transmissible drug resistance of Escherichia coli and Salmonella from humans, animals, and their rural environments. J Infect Dis 13:296-302, 1975.

567. Tompkins LS: Plasmids and transposons in clinical microbiology. *Clin Microbiol* 4:53, 1982.

568. Koterba A et al: Nasocomial infections and bacterial antibiotic resistance in a university equine hospital. *JAVMA* 189:185-191, 1986.

569. Semrad SD et al: Low dose flunixin meglumine: Effects on eicosanoid production and clinical signs induced by experimental entotoxemia in horses. *Equine Vet J* 19:201-206, 1986.

570. Schiefer HB: Equine colitis "X": Still an enigma? *Can Vet J* 22:162-165, 1981.

571. Wierup M: Equine intestinal clostridiosis. *Acta Vet Scand* 62(Suppl):1-182, 1977.

572. Ochoa R and Kern SR: The effects of *Clostridium perfringens* Type A enterotoxin in Shetland ponies-Clinical, morphologic and clinicopathologic changes. *Vet Pathol* 17:738-747, 1980.

573. Wierup M and DiPierto JA: Bacteriologic examination of equine fecal flora as a diagnostic tool for equine intestinal clostridiosis. *Am J Vet Res* 42: 2167-2169, 1981.

574. Anderson G et al: Lethal complications following adminstration of oxytetracycline in the horse. *Nord Vet Med* 23:9, 1971.

575. Weirup M, in Robinson NE: *Current Therapy in Equine Medicine 2.* Saunders, Philadelphia, 1987. p 99.

576. Blackwell NJ: Colitis in equines associated with Strongyle larvae. *Vet Record* 95:401, 1973.

577. Harmon BG et al: Cyathostome colitis and typhlitis. *Compend Cont Ed Pract Vet* 8:S301, 1986.

578. Giles CJ et al: Larval cyathostomiosis (immature tridonema-induced enteropathy): A report of 15 clinical cases. *Equine Vet J* 17:196, 1985.

579. Duncan JL and Pirie HM: The pathogenesis of single experimental infections with *Strongylus vulgaris* in foals. *Res Vet Sci* 18:82-93, 1975.

580. Martens RJ: Non-infectious diarrhea in the foal. *Proc 25th Ann Mtg AAEP*, 1979. p 205.

581. Ogbourne CP and Duncan JL: *Strongylus vulgaris in the Horse: Its Biology and Veterinary Importance.* Commonwealth Agriculture Bureaux, Farnham, England, 1977.

582. Kowles RC et al: Acute equine diarrhea syndrome (AEDS): A preliminary report. *Proc Ann Mtg AAEP*, 1983. p 353.

583. Ristic M et al: Diagnosis of equine monocytic ehrlichiosis (Potomac horse fever) by indirect immunofluorescence. *JAVMA* 189:39-46, 1986.

584. Palmer JE et al: Equine ehrlichial colitis (Potomac horse fever): recognition of the disease in Pennsylvania, New Jersey, New York, Ohio, Idaho and Connecticut. *JAVMA* 189:197-199, 1986.

585. Palmer JE et al: Clinical signs and treatment of equine ehrlichial colitis. *Proc Symp Potomac Horse Fever*, 1988. pp 49-54.

586. Meinersmann RJ et al: Serology for the diagnosis of equine ehrlichial colitis. *Proc Symp Potomac Horse Fever*, 1988. pp 33-36.

587. Benson CE et al: Detection of equine ehrlichial colitis antigen during the acute phase of the disease. *Proc Symp Potomac Horse Fever*, 1988. pp 27-44.

588. Palmer JE: Update on equine diarrheal disease: Salmonellosis and Potomac horse fever. *Proc 12th Ann Mtg ACVIM*, 1984. pp 126-132.

589. Palmer JE et al: Potomac horse fever: Diagnostic criteria and recognition of endemic areas. *Proc 2nd Ann Symp Equine Colic Res*, 1986. pp 157-160.

590. Whitlock RH et al: Potomac horse fever: Clinical characterization and diagnostic features. *Proc 27th Ann Mtg Am Assn Vet Lab Diagnost*, 1984. p 103.

591. Dawson JE et al: Isolation of *Ehrlichia risticii* from the fetus of a mare with Potomac horse fever. *Proc Symp on Potomac Horse Fever*, 1988. pp 107-111.

592. Perry B et al: A case-control study of Potomac Horse Fever. *Prev Vet Med* 4:69-82, 1986.

593. Schmidtmann ET et al: Attempted transmission of *Ehrlichia risticii* by field-captured *Dermacentor variabilis* (Acari: Isodidae). *Am J Vet Res* 47:2393-2395, 1986.

594. Schmidtmann ET et al: Search for an arthropod vector of *Ehrlichia risticii*. *Proc Symp Potomac Horse Fever*, 1988. pp 9-16.

595. Burg JC et al: Potential vectors of Potomac horse fever and future entomological research. *Proc Symp Potomac Horse Fever*, 1988. pp 17-20.

596. Gordon JC et al: Epidemiologic investigations of affected farms. *Proc Symp Potomac Horse Fever*, 1988. pp 21-26.

597. Palmer JE and Benson CE: Unpublished data, 1988.

598. Sessions JE: Potomac horse fever field studies in Maryland and on an endemic farm. *Proc Symp Potomac Horse Fever*, 1988. pp 79-88.

599. Perry BD et al: The epidemiology of Potomac horse fever. *Proc Workshop Diseases Caused by Leukocytic Rickettsiae of Animals and Man*, 1985. p 28.

600. Stephenson EH et al, in Williams JC and Kakoma I: *Ehrlichiosis: A Vector-Borne Disease of Humans and Animals.* Kluwer Academic Publishers, Dordrecht, Holland, 1990.

601. Palmer JE et al: Treatment and control of equine monocytic ehrlichiosis (syn. Potomac horse fever). *Microbiology - American Society for Microbiology*, 1986. pp 203-204.

602. Ziemer EL et al: Clinical and hematologic variables in ponies with experimentally induced equine ehrlichial colitis (Potomac horse fever). *Am J Vet Res* 48:63-67, 1987.

603. Rikihasa Y et al: Immune responses and intestinal pathology of ponies experimentally infected with Potomac horse fever. *Proc Symp Potomac Horse Fever*, 1988. pp 27-32.

604. Palmer JE et al: Equine ehrlichial colitis: effect of oxytetracyline treatment during the incubation period of *Ehrlichia risticii* infection in ponies. *JAVMA* 192:343-345, 1988.

605. Vaughan JT: The acute colitis syndrome - Colitis "X." *Vet Clin No Am* 3:301-314, 1973.

606. Olson NE: Acute diarrheal disease in the horse. *JAVMA* 148:418-421, 1966.

607. Rooney JR: Colitis "X" of horses. *JAVMA* 142:510-511, 1963.

608. Rooney JR et al: Exhaustion shock in the horse. *Cornell Vet* 56:220-235, 1966.

609. Kelly CM: Colitis "X" in the horse. *N Zeal Vet J* 20:190-192, 1972.

610. Dunkin TE: Colitis X. *Proc 15th Ann Mtg AAEP*, 1969. pp 371- 376.

611. Mansmann RA: Equine anaphylaxis. *Fed Proc* 31:661, 1972.

612. Beasley VR et al: Cantharidin toxicosis in horses. JAVMA 182:283-284, 1983.

613. Ray AC et al: Evaluation of an analytical method for the diagnosis of cantharidin toxicosis due to ingestion of blister beetles Epicauta lemniscata by horses and sheep. Am J Vet Res 41:932-933, 1980.

614. Schoeb TR and Panciera RJ: Pathology of blister beetle (Epicauta) poisoning in horses. Vet Pathol 16:18-31, 1979.

615. Oehme FW, in Robinson NE: Current Therapy in Equine Medicine. Saunders, Philadelphia, 1983. p 588.

616. Cook WR: Diarrhoea in the horse associated with stress and tetracycline therapy. Vet Record 93:15-16, 1973.

617. Baker JR and Leyland A: Diarrhoea in the horse associated with stress and tetracycline therapy. Vet Record 93:583-584, 1973.

618. Owen R ap R: Post stress diarrhoea in the horse. Vet Record 96:267-270, 1975.

619. Raisbeck MF et al: Lincomycin-associated colitis in horses. JAVMA 179:362-363, 1981.

620. Knothe H: The effect of trimethoprim-sulphonamide, trimethoprim and sulphonamide on the occurrence of resistant Enterobacteriaceae in human intestinal flora. Infection 7(Suppl 4):S321-S323, 1979.

621. White G and Prior SD: Comparative effects of oral administration of trimethoprim/sulphadiazine or oxytetracycline of the faecal flora of horses. Vet Record 111:316-318, 1982.

622. Borgess MP and Adam WW, in Cooperman M: Intestinal Ischemia. Futura Publishing, Mt Kisko, NY, 1983.

623. Boley SJ et al: Reversible vascular occlusion of the colon. Surg Gyn Obstet 116:53-60, 1963.

624. Keller SA and Horney FD: Diseases of the equine small colon. Compend Cont Ed Pract Vet 7:S113-S118, 1985.

625. Hanson RR et al: Comparison of staple and suture techniques for end-to-end anastomosis of the small colon in horses. Am J Vet Res 49:1621-1628, 1988.

626. Hanson RR et al: Evaluation of three techniques for end-to-end anastomosis of the small colon in horses. Am J Vet Res 49:1613-1620, 1988.

627. Speirs VC et al: Obstruction of the small colon by intramural hematoma in three horses. Aust Vet J 57:88-90, 1981.

628. Livesay MA and Keller SD: Segmental ischemic necrosis following mesocolic rupture in postparturient mares. Compend Cont Ed Pract Vet 8:763-768, 1986.

629. Shires GMH, in Robinson NE: Current Therapy in Equine Medicine 2. Saunders, Philadelphia, 1987. pp 75-79.

630. Sloane DE et al: Non-iatrogenic rectal tears in three horses. JAVMA 180:750-751, 1982.

631. Spensley MS et al: Instrumentation to facilitate surgical repair of rectal tears in the horse: A preliminary report. Proc 31st Ann Mtg AAEP, 1985. pp 553-563.

632. Meagher DM, in White NA and Moore JN: Current Practice of Equine Surgery. Lippincott, Philadelphia, 1990. pp 357-365.

633. Arnold JS and Meagher DM: Management of rectal tears in the horse. J Equine Med Surg 2:55-61, 1978.

634. Stashak TS and Knight AP: Temporary diverting colostomy for the management of small colon tears in the horse: A case report. J Equine Med Surg 2:196-200, 1978.

635. Taylor TS et al: Temporary indwelling rectal liner for use in horses with rectal tears. JAVMA 191:677-680, 1987.

636. Dietz O and Weisner E: Diseases of the Horse. Part I. Karger, New York, 1984. pp 233-237.

637. Rossdale PD and Ricketts SW: Equine Stud Farm Medicine. 2nd ed. Lea & Febiger, Philadelphia, 1980. pp 265-267.

638. Bittermen H et al: Use of hypertonic saline in the treatment of hemorrhagic shock. Circ Shock 21:271-283, 1987.

639. Johnson S: Medical Emergencies. Churchill Livingstone, New York, 1985. pp 234-238.

640. Crane SW: Evaluation and management of abdominal trauma in the dog and cat. Vet Clin No Am 10:655-659, 1980.

641. Posner MC et al: Presumptive antibiotics for penetrating abdominal wounds. Surgery 165:29-32, 1987.

642. Hosgood G: Peritonitis part I: A review of the pathophysiology and diagnosis. Aust Vet Practit 16:184-189, 1986.

643. Schnieder RK, in Mansmann RA, McAllister ES: Equine Medicine and Surgery. 3rd ed. American Veterinary Publications, Goleta, CA, 1982. pp 620-633.

644. Hanselaer JR and Nyland TG: Chyloabdomen and ultrasonographic detection of an intra-abdominal abscess in a foal. JAVMA 12:1465-1467, 1983.

645. Ahrenholz DH and Simmons RL: Surgical Infectious Disease. Appleton-Century-Crofts, New York, 1982. p 796.

646. Guthrie SD: Shock. Churchill Livingstone, New York, 1983. pp 43-63.

647. Zimmerman JJ and Dietrich KA: Current perspectives on septic shock. Emerg Med Clin No Am 4:131-164, 1986.

648. Ellrodt AG: Sepsis and septic shock. Emerg Med Clin No Am 4:809-840, 1986.

649. Dyson S: Review of 30 cases of peritonitis in the horse. Equine Vet J 15:25-30, 1983.

650. West JE: Diagnostic cytology in the equine species: Overview, effusions (peritoneal, pleural, and synovial joint) and transtracheal wash. Proc 30th Ann Mtg AAEP, 1984. pp 169-201.

651. Hosgood G: Peritonitis part II: Principles of treatment. Aust Vet Practit 17:3-9, 1987.

652. Kunesh JP: Therapeutic strategies involving antimicrobial treatment of large animals with peritonitis. JAVMA 10:1222-1225, 1984.

653. Thornhill JA: Therapeutic strategies involving antimicrobial treatment of small animals with peritonitis. JAVMA 10:1181-1184, 1984.

654. Weinstein WM et al: Antimicrobial therapy of experimental intra-abdominal sepsis. J Infect Dis 132:282, 1975.

655. Hau T et al: Secondary bacterial peritonitis: The biological basis of treatment. Curr Prog Surg 16:1, 1979.

656. Orsini JA: Choosing antimicrobial agents in equine practice. Compend Cont Ed Pract Vet 8:671-678, 1986.

657. Adamson PJW *et al:* Susceptibiity of equine bacterial isolates to antimicrobial agents. *Am J Vet Res* 46:447-450, 1985.

658. Valdez H *et al:* Peritoneal lavage in the horse. *JAVMA* 174:388-391, 1979.

659. Kritchevsky JE *et al:* Peritoneal dialysis for presurgical management of ruptured bladder in a foal. *JAVMA* 185:81-82, 1984.

660. DiPietro JA *et al:* Abdominal abscess associated with *Parascaris equorum* infection in a foal. *JAVMA* 182:991, 1983.

661. Koblik PD *et al:* Use of ^{111}In-labelled autologous leukocytes to image an abdominal abscess in a horse. *JAVMA* 186:1319-1322, 1985.

662. Clabough DL and Scrutchfield WL: Ruptured abdominal abscess in a horse. *Southwestern Vet* 37:143-148, 1986.

663. Sweeney CR *et al: Streptococcus equi* infection in horses. Part I. *Compend Cont Ed Pract Vet* 9:689-695, 1987.

664. James DC *et al:* The effect of streptokinase on experimental intraperitoneal adhesion formation. *J Pathol Bacteriol* 90:279-287, 1965.

665. Buckman RF *et al:* A unifying pathogenic mechanism in the etiology of intraperitoneal adhesions. *J Surg Res* 20:1-5, 1976.

666. White NA: Management of postoperative complications in equine colic. *MVP* 64:743-746, 1983.

667. Hackett RP: Rupture of the urinary bladder in neonatal foals. *Compend Cont Ed Pract Vet* 6:S488-S492, 1984.

668. Genetzky RM and Jagemoser WA: Physical and clinical pathological findings associated with experimentally induced rupture of the equine urinary bladder. *Can Vet J* 26:391-395, 1985.

669. Owen J and Slocombe D: Pathogenesis of helminths in equines. *Vet Parasitol* 18:139-153, 1985.

670. Becht JL: Equine colic: Update on recent findings. *Proc Ann Forum ACVIM*, 1984. pp 207-209.

671. Drudge JH: Clinical aspects of *Strongylus vulgaris* infection in the horse: Emphasis on diagnosis, chemotherapy, and prophylaxis. *Vet Clin No Am* 1:251-266, 1979.

672. Schulze JL *et al:* Serum protein electrophoresis as an aid in diagnosis of equine verminous arteritis. *Vet Med* 78:1279-1282, 1983.

673. Hamir AN: Striated muscle tumors in horses. *Vet Record* 111:367-368, 1982.

674. Wright JA and Edwards GB: Adenocarcinoma of the intestine in a horse: An unoccurrence. *Equine Vet J* 16:136-137, 1984.

675. Frye FL *et al:* Hemangiosarcoma in a horse. *JAVMA* 182:287- 289, 1983.

676. Browning AP: Splenic lymphosarcoma in a stallion associated with an acute abdominal crisis. *Vet Record* 119:178-1789, 1986.

677. Crawley GR: Lymphosarcoma resulting in diarrhea, weight loss, and gastrointestinal ulcerations. *Vet Med* 80:66-69, 1985.

678. Humphrey M *et al:* Lymphosarcoma in a horse. *Equine Vet J* 16:547-548, 1984.

679. Mackey VS and Wheat JD: Reflections on the diagnostic approach to multicentric lymphosarcoma in an aged Arabian mare. *Equine Vet J* 17:467-469, 1985.

680. Hambright MB *et al:* Equine lymphosarcoma. *Compend Cont Ed Pract Vet* 5:S53-S56, 1983.

681. Dopson LC *et al:* Immunosuppression associated with lymphosarcoma in 2 horses. *JAVMA* 182:1239-1241, 1983.

682. McCoy DJ and Beasley R: Hypercalcemia associated with malignancy in a horse. *JAVMA* 189:87-89, 1986.

683. Bertone AL *et al:* Surgical resection of intestinal lymphosarcoma in a mare. *Compend Cont Ed Pract Vet* 7:S506-S511, 1985.

684. Guyton AC: *Textbook of Medical Physiology.* 7th ed. Saunders, Philadelphia, 1986. p 342.

685. Markel MD *et al:* Strangulated umbilical hernia in horses: 13 cases (1974-1985). *JAVMA* 190:692-694, 1987.

686. Fretz PB *et al:* Management of umbilical hernias in cattle and horses. *JAVMA* 183:550-552, 1983.

687. Tulleners EP and Fretz PB: Prosthetic repair of large abdominal wall defects in horses and food animals. *JAVMA* 182:258-262, 1983.

688. Tulleners EP and Donawick WJ: Secondary closure of infected abdominal incisions in cattle and horses. *JAVMA* 182:1377-1379, 1983.

689. Adams SB and Fessler JF: Umbilical cord remnant infections in foals: 16 cases (1975-1985). *JAVMA* 190:316-318, 1987.

690. Gibson KT *et al:* Incisional hernias in the horse: Incidence and predisposing factors. *Vet Surg* 18:360-366, 1989.

691. Bristol DG: Diaphragmatic hernias in horses and cattle. *Compend Cont Ed Pract Vet* 8:S407-S412, 1986.

692. Hanson RR and Todhunter RJ: Herniation of abdominal wall in 4 pregnant mares. *JAVMA* 189:790-793, 1986.

693. Tennant BC and Hornbuckle WE, in Anderson NV: *Veterinary Gastroenterology.* Lea & Febiger, Philadelphia, 1980. pp 593-620.

694. Tennant B: Acute hepatitis in horses: Problems of differentiating toxic and infectious causes in the adult. *Proc 24th Ann Mtg AAEP*, 1978. pp 465-471.

695. Tennant BC and Dill SG: in Robinson NE: *Current Therapy in Equine Medicine.* Saunders, Philadelphia, 1983. pp 249-251.

696. Gronwall R: Bilirubin metabolism. *Proc 1st Intl Symp Equine Hematol*, 1975. pp 237-245.

697. Tennant BC *et al:* Clinical signficance of hyperbilirubinemia in the horse. *Proc 1st Intl Symp Equine Hematol*, 1975. pp 246-254.

698. With TK: *Bile Pigments, Chemical, Biological and Clinical Aspects.* Academic Press, New York, 1968.

699. Tennant BC *et al:* Diseases of the equine liver. *Proc 21st Ann Mtg AAEP*, 1975. pp 410-425.

700. Naylor J *et al:* Fasting hyperbilirubinemia and its relationship to free fatty acids and triglycerides in the horse. *Proc Soc Exp Biol Med* 165:86-90, 1980.

701. Fraser CL and Arieff AI: Hepatic encephalopathy. *N Eng J Med* 313:865-872, 1975.

702. Munro HN *et al:* Insulin, plasma amino acid imbalance, and hepatic coma. *Lancet* 1:722-724, 1975.

703. Carlson G, in Mansmann RA and McAllister ES: *Equine Medicine and Surgery.* 3rd ed. American Veterinary Publications, Goleta, CA, 1982. pp 633-643.

704. Cornelius CE, in Kaneko JJ: *Clinical Biochemistry of Domestic Animals.* 3rd ed. Academic Press, Orlando, FL, 1980. pp 201-250.

705. Duncan JR and Prasse KW: *Veterinary Laboratory Medicine: Clinical Pathology.* 2nd ed. Iowa State Univ Press, Ames, 1986. pp 121-144.

706. Bernard W and Divers T: Isoenzyme-5 of lactic dehydrogenase as an indicator of equine hepatocellular disease. *Proc Ann Forum ACVIM,* 1987. p 901.

707. Braun JP et al: Serum gamma glutamyl transferase in equines: Reference papers logic values. *Am J Vet Res* 43:339-340, 1982.

708. Meyer DJ: The liver-Part 1. Biochemical tests for the evaluation of the hepatobiliary system. *Compend Cont Ed Pract Vet* 4:663-674, 1982.

709. Gronwall R et al: Direct measurement of biliary bilirubin excretion in ponies during fasting. *Am J Vet Res* 41:125-126, 1980.

710. Cohn VH, in Goodman LS and Gilman A: *The Pharmacologic Basis of Therapeutics.* 5th ed. MacMillan, New York, 1975. pp 1591-1600.

711. Tennant BC et al: Equine hepatic insufficiency. *Vet Clin No Am* (Large Anim Pract) 3:279-289, 1973.

712. Ford EJH and Godinath C: The excretion of phylloerythrin and bilirubin by the horse. *Res Vet Sci* 16:186, 1974.

713. Pearson EG: Serum bile acids for diagnosis of chronic liver disease in horses. *Proc 5th Ann Forum ACVIM,* 1987. pp 71-76.

714. Frevert CW et al: The ammonia tolerance test may be a clinically useful means of detecting liver disease in hores. *Proc 5th Ann Forum ACVIM,* 1987. p 901.

715. Dodds WJ, in Kaneko JJ: *Chemical Biochemistry of Domestic Animals.* 3rd ed. Academic Press, New York, 1980. pp 671-718.

716. Johnston JK et al: Cholelithiasis in the horse: 10 cases (1982-1986). *JAVMA* 194:405-409, 1989.

717. Engelking LR et al: Hepatobiliary transport of indocyanine green and sulfobromophthalein in fed and fasted horses. *Am J Vet Res* 46:2278-2283, 1985.

718. Pearson EG and Craig AM: The diagnosis of liver disease in equine and food animals. Part I. *MVP* 61:233-237, 1980.

719. Pearson EG and Craig AM: The diagnosis of liver disease in equine and food animals. Part II. *MVP* 61:315-320, 1980.

720. Gibbons WJ: Gibbons' notebook. *MVP* 45:72, 1964.

721. Rantanen NW: Diseases of the liver. *Vet Clin No Am* (Equine Pract) 2:105-114, 1986.

722. Divers TJ: Liver disease and liver failure in horses. *Proc 29th Ann Mtg AAEP,* 1983. pp 213-221.

723. Byars TD: Chronic liver failure in horses. *Compend Cont Ed Pract Vet* 5:S423-S430, 1983.

724. Gulick BA et al: Use of plasma amino acid patterns in liver disease in the horse. *Calif Vet* 34(7):21-23, 1979.

725. Van Der Leur RJT and Kroneman J: Biliary atresia in a foal. *Equine Vet J* 14:91-93, 1982.

726. Turk MAM et al: *Bacillus piliformis* infection (Tyzzer's disease) in foals in northwestern United States: A retrospective study of 21 cases. *JAVMA* 178:279-281, 1981.

727. Swerczek TW et al: Focal bacterial hepatitis in foals: Preliminary report. *MVP* 54:66-67, 1973.

728. Swerczek TW: Multifocal hepatic necrosis and hepatitis in foals caused by *Bacillus piliformis* (Tyzzer's disease). *Vet Annual* 17:130-132, 1977.

729. Pulley LT and Shively JN: Tyzzer's disease in a foal (light- and electron-microscopic observations). *Vet Pathol* 11:203-211, 1974.

730. Hall WC and Van Kruningen HJ: Tyzzer's disease in a horse. *JAVMA* 164:1187-1189, 1974.

731. Harrington DD: Naturally occurring Tyzzer's disease (*Bacillus piliformis* infection) in horse foals. *Vet Record* 96:59-63, 1975.

732. Harringtonn DD: Bacillus piliformis infection (Tyzzer's disease) in two foals. *JAVMA* 168:58-60, 1976.

733. Whitwell KE: Four cases of Tyzzer's disease in foals in England. *Equine Vet J* 8:118-122, 1976.

734. Anderson BC: Tyzzer's disease in foals - Occurrence in California. *Calif Vet* 30(3):36-37, 1976.

735. Thomson GW et al: Tyzzer's disease in the foal: Case reports and review. *Can Vet J* 18:41-43, 1977.

736. Swerczek TW: Experimental focal bacterial hepatitis in foals (Tyzzer's disease). *Proc 55th Conf Res Workers Anim Dis,* 1975. p 13.

737. Ganaway JR et al: Tyzzer's disease. *Am J Pathol* 64:717- 732, 1971.

738. Divers TJ et al: Toxic hepatic failure in newborn foals. *JAVMA* 183:1407-1413, 1983.

739. Acland HM et al: Toxic hepatopathy in neonatal foals. *Vet Pathol* 212:3-9, 1984.

740. Scwerzek TW and Crowe MW: Hepatotoxicosis in neonatal foals. *JAVMA* 183:388, 1983.

741. Gulick BA et al: Effect of pyrrolizidine alkaloid-induced hepatic disease on plasma amino acid patterns in the horse. *Am J Vet Res* 41:1894-1898, 1980.

742. Jubb KVF et al: *Pathology of Domestic Animals.* Vol 2. 3rd ed. Academic Press, New York, 1985. pp 240-313, 313-328.

743. Donawick WJ and Orsini JA, University of Pennsylvania: Personal communication, 1990.

744. Rose JA et al: Serum hepatitis in the horse. *Proc 20th Ann Mtg AAEP,* 1974. p 175-185.

745. Divers TJ, in Robinson NE: *Current Therapy in Equine Medicine 2.* Saunders, Philadelphia, 1987. pp 110-112.

746. Robinson M et al: Histopathology of acute hepatitis in the horse. *J Comp Pathol* 85:111-118, 1975.

747. McDole MG: Cholelithiasis in a horse. *Equine Pract* 2(5):37-40, 1980.

748. Roussel AJ et al: Choledocholithiasis in a horse. *Cornell Vet* 74:166-171, 1984.

749. Scarratt WK and Fessler RL: Cholelithiasis and biliary obstruction in a horse. *Compend Cont Ed Pract Vet* 7:S428- S431, 1985.

750. Traub JL et al: Cholelithiasis in four horses. *JAVMA* 181:59-62, 1982.

751. Tulleners E et al: Choledocholithotripsy in a mare. *JAVMA* 186:1317-1319, 1985.

752. Van Der Leur RJT and Kroneman J: Three cases of cholelithiasis and biliary fibrosis in the horse. *Equine Vet J* 14:251-253, 1982.

753. Reef VB *et al:* Ultrasonographic findings in horses with cholelithiasis: 8 cases (1985-1987). *JAVMA* 196:1836-1840, 1990.

754. Malet PF, in Wyngaarden JB and Smith LH: *Cecil's Textbook of Medicine.* 17th ed. Vol. 2. Saunders, Philadelphia, 1985. pp 852-853.

755. Hickson JCD: The secretion of pancreatic juice in response to stimulation of the vagus nerves in the pig. *J Physiol* 206:275, 1970.

756. Hubel KA: Effect of luminal chloride concentration on bicarbonate secretion in rat ileum. *Am J Physiol* 217:40, 1969.

757. McClure JJ, in Robinson NE: *Current Therapy in Equine Medicine 2.* Saunders, Philadelphia, 1987. pp 46-47.

758. Hardy RM and Johnson GF, in Anderson NV: *Veterinary Gastroenterology.* Lea & Febiger, Philadelphia, 1980. pp 621-647.

759. Avioli L *et al:* Role of the thyroid gland during glucagon-induced hypocalcemia in the dog. *Am J Physiol* 216:939-945, 1969.

760. Juan D: Hypocalcemia: Differential diagnosis and mechanisms. *Arch Intern Med* 139:1166-1171, 1979.

761. Epand RM: Relationships among several different non-homologous polypeptide hormones. *Mol Cell Biochem* 57:41-47, 1983.

762. Kerr OM *et al:* Pancreatic adenocarcinoma in a pony. *Equine Vet J* 14:338-339, 1982.

763. Rico AG *et al:* Tissue distribution and blood levels of gamma glutamyl transferase in the horse. *Equine Vet J* 9:100-101, 1977.

764. Baker RH: Acute necrotizing pancreatitis in a horse. *JAVMA* 172:268-270, 1978.

765. Morris DD, in Robinson NE: *Current Therapy in Equine Medicine.* Saunders, Philadelphia, 1983. pp 253-254.

766. Jeffrey JR: Diabetes mellitus secondary to chonic pancreatitis in a pony. *JAVMA* 153:1168-1175, 1968.

767. Rooney JR: *Autopsy of the Horse. Techniques and Interpretation.* Williams & Wilkins, Baltimore, 1970. pp 70-71.

768. Bulgin MS and Anderson BC: Verminous arteritis and pancreatic necrosis with diabetes mellitus in a pony. *Compend Cont Ed Pract Vet* 5:S482-S485, 1983.

769. Riggs WL: Diabetes mellitus secondary to chronic necrotizing pancreatitis in a pony. *Southwestern Vet* 25:149-151, 1972.

770. Carlson GP, in Mansmann RA and McAllister ES: *Equine Medicine and Surgery.* 3rd ed. American Veterinary Publications, Goleta, CA, 1982. pp 643-644.

771. Palmer JE: Prevention of Potomac horse fever. *Cornell Vet* 79:201-205, 1989.

772. Ross MW *et al:* Myoelctric activity of the cecum and right ventral colon in female ponies. *Am J Vet Res* 50:374-379, 1989.

773. Harrison IW: Cecal torsion in a horse as a consequence of cecocolic fold hypoplasia. *Cornell Vet* 79:315-317, 1989.

774. Steckel RR: Parietal hernia in a horse. *JAVMA* 182:818-819, 1983.

775. Ford TS *et al:* Ileocecal intussusception in horses: 26 cases (1981-1988). *JAVMA* 196:121-126, 1990.

776. DiPietro JA *et al:* Abdominal abscess associated with Parascaris equorum infection in a foal. *JAVMA* 182:991-992, 1983.

777. Herd RP, in Robinson NE: *Current Therapy in Equine Medicine 2.* Saunders, Philadelphia, 1987. pp 332-334.

778. Grant BD and Tennant B: Volvulus associated with Meckel's diverticulum in the horse. *JAVMA* 162:550-551, 1973.

This page is intentionally left blank.

8 Diseases of the Nervous System

R.J. MacKay and I.G. Mayhew

EXAMINATION OF THE NERVOUS SYSTEM[1-7]

Neurologic examination should be performed when a neurologic disorder is suspected from the history and physical examination. Very often it is only after completing a neurologic examination that one can decide whether a neurologic disorder is or is not present. Sometimes an abbreviated examination will suffice to rule out a neurologic disorder, and appropriate inspection of the musculoskeletal and other systems is necessary to define the problem better.

Neurologic examination should start at the head and proceed caudally to the tail. The sequence is the same, whether the patient is standing or recumbent. The anatomic location of a lesion is considered as the examination proceeds. Even if parts of the examination must be omitted because of the nature of the patient, financial constraints or a suspected fracture, the sequence is followed through mentally.

The overall sequence of the neurologic examination is:

1. Head
   - Behavior
   - Mental status
   - Head posture and coordination
   - Cranial nerves
2. Gait and posture
3. Neck and forelimbs
4. Back and hind limbs
5. Tail and anus

Evidence of brain lesions is sought first. If there is no such evidence, then the lesion is caudal to the level of the foramen magnum. If there are signs of brain lesions, then an attempt is made to explain all abnormalities in the rest of the examination by such a lesion. If this cannot be done, then more than one lesion is present.

Examination of limb position and gait gives an overall assessment of sensory and motor control of limbs. This is followed by specific evaluation of the neck and forelimbs. If neurologic signs in the forelimbs cannot be explained by evidence of a lesion rostral to the foramen magnum, then there is a lesion between C_1 and T_2, including peripheral nerves and muscles. The spine and hind limbs are assessed, and if signs in these parts cannot be explained by a lesion cranial to T_3, then a lesion is present between T_3 and S_2 or peripheral nerves or muscles. Finally, the tail, anus and perineum are assessed. If any neurologic abnormality cannot be explained by a lesion cranial to S_2, then a lesion exists between S_3 and the last caudal segment, or in nerves and muscles of these structures.

Results of the neurologic examination must be recorded and not risked to memory. A sample neurologic examination form is shown in Figure 1.

Examination of the Head

Behavior

The owner should be questioned about the patient's behavior and how the patient typically responds. The patient's age, breed and sex may influence behavior. A horse that is recumbent due to cervical spinal cord disease

Figure 1. Sample form for neurologic examination of horses.

VETERINARY MEDICAL TEACHING HOSPITAL
UNIVERSITY OF FLORIDA
NEUROLOGIC EXAMINATION OF LARGE ANIMALS

OUTPAITENT:	STALL NO.:
DATE:	TIME:
CLINICIAN:	CHARGES:
STUDENT:	ACCOUNT:
HISTORY:	

PHYSICAL EXAMINATION:

NEUROLOGIC EXAMINATION

HEAD:
- Behavior:
- Mental Status:
- Head Posture:
- Head Coordination:

Cranial Nerves:

EYES	LEFT	RIGHT
Ophthalmic Examination:		
Vision; II:		
Menace; II-VII, Cerebellum:		
Pupils, PLR; II-III:		
Horners; Symp:		
Strabismus; III, IV, VI, VIII:		

FACE
- Sensation; Vs, cerebrum:
- Muscle mass, jaw tone; Vm:
- Ear, eye, nose, lip reflex; V-VII:
- Expression; VII:
- Sweating, Symp:

VESTIBULAR — EAR
- Eye drop:
- Nystagmus; resting:
- positional:
- vestibular:
- Hearing:
- Special vestibular:

TONGUE
- Tone, mass, fasciculations; XII, cerebrum:

PHARYNX, LARYNX
- Voice; IX, X:
- Swallow; IX, X:
- Endoscopy:
- Slap test:

GAIT:	LEFT		RIGHT	
	FORE	HIND	FORE	HIND
Paresis:				
Ataxia:				
Spasticity:				
Dysmetria:				
Total deficit:				
Other:				

NECK & FORELIMBS	LEFT	RIGHT	TRUNK & HINDLIMBS:	LEFT	RIGHT	TAIL & ANUS:	LEFT	RIGHT
Hoofwear:			Hoofwear:			Strength:		
Posture:			Posture:			Muscle Mass:		
Strength:			Strength:			Tone:		
Muscle Mass:			Muscle Mass:			Reflexes:		
Tone:			Tone:			Sensation:		
Reflexes:			Reflexes:			Rectal:		
Sensation:			Sensation:					
Sweating:			Sweating:					

ASSESSMENT

SITE OF LESION(S): General (circle): cerebrum, brainstem, peripheral cranial nerves, cerebellum, spinal cord, peripheral nerves, muscles, skeleton

Specific:

CAUSE OF LESION(S):

PLAN
- DX:
- RX:
- EX:

SIGNATURE: | DATE:

or musculoskeletal disease usually does not have altered behavior unless it becomes frantic in its struggling. Close observation may be required to observe seizures in an animal with a history of seizures. Auditory and tactile stimulation sometimes elicit seizure activity. Partial seizures in neonatal animals may be seen just as "chewing gum fits," facial twitching or periods of tachypnea.

Bizarre and inappropriate behavior, such as head-pressing, compulsive wandering, circling, change in voice and appetite, licking objects and aggression, usually is easy to recognize and is regarded as a sign of cerebral disease. Though abnormalities usually are symmetric, animals with a cerebral lesion that show compulsive circling behavior tend to circle toward the side of the lesion.

Mental Status

The patient's state of awareness or consciousness is assessed. The animal's level of responsiveness to its internal and external environment is affected by the ascending reticular activating system in the brainstem and by the cerebral hemispheres. These can be affected by stimuli received from the sensory nervous system. Thus, in evaluating the mental status of an animal, the response to visual, tactile, auditory, painful, olfactory and gustatory (nursing) stimuli should be considered.

Coma is a state of complete unresponsiveness to normal stimuli. The deepest comas usually are related to brainstem, particularly midbrain, lesions. Semicoma is a state of partial responsiveness to stimuli. An animal so affected does not respond to the environment nor to minor stimuli, such as visual cues, but usually has an altered response to noxious stimuli. Voluntary movements occur with stimulation. Other less profound levels of loss of awareness are variously described as stupor, obtundation, somnolence, delirium, lethargy and depression.

Horses that are recumbent due to spinal cord diseases usually are bright and alert unless anorectic, dehydrated, exhausted or unduly frightened; they may become frantic, however.

Head Posture and Coordination

All normal animals maintain the head in a certain posture and maneuver it quickly and smoothly to perform certain acts, as prehension of food. Vestibular lesions often result in a head tilt that, when mild, is characterized by a laterally deviated poll, while the caudal neck and muzzle remain on the midline or median plane. In comparison, a horse (with a cerebral lesion) that continually turns in circles often has the head and neck deviated to one side. In this circumstance, the poll is not rotated markedly about the muzzle, and the muzzle deviates from the median plane. A severe vestibular lesion can result in a marked head tilt as well as head and neck turn, usually both toward the side of the lesion (Fig 2).

Animals with bilateral (peripheral) vestibular disease frequently show wide swinging movements of the head and neck.

The cerebellum modulates movements of the head and limbs. With cerebellar disease, fine control of head positioning often is lost, resulting in awkward jerky movements. Even at rest, the lack of control often can be seen as bobbing head movements that can be exaggerated by increasing voluntary effort. The resulting fine jerky movements of the head are called an intention tremor. Such animals "overshoot" when positioning their head, as when moving to eat.

A newborn foal normally holds its head flexed slightly more than an adult horse and moves it in a jerky manner, especially in response to visual or tactile stimuli.

Musculoskeletal disorders must be considered for any asymmetry or deviation of the head and neck.

Cranial Nerves

Abnormalities discovered in the cranial nerve examination are most helpful in diagnosing a lesion of the brainstem. The examination starts with the most rostral nerves and proceeds caudally, assessing the function of each cranial nerve.

I. Olfactory Nerve: Clinical deficit of smell (anosmia) is encountered rarely. Normal function is evaluated by the patient's ability to smell its feed or the hand of the examiner.

II. Optic Nerve: An owner may indicate that a patient has been acting blind; however, a depressed animal or one with loss of balance (vestibular disease) may stumble over objects, thus appearing to be blind without being so.

The visual pathway is tested by the menace (blind or eye preservation) response. A

Figure 2. Comparison of horses with deviation of the head and neck (A) and a head tilt (B). The horse in (A) has a diffuse, symmetric central disease and holds its head and neck to the left. The animal also wanders in circles to the left. The horse in (B) has otitis media-interna, which results in a slight head tilt to the right with the poll held to the right of midline. This is characteristic of vestibular disease. The horse in (B) also has right facial paralysis.

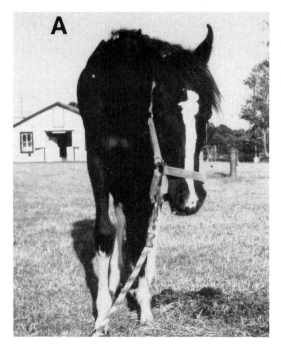
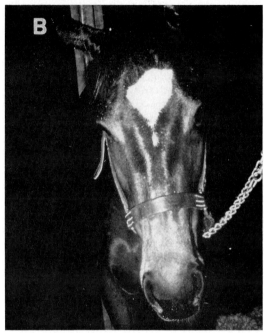

threatening gesture of the hand toward the horse's eye elicits immediate closure of the eyelids, and the head may be jerked away. For all practical purposes, vision in one eye is perceived by the visual cortex of the opposite (contralateral) cerebral hemisphere. The incoming (afferent) pathway for the menace response is the ipsilateral eye and optic nerve, optic chiasm, contralateral optic tract, lateral geniculate nucleus (thalamus), optic radiation and occipital visual cortex. The outgoing (efferent) pathway of the menace response is from this contralateral visual cortex to the ipsilateral facial nucleus, causing closure of the eyelids.

Some stoic, depressed or even excited animals may not respond to a menacing gesture with closure of the eyelids or may keep the eyelids closed. Neonatal foals may not respond to this test until several days of age and may become refractory to repeated menace testing. A true visual deficiency may be detected while the animal moves about its environment, when objects are placed in front of it, or when nonaromatic objects are dropped noiselessly in its visual fields. Unilateral blindness (hemianopia) can be diffi-

cult to assess, and it may take repeated efforts, such as blindfolding each eye in turn, to detect it.

An ophthalmologic examination should be included in the neurologic evaluation. Lesions of the eye and optic nerve result in ipsilateral blindness. Lesions of optic tracts and lateral geniculate nucleus cause contralateral blindness. Space-occupying lesions of the brain frequently produce blindness. This can be due to direct involvement of central visual pathways but, frequently, it is caused by pressure of the mass and cerebral edema forcing the occipital lobes caudally. These lobes are damaged when they herniate under the bony tentorium cerebelli lying between the cerebrum and cerebellum. The resultant blindness is contralateral to the lesion but often bilateral because of associated diffuse brain swelling.

Animals with various diffuse *cerebellar* diseases may have bilaterally deficient menace responses. These animals have not been blind, have not had facial paralysis to explain this finding, and pull their head away from the menacing gesture. Thus, it is assumed that the cerebellum influences the operation of this component of the visual system. Foals appear to see by a few hours of age but do not blink to a menacing gesture until 5-14 days. They blink at a bright light and pull their head away from a menacing gesture, often in a jerky manner. A true menace response usually is present by 1-2 weeks of age.

III. Oculomotor Nerve: Pupil diameter is controlled by 2 muscle groups, the constrictor muscles of the pupil, innervated by the parasympathetic fibers in the oculomotor nerve, and dilator muscles of the pupil, innervated by the sympathetic fibers from the cranial cervical ganglion. These autonomic innervations originate from higher centers in the brainstem and change pupil diameter in response to light (oculomotor nerve) and fear and excitement (sympathetic).

The first observation to be made is the size and symmetry of the pupils, considering the amount of ambient light and emotional status of the patient. The response of the pupils to light directed into the eye (pupillary light response) is noted. The eyeballs are inspected for any lesion that may interfere with pupillary response, such as iritis, iris atrophy or adhesions. The normal response to light directed into one eye is constriction of both pupils; this is called a direct response in the illuminated (ipsilateral) eye and a consensual response in the nonilluminated (contralateral) eye. The incoming (afferent) pathway for this reflex is similar to that for the menace response to the level of the thalamus. The pathway is through the optic nerve, optic chiasm (where crossing occurs), through the optic tracts lateral and dorsal to the thalamus, then ventrally into the midbrain. Crossing occurs at this site also, and axons pass to the parasympathetic oculomotor nuclei in the midbrain on both sides. The motor (efferent) pathway is from these nuclei via the oculomotor nerves to the ciliary ganglia caudal to the eyeball and to the constrictor muscles of the pupils.

This pupillary light reflex is within the brainstem and thus is not affected by lesions of the visual cortex. A widely dilated (mydriatic) pupil in an eye with normal vision suggests an oculomotor nerve lesion. Such an eye is unresponsive to light directed into either eye. The pupil in the contralateral eye with normal oculomotor function responds to light directed into both the ipsilateral (direct response) and contralateral (consensual response) eye. A retrobulbar lesion involving the optic and oculomotor nerves will appear as a mydriatic pupil unresponsive to light shone in either eye; in addition, a visual (menace) deficit is present in that eye.

The oculomotor nerves are subject to damage by edema and space-occupying lesions in the forebrain, causing pressure ventrally on the brainstem. Asymmetric swelling of cerebral tissue may exert greater pressure to one oculomotor nerve, causing unequal pupillary size (anisocoria), usually evident as ipsilateral pupillary dilation. Severe brainstem contusion can produce various pupillary abnormalities in association with coma or semicoma. These can change rapidly in the first few hours following injury. Progressive, bilateral pupillary dilation following cranial injury warrants a grave prognosis.

Nuclei within the brain that control sympathetic nervous system function are located in the hypothalamus, midbrain, pons and medulla. First-order neuronal fibers descend through the midbrain, medulla and cervical spinal cord to synapse on cell bodies in the lateral intermediate gray columns in the thoracolumbar spinal cord. The preganglionic, second-order sympathetic cell bodies supplying the head are situated in the cranial thoracic segments (T_1-T_3). Axons leave these segments of the spinal cord, traverse the thorax, and ascend the neck with the vagus nerve to the cranial cervical ganglion lying on the caudodorsal wall of the medial compartment of the guttural pouch. Postganglionic, third-order sympathetic fibers leave the cranial cervical ganglion to innervate the glands, smooth muscle, and blood vessels of the eyeball, head and cranial cervical area.

Damage to the sympathetic nerves of the eyeball results in Horner's syndrome. This is seen as slight ptosis of the upper eyelid, miosis (constriction of the pupil), and slight protrusion of the nictitating membrane (Fig 3); vision and the pupillary light response are unaffected. In horses, lesions involving the sympathetic supply to the head cause these ophthalmic signs and additional signs, including dilation of facial blood vessels, hyperemia of nasal and conjunctival mucous membranes, and increased surface temperature and sweating of the face. This last sign is most prominent at the base of the ear and is present over the neck caudally to about the level of the axis. These signs have been seen with lesions of the sympathetic pathways in the guttural pouches, in the area of the cervi-

Figure 3. Facial paralysis and Horner's syndrome. The horse in (A) has left facial paralysis involving all branches of the nerve. The left ear, eyelid and lips droop. All of these structures are flaccid and the muzzle is pulled to the right (unaffected side). The foal in (B) has Horner's syndrome on the right side. Ptosis is evident on the right. Sweating is also visible (and hyperthermia palpable) on the right side of the face and cranial aspect of the neck, and is most prominent at the base of the right ear. In (C) and (D), the right, affected (C) and left, unaffected (D) eyes of another horse with Horner's syndrome on the right side are illustrated. Ptosis and slight miosis are evident on the affected (C) side.

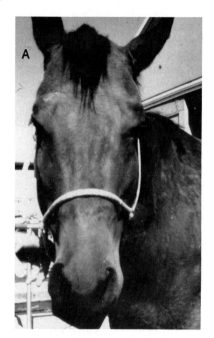
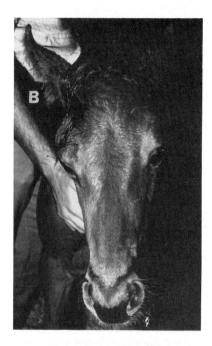
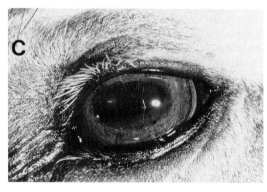
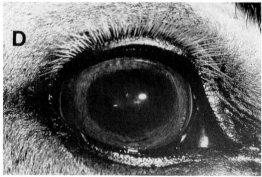

cal vagosympathetic trunk, and at the thoracic inlet.

Horner's syndrome can be expected from large lesions involving the descending sympathetic pathways in the brainstem and cervical spinal cord. Such lesions also cause excessive sweating over the whole affected side of the body, because all the sympathetic pathways leaving the spinal cord have lost their central (upper motor neuron) connections.

III. Oculomotor Nerve, IV. Trochlear Nerve, VI. Abducens Nerve: In addition to innervation of the pupillary constrictor muscles, the oculomotor nerve also innervates the extraocular muscles along with the trochlear and abducens nerves. The functions of these muscles and nerves are tested by observing the position of the eyes within the orbits and observing eye movement. An abnormal position (strabismus) results when these nerves or muscles are damaged.

When evaluating eye position and movement, consideration must be given to the normal response of the eyes to head posture and movement. When a horse's nose is elevated (neck extended), the eyes tend to maintain a horizontal position and thus move ventrally in the orbits. The eyes also respond to head movement in a particular manner. When the head is moved to one side, the eyes move rhythmically instead of remaining fixed in the center of the orbit. There is a slow-phase movement in the direction opposite to the direction the head is moved, followed by a fast phase in the same direction the head is moved. These rhythmic movements continue until the head comes to rest and the eyes return to the center of the orbits. These eye movements are regarded as normal vestibular nystagmus and result from connection between the balance centers (vestibular nuclei) in the medulla and the nuclei of the cranial nerves controlling eye movement (III, IV, VI). Vestibular nystagmus thus requires an intact vestibular system, intact cranial nerves III, IV and VI, and the connection between these.

The exact neurologic signs seen with specific paralysis of each of these 3 cranial nerves are not known in horses. Paralysis of the oculomotor nerve should produce lateral and ventral strabismus, and ptosis of the upper eyelid, mydriasis and absent pupillary light reflex. The mydriasis is seen, and a tendency for lateral eyeball deviation has been observed in horses with midbrain lesions. Paralysis of the trochlear nerve should result in the medial aspect of the pupil rotating dorsally, so-called "dorsomedial" strabismus. Damage to the abducens nerve should produce medial strabismus and decreased ability to retract the globe in the orbit when the cornea is touched at the same time the eyelids are held open (corneal reflex).

The forms of strabismus described for paralysis of each of these cranial nerves should be present in all positions of the head. Such examples of true strabismus are rare. More common is deviation of the eyeballs resulting from disturbance of the vestibular system that alters the normal tonic mechanism controlling eye position. This vestibular strabismus usually is ventral and may be medial. The important difference is that the eyeballs can be moved out of the abnormal position and usually respond with vestibular nystagmus when the head is moved. In unilateral vestibular disease, this vestibular strabismus most often occurs on the same side as the lesion.

Periorbital lesions, particularly due to trauma and neoplasms, often cause mechanical eye deviations. The eyeball position of newborn foals often is ventromedial as compared to that of an adult horse. Also, congenitally blind horses may have abnormal eyeball positioning and movement.

V. Trigeminal Nerve: The large trigeminal nerve contains motor nerve fibers to the muscles of mastication in the mandibular branch and sensory nerve fibers from most of the head in all 3 branches (mandibular, maxillary, ophthalmic).

Loss of motor function of the mandibular nerve bilaterally results in a dropped jaw and inability to chew. The tongue may appear to protrude because it moves rostrally in the mouth. Sialosis results from lack of jaw movement. After 1-2 weeks, the temporal and masseter muscles and the distal belly of the digastricus muscle atrophy. Unilateral lesions (most often due to protozoal myeloencephalitis) result in muscle atrophy on one side without dysphagia. Many normal horses have asymmetric temporal muscles.

Function of the sensory branches of this cranial nerve is tested reflexly and directly by assessing sensation to the head. Lightly pricking the ears, eyelids, external nares and lips tests the ear, eye, nose and lip reflexes. These movements are mediated via the sensory branches of the trigeminal nerve and motor branches of the facial nerve. These reflexes thus require an intact brainstem and trigeminal and facial nuclei but do not require the animal to feel the stimulus. Sensation from the head should be assessed along the distribution of each of the major branches of the trigeminal nerve by observing a cerebral response (withdrawal and shaking of the head, attempts to bite, phonation) to the test. In stoic or depressed animals, sensation may be assessed by lightly pricking the internal nares and nasal septum. Lesions of the sensory nucleus of the trigeminal nerve of the side of the medulla oblongata can cause facial hypalgesia and hyporeflexia without weakness of the muscles of mastication. This may cause feed to become impacted in the rostral cheek pouch because the horse cannot feel the food. Cerebral lesions can produce contralateral facial hypalgesia that is most evident in the nasal septum opposite the lesions, without hyporeflexia. This is thought to be due to involvement of the parietal sensory cortex, with sparing of the trigeminal nuclei and reflex pathways in the brainstem.

VII. Facial Nerve: This is predominantly a motor nerve innervating the muscles of facial expression and the lacrimal and certain salivary glands. It contains the lower motor neurons of many of the reflexes tested previously. Initial evaluation of the facial nerve involves observation of these reflexes that result in closure of the eyelids (menace, palpebral, corneal reflexes) and movement of the ears, lips and nose. Facial paralysis generally is seen as a drooping of the ear, ptosis of the upper eyelid, drooping of the upper lip, and retraction of the nose toward the unaffected side (Fig 3). General inspection for symmetry of facial expression is useful. Some normal horses have a subtle deviation of the nostrils or muzzle to one side. Lack of movement of the nose during inspiration may be one of the earliest findings in partial facial paresis. Comparison of tone in the ears, eyelids and lips on each side may help detect facial weakness. Occasionally a small amount of food may remain in the cheeks on the affected side. This must not be confused with the eating difficulties caused by sensory and/or motor trigeminal paralysis. Because of the lack of muscle tone, saliva may drool from the corners of the lips in facial paralysis. If there is only weakness of the lips and a deviated nasal philtrum without a drooped ear and ptosis, probably there is involvement of only the buccal branches and, perhaps more likely, a peripheral lesion involving the facial nerve along the side of the face.

As with other cranial nerves, central versus peripheral nerve involvement can be diagnosed by identifying involvement of adjacent structures in the medulla oblongata, which produces depression, ataxia and other signs of cranial nerve dysfunction. Lesions of the middle and inner ear causing vestibular signs often cause accompanying facial nerve paralysis. This is because the facial nerve lies in the petrous temporal bone and is separated from the tympanic cavity by only a thin membrane. Absence of signs of involvement of other central pathways is used to differentiate peripheral facial and vestibular nerve disease from involvement of their nuclei and pathways in the medulla oblongata. In horses, the facial nerve lies in the wall of the dorsolateral aspect of the lateral compartment of the guttural pouch and is associated there with the mandibular nerve (V) and maxillary artery.

With various focal thalamic and cerebral lesions, the facial muscles may be hypertonic and hyperreflexic, resulting in spontaneous and reflexly initiated "grimacing." This is due to involvement of the higher motor centers of upper motor neurons controlling facial movement that normally have a calming effect on the facial nucleus. Importantly, the facial reflexes are intact and may be hyperactive. Irritative lesions, such as peracute encephalitides, also can cause grimacing.

VIII. Vestibulocochlear Nerve: The cochlear (auditory) division of this nerve transmits impulses of the sense of hearing. Bilateral middle ear disease causes deafness, but unilateral hearing loss is difficult to detect.

The vestibular division of cranial nerve VIII supplies the major input to the vestibular system and controls balance. Fibers from the inner ear pass through the internal acoustic meatus in the petrosal bone and penetrate the lateral medulla to terminate in the vestibular nuclei. A few fibers pass to small parts of the cerebellum, which are part of the vestibular system. The vestibular system receives input from many higher centers and from the cerebellum, and controls orientation of the head, body, limbs and eyes in space with respect to gravity and motion.

Signs of vestibular disease can be seen from lesions involving any part of the vestibular system. The eyeballs are checked for normal vestibular nystagmus when the head is moved from side to side. Nystagmus with the horse's head in a normal position (spontaneous) and/or with the head held steady by the examiner in various abnormal positions (positional) is abnormal and indicates a disorder of the vestibular system. The direction of nystagmus can help determine the site of vestibular lesions and always is described by referring to the fast phase. In peripheral vestibular disorders, the nystagmus (fast phase) always is directed away from the side of the lesion and from the direction of head tilt. Usually it is horizontal, though it may be rotary or arc-shaped. When lesions involve the central components of the vestibular system in the medulla oblongata, spontaneous and positional nystagmus may be horizontal, vertical or rotary and also may change direction with changes in head posture. Such lesions frequently affect adjacent structures, such as the proprioceptive and motor pathways for voluntary limb movement and the reticular formation, causing ataxia, tetraparesis and depression, respectively.

Signs of peripheral vestibular disease often improve markedly within several days as animals accommodate. Blindfolding an animal that has accommodated to vestibular disease often exacerbates the signs immediately. Conversely, blindness interferes with recovery from vestibular disease. Partly because the vestibular portions of the cerebellum are relatively small, there often is no sign of vestibular disease with cerebellar lesions.

IX. Glossopharyngeal Nerve, X. Vagus Nerve, XI. Accessory Nerve: The major role of these cranial nerves is innervation of the pharynx and larynx with both sensory and motor fibers. The functions of these nerves are tested by listening for normal laryngeal sounds, observing normal swallowing of food and water, assessing the swallowing reflex by passage of a nasogastric tube and, finally, by inspection of the larynx and pharynx with an endoscope, if necessary. The major centers for control of the pharynx and larynx via these 3 cranial nerves are the nucleus ambiguus and nucleus solitarius in the caudal medulla. The most important clinical sign of an abnormality in these regions is paralysis of the pharynx and larynx. The severity of signs depends on whether there is unilateral or bilateral involvement. In pharyngeal paralysis, food and water usually are seen at the nares. Unilateral paralysis of the larynx results in "roaring" at exercise but usually is subclinical in sedentary individuals.

The laryngeal adductor response ("slap test") should be assessed. The skin just caudal to the dorsal scapula is slapped gently with a hand while the larynx is observed through an endoscope or the dorsal larynx is palpated. The normal response is for the *contralateral* arytenoid cartilage to *adduct* briefly, with a palpable twitch at the pharyngeal muscles. The afferent pathway is via segmental thoracic nerves, cranially via the contralateral cervical spinal cord white matter and, finally, to the contralateral vagal nucleus in the medulla oblongata. The efferent pathway is via the vagus nerve to the cranial thorax, then back up the neck in the recurrent laryngeal nerve to the larynx. The reflex can be interrupted at any of these sites.

Lesions in the nucleus ambiguus and swallowing center in the medulla oblongata usually affect adjacent structures, resulting in depression, ataxia, weakness and signs of other cranial nerve involvement. Many severe, diffuse brain diseases cause dysphagia without lesions in the medulla oblongata. This is a result of interference with the higher motor control (voluntary effort) of swallowing. Due to their close association with the guttural pouch, these 3 cranial nerves can become involved with guttural pouch diseases. Dysphagia is seen with the diffuse lower motor neuron and neuromuscular paralysis seen with botulism and with diseases affecting pharyngeal muscles. Stertorous breathing may be detected with diseases causing pharyngeal and laryngeal paralysis.

XI. Accessory Nerve: This nerve provides the motor supply to at least the trapezius and cranial part of the sternocephalicus muscles. Loss of function is difficult to detect without an electromyographic study.

XII. Hypoglossal Nerve: This last cranial nerve has its cell bodies in the hypoglossal nucleus in the caudal medulla oblongata and is the motor nerve to the muscles of the tongue. Thus, the tongue must be inspected for symmetry, normal movement and evidence of atrophy. Normally a horse strongly resists having its tongue withdrawn from the mouth. A unilateral lesion of the hypoglossal nucleus or nerve results in unilateral atrophy of the tongue and weak retraction, though the tongue usually does not remain protruding from the mouth. Bilateral involvement interferes with prehension and swallowing. The tongue usually protrudes, and the animal cannot draw it back into the mouth. Horses that play with their tongues ("tongue chewers") appear to have poor tone in this organ.

With severe cerebral lesions but without focal brainstem involvement, the tongue may remain protruded and is slow to return to its normal position when pulled out of the mouth. This is the result of a lesion in the higher motor centers or upper motor neuron. The voluntary control pathways for function of the tongue are impaired, resulting in weakness without involving hypoglossal nuclei or nerves. Tongue, jaw and lip movement (dystonia) is severely impaired with the upper motor neuron (basal nuclei) lesion in nigropallidal encephalomalacia (yellow-star thistle poisoning).

Evaluating Gait and Posture

After examination of the head, the gait is evaluated as a general assessment of brainstem, cerebellum, spinal cord and peripheral nerve and muscle function. Evaluation of posture and testing postural reactions when appropriate (as in a foal) assesses overall integrity of these areas and the forebrain. If evidence of a lesion has been detected in examination of the head ("head signs"), an attempt is made to explain any abnormalities found in the rest of the examination by the lesion above the level of the atlantooccipital junction. If this cannot be done, there are at least 2 lesions or a diffuse disease. If "head signs" are not found, it is assumed that the lesion(s) are in the spinal cord, peripheral nerves or muscles.

The first observation to be made is which limbs have an abnormal gait and/or posture and, second, whether there is evidence of a musculoskeletal abnormality. The essential components of a neurologic gait abnormality are weakness and ataxia. The latter often is characterized as hypometria and hypermetria. Each limb must be evaluated for evidence of these. Identifying these characteristics of gait abnormality can help localize a lesion in the nervous or musculoskeletal systems (Table 1). This is done while the animal is walking, trotting, turning tightly (pivoting) and backing.

To detect subtle asymmetry in the length of stride, it helps to walk parallel to or behind the animal, matching it step for step. Also, if possible, the gait should be evaluated while the animal is walking up and down a slope, walking with the neck extended, running free in a field, and walking while blindfolded. Subtle signs often are not seen at normal gaits but are seen as consistent mistakes while the animal performs these more involved maneuvers. Postural reactions then can be evaluated where appropriate. With many neurologic disorders causing an abnormal gait, a horse may pace (moving ipsilateral limbs simultaneously) rather than walking (at a 4-beat gait).

Weakness

Weakness or paresis often is manifested by dragging of the limbs, worn hooves and a low arc to the swing phase of the stride. This indicates flexor weakness and often is related to upper motor neuron diseases (brainstem and spinal cord white matter). When an animal bears weight on a weak limb, the limb often trembles and the animal may even collapse on that limb because of lack of support. While circling, walking on a slope and walking with the head elevated, the animal frequently stumbles on a weak limb and knuckles over at the fetlock. Weakness in the pelvic limbs is detected easily by walking next to the horse and pulling the tail laterally to determine the degree of resistance. With severe weakness in all 4 limbs but no ataxia and spasticity, one must strongly consider neuromuscular diseases.

Profound extensor weakness in only one limb suggests a lesion of the spinal cord gray matter, peripheral nerve, or muscle (upper motor neuron) for that limb. Weakness (especially flexor weakness) occurs with descending motor pathway (upper motor neuron) lesions in the brainstem and spinal cord, and is present in the limbs on the same side and caudal to the lesion. A patient with a peracute peripheral vestibular syndrome may appear weak in the limbs on the same side as the lesions due to the tendency to fall in that direction. This "weakness" usually is temporary and overshadowed by the ataxia

Table 1. Types of gait abnormalities with lesions in various locations in the nervous and musculoskeletal systems.

Site of Lesions	Ataxia	Paresis	Hypo-metria	Hyper-metria
Brainstem and spinal cord white matter (UMN & GP)	++	++	+	+
Vestibular system	+		++	
Cerebellum	++		+	++
Peripheral nerve				
Motor-LMN		++		
Sensory	+	+	+	
Musculo-skeletal system			+	+

+ = often present
++ = often very prominent

and by marked hypometria frequently seen in the contralateral limbs.

Ataxia

Ataxia, or proprioceptive deficit, is poor coordination in moving the limbs and body. It is seen as swaying from side to side of the pelvis, trunk and sometimes the whole body, and as weaving of the affected limbs during the swing phase of the stride. This often results in abducted or adducted foot placement, crossing of the limbs or stepping on the opposite foot, especially while the animal is circling or turning tightly. A severely ataxic animal often paces. Circumduction of the outside limbs when turning and circling also is regarded as a proprioceptive deficit. Walking the animal on a slope and with its head elevated often exaggerates ataxia, particularly in the pelvic limbs. When a weak and ataxic animal is turned sharply in circles, the affected limb often is left in one place while the animal pivots around it. This also may occur when backing such an animal.

Blindfolding does not appear to exacerbate weakness and ataxia caused by spinal cord disease. However, the gait abnormality seen with vestibular or cerebellar diseases often worsens with blindfolding. An ataxic gait may be most pronounced when an animal is moving freely in a paddock at a trot or canter, especially when attempting to stop, when the limbs may be wildly adducted or abducted. General proprioceptive deficits are due to lesions of the general proprioceptive sensory pathways that relay information on the position of the limbs and body to the cerebellum (cerebellar proprioception) and to the thalamus and cerebral cortex (conscious proprioception). Conscious proprioceptive deficits are seen by a horse's adopting and maintaining abnormal limb postures when being stopped after turning tightly in circles. Often it is difficult to differentiate weakness from ataxia.

Hypometria

Hypometria, spasticity or stiffness is seen as stiff movement of the limbs with very little flexion of the joints, particularly the carpal and tarsal joints. This generally indicates a lesion affecting the descending motor (upper motor neuron) or vestibular pathways to that limb. A spastic gait, particularly in the thoracic limbs, may be seen best when the animal

is backed or when maneuvering on a slope with its head held elevated. The thoracic limbs may move almost without flexing and resemble a marching tin soldier. Spasticity may be the most obvious sign in the thoracic limbs with cervical spinal cord disease. The short-strided, staggering gait seen in the limbs contralateral to a vestibular lesion may be regarded as hypometria.

Hypermetria

Hypermetria describes a lack of direction and limitation of range of movement and is seen as overreaching of the limbs, with excessive joint movement. This may result in a longer or shorter stride. Hypermetria without paresis (along with other characteristic "head signs") is characteristic of cerebellar disease but also is prominent in some peripheral nerves diseases, such as stringhalt.

Dysmetria

Dysmetria is a term that incorporates hypermetria and hypometria.

Grading Gait Abnormalities

The degree of weakness, ataxia, hypometria and hypermetria should be graded for each limb. An arbitrary scale of 0 to 4+ has been described for the degree of abnormality. A score of 1+ indicates signs that are just detectable in the limb, while 4+ indicates that the patient stumbles and possibly falls at normal gaits. Such grading helps localize a lesion. With focal lesions, particularly compressive lesions in the cranial cervical spinal cord (C_1-C_6) or brainstem, neurologic signs generally are one grade more severe in the pelvic limbs than in the thoracic limbs. With a mild focal cervical spinal cord lesion, there may be a 1+ abnormality in the pelvic limbs but no signs in the thoracic limbs. The anatomic diagnosis in such a case would be a thoracolumbar, cervical or diffuse spinal cord lesion.

A 3+ or 4+ grade in the pelvic limbs and no neurologic abnormality in the thoracic limbs is consistent with a thoracolumbar spinal cord lesion. With a 1+ and 4+ change in the thoracic and pelvic limbs, respectively, one must consider a severe thoracolumbar lesion plus a mild cervical lesion or diffuse spinal cord disease. A 4+ in the thoracic limbs with a 1+ in the pelvic limbs also is not consistent with a single focal C1 to C6 lesion. Such neurologic signs suggest a lesion involving the brachial intumescence (C6-T2), with involvement of the gray matter supplying the thoracic limbs or a diffuse spinal cord lesion. A severe abnormality (3+ or 4+) in one or both thoracic limbs with normal pelvic limbs indicates lower motor neuron involvement of the thoracic limbs (ventral gray columns at C6-T2, peripheral nerves, or muscle).

Gait alterations can occur in all 4 limbs with lesions of the white matter in the caudal brainstem. "Head signs," such as cranial nerve abnormalities, are used to define the site of the lesion. Subacute or chronic lesions of the cerebrum do not alter the gait, though postural reactions, such as hopping, are abnormal and sometimes the gait is regarded as "sluggish."

Evaluating Recumbent Patients

Every effort should be made to assist a recumbent patient to stand and walk, unless there is suspicion of a bone fracture. This is particularly important with heavy animals early in the course of recumbency, before secondary problems of decubital sores, decreased blood supply to the limbs, and dehydration make evaluation difficult and the prognosis worse.

Evaluating the Neck and Forelimbs

Following an overall evaluation of gait, attention is focused on the neck and thoracic limbs. If a gait alteration was detected in the thoracic limbs and there were no signs of brain involvement, this part of the examination attempts to confirm involvement of the spinal cord from C1 to T2 and to localize the lesion within these segments.

Observation and palpation of the neck and forelimbs detect gross skeletal defects, asymmetry in the neck, and muscle atrophy that may be associated with neurologic disease, thus localizing findings. Involvement of the peripheral pre- and postganglionic sympathetic neurons causes local sweating; this can be an extremely helpful localizing sign, as described above in Horner's syndrome.

The neck should be manipulated to assess normal range of movement. Evidence of a stiff neck, such as reluctance to flex the neck or pain on flexing the neck, warrants careful assessment before any conclusions are drawn. Cervical vertebral arthrosis, involvement of cervical nerve roots, and marked cervical spinal cord disease can result in scoliosis and even torticollis.

When the skin of the lateral neck dorsal to the jugular groove is tapped lightly with a probe, contraction of the cutaneous muscle normally results in flicking of the skin. The brachiocephalicus muscle often contracts, causing the shoulder to be pulled cranially. Also there is flicking of the ear rostrally, blinking of eyelids, and contracture of the labial muscles ("smile") with this test. These are termed the local cervical and cervicofacial responses, respectively. The anatomic pathways are not known, though they must involve several cervical segments and the facial nucleus in the medulla. Cervical lesions of the gray and white matter can result in depressed or absent cervical responses.

Sensory perception over the neck and forelimbs can be assessed at the time of observing the cervical responses by continuing the skin tapping over the horse's shoulders and distally on the limbs.

The sway reaction is tested by pushing laterally against the shoulders to force the horse first to attempt to maintain balance and then to take a step laterally, away from the examiner. This test is performed while the animal is standing still and while it is walking forward. One forelimb also may be held up while the patient is forced to hop on the other. This test of postural reaction, used in place of the thoracic limb hopping test (with pelvic limbs also supported), can be performed in smaller patients. Weakness is evidenced by a lack of resistance to lateral shoulder pressure. Weakness and ataxia may cause tripping and stumbling on the forelimbs when taking lateral steps. Pulling laterally on both the tail and the halter simultaneously assesses the resistance (strength) on each side of the body.

Pinching and pressing down with the fingers on the withers of a normal animal result in some ventral movement (lordosis) but then resistance to the downward motion. An animal that is weak in the thoracic limbs or back may not be able to resist this pressure and bows the back more than normal and even buckles in the thoracic limbs.

These tests can help detect an asymmetric thoracic limb abnormality when performed on both sides.

In foals, other postural reactions can be performed. These are of most benefit in detecting subtle proprioceptive and motor pathway lesions when the gait is normal. "Wheelbarrowing" the patient to make it walk on just the thoracic limbs, hopping it to the left and right on each thoracic limb in turn, and hemistanding/hemiwalking the animal by making it stand and then walk sideways on both left, then both right limbs, are 3 useful postural reaction tests. Brainstem, spinal cord and peripheral nerve lesions cause postural reaction deficits on the same side as the lesions, whereas thalamic and cerebral lesions produce contralateral abnormalities.

If an adult horse has a marked gait abnormality and it is feasible to cast the animal, this should be done to assess spinal reflexes. If the patient is ambulating well, it is usual to assume that the spinal reflexes are intact. These reflexes can be studied in all foals.

Evaluating Recumbent Patients

A horse that has recently become recumbent but uses the thoracic limbs well in an attempt to get up most likely has a lesion caudal to T_2. If such an animal cannot attain a dog-sitting posture, the lesion is likely to be in the cervical spinal cord. If only the head but not the neck can be raised off the ground, there probably is a severe cranial cervical lesion. With a severe caudal cervical lesion, say in C_6, the head and neck usually can be raised off the ground, though thoracic limb effort is decreased, and the animal usually cannot maintain sternal recumbency or a dog-sitting posture. Muscular tone can be assessed by manipulating each limb. A flaccid limb with no motor activity is typical of a lesion in the lower motor neurons for that limb. Note that heavy animals that are down for a day or so frequently have poor tone and very little apparent voluntary effort in a limb that has been lain upon. A severe upper motor neuron lesion to the thoracic limbs (cranial to C_6) causes decreased or absent voluntary effort, but there is normal or, more likely, increased muscle tone in the limbs. This is because there is a release of the lower motor neuron that reflexly maintains normal muscle tone from the calming influences of the descending upper motor neuron pathways. Such spastic paralysis can be seen with lesions between C_6 and T_2 if little or no gray matter is affected. A Schiff-Sherrington phenomenon, with excessive extensor tone in the presence of good voluntary activity and normal reflexes in the thoracic limbs, has been seen a few hours following cranial thoracic fractures.

Finally, spinal reflexes are tested in the thoracic limbs. One must remember that a spinal reflex can be intact without the animal's perceiving the stimulus and showing a cerebral response. A spinal reflex requires a peripheral sensory nerve, one or a few segments of spinal cord, a peripheral motor nerve, and effector muscles to be intact. Perception (sensation) of the stimulus used for the reflex requires intact ascending sensory pathways to the forebrain. This sensation usually is seen as a cerebral (conscious) response in the form of changes in facial expression, moving the head or phonating.

The flexor reflex in the thoracic limb involves squeezing the skin of the distal limb with needle holders and observing for flexion of the fetlock, knee, elbow and shoulder. This reflex arc involves sensory fibers in the median and ulnar nerves, spinal cord segments C_6-T_2, and motor fibers in the axillary, median, musculocutaneous and ulnar nerves. Thus, if the flexor reflex is absent and this cannot be accounted for by decubital changes, the lesion likely involves the C_6-T_2 gray matter, peripheral nerves, or flexor muscles of the thoracic limbs. Conscious perception of the stimulus remains intact as long as the afferent fibers in the median and ulnar nerves, dorsal gray columns at C_6-T_2, and ascending sensory pathways in the cervical spinal cord and brainstem are intact. Lesions cranial to C_6 may release this reflex from the calming effect of the upper motor neuron pathways, resulting in an exaggerated reflex. The limb may flex rapidly and remain flexed for some time. Such lesions also may result in a crossed-extensor reflex, with synchronous extension of the opposite limb. This usually occurs only with severe upper motor neuron lesions. Thus, an animal with such a lesion may demonstrate considerable *reflex* (following stimuli) movement but usually has very little voluntary motor activity in the limbs being tested. However, foals up to about 1 month of age have prominent spinal reflexes and a crossed-extensor response.

The biceps reflex is performed by placing 2-3 fingers firmly on the biceps and brachialis muscles on the cranial aspect of the elbow joint, balloting them with a plexor, feeling for contraction of those muscles and observing for flexion of the elbow. On adult horses, the muscle bellies themselves can be percussed with a neurologic hammer or similar plexor. This reflex has its afferent and efferent pathways in the musculocutaneous nerve and involves spinal cord segments C_7 and C_8. This reflex is difficult to evoke except in small foals.

To test the triceps reflex, the relaxed limb is held slightly flexed, and the distal portion of the long head of the triceps and its tendon of insertion are ballotted with a plexor. The examiner observes and palpates for contraction of the triceps muscle, which causes extension of the elbow. The triceps reflex involves the radial nerve's afferent and efferent pathways and spinal cord segments C_7-T_1. The triceps reflex can be difficult to demonstrate in heavy adult horses. If the reflex can be elicited easily in such animals, an upper motor neuron lesion cranial to the spinal cord segments likely is involved.

All of these reflexes are prominent in neonates. The prominent crossed-extensor reflex usually slowly decreases through the first weeks of life.

By this stage of the examination, the clinician should have a clear idea of the presence and location of lesions in the brain, spinal cord cranial to T_2, and peripheral nerves and muscles of the thoracic limbs. The more peripheral the lesion, the better defined the sensory and motor deficits. Lesions of thoracic limb peripheral nerves, such as the suprascapular and radial nerves, cause characteristic gait abnormalities, paralysis of specific muscles with resulting muscle atrophy, specific reflex loss and sensory deficits. The musculocutaneous nerve is sensory to the dorsomedial surface of the metacarpal region. The ulnar nerve has autonomous sensory zones on the skin of the caudal aspect of the proximal arm distal to the olecranon, and on the skin of the lateral forearm. Finally, the skin of the medial pastern region can be used to test the integrity of the sensory fibers in the median nerve.

Evaluating the Trunk and Hind Limbs

If examination of the head, gait, neck and thoracic limbs reveals evidence of a lesion, an attempt should be made to explain any further signs found in the trunk and hind limbs caused by such a lesion. If there are only signs

in the trunk and hind limbs, then the lesion(s) must be between T_2 and S_2, and this part of the examination helps localize the lesion. The examiner must remember, however, that with a grade-1+ gait abnormality in the pelvic limbs, the lesion may be anywhere cranial to the midsacral spinal cord.

The trunk and hind limbs must be observed and palpated for malformation and asymmetry. Lesions of the thoracolumbar gray matter can cause muscle atrophy, which is a very helpful localizing sign. Marked asymmetric myelopathies often cause scoliosis of the thoracolumbar vertebral column, with the concave side opposite the lesion. Sweating over the trunk and hindlimbs is a helpful localizing sign of involvement of the descending sympathetic tracts in the spinal cord. Involvement of specific pre- or postganglionic peripheral sympathetic fibers (second- or third-order neurons) produces patchy strips of sweating. Sensation over the trunk and hind limbs should be evaluated at this stage of the examination. Degrees of hypalgesia and analgesia have been detected caudal to severe thoracolumbar spinal cord lesions.

Gentle pricking of the skin over the trunk, particularly the lateral aspects of the body wall, causes contraction of the cutaneous trunci muscle, seen as flicking of the skin over the trunk (panniculus response). The sensory stimulus travels to the spinal cord in thoracolumbar spinal nerves at the level of the site of stimulation. Impulses travel cranially to C_8-T_1, where the lower motor neuron cell bodies of the lateral thoracic nerves are stimulated, causing contraction of the cutaneous trunci. Lesions anywhere along this pathway may suppress the response. This is easiest to detect with an asymmetric lesion.

The sway reaction for the pelvic limbs involves pushing laterally against the pelvis and pulling laterally on the tail while the horse is standing and while walking, to assess the degree of resistance and to observe the resulting limb movement. Proprioceptive deficits can be observed as marked overabduction and crossing of the limbs when a step is taken to the side. An animal with weak pelvic limbs is easily pulled and pushed laterally. As with the forelimbs, but even more prominently, extensor weakness (notably lower motor neuron disease) results in little resistance to pushing or pulling the hindquarters while the horse is standing still. With a flexor weakness (notably upper motor neuron disease), the horse resists such lateral pressure at rest but is moved off stride very easily when the tail is pulled while the horse is walking. This test can help detect asymmetry in weakness and/or ataxia in the pelvic limbs.

In foals, pelvic limb hopping, "wheelbarrowing," hemistanding and hemiwalking are useful postural reactions that also yield information on cerebellar control, lower motor neurons of the pelvic limbs, the overall integrity of the proprioceptive and motor pathways to and from higher centers. Subacute to chronic lesions involving one cerebral hemisphere only, such as a hematoma or abscess, often cause an abnormal hopping response in the contralateral limbs. This is seen as a slow onset of movement with stumbling; however, there is no observable gait change. Lesions involving the proprioceptive and motor pathways to the pelvic limbs in the brainstem and spinal cord cranial to L3 cause a slow hopping response in the ipsilateral pelvic limb. Lower motor neuron lesions in one pelvic limb result in poor tone, paresis and often an extremely slow or absent hopping response in that limb.

Pinching and pressing down with the fingers on the thoracolumbar or sacral paravertebral muscle cause a normal animal to fix the thoracolumbar vertebral column and resist the ventral motion and not flex the thoracic or pelvic limbs. A weak animal usually cannot resist the pressure by fixing the vertebral column and thus overflexes the back ventrally and begins to buckle in the limbs.

Running a blunt probe along the thoracolumbar and gluteal musculature allows the examiner to evaluate how well a horse can move the thoracolumbosacral vertebrae. A weak horse often buckles in the pelvic limbs when this is done.

Evaluating Recumbent Patients

The pelvic limb spinal reflexes must be evaluated in all animals that can be restrained in lateral recumbency and in all recumbent animals. In addition, the amount of voluntary effort and muscle tone in the pelvic limbs is assessed in recumbent patients. As described for the thoracic limbs, this can be done while watching the animal in its attempt to get up or in its struggling in response to stimuli while lying in lateral recumbency. It is worth reemphasizing that the absence of voluntary movement in a limb that is flaccid and areflexic strongly suggests a lower motor neuron lesion. Asymmetry in voluntary efforts to stand and in muscle tone in the pelvic limbs helps localize a spinal cord lesion to one side or the other. However, consideration must be given to possibly exacerbating a fracture.

The patellar reflex and flexor reflex are the 2 main spinal cord reflexes involving the pelvic limbs. The patellar reflex is performed by supporting the limb in a partly flexed position, tapping the intermediate patellar ligament with a heavy neurologic hammer or a piece of iron pipe, and observing for reflex contraction of the quadriceps muscle and extension of the stifle. The sensory and motor fibers for this reflex are in the femoral nerve, and the spinal cord segments involved are predominantly L4 and L5.

The flexor reflex is performed by pinching the skin of the distal limb with needle holders and observing for flexion of the limb. As with the thoracic limbs, a stronger stimulus, as from an electric prod, may be necessary to elicit this reflex in a heavy horse that has been recumbent on a limb for some time. The stimulus can be increased slowly until a reflex response is obtained or until the patient shows obvious discomfort from the stimulus. The afferent and efferent pathways for this reflex are in the sciatic nerve and involve spinal cord segments L5-S3.

The patellar reflex is hyperactive in newborn foals, and the cranial tibial and gastrocnemius tendon reflexes are performed easily. As with the forelimbs, there are normal, strong, crossed extensor reflexes in the pelvic limbs of foals. In addition, an extensor thrust reflex is obtained, at least in very young foals, by rapidly overextending the animal's toe while the limb is already in extension. This results in forceful extension of the limb.

Sensation of the skin of the pelvic limbs must be assessed independent of reflex activity. The femoral (saphenous) nerve is sensory to the skin of the medial surface of the leg between the stifle and back, the peroneal nerve to the dorsal metatarsus, and the tibial nerve to the plantar surface of the metatarsus and the bulbs of the heels. As for the thoracic limbs, lesions of the peripheral nerves to the pelvic limbs, such as the femoral and peroneal nerves, cause specific motor deficits, though the precise sensory deficits can be difficult to define.

At this stage of the neurologic evaluation, the clinician should have a clear idea of the probable site of any brain or any spinal cord lesion resulting in an abnormal gait or recumbency.

Evaluating the Tail and Anus

This final component of the neurologic examination examines the structures innervated by nerves from the sacral and coccygeal spinal cord segments. If there is evidence of a lesion in the examination up to this point, an attempt is made to explain any abnormalities in this part of the examination by such lesions. If this cannot be done, then there must be a lesion of the sacrococcygeal spinal cord segments, spinal nerves, peripheral nerves or innervated structures.

Tail tone can be assessed just before testing the perineal reflex. A completely flaccid tail with no voluntary movement indicates a lesion of the sacrococcygeal segments or nerves. Decreased voluntary tail movements can be detected with lesions cranial to the coccygeal segments, but usually the spinal cord lesion must be severe if tail weakness is to be apparent. Some horses regarded as natural "tail wringers" flick their tails up and down and laterally while moving. Because this activity also can be observed with painful musculoskeletal disease associated with spinal cord disease, it is not a reliable neurologic finding.

The perineal reflex is elicited by lightly pricking the skin of the perineum and observing reflex contraction of the anal sphincter and flexion (clamping down) of the tail. The sensory fibers are contained within the perineal branches of the pudendal nerve (S_1-S_3). Contraction of the anal sphincter is mediated via the caudal rectal branch of the pudendal nerve, and tail flexion by the sacral and coccygeal segments and nerves (S_1-Co). An animal with a flaccid tail and anus due to a lower motor neuron lesion has no anal (or tail) reflex, though it may still have normal sensation from the anus and tail if the sensory nerves and spinal cord and brainstem white matter pathways to the sensory cortex are intact. Thus, as with all other reflex testing, the sensory perception of the stimulus must

be evaluated separately from the segmental reflex action.

It should be remembered that the spinal cord ends at about the first or second sacral vertebra. Thus, focal lesions of the last lumbar, sacral and coccygeal vertebrae may involve the cauda equina and lower motor neurons (spinal nerves) from many sacrococcygeal spinal cord segments. Depending on the level, this results in varying degrees of hypalgesia, hyporeflexia, hypotonia and muscle atrophy of the tail, anal sphincter, perineum, hips and caudal thighs. Rectal examination may detect a space-occupying lesion and fractures or luxation of the lumbar, sacral and coccygeal vertebrae. In addition, urinary bladder volume and the tone of the bladder wall and rectum should be assessed. Adult animals, especially stallions, that are recumbent for any reason often do not voluntarily urinate and, thus, usually have a distended bladder that eventually "spills over." Manipulating such animals to help them stand, or violent attempts by such animals to stand up, can rupture a bladder wall already weakened by pressure necrosis.

An animal that can walk and has non-obstructive distention of the bladder with urinary incontinence probably has a lesion of the sacral spinal cord segments or pelvic nerves. Such animals usually have excessive feces in the rectum, but usually this does not cause overt constipation unless there is a dense, diffuse, sacral lower motor neuron lesion.

Large paraplegic patients frequently bruise their perineum and tail while dog-sitting and attempting to stand. Use of tail ropes and various forms of sling support frequently causes damage to these areas. Neurologic function must be assessed as soon as possible because perineal and tail contusion result in edema, quickly followed by hypotonia, hyporeflexia and hypalgesia.

Where and What is the Lesion?

After completing the neurologic examination, the clinician should be able to localize the lesion(s) accurately within the cerebrum, brainstem, cerebellum, spinal cord, and/or peripheral nerves and muscles. In doing this, it is helpful to remember the neurologic dictum of trying to explain the signs by one or as few lesions as possible. Also, the clinician should distinguish between definitive abnormal findings, such as severe muscle atrophy and analgesia, and suspected abnormal findings, such as subtle hypalgesia in a stoic patient. To delineate the site and extent of the lesion(s) in question, only the former findings should be used. The latter findings can then be thought of as possible modifiers of a differential diagnosis and initial plan.

After localizing the lesion, possible causes can be considered. The history and physical examination results can be particularly helpful in this exercise. Following is a summary of some characteristics of pathophysiologic categories of disease.

Malformations

With malformations of the calvaria or vertebral column, neurologic signs may not become apparent until later, during growth. Malformations can be caused by infections, trauma and toxins before or after birth.

Infections

Infection by viruses, bacteria, fungi, protozoa and helminth parasites may cause neurologic disease. Characteristically, signs are progressive. They can be acute or insidious, diffuse or multifocal, and often are asymmetric. Outbreaks may occur, and remission is possible.

Trauma

Trauma usually causes sudden onset of signs that become stable within 24 hours. Secondary effects may progress later (eg, hydrocephalus, bony exostoses). Trauma can be focal or multifocal. Signs may fluctuate when there is edema present, particularly with treatment.

Toxic, Nutritional and Metabolic Diseases

These processes usually result in symmetric signs. Often there is diffuse involvement of the nervous system. Signs can fluctuate. The response to early and specific therapy can aid diagnosis, in which case the prognosis may be improved.

Vascular Disease

Vascular disease usually causes an acute onset of signs that stabilize rapidly.

Degenerative Disease

Relentlessly progressive signs characterize degenerative processes. Signs usually are symmetric.

Neoplasia

Neoplasms involving the nervous system are rare in horses. Other organ involvement may be evident. Signs can be peracute but usually are chronic and progressive.

Initial Plan of Management

At this stage, a list of differential etiologic diagnoses can be formulated, and an initial plan appropriate for the clinical circumstances can be proposed. Following consideration of the location of the lesion(s) and the differential diagnosis, an initial plan must be devised. This should include:

- *Diagnostic plan:* This includes using ancillary aids to help confirm and rule out certain disease processes.
- *Therapeutic plan*
- *Client education plan:* Included in this are economic, herd health, public health and prognostic considerations.

Ancillary Diagnostic Aids

Organ biopsy and organ function testing, as well as hematologic, microbiologic, radiographic and serologic examinations assist diagnosis and management of neurologic diseases secondary to diseases of other organ systems. Cerebrospinal fluid analysis, neuroradiographic examinations, electrodiagnostic testing, and histologic study of peripheral nerve and muscle biopsies are very useful in neurologic case management.

Cerebrospinal Fluid Analysis

The procedures for obtaining a CSF sample from the atlantooccipital and lumbosacral sites in horses have been described.[7] Samples of CSF can be obtained from the lumbosacral area in standing horses and from the atlantooccipital and lumbosacral areas in recumbent horses under general anesthesia. Samples of CSF can be obtained at either collection site from foals that are sedated or restrained in lateral recumbency.

A CSF sample can be obtained from the atlantooccipital area by needle insertion on the dorsal midline at the middle of an imaginary line drawn between the cranial borders of the wings of the atlas (Fig 4). The subarach-

Figure 4. For CSF collection from the atlantooccipital site, the horse is placed in lateral recumbency and the head is positioned 90 degrees to the median axis of the neck. The needle is inserted at the intersection of a line drawn between the cranial edges of the wings of the atlas (black circles) and the midline, indicated by the occipital protuberance (black cross). (Courtesy of *Cornell Veterinarian*)

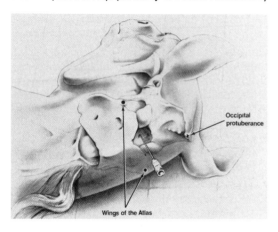

noid space is entered with a 3 1/2-inch, 18- or 20-ga spinal needle at a depth of 1/2 inch (foals) or 2 1/2 inches (adults) and is felt as a sudden loss of resistance to needle passage. A 1 1/2-inch, 19-ga disposable needle with a plastic hub is preferred for use in foals. When the subarachnoid space is entered, CSF immediately is seen in the clear hub of such a needle. A 10-ml CSF sample can be safely removed from an adult horse and 5 ml from a foal.

The area for needle insertion at the lumbosacral site is the palpable depression on the dorsal midline just caudal to the spine of L6, just cranial to the sacral spines, and between the paired tubera sacrale (Figs 5, 6). This site is about level with the highest points of the rump. A 6- to 8-inch, 18-ga spinal needle is required on large horses because the subarachnoid space is at a considerable depth. In foals, a 3 1/2-inch, 18- or 20-ga spinal needle

Figure 6. Lumbosacral CSF collection from the horse. Cranial view of the pelvis, sacrum and area of dissection (insert). In the transverse dissection through the lumbosacral articulations, the spinal needle passes through the skin, thoracolumbar fascia adjacent to the interspinous ligaments, interarcuate ligament, dorsal dura matter and arachnoid, dorsal arachnoid space and conus medullaris. The needle point is in the ventral subarachnoid space. (Courtesy of *Cornell Veterinarian*)

Figure 5. The approximate site of CSF collection from the lumbosacral site is the midpoint of a line joining the caudal borders of the tubera coxarum (black circles). The exact site is a palpable depression bordered craniad by the caudal edge of the sixth lumbar vertebra (black cross), laterad by the tubera sacrale (black squares), and caudad by the cranial edge of the first or second sacral vertebra (black triangle). (Courtesy of *Cornell Veterinarian*)

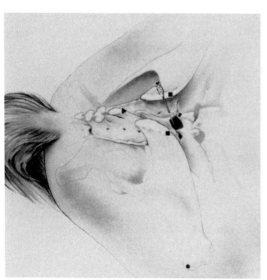

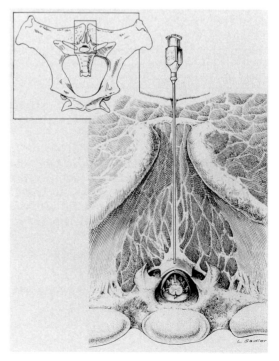

Table 2. Normal CSF values.

Opening pressure (atlanto-occipital site, recumbent)	100-500 mm H₂O
Clarity	clear
Color	colorless
RBC	0/µl
WBC	0-6 /µl
Protein (atlantooccipital or lumbosacral site), 95% confidence limits absolute range	20-85 mg/dl 5-115 mg/dl
Protein, atlantooccipital-lumbo-sacral difference	± 25 mg/dl
Refractive index	1.3347-1.3350

with fitted stylet is used. A change in resistance may be felt when this space is entered, and usually some response by the horse, such as a flick of the tail, indicates correct placement of the needle.

The WBC and RBC are counted using a hemacytometer and diluting fluid, and a differential WBC count is performed if there are >5 WBC/µl CSF. A cytocentrifuge or microfiltration technique may be used to prepare a slide of the cells for this important differential morphologic classification. These methods are not always available and, because WBC in CSF degenerate rapidly, a simple sedimentation chamber can be used (Fig 7).

One ml of CSF is placed in the chamber and allowed to stand for 25 minutes. The supernatant fluid then is aspirated off and saved for protein and other analyses. The glass cylinder is snapped off the slide, the remaining CSF is removed with bibulous paper gently applied to the center of the paraffin ring, and the wax is removed with a scalpel blade. The sample of sedimented cells then is fixed and stained with a blood-smear stain, dried, and covered with a mounting medium and cover glass. The CSF protein content should be determined using a technique that each time standardizes between 0 to 200 mg/dl. Normal values for equine CSF analysis are shown in Table 2.

Increased opening CSF pressure values are not often detected in horses. The CSF pressure can be high due to a space-occupying mass within the calvaria or from obstructed CSF flow within the vertebral canal. Excessive flexion of the neck during measurement may produce falsely elevated readings.

Normal CSF is clear and colorless. Protein contents >150 mg/dl and WBC counts >50/µl result in opacity. Several thousand RBC/µl result in pink discoloration. Xanthochromia (yellow discoloration) is caused by blood pigments or hemoglobin breakdown products in the CSF and usually indicates trauma, leakage of plasma or RBC from damaged vessels, as in vasculitis with EHV-1 myeloencephalitis. A slightly pink discoloration that disappears after centrifugation probably is due to CSF contamination with RBC at the time of collection. Preexisting subarachnoid hemorrhage rapidly results in xanthochromia from RBC breakdown.

The most important factor in determining the significance of excessive RBC in a CSF sample is assessment of the collection procedure. If the first few drops of CSF collected are pink but subsequently collected CSF is clear, the RBC likely are an artifact of collection.

Excessive numbers of WBC are seen in CSF with trauma, infections, neoplasia, and some degenerative, toxic, nutritional and metabolic diseases. Bacterial meningitis results in neutrophilic pleocytosis, whereas most viral CNS diseases produce a lymphocytic to macrocytic response. Neutrophils appear in the CSF in the early stages of EEE virus infection and acute leukoencephalomalacia (moldy corn poisoning). Mononuclear cells, particularly macrophages containing phagocytic vacuoles, are seen in CSF with processes that cause tissue damage. Eosinophils can be expected in the CSF when verminous parasites migrate through the CNS, and occasionally may be found with protozoal myeloencephalitis.

The range of protein content in normal equine CSF is 20-85 mg/dl. Occasionally a

Figure 7. CSF cytology sedimentation chamber.

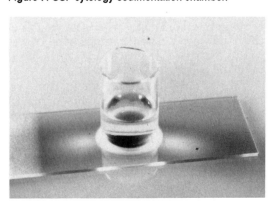

horse without CNS lesions has a CSF protein content outside (up to 110 mg/dl) this wide range (Table 2). It is, therefore, of some help to compare protein contents of CSF obtained from the atlantooccipital and lumbosacral sites. A difference of >20-25 mg/dl is good evidence of a CNS lesion. The source of protein (*ie*, the lesion) is likely closer to the site from which the sample with the higher protein content was obtained. Leakage of blood or plasma into CSF raises the protein content and occurs in traumatic, vascular, inflammatory and some degenerative diseases. Also, globulin production within the CNS can raise the CSF protein content. Usually, this is seen only in chronic infectious and possibly in some immune-mediated diseases.

Refractive index, measured with a hand-held refractometer (American Optical) is a simple measurement roughly related to protein content. A CSF sample with a protein content of ≥300 mg/dl on a urine dipstick test and with a refractive index of ≥1.3350 almost certainly has an elevated protein content.

Radiography

Plain radiography is vital to document fractures, luxation, malformations, and occasionally infections and neoplasms of the skull and vertebral column. Objective measurements of the vertebral canal diameter help determine the probability of spinal cord compression in horses with the wobbler syndrome.[8]

New radiographic contrast media have made positive-contrast myelography feasible for investigating spinal cord disease in horses. Nevertheless, this procedure is not without possible complications. Some expertise is required to perform myelography, and experience is required to interpret the myelograms. Consequently, myelography should be done in a horse only when the results of the study could alter management of the case. This does not detract from the importance and value of this procedure.

Except for some vertebral fracture repairs, vertebral column and spinal cord surgery should not proceed without myelographic confirmation of the site, extent and nature of the lesion(s). Similar comments are offered for vertebral phlebography, which has some value in identifying the cranial extent of cervical spinal cord compression.[8]

Positive-contrast cervical myelography must only be performed under general anesthesia. A technique that has worked well with few or no side effects, is as follows. A needle is positioned to collect lumbosacral CSF and left in place. A CSF sample is submitted for immediate analysis, and myelography is cancelled if evidence of inflammation is found in the CSF sample. After the horse's head and neck are elevated on a wooden plank at about 25 degrees above horizontal, a second needle is positioned in the subarachnoid space at the foramen magnum and a second CSF sample submitted for analysis. About 10-30 ml of CSF are allowed to drip from the lumbosacral site, and 40-60 ml of positive-contrast material (*eg*, iohexol, iopamidol, metrizamide) are administered over 2-5 minutes through the cervical needle, using an extension catheter and manual pressure on the syringe plunger.

Anesthesia is monitored closely, as changes in blood pressure, respiratory rate, pulse rate and even alterations in the depth of anesthesia may occur. An increased flow of CSF at the lumbosacral needle indicates flow of contrast in a caudal direction. At the conclusion of contrast medium injection, the needles are removed and the head is left elevated for a few minutes, at which time the first radiographs are made. Phenylbutazone (2 g IV) is given at the conclusion of the procedure. The horse is allowed to recover from anesthesia and is monitored closely for side effects, such as fever, depression, muscle tremor and convulsions, over the next 24-48 hours.

Electrodiagnostic Testing

Electromyelography: Needle electromyography (EMG) is a useful diagnostic test to help localize a nervous system lesion.[8] With certain gray matter lesions and peripheral nerve diseases, electromyography can provide evidence of the presence, location and extent of a lesion and is helpful in management of such cases. The procedure involves placing needle electrodes in the cranial, paravertebral and limb muscles to detect muscle fibers displaying abnormal electrical activity due to disruption of their nerve supply. With some myopathies and damage to motor neurons in the ventral gray column or in peripheral nerves that innervate muscle fibers, affected muscle fibers develop altered electrical characteristics. After about a week, these denervated muscle fibers develop spontaneous electrical discharges that include excessive insertional activity, positive sharp waves, fibrillation potentials, and bizarre high-frequency discharges. Collectively, these phenomena are termed denervation potentials. The methodology for needle electromyography is the same in all species, and interested readers are referred to other sources for details.[8]

Electroencephalography: Electroencephalography is used to record the electrical activity of the brain as a superficial montage of summated electrical potentials from the cerebrum.[9-11] Once the normal patterns are clearly understood, any abnormal electroencephalographic readings can be identified. Particular changes in electroencephalography tracings are characteristic of hydrocephalus, encephalitis and space-occupying lesions, such as melanomas, abscesses and neoplasms. The reader is referred to other sources for more information on electroencephalography.[9-11]

Several methods of electrodiagnostic testing have been adapted from human neurology for use in small animals.[9-11] Peripheral nerve conduction velocities have been determined for horses.[9-11] Also, auditory brainstem response testing is a good way to assess how intact the peripheral auditory pathways and brainstem are. When refined, these techniques, will help define the extent and nature of certain neurologic disorders.

Thermography and Scintigraphy

These techniques are useful in detecting changes in deep and, particularly, superficial blood flow. Thermographic images can be quite abnormal with myositis, muscle atrophy, and nerve and nerve root irritation and damage. Likewise, scintigraphy can detect deep space-occupying masses and inflammation of the vertebral column in particular. These techniques are discussed in more detail in the chapter on Diseases of the Musculoskeletal System.

Peripheral Nerve and Muscle Biopsy and Necropsy

The reader is referred to other sources for discussions of these procedures.[12] Necropsy technique and tissue sampling procedures are discussed later in this chapter.

DISEASES OF MULTIPLE OR UNKNOWN SITES

Diagnostic and Therapeutic Considerations

Brain-Heart Syndrome

Electrocardiographic abnormalities and myocardial damage have been associated with a variety of CNS disorders in people and experimental animals.[13] These myocardial lesions of necrosis and hemorrhage may result from sympathetic overactivity and local catecholamine release. Parasympathetic overactivity also has been implicated. Myocardial necrosis secondary to CNS disease seldom is fatal; however, it may cause cardiac arrhythmias. Several such cases have been seen in horses.[13,14]

Congenital and Familial Diseases

Hyperkalemic Periodic Paralysis

This condition is discussed in the chapter on Diseases of the Musculoskeletal System.

Diseases With Physical Causes

Lightning Strike

Following lightning storms, horses may be found dead or showing various neurologic syndromes. Scorched, vermiform skin lesions may be present as evidence of lightning strike, but usually these are absent. Two observed syndromes under these circumstances have been coma/semicoma, with epilepsy in the recovery period, and peripheral vestibular disease. It cannot be excluded that such syndromes are the result of secondary head injury (see Diseases of the Forebrain and Diseases of the Brainstem and Cranial Nerves). However, one foal surviving several weeks with vestibular disease that began during a lightning storm in which horses died had severe necrosis of the membranous and osseous labyrinth in the petrosal bone, with no evidence of fractures or sepsis.

Therapy and prognosis of such syndromes are as for head trauma.

Inflammatory, Infectious and Immune Diseases

Outbreaks of encephalomyelitis are usually caused by arboviruses (arthropod-borne viruses) belonging to the genus *Alphavirus,* family Togaviridae. Principal among these are the agents of eastern, western and Venezuelan equine encephalomyelitides.

Borna disease and Near Eastern equine encephalitis (NEEE) are enzootic infections of horses, sheep and goats of regional importance in Germany and the Middle East, respectively.[14] They are caused by similar or identical viruses, as yet unclassified. The clinical signs of infection in either of these diseases are typical of diffuse encephalomyelitis (see below) and, after a course of 1-3 weeks, most affected animals die. At least in the case of NEEE, ticks can serve as vectors for transmission of the disease to horses. Among viral encephalomyelitides of horses, these 2 are considered somewhat unusual in that the incubation periods are very long (1-6 months), inapparent infections are common in enzootic areas, and immune-mediated injury may be involved in the pathogenesis.

Less important are a variety of neurotropic arboviruses that reportedly infect horses, causing seroconversion and occasional clinical disease. These have included Semliki Forest, Russian Spring-Summer, Japanese B, St. Louis, Murray Valley and Ross River encephalitis viruses, and louping ill and Powassan viruses, all members of the family Flaviviridae.[15-20] In addition, California-group viruses and Main Drain virus are Bunyaviridae that may cause neurologic disease in horses.[21,22]

Eastern, Western and Venezuelan Encephalomyelitis

The loss of hundreds of thousands of horses to the major alphaviral encephalomyelitides (WEE, EEE, VEE) during the last 100 years has had considerable economic and social impact on the American continent. In recent years, the importance of these diseases has declined as reliance on horses for transport and agriculture has diminished. As recently as 1971, however, the threatened spread of VEE into the United States was of sufficient importance to warrant declaration of a state of emergency and mobilization of the considerable resources of the Department of Defense. These viruses not only are equine pathogens but also cause disease and even death in people.

In general, the alphaviruses are maintained in nature by incompletely defined sylvatic cycles involving mosquito vectors and bird or rodent reservoirs. Periodically these viruses spill out of their focal reservoirs and infect a wide range of vertebrate hosts, of which the horse is the most severely affected, resulting in epizootics of sometimes devastating proportions.

History and Distribution: The first well-documented cases of WEE in horses occurred in Kansas and adjacent states in 1912.[23] An unrelenting series of outbreaks began in California's San Joaquin Valley in 1931 and culminated in the summer of 1938 with the death of over 180,000 horses.[24] Isolation of the virus and development of a successful vaccine quickly followed. Major outbreaks of WEE have continued in the western and midwestern United States and have occurred in west-central Canada, Mexico and South America.[23] Infection of horses with an eastern variant of WEE (Highlands J virus) has been reported in Florida, and there is serologic evidence of this variant in horses in the Philippines.[25,26]

Eastern equine encephalomyelitis is more restricted within the United States than is WEE, though some geographic overlap of the 2 diseases does occur. Since the first putative descriptions from Massachusetts in 1831 and Long Island in 1845, there have been epizootics in all states on the eastern seaboard and Gulf Coast, and virus isolations in most states east of the Mississippi and in Texas.[23] Though the disease has become less prevalent over the last 30 years because of widespread use of vaccines and the diminishing horse population, significant death losses still occur in some states. In 1982-1983, 319 cases of EEE were diagnosed by or reported to state laboratories in Florida, representing an annual loss to the horse industry of that state at least $1 million.[27] Serious outbreaks also have occurred in eastern Canada, the Caribbean Islands and Central and South America. The EEE virus was first isolated in 1933.

Epizootic VEE virus was first isolated during an epizootic in 1938 in Venezuela.[28] Extremely severe and widespread outbreaks traditionally swept through Venezuela, Colombia, Ecuador and Peru at 6- to 10-year intervals. In 1969, an epizootic erupted on the Pacific coastal plain near the Guatemala-El Salvador border and spread to Costa Rica in 1970 and the southwest corner of Texas in 1971.[29] About 1500 horses died of VEE in Texas before further spread of the disease in the United States was halted by immunization of horses with an attenuated vaccine, resulting in an "immune belt" across the southern United States. No epizootics of VEE have been reported in the United States since the 1971 outbreak, though a focus of enzootic Type-II VEE virus exists in the Everglades region of Florida without associated equine disease (see below).

Epizootiology: Within the EEE virus complex are 2 antigenic variants, characterized as North American or South American types.[30] Three distinct antigenic groups of WEE virus have been demonstrated, with eastern (Highlands J virus), western and central antigenic strains. Considerable geographic overlap occurs.[31] Some cross-reactivity is encountered between WEE and EEE viruses when using hemagglutination inhibition and complement-fixation tests.[32] The prevalence of equine disease due to these agents depends on the size and immune status of the reservoir, vector, and amplifying and "target" (equine) hosts. In nature, WEE and EEE viruses are maintained between epizootics in reservoir hosts that probably include certain birds, rodents and reptiles.[33] Whether these viruses persist as chronic relapsing infections, by occult reservoir host-to-mosquito cycling, or by some other mechanism is not clear. However, infections persist in a variety of birds and reptiles.[23] The viruses periodically spread from rather focal reservoirs out into the general bird population, where they are propagated and amplified by rapid bird-mosquito-bird transmission. The mosquito vector for WEE is usually *Culex tarsalis*, and several species of mosquitoes, including *Culiseta melanura*, transmit EEE among birds. Many avian species become infected and develop high-order viremia and high serum titers to EEE or WEE but usually do not become ill. However, some species, including red-winged blackbirds, cardinals, sparrows, cedar waxwings and Chinese pheasants, may suffer high morbidity and mortality, particularly when infected by EEE virus.[34]

Cases of encephalomyelitis usually begin in susceptible horses 2-3 weeks after virus spreads into the bird population. *Culex tar-salis*, an omnivorous feeder, also is responsible for transferring WEE virus from bird to horse. Different vectors are required for EEE transfer, including *Aedes sollicitans, A vexans, A canadensis* and *Coquillettidia perturbans.*[23,35] The viremia of infected horses is of such low order that further infection of feeding mosquitoes is unlikely.[32] For this reason, horses are often described as "dead-end" hosts. Both EEE and WEE have been associated with naturally occurring and experimentally induced neurologic disease in calves, and EEE has been associated with clinical and experimental infections in cats, dogs, mice, foxes and pigs.[36-39]

Epizootics of EEE and WEE are rather variable with respect to area and time of onset but tend to occur in mid to late summer, when weather conditions (especially warmth and humidity) favor breeding, longevity and mobility of mosquito populations. Standing surface water for mosquito larval development, bush cover for wild hosts, and the immune status of the various hosts also affect the timing and magnitude of equine epizootics. Many of these physical factors are significantly affected by the cultivation, clearing and irrigation of land, and by drainage of swamps. The equine epizootic usually declines with the onset of cool or dry weather unsuitable for mosquito and/or bird activity, and with the depletion of susceptible equine hosts by death or development of immunity among survivors.[23]

Many other vertebrate species become infected and seroconvert during an equine epizootic but rarely with serious disease or viremia sufficient to infect feeding mosquitoes.

It is impossible to discuss VEE as a single entity because of the wide variety of subtypes and variants. The VEE complex of viruses can be separated into enzootic and epizootic groups, according to their natural history and virulence in horses.[40]

The viruses of the enzootic group, though important in the overall view of VEE, are not known pathogens of horses. They persist in focal, isolated wild rodent-mosquito cycles in South and Central America and Florida.[41] The mosquito vectors of enzootic VEE almost exclusively belong to the *Culex (Melanconion)* subgenus.[42,43] Horses living in close proximity to a focus of enzootic VEE activity usually become infected and seroconvert but do not have signs of disease. In fact, horses with serum titers to enzootic VEE virus may be protected from the virulent epizootic virus.[41]

The natural history of epizootic VEE viruses may resemble WEE and EEE in that interepizootic maintenance may depend on silent vertebrate-mosquito cycling, *ie*, possible *Culex*-rodent cycles. Persistent, chronic relapsing, or immune-tolerant infections are likewise possible mechanisms of viral persistence. The fundamental difference between VEE and the North American encephalomyelitides in the evolution of an epizootic is the role of the horse as a powerful amplifying host.[29,41] Because of the very high viremia developed by infected horses, all that is needed to sustain an epizootic once it has begun is a variety of mosquitoes and a population of susceptible horses. There is little evidence yet that birds are important in the dissemination of epizootic VEE, and most avian species are resistant to experimental infection.[41,42] Noncontiguous dispersal is a consistent feature of VEE outbreaks and may be due to movement of apparently healthy infected horses away from the disease center. Transmission by birds or other vertebrates also has been postulated, but most animals do not develop illness or sufficiently high viremia to further distribute the virus to mosquito vectors. Notable exceptions are laboratory rodents, which are extremely susceptible to experimental VEE infection.

Clinical Findings: The sequential clinical and serologic events following infection with EEE, WEE or VEE virus are similar, and differ only in detail and lethality.[23,24,32,40-42] Infected horses respond in any or all of the following ways:

- Inapparent infection with a very low-grade viremia and fever may occur about 2 days after inoculation. Mild lymphopenia and neutropenia usually are present. This sequel may be quite common and probably represents the initial viremia following viral proliferation in regional lymph nodes.
- Generalized febrile illness (up to 41 C), with anorexia, depression, tachycardia, diarrhea (in the case of VEE), and profound lymphopenia and neutropenia may be observed. This stage is associated with the relatively high-grade secondary viremia that follows viral proliferation in various body organs. Though some horses may die during the generalized form, veterinary attention is not usually sought during inapparent or generalized febrile illness.
- Clinical encephalomyelitis is the classic form of the disease. The onset is associated with the febrile crisis described above (Fig 8). The first signs usually occur about 5 days after infection, and most deaths occur 2-3 days later. Biphasic febrile episodes preceding the onset of CNS signs are commonly recorded after experimental EEE infections but are less clearly defined during VEE. Early CNS signs are quite variable and referable to diffuse or multifocal cerebral cortical disease; evidence of brain-

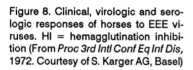
Figure 8. Clinical, virologic and serologic responses of horses to EEE viruses. HI = hemagglutination inhibition (From *Proc 3rd Intl Conf Eq Inf Dis*, 1972. Courtesy of S. Karger AG, Basel)

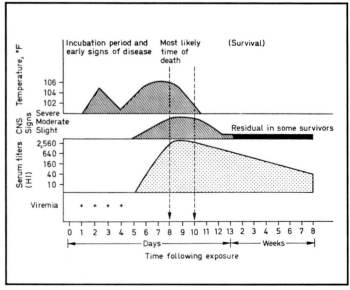

stem and spinal cord involvement becomes more obvious as the illness progresses.

Often the first thing noticed is a change in behavior. Docile animals may become irritable and even bite their handlers; other horses may seem somnolent or fail to respond to their owner's call. Self-mutilation, hyperesthesia and hyperexcitability have also been reported. Food and water usually are refused. Further signs of dementia often follow, including head-pressing, leaning against a wall or fence or compulsive walking, often in a circle (especially around the inside of a stall or small paddock). Blindness and lack of a menace response may be noted at this stage. Signs of cranial nerve disease, including nystagmus, facial paralysis and lingual and pharyngeal paresis, often occur as the disease progresses, and ataxia and paresis of the trunk and limbs result in a progressively unsteady gait.

The rapidity of deterioration and eventual outcome vary among individual horses and among the 3 diseases. Mortality ranges from 75% to 90% for EEE, 19% to 50% for WEE, and 40% to 90% for VEE.[23,29,40] Death, if it occurs, usually is preceded by a period of recumbency during which the horse may be semicomatose and convulsing. Surviving horses gradually recover over a period of weeks but may have residual signs of CNS damage, such as dullness and diminished learning capacity. Such horses are often referred to as "dummies."

Neutralizing, hemagglutination-inhibition and complement-fixation antibodies usually are present at the onset of encephalitic disease and may be present in high levels at death.

Diagnosis: Arboviral encephalomyelitides must be distinguished from other diseases characterized by diffuse cerebral disease with or without signs of brainstem involvement. The most important are hepatoencephalopathy, rabies, protozoal myeloencephalitis, verminous or bacterial meningoencephalomyelitis and leukoencephalomalacia.

A presumptive diagnosis usually is made clinically, especially in areas where these diseases are prevalent during the mosquito season. Characteristic clinicopathologic changes, including increased cell numbers (neutrophils acutely, then mainly lymphocytes) and protein in the CSF, lymphopenia and neutropenia, may contribute to antemortem diagnosis.[41,42]

Both hemagglutination-inhibition and complement-fixation antibody tests have been developed. A 4-fold rise in titer between acute and convalescent serum samples taken 7-10 days apart is considered positive, though a very high single titer in an unvaccinated animal probably is sufficient to establish a diagnosis. Results of acute and single serologic tests must be interpreted very cautiously if there is a history of vaccination against the encephalomyelitides. An enzyme-linked immunosorbent assay (ELISA) can distinguish between vaccinal (IgG only) and virulent virus-induced (IgG and IgM) titers.[44]

Fresh or frozen brain probably is the best tissue for virus isolation. The test inoculum is injected intracerebrally into mice, guinea pigs or wet chicks and produces CNS disease and death in 1-7 days if positive.[23,45] Alternatively, the inoculum is placed directly into cell cultures to test for characteristic cytopathic effects. Neutralization tests with appropriate antisera then are used to identify the virus.[23] Specific viral antigen may be demonstrated in brain tissue (especially pons and medulla) by immunofluorescent techniques.

Characteristic histologic changes in the brain are very strong supportive evidence for the diagnosis. Gross necropsy lesions usually are minimal and nonspecific (see below).

Treatment: Treatment is largely supportive. Affected horses should be placed in a shaded and well-bedded area. Free-choice water and feed should be provided. During the severe stage of the disease, intravenous fluids may be necessary to maintain hydration. An indwelling stomach tube (nasogastric or esophagotomy) may facilitate feeding of dysphagic horses. Recumbent animals should be encouraged to assume a sternal position, and any decubital lesions should be treated vigorously. Intermittent bladder catheterization and manual evacuation of the rectum may be necessary in severe cases. Some veterinarians prefer to use a sling to help the animal remain standing; however, affected horses should not be allowed to hang in the sling.

Treatment for brain edema and inflammation should be instituted in horses that are rapidly deteriorating. This includes all recumbent horses with arboviral encephalitis, as well as those becoming more deeply obtunded or having fluctuating or dilated, unresponsive pupils. A reasonable regimen in these cases is: dimethyl sulfoxide (DMSO) given IV at 1 g/kg as a 20% solution in 5% dextrose every 12 hours for up to 3 days; dexamethasone IM or IV at 0.1-0.2 mg/kg every 6 hours for 1-2 days; and flunixin meglumine IM at 0.5 mg/kg every 12 hours. Mannitol (IV at 0.25-0.5 g/kg as a 20% solution) or furosemide (IV at 0.5-1 mg/kg) also can be considered for control of suspected cerebral edema.

Convulsions can be controlled with diazepam, chloral hydrate, glycerol guaiacolate or barbiturates (pentobarbital or phenobarbital). Severe hyperthermia (40 C) may contribute to convulsions and should be treated vigorously. Antipyretic drugs (corticosteroids or nonsteroidal antiinflammatories) may be ineffective in horses with viral encephalitis; however, alcohol or cold water baths usually are helpful. Specific hyperimmune antisera are of no value in treatment because affected animals usually have high antibody titers at the onset of clinical signs.[32] Vaccination of horses in the early stage of VEE with TC-83 vaccine protects against severe diseases in some cases, possibly because of virus-induced secretion of interferon.[29]

Necropsy Findings: Gross necropsy findings are nonspecific. There is congestion of most organs and a slate-gray discoloration, often with petechial hemorrhage, of the brain and spinal cord, especially obvious on section of formalin-fixed tissue. Often there is brain swelling and evidence of occipital subtentorial herniation, with brainstem compression. Histologically there is evidence of diffuse meningoencephalomyelitis. There is predominant involvement of gray matter, with diffuse neuronal degeneration, gliosis, perivascular and neuroparenchymal infiltrates, and meningitis. Neutrophils are prominent in acute EEE and VEE lesions, whereas lymphocytes predominate in older lesions. On occasion, eosinophils may predominate in EEE. Lymphocytes usually are the primary inflammatory cell in WEE lesions. Previous therapy with potent antiinflammatory agents, particularly corticosteroids, may suppress the inflammatory-cell infiltrates, which then appear very mild.

Control: The EEE and WEE viruses probably will never be eradicated from the United States because reservoirs exist in many areas and do not depend on horse infection for their maintenance. For these reasons, continual vigilance and conscientious immunization programs always will be necessary to minimize and contain epizootics of these diseases in horses. Despite some early work with attenuated viruses, inactivated chick embryo or tissue culture origin vaccines are now used almost exclusively. Monovalent, bivalent (containing EEE and WEE), or trivalent vaccines (containing EEE, WEE, VEE) are available, and choice of the appropriate product for a particular area depends upon the prevalence or likely occurrence of the 3 diseases.

Horses should be given 2 injections 3-4 weeks apart at least a month before the anticipated risk period or before the onset of vector mosquito activity, and then revaccinated annually.[32] The optimal time for vaccination varies with latitude, rainfall and, to some extent, with altitude, ranging from January or February in Florida and Mexico to May or June in parts of Canada and the northern United States. Clinical evidence suggests <6 months of protection following vaccination against EEE or WEE, so revaccination at least once during the summer is necessary in areas with warm climates and long mosquito seasons. Foals of vaccinated mares should be given a series of 2-3 monthly vaccinations beginning at 3 months of age. Foals may be revaccinated at 12 months.[46]

General control measures aimed at reducing mosquito vector populations significantly diminish but do not eliminate the risk of equine infection. These measures include good agricultural and engineering management of cultivated land, drainage and/or insecticide treatment of mosquito-breeding areas, and application of insect repellent to horses, especially at night.[23]

Routine surveillance of the virus pool with sentinel chickens often provides early warning of an impending outbreak and allows time for vaccination of susceptible horses.

The principles of control outlined above generally apply also to epizootics of VEE; however, in marked contrast to EEE and WEE, a VEE outbreak requires quarantine of horses.[29,41] No horse should be considered free of the disease until 3 weeks after vaccination; even this assumes that vaccination is synonymous with immunization. During the 1971 outbreak, the attenuated TC-83 vaccine was used to protect horses in the United States, mainly because a large store of this vaccine had been made available by the government. The attenuated vaccine has the advantage of providing protection within 3 days of vaccination, compared with 7 days for formalin-inactivated vaccines. However, there has been concern that attenuated virus could infect mosquitoes feeding on vaccinated horses and even revert to virulence if passed sufficiently often.[29,47] The TC-83 vaccine now has been replaced by a formalinized product incorporated into a trivalent vaccine with EEE and WEE antigens.[48]

Rabies

Rabies has long been the most feared of all diseases. Though traditionally associated with mad dogs, vampire bats and hydrophobic people, rabies can affect any warmblooded animal and has been reported in horses in most parts of the world.

Cause: The disease is caused by a large neurotropic rhabdovirus. A distinctly different but related rhabdovirus known as Nigerian horse virus has been isolated from the brain of a horse that showed signs resembling those of rabies. In developed countries, the rabies virus pool is largely maintained by transmission among certain wildlife species. Susceptible domestic animals occasionally are infected by contact with sylvan hosts and then have the potential for further transmission of the disease to people and other animals.[49]

The patterns of rabies infection and disease are constantly changed by immunization programs and wildlife population shifts brought about by disease and human-related pressures. In Europe, Russia and Canada, the fox is the most important wildlife reservoir and the most likely vector of equine rabies.[50] Rabid foxes also are found in Alaska and the eastern United States. In the midwestern and southwestern states and in northern California, skunks are the most common vector.[50] The marked aggression and fearlessness shown by rabid skunks make this species especially dangerous.[51] Rabies has been enzootic among raccoons in the southeastern United States for many years. In 1979, an outbreak of raccoon rabies occurred in Virginia and Maryland and, by 1986 it had spread into southern Pennsylvania, West Virginia and the District of Columbia.[50]

In North America, the economic importance of equine rabies is negligible, with only 55 cases reported in the United States and 9 cases in Canada in 1984.[50] Out of 40,561 cases of animal rabies in Canada from 1958 to 1986, only 693 involved horses.[52] However, the disease is still a significant killer of horses (and cattle) in large areas of Central and South America, extending from northern Argentina to northern Mexico and into the Caribbean.[51] In Mexico, tens of thousands of horses died annually of rabies in the early 1960s and at least 1800 horses perished in a small area of Brazil between 1913 and 1918.[51,53] Usually the vector of these rabies epizootics was the blood-sucking vampire bat, though fruit and insect bats also can transmit the disease. Bats also carry rabies in the United States; 44 states reported rabid bats in 1984.[50]

Some measure of rabies control has been achieved in South America over the last 20 years by increased vaccination of livestock.[50,54] Also, the vampire bat population has been effectively controlled in some areas by use of intraruminal anticoagulants (*eg*, diphenadione) in exposed cattle. Continued application of these control methods will decrease the exposure of horses to rabid bats; however, the high prevalence of rabies in dogs in Central and South America is a continuing threat to other domestic animals, including horses. In 1984 alone, 9274 rabid dogs were reported in Mexico.[50]

Several countries, including Australia and New Zealand, have never recorded a case of rabies, and Great Britain, Scandinavia and much of the Caribbean and Pacific Oceania currently are free of the disease.

Pathogenesis: Rabies usually is transmitted by salivary contamination of a bite wound, though infection by inhaled, oral or transplacental routes has been demonstrated in some species.[50] The virus multiplies at the site of infection and, after a variable period of eclipse, moves centrally (centripetally) in the axons of peripheral nerves to reach the sensory or motor neurons in the gray matter of the brainstem or spinal cord.[50] Hematogenous dissemination of virus usually does not occur. Spread throughout the rest of the CNS and sympathetic chain is quite rapid and is due, in part, to multiplication and active spread of the virus in neurons and possibly also passive transport in CSF. The salivary glands usually are infected before the onset of clinical signs by "centrifugal" spread of virus from the CNS via cranial nerves.[50]

The incubation period for rabies in horses seldom has been documented but probably varies from 2 weeks to several months. Rabies virus already is widespread in the CNS by the time the first nervous signs are seen, though the most severe morphologic lesions usually are found in the brainstem or spinal cord at the point of virus entry.[50] Signs observed in horses probably depend on the age, size and immune status of the affected animal, the dose and strain of virus, and the site and source of infection.

Clinical Signs: The signs of rabies, at least terminally, are those of diffuse or multifocal CNS disease. However, even from the small amount of literature describing equine rabies, it is clear that the presenting signs and clinical course are extremely variable.[53,55-58] The reported presenting signs have included the following, singly or in combination: anorexia, depression, blindness, mania, hyperesthesia, muscle-twitching, lameness, paresis and ataxia, urinary incontinence, colic and sudden death. Whatever the presentation, the disease was rapidly progressive and resulted in death 3-10 days after the onset of signs. It is likely that antiinflammatory therapy can prolong the course of the disease. One recovery has been recorded in a presumptive case of experimentally produced rabies in a donkey.[59]

During the course of the disease, rabid horses may have predominantly encephalitic signs or signs primarily referable to spinal cord disease. This distinction is by no means absolute. Horses in the latter group often have ascending flaccid paralysis and ataxia, beginning with knuckling and crossing of one or both pelvic limbs and swaying of the hips. Often there is flaccid paralysis of the tail and anus, retention of urine and feces, and loss of spinal reflexes and sensation as the signs advance. Cutaneous hyperesthesia and self-mutilation may be observed at this stage. The thoracic limbs soon are involved, and affected horses progressively lose the ability to stand and, finally, to remain sternal. There may be no disturbance of behavior or appetite until the final stages, during which signs of encephalitis (mania, dysphagia) frequently appear. The disease transmitted by vampire bats almost invariably is this paralytic form of rabies.[53]

Horses with the encephalitic form of rabies usually manifest some early behavioral changes, such as profound depression ("dumb" rabies) or unprovoked excitement ("furious" rabies). Maniacal horses are particularly dangerous because they may ignore restraint, charge at bystanders, and bite themselves and their surroundings.[60] Other signs of brain disease, such as dysphagia, facial paresis, nystagmus and altered vocalization, often are present. Tetraparesis and ataxia appear early and progress quickly to recumbency. Horses with either form become comatose or convulse and thrash violently before dying.

Cerebrospinal fluid from rabid horses frequently is normal but may show moderate elevations in protein content and mononuclear cell numbers.[61-63]

Diagnosis: Clinical diagnosis of rabies may be difficult but should be considered in any horse showing rapidly progressive CNS signs, especially in areas where rabies is enzootic. Signs of severe gray-matter disease, such as flaccid limbs, tail paralysis, analgesia and loss of spinal reflexes, strongly suggest rabies. Consequently, this disease must be differentiated from other conditions with signs of gray-matter damage, such as neuritis of the cauda equina, EHV-1 myeloencephalitis, protozoal myeloencephalitis and sorghum-Sudan grass poisoning. The encephalitic forms of rabies may resemble arboviral encephalomyelitides, hepatoencephalopathy, brain trauma, protozoal myeloencephalitis or moldy corn poisoning. If rabies is suspected, the brain should be split in half, and one half refrigerated (but not frozen) until it can be transported to a diagnostic laboratory. The other half may be fixed in 10% formalin for later histologic examination if the tests for rabies are negative. Alternatively, the entire head can be refrigerated and submitted to the diagnostic laboratory.[64] The remainder of the carcass should be disposed of by incineration or by burial at a depth deeper than 3 feet.

Histologically, there is diffuse nonsuppurative polioencephalomyelitis, which often is surprisingly mild in horses. The hippocampus, brainstem, cerebellum and spinal cord gray matter frequently are affected, and there is often a ganglionitis, particularly of the trigeminal ganglia. Lesions consist of neuronal degeneration, gliosis and lymphocytic perivascular cuffing. Large eosinophilic cytoplasmic inclusions (Negri bodies) occur in ganglion cells and neurons. Under optimal conditions, histologic examination identified only about 85% of rabies-infected animals and, therefore, is no longer used routinely in the United States as a diagnostic aid.

Fluorescein-conjugated rabies antiserum is used to identify rabies antigen in brain tissue. The fluorescent antibody test is the most widely used test in diagnostic laboratories and identifies at least 98% of rabies-infected brains.[51] The hippocampus and cerebellum most commonly are chosen for examination. Fluorescent antibody staining of the cornea or muzzle hair follicles of suspect horses may be a useful antemortem test for rabies.[65] The results of the fluorescent antibody tests are confirmed in most laboratories by the mouse inoculation test. Homogenates of brain or salivary gland are injected intracerebrally into weanling mice. Mice developing nervous signs after the fifth postinoculation day (and before the 30th day) are killed and the brains examined for evidence of rabies.

Prevention: Horses in high-risk areas may be immunized by annual vaccination (beginning at 3 months of age) with either of 2 inactivated vaccines currently available for equine use (Rabguard-TC: Norden, Imrab: Merieux). However, a partially protected horse bitten by a rabid animal may show signs of rabies that are modified; the horse may not die but may still shed virus. Because of this public health risk factor, considerable thought should go into embarking on a rabies vaccination program for horses.

In 1981 and 1982, a neurologic syndrome consistent with clinical rabies was observed in at least 21 horses following vaccination in the neck musculature (instead of the recommended site, the thigh) with the ERA-strain, tissue culture-origin, vaccine virus.[66] Several of these horses died, while others recovered completely. Modified-live-virus vaccines no longer are recommended for use in horses.

If a previously immunized horse is bitten by a suspect rabid animal, it can be given 3 booster immunizations over 1 week and quarantined for at least 90 days. However, postexposure immunization of an animal not currently vaccinated is thought to be unsafe. Preferably, such animals should be euthanized immediately. A less desirable option, in the event that this is impossible, is confinement and close observation of the animal for 6 months, with primary immunization administered 1 month before release from quarantine.[67]

Equine Herpesvirus Myeloencephalitis

Descriptions of what probably was equine herpesvirus-1 (EHV-1) myeloencephalitis appeared in 1888.[68] However, the first definitive link between the disease and EHV-1 was not made until 1966.[69] Myeloencephalitis associated with EHV-1 infection has since been described in the United States, Canada, continental Europe, Great Britain and Australia.[68] There is no breed or sex selectivity to EHV-1 myeloencephalitis, though pregnant mares in early to midgestation may be more susceptible.[70,71] There is no report of neurologic disease in EHV-1-infected donkeys or mules, though there is evidence that infected mules were the source of a recent outbreak of myeloencephalitis among horses in southern California.[72] Suspected EHV-1 myeloencephalitis has been described in a zebra.[73] Foals may develop the disease, but it is more common in older horses. Though neurologic disease is a much less common sequel to EHV-1 infection than rhinopneumonitis, abortion or birth of weak foals, morbidity may be up to 100% among some groups of horses.[71]

Myeloencephalitis, like other diseases associated with EHV-1, is most common where there are aggregations of horses, as in racing, breeding or boarding establishments.

Clinical Signs: Signs of neurologic disease occur about 7 days after experimental EHV-1 infection by either subcutaneous or nasal routes.[70,71] Fever (up to 41.1 C), with or without a cough and serous nasal discharge, often precedes neurologic signs by several days.[71,74] Respiratory disease or abortion also may be noted among exposed horses. Rarely, pregnant mares abort immediately before, during or sometime after development of neurologic signs, depending upon the stage of pregnancy. In many cases, no antecedent disease is noticed. Horses may be either febrile or normothermic at the onset of neurologic signs.

There is a peracute onset of paresis and ataxia of the trunk and limbs. Gait abnormalities may be noticed initially in one or more limbs; typically the pelvic limbs are severely affected. Signs may be mildly asymmetric. Early involvement varies from subtle signs of clumsiness or stiffness during circling, to "dog-sitting" or recumbency. There often is urinary incontinence and bladder distention at the onset, sometimes accompanied by vulvar or penile flaccidity. Tail elevation, decreased tail tone and perineal hypalgesia are not consistent findings.

In most horses with EHV-1 myeloencephalitis, signs stabilize quickly. Many horses begin to improve within hours, though the neurologic abnormalities in severely affected animals may continue to worsen for several days. If recumbency occurs, it usually is within the first 24 hours, and paralysis may become so complete that the horse cannot lift its head from the ground. Even horses so affected usually are alert and have a good appetite. Clear-cut clinical signs of brain disease are rare, though a few cases of altered behavior or lingual, mandibular or pharyngeal paresis have been described.[74,75] Depression, when it occurs, may be due to complications of fever, secondary bronchopneumonia and recumbency rather than to primary brain disease.

Most horses with EHV-1 myeloencephalitis that remain standing recover completely. Time to recovery depends primarily upon the severity of the initial signs, and ranges from several days to >18 months.[76,77] In horses with protracted convalescence, control of urination returns before gait abnormalities disappear. Many horses that become tetraplegic with EHV-1 myeloencephalitis are euthanized, though there are reports of horses that stand again after being recumbent for several weeks. It is not clear whether any of the spontaneous deaths that occur are due to the direct effects of EHV-1 infection. It is more likely that mortality associated with EHV-1 myeloencephalitis is secondary to complications of paralysis and recumbency, such as dehydration, starvation, ruptured bladder, gastrointestinal obstruction and ulceration, injury or secondary bacterial infection.

A particularly severe form of myeloencephalitis has occurred occasionally after use of a modified-live vaccine of monkey-cell origin.[78] One report described tetraplegia in 3 horses 8-11 days after IM vaccination. The vaccine was withdrawn from the market in 1977.

Etiology and Pathogenesis: DNA "fingerprinting" techniques have confirmed the existence of 2 major subtypes of EHV-1.[68]

These subtypes are very different genetically (<20% homology between subtypes 1 and 2) and antigenically, and have divergent patterns of epizootiology, pathogenesis and clinical disease. On the basis of this genetic dissimilarity, it has been suggested that the subtypes 1 and 2 be reclassified as EHV-1 and EHV-4, respectively.[79] Subtype 2 replicates in respiratory epithelium, is responsible for most outbreaks of upper respiratory disease, and causes occasional abortions. Subtype 1 is more invasive than subtype 2, has a tropism for endothelial cells and lymphocytes, and causes neonatal mortality and myeloencephalitis, abortions, respiratory disease and diarrhea.[68,80] Additional genetic diversity within EHV-1 subtype 1 may partially explain the diverse clinical manifestations of infection with this subtype.[68]

Equine herpesvirus-1, like other herpesviruses, can spread between contiguous cells without an extracellular phase. Therefore, even in the presence of neutralizing antibodies, endothelial cells in the CNS may be infected by contact with virus-bearing leukocytes. It has not yet been determined whether EHV-1 myeloencephalitis is due to direct effects of the virus or to secondary immune-mediated damage. In support of the latter possibility, the lesions of EHV-1 myeloencephalitis are indistinguishable from those induced in experimental animals as a result of an immune-mediated Arthus reaction.[68] Thus, vasculitis in the CNS of infected horses may be due to an immunologic reaction to EHV-1 antigen expressed on the surface of infected endothelial cells.[68]

Diagnosis: A presumptive diagnosis of EHV-1 myeloencephalitis can be made in horses showing both characteristic clinical signs and evidence of active EHV-1 infection. This requires either isolation of the virus from nasopharyngeal swabs and blood buffy coats or demonstration of a 4-fold rise in serum-neutralizing or complement-fixing antibody titers between acute and convalescent serum samples taken 7-10 days apart.[68] Because of the antigenic differences between EHV-1 subtypes, there may be a potential for false-negative results if the reagents and/or viruses used for measuring titers do not include both subtypes.[68]

Because of the association between subtype 1 and neurologic disease, it is important for prognostic reasons to establish early in the course of outbreaks of respiratory disease which of the 2 subtypes of EHV-1 is involved. Monoclonal antibodies that distinguish between EHV-1 subtypes now are available to diagnostic laboratories.[68]

Useful supporting evidence for a diagnosis of EHV-1 myeloencephalitis is finding xanthochromia and marked elevation of protein content (100-500 mg/dl) in samples of CSF. Cell numbers usually are normal.[70] Attempts to isolate the virus from CSF have been unsuccessful. The serum-neutralizing titers in CSF have not been consistently elevated in EHV-1 myeloencephalitis.

Necropsy Findings: A brownish, patchy discoloration may be seen grossly on fresh and fixed sections of brain and especially the spinal cord. These are seen histologically as areas of ischemic and hemorrhagic infarction, with perivascular edema and necrosis of parenchyma. They often are present in a radiating pattern around blood vessels. Such vessels, especially arterioles, often have swelling and hyaline necrosis of the intima and a few mononuclear inflammatory cells within their walls. Perivascular cuffs of lymphocytes, plasma cells and macrophages occur in meninges and parenchyma. Groups of such inflammatory cells associated with neuronal necrosis occur in the trigeminal and sometimes in other ganglia. Lesions consistent with EHV-1 infection, and even intranuclear inclusions, may occur in other areas, such as the respiratory tract, thyroid gland and fetus.

Though the virus has been isolated from the brain or spinal cord of some horses with the characteristic histologic findings of EHV-1 myeloencephalitis, attempts at viral isolation often are unsuccessful.[81] Likewise, isolation of virus from other tissues (except the fetus in pregnant mares) may be difficult in some cases due to the high serum-neutralizing titer at the time of death.

Treatment: Because of the contagious and sometimes devastating nature of all EHV-1-associated syndromes, any horse with suspected EHV-1 infection should be isolated until the diagnosis is ruled out. Most horses with EHV-1 myeloencephalitis can recover if given adequate supportive treatment. The onset of recumbency is no reason for hasty euthanasia. Recumbent horses should be bedded well and encouraged to remain sternal if possible. In moderately affected horses, an abdominal sling may avoid complications of prolonged recumbency. Food and water may have to be fed by hand or via a nasogastric tube. Horses in lateral recumbency must be rolled to the opposite side often to help prevent decubital sores. Administration of laxatives or enemas or manual emptying of the rectum may be necessary. Secondary bacterial infections of the urinary or respiratory tract must be treated vigorously.

Repeated bladder catheterization is unwise, as it may introduce infection; urinary incontinence is seldom a limiting problem. However, recumbent horses with a distended urinary bladder can develop cystitis that can rapidly lead to bladder wall necrosis and septicemia. Consequently, horses should be catheterized judiciously, given assistance to stand and posture for urination, and given appropriate antimicrobial therapy when necessary.

In view of the probable immune-mediated vasculitis, glucocorticoids may be helpful, especially early in the disease. Dexamethasone (or equivalent) may be given at 0.1-0.2 mg/kg every 6 hours the first day and up to several days thereafter, depending upon the response to initial treatment.

It should be remembered that horses that have recovered from clinical EHV-1 infection may remain latently infected, and viral recrudescence and shedding may occur after immunosuppression, as with exogenous corticosteroids or stress.[82]

Prophylaxis: Modified-live and inactivated adjuvant-containing EHV-1 vaccines are available commercially. The efficacy of these vaccines in preventing EHV-1 myeloencephalitis has not been evaluated critically. In a small trial with an inactivated vaccine (Pneumabort-K: Fort Dodge), none of 11 vaccinated pregnant mares developed neurologic disease after EHV-1 infection, whereas 2 of 6 unvaccinated mares developed paresis.[83] However, there is some clinical evidence that prior vaccination does not confer protection against this disease and, in some instances, may actually increase the risk of neurologic disease.[72] If the lesions of EHV-1 myeloencephalitis are immune-mediated, it would be reasonable to assume that vaccination of infected horses could worsen the disease. Therefore, EHV-1 vaccines should not be used in horses already showing signs of EHV-1 myeloencephalitis.

Equine Infectious Anemia

Neuropathologic changes may occur during the course of equine infectious anemia (EIA) infection. These lesions include diffuse or multifocal nonpurulent ependymitis, choroiditis and leptomeningitis. A variety of neurologic signs may be associated with such lesions.[84-86] The most common finding is symmetric ataxia of the trunk and limbs. Occasionally no other clinical and hematologic signs of EIA are present.[86] One mare with EIA had behavioral changes, circling and gait alterations.[84] At necropsy, hydrocephalus was found in addition to the above changes. Cerebrospinal fluid analysis of horses with ataxia due to EIA shows elevated protein content and lymphocytic pleocytosis.

Listeriosis

Clinical disease due to *Listeria monocytogenes* infection seldom has been documented in horses and must be regarded as very rare. When it does occur, listeriosis is manifested as meningoencephalomyelitis, abortion or rapidly fatal septicemia.[87] The latter usually occurs in foals but also has been reported in a herd of mature ponies.[88] In some cases in horses and other livestock, infection has been linked to ingestion of improperly prepared corn silage.[88,89] Immunosuppressed animals are said to be more susceptible to infection by *L monocytogenes*.[90] One report described fatal listeric septicemia in an Arabian foal with combined immunodeficiency.[87] A neurologic form of equine listeriosis that resembled the disease seen in ruminants, with signs primarily referable to brainstem and cauda equina involvement, has been seen.[91] Cerebrospinal fluid analyses in equine cases have not been reported, but elevated protein levels and mononuclear pleocytosis are likely. Blood cultures for *L monocytogenes* may be positive in either form of the disease. Treatment with high levels of potassium penicillin G (50,000 units/kg QID IV) or sodium ampicillin (25 mg/kg QID IV) should be effective if used early in the course of disease. This antibiotic regimen should be continued for at least 7 days and may be followed by an additional 7 days' treatment with IM procaine penicillin G (22,000 units/kg BID) or sodium ampicillin (25 mg/kg QID).

Bacterial Meningoencephalomyelitis

Leptomeningitis (inflammation of the arachnoid and pia mater) occurs as a component of many diffuse, infectious CNS diseases, such as viral and verminous encephalomyelitides. Occult chemical meningitis routinely follows contrast myelography with metrizamide and other contrast solutions. Clinically recognizable meningitis, however, usually is caused by bacteria that spread hematogenously to the meninges, by direct extension of suppurative processes in or around the head (including brain abscesses), or as a result of penetrating wounds of the skull.

The profound neurologic deficits often associated with septic meningitis are a reflection of the diffuse involvement of the superficial parenchyma and nerve roots of the brain and spinal cord. Development of CNS edema or secondary hypertensive obstructive hydrocephalus may complicate the clinical picture further.

Bacterial meningitis most often is seen as a complication of sepsis in neonatal foals. Therefore, the predisposing causes of meningitis are the same as those for other septic conditions of foals, such as maternal uterine infections, early placental separation, unhygienic conditions (*eg,* in the foaling barn), failure of passive transfer of maternal immunoglobulins, and adverse environmental conditions (including extremes of temperature and humidity). The bacteria involved are those most commonly causing neonatal septicemia.[92] Beta-hemolytic streptococci, *Actinobacillus equuli, Escherichia coli* and, more rarely, *Klebsiella pneumoniae* and coagulase-positive staphylococci are likely causes of meningitis during the first month of life. Meningitis caused by *Salmonella* spp, especially *S typhimurium,* occurs more frequently in older foals. In adult horses, sporadic cases of meningitis have been associated with *Streptococcus equi* and *Actinomyces* spp infections.[93,94]

In foals, the prodromal bacteremic phase of meningitis is characterized by fever, lethargy and lack of affinity for the mare. Early meningeal involvement may be suggested by behavioral changes, such as aimless walking, depression and abnormal vocalization ("wanderer," "dummy" and "barker," respectively). Initially there is cutaneous hyperesthesia, muscular rigidity and tremors. Pain often is manifested by trismus and reluctance to move the head or neck. Signs progress rapidly, leading to blindness, loss of the suckling reflex, multiple cranial nerve abnormalities, ataxia and paresis of the limbs. Hyperesthesia is followed by diffusely diminished sensation and reduced spinal reflexes. If the foal is left untreated, recumbency, coma, seizures and death quickly occur.

Bacterial meningitis in foals is an emergency and requires rapid and meticulous management, so early diagnosis is essential. The diagnosis is confirmed by finding bacteria, increased numbers of inflammatory cells (especially neutrophils), and high protein and low glucose concentrations in CSF. Aggressive efforts should be made to identify the causative organism. All accessible sites of sepsis should be sampled and cultured, both aerobically and anaerobically. At a minimum, CSF and blood must be cultured and a CSF sediment Gram-stained. Antimicrobial therapy for bacterial meningitis should be guided initially by CSF Gram stain results and subsequently by bacterial culture and antimicrobial sensitivity tests. If these data are not available, large doses of broad-spectrum antimicrobial or antimicrobial combinations are required (Table 3).

Obviously, antimicrobials for this purpose must reach useful levels in the CSF. Aminoglycosides and penicillins only poorly cross the normal blood-CSF barrier; however, meningeal inflammation considerably improves penetration of these drugs to the CSF.[95] Also, because of the low toxicity of penicillins (but not aminoglycosides), good CSF levels generally can be achieved with large doses of penicillins systemically. Chloramphenicol freely crosses the blood-CSF barrier but has the theoretical disadvantage of bacteriostatic rather than bactericidal action.

Excellent CSF levels of sulfamethoxazole-trimethoprim can be achieved after parenteral administration.[96] Because of their broad antimicrobial activity, potentiated sulfa drugs should be useful as a first treatment of foals with bacterial meningitis when the causative organism is unknown. Neonatal foals may be particularly susceptible to the antifolate actions of sulfa drugs, so it is prudent to give 3 mg of folinic acid (Leucovorin: Lederle) IM twice weekly during sulfa-trimethoprim treatment and for 1 week thereafter to help prevent bone marrow suppression.

Moxalactam and cefotaxime, 2 of the newer third-generation cephalosporins, offer dual advantages of a broad spectrum of action and a high CSF:blood concentration ratio.[97] As these drugs become available to the equine practitioner, they may become the antimicrobials of choice for treatment of Gram-negative meningitis.

A guide to antimicrobial therapy for bacterial meningitis in foals is offered in Table 3. Antimicrobial therapy should be continued for at least 14 days and at least 7 days after resolution of clinical signs.

Gram Stain	Antimicrobial	Dose (/kg)	Interval (hr)
not available	potassium penicillin	50,000 units	6
	or sodium ampicillin	50 mg	6
	sulfa-trimethoprim[1]	25 mg	12
	plus		
	gentamicin sulfate	2.2 mg	8
	or amikacin sulfate	7 mg	8
Gram-pos cocci	potassium penicillin G	50,000 units	6
Gram-neg rods	sodium ampicillin	50 mg	6
	sulfa-trimethoprim[1]	25 mg	12
	gentamicin sulfate	2.2 mg	8
	amikacin sulfate	7 mg	8
	chloramphenicol succinate[2]	25 mg	6

Table 3. Suggested initial antimicrobial therapy for bacterial meningitis in foals.

1 — Supplement foal with folinic acid as described in text.

2 — Should not be combined with aminoglycosides.

Supportive treatment is important and aimed at avoiding or correcting dehydration with oral or intravenous fluids, and treating severe hyperthermia with alcohol baths, fans and cold water enemas. Metabolic derangements, such as azotemia, hyponatremia (<120 mEq Na/L), hyposmolality (<260 mOsm/L), and hypoglycemia (<50 mg/dl), often are present and can exacerbate nervous signs. Such disorders should be identified and corrected. Mild seizures may be controlled by manual restraint. For more severe seizures, a test dose of 5-10 mg diazepam should be given IV and repeated as necessary. Intractable seizures may necessitate sedative to anesthetic doses of chloral hydrate or barbiturate.

In rapidly deteriorating, blind, recumbent or convulsing foals with meningitis, DMSO (1 g/kg given IV as a 20% solution in 5% dextrose) and/or corticosteroids (dexamethasone 0.2-0.5 mg/kg or equivalent) should be given. Rapidly progressive signs often are caused by severe brain edema or obstructive hydrocephalus, which can be fatal unless treated aggressively.

The prognosis for foals with bacterial meningitis is guarded to poor. Even with appropriate treatment, >50% of affected foals die.

Cryptococcosis

Cryptococcal meningoencephalomyelitis is caused by the encapsulated yeast-like fungus *Cryptococcus neoformans,* a saprophyte found commonly in soil and feces, especially in the feces of pigeons and chickens.[98] Several extraneural infections have been recorded in horses, including myxomatous lesions of the lips, nasal cavity, paranasal sinuses, orbits, intestine and lungs.[99] Meningeal localization likely occurs after hematogenous or direct spread from a benign or clinical focus in the respiratory tract. Signs of cryptococcal meningoencephalomyelitis may be acute or insidious in onset but usually progress rather slowly.[99-101] The clinical picture is typical of diffuse meningitis, with dementia, blindness, dysphagia, initial hyperesthesia and rigidity, with progression to ataxia, weakness, recumbency, convulsions, coma and death. An unusual case involved signs localized to spinal cord gray matter, including gluteal muscle atrophy, pelvic limb gait abnormalities, atony, areflexia of the tail and anus, and

perineal hypalgesia. This was due to involvement of the cauda equina and lumbosacral nerve roots and dura.[1]

Antemortem diagnosis is by finding the encapsulated organism in an India ink preparation or routine laboratory stain of CSF sediment, by positive culture on most routine laboratory media, or by a positive latex-agglutination test for cryptococcal antigen in the CSF.[98,103] Clinical evidence of a primary cryptococcal infection should be sought, including culture and India ink preparations of any nasal or tracheal exudates.

Histologically, the characteristic budding, yeast-like organisms are readily found in the meninges, around vessels in the brain parenchyma, or within cavitary lesions in the brain or spinal cord. The cellular reaction to cryptococcal organisms is predominantly mononuclear, characterized by lymphocytes and giant cells.

In people, the disease is treated effectively by combined systemic and intrathecal use of antifungal agents, such as amphotericin B and flucytosine, alone or in combination, for a minimum of 6-10 weeks.[104] A suggested but unproven regimen for a 450-kg horse is 100-150 mg amphotericin B in 4 L of 5% dextrose on alternate days for at least 6 weeks, plus 5-15 mg amphotericin B intrathecally, under anesthesia, once weekly for at least the first 4 weeks.[101] Possible side effects of treatments with amphotericin B are systemic nephrotoxicity and topical neurotoxicity.

Equine Protozoal Myeloencephalitis

Segmental myelitis was identified in Kentucky horses in 1964. In 1970, a study of 52 cases of focal myelitis/encephalitis was reported. Since that time, the same clinical syndromes have been called toxoplasmosis-like encephalomyelitis and protozoan encephalomyelitis. Until the causative agent(s) is identified, it is presumed that all of these disease entities are one, known as equine protozoal myeloencephalitis (EPM).[105]

Equine protozoal myeloencephalitis apparently is confined to horses that have spent time in the Americas. Most cases in the United States have occurred east of the Rocky Mountains; however, in 1984, the disease was documented in 3 horses that had never left California.[106] The same clinical and pathologic syndrome occurs in Brazil, and cases have been seen in the United Kingdom, the latter only occurring in horses transported from North America several months before the onset of signs.[107,108] Many breeds, particularly Standardbreds and Thoroughbreds, are affected at racetracks or at breeding establishments; pleasure horses and ponies appear to be affected less frequently. There is no report of EPM affecting donkeys or mules. Horses of all ages may be affected but most often are 1-6 years old at the onset of signs. More cases occur in the spring and summer than at other times of the year.

Though EPM must be regarded as an infectious disease, it apparently is not contagious from horse to horse. Because the disease occurs in clusters in certain areas and even on single farms over a period of several years, there may be a common source of environmental or animal exposure. Two full-sibling Quarter Horses have been affected within 1 month of each other.[109]

Causes: The putative agent of EPM is a coccidian parasite. Morphologically, the EPM organism is distinct from *Klossiella,* a coccidian found in the kidneys of horses. Both the location of the organism in the host cell and its staining characteristics help differentiate it from *Toxoplasma gondii* and associate it with the genus *Sarcocystis.*[110] Also, serum antibodies specific for *Sarcocystis* spp but not for *Toxoplasma gondii,* are found at a higher rate in horses with EPM than in normal horses.[111] However, the particular species associated with EPM as well as its life cycle and natural history remain unknown, and attempts to reproduce the disease by oral inoculation with a variety of species of *Sarcocystis* have been unsuccessful.[111]

Clinical Signs: The onset of signs is often peracute or acute. Affected horses may stumble and fall during racing or training, with no premonitory signs. Gait abnormalities that are usually interpreted as lameness often are seen early in the course of disease. Ataxia, weakness, recumbency, muscle atrophy and occasionally behavioral changes are other primary signs reported. The neurologic abnormalities are progressive, and almost all infected horses develop various degrees of ataxia, weakness and spasticity in one or more limbs. These signs reflect brainstem or spinal cord involvement. Signs can be symmetric in all limbs, with no evidence of gray-matter lesions; horses with such signs have been called wobblers. However, markedly

asymmetric signs with evidence of gray-matter involvement and multifocal lesion sites frequently become evident. Such signs include sensory deficits, focal sweating, monoplegia (single-limb paralysis), muscle atrophy, reflex loss and cranial nerve dysfunction. These signs are regarded as hallmarks of the disease, especially with evidence of multifocal lesions (Figs 9-11).

Diagnosis: There is no definitive antemortem diagnostic aid. A positive response to antiprotozoal therapy, as described below, is presumptive evidence of EPM. Hematologic, serum biochemical, serologic and radiographic examinations are useful insofar as other diseases may be ruled out. Results of CSF analysis in horses with EPM often are

Figure 9. Left aspect of the head of a 5-year-old Thoroughbred gelding with masseter muscle atrophy. This horse also had atrophy of the temporalis and distal digastricus muscles on the left side. These lesions were the result of an equine protozoal myelitis (EPM) lesion in the motor nucleus of the trigeminal nerve in the brainstem. In addition, the horse had progressive ataxia, atrophy of the right half of the tongue and atrophy of the right gluteal musculature. These additional signs were explained by other focal EPM lesions involving the hypoglossal nucleus, and the gray and white matter of the spinal cord at L_4-S_3.

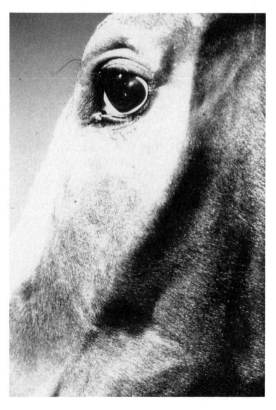

Figure 10. This yearling Standardbred filly had paraparesis worse in the right hind limb than in the left. There was profound weakness in the right hind limb, with constant knuckling of the fetlock and sinking of the pelvis as shown. A decreased panniculus response and depressed sensory perception were evident in the caudal lumbar region. When the animal was recumbent, the patellar reflex was poor in the left limb and almost absent in the right. These signs were caused by an equine protozoal myelitis lesion involving the gray and white matter from L_2 to L_5. The lesion was more severe on the right side.

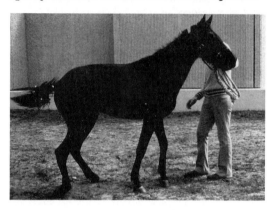

normal; however, abnormal CSF may be found in some horses with large, active lesions. The CSF alterations found include slight to moderate xanthochromia, a few hundred to a few thousand RBC, and up to 100 WBC/μl CSF. Mononuclear cells predominate, but neutrophils are also seen. The protein content is less frequently elevated and usually is not above 150 mg/dl.

Treatment and Prognosis: Treatment is based upon use of antiprotozoal drugs that act by inhibiting folic acid synthesis. These drugs are used routinely in treatment of toxoplasmosis in people. The regimen currently used at the University of Florida is pyrimethamine given at 0.25 mg/kg once daily, in combination with trimethoprim-sulfadiazine (Tribrissen: Coopers) given PO at 15 mg/kg BID. Usually this regimen is continued for 4-6 weeks, then the horse's neurologic status is reevaluated carefully. If there is clinical improvement during this period, or even if previously deteriorating signs are arrested, the presumptive diagnosis is EPM, and antiprotozoal therapy may be maintained for an additional 1-6 months.

Mostly for economic reasons, with this prolonged maintenance therapy, the drugs are given once weekly, with pyrimethamine at 1 mg/kg and trimethoprim-sulfadiazine at 20 mg/kg. Without an objective diagnostic indicator to use as a guide, the decision to discontinue treatment usually is rather arbitrary. To decrease the chance of later relapses, treatment should be reinstituted before and during stressful episodes (*eg,* long-distance transport). This protocol has led to marked improvement of clinical signs in many cases. Some *apparently* complete cures have been seen.

Chronic treatment with folic acid inhibitors can cause bone marrow suppression, with neutropenia, anemia and thrombocytopenia. Fetuses and young animals appear to be particularly susceptible to the toxic effects of these drugs. Therefore, appropriate client education is important if pregnant mares are to be treated. All treated horses should be monitored with WBC counts every 2-4 weeks, and antiprotozoal therapy must be reduced or discontinued if leukopenia develops. Folinic acid (Leucovorin: Lederle) should be given twice weekly (3-10 mg IM) until the WBC count returns to normal.

In severely affected horses with acutely progressive neurologic signs, drugs that decrease inflammation and edema should be

Figure 11. Cranial to caudal view of the back and rump of a 3-year-old Thoroughbred gelding with equine protozoal myelitis. Note the profound atrophy of the left gluteal and caudal longissimus lumborum musculature. Muscular atrophy was due to protozoal myelitis lesions in the gray matter at T_{18}-L_1 and at L_5-L_6 on the left side. The horse also had progressive tetraparesis and asymmetric ataxia. A separate lesion involving gray and white matter at C_1-C_6 accounted for the forelimb signs and probably the hyporeflexia and mild muscle atrophy of the caudal neck region on the right side.

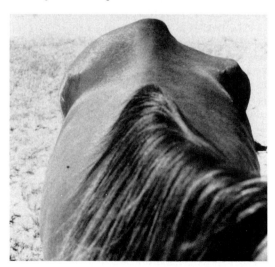

given as needed until signs stabilize. Dimethyl sulfoxide may be administered once daily at 1 g/kg given slowly IV in 3-4 L of 5% dextrose. Dexamethasone given 1-4 times over 24 hours at 0.1-0.2 mg/kg also may be helpful in the short term, though prolonged corticosteroid use may favor protozoal proliferation and further CNS damage.

Necropsy Findings: Gross swelling, discoloration and softening are detected in fresh tissue when a lesion is sectioned. Histologically, the inflammatory lesions consist of prominent lymphoid perivascular cuffing and contain many macrophages, often eosinophils, and occasionally multinucleate giant cells. Large necrotic areas with hemorrhage are present in acute and severe lesions, and astroglial scars occur with chronic lesions. Associated nonsuppurative meningitis is variably present. Consistent with the neurologic signs, lesions often are multifocal within the spinal cord, brainstem, and sometimes the cerebrum and cerebellum. Asymmetry and involvement of gray and white matter also are characteristic. The organisms are seen singly and in groups, free in the tissue but most often within macrophages. Organisms have been seen in neurons, eosinophils, and even within cell nuclei. However, protozoa usually are not seen in CNS lesions of horses treated with antiprotozoal agents as described above. Even when the putative agent is not observed, EPM should be suspected when typical lesions can be defined; such cases are designated EPM (-) in comparison to those in which the organisms are seen, which are designated EPM (+).

In summary, EPM is a relatively frequent cause of progressive spinal cord and brainstem disease in light-breed horses in eastern North America. It can be diagnosed clinically with considerable certainty in many cases and is a potentially treatable disease. The causative agent is closely related to *Sarcocystis* spp, but the life cycle must be defined and an accurate antemortem diagnostic test developed before therapeutic and preventive measures can be fully evaluated.

Verminous Meningoencephalomyelitis

Verminous meningoencephalomyelitis is caused by the meanderings of one or more parasites through the CNS and is, therefore, an extremely variable clinical entity. Depending upon the number, size and location of the parasites and the duration of their migration through the brain or spinal cord, a spectrum of signs is possible, ranging from a nonprogressive localizing neurologic deficit to rapidly fatal, diffuse encephalitis. Verminous meningoencephalomyelitis usually occurs sporadically and has been associated with strongyloid (*Strongylus vulgaris*), filariid (*Setaria* spp), rhabditid (*Halicephalobus deletrix*) and spiruroid (*Draschia megastoma*) nematodes, as well as warble fly larvae (*Hypoderma* spp).[112]

Meningoencephalomyelitis due to *S vulgaris* is a sequel to the aberrant intimal or subintimal migration of fourth-stage larvae to the aorta, left ventricular endocardium, and brachiocephalic, carotid or vertebral arteries. From verminous thrombi at these sites, larvae can be carried by the circulation to any part of the brain or spinal cord to continue migration and development.[113]

Disintegration of a verminous thrombus occasionally results in massive embolic showering, which causes infarction and edema, particularly of the ipsilateral forebrain. Clinical signs are acute in onset in this situation, and progression depends upon further disposition of the nematode(s) that may die or migrate out of the CNS, leaving only residual neurologic impairment. More often, however, the signs progress as further migration occurs. Two reports, one in a horse and one in a donkey, describe migration of *S vulgaris* larvae through almost the entire length of the spinal cord, causing progressive severe limb paralysis and recumbency.[114,115] A series of 6 fatal cases involved clinical courses from 3 hours to 22 days and a variety of neurologic signs that included one to several of the following: depression, limb paresis, ataxia, cranial nerve abnormalities, convulsions and recumbency.[114] Larval migration through the brainstem or cerebellum is likely to cause more severe and progressive signs than is migration through the forebrain. However, massive embolic showering of the cerebrum may cause peracute recumbency, followed by signs of diffuse forebrain disease, such as blindness, circling, head-pressing and dysphagia.

A definitive diagnosis of *S vulgaris* meningoencephalomyelitis usually is made only at necropsy but should be suspected antemortem in any case of acute CNS disease with signs referable to a single lesion, or in any diffuse cerebral syndrome with no history of trauma or intracarotid injection. Changes in CSF are not specific or consistent, but some hemorrhage into the CSF and increased numbers of inflammatory cells, including eosinophils and neutrophils, are expected. Marked CSF xanthochromia and elevated protein concentration accompany the cerebral infarction syndrome.

No data on therapy are available, but treatment of suspected affected horses (with 2 daily treatments of thiabendazole at 440 mg/kg body weight or fenbendazole at 60 mg/kg given once) is justified. Use of anti-inflammatory drugs, such as phenylbutazone at 4.4 mg/kg BID and/or dexamethasone at 0.1-0.25 mg/kg body weight every 6 hours, should begin during the acute phase of the disease. Though ivermectin at 0.2 mg/kg is an effective anthelmintic, parasite killing is delayed because of the drug's GABA-inhibiting method of destroying parasites, so it may not be the drug of choice.

Intracranial myiasis by *Hypoderma* spp in horses was first described in England in 1842 and has since been reported in Europe and the United States.[116,117] The horse is not a normal host for *Hypoderma* (the cattle grub or warble), as successful pupation seldom occurs following tissue migration. Aberrant migration of first-instar larvae occurs through natural skeletal foramina. Fly larvae thus enter the caudal fossa (containing the pons, medulla oblongata and cerebellum) or, less often, the middle and rostral fossae (containing the cerebrum, thalamus and midbrain). Penetration of the cervical spinal cord is very rare. Because of the large size of these larvae, clinical signs of *Hypoderma* migration usually are characterized by sudden onset, a short fulminant course, and death within a week. One such affected horse had severe depression, a dilated left pupil, lingual paresis, left-sided facial paralysis and ataxia and paresis of the left limbs.[116] These signs were caused by extensive migration of a 12.5 x 2-mm *H lineatum* larva through the left side of the brainstem caudally from the region of the oculomotor nucleus.

The diagnostic difficulties described for *S vulgaris* encephalitis apply equally here, but the disease should be considered in areas where cutaneous myiasis by *Hypoderma* is common. If used very early in the course of the disease, treatment of affected horses with organophosphates (*eg*, trichlorfon PO at 40 mg/kg, repeated in 1-3 days; crufomate pour-

on at 75 mg/kg; ronnel PO at 100 mg/kg) may be effective. The possibility of adverse reactions to these systemic insecticides must be considered carefully. In cattle, acute lumbar paralysis may follow such treatment because of destruction of the larvae in the vertebral canal.[118] Antiinflammatory therapy is indicated (see above). The comments offered above regarding ivermectin therapy apply equally here.

Since the first description in 1965, there have been at least 13 reports of *Halicephalobus deletrix* (also known as *Micronema deletrix*) infection of horses in the United States and many other countries.[119] In each instance, there was invasion of cranial tissues. The parasites were found in the brain of 10 horses, in the nasal soft tissues and maxillae of 2 horses, and in the gingiva of another. Seven horses with brain involvement also had renal lesions. Regardless of the tissue involved, the characteristic response to invasion by this parasite was granulomatous inflammation.

Halicephalobus deletrix is a tiny (250-350 μ) rhabditid nematode closely related to several saprophytic species. The natural history of the nematode is not well known, but it is generally thought to be a facultative parasite. Massive invasion of most or all of the brain by hundreds of *H deletrix* adults results in acute signs of diffuse encephalitis, including severe dementia, blindness and incoordination progressing to recumbency, coma and death after a short course. In one unusual case, neurologic disease was preceded by polydipsia and cystitis.[120] Though CSF sampling was not performed in the reported cases, it is reasonable to expect marked pleocytosis with some eosinophils and even larvae or larval fragments in the CSF. All stages of the *H deletrix* life cycle, including gravid females, larvae and ova, may be found in the brain, especially in the Virchow-Robin spaces surrounded by a predominantly mononuclear and giant-cell reaction. The disease is important because of its antemortem similarity to the viral encephalitides; however, the histologic findings at necropsy are diagnostic.

Central nervous system diseases caused by *Setaria* spp are known by a variety of names (*eg*, Kumri and enzootic cerebrospinal nematodiasis) throughout the Orient, India and Sri Lanka and cause significant losses to the horse industry in these countries.[121] Aberrant migration of one or more immature *Se-*

taria nematodes through the brain or spinal cord causes signs indistinguishable from those described above for *S vulgaris* migration. This disease is seasonal in occurrence, corresponding with fly vector activity. In Japan, mosquitoes carry *Setaria digitata* microfilariae from the natural hosts, cattle, to abnormal hosts, including horses, sheep and goats. A case of Kumri has been reported in the United States.[122]

Diethylcarbamazine, given PO at 20-40 mg/kg body weight for 1-3 days, has been successful as a prophylactic or therapeutic microfilaricide during periods of vector activity.[121]

Necropsy Findings: Strongylus vulgaris arteritis, endocarditis and resultant thromboembolic showering of the brain may cause multifocal arterial infarction that may be ischemic or hemorrhagic and may result in diffuse brain edema and swelling. *Strongylus vulgaris, Hypoderma* spp and *Setaria* spp usually create destructive, tortuous, hemorrhagic soft tracts through brain parenchyma. The cellular reaction varies from hemorrhage, with neutrophils in the peracute lesion, to cavitating necrotic areas, with macrophages, eosinophils, lymphocytes and reactive glial cells in the more advanced stages. The more diffuse lesions seen with *H deletrix* infection are characterized by perivascular cuffing with macrophages, plasma cells and eosinophils. Aggressive anti-inflammatory therapy can markedly suppress the associated inflammatory response.

Trypanosomiasis

Fatal infections of equids by various subspecies of the protozoan hemoparasite, *Trypanosoma brucei*, are seen in many parts of the world.[123] Each of these diseases is characterized by fever, anemia, urticaria, lymphadenopathy, dependent edema and emaciation. Signs of meningoencephalomyelitis develop insidiously and are progressive. There reportedly are muscle atrophy, facial nerve paralysis, and limb ataxia and weakness, which is worse in the pelvic limbs. If left untreated, each of the diseases causes death after a course of several weeks to a year.

Trypanosoma brucei infects equids and livestock in tropical Africa, causing the disease known as nagana (also known as African trypanosomiasis). Blood-feeding tsetse flies are the vectors of this organism. A virtually identical disease known as surra is caused by *Trypanosoma evansi*. This disease is found in northern Africa, Turkey, the USSR, India, Indochina, China, the Philippines, Central America and South America. *Trypanosoma evansi* is transmitted mechanically by biting flies, usually horseflies of the genus *Tabanus*. In Central and South America, where the disease is known as murrina or derrengadera, the vampire bat is a vector.

Dourine is a venereal disease of equids, caused by *Trypanosoma equiperdum*. Dourine is found in Asia, South Africa, India and the USSR. It once was common in western Europe and North America but now has been eradicated from these regions. After an initial phase characterized by edema of the external genitalia, dourine resembles other forms of trypanosomiasis.

Diagnosis is by demonstration of the organism in smears of blood, lymph node aspirates or other body fluids. A complement-fixation test has been developed for dourine. Trypanosomicidal therapy is successful if instituted early in the disease. Quinapyramine (5 mg/kg SC) reportedly is effective in eradicating the organism, and quinapyramine prosalt or suramin can be used prophylactically.

Borreliosis

A wide range of neurologic signs has been observed in people infected with the spirochete *Borrelia burgdorferi* (Lyme disease).[124] *Borrelia burgdorferi* was isolated from the brain of a horse in Wisconsin that was euthanized after 1 week with head tilt, dysphagia and flaccid paralysis of the tail.[125] Reports of human cases indicate that neurologic forms of borreliosis can be treated successfully with any of a variety of antibiotics, including penicillin, tetracycline and erythromycin. Antemortem diagnosis can be presumed by demonstration of a rising or high indirect immunofluorescent antibody titer for *B burgdorferi*.[126]

Toxic Diseases

Important nervous system toxicoses are described individually elsewhere in this chapter. The following additional syndromes are rare but occasionally may have local or re-

Chapter 8

gional significance. The reader is referred to other literature for more detailed discussions and bibliographies.[127-131]

Chemical Intoxications

Mercurialism has occurred inadvertently when horses consume grain that has been treated with fungicidal alkylmercury compounds. Chronic ingestion of contaminated feed causes cerebellar and spinal cord neuronal degeneration, with signs of limb ataxia, hypermetria, muscle tremors and coarse head nodding.[132] Central nervous system abnormalities reportedly are not seen in horses poisoned with inorganic mercury compounds or phenylmercuric acetate.[133-135] Emaciation, dermatitis and renal failure are seen consistently in horses chronically poisoned with organic or inorganic mercury compounds.

Horses are much less susceptible to *urea* poisoning than ruminants are; however, signs of ammonia toxicity have been produced experimentally by feeding 450 g to ponies.[128] The earliest signs were aimless wandering and incoordination, followed by severe depression, head-pressing, convulsions and death.

Monensin is a feed additive used as a growth promotant and coccidiostat in cattle and chickens, respectively. Inadvertent consumption by horses of feeds containing monensin has resulted in mortality.[136] Clinical signs in affected horses were depression, anorexia and incoordination and weakness of the pelvic limbs. Diarrhea and excessive sweating also were seen. The LD$_{50}$ of monensin in orally dosed horses has been estimated at 2-3 mg/kg body weight. A related antibiotic, *lasalocid*, also is used as a feed additive for broiler chickens but has a higher therapeutic index than monensin and is unlikely to kill horses that accidentally consume it in treated feed.

Poisoning of horses by *carbamates or organophosphates* usually is due to overzealous application of insecticides, acaricides or anthelmintics, or accidental contamination of food or water with these substances.[128,130] Signs are caused by inhibition of acetylcholinesterase activity, resulting in the uncontrolled muscarinic, nicotinic and central nervous effects of acetylcholine. There are anxiety, hyperexcitability, colic, frequent urination, sweating and muscle tremors, that may be generalized. Muscle hyperactivity and stiffness may be followed by weakness, recumbency and death due to respiratory insufficiency. Organophosphate toxicity can be treated with atropine (0.1 mg/kg, half slowly IV and half IM) and 2-PAM (20 mg/kg IM). Residual organophosphates may be removed by skin washing and saline purgation as appropriate. Horses are said to be highly resistant to delayed neurotoxicity due to organophosphate compounds; however, transient left laryngeal paresis developed in 6 Arabian or part-Arabian foals given the anthelmintic haloxon. Bilateral laryngeal paresis developed in 4 horses after dosing with mineral oil thought to have been contaminated with an organophosphate compound.[137,138]

Chlorinated hydrocarbons once were widely used in industry (polychlorinated biphenyls or PCBs in insulators), horticulture and agriculture.[128,130,131] Accidental exposure of horses to toxic levels of these substances presumably has occurred, but there are few, if any, credible reports in the literature of such incidents. In other animals and people, acute toxicity is associated with excitement interspersed with depression, as well as muscle tremors and severe, unrelenting seizures. Chronic accumulation of chlorinated hydrocarbons may cause a wide array of peripheral or central neuropathies, as well as degeneration of other tissues. Treatment is symptomatic. Use of chlorinated hydrocarbons is now highly restricted due to problems with environmental persistence of both the parent compound and contaminating dioxins. In this regard, it is of interest to note that dioxins also may be neurotoxic. Of 85 horses that were exposed to dioxin in waste oil sludge used to keep down dust, 48 died over a period of weeks to years.[130] In addition to clinical signs of emaciation, colic and laminitis, cerebral edema was noted at necropsy.

It frequently has been stated that a "blind staggers" syndrome seen in the western United States is a form of chronic *selenosis* due to prolonged consumption of selenium-accumulating plants, such as *Astragalus bisculcatus*. However, these signs cannot be duplicated by feeding high levels of selenium and probably are actually a form of locoism.[127-129]

Plant Intoxications[127-131]

Several members of the family Solenaceae cause signs of neurotoxicity when ingested by horses. Poisonous plants contain either the

762

tropone (atropine-like) or solanum groups of alkaloids. Among the former group are *Datura* spp (thorn apple, jimsonweed), *Atropa belladonna* (deadly nightshade) and *Dubosia* spp (corkwoods). These widely distributed species are unpalatable to horses but may cause poisoning when included in hay or grain. Ingestion of jimsonweed caused the death of 11 of 15 ponies. Signs included anorexia, depression, excessive urination and thirst, diarrhea, mydriasis, muscle spasms and convulsions. Physostigmine, a short-acting anticholinesterase, is the treatment of choice and should be used to effect. *Solanum nigram* (black nightshade) appears to be the most toxic of the solanum alkaloid-containing plants. The common potato (*S tuberosum*) may also be toxic when green. Horses poisoned with black nightshade exhibited colic, ataxia, weakness, tremors and convulsions. Solanum alkaloids are cholinesterase inhibitors; therefore, treatment with atropine should be helpful.

Several umbelliferous (hemlock-type) species are among the most poisonous plants known. Those that have caused poisoning in horses are *Oenanthe crocata* (hemlock water drop root), *Circuta* spp (water hemlock), and *Daucus carota* (wild carrot). Those plants are found throughout the United States and many other countries but grow only in wet or swampy areas. The toxic principles, a family of higher alcohols including oenanthotoxin and cicatoxin, are concentrated in the roots and lower stems. A piece of water hemlock root the size of a walnut reportedly was fatal to a horse. Signs of poisoning by umbelliferous plants are reported to be salivation, mydriasis, colic, delirium and convulsions.

Horses are reported to be very susceptible to poisoning by the legume *Laburnum anagyroides* (laburnum). Ingestion of laburnum seeds at 0.6 g/kg caused excitement, incoordination, sweating, convulsions and death. The toxic principle is the alkaloid cystisine. Ingestion of hay heavily contaminated with another legume, *Lathyrus hissolia* (grass vetchling), was associated with severe attacks of ataxia provoked by moving or handling the affected animals. Recovery followed removal of the contaminated feed. Peripheral neuropathy has been associated with *Lathyrus* spp ingestion by horses. The most prominent signs are laryngeal paresis and a stringhalt-type gait.[139]

Robinia pseudoacacia (false acacia, black locust tree) contains the neurotoxin robin and several toxic glycosides. Horses may be poisoned by eating sapling sprouts or bark of mature trees, resulting in anorexia, depression, weakness and posterior paralysis.

Eupatorium rugosum (white snakeroot) and *Aplopappus heterophyllus* (rayless goldenrod) contain the toxic alcohol tremetol that causes a condition known as "trembles" in horses, sheep and cattle. White snakeroot grows in moist areas around ditches and streams in the midwestern and eastern United States, while rayless goldenrod is found primarily in the southwestern United States. After ingestion of these plants for several days, horses exhibit depression, weakness, tremors and dysphagia. Labored breathing and urinary incontinence also are seen. Recovery occurs gradually after removal of horses from the offending plants. A related species, *Artemesia filfifolia* (sand sagebrush), has caused a nervous syndrome called "sage sickness" in horses unused to the plant.

Ingestion of large quantities of *Gomphrena celosioides* (soft khaki weed) causes a syndrome known in Australia as "coastal staggers" and "Bundaberg horse disease." Posterior ataxia, depression and muscle spasms are the usual signs. Horses recover if removed from the causative plant but may die if intake is prolonged.

Descurainia pinnata (tansy mustard), a cruciferous weed found in the United States, has been reported to cause poisoning characterized by blindness and tongue paralysis. Toxicity results after consumption of large quantities of the plant for a prolonged period. *Stipita robusta* (sleepy grass) is a tall perennial needlegrass found in Colorado, New Mexico and Texas. This plant contains high levels of the soporific agent, diacetin alcohol, from which acetone may be liberated in the gut. Signs of ingestion range from mild stupor to recumbency and deep sleep. A catatonic syndrome may be seen in which severely affected horses are "frozen" in unusual positions for long periods. Recovery occurs over several days. It is said that horses that have eaten the plant once will not consume it again.

Meal made from the nuts of the cycad, *Cyas circinalis,* caused ataxia and spinal cord degeneration when fed to horses.

Mycotoxicoses

The syndromes of ryegrass staggers, paspalum staggers and leukoencephalomalacia are examples of mycotoxicoses in horses and are discussed elsewhere in this chapter. Another suspected mycotoxicosis is kikuyu poisoning. Kikuyu grass (*Pennisetum clandestinum*) is a useful forage plant in New Zealand and South America. Signs of toxicity occasionally occur 24-48 hours after horses are given access to pasture damaged by army worm infestation. Circumstantial evidence points to trichothecin mycotoxins produced by *Myrothecium verrucaria* as the causative agents. Clinical signs include anorexia, depression, salivation, colic, muscle tremors, hypermetria and, occasionally, convulsions. Mortality among affected animals is about 80%.

Ingestion of aflatoxin in moldy corn and peanut meal was suspected to have caused the death of 12 horses in Thailand and 2 in the United States.[140] Unfortunately, the clinical signs were not recorded, but necropsy findings were leukoencephalomalacia of the cerebral hemispheres, fatty degeneration of the liver, kidneys and myocardium, and hemorrhagic gastroenteritis.

Snakebite, Tick Paralysis

In the United States, snakebites usually involve viperine snakes, such as the water moccasin or rattlesnake. These snakebites cause intense local reaction but are seldom associated with marked nervous signs. In contrast, the venom of elapine snakes is mainly neurotoxic, with minimal local effects. This group includes cobras, mambas and coral snakes of India, Africa, Asia and Central and South America and the tiger snake, brown snake and Australian death adder of Australia.[128,131] Horses bitten by elapine snakes pass through an initial period of excitement and hyperesthesia, followed by generalized weakness manifested as depression, mydriasis, dysphagia and tremors. Snake bites are seldom fatal in adult horses; however, foals may die within 48 hours after a period of recumbency and convulsions. Treatment with specific antivenin is effective. Broad-spectrum antimicrobials should be given to minimize local infection.

Ixodes holocyclus ticks have been reported to cause a tick paralysis syndrome in foals (and in most other domestic animals and people). Signs of generalized, flaccid paralysis resemble those of botulism. Recovery quickly follows removal of the offending tick(s).[131]

Idiopathic Diseases

Neonatal Maladjustment Syndrome

Neonatal maladjustment syndrome is a noninfectious syndrome of cerebral signs in newborn foals. Attempts to classify the disease according to clinical signs have led to the popular use of such descriptive but nonspecific terms as "barkers," "wanderers," "dummies" and "convulsives." Despite the general acceptance of neonatal maladjustment syndrome as a recognizable clinical entity, the cause of the disease is not yet clear, and there is no consistent association between clinical signs of neonatal maladjustment syndrome and morphologic changes in the CNS.[141] In the brains and spinal cords of some foals dying with neonatal maladjustment syndrome, varying degrees of hemorrhage, edema and necrosis have been observed.[142] However, in at least as many affected foals, no CNS lesions may be identified, either grossly or histologically.[142]

It has been suggested that episodes of brain hypoxia or ischemia during the perinatal period lead to the cerebral dysfunction characteristic of neonatal maladjustment syndrome. Certain obstetric procedures, such as premature clamping of the umbilical cord, have been suggested as causes. Others have speculated that marked changes in intracranial vascular pressure and blood flow during delivery could induce neonatal maladjustment syndrome. Paradoxically, most cases of neonatal maladjustment syndrome occur in foals after a rapid, albeit strenuous, uncomplicated delivery.

Neonatal maladjustment syndrome usually occurs in otherwise normal foals during the first 24 hours postpartum but may be seen at any time during the neonatal period (defined here as the first week of life). Signs are abrupt in onset and referable to diffuse cerebrocortical impairment. Sudden stiff, jerky movements of the head and body progress to extensor spasms of the neck, limbs and tail. Often there is complete loss of the suckling reflex. If able to stand, the foal may wander aimlessly, oblivious to its surroundings and apparently blind. Hyperexcitability, grinding of the teeth, retraction of the lips, exaggerated chewing/sucking movements ("chewing gum" fits) or "gulping" of air and abnormal vocalization ("barking") have been noted during this stage. Many of these signs are caused by partial or mild, generalized seizures.

The rate of progression of signs varies, but affected foals often become recumbent and semicomatose, with paddling and clonic convulsions. Close observation may reveal constricted or dilated, asymmetric pupils. There may be abnormal respiratory patterns and sounds, sometimes associated with hypoxia and respiratory acidosis. Unless there is concurrent sepsis, the hemogram should be relatively normal for foals of this age.

With reasonable care, at least 80% of foals with uncomplicated neonatal maladjustment syndrome without signs of localized or generalized sepsis recover over several hours to several weeks. Neurologic functions return in the reverse of the order in which they were lost, (*ie*, consciousness, standing position, vision and awareness, recognition of dam, and finally suckling ability). Recovery usually is complete if the foal survives, though occasional relapses have been reported.

The management and treatment of foals with neonatal maladjustment syndrome should conform to the principles of neonatal care and should be aimed at maintaining the foal's body temperature, hydration, caloric intake, electrolyte and acid-base balance, and blood glucose concentration. If needed, oxygen may be provided by nasal insufflation. The adequacy of passive transfer of immunity should be assessed. If the serum IgG is <400 mg/dl in the field and <800 mg/dl in a hospital setting, then colostrum and/or plasma should be given.

Unnecessary stimuli, such as bright lights and loud noises, should be avoided. Mild partial or generalized convulsions may be permitted or can be controlled manually without excessive restraint. However, if convulsions are severe enough to cause recumbency, hyperthermia or distress, immediate control can be provided with IV doses of 5-10 mg diazepam. For long-term control, phenobarbital has been used successfully at an initial dosage of 10-20 mg/kg diluted in saline and given IV over 15-20 minutes. Thereafter, adequate levels of phenobarbital may be maintained with a dosage of 5-10 mg/kg given IV

or PO twice daily. Phenytoin at 5-10 mg/kg may control seizures, with maintenance dosages of 1-5 mg/kg BID to QID. However, the therapeutic index of phenytoin is quite low and, under usual circumstances, phenobarbital should be tried first. Dimethyl sulfoxide (500-1000 mg/kg IV in 1 L of 5% dextrose) may rationally be used early in the course of the disease in an effort to combat cerebral edema and scavenge oxygen radicals accumulating secondary to anoxic damage.

Grove Poisoning

In south Florida, a syndrome of ataxia and convulsions occurs in adult horses. The signs fluctuate in severity but are progressive over time and usually result in recumbency and death. Though the clinical syndrome indicates diffuse cerebral, vestibulocerebellar and spinal cord disease, there is no consistent neuropathologic lesion. In addition to neurologic signs, there are ulceration and congestion of the gums, and corneal edema and ulceration. "Grove poisoning" occurs in areas of intensive horticultural activity, though no direct connection has been established with horticultural practices. Therapy with diazepam and atropine, along with saline purgatives, may have resulted in a few cures.

Head-Shaking, Cribbing, Weaving and Other Vices

T.A. Turner

Equine behavioral problems, known as stereotypic behavior or "vices," are undesirable habits caused by removing the horse from its natural environment.[143] They are essentially iatrogenic disorders caused by confinement and artificial feeding. Two characteristics of the feral horse are group or herd living and unlimited grazing time. Horses deprived of these instinctive tendencies may develop displacement behavior that owners and trainers consider vices. The problem can become so severe or annoying to the owner or trainer that veterinary assistance may be sought.

Diagnosis: Stereotypic behaviors may be divided into oral vices and movement vices.[143] Oral vices include cribbing, wood-chewing, coprophagia and biting. Movement vices include stall-walking and weaving, pawing, kicking and head-shaking. Diagnosis is by observing the particular behavior. The most profound of these is self-mutilation, which is covered separately below.

Cribbing is a behavior in which the horse grasps an object with its incisors, flexes its neck and swallows air.[143-150] The horizontal surface of a bucket, fence rail, feed bunk, stall door or even the back of another horse may be used for this purpose. The horse may swallow air without grasping an object, and this is termed *windsucking* or aerophagia. Cribbing occurs most frequently in confined animals but can occur in pastured animals as well.[143,149] It may be a cause as well as a result of gastrointestinal problems.[143] Aerophagia is thought to cause colic. On the other hand, swallowing air may be pleasurable to an animal with abdominal discomfort. A consequence of cribbing is excessive wear of the incisors.

Wood-chewing is similar to cribbing but much more destructive.[143,149] Instead of simply grasping the surface with their teeth, wood-chewing animals ingest the wood. Unlike cribbing, wood-chewing appears to have a specific cause: lack of roughage in the diet.[143] Stereotypic wood-chewing has been associated with low-fiber, high-concentrate pelleted feeds. This may be why feral horses and pastured horses have been observed chewing trees or shrubs when good-quality grass is available. Weather may also be a factor, as wood-chewing increases during cold, wet weather.

Coprophagia is the eating of feces.[149,151] It is normal in foals 1-8 weeks of age and decreases gradually thereafter. Adults avoid eating feces or fecally contaminated feed if they are receiving an adequate diet.[149] Diets deficient in fiber or protein induce coprophagia. Starvation produces a similar result. Horse manure does have some feed value. On a dry-matter basis, it contains 40-60% total digestible nutrients, 8-11% protein, trace minerals, calcium and phosphorus. Aesthetically, coprophagia is very unappealing. It also increases the risk of transmission of parasites and other pathogens and, therefore, could constitute a health hazard.

Biting is perhaps the most undesirable vice.[152] Not only can it be dangerous to the handler or any person around the horse, but it also is a sign of dominance aggression. Biting usually occurs in 2 circumstances. First, it occurs when the horse is trying to exert dominance over people. This is most typically a problem of stallions, and affected animals may be referred to as "rogues." In the second situation, a horse bites because it is trying to get a food treat, such as sugar. Bites from aggressive horses usually occur at or about a person's shoulder.[152] Bites from horses looking for treats usually occur near the pocket where the treats are kept.

Stall-walking and *weaving* are similar vices occurring in closely confined horses.[143,149] Horses that stall-walk usually circle their stall incessantly. Weavers stay in one spot but move constantly from side to side. Restraining the stall-walking horse often converts a stall-walker into a weaver. Both of these vices are forms of self-stimulation and are exacerbated by stress. Horses have been observed to walk or weave more frequently in the evening, before a show, or if they are in pain. Either behavior can adversely affect the horse's condition and performance. Incessant movement may expend more energy than can be ingested in feed. As a result, the animal loses condition or has reduced performance.

Rather than being a form of stimulation, *pawing* is a response to frustration.[143,149] It is a displacement activity that originally served to uncover buried food. Horses paw under a variety of circumstances: while being restrained, eating or waiting for feed. A mare sometimes paws when trying to induce a recumbent foal to stand. Frustration due to confinement and segregation causes the most extreme forms of pawing.[143] Because the horse is a roaming herd animal, it paws to try to escape confinement or establish contact with another horse. This behavior is not inherently detrimental, but it can cause excessive hoof or shoe wear, and it is particularly damaging to dirt and clay floors.

Stall-kicking most likely is a form of self-stimulation.[143] These horses kick the stall walls with their hooves or occasionally with the hocks. The stall-kicker supposedly enjoys the sound its hoof makes as it strikes wood. The resultant concussion and trauma can cause such serious injuries as phalangeal fractures, splint fractures, calcaneal bursitis (capped hock) and plantar desmitis (curb). Stall-kicking, like pawing, may be a conditioned response caused by frustration at feeding time.[143] The horse kicks or paws because of irritation at the delay between when it can first see or smell the feed or feeder and when the feed actually arrives. This behavior is then inadvertently rewarded when the horse is fed.

Head-shaking is a problem of the ridden horse.[153,154] These horses exhibit intermittent, sudden and involuntary head-tossing or nodding movements. Head-shaking is an instinctive behavior associated with the presence of flies.[153] It also can be a normal sign of impatience in an excitable horse. Head-shaking is considered a vice when it occurs in the absence of obvious extraneous stimuli and with such frequency that the horse is difficult to manage or is distressed. Unlike most vices, head-shaking may actually be caused by ill-fitting tack or organic disease.[154] Therefore, a detailed history should be obtained, and a careful clinical examination performed to rule out specific causes, such as rhinitis, hyoid bone lesions, guttural pouch disease, sinusitis, otitis, glossitis, stomatitis, tooth problems, pharyngeal and laryngeal lesions, occipitovertebral injury, myopathies and skin disorders involving the head and neck. This evaluation must include palpation of all superficial structures of the head and neck.[155,156]

The sinuses should be percussed and the oral cavity palpated and visually examined. Endoscopic examination of both nasal passages, the nasopharynx, larynx, guttural pouches and trachea also should be performed. Radiographic examination of the sinuses, dental arcades, occiput and cervical vertebrae should be made. Additionally, otoscopic and ophthalmic examinations should be undertaken.[156] Finally, a series of trigeminal nerve blocks can be performed, because trigeminal neuralgia has been reported as a cause of head-shaking.[157] Other specific causes of head-shaking include ear mite infestation, otitis interna, cranial nerve VII and VIII dysfunction, cervical injury, ocular disease, guttural pouch mycosis, vasomotor rhinitis and periapical dental abscesses.[154]

Treatment: In almost all cases, confinement and artificial feeding must be considered as a cause of a behavioral disorder. An attempt should be made to modify these factors, where practical, to a more natural state. Affected animals should be offered distractions, including toys and companions. Other treatments are varied and range from behavior modification to surgery.[143-152,157] It is not logical to attempt medical or surgical treatment of stereotypic behavior if the horse is to be placed back in exactly the same environmental circumstances.

Treatments to prevent cribbing are diverse.[143,144,148-150] The simplest involves use of a "cribbing strap." The strap is placed around the animal's throat just caudal to the poll so that pressure is exerted when the horse arches its neck and attempts to swallow. This produces negative reinforcement each time the animal tries to crib. If the strap alone is inadequate, spikes can be added as a further hindrance to cribbing. Unfortunately, even though the straps work in most cases, the horse soon learns that the strap causes the discomfort and often resumes cribbing if the strap is removed.

When management methods fail to prevent cribbing, owners often look to medical and surgical treatments.[144-148,150] Narcotic antagonists have stopped cribbing.[144] Treatment regimens used include naloxone at 0.02-0.04 mg/kg body weight, naltrexone at 0.04 mg/kg, nalmefane at 0.08 mg/kg and diprenorphine at 0.02-0.03 mg/kg. Unfortunately, this therapy is palliative but not curative; the behavior returns as blood levels of the drug decline. Not until longer-acting drugs become available will medical treatment be a practical alternative to surgery.

Four surgical procedures have been useful in treatment of cribbing and aerophagia.[145,147,148,150] Bilateral buccostomy is used to treat aerophagia.[155] The procedure is performed by making 5-cm skin incisions bilaterally at the level of the table surface of the first cheek teeth. Each incision is continued through the buccinator muscle and buccal mucosa. The mucosa then is sutured to the skin. The openings prevent the horse from developing the negative pressure in the oral cavity necessary to swallow air. Unfortunately, this procedure is not particularly cosmetic. The remaining 3 procedures are designed to stop cribbing by altering the animal's ability to use the ventral strap muscles of the neck. These muscles, the sternocephalicus, omohyoideus and sternothyrohyoideus, all function in the act of cribbing.[145-147,150]

The least invasive and most cosmetic procedure is bilateral neurectomy of the ventral branches of the spinal accessory nerve (cranial nerve XI).[145,147] The procedure can be performed with the horse standing or under general anesthesia. On each side, an 8-cm incision is made ventral to the jugular vein at the level of the musculotendinous junction of the sternocephalicus muscle. Blunt dissection along the medial aspect of the jugular vein and sternocephalicus muscle helps identify the ventral branch of the accessory nerve. The nerve can be isolated from the fascia on the medial aspect of the sternocephalicus muscle as it runs parallel with the musculotendinous junction for several centimeters. Just distal to this junction, a 3- to 5-cm section of the nerve is removed. Reported success rates for this operation have varied. Most veterinarians agree that the procedure is successful for only a short time, if at all. Therefore, during this time it is important that management changes or behavior modification techniques be implemented to prevent relapse.

The remaining surgical procedures involve resection of the ventral strap muscles of the neck.[146,148,150] This procedure requires general anesthesia. The horse is placed in dorsal recumbency with its neck extended and the ventral neck prepared for aseptic surgery. The skin incision begins along the midline at the level of the thyroid cartilage and is extended caudally for 30-40 cm.[148] The incision is continued by blunt dissection through the deep tissues between the paired sternothyrohyoid muscles until the trachea is reached. Blunt dissection is then continued under the skin around the sternothyrohyoid muscle. The fascia deep to the jugular vein is dissected to facilitate reflection of the vein and skin away from the surgical site.

After the sternothyrohyoid muscles have been dissected free from surrounding tissues, a 15-cm portion of each muscle is removed. If hemorrhage is excessive, a simple-continuous suture pattern through the ventral and dorsal fascia of the muscle can be placed over the transected ends. The dissection is continued around the omohyoid muscle. Particular care is required during this dissection around the dorsal edge of this muscle because of the close proximity of the carotid artery, vagosympathetic trunk and recurrent laryngeal nerve. Next, the sternocephalicus muscle is isolated by blunt dissection from the jugular vein and overlying skin. The caudal aspect of the sternocephalicus is transected and lifted from the incision. With light tension on the muscle, the tendon of insertion is severed. Suction drains are recommended to reduce postoperative seroma formation. Tissues are closed in a routine manner. The drain usually can be removed 48-72 hours postoperatively. This technique has been reported to cause complete remission in 53% of cases and improvement in 15%;[148] however, the result is cosmetically undesirable.

The final procedure is a modification of the above technique.[150] It involves a similar approach except that only small portions of the sternothyrohyoid and omohyoid muscles are resected, while the sternocephalicus is left intact. The ventral branch of the accessory nerve is resected as previously described to partially denervate the sternocephalicus muscle. This procedure is much more cosmetically pleasing than Forsell's technique described above, and has similar results.[150]

Because of the variable results of surgery, a veterinarian cannot depend on surgery alone to cure cribbing. The first line of treatment, and a most important adjunct to surgery, is behavior modification.[143,149] Forms of distraction may involve giving the horse companionship in the form of a goat, pony, chicken or other suitable pet. Often a new habit can be created, such as playing with toys to occupy the animal's time. Most people agree there is no panacea for cribbers, but through management changes, behavior modification and surgery, cribbing at least can be reduced in most horses.

Wood-chewing causes other treatment difficulties.[143,149] Because there is an apparent need or appetite for wood in the horse's diet, use of companions and toys for distraction is not very effective in treating this condition. Many managers attempt to reduce wood-chewing by eliminating wood edges, covering them with metal or wire, or painting them with lead-free taste repellents. Increasing the roughage in a horse's diet reduces its motivation to chew food and is the preferred method of treatment.

Except in the neonate, in which it is normal, coprophagia often indicates a diet that is fiber- or protein-deficient.[149,151] The diet should be examined carefully for content and balance of energy, protein, fiber and trace minerals.[151] If no obvious dietary problems exist, the horse may be eating feces due to boredom. Increasing the horse's exercise or animal contact could be helpful. These horses must be dewormed routinely. Contact with known *Salmonella* shedders should also be avoided.

Horses that bite must be controlled.[152] Immediate punishment is the most effective treatment, and the handler must be persistent in demanding proper behavior. Hitting a biting horse is not an appropriate punishment. Hitting usually only results in a "sneaky" biter. A chain-ended lead rope is extremely useful. The chain can be placed over the nose, under the chin, or around the upper gum. When the horse attempts to bite, punishment is administered by pulling on the chain. Only one punishment cue should be administered at a time. Excessive punishment can result in pain-induced or defensive aggression. It may be necessary to muzzle the biter until the behavior can be changed.

Stall-walking and weaving are best treated by reducing confinement by turning the horse out onto a pasture or into a large run.[143,149] If this is not possible, more frequent periods of work may reduce the behavior. Stall toys also can be helpful in reducing stall-walking or weaving.

Pawing is difficult to control except when it is in anticipation of food.[143,149] To break this vice, the horse must be fed only when it does not paw.[151] The process can be accelerated by feeding small meals throughout the day. Initially the horse must refrain from pawing for only a few seconds before being rewarded by feed. Gradually the amount of time the horse must refrain from pawing is increased before feeding. Training may go faster if a countercommand, such as "Stand," is issued at the same time the feed reward is given. The same technique of retraining can be used for horses that kick in anticipation of the arrival of feed.

Stall-kicking is much more difficult to manage.[153] Turning the horse out in a pasture is an obvious alternative but not always practical. Stall toys and companions may be beneficial in reducing the behavior. When all else fails, the use of a kicking chain usually reduces the behavior. A kicking chain is a light chain that is attached to the pastern of the limb with which the horse kicks. As the horse kicks, the chain hits the horse's leg, causing discomfort and negative reinforcement of the behavior. Unfortunately, kicking chains may cause minor abrasions on the horse's limbs.

Head-shaking can only be considered a vice when all medical causes have been ruled out.[144,154] If a medical reason is not found, retraining may be the only way to stop the behavior. In many of these cases, the horse must be retired because the behavior cannot be changed.

Self-Mutilation Syndrome

This uncommon syndrome usually involves mature, light-breed stallions. Rarely, mares or geldings are affected. The onset of signs often follows a major change in the exercise or breeding regimen, such as returning to stud from racing or being introduced into a new herd.[152,158] The signs begin suddenly and occur intermittently. Typically an affected horse looks at its flank, squeals, grunts, spins, runs in circles, and kicks and bites at its body. With some difficulty, the horse can be distracted with a whip. During an attack, pieces of skin are often ripped off, particularly from the pectoral, flank, stifle and thigh regions.

The pathogenesis is not known. Possibilities include deviant (stereotypic) behavior, focal seizures, myelitis, radiculitis (inflammation of nerve roots), neuritis and hormonal imbalance. Affected breeding stallions require continued, hard exercise.

Sedatives may exacerbate signs, so they should be used with caution. Long-acting sedatives, such as reserpine (Serpasil: CIBA) at 1 mg IM or 4 mg PO or fluphenazine enanthate (Prolixin: Squibb) at 50 mg IM, may be effective but are not licensed for use in horses. Animal companions (sheep, goat, old mare), progesterone therapy (200 mg progesterone in oil IM daily for 10 days) or 8 20-mg megestrol acetate tablets PO daily for 1 month, as well as epidural corticosteroids have been tried with variable success. Special chain muzzles often must be used.

Tics and Localized Tremor Syndromes

A great variety of inherited, inflammatory and infectious conditions can result in generalized tremor or convulsive syndromes. However, tremors or tics confined to one or a pair of limbs are rare in horses. Tics may be either rhythmic or arrhythmic contractions of the proximal or distal muscle of a limb or other body part. They may be initiated by voluntary effort or without conscious input. Theoretically, lesions involving sensory structures (muscle spindles, Golgi tendon organs), sensory nerves, the spinal cord or alpha or gamma motor neurons could be manifested as a focal tic or tremor syndrome.

Stringhalt following trauma to the hock may be regarded as an extreme example of a tic syndrome of this type. In addition, partial seizures or chorea syndromes may be manifested as tics in people.

A thoracic limb tic in a horse has been described.[159] The reader is referred to this article for discussion of a logical approach to the differential diagnosis of tic syndromes using various pharmacologic aids.

DISEASES OF THE FOREBRAIN

R.J. MacKay and I.G. Mayhew

Diagnostic and Therapeutic Considerations

Seizures

Seizures are the result of sudden, abnormal discharging of neurons in part or all of the cerebral cortex. These bursts of cerebrocortical activity cause paroxysmal movements and profound behavioral alterations. On the basis of their clinical appearance and progression, seizures are classified as generalized, partial, or partial with secondary generalization.

Generalized seizures reflect diffuse cerebral disturbance. The onset of a generalized seizure may be signaled by a short period of restlessness and disorientation, with chewing, grinding of the teeth, or other bizarre behavior. This is followed by generalized muscular rigidity (often beginning in the neck), recumbency and unconsciousness. There usually are clonic, paddling movements and signs of autonomic activity, such as salivation, urination and defecation. Diffuse cortical disturbances due to inflammation, metabolic disorders and toxicities may produce generalized seizures.

Signs of a partial seizure depend on the portion of the cerebral cortex discharging. The origin of the abnormal electrical activity is known as the seizure focus. When the seizure focus is in the motor cortex, there may be tremors or involuntary jerking on the contralateral side of the head or body. Seizure foci in other parts of the brain may result in such behavioral abnormalities as exaggerated gulping of air, apparent blindness, confusion, viciousness, unprovoked excitement or unconsciousness. Between seizures, other localizing neurologic deficits may be apparent. Focal lesions in the diencephalon (thalamus, hypothalamus) or cerebral hemispheres from trauma, inflammation, ischemia or compression may initiate partial seizures.

Partial seizures may progress to generalized seizures if the electrical discharge spreads through the entire cerebral cortex. Localizing signs usually are apparent before the onset of such generalized seizures. For example, with a seizure focus in the motor cortex, an animal may turn its head to the side or flick its leg before falling on its side unconscious in a generalized seizure.

Recurrent seizures without evidence of an active underlying disease, known as epilepsy, occur occasionally in horses and are described in detail below.

Seizures are most often the result of some underlying disease. The following conditions may be associated with seizure activity.

- *Inflammation/infection:* Arboviral encephalitis (EEE, WEE, VEE), rabies, meningitis, verminous encephalitis, protozoal myeloencephalitis.
- *Compression:* Cholesterol granuloma, cerebral abscess, hydrocephalus, neoplasm.
- *Vascular disorders/ischemia:* Parasitic thromboembolism, intracarotid injection, neonatal maladjustment syndrome, hypoxemia.
- *Trauma*
- *Toxicity:* Moldy corn poisoning, "grove poisoning."
- *Metabolic disorders:* Hepatoencephalopathy, hypoglycemia, hyposmolality, hyperosmolality, hypocalcemia.

Continual seizures (status epilepticus) should be controlled with glycerol guaiacolate, chloral hydrate or sodium pentobarbital before proceeding with further evaluation (Table 4). Diazepam is expensive but often effective in short-term treatment of seizures. Complications of seizure activity, such as self-inflicted trauma, hyperthermia, acidosis and ventilatory difficulties, can then be managed. Prevention of further seizure episodes depends on identification and successful treatment of underlying disease.

Congenital and Familial Diseases

Hydrocephalus

Though hydrocephalus has a wide variety of causes, it apparently is very rare in horses. Hydrocephalus is an increased CSF volume within the ventricular system (internal hydrocephalus) or subarachnoid space (external hydrocephalus) of the head.[160] It may be congenital or acquired, and normotensive or hypertensive. Normotensive hydrocephalus usually is incidental to hypoplasia or loss of brain parenchyma after destructive prenatal or postnatal infection or injury. The CSF volume passively expands to fill the space normally occupied by brain tissue. Therefore, normotensive compensatory hydrocephalus is the result of, not the cause of, CNS disease. Normotensive hydrocephalus has been seen following massive cerebral destruction in horses surviving such diseases as viral encephalitis, head trauma and neonatal maladjustment syndrome.

In contrast, hypertensive hydrocephalus may cause progressive overt CNS disease by damaging tissue adjacent to expanding ventricles. Generally, hypertensive hydrocephalus is a consequence of obstruction of the CSF conduit (especially the mesencephalic aqueduct and lateral apertures) between the sites of production, in the third and lateral ventricles, and the sites of absorption by the arachnoid villi in the subarachnoid space. Blockage may be due to hypoplasia or aplasia of a conducting or absorbing part or acquired due to inflammation and swelling of, or injury to, the ependymal lining of the aqueduct, lateral apertures or arachnoid villi. Inflammation can be acute, as in neonatal bacterial meningoencephalomyelitis or chronic and proliferative, as in the granulomatous ependymitis of equine infectious anemia. Also, any space-occupying mass, such as a cerebral abscess or large choroid plexus cholesterol granuloma, may result in progressive hypertensive hydrocephalus. Regardless of the etiology, the result usually is increased CSF pressure and dilation of the third and lateral ventricles. However, by the time the animal is evaluated, the pressure may be normal.

Clinical Signs: Hypertensive obstructive hydrocephalus may cause an enlarged calvaria with open sutures in neonates. It should be remembered, however, that normal neonatal foals, especially those born prematurely and those of the Arabian breed, have domed foreheads.

The CNS signs observed are referable to pressure-induced attenuation of cerebral white matter. Most conspicuous are such mental disorders as diminished learning ability, lack of affinity for the dam, and reduced or absent desire or ability to suckle. If the signs progress, the foal may develop menace response deficits, loss of vision and profound depression. Animals that survive for extended periods are regarded as "dummies," and are difficult to train and often unthrifty.[161]

Diagnosis: Plain lateral radiographs may show a characteristic homogeneous, "ground-glass" appearance of the cranial cavity.[161] Direct lateral ventricular centesis may be performed at a point 1-2 cm lateral to the intersection of lines drawn from each bony auditory canal to the lateral canthus of the opposite eye. After surgical preparation, a needle with stylet is introduced through a hole in the skull made by a guarded Steinmann pin. Easily aspirated fluid indicates probable enlargement of the lateral ventricle. Air can be introduced into the ventricle after removal of a small amount (10-20 ml) of CSF to help outline the ventricular system radiographically.

Treatment: In hydrocephalic foals, the brain may be accessible to ultrasound examination through widely open sutures, and computed tomography can define the extent of ventricular enlargement. The treatment of hydrocephalus depends on the cause. Specific medical or surgical treatment for hydrocephalus is not recommended, and euthanasia must be considered, depending on the severity of signs.

Diseases With Physical Causes

Cerebral Trauma

Signs referable to cerebral damage most frequently occur after trauma to the frontal or parietal regions of the head. This may be the fate of an overly inquisitive foal that is kicked by an older animal or of an unruly or frightened horse that runs into a post or wall projection. Unfortunately, it also is seen in horses that have been clubbed by an impatient or brutal handler. Signs that occur acutely after a blow to the head result from mechanical injury to brain tissue, edema that develops around a contusion or hematoma, hemorrhage into brain parenchyma, and ischemia produced by brain swelling and intravascular clotting.[162] In adult horses with cerebral trauma but no skull fracture, mechanical injury and edema are the most important mechanisms causing CNS signs. Neonates are more likely to have significant intracranial bleeding. In all horses, compound fractures of the frontal or parietal bones may cause cerebral laceration and hemorrhage.

There may be an initial period of unconsciousness from which the horse awakens in minutes to hours. Subsequent neurologic signs tend to fluctuate with the degree of intracranial hypertension associated with cerebral edema and hemorrhage. Affected horses usually are depressed and may wander in circles toward the side of the damaged cerebral hemisphere. Characteristically, there is blindness and sometimes decreased facial sensation contralaterally. This latter sign is best appreciated by stimulating the nasal septum or ears. Pupillary light responses should be brisk, though there may be some asymmetry and fluctuation of the pupils, and a tendency toward miosis. Apart from depressed menace responses and apparent lingual paresis, all other cranial nerve responses should be intact. Obvious signs of ataxia usually are not seen. Gait abnormalities suggest progressive involvement of other parts of the brain. Genuine seizure activity or random, uncontrolled thrashing and paddling most often is seen in delirious or semicomatose recumbent horses, and is difficult to accurately correlate with the site of brain lesion. True seizures in horses probably indicate a forebrain lesion. If the cerebral hemispheres swell sufficiently, they can herniate caudally against the midbrain (subtentorial herniation) to cause such signs as dilated, unresponsive pupils.

Development of such a midbrain syndrome is an unfavorable prognostic sign (see Diseases of the Brainstem and Cranial Nerves). In most cases, however, recognition of an uncomplicated cerebral syndrome warrants an optimistic prognosis, once the patient is able to walk. Injury to the cerebral hemispheres is far less critical than brainstem damage, and response to treatment for brain swelling usually is good.

Unless there is clear radiographic evidence of a condition requiring surgical intervention (*eg,* depressed skull fracture), early

Table 4. Anticonvulsant drugs used to treat seizure disorders in horses. Though these drugs have been used with success, several are not licensed for use in horses. These doses should be regarded as guidelines only, and drugs should be given to effect. Smaller doses may be equally effective. It is most appropriate to monitor blood concentrations of all anticonvulsant drugs during maintenance therapy.

	Drug	50-kg Foal	450-kg Horse
Initial Therapy	Diazepam[a]	5-20 mg IV per dose	25-100 mg IV per dose
	Pentobarbital	150-100 mg IV to effect	To effect
	Phenobarbital	250-1000 mg slowly IV	2000-mg doses
	Phenytoin	200-500 mg IV per dose	
	Chloral hydrate (with or without magnesium sulfate and a barbiturate)	3-10 g IV to effect	15-60 g IV to effect
	Xylazine	25-50 mg IV or IM per dose	300-500 mg IV or IM per dose
	Guaifenesin (with or without barbiturate)	IV to effect	40-60 g IV to effect
Maintenance	Phenobarbital	100-500 mg PO, BID to TID	1000-3000 mg PO, BID to TID
	Phenytoin	100-250 mg PO BID	1-5 g PO BID (low therapeutic index)

a — Do not leave in plastic container or syringe for more than a few minutes or drug may become inactivated.

management is supportive and medical. The main objective of medical treatment is to reduce or minimize brain swelling. Life-threatening conditions, such as a blocked airway, severe bleeding, fractured ribs with a ruptured lung or cardiac arrhythmia, should be treated immediately. Seizures may be controlled with 5 mg (foal) to 100 mg (adult) of diazepam, repeated as necessary. Intractable seizures or unmanageable delirious thrashing may require sedative to anesthetic doses of chloral hydrate, glycerol guaiacolate with thiamylal sodium, or sodium pentobarbital. Phenobarbital or phenytoin can be used for long-term control of seizures (Table 4). Xylazine must be used cautiously, as it causes transient hypertension that may exacerbate CNS hemorrhage, and it suppresses ventilation.

Horses with definitive, abnormal CNS signs after cranial trauma should probably receive dexamethasone (or equivalent) at 0.1-0.25 mg/kg body weight within 6 hours of the traumatic incident. This should decrease edema formation and CSF production in several hours. The dose can be repeated every 4-6 hours for 1-4 days. Clinicians should be mindful of the immunosuppressive effects of corticosteroid treatment, especially in foals. Also, it should be recognized that cerebral edema is only one component of head injuries. Many conditions, such as hemorrhage, contusion, laceration, necrosis, associated midbrain lesion and secondary ischemia, are relatively inaccessible to therapy. Nevertheless, horses presented in a coma or semicoma should receive a slow IV infusion of DMSO at 1 g/kg body weight as a 20% solution in 5% dextrose. Intravenous use of DMSO is not approved for horses, and its effects have not been fully evaluated in neonatal foals; however, in research animals, it has decreased CNS edema, reduced platelet aggregation, maintained vascular integrity, scavenged oxygen radicals and increased O_2 availability to the tissues.[163] Improvement may be seen as quickly as 30 minutes after IV infusion.

Dimethyl sulfoxide administration can be repeated every 12-24 hours for up to 4 days, if it results in clinical improvement. Alternatively, hyperosmolar solutions, such as mannitol, can be given to decrease brain edema. Mannitol is given as a 20% solution by slow IV infusion at 0.25 g/kg body weight and can be repeated every 6-12 hours for up to 24 hours. Intracranial bleeding, especially subdural, may be exacerbated by mannitol, so hyperosmolar diuretics probably should be avoided in neonates because of the high incidence of hemorrhage and electrolyte imbalances in this age group. Subdural hematomas are very difficult to diagnose, but fortunately are rare. Furosemide and other renal diuretics may be useful when used in conjunction with dexamethasone, but because of their potential for causing fluid and electrolyte abnormalities, these agents should be used with caution. Continuous pentobarbital-induced anesthesia has shown considerable promise in reducing intracranial hypertension in human patients but has not been evaluated in horses.[164]

Hypoxemia and hypercapnia should be avoided. Reduced arterial pO_2 exacerbates brain swelling, and an elevated pCO_2 increases intracranial blood volume and pressure.[165] The airway must remain patent. Recumbent horses should be rolled to the opposite side often so as to minimize pulmonary arteriovenous shunting and ventilation-perfusion abnormalities. Humidified 100% O_2 may be given via a nasal tube or mask. If possible, the head should be kept at heart-base level or higher to avoid hypostatic intracranial congestion.

Other supportive treatment includes maintenance of hydration and correction of electrolyte and acid-base abnormalities. Overhydration must be avoided, as it can exacerbate brain edema. Fever that may result from violent activity increases brain O_2 consumption and edema. It should be treated with alcohol baths, sedatives and antipyretic drugs. Lubricant ointments should be used on the corneas of recumbent horses.

Monitoring is very important, and constant reevaluation is necessary to assess response to treatment. If there is improvement within 6-8 hours, treatment should be repeated. If there is deterioration or no improvement, more aggressive medical or surgical treatment should be considered. Exploratory craniotomy often is the only way to identify and deal with serious (*eg*, parenchymal or subdural) bleeding. Decompressive procedures can be performed.[166] As decompressive procedures become more widely used in horses, they may become an important early component in management of severe head injuries. If a comatose patient does not improve or continues to deteriorate for 36 hours after injury or surgery, euthanasia usually is indicated.

Intracarotid Injection

The close proximity of the common carotid artery to the jugular vein makes accidental intracarotid injection a very real hazard. The injected material may travel in the carotid distribution to the ipsilateral forebrain to cause acute cerebral disturbance. A violent reaction typically occurs within 5-30 seconds from the time of injection. Initial signs range from apprehension with a wide-eyed expression and sudden facial twitching, head-shaking, kicking and running, to recumbency and loss of consciousness for a variable period.

With xylazine, acepromazine and other water-soluble drugs, horses usually regain consciousness within an hour, and completely recover usually within a week. Marked cardiovascular changes, such as bradycardia, arrhythmias and blood pressure fluctuations, may accompany CNS signs. Consistent but frequently overlooked findings during the recovery period are decreased facial (nasal septum) sensation, blindness and deficient menace response, all contralateral to the injection site. These findings reflect cerebral damage.

Intracarotid injection of procaine penicillin, phenylbutazone and other oil-based or insoluble drugs warrants a much worse prognosis. Intractable seizures, coma or stupor often necessitate euthanasia after intracarotid injection of such drugs.

The morphologic changes caused by accidental injection are typical of acute cerebral ischemia and include marked edema, vascular endothelial damage, hemorrhage and neuronal degeneration.

Treatment is largely symptomatic. Appropriate padding and sedation are indicated for thrashing, delirious horses. With severe cerebral edema and brainstem compression, medical decompression of the CNS should be attempted. Use of mannitol may be contraindicated because of concomitant cerebral hemorrhage, but dexamethasone at 0.1-0.25 mg/kg body weight, DMSO at 1 g/kg and anticonvulsant therapy may be useful. Atropine IV at 0.04 mg/kg may reverse severe bradycardia and arrhythmia accompanying rapid injection of xylazine.

Inflammatory, Infectious and Immune Diseases

Diseases Affecting Multiple Sites

These inflammatory, infectious and immune diseases are discussed above under Diseases of Multiple or Unknown Sites.

Cerebral Abscess

Cerebral abscesses occur sporadically in horses and are most common during epizootics of *Streptococcus equi* (strangles) infection.[167] Such abscesses may be clinically silent, associated with overt meningitis, or cause signs of a space-occupying cerebral lesion. The cerebral hemispheres have a considerable capacity to accommodate slow-growing, large masses but signs of cerebral disease become apparent with sufficient compression and attenuation of cerebral tissue.

The onset of neurologic signs may be acute or insidious, and often the clinical course is characterized by marked fluctuations in the severity of signs. Most obvious are behavioral changes such as depression, head-pressing, aimless wandering or sudden unprovoked excitement. Affected horses may circle or stand with the head and neck directed toward the side of the abscessed cerebral hemisphere. This may progress to episodes of unconsciousness, recumbency and seizures. Consistent early signs are contralateral impaired vision, deficient menace response and decreased facial (nasal septal) sensation. Later there may be signs of brainstem compression, such as asymmetric pupillary constriction, ataxia and weakness.

The condition must be distinguished from other causes of asymmetric cerebral disease, such as protozoal myeloencephalitis, trauma, aberrant parasite migration, parasitic thromboembolism and cholesterol granuloma. Diagnosis is based largely on such aspects as prior strangles infection and the clinical syndrome. Elevations of plasma fibrinogen and globulin concentrations and peripheral WBC count should be expected. Changes in CSF depend on the degree of meningeal or ependymal involvement. In most cases, there is xanthochromia and moderate elevation of CSF protein levels, reflecting cerebral compression and damage.

Numbers of inflammatory cells (particularly neutrophils) in the CSF are elevated only if there is associated meningitis or ependymitis.

If the signs of cerebral abscess are acute, severe and rapidly progressive, brain edema likely is present, and corticosteroids should be given repeatedly until signs stabilize. Otherwise, therapy is based on prolonged use of large doses of appropriate antimicrobial drugs. For a cerebral abscess caused by *Strep equi*, a suggested treatment regimen is potassium or sodium penicillin at 100,000-400,000 IU/kg body weight divided in 4 daily doses for 1-2 weeks, followed by IM procaine penicillin at 22,000 IU/kg body weight every 12 hours for at least 4 more weeks. The addition of rifampin therapy (5-10 mg/kg PO SID) is worth considering.

Though antimicrobial therapy resolves most cases of cerebral abscess in people, results in horses have been poor.[168] An alternative approach is surgical evacuation of the lesion.[166] With careful surgical technique, contents of a cerebral abscess might be aspirated via a small trephine hole if the location of the abscess is known. A *Strep equi* abscess was successfully treated in this way after localization by computed tomography.[169] Recovered horses may have residual deficits, such as impaired vision and decreased facial sensation contralaterally.

Metabolic Diseases

Hepatoencephalopathy

Hepatoencephalopathy (walking disease, walkabout, sleepy staggers) is a clinical syndrome characterized by abnormal mentation in horses with severe hepatic insufficiency due to liver disease or portosystemic shunts. (Other aspects of liver disease in horses, including causes of liver failure, are discussed in detail in the chapter on Diseases of the Alimentary System.)

Numerous abnormalities have been implicated in development of hepatoencephalopathy. Hepatic dysfunction leads to systemic accumulation of ammonia, short-chain fatty acids, mercaptans, indoles, skatoles and gamma amino butyric acid (GABA).[170] Brain levels of these substances may further be increased by altered permeability of the blood-brain barrier. There also is a shift in the ratio in serum of branched-chain amino acids (valine, leucine, isoleucine) to aromatic amino acids (phenylalanine, tryptophan, tyrosine). This ratio normally is about 4.0, but is reduced to 1.0-1.4 in horses with hepatoencephalopathy.[171] Definitive data have not yet been brought forth relating any single abnormality to all cases of hepatoencephalopathy.

The signs of hepatoencephalopathy are referable to diffuse cerebral impairment. Depression and inappetence typically are the first signs. An affected horse may stand for hours with its head hanging, periodically jerking its head upward for no discernible reason. There is repeated yawning, grimacing or twitching of the muzzle and lips. Somnolent periods, marked by head-pressing in a corner or leaning against a stall wall, may alternate with periods of compulsive walking, during which the horse is oblivious to its surroundings and obstacles in its path. Obviously such a horse will not respond appropriately to handling, and occasional horses may even become aggressive or maniacal. As the disease progresses, diminished menace responses and visual impairment are common. Generalized seizures and coma occur terminally after a course of hours to months, depending on the cause.

The diagnosis usually is suspected from the history and clinical signs and can be confirmed by laboratory findings indicative of liver failure. The ammonia tolerance test can be used to confirm a diagnosis of liver failure and hepatoencephalopathy.[172] The prognosis for horses with hepatoencephalopathy is poor to hopeless. Usually there is irreparable hepatic damage at the time of onset of CNS signs; nevertheless, occasional recoveries from hepatoencephalopathy have been recorded.

Treatment generally is empirical and supportive. Correction of hypoglycemia with IV glucose may improve mentation and provide calories. In selected cases, such as in sublethal acute hepatic necrosis (*eg*, Theiler's disease, ferrous fumarate poisoning in foals), it may be worth providing some nutritional support IV to allow time for liver regeneration. Glucose can be infused initially as 10% dextrose in a balanced electrolyte solution. The glucose concentration can be increased in increments over days to a maximum of 40%. Glucose concentration or rate of infusion should be reduced if the blood glucose level exceeds 250 mg/dl or if glucose spills into the urine for more than several hours. These solutions may be supplemented with water-soluble vitamins (especially thiamin). Intravenous amino acids should be used with caution, as they may increase blood ammonia levels. Too little is known about the effects of IV lipids in horses with liver failure to recommend their use.

During the acute phase of the disease, an effort can be made to minimize the gut absorption of protein breakdown products, such as ammonia and mercaptans. At a minimum, mineral oil can be given to help eliminate intestinal contents, which are the substrate for microbial action and production of neuroactive substances (*eg,* ammonia). Use of neomycin (10 g QID in a 450-kg horse) to reduce colonic microflora often has been advocated, but results have been disappointing.[173] In people, nonabsorbable polyalcohols, such as lactulose and sorbitol, are given PO to acidify colonic contents and trap ammonia intraluminally.[174] This form of therapy has not been investigated in horses. If a horse with hepatoencephalopathy survives the acute phase of the disease, it probably is wise to try to provide a palatable diet that is low in protein and high in carbohydrate (*eg,* grass hay/citrus or beet pulp).

Finally, a number of treatments have been reported that either lack adequate rationale or evidence of efficacy. These include IV glutamate, corticosteroids, oral choline and oral branched-chain amino acids.

Hypoglycemia

Blood glucose levels of <40-50 mg/dl may result in weakness, depression and ataxia. Signs may progress to loss of consciousness. In contrast to other species, seizure activity is uncommon in hypoglycemic horses, though seizures occur sometimes in hypoglycemic foals. Untreated hypoglycemia may lead to severe irreversible brain damage. Ischemic neuronal cell change similar to that of cerebral hypoxia is the principal lesion of hypoglycemia.[175] Neurons of the cerebral cortex are most severely affected, resulting in either laminar or focal involvement. Hypoglycemia may result from excessive utilization (sepsis or exhaustion), inadequate intake (starvation), reduced production and mobilization (glycogen depletion or inadequate gluconeogenesis) or disordered regulation of glucose.

In horses, hypoglycemia is encountered most often in neonates, usually as a complication of sepsis or prematurity. Horses with end-stage liver failure or Addisonian syndrome after withdrawal of corticosteroids also may have blood glucose levels of <40 mg/dl.

Signs of hypoglycemia are readily reversed by IV or oral glucose. In neonatal foals, the recommended glucose dosage is 200 mg/kg given initially over 1-2 minutes (90 ml of 10% dextrose in a 45-kg foal), followed by 4-8 mg/kg/minute (100-200 ml of 10% glucose/hour in a 45-kg foal).[176] Bolus administration of hypertonic glucose solutions (*eg,* 50% dextrose) should be avoided, as rapid changes in serum osmolality may exacerbate CNS derangements. Also, rebound hypoglycemia frequently results 40-90 minutes after rapid infusion of concentrated dextrose solutions. Continued IV glucose therapy must be guided by serial measurements of blood glucose levels. Rates of infusion and/or glucose concentration should be reduced incrementally if the blood glucose concentration exceeds 250 mg/dl.

Hypoxemia-Ischemia

The brain (and other nervous tissue) has a high and continuous demand for oxygen. For this reason, nervous tissue is extremely vulnerable to impaired oxygen delivery resulting from hypoxemia or ischemia. The immediate clinical effects of oxygen deprivation probably are due to poorly defined alterations in neurotransmitter function. However, this phase quickly is overshadowed by the effects of altered carbohydrate and energy metabolism.[177] Anaerobic glycolysis depletes brain glucose, reduces energy production, and results in localized lactic acidosis. The ensuing neuronal swelling and edema may exacerbate ischemia and further reduce delivery of oxygen and glucose to cells. Abnormal fluxes of calcium and other ions and accumulation of toxic oxygen radicals precede irreversible cell damage and neuronal death.[177]

Degrees of edema, neuronal necrosis and cavitation occur in particular brain areas of different species. Which areas are preferentially affected by hypoxemia-ischemia in horses is not clear, though the basal nuclei, lateral thalamus, caudal colliculi and frontal parietal and occipital cerebral cortex have been involved in a few cases.[178]

The clinical manifestations of these changes depend on whether all or part of the CNS is affected. Interruption of the blood supply to a portion of the CNS (localized hypoxia) causes signs referable to loss of function of that part. Examples include intracarotid injections, verminous thromboembolism, aortic thrombosis and fibrocartilaginous emboli. These conditions are discussed in detail elsewhere in this book. When the entire CNS is acutely deprived of oxygen (systemic hypoxia), the clinical signs initially are those of impaired cerebral function, *ie*, depression leading to coma and seizures. Depending on the rapidity with which hypoxia develops, horses may lose consciousness when the arterial PO_2 falls below 30 torr.

Systemic hypoxia in horses theoretically may be associated with reduced oxygen tension in inspired air (*eg*, at high altitude). However, most cases of cerebral oxygen deprivation result from respiratory insufficiency. Neonatal respiratory distress syndrome, pulmonary edema, right-to-left cardiac or extracardiac shunts, and pneumonia each may interfere with efficient oxygen exchange at the level of the alveolus. Airway obstruction, pleural effusion, pneumothorax or botulism can cause hypoxemia by reducing pulmonary ventilation. Severe anemia, blood loss, carbon monoxide poisoning and methemoglobinemia (*eg*, red maple leaf poisoning) usually do not affect arterial PO_2 but cause oxygen deprivation by reducing the oxygen-carrying capacity of the blood. Cyanide poisoning (*eg*, some *Sorghum* spp poisoning) prevents oxygen utilization by tissues. Finally, severe hypotension associated with hemorrhagic, septic, anaphylactic or cardiac shock reduces CNS oxygenation by effects on CNS perfusion.

Hypoxic-ischemic brain damage probably is one of the principal factors in development of neonatal maladjustment syndrome discussed above.

Effective treatment of hypoxia-ischemia depends on correction of the underlying problem. Most horses with systemic hypoxia benefit from nasal insufflation of humidified oxygen. Though evidence of their efficacy in this setting still is lacking, use of corticosteroids (dexamethasone at 0.1-0.25 mg/kg) and DMSO (1 g/kg as 20% in 5% dextrose) should be considered for treatment of the edema and inflammation associated with CNS hypoxia-ischemia.

Miscellaneous Metabolic Derangements

Neurologic syndromes associated with hyponatremia (water intoxication) and hypernatremia and other metabolic defects have been described in other species but are not clearly defined in horses. Signs in horses and foals with marked hyponatremia (<110 mEq/L) associated with profound diarrhea, gastroduodenal ulceration, ruptured urinary bladder or acute renal failure occasionally progress from depression to coma and seizures. The sodium shifts may be involved in the neurologic signs in these cases. Marked derangements of other metabolic processes may be associated with coma and seizures in horses, but precise syndromes have not been described.

Toxic Diseases

Metaldehyde Poisoning

Horses may accidentally consume metaldehyde when it is incorporated into bran mash and distributed as a slug bait. Limited clinical evidence indicates that horses are very sensitive to the lethal effects of metaldehyde.[179] Signs of poisoning have included generalized sweating, muscle fasciculations and chronic spasms, incoordination and rapid respiratory and heart rates. Death occurred within 7 hours of metaldehyde ingestion in 3 affected horses.

Miscellaneous Toxicities

See the section entitled Diseases of Multiple or Unknown Sites for a full discussion on this topic.

Leukoencephalomalacia

The syndrome of leukoencephalomalacia (moldy corn poisoning) probably was first described in the United States in 1850 and has since been associated with many sporadic cases and several major outbreaks of fatal disease.[180,181] The best known outbreak occurred in Illinois, Iowa and other midwestern states in 1934 and 1935, and resulted in the death of over 5000 horses, mules and donkeys. Circumstantial clinical evidence and experimental studies during the 1934 outbreak pointed to moldy corn or cornstalk ingestion as the cause of leukoencephalomalacia. Since then, it has been established that contamination of feed by *Fusarium* spp fungi is the usual cause of leukoencephalo-malacia.[180,181] However, the specific causative mycotoxin remains to be identified.

Fusarium moniliforme by far is the most commonly incriminated species, though *F tricinctum* was associated with an episode of leukoencephalomalacia in which 12 horses died.[182-184] Because cool humid conditions favor growth of *Fusarium* spp, leukoencephalomalacia occurs seasonally from late fall to early spring. Though it is commonly associated with water-damaged moldy corn, *F moniliforme* also may contaminate commercially prepared feedstuffs. In a series of cases in North Carolina, the fungus was isolated from both the corn and oat components of pelleted and nonpelleted commercial feeds.[181]

Toxicosis due to *F moniliforme* frequently has components of both leukoencephalo-malacia and hepatic necrosis, with the relative importance of brain or liver lesions depending upon the dosage and duration of intake.[185] Clinical signs of leukoencephalo-malacia are first seen acutely 2-24 weeks (average 3 weeks) after the initial ingestion of moldy corn. In general, the initial signs are referable to cerebral lesions and include depression, unresponsiveness, head-pressing, circling, aimless wandering, blindness and, occasionally, unprovoked excitement and frenzy. The signs frequently are asymmetric. Further progression may be associated with pharyngeal paralysis, incoordination and, finally, recumbency, paddling, coma and death. Mortality in reported outbreaks has varied from 40% to 84%.[180-185] The clinical course usually is one to a few days but may be much longer in horses that recover.

Horses with uncomplicated leukoenceph-alomalacia are not usually febrile, a fact that helps distinguish this disease from arboviral encephalomyelitides. Results of CSF analysis may be normal but may include neutrophilic pleocytosis.[186]

The lesions seen grossly at necropsy usually are diagnostic and consist of focal areas of liquefactive hemorrhagic necrosis in the white matter of one or both cerebral hemispheres (up to several centimeters in diameter). Malacic areas within the gray or white matter of the brainstem and spinal cord are less frequently encountered but may be expected in cases marked by profound weakness and ataxia. Eosinophil infiltration may be an unusual characteristic of the necrotic lesion.

Treatment of affected horses is only supportive. Contaminated feed should be removed from exposed horses and an effort made to eliminate toxin already in the alimentary tract by use of laxatives and activated charcoal. Corticosteroids and nonsteroidal antiinflammatory agents probably should be given, but their effectiveness is not expected to be very good. Anticonvulsant therapy is indicated to control seizure activity.

Neoplasia

Primary Neoplasms

Primary neoplasms of the nervous system are very uncommon in horses. General conclusions regarding the relative incidence and behavior of such tumors cannot be drawn easily. Nervous system neoplasms may be classified according to their origin as tumors of nerve cells, neuroepithelium, glia, peripheral nerves and nerve sheaths, mesodermal structures, and endocrine organs. Readers are referred to the previous edition of this book for references before 1981.[187] More recent reports are cited below within the text.

A single sympathetic ganglioneuroma (also containing cells of glial type) apparently is the only neoplasm of nerve-cell origin reported in horses.[187] Tumors of neuroepithelial origin have included ependymoma, choroid plexus papilloma, neuroepithelial tumor of the optic nerve, malignant medulloepithelioma and pineoblastoma.[187-189] Among glial-cell neoplasms described in horses are optic disc astrocytoma, retinoblastoma and microglioma.[187] Neoplasms of peripheral nerves and nerve sheaths may be more common than CNS neoplasms. In a survey of 11 North American university veterinary hospitals, all nervous tissue tumors found in horses involved peripheral nerves. Most reported peripheral nerve neoplasms have been neurofibromas or neurofibrosarcomas.[187] Neurofibromas often are found cutaneously. The most common sites are the pectoral region, abdomen, neck and face.[187]

The most common mesodermal neoplasm is the meningioma. Neoplastic reticulosis, lipoma in the mesencephalic aqueduct, angioma in the cervical spinal cord, and melanoblastoma of the cerebellar meninges also have been described.[187]

Adenoma of the pars intermedia of the pituitary gland is common; however, any clinical signs observed usually are referable to endocrine dysfunction. Benign neoplasms of the pineal gland (pinealomas) have been reported occasionally.[187]

Secondary Neoplasms

Secondary neoplasms may penetrate the cranial vault or vertebrae, grow through osseous foramina, or reach the nervous system by vascular metastasis. Resulting clinical signs are due to pressure-induced destruction, direct invasion and/or compromise of blood supply to nervous tissue. Extraneural tumors also may infiltrate or encroach upon peripheral nerves.

Lymphosarcoma is the most common secondary neoplasm affecting the nervous system of horses. This tumor has been found in the epidural space (usually thoracic or lumbar) as a cause of compressive myelopathy, in the brain and olfactory tracts, and infiltrated into various peripheral nerves.[187,190] Similar signs of compressive spinal cord disease were caused by metastasis to the epidural space of a malignant pheochromocytoma in a 6-month-old foal.[191]

Melanomas occasionally invade the CNS of white or gray horses. Usually these tumors are found in the epidural space after contiguous spread from melanomatous sublumbar lymph nodes.[187,192] Melanomas of the spinal meninges and brain also have occurred after metastasis of cutaneous melanomas.[187]

Among sarcomas, hemangiosarcomas generally are considered to metastasize more frequently to the brain. Two such cases in horses have been reported.[187] An undifferentiated sarcoma, originating in the mediastinum of an 8-year-old horse, caused signs of spinal cord compression after invasion into the vertebral bodies of T9 and T10.[189]

Adenocarcinomas and carcinomas may invade the brain by direct spread from a primary site, such as the nose or paranasal sinuses, or by metastasis from a distant site, such as the adrenal gland.[187,193] Tumors of bone, such as the osteoma or osteosarcoma, or of bone marrow, such as the plasma-cell myeloma, involving the skull or vertebrae can compress the brain or spinal cord.[187,194]

Malformation Tumors

Malformation tumors include epidermoids, dermoids, teratomas and teratoids. These growths originate from heterotopic tissues that usually lie close to embryonic lines of closure.

Epidermoid cysts (epidermoid cholesteatomas) are slowly enlarging, encapsulated structures that arise from ectopic epithelial tissue during embryonic development. These tumors usually are situated near the midline in the angle between the cerebrum and cerebellum. Epidermoid cysts usually are incidental necropsy findings but occasionally grow large enough to cause CNS signs.[187] There also are a number of reports of intracranial tooth heterotopias, which are not true teratomas. A true teratoma has been described, though the identification was somewhat questionable.[187]

Multifactorial Diseases

Juvenile Epilepsy

This condition occurs in otherwise normal foals from several weeks to several months of age.[195] Seizures begin without warning and occur repeatedly for days or weeks, then abate with or without treatment. Mild generalized seizures with lip retraction and jaw-clamping movements ("chewing gum fits") and sudden deranged physical activity may progress to severe generalized seizures with loss of consciousness, opisthotonus, abnormal head and eye movements, and clonic convulsions. Affected foals typically pitch forward during an attack and traumatize the mucosae of their retracted lips; this finding can be a useful diagnostic aid. Juvenile epilepsy occurs more frequently in Arabians than in foals of other breeds. Rather than being a true inherited epilepsy, juvenile epilepsy may reflect a relatively low seizure threshold that increases sensitivity to many temporary toxic, infectious, metabolic and physical perturbations.

Though affected foals usually "grow out of" juvenile epilepsy without treatment, anticonvulsant therapy (Table 4) should be instituted at the first signs and maintained for several weeks to months. Repeated severe seizures that are not treated can result both in a disturbing postictal cerebral syndrome ("dummy" or "wanderer") and neuronal death, and further, possibly permanent, seizure foci. Any underlying problem that may initiate seizure activity (*eg,* fever) should be corrected. Dummy foals should be fed by nasogastric tube until normal mentation and suckling responses return. In the absence of further seizures, this usually occurs within several days. Central blindness may be a prominent component of the postictal phase and may last up to a week in young affected foals.

Acquired Epilepsy

The term *acquired epilepsy* refers to syndromes of recurrent seizure activity exhibited by horses assumed to have developed an intracranial epileptogenic focus (or foci) during postnatal life. This focus, which may or may not be associated with a morbid lesion, is the nucleating site for the rapidly spreading, paroxysmal neuronal discharges clinically evident as seizures. The epileptogenic site (or sites), located in the cerebral cortex, may become active after the horse has recovered from a cerebral insult due to inflammation, injury or hypoxia. The interval between brain disease and the onset of seizure activity often is months to years; this has been described as the period of "epileptogenic ripening." In affected horses, there is no history of brain damage or evidence of current disease. These cases usually are referred to as *idiopathic epilepsy.*

Seizures may occur without warning or be preceded by a transient change in the horse's behavior (*eg,* wide-eyed apprehension, vocalization). Similar changes are likely before each attack. Seizures may be partial, with signs localizing the lesion to one side, such as facial or limb twitching on one side, or they may be generalized. Generalized seizures usually result in recumbency, rapid eye and jaw movements, opisthotonus and violent paddling or convulsive movements of the limbs. Generalized autonomic discharge causes salivation, pupillary dilation, and uncontrolled urination and defecation. Partial seizures may progress to secondary generalized seizures. Occasionally, just behavioral signs are seen, such as compulsive running in a circle or violent self-mutilation. Seizures generally last no more than a minute and, in the case of generalized seizures, the animal regains its feet within several minutes. Transient postictal signs may range from slight

depression to stupor and blindness, usually lasting a few hours in adults.

It is much more important and usually safer to prevent the next seizure in an epileptic horse than to treat the current one, unless the horse is in *status epilepticus,* or continuous seizure activity. A generalized seizure is violent, potentially dangerous and usually short in duration. An exception is epileptic seizures in foals. These animals can be restrained manually and usually treated medically (Table 4).

A detailed and comprehensive history should be obtained regarding the epileptic horse. The history may indicate activities or conditions that consistently provoke seizures. Estrus, changes in lighting, feeding and other stimuli have provoked seizures in epileptic horses. The history also indicates whether the attacks are becoming more or less frequent and severe. Under controlled conditions, it may be helpful to provoke a seizure. Nonneurologic and neurologic diseases causing seizures or seizure-like signs must be ruled out by a proper diagnostic workup.

Because acquired epilepsy is so varied in its presentation, treatment is individualized. If seizures are very mild, infrequent or declining in frequency, no treatment may be necessary. If a particular activity induces seizures, obviously that activity should be avoided, if practical. With estrus-associated seizures, progesterone treatment or even ovariectomy may be curative. When epileptic seizures cannot be avoided by management changes or are severe or frequent, antiepileptic treatment should be instituted and maintained (Table 4). After a period of at least 3 months without attacks, the drug dose can be reduced gradually over another 3 months, with increases as necessary if seizures recur. Preventive doses of these drugs generally do not cause neurologic side effects but may change the activity of other common drugs, such as phenylbutazone.[196]

Idiopathic Diseases

Cholesterol Granuloma

Cholesterol granulomas (cholesteatomas) are found in the choroid plexuses of 15-20% of old horses.[197] They are more frequent in the plexuses of the fourth ventricle than in the lateral ventricles; however, those in the lateral ventricles are more likely to become large and cause clinical signs. They may represent a chronic granulomatous reaction to cholesterol crystal deposition associated with chronic vascular leakage. Mature cholesterol granulomas generally are circumscribed, firm, granular and yellowish-brown, with a glistening pear-like appearance on cut surface. Most of these masses remain clinically silent, but some grow large enough to compress brain tissue directly or block CSF drainage and cause obstructive hydrocephalus. Cholesterol granulomas often occur bilaterally, but one is usually larger.

Associated clinical signs are very rare and typically insidious in onset. Signs may be intermittent but usually are progressive, asymmetric and referable to impaired cerebral cortical function. Early reports often described affected horses as "stupid" or "confused."[198] One well-documented case was in a 7-year-old Arabian mare that experienced several brief attacks of ataxia, weakness, recumbency and unconsciousness in the previous 2 years.[199] Before a particularly severe episode, the mare circled to the right and had a reduced menace response and facial hypalgesia on the left side. These signs could be explained clinically by a right-sided cerebral lesion. At necropsy, a large (4-cm-diameter) cholesterol granuloma was found within the right lateral ventricle, associated with severe cortical atrophy. A CSF sample was markedly xanthochromic and had a very elevated protein content (322 mg/dl). Temporary improvement of signs may be expected with corticosteroid treatment.

Cholesterol granulomas of the choroid plexus must be distinguished from the much more rare and histologically unrelated epidermoid cholesteatomas.

DISEASES OF THE BRAINSTEM AND CRANIAL NERVES (AUTONOMIC AND SOMATIC)

Diagnostic and Therapeutic Considerations

Dysphagia

Dysphagia is often defined as "difficult swallowing" but, in this section, it is used in its broadest sense to mean difficulty in eating or drinking and includes disorders of prehension, mastication and swallowing. Only primary neurologic dysphagia is discussed; dysphagia from other causes is covered in other chapters.

Central control of eating is mostly by specific medullary centers and their afferent and efferent pathways in the trigeminal (V, muscles of mastication, facial sensation), facial (VII, muscles of the lips and cheeks), glossopharyngeal and vagus (IX and X, pharynx, larynx), and hypoglossal (XII, tongue) nerves. The voluntary effort in eating and drinking is initiated in the cerebral motor cortex and basal nuclei. Therefore, disorders of the forebrain, medulla and cranial nerves V, VII, IX, X and XII can cause dysphagia.

Forebrain diseases do not cause actual paralysis of the muscles involved in eating but can impair voluntary control of these muscles, resulting in uncoordinated, dystonic and/or weak movements of the face, tongue, mouth and pharynx.

Diffuse cerebral disease can cause dysphagia in addition to other gross behavioral and attitudinal abnormalities (*eg,* depression, head-pressing, circling, blindness). Characteristically, there is some weakness and protrusion of the tongue, drooping of the lower lip, and drooling of saliva. Foals lose the suckling reflex. Included in this group are the arboviral encephalitides, rabies, hepatoencephalopathy, diffuse meningitis, neonatal maladjustment syndrome, head trauma with brain swelling, leukoencephalomalacia and hydrocephalus.

Dysphagia caused by lesions of the basal nuclei occurs commonly in the western United States as a result of yellow star thistle or Russian knapweed poisoning (see Nigropallidal Encephalomalacia) but also can be caused by the focal lesions of protozoal myeloencephalitis or migrating nematode larvae. Prehension and mastication are impaired, but affected animals can usually swallow. Other brain signs may be mild or absent.

The signs of dysphagia seen with medullary lesions depend on the specific cranial nerve nuclei affected. Manifestations of various cranial nerve deficits affecting eating are discussed below. There usually are other, often asymmetric signs of medullary disease, such as depression (reticular system), gait deficits (motor and proprioceptive tracts) and other cranial nerve signs (*eg,* vestibular, facial). Specific causes include protozoal myeloencephalitis, migrating parasites, and trauma to the back of the head with medullary hemorrhage. Diffuse brain diseases with a medullary component, such as the togaviral encephalitides, rabies, meningitis, locoweed poisoning and hepatoencephalopathy, also are included here.

Bilateral involvement of the motor branches of the trigeminal nerve (cranial nerve V) causes paralysis and eventually atrophy of the masseter muscles (also of the temporals, pterygoids and distal bellies of the digastricus muscles). The resulting weak jaw tone causes difficulty in mastication and allows the tongue to hang from the mouth. Unilateral trigeminal paralysis does not cause significant dysphagia but may result in slight deviation of the jaw away from the affected side. Damage to the sensory branches of cranial nerve V from the face and mouth does not produce severe dysphagia but may cause food accumulation in the cheeks.

Paralysis of the lips due to facial nerve damage (cranial nerve VII) causes minor problems in prehension of food, especially pasture or grain. Saliva may dribble from the labial commissure, and food often adheres to the gingivae and lips.

Bilateral paralysis of the pharyngeal and palatine muscles, innervated by cranial nerves IX and X (glossopharyngeal and vagus nerves, respectively), makes swallowing impossible. Attempts at eating are followed by choking, dorsal displacement of the soft palate, and food and saliva exiting the nostrils. Unilateral paralysis causes less severe signs. Aspiration of food may lead to necrotic bronchopneumonia and is particularly likely if there is concurrent paralysis of the larynx due to damage of the laryngeal fibers of cranial nerve X. Collapse of the atonic pharyngeal walls, displacement of the soft palate, and poor abduction of the vocal folds cause abnormal respiratory noises, especially during exercise.

Damage to cranial nerve XII (hypoglossal nerve) causes lingual paralysis and eventual atrophy (unilateral or bilateral), with "quidding," drooling and poor tongue retraction. There also may be persistent lingual fasciculations, even when the tongue is relaxed.

Various combinations of cranial nerve deficits may have synergistic effects in producing dysphagia (*eg*, V with XII, VII with XII).

Cranial nerve damage and dysphagia may follow guttural pouch mycosis (IX, X), ruptured rectus capitis ventralis muscle (IX, X),

fractured hyoid bone (V or XII, depending on the site of fracture), excessive traction on the tongue (XII), and retropharyngeal lymph node abscessation (IX, X, XII). All interfere with chewing and swallowing.[200,201] These horses usually have other signs of the primary disease in addition to dysphagia.

Neuritis of the cauda equina (polyneuritis equi) can cause dysphagia by affecting any or all of cranial nerves V, VII, IX, X or XII. Dysphagia also is a common sequel to chronic lead poisoning.

Botulism and diseases resembling botulism (postanesthesia myasthenia, tick paralysis) are associated with generalized paresis of striated muscles, including those of prehension, mastication and swallowing. The toxins produced by *Clostridium botulinum* block neuromuscular transmission by interfering with the action of acetylcholine.

The neurotoxin produced by *Clostridium tetani* facilitates firing of motor neurons throughout the CNS. This toxin has a slight predilection for the medullary nuclei, which control eating. Thus, besides generalized muscle tetany, there is hypertonicity of the muscles that control eating, particularly the masseter muscles, resulting in trismus ("lockjaw").

Diseases With Physical Causes

Brainstem Trauma

Injury to the brainstem usually is associated with trauma to the poll caused by rearing and hitting an obstruction overhead, or falling over backward to strike the head on the ground. Signs of brainstem injury may occur with or without fractures of the skull. Three clinically recognizable neurologic syndromes have been observed following poll trauma in the horse: optic nerve injury, midbrain syndrome and medullary-inner ear syndrome. Each of these syndromes can be seen alone or in combination with each other, or with the cerebral syndrome (above). Injury to the cerebellum, which also may accompany poll trauma, is covered under Medullary Inner Ear Syndrome.

Optic Nerve Injury: This condition is characterized clinically by sudden onset of blindness in one or both eyes.[202,203] Severe optic nerve injury may occur even with blows to the head of insufficient force to cause loss of consciousness. Dilated, fixed pupils and absent menace responses are noted immediately after the traumatic episode. This blindness may be overlooked for awhile, especially if the patient is depressed and not moving around very much. Beginning within days and progressing over 3-4 weeks, there are generalized retinal degeneration and optic nerve atrophy in the affected eye(s).[202,203] This type of injury usually is due to shearing (amputation) of the optic nerve from stretching forces produced by rapid posterior movement of the brain against the fixed canalicular portion of the optic nerves.[204]

Midbrain Syndrome: Closed head injuries (*ie,* no skull fractures) can result in midbrain hemorrhage, and severe cerebral edema can compress this area. Profound neurologic signs and a poor prognosis accompany damage to the midbrain. After an initial period of coma, there is marked depression due to involvement of the rostral part of the ascending reticular activating system. Extensive midbrain injury causes recumbency and "decerebrate" posturing with generalized extensor rigidity. Ambulatory horses have gait deficits of ataxia and weakness.

Affected horses may have vision, but pupillary light responses are sluggish or absent. This is in contrast to horses with the cerebral syndrome, which usually have brisk pupillary light responses. Depending upon the extent of damage and the area of the midbrain involved, the pupils may be "pinpoint-sized" and fluctuant due to involvement of the tectum, or they may be dilated and fixed with damage to the oculomotor nuclei and/or nerves. With unilateral lesions, the ipsilateral pupil is affected initially, and later involvement of the opposite pupil suggests an enlarging lesion. Progression from miosis to bilaterally dilated, unresponsive pupils is a very unfavorable sign. Injury to the nuclei or connections of cranial nerves supplying extrinsic eye muscles can cause eye deviations (strabismus) and abnormal vestibular nystagmus. Spontaneous nystagmus usually is not seen with midbrain lesions.

Bizarre respiratory patterns, cardiac arrhythmias and bradycardia may occur with severe lesions of the midbrain, pons or medulla.

Medullary/Inner Ear Syndrome: Trauma to the back of the head may cause hemorrhage around the medulla and/or into the middle/inner ear. Often this is seriously complicated by fractures of the occipital and petrosal bones, separation of the occipital and petrosal bones, or separation of the basioccipital and basisphenoid bones ventral to the pons and medulla (Fig 12).[205] Preexisting osteochondroarthrosis and ankylosis of the temporohyoid joint(s), which may or may not be associated with otitis media-interna, predispose to fractures through the osseous bulla and adjacent petrous temporal bone.[206] The resulting neurologic signs often are asymmetric and quite variable, depending upon which cranial nerves are affected and the extent of medullary parenchymal damage. Hemorrhage into the middle and inner ear cavities causes vestibular and facial nerve signs, such as head tilt, circling and leaning toward the affected side, ipsilateral facial paralysis, and spontaneous horizontal or ro-

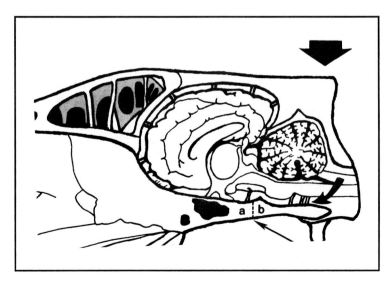

Figure 12. Median section of the equine skull and brain. Trauma to the occipital protuberance (wide arrow) can result in transfer of forces to the temporal bone, with subsequent fractures of its petrosal portion and the basioccipital bone. Separation of the basisphenoid (a) and basioccipital (b) bones often occurs at the suture (long arrow). The facial and vestibulocochlear nerves (curved arrow) are in close proximity to the basioccipital and petrosal bones. Consequently, facial paralysis and/or vestibular signs can result from trauma to the poll and subsequent fracture of these bones or hemorrhage in or around the medulla oblongata.

tary nystagmus, with the fast phase away from the side of the lesion. Vestibular nystagmus may be abnormal or absent. Bleeding may extend into the external ears and guttural pouches.

Hemorrhage in or around the medulla and into the CSF causes additional signs, such as depression, ataxia, weakness, recumbency and other vestibular and cranial nerve signs. Horses with acute vestibular signs often thrash and struggle violently in an effort to stand. Horses with this kind of injury (*eg*, a blow to the poll) occasionally develop a head nod or coarse head tremor that is especially obvious during eating or drinking. This is probably due to direct cerebellar injury.[207]

Prognosis: The prognosis for recovery is fair to guarded for horses showing signs of brainstem damage after closed head injuries. In horses exhibiting the inner ear syndrome without medullary involvement, the prognosis is fair to good for complete recovery. With associated skull fractures, the outlook is guarded to hopeless. Posttraumatic optic nerve atrophy, which may complicate any head injury case, is irreversible. In horses with concurrent vestibular deficits, this form of blindness exacerbates clinical signs by preventing visual compensation.

Treatment: Supportive and medical treatment is as described above for treatment of cerebral trauma. Unfortunately, the response to treatments designed to minimize edema and inflammation usually is minimal, probably because direct mechanical injury and hemorrhage are often more important than edema with this type of injury. Because of the possibility of exacerbating intracranial bleeding by their use, mannitol and other hypertonic solutions are not recommended for treatment of brainstem injury.

Facial Nerve Trauma

The muscles of facial expression are innervated by the facial nerve (VII). This is in distinction to the muscles of mastication, which are supplied by the trigeminal nerve (V). From its nucleus in the medulla oblongata, the facial nerve exits the skull and enters the internal acoustic meatus with cranial nerve VIII (the vestibulo-cochlear nerve), then traverses the petrous temporal bone within the facial canal. During its passage through the facial canal, the nerve courses in the caudal wall of the middle ear and contrib-

utes secretomotor branches to the lacrimal gland via the geniculate nucleus. The facial nerve emerges from the skull through the stylomastoid foramen, then crosses the dorsal aspect of the guttural pouch, where branches originate deep to the parotid salivary gland to supply the caudal ear muscles (caudal auricular nerve), eyelid muscles, and cranial muscles rostral of the ear (auriculopalpebral nerve). The remainder of the nerve crosses the vertical ramus of the mandible about 5 cm ventral to the temporomandibular joint and divides into dorsal and ventral nerves, which supply the cheeks, nose and lips.

Facial paralysis is common in horses. Depending upon the site of damage, some or all of the facial muscles can be affected. Complete unilateral facial paralysis is evident as deviation of the nose toward the normal side, reduced flaring of the ipsilateral nostril during inspiration, and ipsilateral drooping of the lip, eyelid and ear. Reflexes involving cranial nerve VII, such as the lip, eyelid, corneal, menace and ear reflexes, are reduced or absent. Inability to close the eyelid causes exposure keratitis, which may be particularly severe when there is also reduced tear formation from damage to the secretomotor fibers of the facial nerve at or proximal to the geniculate ganglion. Tear production can be evaluated by the Schirmer tear test.[208] Bilateral facial nerve paralysis causes dysphagia, which is evident as dropping of feed and accumulation of feed between the teeth and cheeks. Chronic facial nerve paralysis causes muscle atrophy and fibrous contracture of the face, which often is referred to as (hemi) "facial spasm."

Determination of the site and cause of facial nerve damage is very important in terms of prognosis and therapy. Injury to the facial nerve proximal to the vertical ramus of the mandible causes full facial paresis. Proximal facial nerve trauma usually is caused by fractures of the petrous temporal bone after a blow to the head (see Brainstem Trauma), the stylohyoid bone (usually as a consequence of temporohyoid arthritis and ankylosis), or the vertical ramus of the mandible. Damage within the facial canal often is associated with concurrent signs of vestibular nerve damage, such as head tilt, nystagmus and circling. Tear production also may be reduced. Unilateral facial paralysis due to proximal facial nerve trauma must be differentiated from facial nerve damage or inflammation due to a variety of other causes. These include medullary lesions involving the facial nucleus as well as polyneuritis equi (neuritis of the cauda equina) and idiopathic facial nerve paralysis. Hemorrhage into the middle/inner ear, otitis media/ interna, guttural pouch mycosis and parotid lymph node abscessation each can involve the adjacent facial nerve, causing ipsilateral facial paralysis.

Distal facial nerve damage usually is due to direct injury from a blow or lateral recumbency. The nerve or its branches often are damaged as they cross the mandible and/ or zygomatic arch. Facial paresis following recumbency during general anesthesia is common and usually involves only the nose and lips. Occasionally there also is drooping of the ear and/or eyelid, probably as a result of local damage to the nerve branches supplying these muscles or to damage of the muscles themselves.

The prognosis for return of facial nerve function depends on the site and severity of the causative process. There is a fair chance of recovery with facial nerve deficits caused by trauma to the caudal aspect of the head. In the absence of severe skin laceration, the prognosis for peripheral facial paralysis is good, and recovery takes several days to several months. If there is skin damage with section of the nerve, the nerve ends should be identified and either immediately repaired surgically or tagged (*eg*, with stainless-steel sutures) for future identification and anastomosis.

Inflammatory, Infectious and Immune Diseases

Diseases Affecting Multiple Sites

The section on Diseases of Multiple or Unknown Sites contains a full discussion of such diseases.

Tetanus

Tetanus is a highly fatal, infectious disease caused by the toxin of *Clostridium tetani*. The disease causes muscular rigidity, hyperesthesia and convulsions in horses of all ages. Despite the ready availability of cheap and effective prophylaxis, tetanus continues to cause sporadic equine mortality throughout the world.

The vegetative form of *Cl tetani* is a slender, motile Gram-positive bacillus requiring anaerobic conditions for growth and replication. The organism exists largely in spore form and is commonly found in the intestinal tract and feces of animals and in soils rich in organic material. Spores are resistant to most environmental extremes, chemical disinfectants, and antimicrobial drugs but can be destroyed by heating to 115 C (239 F) for 20 minutes.[131]

The most common route of infection is by wound contamination with *Cl tetani* spores.[131] Disease results when conditions within the contaminated wound favor spore germination, bacterial proliferation and elaboration of toxin. Clostridial growth is favored by a low O_2 tension, which is most often found in the depths of puncture wounds or in wounds with considerable necrosis, impaired blood supply, foreign bodies, or concomitant pyogenic bacterial infection.[209] Neglected puncture wounds are especially dangerous, but any break in the skin or mucous membranes is a potential portal of entry for *Cl tetani*. Castration wounds, metritis following dystocia and/or retained placenta, and use of contaminated hypodermic needles all have been associated with development of tetanus.[131,210] An infected umbilicus is the usual site of *Cl tetani* proliferation and toxin formation in neonates.[211,212] The potential danger of tetanus infection in the normal or inflamed gastrointestinal tract is not known. Spores are viable in tissues for many months and may germinate long after a wound has healed if appropriate conditions are met, such as after reinjury.[131] This accounts in part for the wide variability among individuals in the time between wound contamination and onset of signs of tetanus. The incubation period usually is 1-3 weeks but may range from several days to several months.[131,209]

Clostridium tetani is a noninvasive organism, and signs of tetanus are due to the potent exotoxin tetanospasmin, which is produced locally and acts principally on the CNS. Tetanospasmin is a water-soluble protein that appears to reach the CNS hematogenously and by passage along peripheral nerves.[213,214] The toxin localizes in the ventral horn of the gray matter of the spinal cord and brainstem, binding irreversibly to gangliosides within synaptic membranes.[213] The main action of tetanospasmin is to block the release of inhibitory neurotransmitter. Therefore, reflexes normally inhibited by descending inhibitory motor tracts or by inhibitory interneurons (polysynaptic reflexes) are greatly facilitated, resulting in tetanic contractions of muscles after normal sensory stimulation.[213]

Tetanus toxin has a number of peripheral effects, including sympathetic nervous system stimulation, neuromuscular blockade during the later stages of tetanus, and alterations of catecholamine and adrenocorticoid metabolism.[209,215] The relevance of these findings to tetanus in horses is not known.

Clinical Signs: The severity and rate of progression of clinical signs depend on the dose of toxin and the size, age and immune status of the affected animal. The signs of tetanus reflect spasticity of striated and smooth muscles. The earliest clinical signs depend on the specific muscle groups first affected. In many cases, a slightly stiff gait is the initial sign; some horses are reluctant to feed off the ground due to spasm of cervical muscles. Overreaction to normal external stimuli is another early sign.

Spasm of the muscles of mastication (trismus) may cause difficulty in eating ("lockjaw"). Facial muscle spasm results in an anxious expression with retracted lips, flared nostrils and erect ears. Extraocular muscle contractions cause retraction of the eyeball with resulting prolapse of the nictitating membranes ("flick of the haw"). External stimuli, particularly a hand clap or tap on the forehead, or attempts at eating, often provoke further spasms of facial, masticatory and extraocular muscles. Other striated muscles are progressively affected, causing a very stiff, stilted gait with rigid extension of the neck, limbs and tail ("sawhorse" stance). Spasms of paraspinal musculature often result in ventral or lateral arching of the neck, back or tail. Colic occasionally is the presenting sign or complicates the course of tetanus and may reflect sympathetic overactivity. Spastic paralysis of pharyngeal muscles sometimes results in regurgitation or aspiration of food. Inability to posture appropriately for urination or defecation causes retention of urine and feces.

Once an affected mature horse falls, it generally is unable to regain its feet. Attempts at standing cause further clonic muscle spasms and distress. In lateral recumbency, increased extensor tonus results in rigid extension of extremities and extension of the neck (opisthotonus) and back (lordosis). Foals may be assisted to stand in this remarkably abnormal posture. Even slight stimulation can cause prolonged generalized muscle spasms that may result in vertebral and long bone fractures. Insensible water losses and energy expenditure are greatly increased by this activity, resulting in rapid cachexia, dehydration and metabolic acidosis.

Death usually occurs after 5-7 days and is often caused by asphyxia due to spastic paralysis of respiratory muscles, laryngospasm or aspiration pneumonia. Complications of recumbency and intense muscle spasms, such as decubital sore formation, rhabdomyolysis with myoglobinuria, muscle or tendon rupture, and fractures also can be lethal. If death does not occur, signs usually stabilize after about a week. Recovery is gradual and takes about 6 weeks in most cases.[131,212] If recovery occurs, usually it is complete and without residual signs. Recovered animals are not protected from further episodes of tetanus.

Treatment: The current approach to treatment of tetanus is based on the premise that the toxin-ganglioside bond is chemically irreversible and that recovery is due to gradual replacement of altered gangliosides by normal metabolic processes.[214] For these reasons, treatment is generally symptomatic and supportive, with particular emphasis on good nursing care.

The main objectives of therapy are destruction of *Cl tetani* organisms, neutralization of unbound toxin, control of muscle spasms and general nutrient and metabolic support. Muscular rigidity and reflex spasms first are controlled by placing affected horses in a quiet, dark environment with cotton plugs in the external ear canals to minimize external stimulation.

Destruction of *Cl tetani* organisms and neutralization of the toxin traditionally involve IV, IM or SC administration of large amounts of homologous tetanus antitoxin, plus penicillin or tetracycline therapy and wound debridement to destroy the remaining organisms. The suggested dosages of antitoxin have been rather arbitrary, ranging up to 220 IU/kg body weight every 12 hours.[131] Repeated massive doses are very expensive and probably unnecessary, as circulating toxin levels usually are very low. An IV or IM dose of 5,000-10,000 IU probably is adequate.

In addition, tetanus toxoid is administered at a separate site because protective humoral immunity is not induced by the natural disease. High dosages of penicillin, up to 200,000 IU/kg body weight of potassium penicillin G divided into 4 daily doses, are used for the first 2-4 days to destroy vegetative *Cl tetani* organisms in poorly perfused necrotic tissue. If a wound or infection is found, it should be carefully debrided and irrigated with hydrogen peroxide or another disinfectant solution.

Intrathecal (subarachnoid) administration of tetanus antitoxin has been used with variable success for many years in people and animals with tetanus.[216-218] The rationale for its use has not been clearly defined, but some clinical trials indicate that progression of the disease may be arrested and survival rates improved by this therapy.[216-218] It is worth emphasizing that signs of tetanus may be stabilized but probably not reversed, so intrathecal treatment of affected horses should be most useful if performed early in the disease (*ie,* before recumbency). A dose of 1000-5000 IU homologous tetanus antitoxin should be given at the cisternal or lumbosacral site after slow removal of an equivalent volume of CSF. Addition of 20-100 mg prednisone succinate is optional and has not yet been evaluated in horses.

Ideal chemical control of muscle rigidity and spasms would provide relief of anxiety, muscle relaxation and control of convulsions. However, few commonly used drugs meet these needs. Strong sedatives, such as chloral hydrate, magnesium sulfate and sodium pentobarbital, are useful to diminish anxiety and response to stimulation but cause problems with eating and ambulation when used in doses sufficient to produce muscle relaxation. Ataractics, such as promazine (0.5-1.0 mg/kg body weight every 4-6 hours), chlorpromazine (0.4-0.8 mg/kg body weight every 4-6 hours) and acepromazine (0.05 to 0.1 mg/kg body weight every 4-6 hours), are probably most commonly used in treating tetanus and provide useful muscle relaxation and sedation while allowing the horse to remain standing.[219,220] An effect of repeated use of these ataractics has been splenic enlargement and false anemia. Oil preparations of d-tubocurarrine, given IM at 0.25-0.5 mg/kg body weight daily, have been used successfully in standing animals, but the dangers of overdose and respiratory or limb paralysis are great.[210,221]

Potentially more practical are the centrally acting muscle relaxants, such as methocarbamol and glycerol guaiacolate, which inhibit polysynaptic reflex activity in the brainstem and spinal cord. Glycerol guaiacolate has a relatively short duration of action (25-30 minutes) and is difficult to use in standing animals. However, careful titration of its effects by slow IV drip may produce adequate relaxation without recumbency. Methocarbamol (10-20 mg/kg body weight every 8 hours) is convenient, relieves muscular pain and rigidity in mild cases, and can be used safely in combination with a variety of sedatives. Diazepam has not been properly evaluated in horses with tetanus, but it is the drug of choice in human patients.[217,222] It effectively relieves muscular spasms and anxiety in horses with tetanus but is expensive to use in mature animals (50-200 mg IV every 4-6 hours). Diazepam can be used alone or in combination with sedatives (the dose of diazepam must be reduced accordingly). Xylazine (0.5-1.0 mg/kg body weight) may facilitate brief procedures, such as nasogastric intubation or intravenous catheter placement.

Horses presented in lateral recumbency have very little chance of recovery. Early euthanasia should be considered. Complete paralysis with curariform drugs and total respiratory and nutritional support may be considered for valuable neonates at hospitals with appropriate facilities. Experience with human neonates indicates that paralysis for 4 weeks may be expected.[223]

Good general nursing care is the most important aspect of tetanus treatment. Dysphagic horses can be fed through an indwelling nasoesophageal tube or, conceivably, via a surgically created esophageal fistula. Animals that can eat should be fed and watered from containers placed well above the ground.[212,220] Placement of an indwelling IV catheter minimizes the stress of repeated blood sampling and injections and may be used for total parenteral nutrition of severely affected neonatal foals (see the chapter on Diseases of the Alimentary System). Serum electrolyte concentrations and the hemogram should be monitored regularly and any abnormalities corrected. Such infections as aspiration pneumonia and cystitis must be treated vigorously. Manual rectal evacuation and bladder catheterization may be necessary. Animals in danger of falling should be placed in a sling.[220]

Prophylaxis: Active immunization against tetanus is reliably achieved with potent commercial aluminum hydroxide-adjuvanted toxoids. The usual recommendations are for a second vaccination 3-4 weeks after the first, followed by annual revaccination, with boosters after lacerations or other tetanus-prone wounds. Though annual revaccination often is practiced, there is evidence that protective antibody titers persist for at least 4 years after the first booster.[224]

Equine-origin tetanus antitoxin is widely used to protect unvaccinated horses after injury. The usual prophylactic dose is 1500 IU given SC or IM. There have been occasional reports of acute fatal hepatic necrosis (Theiler's disease) in horses 1-3 months after administration of tetanus antitoxin.[225] In areas where this disease occurs, owners should be advised of the attendant risk when tetanus antitoxin is administered. Nevertheless, wounded, unvaccinated horses everywhere should receive tetanus antitoxin and tetanus toxoid (at separate sites) initially, followed by a toxoid booster 3-4 weeks later and annually thereafter. Circulating tetanus antitoxin may interfere with the immune response to later tetanus toxoid vaccination.[226] For this reason, foals that have received colostrum and/or injected tetanus antitoxin at birth usually are not vaccinated with tetanus toxoid until 4-6 months of age. However, recent evidence suggests that catabolic decay of antitoxin received by either route results in nonprotective titers in most foals by 3-4 months of age.[226] Also, up to 25% of foals receive suboptimal transfer of maternal antibodies, so that even foals of recently vaccinated mares may have low concentrations of circulating tetanus antitoxin.[227]

These data suggest the following regimen for protection of foals against tetanus:

- All foals of mares unvaccinated in the last 30 days of gestation, as well as foals that have not acquired sufficient passive antibodies from colostrum, should receive 1500 IU tetanus antitoxin at birth.
- Tetanus toxoid should be given at 3, 4 and 6 months of age, and then annually.

Botulism

See the section on Diseases of the Neuromuscular Junction in this chapter.

Polyneuritis Equi

See the section on Diseases of the Cauda Equina in this chapter.

Guttural Pouch Diseases

Diseases of the guttural pouches and their etiology, clinical signs and therapy are discussed fully in the chapter on Diseases of the Respiratory System. In this section, only the neurologic consequences of guttural pouch disease will be considered.

Guttural Pouch Mycosis: Most of the clinical signs of guttural pouch mycosis are caused by fungal damage to any of a number of vital structures lying adjacent to the caudodorsal aspect of the medial compartment of the guttural pouch. *Aspergillus* spp, with or without bacteria, usually are incriminated. Pseudomembranous mycotic lesions characteristically arise in this region ventral to the tympanic bulla and medial to the stylohyoid bone.[228] Contained within a fold of the lining of the guttural pouch at this site are the internal carotid artery, glossopharyngeal (IX) and vagus (X) nerves, and cranial cervical sympathetic trunk and ganglion. The spinal accessory (XI) and hypoglossal (XII) nerves also course through this area. Rarely, a mycotic lesion originates in the lateral compartment of the guttural pouch or spreads across the roof from the medial compartment to the area of the internal maxillary artery (a major branch of the external carotid artery) and vein, facial nerve (VII), and mandibular nerve (a branch of cranial nerve V). Fungal plaques also may spread from one guttural pouch to the other by eroding through the apposed medial walls of the pouches.

Though epistaxis is the most common sign of guttural pouch mycosis (discussed fully in the chapter on Diseases of the Respiratory System), there also can be a variety of unfortunate neurologic sequelae. The following is a listing, in approximate order of importance, of the significant neurologic abnormalities that may be associated with guttural pouch mycosis: dysphagia, ranging in severity from occasional coughing during eating to regurgitation of feed, water and saliva through both nostrils (damage to cranial nerves IX and X); abnormal respiratory noises due to soft palate paresis and displacement (IX, X) and/or laryngeal paresis (X); Horner's syndrome (sympathetic trunk and cranial cervical ganglion); facial paralysis (VII); and lingual paresis (XII).[228-233] Inhalation pneumonia is a common complication in severely dysphagic horses. Pharyngeal paresis is usually unilateral; when it is present, bilateral involvement greatly increases the likelihood of feed inhalation and pneumonia.

Various unusual complications of guttural pouch mycosis have been reported. Bony structures adjacent to typical mycotic lesions may become diseased and cause additional cranial nerve involvement. Examples include proliferative osteitis of the stylohyoid bone with or without fracture, avulsion of the insertion of the rectus capitis ventralis muscle (IX, X damage), mycotic lesions of the tympanic bullae that may extend into the middle ear (damage to VII and VIII in or around the middle/inner ear), and osteoarthritis of the temporohyoid or atlantooccipital joints.[201, 228,234-236] It is not clear whether fungal lesions cause or are secondary to bony damage. Fatal fungal encephalitis may occur, by direct extension of a guttural pouch lesion through the basal cranial bones or by embolic dissemination via the internal carotid artery.[237,238]

Persistent dysphagia associated with guttural pouch mycosis warrants a guarded to poor prognosis for long-term survival, even when it occurs without epistaxis. In 3 published series of cases, 5 of 17, 0 of 3 and 1 of 5 dysphagic horses made complete recoveries.[229,232,233] Several other horses survived with persistent low-grade dysphagia. Recovery times ranged up to 18 months and commonly took >1 month. It is not clear whether use of antifungal agents affects the course of disease; thiabendazole, miconazole, griseofulvin, aqueous iodine, gentian violet and nystatin all have been used topically for this purpose, as have systemic iodides, imidazoles and amphotericin B, with varying degrees of success.[232,233] A reasonable but unproven approach to medical treatment of guttural pouch mycosis has been described. An indwelling catheter was used to flush the affected pouch with 250 ml of natamycin solution. Treatments were repeated daily for up

to a month and appeared to cause degeneration of mycotic plaques. Even if the mycotic plaque is eliminated, recovery from dysphagia, if it occurs, may be due to the ability of the deglutition mechanism to accommodate to pharyngeal hemiparesis, rather than to reinnervation of the pharynx. According to published reports, signs caused by damage of other cranial nerve or sympathetic fibers (eg, laryngeal hemiplegia, facial paralysis, Horner's syndrome) are unlikely to improve.

Guttural Pouch Empyema: Guttural pouch empyema per se usually does not cause neurologic deficits, though transient dysphagia that responds to treatment is not uncommon. However, if empyema is persistent and associated with thickening and fibrosis of the guttural pouch mucosa or abscessation of adjacent lymph nodes, various cranial nerve deficits are possible.[239] After the empyema has been resolved medically or surgically (see the chapter on Diseases of the Respiratory System), the neurologic signs may resolve or may be permanent due to strangulation of the nerve(s) in scar tissue.

Guttural Pouch Lavage: Transient or permanent dysphagia may be caused iatrogenically by flushing irritating chemicals into the guttural pouches.[240] In general, physiologic salt solutions, such as normal saline, are the safest and most effective flushing agents. If desired, povidone-iodine, up to 0.01% available iodine (1% Betadine solution), or hydrogen peroxide can be added to the lavage solution safely.

Toxic Diseases

Nigropallidal Encephalomalacia

Prolonged ingestion of yellow star thistle (*Centaurea solstitialis*) or Russian knapweed (*C repens*) produces a neurologic syndrome in horses known as nigropallidal encephalomalacia. Yellow star thistle poisoning was first described in 1954 in northern California and has since been reported in southern California, southern Oregon, Argentina and Australia.[241] In 1969, nigropallidal encephalomalacia due to Russian knapweed ingestion was confirmed in western Colorado, and more recent cases have been reported in eastern Utah and eastern Washington. In a series of 118 cases of nigropallidal encephalomalacia reported in California, 2 peaks of prevalence were observed: one in summer (June-July) and the other in late fall (October-November).[241] Most affected horses were grazing woody or fallow fields.

Clinical signs are peracute in onset and reflect bilateral dystonia of the muscles of prehension and mastication. Affected structures include the masseter, digastricus and facial muscles, and the tongue. Animals with nigropallidal encephalomalacia hold the mouth partly open, with the lips retracted and the tongue partially protruded, resulting in a peculiar "wooden" expression. There is frequently tremor of involved muscles and purposeless, small chewing movements. The tongue may be moved in and out of the mouth or may be curled in the form of a trough. Despite a normal appetite, most affected horses are unable to move food back to the pharynx to be swallowed, and wads of food may be packed around the tongue and gums. Weight loss and debility quickly follow. Many affected horses can drink water by totally immersing their muzzles, and some mildly affected animals maintain condition by adopting unusual eating methods.[242] Behavioral abnormalities, such as circling, depression, yawning or frenzied activity, are common during the first few days after onset of nigropallidal encephalomalacia but can be seen at any time. Most affected horses are readily aroused from a state of drowsiness. The gait is usually normal, though at rest the legs may be placed inappropriately.

There is no effective treatment for nigropallidal encephalomalacia, and most affected horses are euthanized or die within weeks from dehydration, starvation or intercurrent disease. Mildly affected horses sometimes can accommodate adequately and should be provided with pelleted complete feeds or grain that can be scooped into the mouth and swallowed more easily than hay or pasture.

Necropsy findings to which the disease owes its name are quite characteristic and consist of sharply circumscribed areas of coagulative or liquefactive necrosis in the substantia nigra and/or globus pallidus, almost always bilaterally symmetric.

Lead Poisoning

Peripheral neuropathy is a common effect of lead poisoning.[243] Clinically this is apparent as pharyngeal and laryngeal paralysis, with dysphagia, abnormal respiratory noises ("roaring") and inhalation pneumonia.

Horses appear quite susceptible to poisoning by prolonged low-level ingestion of lead. However, acute lead poisoning is rare in horses, apparently because of their selective feeding habits. A daily intake as low as 1.7 mg/kg body weight for several months may cause typical signs of lead intoxication.[244] Generally, affected horses live within the fallout or "smoke" zone of metal mining or smelting industries and are poisoned by eating pasture or hay contaminated by aerial fallout of lead. There is some evidence that cadmium, which often is found in association with lead in smelter fallout, can contribute to the signs of lead poisoning of horses. In addition to these sources, lead-based herbicide orchard sprays and flaking or peeling paint occasionally have been associated with lead toxicosis in horses.

The earliest clinical signs of lead poisoning may be an abnormal inspiratory noise during exercise or coughing during feeding, with persistent "choke" and reflux of food through the nostrils. Pneumonia often occurs due to food inhalation. All of these signs are referable to dysfunction of cranial nerves IX and X. Other signs of peripheral neuropathy have been recorded, including dysmetria of the lips and tongue, facial paralysis, limb weakness and ataxia, and paralysis of the anal sphincter.

Anorexia, depression, weight loss and a poor haircoat soon follow. Other rather variable clinical signs have been reported, including transient colic, lameness, protein-losing nephropathy with ventral edema, and a blue "lead line" along the gingival margins of the teeth.[245] Anemia is a common finding and occasionally is accompanied by immature RBC and basophilic stippling of RBC.

The diagnosis usually is based on clinical signs and history, but lead assays of blood and urine may be diagnostic.[243] Because 90% of lead in blood is bound to RBC in an inactive form, blood lead levels of anemic or hemoconcentrated animals should be interpreted cautiously.[246] Blood levels do not always reflect the total body content of lead in chronic poisoning because the distribution in and mobilization from tissues are affected by the status of other substances, including Ca, P, vitamin D and Zn.[243,245,247] Urine lead levels are rather variable, but the concentration of lead in the urine of affected animals may dramatically increase to >1 ppm after chelation treatment with Ca versenate

(EDTA). The diagnostic value of this finding is uncertain. Other assays of the biochemical activity of lead, such as serum delta-amino-levulinic acid dehydrase activity and urine delta-aminolevulinic acid or porphyrin concentrations, have not been evaluated adequately in horses.

Tissue levels of lead are consistently elevated in horses with chronic lead poisoning. The best tissues for analysis are bone, liver and kidney.[243]

Chelation of the lead in soft tissues with Ca versenate appears to be the most effective treatment.[243] Intermittent dosage may be more effective than constant administration. A daily dosage of 2% Ca versenate at 50-100 mg/kg body weight in a slow IV drip has been used successfully. This was repeated daily for 3 days, then repeated for 3 days again after an interval of 4 days. Concurrent use of acidifying agents may promote resorption of lead from bone.

Neoplasia

See the section on Diseases of the Forebrain for information on this topic.

Multifactorial Diseases

Narcolepsy-Cataplexy

Sleep attacks (narcolepsy) with profound loss of muscle tone (cataplexy) have been described in horses.[248-250] There appear to be 2 different syndromes of narcolepsy-cataplexy: a rare but persistent form affecting horses of many breeds, and a fairly common transient condition affecting foals and yearlings. The former syndrome, seen in most light breeds and in Miniature Horse foals and crossbred ponies, may occur as a familial disorder in Shetland pony foals and Suffolk horses. Between attacks, there is no neurologic abnormality. The signs may range from drowsiness with hanging of the head (narcolepsy) and buckling at the knees, to sudden and total collapse (cataplexy). When forced to walk, affected horses may appear incoordinated. The unconscious state is typical of rapid eye movement sleep with generalized atonia and areflexia, usually with maintenance of some eye and facial responses and normal cardiopulmonary function. While a horse is recumbent due to a cataplectic attack, no spinal reflexes can be elicited. The

animal can be roused from this state with varying degrees of difficulty and regains its feet quietly. Some form of stimulation, such as grooming or petting, washing with a hose, or leading the horse out of a stall, usually precedes an attack. For each individual, the precipitating stimulus is very consistent. The condition usually does not worsen, though some affected aged mares have relentless progression of signs to the point of severe knee and face trauma.

Narcolepsy-cataplexy is quite common in newborn light-breed foals. Usually these affected foals have only one or a few episodes and then "grow" out of the condition. In weanling foals and yearling horses of light breeds, one or several episodes may occur, occasionally triggered by specific stimuli (eg, being hosed down). Some of these syndromes appear to resolve and others persist.

Attacks can reliably be induced with the cholinesterase inhibitor, physostigmine (0.06-0.08 mg/kg IV). Narcolepsy-cataplexy is induced within minutes of physostigmine administration.[250] Caution is required in carrying out the provocative test, as the drug can cause colic. Atropine (0.08 mg/kg IV) resolves signs of narcolepsy-cataplexy for up to 30 hours following administration.[250] For longer-term control, the tricyclic antidepressant drug, imipramine, may be useful. This can be given IV or IM at 0.55 mg/kg. Signs are relieved for 5-10 hours without side effects. Unfortunately, administration of imipramine PO is not reliable.[250]

Idiopathic Diseases

Temporohyoid Osteoarthropathy

By the time the neurologic abnormalities associated with otitis media/interna become apparent, usually there are extensive radiographic changes involving the stylohyoid bone, tympanic bulla, and petrous portion of the temporal bone.[206,251] The predominant changes are proliferative, consisting of periosteal reaction, enlargement and sclerosis of the affected bones. These abnormalities are best appreciated on ventrodorsal views of the skull, obtained under general anesthesia. Corresponding with these radiographic findings, there is exuberant subperiosteal bone proliferation, with fusion between the temporal and hyoid bones and degrees of stricture of the external ear canal and obliteration of the lumen of the tympanic bulla. Extension of the proliferative process to involve the vestibular labyrinths and facial canal causes signs of peripheral vestibular and facial nerve disease, respectively.[206]

It generally has been assumed that bony reaction to chronic middle ear infection or guttural pouch disease results in temporohyoid osteoarthropathy. Another possibility is that osteochondroarthrosis of the temporohyoid joint precedes other changes, and that involvement of the osseous bulla and proximal stylohyoid bone occurs by extension of the primary arthrosis. Regardless of cause, ankylosis of the temporohyoid joint interferes with the interdependent coordinated movements of the tongue, hyoid apparatus and larynx during swallowing, vocalizing, and combined head and neck movements.[206] Sudden mechanical forces applied to this immobilized joint may result in bony fractures, usually through the adjacent petrous part of the temporal bone. Further damage to the vestibular and facial nerves often accompanies such fractures. Other cranial nerves, especially IX and X, or adjacent areas of the medulla also may be affected, causing additional nervous abnormalities, such as dysphagia and depression. Infection of the fracture site may lead to secondary otitis media/interna and leptomeningitis.

The medical treatment of otitis media/interna has been described elsewhere in this chapter. Removal of a section of the affected stylohyoid bone is well tolerated and, therefore, it may be a useful adjunctive form of therapy designed to relieve the mechanical stresses on an ankylosed temporohyoid joint.[252]

DISEASES OF VESTIBULAR AND CEREBELLAR STRUCTURES

Diagnostic and Therapeutic Considerations

Vestibular Disorders

Each side of the vestibular system consists of a receptor, cranial nerve and central nuclei. The labyrinthine vestibular receptor occupies the inner ear with the auditory receptor (cochlea) and is contained within the petrous temporal bone. The vestibular nerve passes from the receptor to the medulla through the internal acoustic meatus with the cochlear (auditory) division of cranial nerve VIII. In each side of the medulla are 4 vestibular nuclei with major connections to the cranial nerves controlling eye movements (III, IV, VI) and to spinal nerves affecting muscle tone of the neck, trunk and limbs. Connections also are made with small parts of the cerebellum.

The function of the vestibular system is to maintain appropriate orientation of the trunk, limbs and eyes with respect to the position and movements of the head. Therefore, vestibular disease results in disturbed equilibrium and ataxia, usually without paresis. Vestibular disorders tend to be unilateral or asymmetric and are caused by either peripheral or central lesions. Peripheral disease causes a head tilt toward the affected side, abnormal vestibular nystagmus, spontaneous horizontal or rotatory nystagmus with the fast phase away from the affected side and, with elevation of the head, exaggerated eye drop ipsilaterally. There usually is a staggering, dysmetric gait, with a tendency to lean or circle toward the affected side because of increased extension of the contralateral limbs.

Horses with any acute peripheral or central vestibular disease sometimes fall or even roll to the side of the lesion and may panic and thrash wildly in an effort to stand. Central lesions generally cause pronounced gait deficits, and nystagmus may be variably horizontal, vertical or rotatory. The fast phase of the nystagmus can be away from or toward the side of the lesion and may alter direction with changes in head position. Bilateral vestibular disease causes dysmetria, severe ataxia, and complete absence of normal vestibular nystagmus. The horse may have wide swinging movements of the head. As with any vestibular disorder, signs are markedly exacerbated by blindfolding. Deafness is also apparent with bilateral involvement of the cochlear division of cranial nerve VIII.

In addition to vestibular signs, central vestibular disease frequently involves adjacent brainstem structures to cause depression (reticular system), paresis (motor tracts), and other cranial nerve deficits (*eg*, cranial nerve VIII). With severe depression and recumbency, abnormal eye positions and movements may be the only indicators of vestibular disease.

Conditions causing central vestibular signs include diffuse brain disease caused by head trauma, infectious meningoencephalitides and metabolic encephalopathies, and focal brain stem diseases, such as protozoal myeloencephalitis and aberrant parasite migration. Tremorgenic mycotoxins have a predilection for the central vestibulocerebellar system and are responsible for the signs seen in ryegrass staggers and Dallis grass poisoning.

Signs of peripheral vestibular disease usually are unilateral and acute in onset. Central accommodation often occurs over a period of weeks, and affected animals may even return to racing. Signs of vestibular disease may still be elicited by blindfolding, however. Peripheral vestibular disease may be associated with trauma to the head, polyneuritis equi (neuritis of the cauda equina) or temporohyoid osteoarthropathy/otitis media-interna, or may be idiopathic. These conditions are discussed in detail elsewhere in this chapter.

Cerebellar Disorders

The cerebellum receives proprioceptive information from all parts of the body and projections from the brainstem motor centers. By continuous assimilation of this and other information, the cerebellum regulates the quality of motor activity via its efferent pathways. Therefore, cerebellar disorders generally are expressed as errors in the rate, range and force of movement. These errors are most obvious as delayed and exaggerated (hypermetric) movements, increased extensor tonus (spasticity) and intention tremors. Despite profound dysmetria, normal strength is preserved. Sensorium and vision are normal, though the menace response may be absent due to interruption of the pathway from the occipital cortex to the facial nucleus as it passes through the cerebellum.

Congenital and Familial Diseases

Cerebellar Hypoplasia

Congenital and/or hereditary cerebellar disorders of domestic animals have been grouped into diseases caused by *in-utero* or neonatal viral infection, malformations of genetic, toxic or unknown etiology, and degenerative diseases referred to as abiotrophies, many of which are genetic in origin (see below).[253] To date, no toxin or virus has been linked with abnormalities of cerebellar development in foals, and congenital malformation/hypoplasia of the cerebellum appears to be extremely rare. Occasional cerebellar syndromes and degenerative lesions are seen in newborn foals, at least in Thoroughbred and Paso Fino breeds. Signs of dysmetria and ataxia are evident as soon as the foal attempts to stand and walk.[254]

Cerebellar Abiotrophy

Cerebellar abiotrophy is assumed to reflect an inherited metabolic defect of cortical cerebellar neurons, which results in the premature death of these neurons during late fetal or early neonatal life. Well-defined syndromes of familial cerebellar abiotrophy have been reported in the Arabian horse and Gotland pony breeds.[255,256]

Among some lines of Arabian horses, up to 8% of foals of either sex may be clinically affected.[257] In a study of 6 foals with cerebellar abiotrophy, one stallion was represented in the lineage of each foal within the previous 7-8 generations.[256] The disease is inherited in Gotland ponies as an autosomal recessive gene.[255]

Signs of cerebellar disease may be present at birth but usually develop during the first 6 months after birth. Progression of signs is variable but often slow or inapparent, after an initial rapid deterioration. Affected foals develop a spastic ataxic gait and pronounced dysmetria ("goose-stepping"), especially of the front limbs. At rest they may stand basewide, with rhythmic swaying of the trunk and neck from side to side or backward and forward. These signs are exaggerated during walking or excitement. Blindfolding has no effect on posture or gait.

Hopping responses are delayed and hypermetric. Spinal reflexes are normal or hyperactive. If the head is elevated, the foal may buckle in the rear limbs or fall over backward. There usually is a head tremor exaggerated by voluntary movements, such as reaching to suckle the mare or to sniff at feed offered by the examiner. Head tremor often is the first sign noticed in affected foals and is prominent thereafter. Careful observation may reveal an intention tremor of the eyes and tongue. As expected in a diffuse cerebellar disorder (see the section on Neurologic Examination in this chapter), the menace response usually is absent or suppressed bilaterally, though vision is unaffected. In contrast to those diseases caused by lesions of the spinal cord or brainstem, there is no paresis.

A tentative diagnosis can be made from the characteristic history and clinical signs. Specific abnormalities usually have not been detected using ancillary examinations. However, CSF protein concentrations were elevated in 3 of 6 foals and CSF creatine kinase activity elevated in 3 of 4 foals.[258]

Though some animals have reportedly improved to varying degrees, there is no effective treatment. Gross necropsy findings usually are unremarkable, though the cerebellum:whole brain weight ratio may be ≤0.08, as compared to that in normal age-matched foals.[259] Histologic abnormalities are confined to the cerebellar cortex and thalamus. There is diffuse reduction in numbers as well as degeneration and disorientation of Purkinje cells, often accompanied by thinning and depletion of the granular and molecular layers. In addition, mineralized neuronal cell bodies have been identified in the thalamus of each of 30 brains examined histologically at the University of Kansas.[256] Though the significance of these thalamic changes is not yet known, their occurrence appears to be specific for the condition of Arabian horse cerebellar abiotrophy.

Diseases With Physical Causes

Injury

See the section on Diseases of the Brainstem and Cranial Nerves for information on this topic.

Inflammatory, Infectious and Immune Diseases

Otitis Media-Interna

Compared to other species, horses are afflicted by otitis media-interna only rarely. Though there is no information regarding the source of otitis media-interna, it is reasonable to assume that the middle ear can be infected by direct spread of processes in the pharynx, guttural pouch or external ear, or by hematogenous spread from a distant site. In addition to vestibular signs of head tilt, circling and ataxia, there may be fever and a hemogram indicating bacterial infection (leukocytosis, neutrophilia), with an elevated plasma fibrinogen concentration. Concurrent ipsilateral facial paralysis is common due to extension of the suppurative process from the middle ear into the adjacent facial canal or internal acoustic meatus containing cranial nerve VII. Signs of facial nerve damage may precede vestibular signs. Rupture of the tympanic membrane occasionally causes discharge from the external ear. Rhinolaryngoscopy may disclose pharyngitis or guttural pouch disease, and ventrodorsal skull radiographs usually show sclerosis of the affected tympanic bulla, even in acute cases of suspected otitis media-interna.

There also is thickening and sclerosis of the stylohyoid and petrous temporal bones, and fusion of the temporohyoid joint on the affected side. The relationship between the rather dramatic bony changes present at the onset of vestibulofacial signs and middle ear infection is unclear (see Temporohyoid Osteoarthropathy). Some or most cases diagnosed as otitis media-interna actually may be secondary manifestations of temporohyoid joint disease in the absence of middle ear infection. Regardless of such infection, they may result in sudden fracture of the petrous bone in the absence of external trauma. Typically such fractures involve the internal acoustic meatus, causing acute signs of vestibular and facial nerve dysfunction. Bacterial meningitis may be a complicating factor.

Any ear, guttural pouch, or pharyngeal exudates or abnormal CSF must be cultured. Beta-hemolytic streptococci, penicillin-resistant staphylococci, and *Actinobacillus equuli* have been cultured from middle ear infections, but other organisms may be cultured, including *Aspergillus* spp, with extension of guttural pouch mycosis. Cerebrospinal fluid analyses may be normal in horses with otitis media/interna, or there may be elevated concentrations of protein and RBC or of WBC with secondary fractures or infections, respectively.

Though the specific causative agent, or even the presence of infection, cannot always be established, prolonged antimicrobial therapy is justified in all cases of otitis media-interna. If streptococcal infection is suspected or if signs improve with penicillin therapy, high levels of penicillin should be maintained for 2-6 weeks. Other appropriate drugs are ampicillin, sulfonamides, trimethoprim-sulfa combinations and oxacillin for penicillin-resistant staphylococci. There may be an indication for short-term (12-48 hours) use of corticosteroids at initiation of therapy for acute otitis interna. Medical treatment of exposure keratitis, maintenance of a tarsorrhaphy or, in extreme cases, eyeball enucleation may be necessary in management of chronic facial nerve paralysis associated with this condition. Surgical drainage of empyema of a tympanic bulla should be considered in cases resistant to medical therapy. To minimize the mechanical stresses resulting from ankylosis of the temporohyoid joint, particularly in cases complicated by fracture of the petrous temporal bone, consideration should be given to removing a section of the affected stylohyoid bone.

The prognosis for functional recovery is fair to good, even though facial nerve and compensated vestibular dysfunction may remain. Central accommodation often occurs over a period of weeks, and affected animals may even return to racing. Signs of vestibular disease may still be elicited by blindfolding, however, and associated facial nerve paralysis may not resolve.

Metabolic Disease

Hypocalcemia

The chapter on Diseases of the Musculoskeletal System contains a full discussion of hypocalcemia (transit tetany).

Toxic Diseases

Ryegrass Staggers, Dallis Grass Poisoning and Other Tremorgenic Mycotoxicoses

Several "staggers" syndromes of horses (and other livestock) are known or thought to be caused by ingestion of tremorgenic mycotoxins. The best described is ryegrass staggers, which affects horses grazing perennial ryegrass (*Lolium perenne*) pastures in the summer or fall. It occurs most commonly in New Zealand but has also been reported in the United States, England and Australia.[260] The causative mycotoxin, identified as lolitrem B, is produced by fungal endophytes that parasitize ryegrass plants and seeds.[261] Dallis grass poisoning (paspalum staggers) also occurs in New Zealand, Australia, the United States and Europe. The signs are caused by a toxin contained in the sclerotia (ergots) of *Claviceps paspali* that parasitize Dallis grass (*Paspalum dilitatum*). Less well defined are "staggers" outbreaks in horses that may not have access to pasture.[262] Several such outbreaks have been seen in Florida in groups of horses that were fed coastal Bermuda grass hay. These cases in horses may be comparable to "Bermuda grass tremor" of ruminants which occurs throughout the southern United States.[263] The toxic principle is not known; however, it is reasonable to speculate that fungal tremorgens, such as those produced by *Penicillium* spp and *Aspergillus* spp, might be involved.

In each case, the clinical signs are those of a vestibulocerebellar disorder with evidence of diffuse spinal or peripheral nerve involvement. Initially there is diffuse, intermittent, mild muscle tremor that progresses to varying degrees of ataxia, with a head nod, swaying, an uncoordinated gait, and a wide-based, rocking stance. Severely affected animals may stumble and fall, causing severe tetanic muscle spasms. If left undisturbed, recumbent horses usually recover and regain their feet within a short time. Excitement or blindfolding markedly exacerbates all signs. The condition is not usually fatal, except where accidents result in injury or drowning. Definitive neuropathologic changes are not seen at necropsy.[260]

Careful removal of affected horses from the contaminated feedstuff results in resolution of signs in 1 to several weeks. Affected animals should be placed in a flat area, free of obstacles and handled as little as possible until they recover. If chemical restraint is necessary, diazepam (50 mg IV in a 450-kg horse) is the drug of choice.

Locoism and Darling Pea Toxicity

Locoweed toxicity (locoism) is a chronic, progressive neurologic disorder of horses, cattle and sheep grazing the range lands of western North America.[264,265] It is caused by prolonged ingestion of certain species of *Astragalus* and *Oxytropis* legumes (locoweeds).

Outbreaks of locoweed poisoning occur when normal forage is scarce, in conditions of overgrazing or during drought. Horses eating locoweed tend to develop a craving for them, even to the exclusion of other feeds. Clinical signs begin abruptly and indicate a diffuse CNS disorder. There are marked dementia and periods of depression alternating with frenzied excitement when affected horses are disturbed. Variable visual impairment, head-nodding and dysphagia with lingual and labial paresis also are observed. Gait abnormalities may be severe and characterized by high-stepping, toe-scuffing, stumbling and swaying. These signs are exacerbated by excitement, and mildly affected horses may seem normal until disturbed or handled. Weight loss occurs quickly and often progresses to emaciation and death. In addition to the neurotoxic effects, locoweed ingestion by pregnant mares has been associated with increased incidence of abortions and limb deformities in term foals.[266]

Mildly affected horses recover within 1-2 weeks if promptly removed from the source of locoweeds. However, there is said to be no recovery from chronic locoweed poisoning, even following removal of the offending plants from the horses' diet. Slightly affected animals remain unsafe for riding and show nervous signs when excited.

Horses generally will not eat toxic quantities of locoweeds if other good forages are available. Because locoweeds emerge early in the spring before most pasture or range grasses, feed should be supplemented at that time until normal forages become available.

Gross necropsy findings are unremarkable but histologically there is widespread neurovisceral cytoplasmic vacuolation.[267] These changes affect most organs and virtually all neurons of the CNS. In protracted cases, there is neuroaxonal dystrophy.

The indolizidine alkaloids swainsonine and swainsonine N-oxide have been identified as the cause of locoism.[268] They act by inhibiting the lysosomal enzyme, mannosidase, resulting in lysosomal accumulation of mannose-rich oligosaccharides. The resultant cellular vacuolation impairs cellular function and accounts for the signs of locoism. Locoism, therefore, is comparable to hereditary mannosidosis of people and cattle.

Swainsonine is also the toxic principle of Darling pea (*Swainsona* spp) poisoning of horses in Australia.[269] Not surprisingly, the clinical and pathologic features of Darling pea toxicity are very similar to those described above for locoism in North America.

Neoplasia

See the section on Diseases of the Forebrain for a complete discussion of this topic.

Idiopathic Diseases

Temporohyoid Osteoarthropathy

The section on Diseases of the Brainstem and Cranial Nerves contains a discussion of this topic.

Idiopathic Vestibular Syndrome

Horses occasionally show acute signs consistent with unilateral peripheral vestibular disease, with no other neurologic sign and no history or evidence of trauma. These animals can be treated as for occult head trauma. Irrespective of therapy, the signs resolve completely in 1-3 weeks. This may be the result of a transient disease of the vestibular nerve, possibly viral or immune-mediated neuritis or labyrinthitis.

Gomen Disease

For more than 40 years, a neurologic syndrome of horses has been observed in a localized region of the South Pacific island of New Caledonia.[270] The disease has never been recorded in indigenous horses < 1 year old. In horses brought in from outside the area, signs take at least 1-2 years to become apparent. First seen is mild toe-dragging in the pelvic limbs, progressing over several years to severe incoordination. Signs are worse in the pelvic limbs than in the thoracic limbs. The involvement usually is bilateral but may be asymmetric. The degree of ataxia is exacerbated by forcing the animal to run or by blindfolding it. Continued progression of signs invariably leads to recumbency and death by starvation, accident or euthanasia. Necropsy reveals gross atrophy of the cerebellar vermis, with thinning of the molecular cell layer of the cerebellum, and loss of Purkinje and granule cells.[271] There also is widespread pigment accumulation (lipofucsin-like) in neurons throughout the CNS. The disease is thought to be environmental

DISEASES OF THE SPINAL CORD

Congenital and Familial Diseases

Occipitoatlantoaxial Malformation

Occipitoatlantoaxial malformation describes a group of congenital disorders involving the occipital bones, atlas and axis.[272,273] The basic malformations include fusion of the atlas to the occiput, hypoplasia of the atlas, hypoplasia of the dens, and modification of the atlantoaxial joint surfaces (Fig 13). There may be ventral luxation of the axis on the atlas, and some of the malformations include cervical scoliosis associated with an extra bony piece on the caudal axis.

Four subtypes of occipitoatlantoaxial malformation have been reported: familial occipitalization of the atlas and atlantization of the axis in Arabian horses; asymmetric occipitoatlantoaxial malformation; asymmetric atlantooccipital fusion; and occipitoatlantoaxial malformation with 2 atlases. The inherited condition of Arabians is by far the most commonly reported occipitoatlantoaxial malformation (19 cases thus far). A similar occipitoatlantoaxial malformation syndrome has been seen in horses not of the Arabian breed, a 19-month-old Appaloosa and a 3-year-old Quarter Horse.[274] In these cases, the structural abnormalities appeared to be present at birth, but perinatal injury to the neck with subsequent vertebral remodeling could not be ruled out.

Affected animals may manifest a wide variety of syndromes. Foals may be born dead because of severe parturient compression of the medulla oblongata and spinal cord by the unstable craniovertebral bones. With mild compression of the CNS during parturition, foals may show tetraparesis or tetraplegia. Close inspection of the craniovertebral region often reveals a clicking noise when the head is moved. The clicking presumably is due to continual luxation-relocation of the axis and dens on the atlas (which is fused to the skull). Reduced atlantooccipital movement can be detected in affected animals. The atlas is palpably abnormal and, in particular, the

Figure 13. Right lateral view of the skull and first 4 cervical vertebrae from a newborn Arabian foal with OAAM. The hypoplastic atlas is fused to the occipital bones. The normally broad wings of the atlas are present as rudimentary peg-like processes. The atlantoaxial joint resembles a normal occipitoatlantal joint. Therefore, the assimilated atlas is occipitalized and the axis is atlantalized. The dens (not visible) is hypoplastic and the wings of the axis are broad.

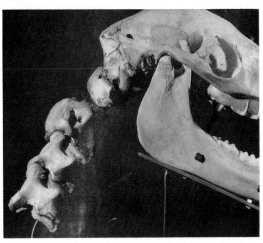

normally broad wings are reduced in size and can be palpated beneath the skin as small bony pegs (Fig 14). In addition, these horses usually have an abnormal head and neck carriage, with the neck extended. Some cases of occipitoatlantoaxial malformation are presented as wobblers, with progressive ataxia and tetraparesis in weanlings or yearlings. This usually is due to spinal cord compression

Figure 14. Closeup view of the right craniovertebral region of an Arabian yearling with OAAM and the wobbler syndrome. A bump is visible just caudal to the ear (arrows) and a bony, peg-like wing of the atlas was palpated at this site on each side. The animal had very restricted movement of the head on the neck.

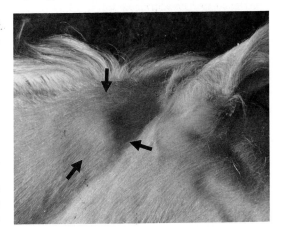

caused by accumulation of fibrous tissue associated with the unstable atlantoaxial joint. One affected Arabian filly had abnormal head posture and a palpably abnormal atlas but no neurologic signs by 5 years of age; radiographs confirmed the diagnosis of occipitoatlantoaxial malformation. Horses with prominent asymmetry (subtypes 2 and 4) often have cervical scoliosis, which may be the only clinical sign.

Clinical diagnosis of an occipitoatlantoaxial malformation can be confirmed by radiography of the head and neck (Fig 15). It is extremely helpful to have radiographs of the same regions from normal horses of a similar age for comparison (Fig 16).

Surgical stabilization of the malformation may be considered in cases of occipitoatlantoaxial malformation to prevent further compression of the spinal cord. Fusion of the axis to the atlas, perhaps with a dorsal laminectomy of the atlas if the vertebral canal is severely compromised at that site, may be successful. It should be remembered, however, that surgical interference is only palliative and results in further neck rigidity that may be unsightly and may promote malarticulations in the 2nd through the 7th cervical vertebrae.

Careful dissection of the craniovertebral region at necropsy is required to accurately define the exact morphology of an occipitoatlantoaxial malformation (Fig 13). The entire vertebral column should be studied and, as with any congenital anomaly, other organs scrutinized for coexisting malformation.

It is almost certain that occipitoatlantoaxial malformation is hereditary in Arabians and may have a simple autosomal recessive mode of inheritance. Consequently, breeding affected animals and rebreeding their parents should be discouraged. The basis for the other subtypes of occipitoatlantoaxial malformation is not known.

Myelodysplasia and Vertebral Anomalies

In addition to cervical vertebral and occipitoatlantoaxial malformations, other congenital and developmental anomalies of the spinal cord (myelodysplasias) may result in clinical neurologic disease. The skeletal investment of the developing spinal cord is dependent on the developmental integrity of the neural tube. For this reason, gross malformations of the axial skeleton tend to accompany severe anomalies of the spinal cord.[197] An anomaly of this type, occasionally seen in horses, is spina bifida.[275] This condition results from failure of fusion of the halves of the dorsal arch, which thus includes the spinous processes. This may or may not be associated with protrusion through the vertebral defect of cystic dilatations of the spinal cord (myelocele), meninges (meningocele), or both (meningomyelocele). Severe myelodysplasia, especially of the dorsal regions of the cord, accompanies spina bifida.

Other forms of myelodysplasia may occur with or without vertebral anomalies. These may include varying degrees of syringomyelia (tubular cavitations), hydromyelia (dilation of the central canal) or diplomyelia (spinal cord duplication). Congenital vertebral

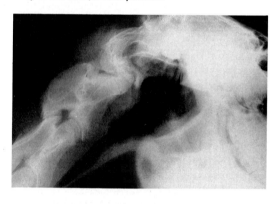

Figure 15. Plain left lateral radiograph of the yearling Arabian with OAAM shown in Figure 14, showing atlantooccipital fusion, hypoplasia of the atlas and dens, and modification of the atlantoaxial joint. Ventral luxation of the axis on the atlas, with impaction of the dens on the body of the atlas, is also present.

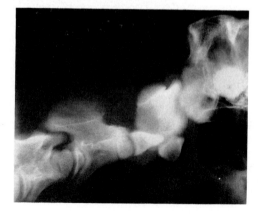

Figure 16. Plain left lateral radiograph of a normal neonatal foal for comparison with Figure 15.

anomalies may occur with or without myelodysplasia. Some of these reported in species other than the horse include block vertebrae, butterfly vertebrae and hemivertebrae. Congenital deviations and contractures of the axial skeleton occur as part of the "contracted foal syndrome" (see below under Arthrogryposis). Vertebral column defects include scoliosis, lordosis, kyphosis and torticollis. Variations in the number of regional vertebrae and developmental vertebral ankyloses have been reported.[276,277] Morphologic variations, including cervical ribs and transposition of one or both ventral processes from the 6th to the 7th cervical vertebrae, also have been seen.[278,279]

Myelodysplasia may be clinically apparent at birth or manifested soon after birth as stable neurologic abnormalities such as paraparesis. A prominent component of the syndrome is a bunny-hopping gait and bilaterally active reflexes in the limbs at the level of the defect.[280] Thus, in a case of lumbar myelodysplasia, the flexor and patellar reflexes in the pelvic limbs both operate when the reflex is initiated in one limb.[281]

Associated severe vertebral anomalies, such as a bifid spine, may cause spinal cord compression and progressive neurologic deficits. Vertebral column contractures, deviations, vertebral transpositions and vertebral fusions generally do not cause neurologic signs.

Diseases With Physical Causes

Spinal Cord Trauma

Equine practitioners probably see more cases of suspected spinal cord and brain trauma than any other neurologic disorder. At least 90 cases of vertebral trauma, with or without associated neurologic signs, are described in the literature.[282-292] In a 3-year study of fatal fractures in 125 horses at racing events in Britain, 23% involved the cervical vertebrae, while the remainder involved the thoracolumbar vertebrae.[291]

The incidence of injuries to the vertebrae is not known. However, in an evaluation of 2170 radiographic and necropsy referral cases, 16 fractures involved cervical vertebrae, 22 involved thoracolumbar vertebrae, and 4 involved sacral and coccygeal vertebrae.[285] Of the 42 fractures involving vertebrae, 21 horses had neurologic signs. All 21 horses sustained fractures of the vertebral body, arch and/or articular processes, whereas none of the 7 horses with fractured thoracic dorsal spinous processes had neurologic signs. From the cases described in the literature and general descriptions of vertebral fractures, as well as from the authors' personal experience, cervical vertebrae are more prone to fractures than the rest of the vertebral column.[287-292] The occipitoatlantoaxial region is most often involved with cervical trauma.[282-284,288-291] Excluding fractures of the dorsal spinous processes that involve T_1-T_{12}, several sites apparently are predisposed to thoracolumbar vertebral fractures.[285-287,291] These sites are the cranial thoracic (T_1-T_3), midthoracic (T_9-T_{16}) and lumbar vertebrae (T_{18}-L_6). These sites probably correspond to the anchor points of the vertebral column, the site of most dorsoventral vertebral movement (T_{12}), and the site that bears the most weight.

Cervical vertebral fractures probably are more common in foals, whereas fractures in the thoracolumbar region are more prevalent in adults.[285] Horses in jumping events apparently sustain neck and back injuries quite frequently. The possibly increased susceptibility for back injury in heavily lactating brood mares could be related to vertebral osteoporosis.[285,291] Foals that pull back against a halter during handling and those that fall over backward are more likely to injure the occipitoatlantoaxial region.[284,290] Any horse that rears up and falls may sustain head trauma, and this likely is the mechanism for sacrococcygeal fractures, with damage to the cauda equina, all of which may occur simultaneously.[292] Younger horses, easily frightened by such things as thunderstorms, run into all sorts of objects and fall over while running, injuring their vertebrae and spinal cord. Cervical hyperflexion and hyperextension injuries result from such falls, and cranial thoracic and midback fractures result from striking solid objects (Figs 17, 18).[285]

Clinical Signs: An extremely important aspect of all cases of trauma to the vertebral column is whether neurologic signs are present. Surprisingly, not all horses with a fractured vertebral body, arch or articular process have signs of spinal cord damage. The syndromes that result are quite variable.

Fractures of C_1-T_2 may result in degrees of tetraplegia or tetraparesis with ataxia. Those of T_3-L_6 may cause paraplegia or paraparesis and ataxia. Fractures of the sacrum may produce urinary and fecal incontinence and, sometimes, muscle atrophy and a gait abnormality in the pelvic limbs. Fractures of the sacrum and coccygeal vertebrae are discussed below.

Classically, neurologic signs appear suddenly at the time of injury. There also may be other signs due to the injury, such as lacera-

Figure 17. Radiograph of the cervical vertebrae of a mature Thoroughbred stallion that suffered a severe hyperflexion injury of the neck. Acute tetraplegia quickly resolved and, at the time the radiograph was made, the stallion had a normal gait despite a slight cervical kyphosis. Multiple vertebral fractures have healed by apparent fusion of the fifth and sixth vertebrae.

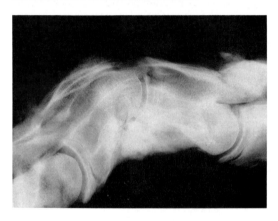

Figure 18. The fifth, sixth and seventh cervical vertebrae, shown here in median section, from a yearling Thoroughbred colt that sustained a hyperextension injury to the neck. There is dorsal luxation of C_5 on C_6, with a slightly displaced fragment off the ventral aspect of C_5. The spinal cord was moderately contused at the C_5-C_6 region, with resulting tetraplegia.

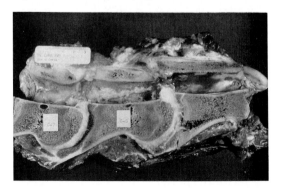

tions or hemorrhage into and from body cavities, and particularly signs of pain and distress, including tachypnea, tachycardia, profuse sweating, mydriasis and splinting or rigid posturing to protect body parts. Traumatized patients may become frantic from pain or the inability to stand. Such struggling can exacerbate trauma to the spinal cord. Sometimes there is a brief period of recumbency, followed by staggering for some time, and then recovery from neurologic signs in hours to days. This can occur even with profound vertebral trauma. Such patients may still require treatment and/or rest. Neurologic signs may be delayed for hours or even days to months after vertebral trauma.[285] Such cases usually involve various combinations of vertebral instability, progressive hemorrhage, callus formation and secondary degenerative joint disease involving damaged articular processes. The last 2 have resulted in the wobbler syndrome, with progressive signs of tetraparesis and ataxia in young horses.[8]

Diagnosis: To complete a physical examination, it may be necessary to sedate a frantic horse with suspected spinal cord trauma. Diazepam at 0.1 mg/kg or xylazine at 1 mg/kg may be useful because of ease of administration, but chloral hydrate or pentobarbital may be more useful as longer-acting hypnotics. Any respiratory difficulty, blood loss or gross instability of the limbs or neck must be attended to immediately. Signs of head trauma, long-bone fracture and bleeding from body orifices should be sought. A rectal examination should be performed whenever possible to assess retention of urine and feces and to palpate the pelvis, sacrum and caudal vertebral column. Efforts should be made to reduce movement in all horses with suspected spinal cord trauma.

A thorough neurologic examination should allow localization of the lesion(s) within the spinal cord. Horses with spinal cord trauma from C_1 to T_2 usually have tetraparesis and ataxia or tetraplegia. A recumbent horse with a lesion at C_1-C_3 has difficulty raising its head off the ground. In comparison, a horse rendered recumbent by trauma at C_4-T_2 should be able to lift its head and cranial neck (Figs 19, 20). A paraplegic horse that "dog-sits" usually has a lesion caudal to T_2. Some degree of asymmetry may be present with spinal cord trauma, but signs are almost always bilateral.

Such localizing signs as hyporeflexia, hypotonia, sensory defects and sweating are extremely helpful findings (Fig 19). The level of hypalgesia on the neck or back indicates the cranial limit of a lesion. Partial depression of the local cervical responses may occur with midcervical and caudal cervical lesions. A depressed cutaneous trunci response occurs frequently with caudal cervical-cranial thoracic spinal cord damage. A line of hyporeflexia may be evident across the trunk, approximating the cranial extent of a lesion. Particularly in the early posttrauma phase, a region of hyperesthesia may be detected just cranial to the lesion. Strip patches of sweating may occur when thoracolumbar spinal nerve roots are damaged. Excessive whole-body sweating, seen frequently in horses with a broken neck or back, may be due to involvement of pain pathways and sympathetic spinal cord pathways. This may include sweating on the neck and Horner's syndrome, if the lesion is cranial to the cranial thoracic spinal cord segments.

If spinal shock occurs, with suppression of all reflexes caudal to a massive spinal cord lesion, it probably only lasts for minutes or hours. The Schiff-Sherrington phenomenon, with extensor hypertonia of the thoracic limbs, may occur after severe thoracic spinal cord damage. The important factor differentiating this from a severe cervical lesion is that in the former, voluntary effort and pain perception are good in the thoracic limbs, whereas in the latter, voluntary effort and pain perception are depressed (or absent) in all 4 limbs. The prognosis with either condition still is poor.

At this stage of evaluation, an initial prognosis must be given; the outlook must be guarded for all recumbent horses. However, much may be gained and little lost if final judgment is withheld for one to several hours, providing the horse is not suffering unduly. During the acute phase of spinal cord trauma, functional loss is far more profound than would be expected from the morphologic changes.[293,294] Consequently, if further damage is prevented, return of functional integrity can be remarkable, even in animals receiving no therapy (Fig 17).[285,288,295,296]

The most helpful aid in confirming vertebral trauma is plain radiography. However, this procedure does not directly evaluate the presence and extent of spinal cord damage. Vertebral components may be in very differ-

ent positions with no respect to displacements that may have occurred at the time of injury. Even vertebral canal diameter can give a false impression of the degree of spinal cord compromise (Fig 17). The possible combinations of epiphyseal separations, fractured vertebral bodies, luxations, separated articular pedicles and nondisplaced fractures are endless. However, the neurologic examination usually is of greater significance in determining prognosis and response to therapy, and radiographs are of more significance in deciding whether or not surgery is indicated.

If there is a suggestion of increased intracranial pressure in a horse that may have

Figure 19.Ventral view of the head and neck of a tetraplegic 3-month-old Quarter Horse filly that sustained a neck injury while exercising on a mechanical walker. Signs of ataxia progressed to tetraplegia over 24 hours. The filly was unable to raise its head or neck off the ground. There was a strip of analgesia on the neck caudal to the ears, as shown, with absence of the local cervical responses in this region, and hypalgesia of the whole body caudal to this site.

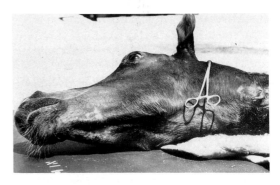

Figure 20. A fractured dens with atlantoaxial luxation was diagnosed radiographically in the horse in Figure 19. Lack of response to therapy and a bad prognosis necessitated euthanasia. Severe spinal cord contusion was confirmed at necropsy.

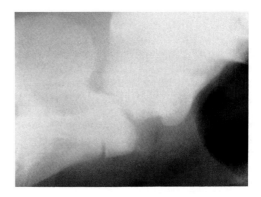

sustained an injury, it is unwise to collect a large volume of CSF from the atlantooccipital site because of the risk of caudal herniation of the occipital lobes of the cerebrum and cerebellum. However, collection of CSF from horses with spinal cord trauma and no head signs is quite safe, particularly from the lumbosacral site. A CSF analysis is sometimes useful in ruling out other causes of peracute spinal cord disease, such as EHV-1 myeloencephalitis, larval migration and protozoal myeloencephalitis. Firm evidence of subarachnoid hemorrhage, however, may not always be found on analysis of CSF from horses with spinal cord trauma; in fact, results of CSF analysis in such animals often are normal.

Electromyography can be valuable in helping localize the site of spinal cord trauma and can direct radiographic attention. Evidence of denervation of muscles first appears a week or so after damage to the ventral gray matter or nerve roots. Prominent multifocal or diffuse denervation potentials found by electromyography on a horse with spinal cord disease would be strong evidence for some (multifocal) mechanism other than injury.

A hematologic stress pattern, unconjugated hyperbilirubinemia, perineal azotemia and chemical and enzymatic evidence of soft tissue and possibly bone damage may be expected in recumbent animals.

Treatment: The logical medical management of spinal cord trauma, based upon recent research into the pathophysiologic mechanisms involved, continues to be debated.[284,290,297,298] The initial events in spinal cord trauma almost certainly are mechanical.[294] The explanation for profound functional loss from minimal anatomic derangement is possibly related to primary extrusion of K ions from cells, with extensive local depolarization (block) of neurons.[293] An immediate systemic arterial pressor response probably is mediated by vascular and adrenergic receptors.[293] Suppression of this pressor response may markedly decrease the number of resulting spinal cord hemorrhages.[293,299] A dramatic change in spinal cord blood flow apparently occurs within 1-2 hours.[300] The rate at which spinal cord compression occurs is probably important; slow compression is associated with fewer permanent deficits than rapid compression to the same degree.[301] This leads to the suggestion that changes in blood flow are less important than primary mechanical factors, though time is probably important.[301]

One report indicated that local catecholamine levels rise sharply in contused spinal cords and anticatecholamine (alphamethyltyrosine, reserpine, levodopa, phenoxybenzamine) therapy drastically reduces the consequences of spinal cord trauma.[298] Other authors were not able to reproduce these results, though the role of vasoactive substances in spinal cord trauma has not been dismissed.[293,294,298,302]

One interesting hypothesis states that platelet activation and resulting thrombi and emboli were a vital component of the cascade resulting in hemorrhage, edema and necrosis.[295] Suppression of platelet aggregation and block of vasospasm were thus logical treatment suggestions. Manipulation of vasoconstriction and clotting mechanisms with dimethyl sulfoxide and epsilon aminocaproic acid were purportedly very beneficial in spinal cord trauma.[303] However, in at least one controlled experiment, neither DMSO nor epsilon aminocaproic acid significantly improved functional recovery of contused canine spinal cords.[298] Clinical modulation of platelet function in spinal cord trauma patients is in its infancy, and exciting results may be forthcoming. Also, recent interest has been revived in use of compounds that decrease metabolic requirements, such as gamma hydroxybutyrate and barbiturates, and in loop diuretics, such as furosemide, in treatment of nervous system trauma.[164] The role of such therapy for spinal cord disease remains questionable.

A discussion of medical management of spinal cord trauma would be incomplete without reference to use of hyperosmolar diuretics, such as mannitol, and glucocorticoids. A large proportion of spinal cord trauma patients of all species probably receive these compounds. Frequently used regimens include 20% mannitol given IV at 0.25-2 g/kg and dexamethasone given IV at 0.1-2.2 mg/kg, both repeated up to 4 times daily. There is little proof demonstrating the effectiveness of these compounds. Some reports suggest that, in experimental spinal cord trauma in dogs, these compounds were not very effective in protecting long-term spinal cord function.[298,304] It is possible, however, that glucocorticoids help reduce the severity of the damage in experimental spinal cord edema.[293]

There is not full agreement on medical management of spinal cord trauma. The following remarks are based on the literature cited, on the experience of others, and on personal experience with horses suffering from spinal cord trauma. In the peracute stages, IV dexamethasone at 0.1-0.2 mg/kg may be given up to 4 times daily for 2-4 days. After the first 24-48 hours, the benefit of corticosteroids probably is reduced, and problems with decubital infections, cystitis, laminitis, delayed bone healing and occasional systemic infection can be so marked that they are best avoided.

If continued bleeding is suspected or if systemic blood pressure is likely to be elevated in the peracute phase following injury, 1-2 standard doses of furosemide are useful. The horse must be kept calm or sedated with chlorpromazine, acepromazine, chloral hydrate, pentobarbital or other agents. Use of 20% mannitol, given IV at 0.25-1 g/kg, and glycerol in water, given PO at 1 g/kg, has not been very successful in our hands. Severe prerenal azotemia results from overuse of furosemide and mannitol in recumbent patients. The effectiveness of DMSO in equine spinal cord trauma has been difficult to establish, though in acute cases, we sometimes use 20% DMSO in 5% dextrose, given slowly IV at 1 g/kg at 12- to 24-hour intervals for up to 4 doses. Antibiotics probably are not required for vertebral fractures or spinal cord trauma but may be necessary to treat concurrent skin lesions, cystitis and pneumonitis, especially in recumbent patients. If, in the final analysis, specific neurologic deficits caused by spinal cord trauma improve dramatically after a particular treatment, consideration should be given to repeating that treatment.

External manipulation, external and internal fixation, and surgical decompression and fusion have not been employed very extensively in horses with vertebral damage. Manipulation of cervical vertebral luxations and torticollis, preferably under general anesthesia, with use of external support in the form of a cradle or neck cast, is a reasonable consideration.[283] Great care must be taken when manipulating damaged vertebrae under anesthesia to prevent further spinal cord trauma. Excellent results have been reported with surgical immobilization of a fractured dens in a 3-week-old Appaloosa colt and a 4-week-old Thoroughbred filly.[288,289] Com-

plete remission of signs was obtained by surgical correction of a complete ventral luxation of the axis on the atlas in an 11-day-old Arabian colt.[305] The Appaloosa received oxytetracycline but no other drugs postoperatively, and the Arabian colt received no drugs postoperatively.

Critical selection of candidates for surgery is vital. Surgery probably is indicated if a horse's neurologic condition deteriorates after appropriate medical therapy for spinal cord trauma, and decompression of the spinal cord and stabilization of luxations or fractures are feasible. The techniques of cervical dorsal decompressive laminectomy described for horses may be modified for decompression of a spinal cord that is compromised by hematoma, displaced soft tissues or bone. Surgical hardware often is not strong enough to withstand the forces within the middle of the equine cervical vertebral column. Therefore, intervertebral fusion may be a promising technique to stabilize fractures of the arch and articular processes of cervical vertebrae in horses, as it is in people. Other techniques using vertebral plates, screws or wires must be modified from standard small animal or human methods.

Prognosis: The prognosis for horses with spinal cord trauma associated with luxations or fractures of the vertebral body, arch or articular processes must remain guarded to poor for return to use. Healing of such fractures frequently results in some degree of vertebral malalignment, sometimes with lordosis, kyphosis, scoliosis or torticollis (Fig 17). Even after apparent healing and resolution of neurologic signs, delayed callus formation and degenerative changes in adjacent articulations can result in delayed permanent spinal cord compression.

No simple rules can be given for management of horses with spinal cord trauma. In our experience, 2 points are worthy of emphasis. First, thorough and repeated neurologic examinations help in arriving at a prognosis and evaluating progress of the animal. Second, no individual medical therapeutic regimen is more singularly beneficial in healing spinal cord injuries than the passage of time.

Fibrocartilaginous Emboli

Focal spinal cord infarction due to multiple fibrocartilaginous emboli has been reported in an 8-year-old Quarter Horse.[306]

The fibrocartilaginous material was thought to originate from a degenerated intervertebral disk. The ischemic lesion involved both gray and white matter in the caudal cervical spinal cord and resulted in peracute quadriplegia.

In a similar case, an 11-year-old horse had peracute hemiplegia of the limbs on the right side and ipsilateral sweating. Considerable improvement occurred over 6 months, though residual thoracic limb abnormalities led to euthanasia of the horse.[307] The prognosis for this condition occurring in other species is good to excellent. Therefore, should this disease be suspected, hasty euthanasia should be discouraged.

Inflammatory, Infectious and Immune Diseases

Diseases Affecting Multiple Sites

The section on Diseases of Multiple or Unknown Sites contains a discussion of such conditions.

Vertebral Osteomyelitis

Infection of the vertebrae or intervertebral disks may result in compression of the spinal cord and paraparesis or tetraparesis. The causes and associations of vertebral osteomyelitis are the same as those for infections of the appendicular skeleton. Most vertebral infections occur hematogenously during a bacteremic episode. In this regard, inadequate transfer of maternal antibody is an important risk factor for foals. A pre-existing site of infection, such as an umbilical or lung abscess, is a likely source for hematogenous spread to the vertebrae. In young animals, blood-borne bacteria frequently lodge near physeal growth plates.[308] Thus, in the vertebral column, osteomyelitis begins in the vertebral bodies, spinous or transverse processes, or in the vertebral ends of ribs. Less frequently, vertebrae are infected by direct implantation via a penetrating wound or by direct extension of adjacent processes such as lymph node, intrathoracic or injection abscesses.[197,309]

As the site of sepsis becomes established, there is localized pain manifested as resistance to palpation, stiffness and reluctance to move the affected vertebrae. Fever, neutrophilia and an elevated plasma fibrinogen concentration also may be expected at this stage. Further enlargement of the lesion causes both destruction and remodelling of bone. These changes may be apparent radiographically. Compression fractures of weakened vertebral bodies may be noted incidentally on radiographs or, if the fractured ends are severely displaced, cause acute onset of neurologic signs.

Once the septic process invades through cortical bone, it may expand to involve intervertebral disks and adjacent vertebrae. Infection also can spread into the paravertebral region, forming an expanding abscess that eventually may fistulate to outside the body. A more serious development is spread of the lesion into the epidural space, causing local compression of the spinal cord and involvement of nerve roots. The epidural space also occasionally is seeded hematogenously with bacteria, without primary vertebral involvement.[310] Signs are typical of a focal spinal cord lesion. Depending on site and severity of compression, these may range from localized cutaneous hyperesthesia without gait abnormalities, to paresis of one or more limbs, and hypalgesia, localized sweating, hyporeflexia and muscle atrophy. Neurologic signs of compression may be acute or begin insidiously and progress. Rarely, an epidural abscess penetrates the dura to cause leptomeningitis.

The intervertebral disk seldom is a primary site of infection in horses, though the pyogenic process of osteomyelitis may secondarily invade the intervertebral space. Diskospondylopathy, defined radiographically by narrowing of the disk space, and lysis and sclerosis of adjacent vertebral parts have been described in horses.[311] This syndrome was similar clinically to vertebral osteomyelitis as described above but bacteria usually either could not be isolated from the lesions or were nonpathogenic types of doubtful significance. An association with trauma or a degenerative process was suggested as the inciting cause, as most cases involved the disk space between C_7 and T_1.

Cause: Various organisms have caused vertebral osteomyelitis in horses. In neonatal foals, the likely agents are bacteria most commonly associated with sepsis: beta-hemolytic streptococci, *Actinobacillus equuli* and *E coli*. In older foals, *Rhodococcus equi*, *Klebsiella* spp or *Salmonella* spp also may be found. Any of these organisms may cause the disease in adults, and coagulase-positive staphylococci, *Actinobacillus lignieresii, Rhodococcus equi, Mycobacterium bovis, Brucella abortus, Eikenella corrodens* and *Aspergillus* spp all have been found.[309,310,312]

Diagnosis: The clinical signs, when combined with a hemogram, indicate inflammation and are highly suggestive of the diagnosis. Radiography is an important aid to diagnosis, but radiographic changes may not be present at the first sign of clinical disease. Also, thoracic and lumbar vertebrae cannot be radiographed satisfactorily with small portable units. Specialized techniques, such as nuclear scintigraphic bone scans and cutaneous thermography, may help localize the affected segment. If associated leptomeningitis is present, pleocytosis and elevated protein content may be expected on CSF analysis. More often, results of CSF analysis are normal or consistent with spinal cord compression. Finally, a card test for serologic evidence of *Brucella abortus* infection or skin tests for tuberculosis may be considered if vertebral osteomyelitis is diagnosed in adult horses.

Treatment: Every effort should be made to obtain cultures of the causative organism before antimicrobial treatment. This may include sampling by one or all of the following techniques: needle aspiration, percutaneous biopsy or excision of a specimen of infected bone, aspiration of paravertebral or other abscesses, and blood and urine cultures. Samples should be submitted for both aerobic and anaerobic cultures. Depending on the results of sensitivity testing, appropriate antimicrobial treatment should be continued for at least 6 weeks (see Osteomyelitis in the chapter on Diseases of the Musculoskeletal System). If sensitivity data are not available, treatment should be with large doses of a broad-spectrum antimicrobial, at least initially. The public health aspects of tuberculosis and brucellosis should be considered before treatment is undertaken.

Another aspect of therapy of vertebral osteomyelitis and epidural abscess in horses is surgical exploration and drainage. This was successfully performed in a horse with osteomyelitis of C2, using a dorsal approach, removal of the infected dorsal spinous process and vertebral arch, suction drainage and systemic antimicrobial therapy.[312] If neurologic signs have been rapidly progressive or if there is profound spinal cord compression, indicated by recumbency, poor voluntary effort

and hypalgesia caudal to the lesion, surgical relief of pressure on the spinal cord probably should be attempted. Surgical drainage is also appropriate if large volumes of purulent material are associated with damage to the spinal cord. Finally, surgical exploration, biopsy, culture and drainage are extremely helpful if antimicrobial therapy has been unsuccessful, particularly if no positive cultures have been obtained.

Prognosis: The prognosis for pyogenic vertebral osteomyelitis and epidural abscess is guarded to poor. However, if patients can be treated before neurologic signs are marked and if appropriate long-term antimicrobial therapy is economically feasible, the outlook for improvement or resolution of neurologic signs is fair.

Tetanus

The section on Diseases of the Brainstem and Cranial Nerves in this chapter contains a discussion of Tetanus.

Ehrlichiosis

Horses infected with the rickettsia *Ehrlichia equi* often have transient truncal and limb ataxia.[313] A morphologic basis for these signs has not been demonstrated.

Metabolic Disease

Hypocalcemia

The chapter on Diseases of the Musculoskeletal System contains a discussion of hypocalcemia (transit tetany).

Toxic Diseases

Bracken Fern and Horsetail Poisoning

Ingestion of either *Pteridium* (bracken fern) or *Equiperdum* (horsetail) species causes neurologic disease in horses.[314-316] Poisoning is due to thiaminase that, after repeated ingestion, causes thiamin deficiency. Horses usually do not eat these plants but may if other forage is scarce. Most cases of poisoning are due to incorporation of bracken fern or horsetail into hay, where it is rendered more palatable. Signs begin insidiously several weeks after ingestion begins and may even develop after removal of the contaminated hay. The most apparent clinical abnormality is ataxia, which may be severe and involve all 4 limbs. In addition, there are anorexia and bradycardia. Affected horses may have a "tucked-up" appearance. Signs of forebrain disease are seldom seen, though head-pressing was noted in one horse and blindness in another. Terminally there are convulsions and opisthotonus. In a group of experimentally poisoned horses, blood thiamin levels fell from 8.5 to 1.5 μg/dl and blood pyruvate levels increased from 2.2 to 6.25 mg/dl.[130] Thiamin administration, PO at 0.5-1 g BID, results in rapid resolution of signs.[315] Virtually identical signs were induced in 4 horses by prolonged feeding of the thiamin analogue, amprolium.[317]

Birdsville Indigo Poisoning

Birdsville indigo (*Indigofera linnaei*, previously called *I enneaphylla*), grows throughout northern Australia but causes toxicity problems only in inland areas, particularly around Alice Springs and Birdsville.[130,318] Poisoning occurs only in horses and is known as Birdsville disease. Signs of poisoning can be induced in horses after about 3 weeks' consumption of 4.5 kg of green plant daily. Affected horses first become dull and lethargic. Later they develop signs of limb ataxia and weakness, most prominent in the pelvic limbs. There is marked weight loss and terminally there may be convulsions and struggling. Less severely affected horses that are removed from the offending plants may recover completely, but more often there are persistent gait abnormalities. No pathologic changes have been described in either experimentally or naturally affected horses. The toxic principles of *I linnaei* seeds and pods are the arginine-antagonists indospicine and canavanine. Dietary supplementation with arginine-rich materials, such as peanut meal, gelatin and alfalfa chaff, protects against experimental forms of *I linnaei* toxicity. Such supplementary feeding now is the recommended practice for control of naturally occurring Birdsville disease.

Neoplasia

The section on Diseases of the Forebrain contains a discussion on Neoplasia.

Multifactorial Diseases

Equine Degenerative Myeloencephalopathy

Equine degenerative myeloencephalopathy (EDM) is a diffuse degenerative disease of the spinal cord and brainstem of domesticated and captive equids in North America and England.[319-321] A familial tendency is suspected, and clusters of cases have been observed in most light-breed horses and in Grant's zebras. A similar condition has been seen in captive Mongolian wild horses (*Equus przewalskii*). Recent evidence supports the hypothesis that some cases of EDM are associated with vitamin E deficiency.[321] The role of vitamin E in the pathogenesis of these myelopathies must be confirmed by controlled trials.

Cause: On each of 2 breeding farms with a high incidence of EDM among foals, there appeared to be a familial predisposition toward the disease. More important, horses on both farms had low serum concentrations of vitamin E.[321] The latter finding apparently reflected vitamin E-poor diets, which consisted of sun-bleached grass hay, yellow-grain based rations and pelleted feeds. There was no access to grass pastures. Dietary supplementation with vitamin E dramatically reduced new cases of EDM at both farms and led to significantly increased serum vitamin E concentrations. A previous EDM cluster in Mongolian wild horses also revealed an association with vitamin E-deficient feed or low serum vitamin E concentrations.[322] Not all foals with low serum vitamin E concentrations at the time of sampling showed neurologic signs, perhaps reflecting varied individual susceptibility to the disease. Also, serum concentrations of vitamin E in several chronically affected horses, each of which occurred as a single case, have been normal.

In most outbreaks in which multiple horses are affected, vitamin E deficiency in association with familial predisposition to the disease are likely contributing factors. However, other nutritional, toxic, metabolic or hereditary processes should also be considered, especially with isolated, single cases.[319]

Clinical Signs: Equine degenerative myeloencephalopathy usually occurs in foals of either sex but may affect horses up to about 3 years of age. The disease may occur in a single animal or affect whole groups of young horses that frequently are related. Signs of EDM are restricted to the nervous system. There is an insidious or abrupt onset of symmetric ataxia, paresis and dysmetria of the limbs. Typically, pelvic limb signs are worse than thoracic limb signs by at least one grade. These horses often are described as "wobblers."

Clinical signs may progress to the point of causing recumbency or may be stable for many months. A common finding, particularly in those with neurologic signs for >6 months, hyporeflexia over the neck and trunk. Cervical, cervicofacial and cutaneous trunci reflexes all may be affected, as well as the laryngeal adduction ("slap") test. However, specific signs of gray-matter disease, such as muscle atrophy and lack of sensation, are not seen in horses with EDM.

Equine degenerative myeloencephalopathy is not associated with hematologic, serum biochemical or CSF abnormalities.

Diagnosis and Prevention: A presumptive diagnosis of EDM usually can be made by careful evaluation of the history and clinical signs. Cervical radiographs should be made to help rule out cervical vertebral malformation. If EDM is suspected, the vitamin E status of the affected horse(s), as well as any stable- or pasturemates, should be determined. Serum vitamin E concentrations accurately reflect vitamin E status at the time of analysis; horses normally have at least 1.5 μg/ml serum. Serum vitamin E levels <1 μg/ml have been associated with EDM. By reference to standard nutrition manuals, the daily vitamin E intake can be estimated and compared to the recommended dietary level.

If vitamin E intake is found to be suboptimal on farms where EDM has occurred, all horses on those farms should receive vitamin E supplementation at 1.5 mg (2.25 IU)/kg body weight per day. In addition, affected horses may be treated with 1000-3000 IU vitamin E in oil IM daily for up to 1 week. Serum vitamin E concentrations should be determined periodically to assess the effectiveness of these measures. It is not yet known whether it is possible to alter the clinical course of EDM with supplemental vitamin E; this probably would be effective only in the early stage of the disease. Because EDM tends to be familial, the presence of the disorder within a family should be considered when breeding stock is selected.

Necropsy Findings: No significant gross findings are evident. Histologic lesions apparently are restricted to the CNS, though the peripheral nervous system has not been scrutinized.[319] Degenerative lesions occur throughout the spinal cord and caudal brainstem white matter and in many nuclei in the gray matter of the spinal cord and brainstem; hence the name of the condition.

Neuronal fiber degeneration is present in all funiculi of the spinal cord. This is most prominent in the dorsolateral (ascending spinocerebellar) tracts and ventromedial (descending) tracts of the cranial cervical and midthoracic segments. An added component of demyelination also can be detected in these particular tracts. Neurochemical analyses also have corroborated loss of spinal cord myelin lipids in EDM, as compared with levels in spinal cord tissue from control horses and horses with other spinal cord diseases.

Neuroaxonal dystrophy with florid spheroid formation characterizes the gray matter lesions most prominent in the nucleus thoracicus and lateral cuneate nucleus in early cases. This lesion may not be prominent in chronic cases and can easily be overlooked in very chronic cases that have been treated with vitamin E supplementation.

Cervical Vertebral Malformation – Malarticulation

A.J. Nixon

Cervical vertebral malformation (CVM) describes a group of malformation-malarticulation anomalies involving the cervical vertebrae of ataxic horses ("wobblers"). The term "wobbler" has been largely superseded by more descriptive categorization. Though 2 subdivisions of CVM have been described, cervical static stenosis and cervical vertebral instability, both groups generally result from bone and joint malformation of some type.[2,166,187,307,323-328]

Cervical vertebral instability typically involves deformation of the vertebral bodies, with malarticulation and subluxation on flexion of the vertebrae. The size, shape and integrity of the articular facets frequently are abnormal. Cervical static stenosis, a separate entity generally involving the caudal cervical vertebrae, results from degenerative joint disease of the articular facets, with bony and occasionally soft tissue impingement into the vertebral canal. Secondary changes in the dorsal laminae and ligamentum flavum frequently contribute to spinal cord compression.[8,327] The initiating factors in degenerative joint disease and cervical static stenosis probably involve aberrations in cartilage and bone development, and may precede clinical ataxia by many months to years.[8]

Pathogenesis: The precise abnormalities in bone and joint development resulting in CVM still are not completely known. Many factors are likely interacting to modify regular development of the cervical vertebrae. These include nutrition, genetics, biomechanical forces (possibly due to conformation), and exercise (including trauma). Cervical vertebral malformation is only one clinical entity in the group of developmental orthopedic diseases that include physitis, acquired contracted tendons, osteochondritis dissecans, malformation of the cuboidal bones of the carpus and tarsus, and juvenile arthritis.

A genetic study of wobbler matings revealed that none of the offspring was a clinical wobbler; however, the offspring had an extraordinarily high incidence of contracted tendons, osteochondritis dissecans and physitis.[329] An earlier study implicated a genetic propensity for rapid growth and superior performance, but another more recent survey found no evidence that CVM was genetically predetermined.[330,331]

The importance of dietary factors, particularly trace minerals, in the pathogenesis of developmental orthopedic diseases has been investigated.[332] Feeding trials have implicated copper deficiency as a major determinant of aberrant endochondral ossification.[333,334] Necropsy of copper-deficient animals showed an extraordinarily high incidence of vertebral osteochondrosis lesions.[335] Longer-term nutritional studies are needed to adequately demonstrate that these osteochondritis dissecans lesions develop into spinal cord compressive syndromes. Complicating dietary factors probably are also involved, including high protein levels and high caloric intake.[8,187,323,324,326,336] Marginally low levels of trace minerals may only be of metabolic importance under circumstances of maximum need, as during rapid growth. Young horses with CVM are frequently reported to have a large body size for their age.[2,8,187,323,326-328,337,338] A study in 1942 drew the analogy of CVM in horses to copper deficiency (sway-

back) in lambs, and suggested that pregnant mares be treated with copper sulfate.[339] The interplay of other dietary components in the etiology of developmental orthopedic diseases and CVM still is under investigation.

A study of bone formation, bone remodelling and total bone volume showed that horses with CVM and osteochondritis dissecans had significantly decreased bone modelling and remodelling as yearlings.[340] As these horses matured to 3 years of age, quantitative bone turnover and total bone volume increased over age-matched normals. Decreased bone formation and turnover in affected yearlings support the finding of articular and physeal chondronecrosis associated with delayed endochondral ossification.[8,330,336,341,342] Control of bone formation by hormones, growth factors and local regulatory factors is complex, but these factors may play an intermediary role between some of the dietary inadequacies and the final cartilage and bone deformations of CVM.

Osteochondrosis of the articular facets and metaphyseal growth plates was present in many 3-month-old foals fed a copper-deficient diet.[335] Gross articular lesions of osteochondritis dissecans usually became evident at 3-6 months of age.[335,342] Osteochondrosis of the articular facets in itself rarely results in compression of the spinal cord but may later result in degenerative joint disease and vertebral stenosis.[8,187,323,327] Abnormalities in endochondral ossification at the vertebral physes (osteochondrosis) are more clinically significant and result in instability.[8,323,324,336,341,343] Typical developmental defects include flaring and enlargement of the caudal epiphyses and metaphyses, irregular metaphyseal growth plates with occasional areas of retained cartilage or osteosclerotic plaques, and disparity of longitudinal growth of the vertebral body and dorsal lamina (Fig 21).[8,187,323,344] Reduced growth of the caudal physis in the more cranial of 2 adjacent vertebrae at an affected articulation results in a short vertebral body as compared to the dorsal lamina, and partial flexion of the articulation in the standing animal. Because the fibrous intervertebral disk firmly unites adjacent vertebrae, deformation of the caudal metaphysis-epiphysis unit allows subluxation on flexion, with compression of the spinal cord between the cranial end of one vertebra and the dorsal lamina of the cranially adjacent vertebra (Fig

22). The deformations of the metaphyseal-epiphyseal units contribute to the narrow caudal foramina commonly seen in cervical vertebral instability.[8,187,323,345] The contribu-

Figure 21. Third and fourth cervical vertebrae in the extended position from a 10-month-old horse with cervical vertebral instability. The metaphyses and epiphyses of the vertebral bodies are flared, narrowing the vertebral canal. Other lesions consistent with aberrant bone development include physes that are irregular and contain osteosclerotic plaques, and a disparity of vertebral body and dorsal lamina lengths. This disparity results in caudal displacement of the dorsal intervertebral space (arrows) with respect to the intervertebral disk and predisposes the spinal cord to compression between the cranial portion of C_4 and the lamina of C_3.

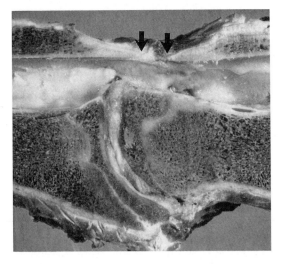

Figure 22. Third and fourth cervical vertebrae in the flexed position from the same horse as in Figure 21. Note the increased narrowing between the cranial vertebral epiphysis of C_4 and dorsal lamina of C_3, typical for cervical vertebral instability.

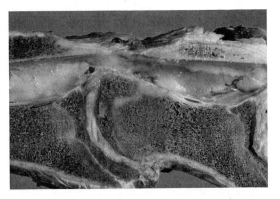

tion of the lateral vertebral arches and articular processes to vertebral narrowing is less important.[307,342,345-347]

Simple malformation and cartilage defects of the articular facets are commonly observed at sites of spinal cord compression and other noncompressive articulations in cervical vertebrae (Fig 23).[8,187,342,345,347,348] Articular facet lesions are not pathognomonic for spinal cord compression, nor is there a correlation between severity of articular facet changes and severity of spinal cord lesions.[348] A study of the cervical vertebrae of 300 fetuses and foals revealed that facet malformation and asymmetries developed in the third and fourth postnatal months.[342] Facet overgrowth and asymmetry were thought to begin with an osteochondrosis cleft in the last portions of the facet to ossify (*ie*, the cranioaxial portions of the cranial facets and caudal, abaxial portions of the caudal facets).[342,344] Cranial facets more often are involved in spinal cord compression due to this axial proliferation of the facet perimeter. Vascularization and ossification of this enlarged and semidetached cartilage fragment result in reattachment, often forming a secondary center of ossification with a deep cartilage fold demarcating the original facet from later developing tissue (Fig 24). If the cartilage fragment completely detaches, a free osteocartilaginous body develops. These osteochondritic joints are confined to weanlings and yearlings and, in concert with

Figure 23. Osteochondritis dissecans of the articular facet at C_3-C_4, with a semidetached cartilage flap and a deeply cleft facet perimeter.

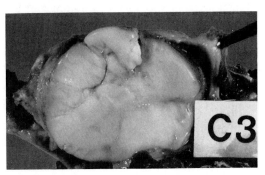

Figure 24. Standing lateral radiograph of a 7-month-old Thoroughbred filly with osteochondrosis of the facet joints at C_3-C_4, C_4-C_5 and C_5-C_6 (arrows). Only the C_3-C_4 junction was determined by myelography and necropsy to be a site of spinal cord compression. Osteochondrosis lesions of the facet often occur at multiple intervertebral junctions in the cervical vertebrae of young horses. Unless there are accompanying lesions in the vertebral bodies, as seen in Figure 21, these facet lesions do not always result in spinal cord compression.

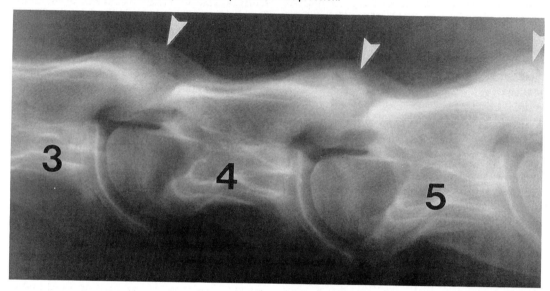

osteochondrosis changes in the vertebral body, result in cervical vertebral instability.[323,324,341,344]

Articular osteochondrosis lesions can result in degenerative joint disease by the time a horse is 2-3 years old. Similarly, trauma to the immature cartilage surfaces of the facets may result in degenerative joint disease. Associated with degenerative joint disease of the articular facets are further gross and occasionally massive enlargements of the perimeter of the facets due to osteophyte development (Fig 25). Compounding this enlargement are hypertrophy and fibrosis of the synovial membrane and joint capsule. Encroachment on the vertebral canal and lateral foramina can occur from either or both of these tissues.[8,187,307,323,349,350] Subsequent degeneration of cervical spinal nerves was recorded as early as 1939.[349] Why osteochondrosis and osteochondritis dissecans result in cervical vertebral instability in the midcervical vertebrae of weanlings and yearlings but not the caudal vertebrae is unknown. Osteochondrosis lesions occur in the caudal vertebrae but rarely result in clinical disease unless they cause degenerative joint disease. Additionally, it is not known why degenerative joint disease in the midcervical vertebrae is so uncommon.

Changes in the joint capsules, including fibrosis and fibrovascular proliferation, extend axially to blend imperceptibly with the ligamentum flavum, which frequently contains areas of hemorrhage, fibrovascular proliferation and occasionally foci of fibrocartilage.[8,327,351] Proliferation in these soft tissues is thought to result from stretching and tearing secondary to the instability asso-

Figure 25. Cranial view of the sixth cervical vertebra from a 2-year-old horse with degenerative joint disease involving the right facet joint at C_5-C_6. The facet is markedly enlarged due to periarticular osteophytes and joint capsule hypertrophy. The result has been bony encroachment on the vertebral canal and right-sided vertebral stenosis.

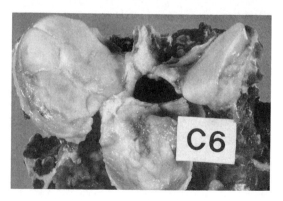

ciated with degenerative joint disease of the facet joints.[327,352] Such a mechanism is described for paravertebral ligament enlargements of the human spine.[353,354] These soft tissue enlargements secondary to degenerative joint disease of the facet joints are involved more frequently in development of spinal cord compression than the cartilage and bone proliferations of degenerative joint disease.[352]

Osteosclerosis of the dorsal laminae of the caudal cervical vertebrae is common and results from increased tension on the laminae by the ligamentum flavum.[327] Increased fibrocartilage and later endochondral ossification at the insertion of the ligamentum flavum on the dorsal lamina possibly result from tension on and stretching of the ligamentum flavum.[327]

Epidural synovial cysts have been reported as herniations (ganglia) or simple attachments to the synovial membrane of degenerate facet joints.[2,307,323-327,352,355,356] They can be multiple, frequently involve C6-C7, can compress the cord dorsolaterally, and rarely compress the spinal nerves as they exit the lateral vertebral foramina (Fig 26). Those directly communicating with a facet joint frequently collapse on flexion of the neck when spinal cord compression is relieved.

Figure 26. Epidural synovial cyst at C_6-C_7 (white arrows) associated with degenerative joint disease and chronic hypertrophy of the joint capsule. The enlarged joint capsule can also be seen more laterally in the vertebral canal (black arrow). These soft tissue structures are often partially retracted from the vertebral canal by flexion of the vertebral junction.

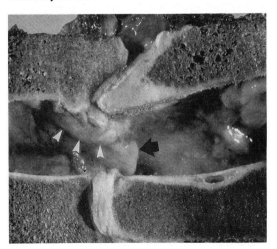

The cervical disks rarely contribute to the pathogenesis of stenosis. Only 2 reports of cervical disk herniation with spinal cord compression exist.[357,358] Disruption of the dorsal anulus fibrosus and protrusion of nucleus fibrocartilage also have been described in 5 normal horses studied in a review of normal cervical disks from 17 horses.[359] None of these animals had spinal cord compression associated with the protrusion. Degeneration of the nucleus pulposus in equine cervical disks is extremely uncommon due to their fibrous nature, as compared to the viscous collagen and mucoprotein material found in the nucleus of disks in people and other species.[357,359]

Histopathologic Findings: Horses with CVM have one or more focal compression-type lesions in the cervical spinal cord. Grossly, such lesions may appear as flattening of the cord. Histologically, they are characterized by swollen and disrupted axons and phagocytosis of myelin in white matter. Mild hemorrhages sometimes are seen in acute lesions. In the white matter of chronically affected animals, there are continued degeneration of neuronal fibers, proliferation of capillaries with prominent fibrous coats and astrofibrosis. More severely affected horses also have neuronal necrosis, loss of cell bodies and sometimes astrofibrosis in the gray matter. Massive focal lesions also occur with cavitating necrosis of white matter, particularly in lateral funiculi and occasionally in gray matter. Markedly asymmetric lesions are found in horses with prominently asymmetric signs. Cranial to the focal lesions, there is secondary degeneration of neuronal fibers (axons and myelin) in ascending tracts for variable distances, depending on the extent and age of the focal lesion. Caudal to the lesion, there is secondary fiber degeneration in descending tracts. This fiber degeneration is the result of neuronal fibers being severed from their cell bodies by the focal lesion. It is most prominent in dorsolateral funiculi cranial to the lesion, and deep lateral and ventromedial funiculi caudal to the lesion (Fig 27).

Clinical Signs: Cervical vertebral malformation is a common cause of ataxia in young horses. Most animals with instability are 6-18 months old, while those developing static stenosis are 18 months to 3 years old before signs appear.[323,326,328,340] Thoroughbreds and Quarter Horses have a high incidence of CVM.[323,324,326] The conditions occur in all

Figure 27. The histopathologic lesions of cervical vertebral malformation consist of a focal compression-type
lesion in the cervical spinal cord, and secondary neuronal
fiber degeneration in ascending tracts cranial to the lesion
and in descending tracts caudal to the lesion. (Courtesy
of *Cornell Veterinarian*)

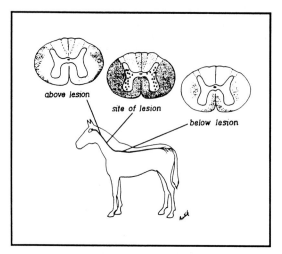

breeds, however, including the Arabian, Tennessee Walking Horse, American Saddlebred
and draft horse breeds.[324,326] Both sexes can
be affected, though most sources say males
are overrepresented.[2,8,187,326,330,336,338] Many
horses are well grown, and some have a history or signs of other developmental orthopedic disease, such as osteochondritis dissecans
and physitis.[8,343] Many affected horses have
a history of some minor fall or training incident that confuses the diagnosis with the
possibility of a fracture rather than a developmental vertebral malformation. Further, the
possibility that the horse was exhibiting mild
and unsuspected signs before the fall can
never be ruled out.

Clinical signs of ataxia and paresis usually
begin acutely, progress and then may stabilize or regress.[187,323,326,328] Complete recovery is very uncommon, though cycles of
improvement and later deterioration are frequent. Most affected horses appear out-
wardly normal; however, palpable swellings
of the cervical vertebrae are detected occasionally, particularly if the facet joints of the
midcervical vertebrae are involved in a degenerative process. Obvious cervical mal-
alignments are not generally a feature of
CVM; however, angular fixations do occur,
particularly at C2-C3, and occasionally are
visible and palpable. Ankylosed vertebrae
frequently result in instability at the adjacent

intervertebral junctions and may not be a site
of focal spinal cord compression. Pain on
palpation or lateral bending of the neck is
frequent, and reduced range of lateral motion often results from malformation or degenerative joint disease of the facet joints.

The principal neurologic signs include
ataxia, weakness and spasticity.[2,8,187,326]
Generally the pelvic limbs are most affected,
with thoracic limb signs being less obvious
(usually one grade less) and, occasionally,
developing later in the course of the disease.
Some affected horses may even show an apparent single pelvic limb lameness. Careful
neurologic evaluation is needed to identify
abnormalities in other limbs. Slight asymmetry of signs is common and may be marked,
depending on the lateralized nature of the
compression.[187,323,325,349,350,355] Extraordinarily severe thoracic limb signs, including
poor ability to step backward, can result from
malformation of the C6-C7 or C7-T1 junctions, where focal compression is applied to
the cervical intumescence.[323] Synovial cysts
or lateral foraminal stenosis due to bony osteophytes can exert pressure on the exiting
nerve roots and spinal nerves, resulting in
significant neck pain and a stilted, choppy
thoracic limb gait.[187,324] Severe lateral stenosis can result in unilateral pectoral and thoracic limb muscle atrophy; however, this is
considered uncharacteristic for CVM.[323]

Clearly, the neurologic signs of wobblers
with CVM are little different from those of
other diseases included in the differential
diagnosis, especially protozoal myeloencephalitis, degenerative myeloencephalopathy
and vertebral trauma.[2,8,187,326,328] A detailed
analysis of the history and careful neurologic
examination are helpful in establishing a tentative diagnosis, but radiography and myelography are most useful in confirming CVM.

Diagnosis: Radiographic and myelographic examinations are the most definitive
and valuable diagnostic tools in differentiating animals with CVM from those with other
spinal cord diseases. However, interpretation
of plain cervical radiographs can be difficult,
and the presence of obvious bony change does
not necessarily indicate a compressive spinal
cord lesion.[8,187,324,326] Myelography currently
is the best means of positively demonstrating
spinal cord compression.[323,324,328,361]

A tentative diagnosis usually can be obtained with plain cervical radiographs, based
on narrowing of the vertebral canal, degen-

erative joint disease of the facet joints, or malalignment of vertebrae. Plain radiographs of the midcervical area should be scrutinized carefully for evidence of malalignment associated with metaphyseal and epiphyseal flaring, disparate lengths of the vertebral body and dorsal laminae, and malformation and osteochondritis dissecans of the articular facets (Fig 28). Flexion and extension under general anesthesia also may reveal a tendency for an intervertebral junction to subluxate on flexion; however, because anesthesia is required for these manipulative tests, they are rarely used without myelography, as they are repeated at the time of myelography and then give a more precise indication of compression.

Measuring the vertebral canal diameter on plain radiographs has been advocated as a more objective measure of canal stenosis and spinal cord compression.[8,187] The values for minimal sagittal diameter for a particular horse can be compared to published normals for horses of similar size (Table 5). A value for minimal flexed diameter and minimal dural space diameter can be obtained at the time of myelography and compared to normal values. Horses with values less than normal minimums are almost certain to have vertebral canal stenosis. However, care must be used in duplication of the radiographic technique, especially in the object-film distance, as failure to keep the radiographic plate against the horse's neck results in magnification of the image, with resultant false-negative diagnoses. False-positive diagnoses, on the other hand, appear to be rare. Animals with lateral compression of the spinal cord and those with significant soft tissue components to the compression may be missed. In these horses, dorsoventral views obtained

during myelography allow accurate diagnosis.

The caudal cervical vertebrae should also be examined for additional radiographic features consistent with the purely stenotic form of CVM. Signs of degenerative joint disease, such as osteophytosis, subchondral bone sclerosis, and narrowed, roughened or obliterated joint spaces, can be significant (Fig 29).[2,187,324,361,362] Sclerosis and increased dorsoventral thickness of the dorsal laminae also are common findings in the form of CVM with static stenosis of the vertebral canal. In

Figure 29. Standing lateral radiograph of a 2-year-old horse with cervical static stenosis at C_6-C_7. Prominent osteophytosis and subchondral bone sclerosis have resulted in a roughened facet joint space. Sclerosis of the dorsal lamina of the seventh cervical veterebra is also evident, particularly the cranial border. Under anesthesia there was little motion at this level, suggesting the vertebral junction was partially ankylosed. Necropsy revealed spinal cord compression due to bony osteophytosis of the right facet joints and thickening of the dorsal lamina.

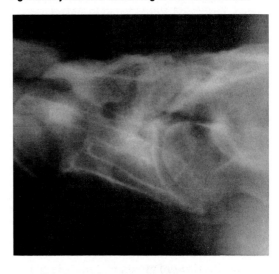

Figure 28. Standing lateral radiograph from a 10-month-old Thoroughbred colt with cervical vertebral instability (same horse as Figures 21 and 22). Note the typical flaring of the caudal metaphyses and epiphyses of the third and fourth cervical vertebrae, resulting in narrowing of the vertebral canal. The vertebrae are also aligned in a slightly flexed position.

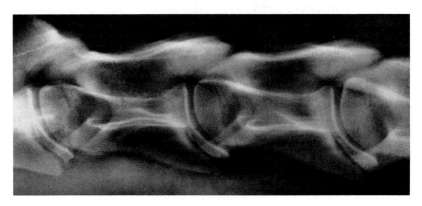

advanced stages, vertebral ankylosis and, rarely, narrowed disk spaces can be seen.

When plain radiographs demonstrate a suspicious area within the cervical spine, positive-contrast myelography is necessary to confirm the diagnosis, establish the number of intervertebral junctions involved and the severity of lesions in each, and to define the soft tissue contribution to spinal cord compression.[166,324,361] These factors are especially important if surgical decompression is being contemplated. Plain radiographs provide insufficient information. In a series of 306 myelographic studies in horses, false-positive diagnoses had been based on previous plain radiographs in 121 animals (40%), while false-negative diagnoses were made in 66 cases (22%).[362] This demonstrates how inaccurate and, at times, misleading survey radiographs can be. Techniques for myelography in horses are described in the literature.[361-364] The procedure should be performed under general anesthesia to allow for flexed, extended and ventrodorsal views of the cervical vertebrae. One report describes standing myelography and the associated complications.[365] Only water-soluble, nonionic contrast agents are suitable for use in equine myelography. Iohexol (Omnipaque: Winthrop), iopamidol (Isovue: Squibb) and metrizamide (Amipaque: Winthrop) are the most popular.

The horse is positioned in right lateral recumbency, and the head and neck are elevated on an inclined board. The lumbosacral subarachnoid space is punctured on the dorsal midline with a 6-in, 18-ga spinal needle, using the caudal limits of the tuber coxae as transverse landmarks. A sample of cerebrospinal fluid is collected and the stylet replaced. The atlantooccipital subarachnoid space is penetrated with a 3-in, 18-ga needle and another sample of CSF collected. Both samples of CSF can be submitted for laboratory analysis. Then, 30-50 ml of the contrast medium are injected slowly into the atlantooccipital subarachnoid space while CSF is allowed to flow freely from the lumbosacral needle. The lumbosacral exit port is not essential, nor is removal of CSF before introduction of the contrast medium. However, these procedures enhance the speed of caudal

Table 5. Reference values of measurements from radiographs made with the horse in lateral recumbency on the radiographic plate, with a 90-cm focal-film distance. These ranges are for the minimum sagittal diameter and minimum flexed diameter of the vertebral canal and for the minimum sagittal diameter of the myelographic dural space. These values are useful in identifying horses with CVM. Caution should be used when comparing values obtained with other radiographic techniques.

Radiographic Measurement	Horse's Weight	Cervical Vertebrae										
		C2	C2-C3	C3	C3-C4	C4	C4-C5	C5	C5-C6	C6	C6-C7	C7
Minimum sagittal diameter (mm)	<320 kg	20.8-26.8	—	18.1-21.5	—	16.7-20.7	—	17.3 22.1	—	18.3-23.9	—	19.8-26.1
	>320 kg	22.1-31.3	—	18.5-25.9	—	17.7-24.9	—	18.7-26.1	—	19.0-29.1	—	22.2-32.6
Minimum flexed diameter (mm)	<320 kg	—	19.3-29.7	—	13.4-22.0	—	13.2-22.5	—	16.1-25.7	—	21.6 36.7	
	>320 kg	—	22.8-36.5	—	15.6-27.8	—	14.8-28.2	—	17.9-32.9	—	28.5-45.6	
Minimum flexed dural space diameter (mm)	<320 kg	15.8-25.2	11.3-23.1	13.8-20.4	9.0-16.8	14.5-19.5	9.9-15.7	14.6-20.0	11.9-17.7	16.3-21.7	17.3-22.7	20.0-27.0
	>320 kg	16.9-27.9	12.9-27.9	15.5-24.1	10.5-20.9	15.1-23.3	10.8-19.0	15.4-24.8	11.4-20.8	18.0-26.2	17.6-25.6	16.2-34.6

814

migration of the contrast column. It is imperative that the contrast medium be introduced slowly.

Analytical-grade metrizamide (Accurate Chemical) in a dose of 12-20 g, mixed with 30-50 ml of sterile water, is the most commonly used contrast agent.[361-364] It is inexpensive compared to the medical-grade compound (Amipaque: Winthrop) but has the disadvantages of poor stability following reconstitution and is a nonsterile product, needing to be passed through a 0.2-μ millipore filter (Acrodisc: Gelman) before injection. Use of other new non-ionic, water-soluble, iso-osmolar contrast agents has been described.[366,367] These products are more expensive but are sterile, stable in solution, and convenient to use, and result in less muscle fasciculation and hyperthermia in the postmyelography recovery period. They are preferred over metrizamide for human myelography.[368]

The horse's head and neck are maintained in the elevated position for 3-5 minutes following contrast medium injection. The inclined board is removed and a series of radiographs obtained with the cervical vertebrae neutrally positioned and later in the flexed position. Hyperextended views rarely contribute further to the diagnosis and are not routinely obtained. If a lesion is present on the lateral examination, a ventrodorsal projection is recommended to determine the lateral component of compression (Fig 30). Soft tissue compression of the spinal cord, such as from a synovial cyst, is easily missed without a ventrodorsal projection. This projection can be reliably obtained for the vertebral junctions cranial to C_6-C_7 but generally is of poor quality for C_6-C_7 and C_7-T_1.[324,362,364]

Unstable vertebral articulations generally appear normal on the neutrally positioned myelographic projection (Fig 31). On flexion, however, a focal lesion is readily apparent as the vertebrae subluxate and compress the dorsal and ventral contrast columns (Fig 32). Compression of only the ventral contrast column when the vertebrae flex is a normal finding. Narrowing of the dorsal contrast column by >50% is considered to indicate significant compression; however, false positives and negatives still can occur, regardless of the examiner's experience.[8,323,324,361,362] Interpretation becomes increasingly difficult when the degree of contrast column narrowing approaches 50%. It is critical that the

narrowed areas of the dorsal and ventral contrast columns are diametrically opposed.

The site most frequently affected by vertebral instability is C_3-C_4.[2,8,166,187,307,323,324,338,361,362] Other sites frequently involved include C_4-C_5 and C_5-C_6. Multiple-level instability has been described at up to 3 consecutive levels.[348,362,369] A study of myelograms in 306 horses showed that 29% of horses with evidence of spinal cord compression had multiple sites affected.[362] The most frequent combination was C_3-C_4 and C_5-C_6. Cases of combinations of instability in the midcervical vertebrae and static stenosis caudal to this also appear in the literature, and demonstrate the importance of a complete myelographic study.[324,338]

Evidence of degenerative joint disease and thickened sclerotic dorsal laminae in the caudal cervical vertebrae can lead to a tentative diagnosis of CVM with static stenosis. Myelography confirms the diagnosis. Nevertheless, severe degenerative joint disease or lam-

Figure 30. Ventrodorsal myelogram at C_5 and C_6 from a yearling with cervical vertebral instability. There is marked compression of the contrast column from the left side (arrows), though only mild narrowing of the dorsal and ventral contrast columns was noted on the lateral myelogram.

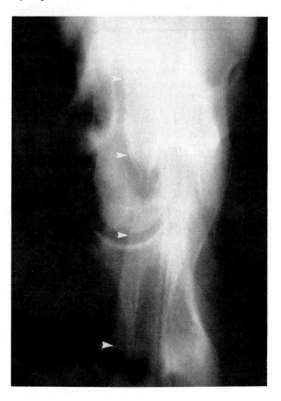

ina changes can be incidental findings, and not a source of spinal cord compression at all. The typical myelographic feature of cervical static stenosis is spinal cord compression throughout the full range of vertebral motion (Fig 33). Early in the disease, especially when the compression is predominantly due to exuberant joint capsule and ligamentum flavum, variable relief of the spinal cord compression can result from flexion (Fig 34). Later, bony changes become more severe, ankylosis of the vertebral junction develops, and spinal cord compression is continual.[324] The C6-C7 articulation most frequently is involved, and C5-C6 to a lesser extent. Compression at both levels has been described.[187,] [323,327,338,361,362,370] Compression involving C7-T1 also has been described in 2 horses.[370]

Complications of metrizamide myelography include fever, hyperesthesia, neck muscle fasciculations and exacerbation of neurologic signs.[361,362] Most postmyelography signs are mild and resolve within 24-48 hours, though increased ataxia may be more prolonged. No generalized seizures have been described using sterile water as a diluent with metrizamide. These side effects appear to be reduced further by use of iopamidol or iohexol, rather than metrizamide.[366,371]

Ancillary Testing: Analysis of cisternal and lumbosacral CSF samples is routine

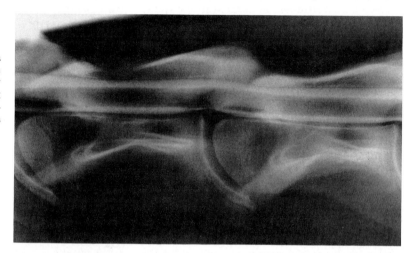

Figure 31. Myelogram of a Thoroughbred yearling with cervical vertebral instability at C_3-C_4. With the neck neutrally positioned, no spinal cord compression is present.

Figure 32. Flexion of the cervical vertebrae of the horse in Figure 31 results in subluxation of the vertebral articulation and compression of the spinal cord. Dorsal and ventral contrast columns are attenuated at the same level. Narrowing of only the ventral contrast column as the cervical vertebrae are flexed is a normal finding.

Figure 33. Myelogram from a 3-year-old horse with cervical static stenosis with the vertebrae in neutral position. Spinal cord compression is marked, as demonstrated by the narrowed dorsal and ventral contrast columns.

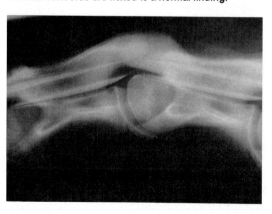

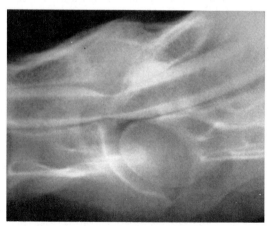

when sampled at the time of myelography. Laboratory analysis of CSF from animals with CVM generally is normal.[2,8,187,324,326] Any changes are mild and often include xanthochromia and an elevated protein content (70-130 mg/dl). Ruling out other neurologic conditions in the differential diagnosis of CVM is often the most useful purpose of CSF collection.[2,187]

Electromyography is rarely of assistance in diagnosis of CVM.[8,187] It is more helpful in detection of other neurologic diseases included in the differential diagnosis. Changes in the electromyographic patterns occasionally can be detected when articular osteophytes, joint capsule thickenings or synovial cysts exert sufficient pressure on the nerve roots to produce signs of lower motor neuron disease.[324]

Conduction velocity and amplitude of sensory impulses from peripheral nerves to the spinal cord (*spinal somatosensory evoked potentials*) and to the brain (*cortical somatosensory evoked potentials*) are altered in cases of CVM. Though normal values for several peripheral nerves in the pelvic and thoracic limbs of the horse have been established, the variability in results so far precludes use of spinal or cortical evoked potentials as an accurate means of defining the site and severity of the lesion.[372] Spinal recorded somatosensory evoked potentials have been valuable for diagnosis and prognosis in acute compressive spinal cord diseases in dogs.[373]

Treatment: Medical treatment of CVM is aimed at reducing edema and inflammation within the spinal cord. Most horses temporarily respond to medical therapy but regress when treatment ceases. Chronic spinal cord compression responds less definitively to medical management. Many horses with neurologic signs of short duration continue to deteriorate, and few ever improve and return to athletic activity.[187,324,326,328] Some mildly affected horses may stabilize and be suitable for breeding.

In the acute stages of the disease, phenylbutazone, corticosteroids and dimethyl sulfoxide (DMSO) are the most frequently used drugs. Dexamethasone at dosages up to 2 mg/kg IV or methylprednisolone sodium succinate (Solu-Delta-Cortef: Upjohn) in acute cases have been most popular. The effects usually are positive, but signs frequently deteriorate on drug withdrawal. The dangers of corticosteroid-induced laminitis, especially following use of large doses of dexamethasone, must be explained to the client before use. Dimethyl sulfoxide frequently is given in conjunction with or in lieu of corticosteroids. The usual dosage is 1 g/kg given slowly IV, using a maximum concentration of 20%. Dimethyl sulfoxide reportedly has diuretic, vasodilatory, antiinflammatory and membrane-stabilizing capabilities, in addition to being a potent scavenger of superoxide radicals.[374] Further, it increases cellular resistance to hypoxia and ischemia.[374] Diuretics, such as furosemide, can be given but rarely result in clinical improvement. Stall rest combined with antiinflammatory therapy is recommended to minimize spinal cord damage. Animals whose neurologic signs stabilize during stall rest eventually may be turned out to a small pasture.

Surgical therapy aimed at decompressing the spinal cord was first described in 1979.[375,376] This allowed an improved prog-

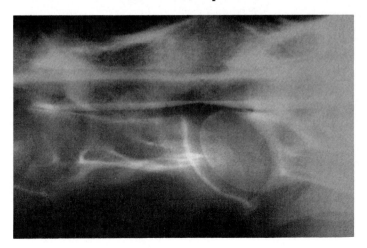

Figure 34. Myelogram from a horse with cervical static stenosis, with partial relief of the spinal cord compression by flexion of the articulation. The major compressive tissues were the ligamentum flavum and joint capsules. With increasing duration of clinical signs, the compressive tissues are more commonly the dorsal lamina and new bone production on the medial aspects of the facets. In these later stages, flexion offers little or no relief of compression.

nosis for survival but the prognosis for resumption of work still was not very good.

Stabilization of vertebrae by interbody fusion or arthrodesis is indicated in horses with instability.[375,377] The technique was adapted for use in horses from the original Cloward method of cervical intervertebral fusion in people.[378] The decompressive effect of ventral interbody fusion results from bony union of the 2 affected vertebrae, fixing them in extension. Because compression of the spinal cord usually is maximal during flexion, fusion prevents further compression and allows remodelling of the vertebral canal. The technique is well described in the literature.[166, 324,325,375,379-381] All descriptions involve a ventral approach, with removal of a major portion of the intervertebral disk and associated vertebral epiphyses. A frozen allograft bone dowel or various types of stainless-steel cylinders are then tamped into the drill hole to provide immediate fixation and promote eventual bony union of the 2 affected vertebrae.

Horses are positioned in dorsal recumbency with a narrow brace or leg stand beneath the affected intervertebral junction (Fig 35). The ventral surface of the neck from the mandible to the thoracic inlet is prepared for surgery. A 30-cm ventral midline skin incision, centered on the affected intervertebral junction, allows exposure of the omohyoideus and sternothyrohyoideus muscles. These are separated on the midline, and the deep fascia over the trachea is incised to allow the trachea to be retracted to the left. The right carotid artery and vagosympathetic trunk are retracted carefully to the right by tension on the adjacent sternocephalicus muscle. The ventral crest of the cranial vertebra at the affected junction is exposed by severing the insertions of the longus colli muscles. The ventral crest is then removed with a curved osteotome and its cancellous bone harvested for later use as a bone graft. The level bed thus formed extends cranially from the intervertebral disk, and the caudal physis of the vertebra is readily identified (Fig 36).

An 18-mm drill guide is centered over this physis and locked into the vertebral bone. The 18-mm drill is used to penetrate the disk space to within 10 mm of the vertebral canal. If this guide hole is suitably placed, a 25-mm hole is made to a similar depth using a larger drill and guide. The disk should be centered in the depths of the completed drill hole (Fig 37). Debris is removed from the site, and a fenestrated stainless-steel cylinder 22 mm long is packed with the drillings and with cancellous bone from the ventral crest, then driven into the hole. A corticocancellous bone graft can be used as an alternative but must be previously aseptically harvested from a donor, frozen, and then thawed for use. Complications with the graft's backing out, fracturing or collapsing have been described.[370, 382] The stainless-steel basket is placed below the level of the ventral surface of the vertebra and tends to lock in place when the horse stands postoperatively (Fig 38). If the caudal cervical vertebrae are being fused, a plastic

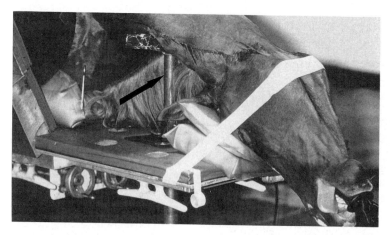

Figure 35. Horse positioned for cervical intervertebral fusion. The cervical vertebrae are extended by a support stand (arrow) at the approximate level of fusion.

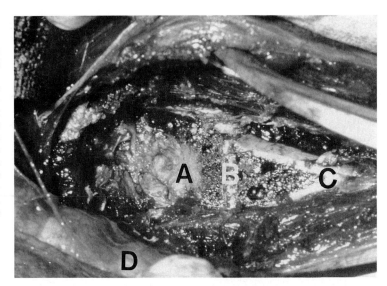

Figure 36. Ventral surface of an intervertebral junction exposed for fusion. The ventral crest (C) has been removed to expose the caudal physis of the cranial vertebra (B) and the intervertebral disk (A). The caudal physis is used to locate the drill site cranial to the disk, which compensates for the cranial curvature of the disk as the drill penetrates toward the vertebral canal. A retractor separates the longus colli muscles, and the trachea (D) is reflected to the left.

spinal plate is secured over the implant with cancellous bone screws to prevent the cylinder's backing out.

The longus colli muscles are reapposed over the implant and vertebrae with absorbable suture, and a suction drain placed immediately ventral to these muscles and exteriorized ventral to the jugular vein. The omohyoid and sternothyrohyoid muscles and subcutaneous tissues are sutured in continuous horizontal mattress patterns and the skin apposed with staples. The wound is protected by a stent bandage and the neck is wrapped with adhesive tape. Antibiotics and phenylbutazone are given preoperatively and continued for 3-5 days after surgery. The

Figure 37. Ventral fusion procedure with a 25-mm hole drilled over the intervertebral disk. A bone dowel or stainless-steel cylinder is then driven into the hole to provide immediate stabilization in extension.

drain and stent bandage are removed on day 5-6. The horse is confined to a stall for 8 weeks after surgery and then turned out for gradually increasing exercise.

Long-term results of cervical fusion are fair.[338,370] In a series of 27 horses, 15 returned to normal, and most of these were used for some athletic endeavor.[370] Those with residual neurologic signs were mildly affected (grade 1) and were satisfactory breeding animals. In another series, 72 of 89 horses improved 1 or more grades following

Figure 38. Standing lateral radiograph of a horse 4 days after cervical intervertebral fusion. The stainless-steel cylinder has been packed with cancellous bone, and maintains the affected vertebrae in extension until bony union occurs.

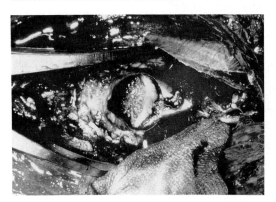

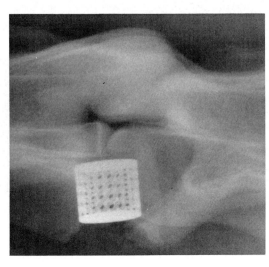

cervical fusion, with 9 improving 3 grades (on a scale of 4).[338] Many horses were assessed as normal on followup examination. Nevertheless, only 11 (12%) were able to perform as athletes; 7 (8%) of these raced and won. Twenty-four others (27%) were suitable for other riding activities or breeding.

Dorsal laminectomy has been the procedure of choice for decompression of cervical static stenosis lesions. The caudal cervical vertebrae are usually affected, especially C_6-C_7. Due to the consistent compression of the spinal cord irrespective of neck position, laminectomy is recommended for immediate decompression. The compression usually is quite focal, and a short laminectomy adequately removes the thickened laminae and associated exuberant soft tissues. It also provides access to the inner aspects of the neural canal for removal of encroaching articular facets, osteophytes and joint capsule. The approach to the caudal cervical vertebrae is relatively deep, and the surgery is a lengthy, demanding procedure. Several different descriptions appear in the literature.[166,379,383]

Selection of horses for laminectomy should eliminate particularly excitable animals and horses with any tendency for vertebral subluxation at C_6-C_7. These animals are better treated by interbody fusion.[370] Horses that have been recumbent for several days are the very worst candidates for any type of surgery, particularly laminectomy.

The horse is positioned in left lateral oblique recumbency, with the neck flexed and the dorsal surface extended beyond the edge

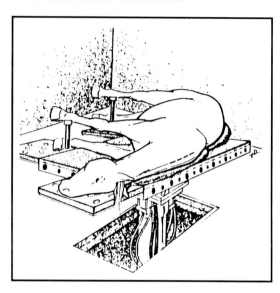

Figure 39. Left lateral oblique positioning used for dorsal laminectomy. The neck is flexed to reduce the depth of the vertebrae from the dorsal midline.

of the surgery table (Fig 39). After sterile preparation and draping, a 35- to 40-cm dorsal midline skin incision is made, commencing at the withers and extending cranially. The incision is extended through the nuchal fat, and the funicular ligamentum nuchae is separated on the midline. The lamellar portions of the ligamentum nuchae and adjacent spinalis and semispinalis muscles are separated and retracted with long-bladed retractors (Finochietto: Scanlan) (Fig 40). The dorsal spinous process of the 7th cervical and 1st thoracic vertebrae is used to identify the level

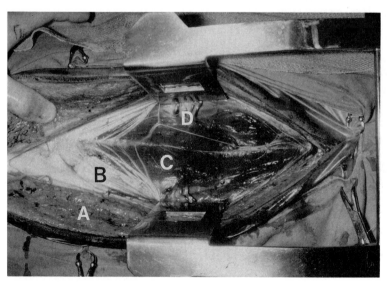

Figure 40. Dorsal approach to expose the caudal cervical vertebrae for laminectomy. Subcutaneous nuchal fat (A), lamellar ligamentum nuchae (B), spinalis muscles (C), and deep cervical blood vessels (D). Retraction is provided by large Finochietto self-retaining retractors. (Courtesy of J.B. Lippincott)

of dissection. The exposed multifidus muscles are elevated from the affected dorsal laminae with periosteal elevators. The joint capsules are carefully incised and reflected, and the ligamentum flavum excised with scissors. The dura mater should then be visible (Fig 41).

A short elliptic laminectomy is performed by forming a full-thickness channel through the lamina with a high-speed air drill. The cranial vertebra is decompressed first. The free piece of bone so formed is grasped in bone-holding forceps and freed of its soft tissue attachments with scissors. The caudal vertebra then is decompressed, resulting in an elliptic defect (Fig 42). If there is lateral compression from the joint capsules or bony in-growth of the facets, the dura is retracted gently and excess tissue removed with rongeurs and a diamond bur. When the spinal cord has been sufficiently decompressed, the laminectomy defect is lavaged copiously with saline and a free-fat graft is harvested from the nuchal fat and placed snugly into the defect. The multifidus muscles are sutured over the graft and a fenestrated suction drain placed dorsal to these muscles and exteriorized through the skin laterally. The funicular portion of the ligamentum nuchae, nuchal fat and subcutaneous tissues are closed with continuous patterns of absorbable suture material and the skin is apposed with monofilament nylon. A stent bandage is sutured in place. The horse should be assisted during recovery from anesthesia as it attempts to stand.

Preoperative antibiotics and phenylbutazone are continued for 3-5 days after surgery, and the drain and stent removed on day 5-7.

Of 30 horses followed for 5-7 years after laminectomy, 17 returned to normal neurologic status within 2 years, though the age of these horses at the end of their recuperative period usually excluded them from racing.[370,384] Most horses in that series, however, were Quarter Horses not bred for racing, but many performed in their intended use, such as rodeo eventing, Western pleasure or show ring eventing. Three horses had double-level laminectomies; 2 of these horses

Figure 42. A short elliptic laminectomy extends 2-3 cm from the free border into the lamina of each vertebra. The elliptic shape reduces concentration of stress by eliminating the corners of a rectangle.

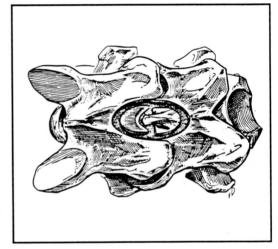

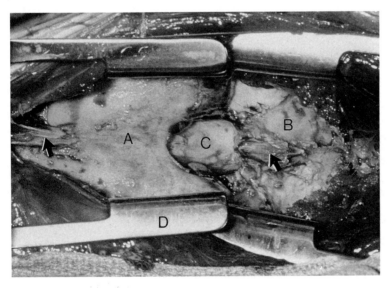

Figure 41. Dorsal laminae exposed for removal. The lamina of the cranial vertebrae (A) and caudal vertebra (B) have been cleared of the multifidus muscles and ligamentum flavum to expose the dura mater (C). The multifidus muscles are retracted with hinged self-retaining rake retractors (D). Arrows point to the dorsal spinous processes. (Courtesy of J.B. Lippincott)

returned to normal and intended use, and the other, a breeding stallion, improved neurologically but had a persistent stiff neck and eventually was euthanized.

An alternative surgical technique for horses with a stenotic vertebral canal involves interbody fusion of the caudal cervical vertebrae.[385] The surgical procedure is similar to intervertebral fusion of midcervical vertebrae; the rationale is different, however, as the spinal cord remains compressed for some time after surgery. Experimental studies demonstrated that articular facets and soft tissues atrophy after midcervical fusion.[382] This finding was used to theorize that atrophy of enlarged facets, joint capsules, ligamentum flavum and laminae might be expected after vertebral fusion. Of 8 horses in a preliminary report, 7 improved at least one grade within 10 months.[385] Followup myelography demonstrated considerable decompression of the spinal cord. The major disadvantage with this technique of self-decompression is the delay in relief of spinal cord compression by as long as 6 months. Long-term results are unavailable.

Prognosis: The prognosis appears improved after surgical therapy, though surgery by no means returns all animals to its intended use. The severity and duration of clinical signs and the adequacy of the diagnostic workup and surgical decompression often dictate the eventual outcome. Conservative therapy, for the most part, rarely returns a horse to useful purposes, even breeding. Many are destroyed for humane reasons. The generally poor outlook continues to stimulate study of the etiology of CVM and related diseases in horses.

Idiopathic Diseases

R.J. MacKay and I.G. Mayhew

Arthrogryposis (Contracted Foal Syndrome)

This term describes a wide range of contractures and curvatures of the limbs and vertebral column of neonatal foals. These defects resemble a syndrome in calves for which genetic factors, toxin ingestion during pregnancy, and prenatal viral infection are incriminated as causes. Affected calves have microscopic lesions in the spinal cord, peripheral nerves and muscles.[386] Despite the frequency of the mild forms of limb contracture and curvature in neonatal foals, the cause and pathogenesis usually are not known. An outbreak of limb deformities in foals born to mares that grazed on locoweed (*Astragalus mollismus*) while pregnant occurred in New Mexico.[266] In the southwestern United States, a high incidence of arthrogrypotic limb abnormalities has been seen in foals born to mares that grazed sorghum-Sudan grass or other *Sorghum* spp grasses between the 20th and 50th days of gestation.[387]

Symptomatic treatment of limb contractures and deformities with splints, casts, physical therapy and surgical intervention is discussed in the chapter on Diseases of the Musculoskeletal System. The success or failure of these treatments may depend, in a large part, on the degree of involvement of the central and peripheral nervous systems. A foal born with a single hind limb fixed in a flexed position had a depletion of lower motor neuron cell bodies in the ventral horn of the spinal cord in segments L_3 to S_4, as well as lesions in the peripheral nerves and muscles of that limb.[281] Such cases will not be cured by symptomatic management.

Vascular Abnormalities

Tumors, hamartomas, malformations or dilatations of vascular tissue may cause compression of neural tissue as they enlarge within the CNS. Lesions increase in size by growth or vascular degeneration and hemorrhage. Rare vascular abnormalities that have caused signs of focal spinal cord compression in horses are hemangioma, hematoma, hamartoma and aneurysm.[8,388-390]

Postanesthetic Myelopathy

A syndrome of postanesthetic hemorrhagic myelopathy has been reported in 6 horses.[391-395] Each of the affected horses was young (6-24 months) but heavy (300 kg). Neurologic abnormalities occurred after periods of anesthesia in dorsal recumbency of 45-105 minutes. Anesthesia was maintained with halothane-oxygen mixtures in all cases. Of the 6 affected horses, 3 were anesthetized for repair of umbilical hernias and 2 for removal of retained testes. Excision of chronically abscessed mandibular lymph nodes was the reason for anesthesia in the other horse. What appears to be an unusual preponderance of 2 abdominal procedures among this group may merely reflect the high frequency of such surgeries in young horses. In most cases, anesthesia and the initial period of recovery were uneventful. However, degrees of limb weakness were evident soon after recovery.

Initial signs ranged from difficulty standing, to tetraplegia with flaccid paralysis and anesthesia of the pelvic limbs. A characteristic clinical sign was depression of sensation and spinal reflexes over several contiguous segments. This is in contrast to the signs expected with focal spinal cord disease (*eg*, equine protozoal myeloencephalitis, vertebral fracture), in which there often is only a narrow strip of hypalgesia. Affected horses became recumbent or remained in lateral recumbency until euthanasia 1-8 days after surgery. At necropsy, there were hemorrhage and congestion of the meninges and spinal cord, and degrees of malacia of gray matter over at least several spinal cord segments at sites anywhere from the caudal cervical to caudal sacral spinal cord. Histologically, there were hemorrhage, venous distension and variable neuronal degeneration. These changes are consistent with hypoxic-ischemic neuronal damage of unknown cause.

There is speculation that the syndrome is due to systemic arterial hypotension and local venous congestion caused by halothane anesthesia, and compression of the caudal cava by abdominal viscera, respectively. Obviously, other contributory factors are involved, as the great majority of horses anesthetized in dorsal recumbency have no untoward sequelae.

The prognosis is hopeless in cases such as those described in the literature. However, it is likely that milder cases are not recognized. Those horses may benefit from supportive care and treatment for edema and toxic damage with corticosteroids and DMSO.

DISEASES OF THE CAUDA EQUINA

Diseases With Physical Causes

Sacral Fractures

Sacral fractures and sacrococcygeal luxations occur quite commonly. These injuries occur more often in mature horses than in foals. Sometimes there is a history of the horse's falling backward and striking its rump on the ground. In other cases, sacral injury was caused when the horse's rump was dragged under an overhead obstruction, such as the top half of a stall door. The neurologic signs of sacral fracture result from damage to the sacral and caudal nerve roots of the cauda equina as they course through the sacral vertebral canal. Arising from these nerve roots are the pudendal and caudal nerves and the parasympathetic pelvic nerves.[396] Thus, cauda equina injury results in varying degrees of paralysis, hypalgesia and hyporeflexia of the bladder, rectum, anus, vulva, tail and perineal skin as far ventrally as the udder or prepuce (Figs 43, 44). Fecal obstipation, bladder distention and urinary incontinence result. Neurologic signs may be evident immediately after injury or may occur days to weeks later due to delayed displacement of the fracture site. Once present, signs usually do not worsen. Rarely, exuberant callus formation at the fracture site may further compress sacral roots and exacerbate neurologic signs.

Sacral fracture is suggested by a history of trauma. Palpation of the sacrum per rectum can reveal a fracture with or without callus formation. Radiographs of the area are difficult to make and interpret. Ultrasound examination of the sacrum per rectum may be worth trying. Cauda equina syndrome due to sacral fracture must be differentiated from other diseases with similar clinical signs. Consideration should be given to neuritis of the cauda equina, sorghum-Sudan grass toxicity, EHV-1 myeloencephalitis, epidural empyema and other caudal meningomyelitides, such as cryptococcosis and listeriosis.

Conservative treatment usually is undertaken, and signs are monitored as in any peripheral nerve disorder. Particular attention must be given to evacuation of the rectum and urinary bladder. Antiinflammatory treatment (corticosteroids, nonsteroidal antiinflammatories) can be given for the first 3 days to minimize swelling due to trauma. Without clinical improvement in 6-12 weeks, the prognosis for long-term improvement is very poor. At least in other species, sacral fracture and displacement result in degrees of contusion, rather than in amputation, of sacrocaudal nerve roots. Assuming this is also true in horses, it probably is worth considering dorsal laminectomy of the sacrum to relieve compression of the cauda equina in horses with sacral fractures and cauda equina syndrome.

Figure 43. View of the tail, anus and perineum of a filly that suffered a fracture of the second sacral vertebra. Analgesia, areflexia and hypotonia were present in the tail, anus and perineal area, and there was fecal and urinary incontinence. These signs mimic those of neuritis of the cauda equina. An abnormal bulge, palpable on the ventral aspect of the sacrum, probably corresponded to the luxation at the fracture site.

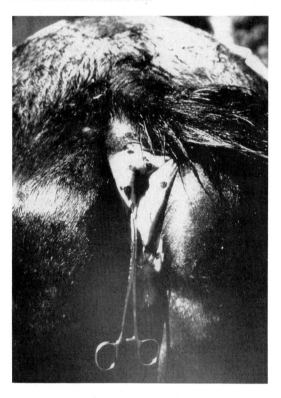

Figure 44. Right lateral view of the median section of the sacrum of the horse in Figure 43. (Courtesy of Dr. G.P. Carlson)

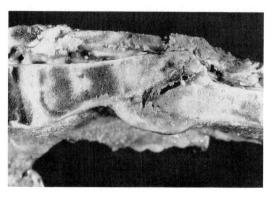

Tail Injuries

Cauda equina nerve roots may be damaged when heavy horses are lifted by the tail (usually with the aid of a tail rope). If there is sacrococcygeal dislocation, severe stretching and tearing of the cauda equina likely will result in permanent neurologic dysfunction. If there is no luxation of the tail, the neuronal lesion probably is a neurapraxia (functional and not structural) and can resolve with time and supportive care.

Though prohibited by the American Quarter Horse Association, tail injection of show horses of this breed is a common practice. The aim of the procedure is to minimize undesirable tail movement and carriage by partially or completely paralyzing the dorsal coccygeal musculature. Several intramuscular sites on each side of the tail head usually are injected with solutions of alcohol. Injections are often repeated to maintain the effect, resulting eventually in degrees of denervation and scarring that may be detectable by electromyography and cutaneous thermography, respectively. Guidelines for electromyographic detection of tail injections have been described.[397]

Inflammatory, Infectious and Immune Diseases

Neuritis of the Cauda Equina

A distinct pathologic syndrome characterized by chronic inflammation of the extradural roots of the cauda equina is seen in horses and ponies of both sexes.[398-402] Affected animals usually are mature or aged. The disease has not been reported in foals or yearlings. Cases of neuritis of the cauda equina have followed outbreaks of respiratory disease.

Cause: Most attempts to isolate an etiologic agent or to transmit the disease to other horses have been unrewarding. An equine adenovirus has been isolated from the cauda equina of 2 of 3 affected horses, though the role of virus in the pathogenesis of the disease is not understood.[396] The lesions are strongly suggestive of an immune-mediated process similar to experimental allergic neuritis of laboratory animals.[405] Experimental allergic neuritis is induced in rats by repeated immunization with homogenates of peripheral nerves, or with a specific protein purified from peripheral nerves, P2 myelin protein.[405]

That neuritis of the cauda equina indeed may be a spontaneous form of experimental allergic neuritis is suggested by studies that have demonstrated anti-P2 serum antibodies in horses with confirmed neuritis of the cauda equina but not in normal horses or in horses with neurologic diseases other than neuritis of the cauda equina.[406,407] Use of an enzyme-linked immunosorbent assay to detect anti-P2 antibodies helps differentiate this disease from other peripheral neuropathies.[407]

Clinical Signs: Because of the frequent multifocal or diffuse character of the disease, the name *polyneuritis equi* has been proposed. The presenting signs are quite variable, though usually referable to sacrococcygeal nerve root involvement. There usually is an insidious onset and progression over several weeks, though the signs may be noticed acutely by the owner. Often there is a recent history of rubbing and abrasion of the tail head and perineum, colic due to obstipation, or hypersensitivity to pressure over the gluteal area. By the time veterinary attention is sought, there usually is a well-demarcated area of cutaneous analgesia and areflexia involving the tail, perineum, caudal gluteal area, and the penis but not the prepuce. Frequently the area of cutaneous analgesia is surrounded by a band of hyperesthesia. The tail hangs limply without tone, and the anal sphincter, rectum, bladder, urethral sphincter and vulva or penis are paralyzed. This leads to fecal retention, and feces may appear at the orifice of the flaccid, dilated anus. After 1-2 weeks, there are marked atrophy of coccygeal muscles, urinary incontinence with bladder distention, and continual dribbling of urine from a gaping vulva or prolapsed penis, resulting in urine scalding of the perineum and legs. Appetite and vital signs usually are normal at this stage unless there is severe secondary cystitis.

Pelvic limb weakness may occur, especially as the disease progresses, due to inflammation of the sacral and even lumbar nerve roots and extension of perineuritis to the lumbosacral plexus supplying the gluteal, sciatic and, rarely, the femoral nerves. Gait abnormalities often are subtle and asymmetric, at least initially, with slight swaying of the hips, stumbling, and toe-dragging in the pelvic limbs. Depending on nerves affected, there may be atrophy of the gluteal, biceps femoris or other muscles on one or both sides. Examination of CSF collected by lumbosacral puncture usually reveals moderate elevations in protein concentration and numbers of mixed populations of WBC.[402]

Though signs of sacrococcygeal nerve root disease are most obvious, involvement of other nerve roots and peripheral nerves is not uncommon. Many affected horses thus have evidence of cranial nerve abnormalities, including masseter atrophy and weakness (motor V), facial paralysis (VII), head tilt, nystagmus and staggering gait (VIII), tongue weakness (XII), difficult swallowing (IX, X), depressed pupillary light reflex (III), and blindness (II).[398-400,402,403] Cranial nerves V, VII and VIII are affected most commonly, usually asymmetrically. There are rare reports of thoracic limb weakness and ataxia due to involvement of the nerve roots and nerves of the brachial outflow and plexus. Histologically, the autonomic nervous system is involved.[404]

Treatment: Despite clinical fluctuations during the course of the disease, neuritis of the cauda equina invariably persists and is fatal without treatment. However, regular manual evacuation of the rectum, catheterization of the bladder, and monitoring for and treatment of urinary tract infection may prolong the life of the horse for many months. The reproductive productivity of affected horses is not likely to be rewarding. Treatment with various antibiotics, and systemic, epidural and subarachnoid administration of corticosteroids all have been ineffective.

Necropsy Findings: Grossly, the epidural nerve roots of the cauda equina are discolored and coated with a thick, fibrous material. This perineural material extends intradurally and through intervertebral foramina, then along the lumbar, sacral and coccygeal nerves. Histologically, in the acute stage, there is lymphocytic neuritis with evidence of demyelination.[408] Later there is chronic granulomatous neuritis that extends extradurally, with mononuclear cellular inflammation, sometimes hemorrhage, and marked collagen deposition in the epineurium.

Toxic Diseases

Sorghum Poisoning

A syndrome characterized by ataxia and cystitis has been reported in horses grazing *Sorghum* spp plants.[409,410] Cases have been observed in Texas, Oklahoma, New Mexico,

Arizona, California, Kansas and Colorado. A similar syndrome has been seen in horses, cattle and sheep in northern and western Australia.[411,412] The disease most commonly has been seen in horses grazing hybrid crosses of sorghum (*S vulgare*) and Sudan grass (*S vulgare* var *sudanense*); however, other species, including Johnson grass (*S halepense*), have been incriminated. Well-cured *Sorghum* hay apparently does not cause the disease.

There is no breed or sex predilection, and horses ≥5 months of age have been affected. Symmetric ataxia and weakness of the pelvic limbs usually are the first signs noted. Flaccid paralysis of both pelvic limbs and the tail occasionally develops within 24 hours after the onset of neurologic signs. Urinary incontinence develops soon after nervous signs in most horses, manifested as continual dribbling from a "relaxed" vulva or penis. When affected horses are removed from sorghum-Sudan pasture, they usually improve but do not fully recover. In a series of cases involving 36 affected horses from various areas in the southwestern United States, the average morbidity was 25%; mortality was <2%.[409,410] Death, when it does occur, usually is due to severe cystitis. Lesions found at necropsy are varying degrees of cystitis and, microscopically, axonal degeneration and demyelination at all levels of the spinal cord, with the most severe changes found in the lumbosacral segments. The toxic principle in sorghum-Sudan is not known, but causal roles have been suggested both for cyanogenic glycosides and lathyrogenic precursors in *Sorghum* plants.[410-412]

DISEASES OF THE PERIPHERAL (SPINAL) NERVES

Diseases With Physical Causes

Peripheral Nerve Injuries

Suprascapular Nerve: Surgical transection of the suprascapular nerve at the cranial border of the scapula results in atrophy of the supraspinatus and infraspinatus muscles (sweeney) but no persistent gait abnormality.[413,414] This must be contrasted with the condition that commonly results from shoulder trauma.[415,416] Typically, this occurs when galloping horses collide with other horses or with inanimate objects, such as fences. Suprascapular nerve injury also may be caused by tension on the nerve as the animal stumbles with the limb stretched back. Injury, therefore, is most frequent in horses worked over uneven ground.

The forces of impact and/or stretching apparently damage some to all of the nerve roots of the brachial plexus that contribute to the subscapular, pectoral and probably other nerves supplying the thoracic limb, as well as directly injuring the suprascapular nerve. Consequently, many of the supporting structures of the shoulder, including the subscapularis, supraspinatus and infraspinatus muscles, are effectively denervated. This causes laxity or instability of the shoulder joint, which allows the shoulder to subluxate or "pop" laterally ("shoulder slip") as the affected limb bears weight. Some horses circumduct the affected limb during protraction to avoid dragging the toe. The resultant lameness renders the horse unsound for athletic events.

Treatment of uncomplicated suprascapular nerve paralysis due to trauma is unnecessary if the horse is not used for performance. However, for cosmetic purposes and for horses expected to exercise satisfactorily, therapy should be considered at the time of injury and again in 2-12 weeks. Ideally, the severed stumps of the nerve should be anastomosed if the suprascapular nerve is severed at the time of injury.[416] If this is not feasible because of related soft tissue trauma, the stumps of the nerve may be freed from adjacent tissues and identified using stainless-steel sutures to allow exploration and anastomosis after other soft tissue healing is complete. It is reasonable to assume that at least the fibrous nerve sheath is still intact in cases of closed trauma resulting in suprascapular nerve paralysis. Under these circumstances, systemic administration of anti-inflammatory agents for a short time (*eg*, dexamethasone IM at 0.05 mg/kg BID, flunixin meglumine IM at 0.5 mg/kg BID, or phenylbutazone PO at 2.2 mg/kg BID for 3 days) may help suppress local swelling and inflammation that can further damage nerve fibers. Stall confinement also is appropriate. Immediate application of icepacks to the area also should be considered.

Function returns in days to weeks in cases of neurapraxia (loss of function due to concussion to the nerve). If there has been severance of axons (axonotmesis) or whole fibers (neurotmesis), with relative preservation of the endoneurium, perineurium and epineurium, the nerve fibers distal to the injury site undergo Wallerian degeneration. Proximal axons may then regrow down the distal fibrous framework at about 1 inch/ month to reinnervate the atrophied muscles. Consequently, enough time should be allowed for this process (*ie*, reversal of muscle atrophy) to occur. However, allowing too much time to elapse can result in permanent fibrosis and contracture of atrophied muscles. Therefore, if treatment of a horse with chronic, traumatic suprascapular paralysis is necessary, surgical decompression probably should be performed within 8-12 weeks of injury.[417]

A surgical procedure has been designed to relieve compression of the suprascapular nerve as it winds around the front of the scapula.[418] Even in normal horses, the nerve at this site is subject to compression sufficient to cause continual mild demyelination and repair.[419] Therefore, in horses with sweeny, there may be improved likelihood both of recovery from nerve concussion (neurapraxia) and of regeneration of severed axons along nerve sheaths if a decompressive procedure is performed at this site. Results of the surgery have been excellent, with each of 12 treated horses recovering part or all of the mass of infraspinatus and supraspinatus muscles.[418] Somewhat surprisingly, the gait abnormalities associated with shoulder instability were completely resolved in all 12 horses, even though nothing was done to restore function of the subscapularis muscle. The reader is referred to another publication for details of the scapular notch resection procedure for decompression of the suprascapular nerve.[418] The essential element of the procedure is removal of a 1.5-cm section of bone immediately underlying the nerve at the cranial margin of the scapula.

Attempts at camouflaging signs of sweeney, such as injecting air under the skin of the shoulder or creating a foreign body reaction over the shoulder by implanting a coin, have been employed.[417] Results of such "treatments" are less than satisfactory.

Radial Nerve and Brachial Plexus: Failure to bear weight on a thoracic limb because of inability to extend the limb and flex the shoulder joint reflects total radial paralysis.[414,417] Affected horses have great difficulty getting up and down, and stand with the shoulder extended. The elbow, knee, fetlock and interphalangeal joints are flexed, and the dorsum of the toe rests on the ground.[420] The elbow is maintained in the "dropped" position during locomotion, and the limb is advanced only half a stride, usually with the toe dragging; the horse collapses on the limb when forced to bear weight on it. With partial paralysis, the horse may be able to advance the limb by jerking the shoulder and limb craniad to support some weight and may back up reasonably well.[420] This may reflect some function in the extensor carpi radialis and common digital extensor muscles. Interestingly, horses with partial radial paralysis often can bear weight on the limb and paw the ground, especially if supported in a body sling. This probably is due to function of the flexor muscles of the elbow (and musculocutaneous nerve), allowing elevation of the limb, passive striking of the ground, then flexion of the carpus and digits via ulnar and median innervation. Areas of analgesia of the skin of the leg have been defined in radial paralysis cases.[6] However, these are not easily defined in clinical cases, and electrophysiologic studies have failed to reveal a clinically testable autonomous zone for the cutaneous branches of the radial nerve.[421] Radial paralysis of more than 2 weeks' duration results in degrees of atrophy of the triceps, extensor carpi radialis, ulnaris lateralis and digital extensor muscles.

The radial nerve is well protected by surrounding muscle but can be damaged by direct trauma and prolonged lateral recumbency, particularly with malpositioning of the limb. The radial-type paralysis seen frequently in the dependent and occasionally in the upper (nondependent) forelimb after anesthesia in lateral recumbency originally was thought to be the result of pressure on and stretching of the radial nerve.[422] This form of postanesthetic lameness is most probably the result of ischemic myopathy, with a component of ischemic neurapraxia (see the chapter on Diseases of the Musculo-skeletal System).[423] Severe trauma to the cranial shoulder region may result in signs of radial paralysis as a component of presumed compression of the nerves of the brachial plexus, as described under Suprascapular Paralysis. Fractures of the first rib also can result in paralysis of the radial nerve and other nerves of the brachial plexus.

Radial paralysis may accompany humeral fractures. Function of this nerve should be evaluated before fracture repair because of the poorer prognosis that accompanies radial damage.[417] If traumatic radial paralysis has occurred more than 1-2 weeks before evaluation, needle electromyography may help define the extent of muscular denervation. The radial nerve should be examined at the time of any humeral fracture fixation, and appropriate debridement and re-anastomosis performed as described under Suprascapular Paralysis. The forelimb should be placed in a light plaster cast to avoid trauma and flexion contracture.[417] Because the rate of regrowth of severed axons is about 1 inch per month, regrowth of more than about 12 inches cannot be expected, as irreversible fibrotic contracture will likely intervene.

Tumors and abscesses in the cranial thorax and tumors of the brachial plexus and radial nerve may rarely result in radial paralysis. Spinal cord lesions, such as protozoal myelitis involving the caudal cervical and cranial thoracic ventral gray matter, can produce the syndrome, though additional signs of myelopathy usually are seen. Horner's syndrome may be expected with cranial thoracic gray matter or nerve root involvement.

Musculocutaneous, Median and Ulnar Nerves: Paralysis of any of these nerves rarely occurs as a singular event, and the resulting syndromes are not well documented.[414] However, brachial plexus injuries and spinal cord lesions involving gray matter of the brachial intumescence may cause signs related to involvement of some or all of these nerves. The nerves are well protected under the shoulder girdle and not often involved in long-bone fractures, though elbow fractures may affect the ulnar and median nerves.

Section of the proximal musculocutaneous nerve results in a gait alteration that may disappear within 3 months.[414] Toe dragging is associated with decreased elbow flexion.

Needle electromyography can disclose denervation potentials in the biceps and brachialis muscles. Partial sensory loss is expected in the skin over the craniomedial aspect of the knee and metatarsal region, possibly distally to the coronet.[421]

Median neurectomy results in a stiff gait in the limb, with toe dragging due to decreased flexion of carpus and fetlock, and hypalgesia of the medial aspect of the distal limb. Within 2 months, there is little or no gait abnormality.[414]

The remarkable subtlety of gait alteration with paralysis of the individual nerves after a period of adaptation (3 months) may be explained in part by crossing of fibers from one nerve to the other. Decussation occurs at least between the musculocutaneous and median nerves.[414] Ulnar neurectomy results in a gait change that is similar, though more pronounced, to that seen in median neurectomy. There is decreased flexion of the carpus and fetlock, and the foot may be projected in a jerky fashion. There is said to be marked hypalgesia of the lateral aspect of the metacarpus and foot, and probably of the caudal aspect of the forearm.[421] Residual gait abnormalities include stumbling on the limb and decreased flexion of the fetlock. Obvious atrophy of the digital flexors should be apparent. All these findings may be variable.

Combined ulnar and median neurectomy apparently results in signs very similar to those of ulnar neurectomy alone.[414]

Therapy for paralyses involving these nerves is the same as described above for peripheral nerve injuries, though aggressive therapy may be unnecessary because of the remarkable improvement of any gait alteration with the passage of time.

Femoral Nerve: The femoral nerve innervates the major extensor muscles of the stifle, and paralysis of this nerve results in inability to extend the stifle. Because of reciprocal flexion of the tarsus and digits when the stifle flexes, femoral nerve damage results in extensor paralysis, with the affected limb held in an overflexed position and the ipsilateral hip lower than the other. Essentially, no weight is supported on the affected limb during locomotion. Bilateral involvement causes the horse to have great difficulty in rising from the recumbent position. Once standing, the horse assumes a "crouched" position because of flexion of the joints of both pelvic limbs. If the horse is recumbent, the patellar reflex is depressed or absent, though there is a normal flexor reflex if the sciatic nerve is intact. There may be hypalgesia of the medial thigh if the lesion involves the saphenous nerve or the femoral nerve proximal to where this sensory branch bifurcates. Ultimately, there is atrophy of the quadriceps muscles.[417] The horse's gait abnormality may eventually improve slightly, presumably by the action of the proximal abductor and adductor muscles' fixing the stifle joint, allowing weight-bearing on the limb.[420]

The femoral nerve is well protected from external injury during its course but may be damaged by penetrating wounds in the caudal flank. Femoral paralysis has occurred with abscesses, tumors and aneurysms in the region of the external iliac arteries. Fractures of the pelvis and femur may be associated with damage to the femoral nerve; integrity of the nerve should be determined before fracture repair is attempted in such cases.

Femoral nerve injury was suspected in 2 adult horses that had difficulty standing after a period of anesthesia in dorsal recumbency. Signs of postanesthetic myopathy complicated the clinical picture in both horses. In a horse that died, necropsy revealed bruising over both femoral nerves over the insertion of the psoas minor muscles.[424] Overextension of a pelvic limb (or limbs) in a recumbent horse has resulted in femoral paralysis.[417] Exertional rhabdomyolysis and postanesthetic myopathy syndromes may cause unilateral or bilateral extensor weakness in the pelvic limbs that clinically resembles femoral nerve damage because of involvement of the quadriceps musculature (see the chapter on Diseases of the Musculoskeletal System).

Spinal cord lesions of the ventral gray matter or nerve roots at L_4 and L_5 can result in femoral paralysis and must be differentiated from paralysis due to injury to the femoral nerve. Equine protozoal myeloencephalitis has caused this, though helminths and trauma also could do the same.

Despite hope for improvement, the prognosis must be guarded unless the nerve can be repaired. A light horse with unilateral femoral paralysis may get around satisfactorily without breaking down in the contralateral limb. The principles of medical and surgical management of peripheral nerve injuries are discussed under Suprascapular Paralysis.

Peroneal Nerve: This branch of the sciatic nerve supplies the flexor muscles of the tarsus and extensor muscles of the digits. Paralysis thus results in extension of the tarsus, and flexion of the fetlock and interphalangeal joints. At rest, an affected horse holds the limb somewhat extended caudad, with the dorsum of the hoof resting on the ground. During locomotion, the foot is dragged along the ground, then jerked caudad when an attempt is made to bear weight on the limb, after which the limb is pulled partly craniad again. This caudal jerking of the limb and sliding of the hoof on the ground may be repeated several times. If the limb is advanced manually and the toe extended, the horse can bear weight on the limb.[420] Hypalgesia reportedly occurs on the craniolateral aspect of the gaskin, hock and metatarsal regions.[6,420] Atrophy of the craniolateral aspect of the gaskin may be expected.

The peroneal nerve is most vulnerable to external injury where it crosses the lateral condyle of the femur. Injury from kicks by other horses and from lateral recumbency usually does not sever the nerve, and many affected horses eventually improve.

The limb should be supported and protected. Other aspects of therapy are as described for suprascapular nerve injury.

Tibial Nerve: The tibial branch of the sciatic nerve innervates the gastrocnemius and digital flexor muscles. Paralysis causes the limb to be held with the tarsus flexed and the fetlock resting in a flexed or partly knuckled position. Consequently, the hip is held lower on the affected side. Flexion of the hock and extension of the digits are unopposed; therefore, the horse overflexes the limb when walking, and the foot is raised higher than normal. In addition, controlled extension of the hock cannot occur at completion of the advancing phase of the stride, and the foot is dropped straight to the ground. The overall stride is similar to that seen with stringhalt.[420] Atrophy of the gastrocnemius muscle and anesthesia of the caudal metatarsal region and medial and caudal coronary region also occur.[6]

Tibial paralysis is very uncommon, partly because the nerve is well protected by the muscles and bones of the limb.

Sciatic Nerve: The sciatic nerve supplies the main extensor muscles of the hip and flexor muscles of the stifle, and divides into peroneal and tibial branches. Total sciatic paralysis results in a profoundly abnormal gait and posture, mainly from flexor weakness. At rest, the limb hangs behind the horse, with the stifle and hock extended, the fetlock and interphalangeal joints partly flexed, and the dorsum of the hoof on the ground. During locomotion, the foot is dragged, or the distal limb is jerked dorsad and somewhat craniad by the flexor muscles of the hip and the extensor muscles of the stifle (femoral nerve innervation). If the foot is manually advanced and placed on the ground ventral to the pelvis, the horse can support weight with some flexion of the hock and take a stride.[420,422] Muscles of the caudal thigh and all of the limb distal to the stifle atrophy.[6] Degrees of hypalgesia over most of the limb except for the medial thigh have been reported.[420]

The proximal sciatic nerve is well protected, though, because of its close relationship with the pelvis, it may be damaged by fractures of the pelvis, especially of the ischium. In young foals, deep injection reactions caudal to the proximal femur and *Salmonella* osteomyelitis of the sacrum and pelvis have resulted in sciatic paralysis. Treatment of such primary problems may resolve sciatic paralysis, but if the nerve is severed, the prognosis is unfavorable, even with surgical anastomosis. This is because of the great distance over which nerve fiber regeneration must proceed. Support and protection should be given to the distal limb. Other aspects of therapy of peripheral neuropathies are covered above.

Syndromes of sciatic palsy and flexor weakness can occur with spinal cord lesions, such as equine protozoal myeloencephalitis affecting the L_5-S_3 ventral gray matter or nerve roots. Other signs, such as urinary bladder paralysis, gluteal atrophy and degrees of extensor weakness, also may be present.

Postfoaling Paralysis

"Obturator" paralysis is an infrequent sequel to foaling. Signs may occur even without a history of dystocia.[425] Because of its course along the medial aspect of the shaft of the ilium, the obturator nerve is vulnerable to compression by the bony prominences of the foal during the birth process.[426] The nervous web from which the cranial gluteal, sciatic and caudal gluteal nerves arise also is exposed to parturient compression where it lies against the ventral aspect of the sacrum.

Depending on the severity of nerve and nerve root contusion, signs may range from mild stiffness to paraplegia. In mild cases, unilateral obturator nerve involvement may be apparent as abduction and circumduction of the ipsilateral limb at a walk. The affected limb may slip laterally on slippery surfaces, especially when the mare attempts to rise. Occasionally hemorrhage in and around the femoral nerves results in extensor weakness, patellar hyporeflexia, and analgesia of the medial thigh. Antiinflammatory therapy (corticosteroids, phenylbutazone) is indicated, as well as basic nursing care in recumbent horses. Individual nerve roots usually are not severed, and function should return over a period of weeks, providing that complications of prolonged recumbency (ischemic myoneuropathy, decubital ulcers) do not necessitate the horse's destruction. Use of a body sling should be considered in horses that can support most of their own weight at least part of the time. The prognosis for survival in postfoaling paralysis is fair, with about 50% recovering.

Inflammatory, Infectious and Immune Diseases

Polyneuritis Equi

The section on Diseases of the Cauda Equina contains a discussion of this subject.

Neoplasia

Neoplastic conditions are discussed in this chapter under Diseases of the Forebrain.

Idiopathic Diseases

Stringhalt, Shivering

Stringhalt is characterized by an abnormal gait, with involuntary and exaggerated flexion of the hock of one or both pelvic limbs during attempted movement.[427] Intoxication from hay containing *Lathyrus hirsutus* (caley pea) plants results in a syndrome (neurolathyrism) of pelvic limb dysmetria that, in its chronic form, is very similar to stringhalt.[139] A clinically related condition of draft breeds, known as "shivers," is characterized by tremors of the musculature of the pelvic limbs and elevation of the tail.[428] The condition is most pronounced when the affected animal is forced to move backward or to exercise. "Shivers" is thought to be hereditary and usually is progressive.

Stringhalt occurs in both outbreak and sporadic forms. The cause has not been identified in either type, but outbreaks of stringhalt (Australian stringhalt) have been associated with particular pasture and climatic conditions.[427,429] Horses grazing weed-infested pastures during periods of drought most often are affected. *Hypochaeris radicata* (dandelion, cat's ear, flatweed) plants frequently dominate pastures of this type. Outbreaks of Australian stringhalt also have been seen in horses grazing European dandelion (*Taraxacum officinale*) or mallow plants (*Malva parviflora*). Feeding dandelion plants or plant extracts to horses has not reproduced the disease. Because Australian stringhalt occurs when climatic conditions favor mycotoxicoses of grazing animals (*eg*, facial eczema, ryegrass staggers, paspalum staggers), a mycotoxic cause is suspected.[429] Sporadic cases of stringhalt have been linked to various musculoskeletal disorders of the pelvic limb, as well as to lumbosacral spinal cord disease. No consistent cause and effect have been demonstrated.

Signs of stringhalt often develop suddenly. In mild cases, exaggerated hock flexion is seen only during turning or backing and may disappear with exercise. In its most severe form, however, stringhalt is disabling. In such horses, the affected limb is flexed so violently that the fetlock slaps the abdomen with each step. The limb may remain flexed for several minutes. When both pelvic limbs are severely involved, forward movement is only possible by a bizarre "bunny-hopping" action. In extreme cases, the horse may be unable to stand. With chronic stringhalt, there may be atrophy of distal limb muscles. Some horses with Australian stringhalt also have thoracic limb involvement, evident as spasticity, toe-scuffing and stumbling.[427,429] Inspiratory stridor due to left laryngeal hemi-

paresis also is a complication of some cases of Australian stringhalt (and of lathyrism).

The signs of stringhalt likely result from interference with the reflex arcs and connections that maintain postural tone and coordinate muscle contraction in the pelvic limbs. Thus, stringhalt may result from a sensory or motor neuropathy, myopathy or spinal cord disease, and there is some evidence for cases occurring with lesions at each of these sites. Tibial neurectomy produces stringhalt-like signs, with unopposed hock flexion and digital extension (peroneal nerve) predominant. In lathyrism and Australian stringhalt, there is nerve fiber degeneration in at least the distal sciatic nerve, with evidence of neurogenic muscle atrophy in severe cases.[139,430] Degeneration of the left recurrent laryngeal nerve is seen in cases showing laryngeal hemiparesis. Equine protozoal myeloencephalitis and other spinal cord diseases occasionally result in a stringhalt-like gait. Some sporadic cases are associated with previous injury to the hock and could represent an acquired resetting of the neuromuscular spindle trigger mechanism.

Horses with Australian stringhalt usually recover over a period of weeks to more than a year. Treatment in these cases is supportive. Horses should be removed from the offending pasture and given stall or paddock rest until signs resolve. Other livestock apparently can graze such pasture with impunity. Some cases of sporadic stringhalt also improve with rest, though this is not a consistent finding.

Mildly to moderately affected horses may improve after tenectomy of the lateral digital extensor tendon.[417] This procedure usually is performed in the standing horse but may be done on a recumbent animal. After surgical preparation of the lateral aspect of the hock, local anesthetic is infiltrated subcutaneously at the musculotendinous junction about an inch proximal to the lateral malleolus and distal to the hock, just before the tendon unites with that of the long digital extensor. A 3-cm skin incision is made at each site, and the tendon is identified. In the distal incision, forceps are passed under the tendon, which then is cut. Next, forceps are passed under the tendon at the proximal site and traction exerted to draw the transected end of the tendon through the tendon sheath and out of the proximal incision. The tendon is then cut, removing about 5 cm of muscle with it. The subcutaneous and skin incisions are sutured routinely. Bandaging is not necessary. Some horses show immediate improvement. Others show a gradual improvement over weeks to months.

DISEASES OF THE NEUROMUSCULAR JUNCTION

Congenital and Familial Diseases

Hyperkalemic Periodic Paralysis

This topic is covered in the chapter on Diseases of the Musculoskeletal System.

Myotonia

This topic is covered in the chapter on Diseases of the Musculoskeletal System.

Inflammatory, Infectious and Immune Diseases

Botulism

Signs of botulism are due to actions of the extremely potent exotoxins elaborated by vegetative *Clostridium botulinum* organisms.[431] These toxins interfere with release of acetylcholine at nerve endings, causing widespread neuromuscular blockade and weakness.[432]

Clostridium botulinum is a Gram-positive bacillus that requires anaerobic conditions for multiplication. Eight toxigenic culture types are recognized, each producing toxins of different antigenicity and potency;[432] these are designated A to G and include C_1 and C_2. Types B, C and D have been incriminated in naturally occurring cases of equine botulism.[433-447] *Clostridium botulinum* occurs commonly in soil and in the intestinal contents of normal birds and mammals.[431] The prevalence of each serotype in soil and intestinal contents varies greatly with geographic location.

The most common cause of botulism is ingestion of preformed toxin in contaminated or spoiled feedstuffs.[431] Toxin can also be elaborated by *Cl botulinum* organisms in necrotic tissue (wound botulism, toxicoinfectious botulism), and there is evidence that toxin can be produced by organisms in the gastrointestinal tract of human infants.[177] Wound contamination (toxicoinfectious botulism) and ingestion of preformed toxin have caused botulism in horses.

Ingestion of Toxin: The type of toxin contaminating a feedstuff in a particular area often reflects the variety of *Cl botulinum* most commonly found in the local soil. Type-B toxin was identified in samples of potatoes and oats that caused outbreaks of botulism in horses in Israel and Canada, respectively.[440,442] An English outbreak of botulism was thought to result from type-B toxin contamination of "big bale" silage.[446] Poor ensiling techniques may have prevented acidification of the feedstuff, allowing soil-origin *Cl botulinum* to proliferate and produce toxin. In many countries of Europe, where the disease has been enzootic among horses, botulism due to type-C toxin is apparently most important (especially in France, Yugoslavia, Scandinavia and Spain), with type D occurring less frequently.[438] Many significant outbreaks in Europe have been traced to feed contaminated by the putrefied carcasses of cats, rodents or birds.[434,438-440] In Spain, 34 mules on 24 farms died with signs of botulism over 8 months. The source of toxin in these cases was a macerated cat skull found in a village granary.[434] In a similar outbreak in Yugoslavia, 46 of 115 horses on one property showed signs of botulism after eating silage contaminated by a decomposed cat carcass; 29 of these horses died.[440] As little as 50-100 g of hay around such a carcass could be lethal if ingested by a horse.[439] One author found high levels of type-C toxin in feces of normal cats and considered contamination of horse feed by cat feces a possible hazard.[434]

Regardless of the route of administration and type of toxin, the clinical picture is rather consistent, varying only in severity. The mortality in naturally occurring equine cases has been estimated at 69% to >90%.[434,439,440,446] Death may occur within several hours of the appearance of clinical signs or may take up to a week. One experimental horse showed typical signs of paralysis for 16 days before dying. Recovery may take weeks or even months but is complete if it occurs.

Locomotor abnormalities usually are noticed first. A slight drop in temperature may precede other signs. Affected horses move with a shuffling, stilted gait, drag their toes along the ground, and may stand with head and neck hanging below the horizontal position. Complete absence of facial expression creates a dull, sleepy appearance. Saliva frequently drools from the corners of the mouth (Fig 45). Though the appetite is unaffected, mastication and lingual movements may be so feeble that partly chewed food drops from the mouth. Difficulty in swallowing often causes water and feed material to the nostrils (Fig 45). There may be muffled vocalization (dysphonia) and respiratory stridor, the latter caused by dorsal displacement of the soft palate. Mydriasis and sluggish pupillary reflexes usually appear early in the disease, as does flaccid paresis of the tongue.

Some affected horses turn to look at their flanks, suggesting abdominal pain. Often there is complete cessation of intestinal sounds, and rectal examination may reveal dry, mucus-covered feces. Decreased tail tone may be noticed during rectal examination. The urinary bladder often is distended, and there may be frequent passage of small amounts of urine, accompanied by penile protrusion and paralysis in males.

As weakness becomes more profound, there is muscular trembling and generalized sweating. Breathing becomes labored, with a prominent abdominal effort. Once adult horses with botulism become recumbent, they seldom rise again. Such horses soon be-

Figure 45. Adult horse with a botulism-like syndrome, showing the expressionless, flaccid muzzle and lips. Saliva drooling from the lips and food material in the nares are evidence of dysphagia. The nostrils fail to flare with inspiration.

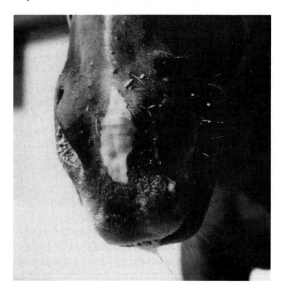

come too weak to maintain a sternal position. Respiratory arrest and death occur after a variable period of lateral recumbency, during which there are weak paddling movements and increasing dyspnea. Skin sensation is normal throughout the disease, though spinal and cranial nerve reflexes generally are depressed. There is no abnormality of sensorium, though weakness and lack of facial expression convey an impression of stupor. The clinical course in less severely affected animals may be complicated by inhalation pneumonia or necrotic cystitis.

Clostridium botulinum toxin is very rarely detected in the serum of horses with naturally occurring botulism. However, toxin was detected in the serum of 1 clinical case and in several experimentally poisoned horses after the onset of clinical signs.[436,446]

Necropsy findings generally are unremarkable in cases of botulism. Toxin occasionally is found in liver or gastrointestinal contents. It is important to remember that *Cl botulinum* organisms normally present in the intestine may elaborate toxin postmortem if sufficient putrefaction occurs. Only fresh or frozen samples should be submitted for toxin detection.

Toxicoinfectious Botulism: Toxicoinfectious botulism is the likely cause of both the "shaker foal syndrome" and sporadic deaths in older horses.[444,447,448] The shaker foal syndrome has been enzootic in central Kentucky for more than 40 years. The widespread use of type-B toxoid vaccination has greatly reduced the incidence of this disease in recent years.[449,450] The disease most often affects fast-growing foals 1-2 months of age. However, cases have been seen as early as 14 days and as late as 180 days of age. Clinical signs are typical of botulism, as described in the previous section. Initially there is a stilted gait, muscle tremor and inability to stand for more than a few minutes. Dysphagia, nasal reflux of milk, constipation, mydriasis and sluggish pupillary light responses, frequent urination and dyspnea are also seen. Without intensive nursing care and specific serotherapy, mortality exceeds 50%, with death usually occurring 1-3 days after onset of signs. Intensive treatment instituted early in the disease has reduced mortality to ≤15% (see treatment section below).[450]

In 8 shaker foals, *Cl botulinum* type B was isolated from foci of tissue necrosis in a variety of sites, including gastric ulcers, foci of hepatic necrosis, abscesses in the navel or lungs, and wounds in skin and muscle.[444] Proliferation of *Cl botulinum* type-B organisms in these sites probably resulted in toxicoinfectious botulism. The shaker foal syndrome has since been reproduced by inoculation of *Cl botulinum* type-B spores into experimentally created areas of muscle necrosis.[448]

There may be a higher incidence of shaker foal syndrome in foals of mares fed an excessively nutritious diet and exposed to stress. High levels of glucocorticoids in the milk of such mares may facilitate dissemination of *Cl botulinum* organisms in the foal from the gut to areas of tissue necrosis.[444,448] Extremely small amounts of type-B toxin can be lethal in this situation, and attempts to detect toxin in the serum of affected foals are unlikely to be successful. A 2-month-old foal had type-C toxicoinfectious botulism.[443] The site of *Cl botulinum* infection was thought to be the large intestine, which was irritated by sand.

Diagnosis: A definitive diagnosis of botulism, either ingestive or toxicoinfectious, is seldom made antemortem, but clinical signs are highly suggestive. Nevertheless, serum samples from horses with the first signs of disease should be frozen and submitted to a diagnostic laboratory for toxin detection. At necropsy, stomach and intestinal contents, feces, liver, suspect feed or carrion, and areas of tissue necrosis should be submitted for anaerobic culture and biologic assay for *Cl botulinum* toxin. The results of such tests must be interpreted in light of the foregoing discussion. Isolation of *Cl botulinum* organisms and identification of the necrotoxin from wounds can be undertaken to confirm cases of wound botulism.[444,448] Finding brief, small-amplitude, overly abundant motor-unit action potentials on needle electromyographic examination of a paralyzed flaccid horse or foal is presumptive evidence of botulism.[451]

Treatment: Death from botulism usually is due to respiratory failure. Unfortunately, prolonged artificial respiration of adult horses seldom is practical; however, shaker foals have successfully been ventilated for up to a week in neonatal intensive-care units of teaching hospitals and specialized practices. Such foals also must receive parenteral nutrition. Less severely affected horses may need intensive support for several weeks during recovery. If gastric emptying and intestinal motility are adequate, placement of an indwelling nasoesophageal tube ensures adequate hydration and nutrition, and reduces the likelihood of aspiration pneumonia. Mineral oil should be given initially and thereafter as needed to avoid or treat constipation.[450] Recumbent horses should be encouraged to remain sternal and, if possible, assisted to stand for short periods and to posture for urination. Recumbent horses may require careful catheterization to prevent serious bladder distention and necrosis. Bacterial urinary and respiratory tract infections must be treated vigorously with appropriate antimicrobial drugs. Drugs that may potentiate neuromuscular blockage, such as aminoglycoside antibiotics, tetracyclines and procaine penicillin, must be avoided.

If toxicoinfectious botulism is suspected, as in the shaker foal syndrome, high levels of K penicillin (100,000-400,000 IU/kg body weight divided into 4 daily doses) may be given IV to destroy vegetative *Cl botulinum* organisms proliferating in necrotic tissue. However, use of antibiotics in people with wound botulism has been of questionable value. Wounds should be debrided and irrigated meticulously. Likewise, any abscess should be cultured and drained.

Specific serotherapy has been used for many years in Europe with moderate success.[438] One investigator reported a reduction in mortality from 90% to 25% due to use of specific antitoxin in field outbreaks of botulism.[434] Use of a homologous type-B antiserum, produced at the University of Pennsylvania (200 ml given slowly IV, providing about 28,000 neutralizing units of antitoxin), may have improved survival rates when given early in the course of the shaker foal syndrome.[450,451] A dosage of about 140 units of type-B antitoxin/kg body weight (total of 500 ml) may have been beneficial in an adult horse with toxicoinfectious botulism.[447]

Edrophonium, 4-aminopyridine and acetylcholine-potentiating drugs are used to help reverse the neuromuscular blockade of botulism in other species; the safety of their use in horses is yet to be determined. Neostigmine has been used often in horses with botulism-like syndromes. Doses vary from 2 mg IM to 20 mg in 500 ml 5% dextrose in water, given IV over 30 minutes. Parasympathomimetic effects are seen often, but the value of such therapy in equine botulism is not certain and has been said to be detrimental.[447] However, such agents might be worth using to determine whether the particular myasthenic syndrome is neostigmine-responsive.

Prevention: Type-C toxoid is commercially available in the United States. Type-B toxoid (Bot Tox-B: Neogen) may be quite effective at preventing shaker foal syndrome.[449] In Kentucky, pregnant mares initially are vaccinated with type-B toxoid at the 8th, 9th and 10th month of gestation, and thereafter at the 10th month of each pregnancy.[450]

Postanesthetic Myasthenia

At least 3 horses have been encountered with a botulism-like syndrome immediately following general anesthesia.[187] Difficult recovery from anesthesia, lack of facial expression, flaccid tongue, dysphagia, mydriasis, and inability to elevate the head were characteristic signs. Other signs of botulism, such as flaccid tail, reduced patellar reflex, megaesophagus, and even periods of several days of recumbency, were variably present. Whether this syndrome is a form of botulism or myasthenia resulting from neuromuscular blockage due to certain drug-anesthetic agent combinations has not been determined. Each of the 3 affected horses was able to walk within 5-7 days, and totally recovered within a month with supportive care.

References

1. Adams R and Mayhew IG: Neurological examination of newborn foals. *Equine Vet J* 16:306-312, 1984.

2. deLahunta A: *Veterinary Neuroanatomy and Clinical Neurology.* 2nd ed. Saunders, Philadelphia, 1983.

3. Oliver JE *et al: Veterinary Neurology.* Saunders, Philadelphia, 1983.

4. Palmer AC: *Introduction to Animal Neurology.* Blackwell Scientific, Oxford, 1976.

5. Blythe LL: Neurologic examination of the horse. *Vet Clin No Am* 3:255-281, 1987.

6. Rooney JR: *Clinical Neurology of the Horse.* KNA Press, Kennett Square, PA, 1971.

7. Mayhew IG: Collection of cerebrospinal fluid from the horse. *Cornell Vet* 65:500-511, 1975.

8. Mayhew IG *et al:* Spinal cord disease in the horse. *Cornell Vet* 68:11-207, 1978.

9. Redding RW, in Oliver JE *et al: Veterinary Neurology.* Saunders, Philadelphia, 1987. pp 111-145,

10. Bowen JM, in Oliver JE *et al: Veterinary Neurology.* Saunders, Philadelphia, 1987. pp 145-168.

11. Redding RW and Myers LJ, in Oliver JE *et al: Veterinary Neurology.* Saunders, Philadelphia, 1987. pp 168-177.

12. Swaim SF, in Oliver JE *et al: Veterinary Neurology.* Saunders, Philadelphia, 1987. pp 493-512.

13. King JM *et al:* Myocardial necrosis secondary to neural lesions in domestic animals. *JAVMA* 180:144-148, 1982.

14. Daubney R and Mahalu EA: Viral encephalomyelitis of equines and domestic ruminants in the Near East-Part I. *Res Vet Sci* 8:375-397, 1967.

15. Robin Y *et al:* Virus de la foret de Semliki et encephalomyelites equines au Senegal. *Ann Microbiol (Inst Pasteur)* 125A:235-241, 1974.

16. Nakamura H: Japanese encephalitis in horses in Japan. *Equine Vet J* 4:155-156, 1974.

17. Hammon WM *et al:* Infection of horses with St. Louis encephalitis virus, experimental and natural. *Proc Soc Exp Biol Med* 49:335-340, 1942.

18. Gard GP *et al:* Association of Australian arboviruses with nervous disease in horses. *Aust Vet J* 53:61-66, 1977.

19. Timoney PJ *et al:* Encephalitis caused by louping ill virus in a group of horses in Ireland. *Equine Vet J* 8:113-117, 1976.

20. Little PB *et al:* Powassan viral encephalitis: A review and experimental studies in the horse and rabbit. *Vet Pathol* 22:500-507, 1985.

21. Lynch JA *et al:* California serogroup virus infection in a horse with encephalitis. *JAVMA* 186:389, 1985.

22. Emmons RW *et al:* Main Drain virus as a cause of equine encephalomyelitis. *JAVMA* 183:555-558, 1983.

23. Hanson RP: American arboviral encephalomyelitides of equidae. Virology and epidemiology of eastern and western arboviral encephalomyelitis of horses. *Proc 3rd Int Conf Eq Inf Dis,* 1972. Karger, Basel, 1973. pp 100-114.

24. Haring CM *et al:* An infectious brain disease of horses and mules (encephalomyelitis). *Univ Calif Coll Agr Exp Stn Circular* 332:1-14, 1931.

25. Hoff GL *et al:* Occurrence and distribution of western equine encephalomyelitis in Florida. *JAVMA* 172:351-352, 1978.

26. Mace DL *et al:* Evidence of the presence of equine encephalomyelitis in Philippine animals. *Bull US Army Med Dept* 9:504-507, 1949.

27. Wilson JH *et al:* A survey of eastern equine encephalomyelitis in Florida horses: Prevalence, economic impact, and management practices, 1982-1983. *Prev Vet Med* 4:261-271, 1986.

28. Kubes V and Rios FA: The causative agent of infectious equine encephalomyelitis in Venezuela. *Science* 90:20-21, 1939.

29. Spertzel RO: Venezuelan equine encephalomyelitis vaccination and control. *Proc 3rd Int Conf Eq Inf Dis,* 1972. Karger, Basel, 1973. pp 146-156.

30. Casals J: Antigenic variants of equine encephalitis virus. *J Exp Med* 119:547-565, 1964.

31. Henderson JR: Immunologic characterization of western equine encephalomyelitis strains. *J Immunol* 93:452-461, 1964.

32. Byrne RJ: The control of eastern and western arboviral encephalomyelitis of horses. *Proc 3rd Int Conf Eq Inf Dis*, 1972. Karger, Basel, 1973. pp 115-123.

33. Lillie LE *et al*: IV. Equine epizootic of western encephalomyelitis in Manitoba–1975. *Can J Pub Hlth* 67:21-27, 1976.

34. Hess AD and Holden P: The natural history of arthropod-borne encephalitides in the United States. *Ann NY Acad Sci* 70:294-311, 1958.

35. Edman JD *et al*: Host feeding patterns of Florida mosquitoes. II. Culiseta. *J Med Entomol* 9:429-434, 1972.

36. Libikova H: Natural foci of the western type of North American equine encephalomyelitis (WEE) in Czechoslovakia. 2. Experimental pathogenicity of viruses of WEE from Slovakia for laboratory, domestic, and wild animals. *Acta Virol* 1:93-101, 1957.

37. Pursell AR *et al*: Naturally occurring and experimentally induced eastern encephalomyelitis in calves. *JAVMA* 169:1101-1103, 1976.

38. Karstad L and Hanson RP: Natural and experimental infections in swine with the virus of eastern equine encephalitis. *J Infect Dis* 105:293-296, 1959.

39. Goldfield M *et al*: Arbovirus infection of animals in New Jersey. *JAVMA* 153:1780-1787, 1968.

40. Gibbs EPJ: Equine viral encephalitis. *Equine Vet J* 8:66-71, 1976.

41. Johnson KM and Martin DH: Venezuelan equine encephalitis. *Adv Vet Sci Comp Med* 18:79-116, 1974.

42. Kissling RE and Chamberlain RW: Venezuelan equine encephalitis. *Adv Vet Sci Comp Med* 11:65-84, 1967.

43. Galindo P: *Venezuelan Encephalitis*. Scientific Publication No. 243, Pan Am Hlth Org, Washington, 1972. pp 249-253.

44. Calisher CH *et al*: Rapid and specific sero-diagnosis of western equine encephalitis virus infection in horses. *Am J Vet Res* 47:1296-1299, 1986.

45. Sudia WD and Newhouse VF: Epidemic Venezuelan equine encephalitis in North America: A summary of virus-vector-host relationships. *Am J Epidem* 101:1-13, 1975.

46. Wilson JH, in Robinson NE: *Current Therapy in Equine Medicine*. 2nd ed. Saunders, Phildelphia, 1987. pp 345-347.

47. Taylor WM and Buff E: Transmissibility of an attenuated Venezuelan equine encephalomyelitis vaccine virus. *JAVMA* 161:159-163, 1972.

48. Vanderwagen LC *et al*: A field study of persistence of antibodies in California horses vaccinated against western, eastern and Venezuelan equine encephalomyelitis. *Am J Vet Res* 36:1567-1571, 1975.

49. Crick J and Brown F: Rabies vaccine for animals and man. *Vet Record* 99:162-167, 1976.

50. Anon: *Rabies Surveillance Annual Summary 1984*. US Dept of Health and Human Services, Centers for Disease Control, Atlanta, 1985.

51. Baer GM: *The Natural History of Rabies*. Academic Press, New York, 1975.

52. Rosatte R: Rabies in Canada: History, epidemiology and control. *Can Vet J* 29:362-365, 1988.

53. Ornelas OV and Aranalde UA: Bat rabies in Mexico. *Southwestern Vet* 1:13-16, 1964.

54. Taylor D: Rabies: Epizootic aspects; diagnosis; vaccines; notes for guidance; offical policy. *Vet Record* 99:157-160, 1976.

55. Joyce JR and Russell LH: Clinical signs of rabies in horses. *Compend Cont Ed Pract Vet* 3:S56-S61, 1981.

56. Hahn DG: A case of equine rabies with human and bovine exposure. *VM/SAC* 78:1409-1410, 1982.

57. West GP: Equine rabies. *Equine Vet J* 17:280-282, 1985.

58. Meyer EE *et al*: Hindlimb hyperesthesia associated with rabies in two horses. *JAVMA* 188:629-632, 1986.

59. Ferris DH *et al*: A note on experimental rabies in the donkey. *Cornell Vet* 58:270-277, 1968.

60. Schroeder WG: Suggestions for handling horses exposed to rabies. *JAVMA* 155:1842-1843, 1969.

61. Marler RJ *et al*: Rabies in a horse. *JAVMA* 175:293-294, 1979.

62. Carlson GP, Davis, CA: Unpublished observations, 1989.

63. Merritt AM and Mayhew IG, Gainesville, FL: Unpublished observations, 1989.

64. Abelseth MK and Trimarchi CV: *Report on Rabies*. Vet Learning Systems, Somerville, NJ, 1983. pp 11-16.

65. Smith WB *et al*: Diagnosis of rabies by immunofluorescent staining of frozen sections of skin. *JAVMA* 161:1495-1501, 1972.

66. Mayhew IG, Gainesville, FL, Carlson G, Davis, CA: Unpublished observations, 1989.

67. Nat Assoc State Publ Health Vet: Compendium of Animal Rabies Control, 1988. *JAVMA* 192:18-22, 1988.

68. Allen GP and Bryans JT, in Pandey R: *Progress in Veterinary Microbiology and Immunology*. Karger, Basel, 1986. pp 78-144.

69. Saxegaard F: Isolation and identification of equine rhinopneumonitis virus (equine abortion virus) from cases of abortion and paralysis. *Nord Vet Med* 18:504-512, 1966.

70. Jackson TA *et al*: Equine herpesvirus-1 infection of horses: Studies on the experimentally induced neurologic disease. *Am J Vet Res* 38:709-719, 1977.

71. Greenwood RES and Simson ARB: Clinical report of a paralytic syndrome affecting stallions, mares and foals on a Thoroughbred stud farm. *Equine Vet J* 12:113-117, 1980.

72. Carlson GP, Davis, CA: Personal communication, 1989.

73. Montali RJ *et al*: Equine herpesvirus type 1 abortion in an onager and suspected herpesvirus myelitis in a zebra. *JAVMA* 187:1248-1249, 1985.

74. Roberts RS: A paralytic syndrome in horses. *Vet Record* 77: 404, 1965.

75. Thein P: Infection of the central nervous system of horses with equine herpesvirus serotype 1. *J So Afr Vet Assn* 52:239-241, 1981.

76. Bitsch V and Dam A: Nervous disturbances in horses in relation to infection with equine rhinopneumonitis virus. *Acta Vet Scand* 12:134-136, 1971.

77. Pursell AR et al: Neurologic disease due to equine herpesvirus 1. *JAVMA* 175:473-474, 1979.

78. Liu IKM and Castleman W: Equine posterior paresis associated with equine herpesvirus 1 vaccine in California: A preliminary report. *J Equine Med Surg* 1:397, 1977.

79. Studdert MJ et al: Differentiation of respiratory and abortigenic isolates of equine herpesvirus 1 by restriction endonucleases. *Science* 241:562-565, 1981.

80. Patel JR et al: Variation in cellular tropism between isolates of equine herpesvirus-1 in foals. *Arch Virol* 74:41-51, 1982.

81. Thorsen J and Little PB: Isolation of equine herpesvirus type 1 from a horse with an acute paralytic disease. *Can J Comp Med* 39:358-359, 1975.

82. Edington N et al: Experimental reactivation of equid herpesvirus-1 (EHV1) following the administration of corticosteroids. *Equine Vet J* 17:369-372, 1985.

83. Moore BO and Koonse HJ: Inactivated equine herpesvirus-1 vaccine Pneumabort K. *Proc 24th Ann Mtg AAEP*, 1978. pp 75-88.

84. McIlwraith W and Kitchen ND: Neurological signs and neuropathy associated with a case of equine infectious anemia. *Cornell Vet* 68:238-249, 1978.

85. McClure J et al: Ataxia in four horses with equine infectious anemia. *JAVMA* 180:279-283, 1982.

86. Held JP et al: Ataxia as the only clinical sign of cerebrospinal meningitis in a horse with equine infectious anemia. *JAVMA* 183:324-325, 1985.

87. Clark ED et al: Listeriosis in an Arabian foal with combined immunodeficiency. *JAVMA* 172:363-366, 1978.

88. Emerson FG and Jarvis AA: Listeriosis in ponies. *JAVMA* 152:1645-1646, 1968.

89. Gillespie JH and Timoney JH: *Hagan and Bruner's Infectious Diseases of Domestic Animals.* 7th ed. Comstock Publishing, Ithaca, NY, 1981.

90. Gantz NM et al: Listeriosis in immunosuppressed patients. *Am J Med* 58:637-643, 1975.

91. Mayhew IG and MacKay RJ, Gainesville, FL: Unpublished case report, 1989.

92. Koterba AM et al: Prevention and control of infection. *Vet Clin No Am* 1:41-50, 1985.

93. Jones TC and Mayrer FD: The pathology of equine influenza. *Am J Vet Res* 4:15-31, 1943.

94. Rumbaugh GE: Disseminated septic meningitis in a mare. *JAVMA* 171:452-454, 1977.

95. Brewer BD: Therapeutic strategies involving antimicrobial treatment of the central nervous system in large animals. *JAVMA* 10:1217-1221, 1984.

96. Green SL et al, Gainesville, FL: Unpublished data, 1989.

97. Cherubin CE et al: Treatment of gram-negative bacillary meningitis: Role of the new cephalosporin antibiotics. *Rev Infect Dis* 4:S453-S464, 1982.

98. Jungerman PR and Schwartzman RM: *Veterinary Medical Mycology.* Lea & Febiger, Philadelphia, 1972.

99. Cho D-Y et al: Cerebral cryptococcosis in a horse. *Vet Pathol* 23:207-209, 1986.

100. Barron CN: Cryptococcosis in animals *JAVMA* 124:125-127, 1955.

101. Steckel RR et al: Antemortem diagnosis and treatment of cryptococcal meningitis in a horse. *JAVMA* 180:1085-1089, 1982.

102. Barclay WP and deLahunta A: Cryptococcal meningitis in a horse. *JAVMA* 174:1236-1238, 1979.

103. Bennett JE et al: A comparison of amphotericin B alone and combined with flucytosine in the treatment of cryptococcal meningitis. *N Eng J Med* 301:126-131,1979.

104. Bell WE: Treatment of fungal infections of the central nervous system. *Ann Neurology* 9:417-422, 1981.

105. Mayhew IG et al: Equine protozoal myeloencephalitis. *Proc 22nd Ann Mtg AAEP*, 107-114, 1976. pp 107-114.

106. Dorr TE et al: Protozoal myeloencephalitis in horses in California. *JAVMA* 185:801-802, 1984.

107. Lombardo de Barros CS, Santa Maria, Brazil: Personal communication, 1989.

108. Whitwell KE, Newmarket, England: Personal communication, 1989.

109. Traver DS et al: Protozoal myeloencephalitis in sibling horses. *J Equine Med Surg* 2:425-428, 1978.

110. Simpson CF and Mayhew IG: Evidence for *Sarcocystis* as the etiologic agent of equine protozoal myeloencephalitis. *J Protozool* 27:288-292, 1980.

111. Fayer R and Dubey JP: Comparative epidemiology of equine protozoal myelitis. *Proc 6th Intl Cong Parasitol.* Australian Academy of Science, Canberra, 1986. p 615.

112. Mayhew IG et al: Migration of a spiruroid nematode through the brain of a horse. *JAVMA* 180: 1306-1311, 1982.

113. Little PB et al: Verminous encephalitis of horses: Experimental induction with *Strongylus vulgaris* larvae. *Am J Vet Res* 35:1501-1510, 1974.

114. Little PB: Cerebrospinal nematodiasis of equidae. *JAVMA* 160:1407-1413, 1972.

115. Mayhew IG et al: Verminous (*Strongylus vulgaris*) myelitis in a donkey. *Cornell Vet* 74:30-37, 1984.

116. Olander HJ: The migration of *Hypoderma lineatum* in the brain of a horse. *Vet Pathol* 4:477-483, 1967.

117. Hadlow WJ et al: Intracranial myiasis by *Hypoderma bovis* (Linnaeus) in a horse. *Cornell Vet* 67:272-281, 1977.

118. Anon: Side effects of treating warble fly with systemic insecticides. *Vet Record* 103:355-356, 1978.

119. Blunden AS *et al*: *Halicephalobus deletrix* infection in a horse. *Equine Vet J* 19:255-260, 1987.

120. Alstad AD *et al*: Disseminated *Micronema deletrix* infection in the horse. *JAVMA* 174:264-266, 1979.

121. Innes JRM and Pillai CP: Kumri-so-called lumbar paralysis-of horses in Ceylon (India and Burma) and its identification with cerebrospinal nematodiasis. *Brit Vet J* 3:233-235, 1955.

122. Frauenfelder HC *et al*: Cerebrospinal nematodiasis caused by a filariid in a horse. *JAVMA* 177:359-362, 1980.

123. Levine ND: *Veterinary Protozoology*. Iowa State Univ Press, Ames, 1985.

124. Reik LR *et al*: Neurologic abnormalities in Lyme disease without erythema chronicum migrans. *Am J Med* 81:73-78, 1986.

125. Burgess EC and Mattison M: Encephalitis associated with *Borrelia burgdorferi* infection in a horse. *JAVMA* 191:1457-1458, 1987.

126. Bosler EM *et al*: Natural distribution of the *Ixodes dammini* spirochete. *Science* 220:321-322, 1983.

127. Cheeke PR and Shull LR: *Natural Toxicants in Feeds and Poisonous Plants*. AVI Publishing, Westport, RI, 1985.

128. Clarke EGC and Clarke ML: *Veterinary Toxicology*. Balliere-Tindall, London, 1975.

129. Keeler RF *et al*: *Effects of Poisonous Plants on Livestock*. Academic Press, New York, 1978.

130. Seawright AA: *Animal Health in Australia. Vol 2: Chemical and Plant Poisons*. Aust Govt Publishing Service, Canberra, 1982.

131. Blood DC *et al*: *Veterinary Medicine*. 6th ed. Bailliere-Tindall, London, 1983.

132. Seawright AA and Costigan P: Chronic methylmercurialism in a horse. *Vet Human Toxicol* 20:6-9, 1978.

133. Roberts MC *et al*: The effects of prolonged daily low level mercuric chloride dosing in a horse. *Vet Human Toxicol* 20: 410-415, 1978.

134. Schuh JCL *et al*: Concurrent mercuric blister and dimethyl sulfoxide (DMSO) application as a cause of mercury toxicity in two horses. *Equine Vet J* 20:68-71, 1988.

135. Roberts MC *et al*: Chronic phenylmercuric acetate toxicity in a horse. *Vet Human Toxicol* 21:321-327, 1979.

136. Hanson LJ *et al*: Toxic effects of lasalocid in horses. *Am J Vet Res* 42:456-461, 1981.

137. Rose RJ *et al*: Laryngeal paralysis in Arabian foals associated with oral haloxon administration. *Equine Vet J* 13:171-176, 1981.

138. Duncan ID and Brook D: Bilateral laryngeal paralysis in the horse. *Equine Vet J* 17:228-233, 1985.

139. Fowler ME, in Mansmann RA and McAllister ES: *Equine Medicine and Surgery*. 3rd ed. American Veterinary Publications, Goleta, CA, 1982. pp 207-208.

140. Angsubhakron S *et al*: Aflatoxicosis in the horse. *JAVMA* 178:274-278, 1981.

141. Mayhew IG: Observations on vascular accidents in the central nervous system of neonatal foals. *J Reprod Fert* 32:569-575, 1982.

142. Palmer AC and Rossdale PD: Neuropathological changes associated with the neonatal maladjustment syndrome in the Thoroughbred foal. *Res Vet Sci* 20:267-275, 1976.

143. Houpt KA: Stable vices and trailer problems. *Vet Clin No Am* 2:623-633, 1986.

144. Dodman NH *et al*: Investigation into the use of narcotic antagonists in the treatment of a sterotypic behavior pattern (crib biting) in the horse. *Am J Vet Res* 48:311-319, 1987.

145. Firth EC: Bilateral ventral accessory neurectomy in windsucking horses. *Vet Record* 106:30-32, 1980.

146. Forsell G: The new surgical treatment against crib-biting. *Vet J* 82:538-548, 1926.

147. Frauenfelder H: Treatment of crib biting: A surgical approach in the standing horse. *Equine Vet J* 13:62-63, 1981.

148. Morin T: Surgical management of crib biting in the horse. *Compend Cont Ed Pract Vet* 4:S69-S74, 1982.

149. Ralston SL: Common behavioral problems of horses. *Compend Cont Ed Pract Vet* 4:S152-S160, 1982.

150. Turner AS *et al*: Modified Forssell's operation for crib biting in the horse. *JAVMA* 184:309-312, 1984.

151. Ralston SL: Feeding behavior. *Vet Clin No Am* 2:609-621, 1986.

152. Beaver BV: Aggressive behavior problems. *Vet Clin No Am* 2:635-644, 1986.

153. Cook WR: Head shaking in horses. *Equine Pract* 1(5):9-17, 1979.

154. Lane JG and Mair TS: Observations on head shaking in the horse. *Equine Vet J* 19:331-336, 1987.

155. Cook WR: Head shaking in horses: History and management tests. *Equine Pract* 1(6):36-39, 1979.

156. Cook WR: Head shaking in horses: Diagnostic tests. *Equine Pract* 2(1):31-40, 1980.

157. Cook WR: Head shaking in horses: Special diagnostic procedures. *Equine Pract* 2(2):7-15, 1980.

158. Houpt KA: Behavioral problems in horses. *Proc 31st Ann Mtg AAEP*, 1985. pp 113-124.

159. Beech J: Forelimb tic in a horse. *JAVMA* 180:258-260, 1982.

160. Foreman JH *et al*: Congenital internal hydrocephalus in a Quarter Horse foal. *J Equine Vet Sci* 3:154-164, 1983.

161. Bester RC *et al*: Hydrocephalus in an 18-month-old colt. *JAVMA* 168:1041-1042, 1976.

162. Stewart RH: Central nervous system trauma. *Vet Clin No Am* 3:371-377, 1987.

163. Brayton CF: Dimethyl sulfoxide (DMSO): A review. *Cornell Vet* 76:61-90, 1986.

164. Miller SM *et al*: Cerebral protection by barbiturates and loop diuretics in head trauma: Possible modes of action. *Bull NY Acad Med* 56:305-313, 1980.

165. Reulen HJ and Schurmann K: Nonsurgical management of severe head injuries. *Prog Neurol Surg* 10:291-322, 1981.

166. Stashak TS and Mayhew IG, in Jennings PB: *The Practice of Large Animal Surgery*. Saunders, Philadelphia, 1984. pp 983-1041.

167. Ford J and Lokai MD: Complications of *Streptococcus equi* infection. *Equine Pract* 2(3):41-44, 1980.

168. Raphel CR: Brain abscess in three horses. *JAVMA* 180:874-877, 1982.

169. Allen JR *et al*: Brain abscess in a horse: Diagnosis by computed tomography and successful surgical treatment. *Equine Vet J* 19:552-555, 1987.

170. Zieve L, in Popper H and Schaffner F: *Progress in Liver Diseases*. Grune & Stratton, New York, 1979. pp 327-341.

171. Gulick BA *et al*: Effect of pyrrolizidine alkaloid-induced hepatic disease on plasma amino acid patterns in the horse. *Am J Vet Res* 41:1894-1898, 1980.

172. Frevert CW *et al*: The ammonia tolerance test may be a clinically useful means of detecting liver disease in horses. *Proc 5th Ann Vet Med Forum Am Coll Vet Intern Med*, 1987. pp 901.

173. Tennant BC *et al*: Equine hepatic insufficiency. *Vet Clin No Am* 3:279-289, 1973.

174. Tennant BC and Hornbuckle WE, in Anderson NV: *Veterinary Gastroenterology*. Lea & Febiger, Philadelphia, 1980. pp 593-620.

175. Brierly JB, in Blackwood W and Cosellis JAN: *Greenfield's Neuropathology*. Edward Arnold, London, 1976. pp 43-85.

176. Koterba AM: Some aspects of fluid therapy in the neonatal foal. *Proc 9th Bain-Fallon Mem Lectures*, 1987. pp 153-156.

177. Volpe JJ: *Neurology of the Newborn*. 2nd ed. Saunders, Philadelphia, 1987.

178. MacKay RJ and Mayhew IG, Gainesville, FL: Unpublished data, 1989.

179. Auer JA and Watkins JP: Treatment of radial fractures in adult horses: An analysis of 15 clinical cases. *Equine Vet J* 19:103-110, 1987.

180. Wilson BJ *et al*: Equine leukoencephalomalacia. *JAVMA* 163:1293-1294, 1973.

181. Wilson TM *et al*: Linking leukoencephalomalacia to commercial horse rations.*Vet Med* 80:63-69, 1985.

182. Marasas WFO *et al*: Leukoencephalomalacia: A mycotoxicosis of equidae caused by *Fusarium moniliforme* Sheldon. *Onderstepoort J Vet Res* 43:113-121, 1976.

183. Domench J *et al*: Equine leucoencephalomalacia in New Caledonia. *Aust Vet J* 62:422-423, 1985.

184. Gabal MA *et al*: Fusariotoxicoses of farm animals and mycotoxic leukoencephalomalacia of the equine associated with the finding of tricothecenes in feedstuffs. *Vet Human Toxicol* 28:207-212, 1986.

185. Haliburton JC *et al*: (ELEM): A study of *Fusarium moniliforme* as an etiologic agent. *Vet Human Toxicol* 21:348-351, 1979.

186. Masri MD: Clinical, epidemiologic and pathologic evaluation of an outbreak of mycotoxic encephalomalacia (MEM) in South Louisiana horses. *Proc 33rd Ann Mtg AAEP*, 1987.

187. Mayhew IG and MacKay RJ, in Mansmann RA and McAllister ES: *Equine Medicine and Surgery*. 3rd ed. American Veterinary Publications, Goleta, CA, 1982. pp 1159-1252.

188. Holshus HJ and Howard EB: Pineoblastoma, a primitive neuroectodermal tumor in the brain of a horse. *Vet Pathol* 19:567-569, 1982.

189. Bistner S *et al*: Neuroepithelial tumor of the optic nerve in a horse. *Cornell Vet* 73:30-40, 1983.

190. Shamis LB *et al*: Lymphosarcoma as the cause of ataxia in a horse. *JAVMA* 184:1517-1518, 1984.

191. Froscher BG and Power HT: Malignant pheochromocytoma in a foal. *JAVMA* 181:494-496, 1982.

192. Kirker-Head CA *et al*: Pelvic limb lameness due to malignant melanoma in a horse. *JAVMA* 186:1215-1217, 1985.

193. Wright JA and Giles CJ: Diffuse carcinomatosis involving the meninges of a horse. *Equine Vet J* 18:147-150, 1986.

194. Livesey MA and Wilkie IW: Focal and multifocal osteosarcoma in two foals. *Equine Vet J* 18:407-410, 1986.

195. Sweeney CR and Hansen TO, in Robinson NE: *Current Therapy in Equine Medicine*. 2nd ed. Saunders, Philadelphia, 1987. pp 349-353.

196. Rall TW and Schleifer LS, in Gilman AG *et al*: *Goodman and Gilman's The Pharmacological Basis of Therapeutics*. 7th ed. Macmillan, New York, 1985. pp 446-472.

197. Sullivan ND, in Jubb KVF *et al*: *Pathology of Domestic Animals*. 3rd ed. Academic Press, Orlando, FL, 1985. pp 201-338.

198. Critchley M and Ferguson FR: The cerebrospinal epidermoids (cholesteatomata). *Brain* 51:334-384, 1928.

199. Carlson GP, Davis, CA: Personal communication, 1978.

200. deLahunta A: *Veterinary Neuroanatomy and Clinical Neurology*. Saunders, Philadelphia, 1977.

201. Knight AP: Dysphagia resulting from unilateral rupture of the rectus capitis ventralis muscles in a horse. *JAVMA* 17:735-738, 1977.

202. Martin L *et al*: Four cases of traumatic optic nerve blindness in the horse. *Equine Vet J* 18:133-137, 1986.

203. Rebhun WC: Traumatic optic neuropathy: How to prevent permanent blindness. *VM/SAC* 81: 350-353, 1986.

204. Matsuzaki H *et al*: Optic nerve damage in head trauma: Clinical and experimental studies. *Jpn J Ophthalmol* 26:447-461, 1982.

205. Stick JA *et al*: Basilar skull fractures in three horses. *JAVMA* 176:228-231, 1980.

206. Blythe LL *et al*: Vestibular syndrome associated with temporohyoid fusion and temporal bone fractures in three horses. *JAVMA* 185:775-781, 1984.

207. Shideler RK and Perce RB: Occipital fracture in a foal. *VM/SAC* 71:218-219, 1976.

208. Gelatt KN: *Veterinary Ophthalmology*. Lea & Febiger, Philadelphia, 1981. pp 206-261.

209. Tillman DB: Tetanus. *West J Med* 129:107-109, 1978.

210. Booth NH and Pierson RE: Treatment of tetanus with d-tubocurarine chloride. *JAVMA* 128: 257-261, 1956.

211. Gibbons WJ: Case report: Tetanus. *Cornell Vet* 30:533-537, 1940.

212. Donaldson RS: Multivitamins and tetanus. *Vet Record* 101:353, 1977.

213. Mellanby J: Comparative activities of tetanus and botulinum toxins. *Neuroscience* 11:29-34, 1984.

214. Furste WJ: Tetanus. *J Trauma* 16:755-757, 1976.

215. Rie MA and Wilson RS: Morphine therapy controls autonomic hyperactivity in tetanus. *Ann Intern Med* 88:653-654, 1978.

216. Sedaghatian MR: Intrathecal serotherapy in neonatal tetanus: A controlled trial. *Arch Dis Child* 54:623-625, 1979.

217. Sanders RKM et al: Intrathecal antitetanus serum (horse) in the treatment of tetanus. *Lancet* 1:974-977, 1977.

218. Muylle E et al: Treatment of tetanus in the horse by injection of tetanus antitoxin into the subarachnoid space. *JAVMA* 167:47-48, 1975.

219. Lundvall RL: Chlorpromazine hydrochloride for tetanus in the horse. *JAVMA* 132:254-255, 1958.

220. Owen IN et al: The treatment of tetanus with particular reference to chlorpromazine. *Vet Record* 71:61-65, 1959.

221. Smithcors JF: The treatment of tetanus with curare-a little known chapter in veterinary history. *JAVMA* 132:303-305, 1958.

222. Odusote KA et al: Favorable prognosis of prolonged coma associated with large doses of diazepam in severe tetanus. *Trop Geogr Med* 28:194-198, 1976.

223. Adams JM et al: Modern management of tetanus neonatorum. *Pediatrics* 64:472-477, 1979.

224. Wintzer HJ et al: Zur Tetanusprophylaxe beim Pferd. *Berl Munch Tierarztl Wochenschr* 88:181-183, 1975.

225. Tennant BC: Acute hepatitis in horses: Problems of differentiating toxic and infectious causes in the adult. *Proc 24th Ann Mtg AAEP*, 1978. pp 465-471.

226. Liu IK et al: Duration of maternally derived immunity to tetanus and response in newborn foals given tetanus antitoxin. *Am J Vet Res* 43:2019-2022, 1982.

227. McGuire TC et al: Failure of colostral immunoglobulin transfer as an explanation for most infections and deaths of neonatal foals. *JAVMA* 170:1302-1304, 1977.

228. Cook WR et al: The pathology and aetiology of guttural pouch mycosis in the horse. *Vet Record* 83:422-428, 1968.

229. Cook WR: The clinical features of guttural pouch mycosis in the horse. *Vet Record* 83:336-345, 1968.

230. Freeman DE: Diagnosis and treatment of diseases of the guttural pouch. *Compend Cont Ed Pract Vet* 2:S3-S11, 1980.

231. Freeman DE: Diagnosis and treatment of diseases of the guttural pouch. *Compend Cont Ed Pract Vet* 2:S25-S32, 1980.

232. Church S et al: Treatment of guttural pouch mycosis. *Equine Vet J* 18:362-365, 1986.

233. Greet TRC: Outcome of treatment in 35 cases of guttural pouch mycosis. *Equine Vet J* 19:483-487, 1987.

234. Firth EC: Vestibular disease and its relationship to facial paralysis in the horse: A clinical study of 7 cases. *Aust Vet J* 53:560-565, 1977.

235. Bjorklund NE and Palsson G: Guttural pouch mycosis in the horse. A survey of 7 cases and a case report. *Nord Vet Med* 22:65-74, 1970.

236. Dixon PM and Rowland S: Atlanto-occipital joint infection associated with guttural pouch infection in a horse. *Equine Vet J* 13:260-262, 1981.

237. Wagner PC et al: Mycotic encephalitis associated with a guttural pouch mycosis. *J Equine Med Surg* 2: 355-359, 1978.

238. McLaughlin BG and O'Brien JL: Guttural pouch mycosis and mycotic encephalitis in a horse. *Can Vet J* 27:109-111, 1986.

239. Modransky PD et al: Dysphagia associated with guttural pouch empyema and dorsal displacement of the soft palate. *Equine Pract* 4(8):34-38, 1982.

240. Wilson JH: Effects of indwelling catheters and povidone iodine flushes on the guttural pouches of the horse. *Equine Vet J* 17:242-244, 1985.

241. Cordy DR, in Keeler RG et al: *Effects of Poisonous Plants on Livestock*. Academic Press, Orlando, FL, 1978. pp 327-336.

242. Young S et al: Nigropallidal encephalomalacia in horses caused by ingestion of weeds of the genus *Centaura*. *JAVMA* 157:1602-1605, 1970.

243. Burrows GE: Lead poisoning in the horse. *Equine Pract* 4(6):30-36, 1982.

244. Aronson AL: Lead poisoning in cattle and horses following long-term exposure to lead. *Am J Vet Res* 33:627-629, 1972.

245. Holm LW et al: The treatment of chronic lead poisoning in horses with calcium disodium ethylenediaminetetraacetate. *JAVMA* 123:383-388, 1953.

246. Goyer RA and Rhyne BC: Pathological effects of lead. *Int Rev Exptl Path* 12:1-77, 1973.

247. Willoughby RA et al: Lead and zinc poisoning and the interaction between Pb and Zn poisoning in the foal. *Can J Comp Med* 36:348-359, 1972.

248. Sheather AL: Fainting in foals. *J Comp Path Ther* 37:106-113, 1924.

249. McGrath JT: Some nervous disorders of the horse. *Proc 8th Ann Mtg AAEP*, 1962. pp 157-163.

250. Sweeney CR et al: Narcolepsy in a horse. *JAVMA* 183:126-128, 1983.

251. Power HT et al: Facial and vestibulocochlear nerve disease in six horses. *JAVMA* 183:1076-1080, 1983.

252. Blythe LL, Corvallis, OR: Personal communication, 1987.

253. deLahunta A: Comparative cerebellar disease in domestic animals. *Compend Cont Ed Pract Vet* 11:8-19, 1980.

254. Mayhew IG and MacKay R, Gainesville, FL: Unpublished observations.

255. Bjorck G et al: Congenital cerebellar ataxia in the Gotland pony breed. *Zentralbl Veterinarmed* 20A:341-354, 1973.

256. deBowes RM et al: Cerebellar abiotrophy. *Vet Clin No Am* 3:345-352, 1987.

257. Sponseller ML: Equine cerebellar hypoplasia and degeneration. *Proc 13th Ann Mtg AAEP*, 1967. pp 123-126.

258. Beatty MT *et al*: Cerebellar disease in Arabian horses. *Proc 31st Ann Mtg AAEP*, 1985. pp 241-245.

259. Mayhew IG: Clinical neurology and neuropathology in the large animal neonate. *Proc 1st Ann Conf Intl Soc Vet Perinatol*, 1988.

260. Mortimer PH, in Keeler RF *et al*: *Effects of Poisonous Plants on Livestock*. Academic Press, Orlando, FL, 1978. pp 353-361.

261. Munday BL *et al*: Intoxication of horses by lolitrem B in ryegrass seed cleanings. *Aust Vet J* 62(6):207, 1985.

262. Cysweski SJ: *Paspalum* staggers and tremorgen intoxication in animals. *JAVMA* 163:1291-1292, 1973.

263. Strain GM *et al*: Toxic Bermuda grass tremor in the goat: An electroencephalographic study. *Am J Vet Res* 43:158-162, 1982.

264. vanKampen KR *et al*, in Keeler RF *et al*: *Effects of Poisonous Plants on Livestock*. Academic Press, Orlando, FL, 1978. pp 465-471.

265. Harries WN *et al*: An outbreak of locoweed poisoning in horses in Southwestern Alberta. *Can Vet J* 13:141-145, 1972.

266. McIlwraith CW and James LF: Limb deformities in foals associated with ingestion of locoweed by mares. *JAVMA* 181:255-258, 1982.

267. James LF and vanKampen KR: Acute and residual lesions of locoweed poisoning in cattle and horses. *JAVMA* 158:614-618, 1971.

268. Molyneux RJ and James LF: Loco intoxication: Indolizidine alkaloids of spotted locoweed (Astragalus lentiginosus). *Science* 216:190-193, 1982.

269. Huxtable CR and Dorling PR: Poisoning of livestock by *Swainsona* spp: Current status. *Aust Vet J* 59:50-53, 1982.

270. LeGonidec G *et al*: A neurologic disease of horses in New Caledonia. *Aust Vet J* 57:194-195, 1981.

271. Hartley WJ *et al*: The pathology of Gomen disease: A cerebellar disorder of horses in New Caledonia. *Vet Pathol* 19:399-405, 1982.

272. Mayhew IG *et al*: Congenital occipitoatlantoaxial malformation in the horse. *Equine Vet J* 10:103-113, 1978.

273. Watson AG and Mayhew IG: Familial congenital occipitoatlantoaxial malformation (OAAM) in the Arabian horse. *Spine* 11:334-339, 1986.

274. Wilson WD *et al*: Occipitoatlantoaxial malformation in two non-Arabian horses. *JAVMA* 187: 36-40, 1985.

275. Leathers CW *et al*: Cervical spina bifida with meningocele in an Appaloosa foal. *J Vet Orthop* 1:55-58, 1979.

276. Stecher RM and Goss LJ: Ankylosing lesions of the spine: pathologic or biologic. *JAVMA* 138:248-255, 1961.

277. Stecher RM: Anatomical variations of the spine of the horse. *J Mammology* 43:205-219, 1962.

278. Klaasen JK and Wagner PC: Congenital vertebral abnormalities in a foal. *Equine Pract* 3(4):11-18, 1981.

279. Whitwell KE and Dyson S: Interpreting radiographs. 8: Equine cervical vertebrae. *Equine Vet J* 19:8-14, 1987.

280. Cho DY and Leipold HW: Syringomyelia in a Thoroughbred foal. *Equine Vet J* 9:195-197, 1977.

281. Mayhew IG: Neuromuscular arthrogryposis multiplex congenita in a Thoroughbred foal. *Vet Pathol* 21:187-192, 1984.

282. Baker GJ: Comminuted fracture of the axis. *Equine Vet J* 2:37-38, 1970.

283. Funk KA and Erickson ED: A case of atlantoaxial subluxation in a horse. *Can Vet J* 9:120-123, 1968.

284. Guffy MM *et al*: Atlantoaxial luxation in a foal. *JAVMA* 155:754-757, 1969.

285. Jeffcott LB and Whitwell KE: Fracture of the thorocolumbar spine of the horse. *Proc 22nd Ann Mtg AAEP*, 1976. pp 91-102.

286. Mason BJE: A spinal cord compression causing paraplegia in a foal. *Equine Vet J* 3:155-157, 1971.

287. Moyer WA and Rooney JR: Vertebral fracture in a horse. *JAVMA* 159:1022-1024, 1971.

288. Owen Rh ap Rh and Smith-Maxie LL: Repair of fractured dens of the axis in a foal. *JAVMA* 173:854-856, 1978.

289. McCoy DJ *et al*: Ventral approach for stabilization of atlanto-occipital subluxation secondary to odontoid fracture in a foal. *JAVMA* 185:545-549, 1984.

290. Stone DE *et al*: Surgical decompression for traumatic atlantoaxial subluxation in a weanling filly. *JAVMA* 174:1234-1236, 1979.

291. Vaughan JT and Mason MBJ: *A Clinico-pathological Study of Racing Accidents in Horses*. Royal Veterinary College, North Mymms, Hatfield, Herts, England, 1976.

292. Wagner PC *et al*: Traumatic injury of the cauda equina in the horse: A case report. *J Equine Med Surg* 1:282-285, 1977.

293. Eidelberg E: The pathophysiology of spinal cord injury. *Radiol Clin No Am* 15:241-246, 1977.

294. Griffiths IR *et al*: Early vascular changes in the spinal grey matter following impact injury. *Acta Neuropath* 41:33-39, 1978.

295. Nelson E *et al*: Spinal cord injury: The role of vascular damage in the pathogenesis of central hemorrhagic necrosis. *Arch Neurol* 34:332-333, 1977.

296. Parker AJ and Smith CS: Functional recovery from spinal cord trauma following dexamethasone and chlorpromazine therapy in dogs. *Res Vet Sci* 21:246-247, 1976.

297. Osterholm JL: The pathophysiological response to spinal cord injury. The current state of related research. *J Neurosurg* 40:5-33, 1974.

298. Parker AJ and Smith CW: Lack of functional recovery from spinal cord trauma following dimethylsulfoxide and epsilon amino caproic acid therapy in dogs. *Res Vet Sci* 27:253-255, 1979.

299. Rawe SE *et al*: The histopathology of experimental spinal cord trauma. The effect of systemic blood pressure. *J Neurosurg* 48:1002-1007, 1978.

300. Rivlin AS and Tator CH: Regional spinal cord blood flow in rats after severe cord trauma. *J Neurosurg* 49:844-853, 1978.

301. Kobrine AI *et al:* Experimental acute balloon compression of the spinal cord. Factors affecting disappearance and return of the spinal evoked response. *J Neurosurg* 51:841-845, 1979.

302. Senter HJ *et al:* Alteration of posttraumatic ischemia in experimental spinal cord trauma by a central nervous system depressant. *J Neurosurg* 50: 207-216, 1979.

303. Mendenhall HV *et al:* Aggressive pharmacologic and surgical treatment of spinal cord injuries in dogs and cats. *JAVMA* 168:1026-1031, 1976.

304. De la Torre JC: Spinal cord injury: Review of basic and applied research. *Spine* 6:315-355, 1981.

305. Holliday TA, Davis, CA: Unpublished data, 1973.

306. Taylor HW *et al:* Ischemic myelopathy caused by fibrocartilaginous emboli in a horse. *Vet Pathol* 14:479, 1977.

307. Whitwell KE: Causes of ataxia in horses. *In Practice* 2:17-24, 1980.

308. Waldvogel FA and Vasey H: Osteomyelitis: the past decade. *N Eng J Med* 303:360-370, 1980.

309. Markel MD *et al:* Vertebral body osteomyelitis in the horse. *JAVMA* 188:632-634, 1986.

310. Chaldek DW and Ruth GR: Isolation of *Actinobacillus lignieresi* from an epidural abscess in a horse with progressive paralysis. *JAVMA* 178:64-66, 1976.

311. Adams SB *et al:* Diskospondylitis in 5 horses. *JAVMA* 186:270-272, 1985.

312. Richardson DW: *Eikenella corrodens* osteomyelitis of the axis in a foal. *JAVMA* 188:298-299, 1986.

313. Madigan JE and Gribble D: Equine ehrlichiosis in northern California. *JAVMA* 190:445-448, 1987.

314. Evans ETR *et al:* Studies on bracken poisoning in the horse. *Brit Vet J* 107:364-371, 1951.

315. Evans ETR *et al:* Studies on bracken poisoning in the horse. Part II. *Brit Vet J* 107:399-411, 1951.

316. Henderson JA *et al:* The antithiamine action of *Equisetum. JAVMA* 120:375-378, 1952.

317. Cymbaluk NF *et al:*Amprolium-induced thiamin deficiency in horses: clinical features. *Am J Vet Res* 39:255-261, 1978.

318. Rose AL *et al:* Birdsville disease in the Northern territory. *Aust Vet J* 27:189-196, 1951.

319. Mayhew IG *et al:*Equine degenerative myeloencephalopathy. *JAVMA* 170:195-201, 1977.

320. Beech J: Equine degenerative myeloencephalopathy. *Vet Clin No Am* 3:353-355, 1987.

321. Mayhew IG *et al:* Equine degenerative myeloencephalopathy: A vitamin E deficiency that may be familial. *J Vet Int Med* 1:45-50, 1987.

322. Liu IK *et al:* Myelopathy and vitamin E deficiency in six Mongolian wild horses. *JAVMA* 183:1266-1268, 1983.

323. Nixon AJ *et al:* Diagnosis of cervical vertebral malformation in the horse. *Proc 28th Ann Mtg AAEP,* 1982. pp 253-266.

324. Nixon AJ, in Stashak TS: *Adams' Lameness in Horses.* 4th ed. Lea & Febiger, Philadelphia, 1987. pp 772-784.

325. Wagner PC, in Mansmann RA and McAllister ES: *Equine Medicine and Surgery.* 3rd ed. American Veterinary Publications, Goleta, CA, 1982. pp 1145-1158.

326. Reed SM *et al:*Ataxia and paresis in horses. Part I. Differential diagnosis. *Compend Cont Ed Pract Vet* 3:S88-S99, 1981.

327. Powers BE *et al:* Pathology of the vertebral column of horses with cervical static stenosis. *Vet Pathol* 23:392-399, 1986.

328. Smith JM *et al:* Central nervous system disease in adult horses. Part II. Differential diagnosis. *Compend Cont Ed Pract Vet* 9:772-780, 1987.

329. Wagner PC *et al:* A study of the heritability of cervical vertebral malformation in horses. *Proc 31st Ann Mtg AAEP,* 1985. pp 43-50.

330. Dimock WW: "Wobbles": an hereditary disease in horses. *J Hered* 41:319-323, 1950.

331. Falco MJ *et al:* An investigation into the genetics of "wobbler" disease in Thoroughbred horses in Britain. *Equine Vet J* 8:165-169, 1976.

332. Knight DA *et al:* Correlation of dietary mineral to incidence and severity of metabolic bone disease in Ohio and Kentucky. *Proc 31st Ann Mtg AAEP,* 1985. pp 445-461.

333. Knight DA *et al:* Copper supplementation and cartilage lesions in foals. *Proc 33rd Ann Mtg AAEP,* 1987. pp 191-194.

334. Gabel AA *et al:* Comparison of incidence and severity of developmental orthopedic disease on 17 farms before and after adjustment of ration. *Proc 33rd Ann Mtg AAEP,* 1987. pp 163-170.

335. Reed SM *et al:* The relationship of cervical vertebral malformation to developmental orthopedic disease. *Proc 33rd Ann Mtg AAEP,* 1987. pp 139-142.

336. Alitalo I and Karkkainen M: Osteochondrotic changes in the vertebrae of four ataxic horses suffering from cervical vertebral malformation. *Nord Vet Med* 35:468-474, 1983.

337. Dimock WW: Incoordination of horses (wobbles). *Bull Kentucky Agri Exp Stn* 553:1-36, 1950.

338. Grant BD *et al:* Long-term results of surgery for equine cervical vertebral malformation. *Proc 31st Ann Mtg AAEP,* 1985. pp 91-96.

339. Olafson P: "Wobblers" compared with ataxia ("swingback") lambs. *Cornell Vet* 32:301-314, 1942.

340. Reed SM *et al:* Pathogenesis of cervical vertebral malformation. *Proc 31st Ann Mtg AAEP,* 1985. pp 37-42.

341. Schebitz H and Dahme E: Spinal ataxia in the horse. *Proc 13th Ann Mtg AAEP,* 1967. pp 133-148.

342. Rooney JR: *Biomechanics of Lameness in Horses.* Kreiger Publishing, Huntington, NY, 1977.

343. Reiland S *et al:* Osteochondrosis of the spine of the horse. *Svensk Veterinartidning* 35:63-65, 1983.

344. Prickett ME: Equine spinal ataxia. *Proc 14th Ann Conv AAEP,* 1968. pp 147-158.

345. Rooney JR: Equine incoordination. I. Gross morphology. *Cornell Vet* 53:411-422, 1963.

346. Ruppanner R *et al:* Equine incoordination. *Can Vet J* 13:180-183, 1972.

347. Yamagiwa J *et al:* Pathological studies on equine spinal ataxia in Japan. *Jpn J Vet Sci* 42:681-694, 1980.

348. Milne DW *et al*: Diagnosis and pathology of the wobbler syndrome (spondylolisthesis): A preliminary study. *Proc 19th Ann Mtg AAEP*, 1973. pp 303-309.

349. Dimock WW and Errington BJ: Incoordination of Equidae: Wobblers. *JAVMA* 95:261-267, 1939.

350. Schulz LC *et al*: Zur Pathogenese der spinalen Ataxie des Pferdes. Spondyloarthrosis. Pathologisch-anatomische Untersuchungen. *Dtsch Tierrztl Wochenschr* 72:502-506, 1965.

351. Stickle R *et al*: Radiographic diagnosis. *Vet Radiol* 29:28-30, 1988.

352. Dahme E and Schebitz H: Zur Pathogenese der spinalen Ataxie des Pferdes unter Zugrundelegung neuerer Befunde. *Zbl Vet Med* 17:120-143, 1970.

353. Beamer YB *et al*: Hypertrophied ligamentum flavum. *Arch Surgery* 106:289-292, 1973.

354. Hirsh LF: Cervical degenerative arthritis. *Postgrad Med J* 74:123-130, 1983.

355. Gerber H *et al*: Spinale Ataxie beim Pferd, verursacht durch synoviale Cysten in der Halswirbelsaule. *Schweiz Arch Tierheilk* 122:95-106, 1980.

356. Fisher LF *et al*: Spinal ataxia in a horse caused by a synovial cyst. *Vet Pathol* 18:407-410, 1981.

357. Nixon AJ *et al*: Cervical intervertebral disk protrusion in a horse. *Vet Surg* 13:154-158, 1984.

358. Foss RR *et al*: Cervical intervertebral disc protrusion in two horses. *Can Vet J* 24:188-191, 1983.

359. Yovich JV *et al*: Morphologic features of the cervical intervertebral disks and adjacent vertebral bodies of horses. *Am J Vet Res* 46:2372-2377, 1985.

360. Clare NT: The metabolism of phenothiazine in ruminants. *Aust Vet J* 23:340-344, 1947.

361. Rantanen NW *et al*: Ataxia and paresis in horses. Part II. Radiographic and myelographic examination of the cervical vertebral column. *Compend Cont Ed Pract Vet* 3:S161-S171, 1981.

362. Papageorges M *et al*: Radiographic and myelographic examination of the cervical vertebral column in 306 ataxic horses. *Vet Radiol* 28:53-59, 1987.

363. Beech J: Metrizamide myelography in horses. *J Am Vet Radiol Soc* 20:22-32, 1979.

364. Nyland TG *et al*: Metrizamide myelography in the horse: Clinical, radiographic and pathologic changes. *Am J Vet Res* 41:204-211, 1980.

365. Foley JP *et al*: Standing myelography in six adult horses. *Vet Radiol* 27:54-57, 1986.

366. May SA *et al*: Iopamidol myelography in the horse. *Equine Vet J* 18:199-202, 1986.

367. Puglisi TA *et al*: Comparison of metrizamide and iohexol for cisternal myelographic examination of dogs. *Am J Vet Res* 47:1863-1869, 1986.

368. Shaw DD *et al*: Iohexol: Summary of North American and European trials in adult lumbar, thoracic and cervical myelography with a new nonionic contrast medium. *Invest Radiol* 20:S44-S50, 1985.

369. Grant BD *et al*: Surgical treatment of multiple level cord compression in the horse. *Equine Pract* 7(2): 19-24, 1985.

370. Nixon AJ and Stashak TS: Surgical therapy for spinal cord disease in the horse. *Proc 31st Ann Mtg AAEP*, 1985. pp 61-74.

371. MacLean AA *et al*: Use of iohexol for myelography in the horse. *Equine Vet J* 20:286-290, 1988.

372. Strain GM *et al*: Cortical somatosensory-evoked potentials in the horse. *Am J Vet Res* 49:1869-1872, 1988.

373. Shores A *et al*: Spinal-evoked potentials in dogs with acute compressive thoracolumbar spinal cord disease. *Am J Vet Res* 48:1525-1530, 1987.

374. De la Torre JC *et al*: Dimethyl sulfoxide in central nervous system trauma. *Ann NY Acad Sci* 243:362-389, 1975.

375. Wagner PC *et al*: Surgical stabilization of the equine cervical spine. *Vet Surg* 8:7-12, 1979.

376. Stashak TS: A surgical technique for correction of cervical vertebral stenosis in the horse. *Proc 116th Ann Mtg AVMA*, 1979. pp 1-4.

377. Wagner PC *et al*: Evaluation of cervical spinal fusion as a treatment in the equine "wobbler" syndrome. *Vet Surg* 8:84-88, 1979.

378. Cloward RB: The anterior approach for removal of ruptured cervical discs. *J Neurosurg* 5:602-617, 1958.

379. Wagner PC *et al*: Ataxia and paresis in horses. Part III. Surgical treatment of cervical spinal cord compression. *Compend Cont Ed Pract Vet* 3:S192-S202, 1981.

380. Wagner PC *et al*: Treatment of cervical vertebral instability by interbody fusion in the horse. *Proc 31st Ann Mtg AAEP*, 1985. pp 51-60.

381. Nixon AJ and Stashak TS: Surgical management of cervical vertebral malformation in the horse. *Proc 28th Ann Mtg AAEP*, 1982. pp 267-276.

382. DeBowes RM *et al*: Cervical vertebral interbody fusion in the horse: A comparative study of bovine xenografts and autografts supported by stainless steel baskets. *Am J Vet Res* 45:191-199, 1984.

383. Nixon AJ and Stashak TS: Dorsal laminectomy in the horse. 1. Review of the literature and description of a new procedure. *Vet Surg* 12:172-176, 1983.

384. Nixon AJ *et al*: Dorsal laminectomy in the horse. III. Results in horses with cervical vertebral malformation. *Vet Surg* 12:184-188, 1983.

385. Grant BD *et al*: Ventral stabilization for decompression of caudal cervical spinal cord compression in the horse. *Proc 31st Ann Mtg AAEP*, 1985. pp 75-90.

386. Huston R *et al*: Congenital defects in foals. *J Equine Med Surg* 1:146-161, 1977.

387. Pritchard JT and Voss JL: Fetal ankylosis in horses associated with hybrid Sudan pasture. *JAVMA* 150:871-873, 1967.

388. Palmer AC and Hickman J: Ataxia in a horse due to an angioma of the spinal cord. *Vet Record* 72:611-613, 1960.

389. Miller LM *et al*: Ataxia and weakness associated with fourth ventricle vascular anomalies in two horses. *JAVMA* 186:601-603, 1985.

390. Gilmour JS and Fraser JA: Ataxia in a Welsh Cob filly due to a venous malformation in the thoracic spinal cord. *Equine Vet J* 9:40-42, 1977.

391. Schatzmann U *et al*: Akute Hematomyelie nach langerer Ruckenlage beim Pferd. *Schweiz Arch Tierheilk* 121:149-155, 1979.

392. Zink MC: Postanesthetic poliomyelomalacia in a horse. *Can Vet J* 26:275-277, 1985.

393. Yovich JV et al: Postanesthetic hemorrhagic myelopathy in a horse. *JAVMA* 188:300-301, 1986.

394. Brearley JC et al: Spinal cord degeneration following general anesthesia in a Shire horse. *Equine Vet J* 18:222-224, 1986.

395. Blakemore WF et al: Spinal cord malacia following general anesthetic in the horse. *Vet Record* 114:569-570, 1984.

396. Edington N et al: Equine adenovirus 1 isolated from cauda equina neuritis. *Res Vet Sci* 37:252-254, 1984.

397. Colter SB: Electromyographic detection and evaluation of tail alterations in show ring horses. *Proc 6th Ann Forum Am Coll Vet Int Med*, 1988. pp 421-426.

398. Greenwood AG et al: Neuritis of the cauda equina in a horse. *Equine Vet J* 5:141-145, 1973.

399. Rimaila-Parnanen E: Neuritis of the cauda equina in a horse. *Nord Vet Med* 28:464-467, 1976.

400. Rousseaux CG et al: Cauda equina neuritis: A chronic idiopathic polyneuritis in two horses. *Can Vet J* 25: 214-218, 1984.

401. White NA et al: Scanning electron microscopic study of *Strongylus vulgaris* larva-induced arteritis in the pony. *Equine Vet J* 15:349-353, 1983.

402. Scarratt WK and Jortner BS: Neuritis of the cauda equina in a yearling filly. *Compend Cont Ed Pract Vet* 7:S197-S202, 1985.

403. White PL et al: Neuritis of the cauda equina in a horse. *Compend Cont Ed Pract Vet* 6:S217-S222, 1984.

404. Wright JP et al: Neuritis of the cauda equina in the horse. *J Comp Pathol* 97:667-675, 1987.

405. Kadlubowski M et al: Experimental allergic neuritis in the Lewis rat: Characterization of the activity of peripheral nerve myelin and its major basic protein P2. *Brain Res* 184:439-454, 1980.

406. Kadlubowski M and Ingram PL: Circulating antibodies to the neuritogenic myelin protein, P2, in neuritis of the cauda equina of the horse. *Nature* 293:299-300, 1981.

407. Fordyce PS et al: Use of an ELISA in the differential diagnosis of cauda equina neuritis and other equine neuropathies. *Equine Vet J* 19:55-59, 1987.

408. Cummings JF et al: Neuritis of the cauda equina, a chronic idiopathic polyradiculoneuritis in the horse. *Acta Neuropath* 46:17-24, 1979.

409. Adams LG et al: Cystitis and ataxia associated with sorghum ingestion by horses. *JAVMA* 155:518-524, 1969.

410. vanKampen KR: Sudan grass and sorghum poisoning of horses: A possible lathyrogenic disease. *JAVMA* 156:629-630, 1970.

411. Knight PR: Equine cystitis and ataxia associated with grazing on pastures dominated by sorghum species. *Aust Vet J* 44:257, 1968.

412. McKenzie RA and McMicking LI: Ataxia and urinary incontinence in cattle grazing sorghum. *Aust Vet J* 53:496-497, 1977.

413. Dyson S: *The Differential Diagnosis of Shoulder Lameness in the Horse*. Fellowship thesis: Royal College of Veterinary Surgeons, 1986.

414. Henry RW: *Gait Alteration in the Equine Pectoral Limb Produced by Neurectomies*. Master's thesis, Oklahoma State Univ, 1976.

415. Duncan ID and Schneider RK: Equine suprascapular neuropathy (sweeny): Clinical and pathologic observations. *Proc 31st Ann Mtg AAEP*, 1985. pp 415-428.

416. Swaim SF: Peripheral nerve surgery in the dog. *JAVMA* 161:905-911, 1972.

417. Adams OR: *Lameness in Horses*. 3rd ed. Lea & Febiger, Philadelphia, 1974.

418. Schneider JE et al: Scapular notch resection for suprascapular nerve decompression in 12 horses. *JAVMA* 187:1019-1020, 1985.

419. Hammang JP and Duncan ID: Subclinical entrapment neuropathy of the equine suprascapular nerve. *J Neuropathol Exp Neurol* 45:370, 1986.

420. Hickman J: *Veterinary Orthopedics*. Oliver and Boyd, Edinburgh, Scotland, 1964.

421. Blythe LL and Kitchell RL: Electrophysiologic studies of the thoracic limb of the horse. *Am J Vet Res* 43:1511-1524, 1982.

422. Rooney JR: Radial paralysis in the horse. *Cornell Vet* 53:328-338, 1963.

423. Trim CM and Mason J: Post-anaesthetic forelimb lameness in horses. *Equine Vet J* 5:71-76, 1973.

424. Dyson S et al: Femoral nerve paralysis after general anaesthesia. *Equine Vet J* 20:376-379, 1988.

425. Roberts SJ: *Veterinary Obstetrics and Genital Diseases (Theriogenology)*. 3rd ed. David & Charles, N Pomfret, VT, 1986.

426. Dyce CM et al: *Textbook of Veterinary Anatomy*. Saunders, Philadelphia, 1987.

427. Cahill JI et al: A review and some observations on stringhalt. *N Zeal Vet J* 33:101, 1985.

428. Mitchell WM: Some further observations on pathological changes found in horses affected with "shivering" and their significance. *Vet Record* 10:535-537, 1930.

429. Pemberton DH and Caple IW: Australian stringhalt in horses. *Vet Annual* 20:167, 1980.

430. Cahill JI et al: Stringhalt in horses: a distal axonopathy. *Neuropath Appl Neurobiol* 12:459-475, 1986.

431. Smith LDS: *Botulism: The Organism, Its Toxin, the Disease*. Charles C Thomas, Springfield, IL, 1977.

432. Gunderson CB: The effects of botulinum toxin on the synthesis, storage and release of acetylcholine. *Prog Neurobiol* 14:99-119, 1980.

433. Mohler JR: Cerebrospinal meningitis ("forage poisoning"). *Bull USDA* 65, 1914.

434. Botija CS: Le botulisme des equides en Espagne (epizootologie clinique, traitement et prevention). *Bull Off Intl Epizoot* 42:759-764, 1954.

435. Tamarin R and Neeman L: The identification of *Clostridium botulinum* type B toxin as the cause of an outbreak of botulism in equines. *Refuah Vet* 19:14-15, 1962.

436. Lemetayer E et al: Recherches sur le botulisme experimental chez le cheval. *Bull Acad Vet* 26:391-399, 1953.

437. Legroux R *et al:* Le botulisme experimental de cheval et la question du botulisme naturel. *Ann Inst Pasteur* 72:545-552, 1946.

438. Jacquet J: Sur le botulisme equin et notamment le botulisme experimental provoque a l'aide de la toxine. *Bull Off Intl Epizoot* 42:473-481, 1954.

439. Muller J:Equine and bovine botulism in Denmark. *Bull Off Intl Epizoot* 59:1379-1390, 1963.

440. Lapcevic E: L'intoxication des chevaux par le botulisme. *Bull Off Intl Epizoot* 42:507-513, 1954.

441. DeFagonde AP: Botulismo animal. *Bull Off Intl Epizoot* 59:1361-1377, 1963.

442. Mitchell CA *et al*: Isolation of *Cl botulinus* from oat grain. *Can J Comp Med* 3:245-247, 1939.

443. MacKay RJ and Berkhoff GA: Type C toxicoinfectious botulism in a foal. *JAVMA* 180:163-164, 1982.

444. Swerczek TW. Toxicoinfectious botulism in foals and adult horses. *JAVMA* 176:217-220, 1980.

445. Divers TJ *et al: Clostridium botulinum* type B toxicosis in a herd of cattle and a group of mules. *JAVMA* 188:382-386, 1986.

446. Ricketts SW *et al*: Thirteen cases of botulism in horses fed big bale silage. *Equine Vet J* 16:515-518, 1984.

447. Bernard W *et al*: Botulism as a sequel to open castration in a horse. *JAVMA* 191:73-74, 1987.

448. Swerczek TW: Experimentally induced toxico-infectious botulism in horses and foals. *Am J Vet Res* 41:348-350, 1980.

449. Lewis CE *et al*: Evaluation of *Clostridium botulinum* toxoid, type B, for the prevention of shaker foal syndrome. *Proc 27th Ann Mtg AAEP,* 1981. pp 233-237.

450. Cudd TA, Lexington, KY: Personal communication, 1988.

451. Johnston J and Whitlock RH, in Robinson NE: *Current Therapy in Equine Medicine 2.* Saunders, Philadelphia, 1987. pp 367-370.

This page is intentionally left blank.

Index

A

abdomen, acute distention, 1, 2
  examination, 68, 69
  abdominocentesis, 486-489
abdominal crisis, see colic
abdominal distention, 1, 2
abdominal hernia, 690-692
abdominocentesis, 486-489, 516, 674, **1541**
abiotrophy, cerebellar, 793, 794
abortion, 2, 3, **1066-1071**
  fetal examination, **1067**
  fetal mummification, **1071**
  herpesvirus-1, **1069, 1070**
  maternal illness, **1068**
  prevention, **1068**
  therapeutic, **1069**
  twinning, **1059, 1060**
  umbilical cord torsion, **1069**
  viral arteritis, **1070, 1071**
abrasions, **1584, 1590**
abscess, abdominal, 674-677
  cerebral, 774, 775
  corynebacterial, **1325, 1326, 1665**
  pectoral, **1325, 1326, 1665**
  retrobulbar, **1096**
  spleen, **1845**
  stromal, corneal, **1115-1117**
  subsolar, **1343, 1344**
  treatment, **1608, 1609**
  umbilical, **1564, 1565**
  ureachal, **1564, 1565**
  vitreal, **1127**
accessory carpal bone fracture, **1429**
accessory genital glands, **916-918**
acetabular fractures, **1502, 1503**
Achilles tendon rupture, **1488**
acid-base therapy, 139-142
acidosis, renal tubular, **1556, 1557**
actinomycosis, **1666, 1667**
Addison's disease, **1748, 1749**
adenovirus infection, 385
adhesions, abdominal, 609, 610, 677, 678
adrenal glands, diseases, **1748, 1749**
African horse sickness, 378-380
agammaglobulinemia, **1822**
aggression, **887, 888**
alar folds, redundant, 391, 392
alimentary system, 473-704
  abdominal surgery, 514-532
  abdominal wall hernia, 690-692
  abdominocentesis, 486-489, 516, 674
  abscesses, abdominal, 674-677
  adhesions, 609, 610, 677, 678
  anastomosis, bowel, 523-530
  Anoplocephala perfoliata, 618
  antacids, 506, 507
  anthrax, 532, 533
  ascariasis, 617, 618, 621

ascarid impaction, 621
ascites, 682
atresia ani, 664
basophilic enterocolitis, 625
bezoars, 635, 636, 661, 662
biliary atresia, 698
blister beetle poisoning, 324, 483, 533-535, 655, 656
bowel motility, 503, 504
bowel surgery, 514-532
catharidin toxicity, 324, 483, 533-535, 655, 656
cecum, 627-633
choke, 572, 573, 583-586
cholelithiasis, 701
clinical pathology tests, 482-489
clostridiosis, 648, 649
colic, 10, 11, 120, 486-489, 499-502, 514-532, 541, 542
colitis X, 653-655
decay, dental, 568, 569
dental problems, 550-570
dentigerous cysts, 562
diaphragmatic hernia, 689, 690
diarrhea, 498, 499, 649-651, 657
dysphagia, 15, 16, 781, 782
eating difficulties, 15, 16, 781, 782
ehrlichial colitis, 651-653
Eimeria leukarti, 618, 619
endoscopy, 479, 480
enteritis, clostridial, 620, 621
enteritis, granulomatous, 620, 624
enteritis, nongranulomatous, 541
enteritis, proximal, 626, 627
enteritis, viral, 619, 620
enteroliths, 635, 636, 661, 662
eosinophilic gastroenteritis, 625
epiploic foramen hernia, 611
esophagitis, 587
esophagus, 572-593
  examination, 473-489
fecal consistency, 504-506
feces, abnormal, 21, 22
gastric dilatation, 600
gastric impaction, 600
gastric rupture, 600, 601
gastritis, 604
gastroduodenal ulcers, 605, 606
granulomatous colitis, 649
grass sickness, 540
hemoperitoneum, 667-669
hepatitis, 700, 701
hyoid apparatus, 548-550
hyperalimentation, 510, 511
ileal impaction, 623
ileus, 516, 539, 540
incisional hernias, 685-689
infarction, bowel, 496, 538, 539
inguinal hernia, 612, 613, 684, 685
intraabdominal hemorrhage, 667-669

intubation, nasogastric, 475, 516
intussusception, 613, 614, 632, 663
lactase deficiency, 622
lampus, 547
laparoscopy, 489
laparotomy, 489, 518-520
large colon, 633-659
lethal white syndrome, 532, **1716**
liver, diseases, 692-702
malabsorption, 607, 609
malassimilation, 607
maldigestion, 607
mandibular cysts, 563
Meckel's diverticulum, 608
meconium impaction, 659, 660
medical therapy, 499-514
megaesophagus, 581, 582
mesenteric hernia, 611, 612
mesodiverticular band, 608, 609
mouth, diseases, 543-548
mycotoxicosis, 700
neoplasia, 536-538
nonsteroidal antiinflammatory toxicity, 535, 536, 602, 603
nutritional support, 507-510
obstruction, bowel, 490-498
oligodontia, 564
oral cavity, diseases, 543-548
palate, cleft, 544-546
pancreas, 702-704
pancreatitis, 703, 704
Parascaris equorum, 617, 618, 621
parrot mouth, 561
penetrating wounds, 669, 670
pedunculated lipoma, 615, 616, 662, 666
periodontal disease, 567
periostitis, alveolar, 567
peritonitis, 670-674
Potomac horse fever, 651-653, **1765**
prepubic tendon rupture, 690-692
protein-losing enteropathy, 607, 608
pruritus ani, 666
pyloric stenosis, 599, 600, 602
pyrrolizidine toxicity, 699
radiography, 480, 481
rectal examination, 70, 476-479, 516
rectal prolapse, 666, 667
rectovaginal laceration, 667
rectum, 663-667
roundworms, 617, 618, 621
salivary glands, 570-572
salivation, excessive, 37, 38
salmonellosis, 120, 483, 643-647
shear mouth, 562
small colon, 659-663
small intestine, 606-627
smooth mouth, 566
sounds, intestinal, 516, 539, 540
sow mouth, 561
step mouth, 566

(A continued)

stomach, 593-606
stomatitis, 547, **1707**
strangulation, bowel, 490-498
strangles,674-677
Streptococcus equi, 674-677
Strongyloides westeri, 616
Strongylus vulgaris, 496, 538, 539, 649, 650
tapeworms, 618
teeth, 550-570
tenesmus, 39, 40
Theiler's disease, 700, 701
thread worms, 616
transfaunation, 511
traumatic hernias, 687
typhlitis, 629
Tyzzer's disease, 698
umbilical hernia, 613, 683, 684
umbilical infection, 687
ultrasonography, 481, 482
uroperitoneum, 678, 679
verminous arteritis, 679-681
volvulus, small colon, 662
wave mouth, 565
weight loss, 46-48
wolf teeth, 557, 564
xylose absorption test, 485
alopecia, **1683-1694**, 1685-1694
aminoglycoside toxicity, **1553**
amputation, limb, **1253**
penile, **925-927**
Amsinckia intermedia, 699
amyloidosis, cutaneous, **1663**
nasal, 395
renal, **1556**
anagen defluxion, **1683**
analgesics, 81-86, 499-502, 516
anemia, aplastic, **1795-1797**
autoimmune hemolysis, **1805**
babesiosis, **1765, 1806**
blood loss, **1807, 1808**
blood transfusion, **1791-1793, 1805, 1808**
causes, **1802, 1803**
chronic disease, **1808**
clostridiosis, **1806**
ehrlichiosis, **1763, 1765, 1780, 1806**
equine infectious, **1764, 1765, 1804, 1837**
neonatal isoerythrolysis, **1804, 1805**
hemolytic, **1803-1806**
iron deficiency, **1809**
onion poisoning, **1807**
phenothiazine toxicity, **1807**
piroplasmosis, **1765, 1806**
red maple leaf toxicity, **1806**
transfusion reactions, **1805**
anesthesia, 81-120
agents, induction, 97-103
apparatus, 103-105
auriculopalebral block, **1085, 1086**
complications, 117-120
controlled ventilation, 114-116
epidural, **1168**
eyeball, **1085, 1086**
eyelid, **1085, 1086**
forelimb, **1163-1167**
induction, 97-103
inhalation, 105-109
joints, **1166-1168**
local anesthesia, **1163-1168**
monitoring, 111-114
nerve blocks, **1163-1168**
orbit, **1085, 1086**
postanesthetic myasthenia, 120, 835, **1319**

postanesthetic myelopathy, 822, 823
postanesthetic myopathy, 117-119, **1319-1321**
preanesthetics, 93-97
recovery, 116, 117
sedatives, 81-86, 93-97
shoulder, **1452**
standing restraint, 81-86
tranquilizers, 81-86, 93-97
ventilation, controlled, 114-116
anestrus, **1028**
angular deformities, **1298-1307**
carpus, **1435, 1436**
fetlock, **1397-1399**
hock, **1478, 1479**
metacarpus, **1420, 1421**
angiocardiography, 210, 211
angioedema, **1679**
anhidrosis, 42, 43, **1683, 1684**
aniridia, **1119**
Anoplocephala perfoliata, 618
antacids, 506, 507
anthelmintics, 510, 511
anthrax, 532, 533
antibiotics, see drugs
aortic insufficiency, 301, 310-314
aortic rupture, 284
aortoiliac thrombosis, 287-291
aplasia cutis, **1720**
aplastic anemia, **1795-1797**
Arabian fading syndrome, **1716**
arrhythmias, cardiac, 213, 214, 230-260
arsenic poisoning, **1714**
arteries, diseases, 277-291
aortic rupture, 284
aortoiliac thrombosis, 287-291
arteritis, parasitic, 281, 282
arteritis, viral, 384, 385
arteritis, verminous, 679-681
neoplasia, 282, 283
persistent ductus arteriosus, 278, 279
persistent right aortic arch, 279
persistent truncus arteriosus, 279, 280
pulmonary artery rupture, 285, 286
pulmonic atresia, 280
tetralogy of Fallot, 280, 281
thrombosis, 287-291
uterine artery rupture, 285, **1014**
vasculitis, 281
arteritis, parasitic, 281, 282
verminous, 679-681
viral, 384, 385, **918, 1678, 1836**
arthritis, see joints
arthrodesis, **1253-1258**
arthrography, **1175**
arthrogryposis, 822
artificial insemination, **870, 871**
artificial lighting, **866, 999**
artificial vagina, **871-873**
arytenoid chondritis, 412-414
arytenoidectomy, 412-414
ascarids, 617, 618, 621
impaction, 621
ascites, 682
Aspergillus, 394, 408-410
aspiration pneumonia, 431, 432
asteroid hyalosis, **1128**
astringents, topical, **1644**
ataxia, 733
atheroma, 395, 396
atopy, **1653**
atresia ani, 664
atrial fibrillation, 241-246
atrial flutter, 246, 247
atrial septal defects, 319, 320
atrial tachycardia, 246, 247

atrioventricular block, 236-240
atrioventricular dissociation, 252-254
atrioventricular insufficiency, 301, 305-310
atrioventricular stenosis, 308-310, 313, 314
aural plaques, **1720**
auriculopalpebral nerve block, **1085, 1086**
autoimmune diseases, **1770, 1804, 1805**
autoimmune hemolytic anemia, **1805**
avulsions, **1586**
axillary nodular necrosis, **1664**
azoospermia, **942, 943**
azotemia, **1545, 1546**
azoturia, 327, **1321-1324**

B

babesiosis, **1765, 1806**
back problems, 3-5, **1154-1160**
bacterial meningoencephalomyelitis, 754-756
bacteriospermia, **941**
balanitis, **934**
bandaging, **1603, 1604**
barker foals, 754-756, 764
basophilia, **1815**
basophilic enterocolitis, 625
bee stings, **1678**
behavior, abnormal, 5-7
aggression, **887, 888**
biting, 766
cribbing, 766
coprophagia, 766
depression, 13, 14
head-shaking, 767
pawing,, 766
self-mutilation, 769
sexual, mare, **982-988, 1008-1010**
sexual, stallion, **883-888**
stallion-like, **882**
stall-walking, 766
vices, 765-769
besnoitiosis, **1713**
bezoars, 635, 636, 661, 662
bicipital bursitis, **1456, 1457**
biliary atresia, 698
biopsy, endometrial, **960-963**
kidney, **1543**
liver, 696
muscle, **1163**
skin, **1577, 1578**
testicular, **856, 907**
Birdsville indigo poisoning, 806
black flies, **1690, 1691**
bladder, urinary, calculi, **1562, 1563**
cystitis, **1560**
cystotomy, **1562**
neoplasia, **1561**
paralysis, **1561**
rupture, **1559, 1560**
blastomycosis, **1672, 1673**
bleeder syndrome, 451-454
bleeding, 7-9
blepharitis, **1101, 1102**
blindness, 9, 10
moon blindness, **1121-1124**
night blindness, **1129-1131**
pituitary tumor, **1738**
blind staggers, 762
blister beetle toxicity, 324, 483, 533-535, 655, 656, **920, 1555, 1561**
blood, see also hemolymphatic system
cell counts, **1756-1759**

(B continued)

cell morphology, 1757, 1762, 1763
collection, 1755, 1756
gas analysis, 206-208, 360
loss, 1807, 1808
pressure, 218, 219, 262
reference intervals, 1774
transfusions, 1791-1793, 1805, 1808
blowflies, 1676
bog spavin, 1476
Bolz operation, 924, 925
bone, angular deformities, 1298-1307, 1397-1399
arthrodesis, 1253-1258
bone spavin, 1474-1476
bucked shins, 1410-1413
casts, 1229-1234
cysts, 1402, 1459, 1494-1499
distal interphalangeal osteochondrosis, 1369
exostoses, 1281, 1414-1416, 1449
flexural deformities, 1307, 1308, 1399-1401
fluoride toxicosis, 1293-1296
fractures, 1200-1248
grafts, 1243-1246
healing, 1204-1211
hypertrophic osteopathy, 1316, 1317
implants, 1236-1242
marrow aplasia, 1795-1797
marrow collection, 1756
marrow evaluation, 1760, 1774-1787
navicular disease, 1346-1354
nuclear imaging, 743, 1185-1191
nutritional deficiencies, 1296-1298, 1301
osteochondritis dissecans, see osteochondrosis
osteochondroma, 1449
osteochondrosis, 1308-1316, 1369, 1378, 1401, 1402, 1438, 1480, 1481, 1494
osteomyelitis, 804, 805, 1289-1292, 1419, 1420
osteopetrosis, 1281
osteotomy, 1248-1253
pastern osteochondrosis, 1378
patellar chondromalacia, 1491
pedal oseitis, 1340, 1341
physitis, 1315, 1316
pins, 1241
plates, 1238-1241
radiography, 1170-1178
scintigraphy, 743, 1185-1191
screws, 1236-1238
splints, 1225-1235
"splints," 1414-1416
tarsitis, 1474-1476
thermography, 743, 1191-1194
bone marrow, aplasia, 1795-1797
collection, 1756
evaluation, 1760, 1774-1787
bone spavin, 1474-1476
Bordetella bronchiseptica, 438
Borna disease, 744
borreliosis, 1292, 1293
botryomycosis, 1665
bots, 601, 602
botulism, 782, 832
bowed tendons, 1416, 1417
brachygnathia, 561, 1460
bracken fern poisoning, 805, 806
bradycardia, 229, 230
brain-heart syndrome, 743
breeding, see reproductive system
bronchoalveolar lavage, 359
BSP clearance, 695, 696

bucked shins, 1410-1413
buffy coat analysis, 1759
bulbourethral gland, 916, 917
bullous pemphigoid, 1708
bundle branch block, 255
buphthalmos, 1095, 1096
burns, 1625-1630
bursitis, bacterial, 1667
bicipital, 1456, 1457
cunean, 1474

C

calcinosis circumscripta, 1664
calculi, cystic, 1562, 1563
renal, 1550
salivary, 571
ureteral, 1558
calluses, 1721
candidiasis, 1706
canker, 1371, 1372
cantharidin toxicity, 324, 483, 533-535, 655, 656, 920, 1555, 1561
capped elbow, 1446
capped hock, 1471
capped knee, 1433
carcinoma, renal
cardiomyopathy, 329
cardiovascular system, 135-334
anatomy, 166-168
angiocardiography, 210, 211
aortic insufficiency, 301, 310-314
aortic rupture, 284
arrhythmias, 213, 214, 230-260
arteries, diseases, 277-291
arteritis, parasitic, 281, 282, 384, 385, 679-681, 918, 1678, 1836
atrial fibrillation, 241-246
atrial flutter, 246, 247
atrial septal defect, 319, 320
atrial tachycardia, 246, 247
atrioventricular block, 236-240
atrioventricular dissociation, 252-254
atrioventricular insufficiency, 301, 305-310
atrioventricular stenosis, 308-310
auscultation, 182-186, 220-228
blood pressure, 218, 219, 262
blood gas analysis, 206-208
bradycardia, 229, 230
bundle branch block, 255
cardiac catheterization, 210, 211
cardiac radiography, 209-212
cardiomyopathy, 329
congenital heart disease, 262-268
congestive heart failure, 268-277
cor pulmonale, 273, 274
digitalization, 276, 277
echocardiography, 206, 214-217
electrocardiography, 187-198
endocardial fibroelastosis, 298, 299
endocarditis, 302-305
examination, 165-219
exercise testing, 198-206
heart failure, 268-277
heart sounds, 182-186, 220-228
idioventricular rhythm, 255
jugular pulse, 173-175
jugular thrombophlebitis, 293-295
murmurs, 220-228
myocardial fibrosis, 324-327
myocardial hypertrophy, 329
myocarditis, 320, 321
parasystole, 252-254
paroxysmal atrial fibrillation, 246

pericardiocentesis, 332, 333
pericarditis, 330-333
persistent ductus arteriosus, 278-279
persistent foramen ovale, 319, 320
persistent right aortic arch, 279
persistent truncus arteriosus, 279, 280
phonocardiography, 208, 209
premature atrial contractions, 247, 248
premature ventricular contractions, 251
pulmonic stenosis, 313, 314
pulse, evaluation, 176-179
radiography, 209-212
sinoatrial block, 234-236
sinus arrhythmia, 233, 234
sounds, heart, 182-186, 220-228
syncope, 260, 261
tachycardia, 229
tetralogy of Fallot, 280, 281
thrombosis, 287-293
tricuspid atresia, 299-301
vasculitis, 281
vectorcardiography, 191-196
veins, diseases, 291-295
ventricular arrhythmias, 249-255
ventricular fibrillation, 254
ventricular septal defect, 315-319
ventricular tachycardia, 251, 252
wandering pacemaker, 234
Wolff-Parkinson-White syndrome, 248, 249
caries, 568, 569
carpal canal syndrome, 1430, 1431
carpal fractures, 1420-1430
carpal joint infection, 1434
carpus
accessory carpal bone fractures, 1429
angular deformities, 1435, 1436
capped knee, 1433
carpal canal syndrome, 1430, 1431
comminuted fractures, 1430
common digital extensor tendon rupture, 1432
degenerative joint disease, 1438-1440
extensor carpi radialis muscle rupture, 1431
flexural deformities, 1436-1438
fractures, 1420-1430
hygroma, 1433
joint infection, 1434
osteochondrosis, 1438
slab fractures, 1425-1429
Caslick's procedure, 1040
castration, 877-883
cryptorchidectomy, 898-900
casts, 1229-1234
cataracts, 1125-1128
catheterization, cardiac, 210, 211
intravenous, 139, 140
cauda equina disorders, 823-826
cauda equina neuritis, 824, 825
cecum, 627-633
anatomy, 627
examination, 627, 628
fistula, 628
impaction, 629, 630
infarction, 633
intussusception, 632
perforation, 631
tapeworms, 629
torsion, 628
tympany, 632
typhlitis, 629
cellulitis, 1608, 1609, 1677, 1678
cerebellar abiotrophy, 793, 794
cerebellar hypoplasia, 793, 794
cerebral abscess, 774, 775

(C continued)

cerebrospinal fluid analysis, 739-742
cervical vertebral malformation, 807-822
cervix, diseases, **1037-1039**
cesarean section, **1020-1022**
champignon, **881**
chlorinated hydrocarbon poisoning, 762
choke, 572, 573, 583-586
cholelithiasis, 701
cholesteatoma, 780, 781
cholesterol granuloma, 780, 781
chorioptic mange, **1693**
chorioretinitis, **1131, 1132**
chromomycosis, **1671**
chromosomal analysis, **856**
chronic obstructive pulmonary disease,
 443-449
cilia, distichiasis, **1100**
 ectopic, **1100**
 trichiasis, **1100**
cinematography, **1196, 1197**
circumcision, **936, 937**
Claviceps purpurea, **1711**
cleft palate, 544-546
clostridial myonecrosis, **1324, 1325**
clostridiosis, 648, 649, **1806**
Clostridium botulinum, 782, 832
Clostridium perfringens, 648, 649,
 1325, 1806
Clostridium tetani, 782, 785-788
clotting, **1771, 1772, 1787-1789,
 1831-1843**
coagulation, **1771, 1772, 1787-1789,
 1831-1843**
coccidioidomycosis, 394, 451, **1673**
coccygeal paralysis, 824
coital exanthema, **1058, 1706, 1707**
colic, 10, 11
 abdominocentesis, 486-489, 516
 analgesia, 499-502
 flatulent, 542
 postanesthetic, 120
 spasmodic, 541
 surgery, 514-532
colitis X, 653-655
collapse, 11-13
collateral cartilage, necrosis, **1339**
 ossification, **1340**
coloboma, **1098, 1119, 1129**
colon, large, 633-659
 atresia coli, 634
 bezoars, 635, 636
 blister beetle poisoning, 655, 656
 cantharidin toxicosis, 655, 656
 clostridiosis, 648, 649
 colitis X, 653-655
 diarrhea, antimicrobial-associated, 657
 diarrhea, parasitic, 649, 650
 displacement, 640-642
 ehrlichial colitis, 651-653, **1765**
 enteroliths, 635, 636
 fecaliths, 635, 636
 granulomatous colitis, 649
 impaction, 634, 635
 infarction, 658
 intussusception, 642
 parasitism, 649-650
 Potomac horse fever, 651-653
 salmonellosis, 643-647
 Strongylus vulgaris, 496, 538, 539, 649,
  650
 tympany, 658
 volvulus, 637-640
colon, small, 659-663
 bezoars, 661, 662
 enteroliths, 661, 662

fecaliths, 661, 662
 impaction, 660, 661
 intussusception, 663
 meconium impaction, 659, 660
 pedunculated lipoma, 662
 volvulus, 662
Colorado strangles, **1325, 1326, 1665**
colostrum, immunoglobulins, **1790,
 1791, 1824**
combined immunodeficiency, **1814,
 1819-1822**
compression plates, bone, **1238-1241**
congenital defects, 28, 29
congestive heart failure, 268-277
conjunctival hypertrophy, **1109**
conjunctivitis, **1106, 1107**
contact dermatitis, **1702-1704**
contagious equine metritis, **922, 923,
 938, 1034-1036**
contracted foal syndrome, 822
contracted heels, **1371**
contusions, **1585, 1590**
convulsions, 770, 779, 780
Coombs' test, **1770**
coprophagia, 766
copulation, see reproductive system
cornea, see also eye
 dystrophy, **1118, 1119**
 fluorescein staining, **1085**
 keratitis, **1110, 1114, 1115, 1117**
 ulcers, **1111, 1113, 1114**
Corynebacterium equi, 436-438
Corynebacterium pseudotuberculosis,
 1325, 1326, 1665
coughing, 13, 14
coupage, 378
coxofemoral luxation, **1504, 1505**
cramping, muscle, **1328, 1329**
cranial nerves, 725-731
cranial trauma, 771-774
cribbing, 766
cryosurgery, **1635-1637**
cryptococcosis, 394, 756, **1673**
cryptorchidectomy, **898-900**
Cryptosporidium, 618, 619
CSF analysis, 739-742
Culicoides dermatitis, **1685-1687**
cultures, eye, **1086**
 reproductive tract, **850, 958-960**
 skin, **1575, 1576**
cunean bursitis, **1474**
curb, **1474**
curly coat, **1718, 1741**
Cyathostoma, 649, 650
cyst, bone, **1402, 1459, 1494-1499**
 dentigerous, 562, **1654**
 dermoid, **1654**
 endometrial, **1037**
 esophageal, 580
 iridal, **1125**
 mandibular, 563
 Morgagni, **969**
 ovarian, **1025**
 paranasal sinus, follicular, 396
 pharyngeal, 398, 399
 uterine, **1037**
cystic calculi, **1562, 1563**
cystitis, **1560**
cystotomy, **1562**
cytologic examination
 blood cells, **1757, 1762, 1763**
 bone marrow, **1760, 1774-1787**
 reproductive tract, **957, 958**
 skin, **1578**

D

dacryocystitis, **1107**
Dallis grass poisoning, 795
darling pea poisoning, 795, 796
death, sudden, 40-42, 260, 261
debridement, wound, **1597, 1598**
decay, dental, 568, 569
decubital ulcers, **1721**
degenerative joint disease, **1216-1220**
 carpus, **1438-1440**
 fetlock, **1402-1405**
 hock, **1476**
 pastern, **1378, 1379**
 treatment, **1258-1261**
degenerative myeloencephalopathy, 806,
 807
dehiscence, wound, 685-689, **882**
demodectic mange, **1680, 1681**
dental, see teeth
dentigerous cysts, 562, **1654**
depression, 14, 15
dermatitis, see skin
dermatophilosis, **1575, 1694-1696**
dermatophytosis, **1698-1700**
dermographism, **1652**
dermoid, **1105, 1110**
dermoid cysts, **1654**
desmitis, distal sesamoidean, **1394**
 inferior cheek, **1417, 1418**
 plantar, **1474**
 suspensory, **1418, 1419**
deworming, 510, 511
diabetes insipidus, **1557**
diabetes mellitus, **1739, 1741, 1749**
diaphragmatic flutter, **1327**
diaphragmatic hernia, 456, 457, 689, 690
diarrhea, 498, 499, 649-651, 657
Dictyocaulus arnfieldi, 442, 443
diestrus, prolonged, **1027**
digitalization, 276, 277
dimethylsulfoxide, 148, 149, **1259**
disseminated intravascular coagulation,
 162, 163, **1022, 1838-1842**
distichiasis, **1100**
diverticulum, Meckel's, 608
DMSO, 148, 149, **1259**
Dohle bodies, **1780**
dourine, **851, 892, 920, 938, 1800, 1801**
dracunculiasis, **1676**
drainage, wound, **1600-1602**
Draschia megastoma, 601, 602, **938**
drug eruption, **1653**
drugs, anabolic steroids, **903**
 analgesia, 81-86, 499-502, 516
 antacids, 506, 507, 595, 597
 anthelmintics, 510, 511
 antifungals, **1645, 1647**
 antiinflammatories, 142-145, **1645,
  1646**
 antimicrobials, 142-145, 511-513,
  1087-1089, 1602, 1603, 1645-1647
 antipyretics, 145-150
 aplastic anemia, **1795**
 bowel motility, 503, 504
 corticosteroids, 149, 150, **1259, 1645,
  1646**
 digitalization, 276, 277
 dimethylsulfoxide, 148, 149, **1259**
 drug eruption, **1653**
 electrolytes, 139-142
 fecal consistency, 504-506
 fluids, 139-142
 gold salts, **1647**

(D continued)

hyaluronic acid, **1260**
immunostimulants, **1648**
immunosuppressants, **1647**
nonsteroidal antiinflammatories,
    145-148, 535, **1090, 1258**
polysulfated glycosaminoglycan, **1261**
superoxide dismutase, **1259**
dummy foals, 754-756, 764
dysphagia, 15, 16, 781, 782
dystocia, **1015-1022**

E

ear, aural plaques, **1720**
    ear-tick infestation, **1650, 1719**
    hematoma, **1655**
    otitis interna, 794, 795
    psoroptic otitis, **1719**
Eastern equine encephalomyelitis,
    744-749
eating difficulties, 15, 16, 781, 782
echocardiography, 206, 214-217
ectoparasitism, bee stings, **1678**
    black flies, **1690, 1691**
    blowflies, **1676**
    Culiculoides, **1685-1687**
    dracunculiasis, **1676**
    face flies, **1722**
    fire ant stings, **1704**
    gasterophiliasis, **1676**
    Habronema, 601, 602, **894, 934, 935,**
        938, 1101, 1613, 1673-1675
    horn flies, **1690**
    Hypoderma, **1655**
    louse infestation, **1692**
    mange, **1692, 1693**
    mosquito bites, **1649, 1650**
    myiasis, **1675, 1676**
    Onchocerca, **938, 1102, 1107, 1115,**
        1121-1124, 1687-1690
    Oxyuris equi, **1575, 1691**
    parafilariasis, **1676**
    pediculosis, **1692**
    Pelodera, **1709**
    pinworms, **1575, 1691**
    screwworms, **1675**
    Simulium, **1690, 1691**
    spider bites, **1679**
    summer sores, 601, 602, **894, 934, 935,**
        938, 1101, 1613, 1673-1675
    tabanid flies, **1649**
    Thelazia, **1107**
    tick infestation, 764, **1650, 1719**
    tick paralysis, 764
    trombiculid mites, **1694**
    warbles, **1655**
ectopic ureters, **1558**
ehrlichial colitis, 651-653, **1765**
ehrlichiosis, **1763, 1765, 1780, 1806,**
    1837
ehrlichiosis, monocytic, **1765**
Eimeria leukarti, 618, 619
ejaculation, **863-865, 885-887, 940**
elbow joint, **1440-1450**
electrocardiography, 187-198
electroencephalography, 743
electrolyte excretion, urinary, **1541**
electromyelography, 742
electromyography, **1162**
electroretinography, **1087**
embryonic death, 1063-1066
emergencies, 51, 52
emphysema, subcutaneous, **1677**
empyema, guttural pouch, 406-408, 789
    paranasal sinus, 392-394

encephalitis, verminous, 759-761
encephalomalacia, nigropallidal, 789,
    790
encephalomyelitis, Eastern, 744-749
    herpesvirus-1, 751-753
    immunization, 748
    Near Eastern, 744
    protozoal, 756-759
    Venezuelan, 744-749
    Western, 744-749
endocardial fibroelastosis, 298, 299
endocarditis, 302-305
endocrine system, Addison's disease,
    1748, 1749
    adrenal gland disorders, **1748, 1749**
    diabetes mellitus, **1739, 1741, 1749**
    examination, **1737-1739**
    function tests, **1581, 1743**
    glucose metabolism, disorders, **1739,**
        1740
    hyperglycemia, **1739**
    hyperlipidermia syndrome, **1740**
    hypoadrenocorticism, **1748, 1749**
    hypothyroidism, **1648, 1686, 1741,**
        1745-1748
    neoplasia, 703, **1718, 1740-1745, 1749**
    pancreatitis, chronic, 703, 704, **1749**
    pituitary adenoma, **1718, 1740-1745**
    thyroid diseases, **1745-1748**
endometrial cups, **993**
endometrial fibrosis, **1036, 1037, 1065**
endometritis, **1029-1033, 1036, 1065**
endoparasitism, *Anoplocephala*
    perfoliata, 618, 619
    anthelmintics, 510, 511
    ascariasis, 617, 618, 621
    Cryptosporidium, 618, 619
    Cyathostoma, 649, 650
    Draschia megastoma, 601, 602
    Eimeria leukarti, 618, 619
    Gasterophilus, 601, 602, **1676**
    gastric, 601, 602
    Habronema, 601, 602
    Halicephalobus deletrix, 760
    Hypoderma, 760, 761
    Parascaris equorum, 442, 617, 618, 621
    protozoans, 618, 619
    roundworms, 617, 618, 621
    Setaria, 760, 761, **938**
    Strongyloides westeri, 616
    Strongylus vulgaris, 496, 538
    tapeworms, 618, 629
    thread worms, 616
    Trichostrongylus axei, 601, 602
endophthalmitis, **1124**
enteritis, clostridial, 620, 621
    granulomatous, 620, 624
    proximal, 626, 627
    nongranulomatous, 541
    viral, 619, 620
enterolith, 635, 636, 661, 662
entropion, **1097, 1098**
enzymology, endocrine disease, **1738,**
    1739
    heart disease, 212, 213
    liver disease, 694
    muscle disease, **1161, 1162**
    urinary disease, **1541**
eosinopenia, **1815**
eosinophilia, **1814**
eosinophilic dermatitis, **1713**
eosinophilic gastroenteritis, 625
epididymis, **908-910**
epididymitis, **909**
epidural anesthesia, **1168**
epiglottic entrapment, 421-424

epilepsy, 779, 780
epiploic foramen hernia, 611
epistaxis, 451-454
epitheliogenesis imperfecta, **1720**
equine degenerative
    myeloencephalopathy, 806, 807
equine infectious anemia, 754, **1764,**
    1765, 1804, 1837
equine protozoal myeloencephalitis,
    756-759
equine viral arteritis, 384, 385, **918,**
    1678, 1836
erection, **863-865, 884, 885**
ergotism, **1711**
erythema multiforme, **1653**
erythematosus, discoid, **1717**
    systemic, **1713**
erythrocytosis, **1808, 1819**
esophagus, 572-593
    choke, 572, 573, **583-585**
    cysts, 580, 581
    diverticulum, 582, 583
    endoscopy, 574, 575
    esophagitis, 587
    examination, 572-577
    foreign body, 585, 586
    impaction, 572, 573, 583-586
    megaesophagus, 581, 582
    perforation, 587-589
    radiography, 573, 574
    rupture, 587
    stricture, 589-593
    surgery, 577-580
estrous cycle, **982-988**
estrus synchronization, **1003**
ethmoid hematoma, 397
evisceration, **882, 1611**
examination, alimentary, 473-489
    blood, **1753-1774**
    breeding soundness, **847-856, 866**
    cardiovascular, 165-219
    certificate, 16-19, 70-79
    electrocardiographic, 187-198
    endocrine, **1581, 1737-1739**
    eye, **1083-1087**
    hemolymphatic, **1753-1774**
    insurance, 16-19, 78, 79
    musculoskeletal, **1143-1200**
    necropsy, 123-137
    neurologic, 723-743
    ophthalmologic, **1083-1087**
    physical, 64-80
    postmortem, 123-137
    procedures, 51-81
    purchase, 16-19, 70-78
    rectal, 70, 476-479, 516, **952-954, 1539**
    reproductive, mare, **949-979**
    reproductive, stallion, **847-856**
    respiratory, 353-361
    restraint, physical, 55-63
    urinary, **1539-1545**
exanthema, coital, **1058**
exercise-induced pulmonary
    hemorrhage, 451-454
exercise testing, 198-206
    heart rate meter, 204
    heart score, 206
    telemetry, 204, 205
exostoses, **1281, 1414-1416, 1449**
eye, **1083-1133**
    anatomy, **1083, 1084**
    anesthesia, **1085, 1086**
    aniridia, **1119**
    antifungals, **1090, 1091**
    antimicrobials, **1087-1089**
    asteroid hyalosis, **1128**

(E continued)

atropine, 1090
auriculopalpebral nerve block, 1085, 1086
blepharitis, 1101, 1102
buphthalmos, 1095, 1096
cataracts, 1125, 1128
chemosis, 1108
chorioretinitis, 1131, 1132
coloboma, 1098, 1119, 1129
conjunctival hypertrophy, 1109
conjunctivitis, 1106, 1107
cornea, diseases, 1109-1119
corneal dystrophy, 1118, 1119
corneal ulcers, 1111, 1113, 1114
corticosteroids, 1089
culture, 1086
dacryocystitis, 1107
dermoid, 1105, 1110
distichiasis, 1100
ectopic cilia, 1100
electroretinography, 1087
enophthalmia, 1124
entropion, 1097, 1098
examination, 1083-1087
eyelids, 1097-1105
fluorescein dye, 1085
foreign bodies, 1106, 1112
habronemiasis, 1101
heterochromia, 1120
iris cysts, 1120
iris prolapse, 1120
keratitis, 1110, 1114, 1115, 1117
lacerations, 1099, 1112
lens luxation, 1126
Leptospira, 1121-1124
microphthalmia, 1094
moonblindness, 1121-1124
nasolacrimal duct obstruction, 1106
nasolacrimal punctum, absence, 1105
nasolacrimal lavage, 1093
neoplasia, 1097, 1102, 1109, 1117, 1125
night blindness, 1129-1131
nonsteroidal antiinflammatories, 1090
nyctalopia, 1129-1131
Onchocerca, 1102, 1107, 1115, 1121-1124
ophthalmoscopy, 1085
optic nerve hypoplasia, 1132
optic nerve injury, 782, 1133
optic neuritis, 1133
optic neuropathy, proliferative, 1133
orbital cellulitis, 1096
panophthalmitis, 1125
paracentesis, 1086
pemphigus, 1108
periodic ophthalmia, 1121-1124
phacoanaphylactic uveitis, 1127
phthisis bulbi, 1096
problems, 19, 21
recurrent uveitis, 1121-1124
retinal detachment, 1131, 1132
retrobulbar abscess, 1096
sarcoid, 1103-1105
slit lamp examination, 1087
stromal abscesses, 1115-1117
subconjunctival injection, 1088, 1089
subpalpebral lavage, 1092
synchysis scintillans, 1128
therapy, 1087-1094
tonometry, 1085, 1087
trauma, 1095
trichiasis, 1100
uveitis, 1120-1124
vitrial abscesses, 1127
vitritis, 1127

vitreous floaters, 1127, 1128
warts, 1105

F

face flies, 1722
facial fractures, 1464-1466
facial nerve paralysis, 784
farcy, 1667
feces, abnormal, 20, 21
feed, see nutrition
femoral fractures, 1499-1502
femoral nerve paralysis, 828, 829
fetal mummification, 1071
fetlock, angular deformities, 1397-1399
  bone cysts, 1402
  degenerative joint disease, 1402-1405
  distal sesamoidean desmitis, 1394
  distal sesamoidean ligament rupture, 1394
  flexural deformities, 1399-1401
  joint infection, 1395, 1396
  luxation, 1391, 1392
  osselets, 1403
  osteochondritis dissecans, 1401, 1402
  osteochondrosis, 1401, 1402
  proximal phalanx fractures, 1379-1385
  proximal sesamoid fractures, 1385-1391
  sesamoiditis, 1404, 1405
  tenosynovitis, 1396, 1397
  villonodular synovitis, 1392-1394, 1403
fever, 22, 23
  treatment, 145-150
fibrillation, atrial, 241-246
  ventricular, 254
fibroma, 1663
fibrosarcoma, 1663
fire ant stings, 1704
first aid, fractures, 1224-1229
fistulous withers, 1667
flexural deformities, 1307, 1308
  carpus, 1435, 1436
  fetlock, 1399-1401
floaters, vitreal, 1127, 1128
fluid therapy, 139-142
fluorescein staining, cornea, 1085
fluoride toxicosis, 1293-1296
fly bites, tabanid, 1649
foal-heat diarrhea, 498, 499
foaling, see parturition
foals, abnormalities, 30-33
  agammaglobulinemia, 1822
  angular deformities, 1298-1307, 1397-1399, 1420, 1421, 1435, 1436, 1478, 1479
  arthrogryposis, 822
  ascarid impaction, 621
  barker foals, 754-756, 764
  cataracts, 1125, 1126
  cerebellar disorders, 793, 794
  combined immunodeficiency, 1814, 1819-1822
  contracted foal syndrome, 822
  convulsions, 770, 779, 780
  diarrhea, 498, 499
  dummy foals, 754-756, 764
  epilepsy, 770, 779, 780
  failure of passive transfer, 1767, 1789, 1790, 1824-1826
  flexural deformities, 1307, 1308, 1399-1401, 1435, 1436
  gastric ulcers, 605, 606
  genetic defects, 28, 29
  hepatopathy, toxic, 699
  hydrocephalus, 771

hyperalimentation, 507-510
hypogammaglobulinemia, 1823
IgM deficiency, 1823
immune response, 1767, 1789, 1790
immunodeficiency, combined, 1814, 1819-1822
malformations, 28, 29
meconium aspiration, 430
meconium impaction, 659, 660
meningitis, 754-756
neonatal isoerythrolysis, 1804
neonatal maladjustment syndrome, 764, 765
nutritional support, 507-510
omphalitis, 687, 1564, 1565
parrot mouth, 561, 1460
persistent pulmonary hypertension, 430
pneumonia, 386, 441, 454, 455
pneumothorax, 457, 458
polydactylism, 1405, 1406
respiratory disease, 356, 360, 361, 377, 378, 386, 429, 430, 441, 454-458
respiratory distress syndrome, 429, 430
restraint, 62
seizures, 770, 779, 780
septicemia, 159-161, 1812
twins, 971, 1012, 1013, 1059, 1060
umbilical infection, 687, 1564, 1565
viral enteritis, 619, 620
wry nose, 391, 1460, 1461
folliculitis, 1696, 1697
food allergy, 1653
foot, canker, 1371, 1372
  collateral cartilage necrosis, 1339
  collateral cartilage ossification, 1340
  contracted heels, 1371
  deep digital flexor tendon rupture, 1338, 1339
  distal interphalangeal flexural deformity, 1366-1369
  distal interphalangeal joint infection, 1345 1346
  distal interphalangeal osteochondrosis, 1369
  distal phalanx fracture, 1335-1338
  founder, 1354-1366, 1843
  keratoma, 1332, 1333
  laminitis, 1354-1366, 1843
  long toe, 1342, 1343
  navicular disease, 1346-1354
  pedal osteitis, 1340, 1341
  pododermatitis, 1344, 1345
  quittor, 1339
  sheared heels, 1341, 1342
  sidebone, 1340
  sole bruising, 1333-1335
  subsolar abscess, 1343, 1344
  thrush, 1344, 1345
  underrun heels, 1342, 1343
  wall cracks, 1331
foreign bodies, 399, 426, 427, 546, 547, 1648
founder, 1354-1366, 1843
fractures, accessory carpal bone, 1429
  acetabular, 1503, 1504
  arthrodesis, 1253-1258
  arthroscopy, 1262, 1263
  arthrotomy, 1262
  biomechanics, 1200-1204
  bone grafts, 1243-1246
  carpal bones, 1420-1430
  casts, 1229-1234
  distal phalanx, 1335-1338
  distal tarsal, 1470
  external coaptation, 1225-1235
  facial, 1464-1466

(F continued)

femoral, 1499-1502
first aid, 1224-1229
healing, 1204-1211
implants, 1236-1242
internal fixation, 1235-1243
lumbar, 1515
malleolus of distal tibia, 1470
mandibular, 1461-1464
maxillary, 1461-1464
middle phalanx, 1372-1375
osteotomy, 1248-1253
patellar, 1489-1491
pelvic, 1503, 1504
periorbital, 1466, 1467
physeal, 1211-1215, 1246-1248
proximal phalanx, 1379-1385
proximal sesamoid, 1385-1391
pins, intramedullary, 1241
plates, bone, 1238-1241
radial, 1440-1442
sacral, 823
Salter-Harris types, 1213-1215
screws, bone, 1236-1238
second, fourth metacarpal, metatarsal, 1413, 1414
splint bone, 1413, 1414
splint application, 1225-1235
stress fractures, metacarpal/metatarsal, 1410-1413
tarsal bone, 1468-1470
third metacarpal/metatarsal, 1406-1410
thoracolumbar, 1509
tibial, 1482-1487
transport, patient, 1228, 1229
ulnar, 1442-1446
frontal sinus, see sinuses, paranasal
frostbite, 1709
fungal granulomas, 1668-1673
funiculitis, 881, 914

G

gait evaluation, 732-734, 1151, 1152, 1194-1200
Gasterophilus spp, 601, 602, 1676
gastric, see stomach
gastrocnemius rupture, 1488
gastrointestinal system, see alimentary system
genetics, defects, 28, 29
  gonadal dysgenesis, 1024
  hermaphroditism, 889
  intersexuality, 889, 890
  lethal white syndrome, 532, 1716
  pseudohermaphroditism, 889
  sex reversal syndrome, 889
genital system, see reproductive system
gestation, see reproductive system
girth galls, 1664
glanders, 440, 441, 1667
glomerulonephritis, 1550-1552
gold therapy, 1647
Gomen disease, 796
gonadal dysgenesis, 1024
grafting, bone, 1243-1246
  skin, 1613-1625
granulation tissue, 1594, 1595, 1604-1607, 1676
granulosa-cell tumor, 1025
  grass sickness, 540
grease heel, 1711, 1712
grove poisoning, 765
guttural pouches, 402-411
  anatomy, 402
  empyema, 406-408, 789

mycosis, 408-411, 788
surgery, 402-404
tympany, 404-406

H

habronemiasis, 601, 602, **894, 934, 935,** 1101, 1613, 1673-1675
hair, abnormalities, 23, 24, **1680, 1683,** 1716-1719
hair follicle dystrophy, **1680**
hair loss, **1683-1694**
hairy vetch poisoning, **1680**
Halicephalobus deletrix, 760
head-shaking, 767
head trauma, 771-774
health certificates, 16-19, 70-79
heart, see cardiovascular system
heaves, 443-449
heavy metal poisoning, **1553**
Heinz bodies, **1761**
hematidrosis, **1722**
Hematobia, **1690**
hematology, see blood
hematoma, **929, 930, 1585, 1591, 1655**
hematopoiesis, **1774-1787**
hemilymphatic system, **1753-1846**
  agammaglobulinemia, **1822**
  anemia, **1795-1797, 1802-1809**
  aplastic anemia, **1795-1797**
  arteritis, 281, 282, 384, 385, 679-681, **918, 1678, 1836**
  autoimmune disease, **1770, 1804, 1805**
  autoimmune hemolytic anemia, **1805**
  babesiosis, **1765, 1806**
  basophilia, **1815**
  blood cell counts, **1756-1759**
  blood cell morphology, **1757, 1762, 1763**
  blood collection, **1755, 1756**
  blood gas analysis, 206-208, 360
  blood loss, **1807, 1808**
  blood pressure, 218, 219, 262
  blood transfusion, **1791-1793, 1805, 1808**
  bone marrow aplasia, **1795-1797**
  bone marrow collection, **1756**
  bone marrow evaluation, **1760, 1774-1787**
  buffy coat analysis, **1759**
  clotting, **1771, 1772, 1787-1789, 1831-1843**
  coagulation, **1771, 1772, 1787-1789, 1831-1843**
  colostral immunoglobulins, **1790, 1791, 1824**
  combined immunodeficiency, **1814, 1819-1822**
  Coombs' test, **1770**
  differential cell counts, **1762, 1763**
  disseminated intravascular coagulation, 162, 163, **1022, 1838-1842**
  Dohle bodies, **1780**
  drug toxicity, **1795**
  ehrlichiosis, **1763, 1765, 1780, 1806, 1837**
  ehrlichiosis, monocytic, **1765**
  eosinopenia, **1815**
  eosinophilia, **1814**
  equine infectious anemia, **1764, 1765, 1804, 1837**
  erythrocyte evaluation, **1759, 1774-1777**
  erythrocytosis, **1808, 1819**
  examination, **1753-1774**

Heinz bodies, **1761**
hematopoiesis, **1774-1787**
hemolytic anemia, **1803-1806**
hemophilia A, **1831**
hemostasis, **1771, 1772, 1787-1789, 1831-1843**
hypogammaglobulinemia, **1823**
hypoproteinemia, **1826, 1827, 1843**
IgM deficiency, **1823**
immune system evaluation, **1765-1771**
immunodeficiency, combined, **1814, 1819-1822**
immunoglobulins, colostral, **1790, 1791, 1824**
iron deficiency, **1809**
leukemia, **1798, 1800, 1815-1819**
leukocyte evaluation, **1761, 1777-**
leukocytes, numbers, **1774, 1809-1819**
liver disease, clotting, **1842**
lymphangitis, epizootic, **1672, 1843, 1844**
lymphosarcoma, **1797-1799, 1845**
lymphocytosis, **1813**
lymphopenia, **1813**
mal de caderas, **1802**
monocytosis, **1813**
multiple myeloma, **1800, 1819**
murrina de caderas, **1802**
myeloproliferative disorders, **1800, 1815-1819**
nagana, **1802**
neonatal isoerythrolysis, **1804, 1805**
neoplasia, **1797-1800, 1815, 1845**
neutropenia, **1811**
neutrophilia, **1809-1811**
normal values, **1774**
onion poisoning, **1807**
phenothiazine toxicity, **1807**
piroplasmosis, **1765, 1806**
plasma-cell myeloma, **1800, 1819**
plasma transfusion, **1793, 1794**
platelet evaluation, **1764**
polycythemia, **1808, 1819**
protein-losing enteropathy, 607, 608, **1828-1831**
proteins, plasma, **1771-1774, 1826-1831**
purpura hemorrhagica, **1710, 1836**
red maple leaf toxicity, **1806**
reference intervals, **1774**
serologic evaluation, **1764, 1765**
spleen, diseases, **1844-1846**
splenic abscess, **1845**
splenic puncture, **1845**
splenic rupture, **1845**
splenomegaly, **1845**
surra, **1801, 1802**
sweet clover poisoning, **1838**
therapy, **1791-1794**
thrombocytopenia, immune-mediated, **1832-1835**
transfusion reactions, **1805**
trypanosomiasis, **1800-1802**
vasculitis, **1835, 1836**
warfarin poisoning, **1837, 1838**
hemolytic anemia, **1803-1806**
hemoperitoneum, 667-669
hemophilia A, **1831**
Hemophilus equigenitalis, **922, 923, 938, 1034-1036**
hemorrhage, ejaculatory, **939**
  intraabdominal, 667-669
  postpartum, 285, **1014**
hemospermia, **939**
hemostasis, **1771, 1772, 1787-1789, 1831-1843**
hemothorax, 458

(H continued)

hepatic, see liver
hepatitis, 700, 701
hepatoencephalopathy, 693, 775, 776
hermaphroditism, **889**
hernia, abdominal, 690-692
　diaphragmatic, 456, 457, 689, 690
　epiploic foramen, 611
　incisional, 685-689
　inguinal, 612, 613, 684, 685, **911-914**
　mesenteric, 611, 612
　traumatic, 687
　umbilical, 613, 683, 684
herpesvirus-1, 382-384
　abortion, **1069, 1070**
　encephalomyelitis, 751-753
　immunization, 384
herpesvirus-2, 382-384
heterochromia iridis, **1120**
hip, acetabular fractures, **1503, 1504**
　joint infection, **1505, 1506**
　luxation, **1504, 1505**
　pelvic fractures, **1503, 1504**
　round ligament rupture, **1505**
histoplasmosis, **1672, 1843, 1844**
Histoplasma farciminosum, **1672,**
　1843, 1844
hives, **1651, 1652**
hock, angular deformities, **1478, 1479**
　bog spavin, **1476**
　bone spavin, **1474-1476**
　capped hock, **1471**
　cunean tendinitis/bursitis, **1474**
　curb, **1474**
　deep digital flexor tenosynovitis, **1476**
　degenerative joint disease, **1476**
　distal tarsal joint luxation, **1470**
　extensor tendon laceration, **1471-1473**
　hygroma, **1471**
　joint infection, **1477, 1478**
　malleolus, distal tibia fracture, **1470,**
　　1471
　osteochondrosis, **1480, 1481**
　plantar desmitis, **1474**
　stringhalt, **1481, 1482**
　superficial digital flexor tendon
　　luxation, **1473**
　tarsal bone fractures, **1468-1470**
　tarsitis, **1474-1476**
　tarsocrural synovitis, **1476**
　thoroughpin, **1476**
hoof, see foot
hormonal therapy, **998-1004**
horn flies, **1690**
horse pox, **1701**
horseflies, **1649**
horsetail poisoning, 805, 806
humeral fractures, **1450, 1451, 1454**
hunters' bumps, **1157, 1515**
hydramnios, **1063**
hydroallantois, **1063**
hydrocele, **881, 911**
hydronephrosis, **1556**
hydrocephalus, 771
hydrotherapy, **1273**
hygroma, **1433, 1446, 1471**
hyoid fractures, 548-550
hyperalimentation, 507-510
hyperelastosis, **1720, 1721**
hyperglycemia, **1739**
hyperhidrosis, 42, 43, **1722**
hyperkalemic periodic paralysis, **1318,**
　1319
hyperlipidemia syndrome, **1740**
hypermetria, 733
hyperproteinemia, **1827, 1828**
hypertrichosis, **1719**

hypertrophic osteopathy, **1316, 1317**
hypoallergenic diets, **1581**
Hypoderma, encephalitis, 760, 761
　nodules, **1655**
hypogammaglobulinemia, **1823**
hypoglycemia, 776
hypometria, 733
hypoproteinemia, **1827, 1828**
hypothyroidism, **1648, 1681, 1741,**
　1745-1748
hypoxemia, 776, 777

I

icterus, 692, 693
IgM deficiency, **1823**
ileum, impaction, 623
ileus, 516, 539, 540
immune system,
　autoimmune disease, **1770, 1804, 1805**
　cellular immunity, **1768, 1769**
　colostral immunoglobulins, **1790, 1791,**
　　1824
　combined immunodeficiency, **1814,**
　　1819-1822
　Coombs' test, **1770**
　functional evaluation, **1765-1771**
　humoral immunity, **1766-1768**
　hypogammaglobulinemia, **1823**
　IgM deficiency, **1823**
　immunodeficiency, combined, **1814,**
　　1819-1822
　immunoglobulins, colostral, **1790,**
　　1791, 1824
　passive transfer in foals, **1767, 1789,**
　　1790, 1824-1826
　serologic evaluation, **1764, 1765**
　thrombocytopenia, immune-mediated,
　　1832-1835
　transfusion reactions, **1805**
immunodeficiency, combined, **1814,**
　1819-1822
immunoglobulins, colostral, **1790,**
　1791, 1824
implants, bone, **1236-1242**
incisions, **1585, 1591-1596**
infarction, bowel, 496, 538, 539
infertility, see reproductive system
influenza, equine, 380-382
infraspinatus bursitis, **1457**
inguinal hernia, 612, 613, 684, 685,
　911-914
inhalation therapy, 374, 375
injection, intracarotid, 774
inner ear syndrome, 783
insemination, artificial, **870, 871**
intersexuality, **889, 890**
intertrigo, **1704**
intestines, small, 606-627
　adhesions, 609, 610
　Anoplocephala perfoliata, 618
　ascariasis, 617, 618, 621
　ascarid impaction, 621
　basophilic enteritis, 625
　clostridial enteritis, 620, 621
　Cryptosporidium, 618, 619
　Eimeria leukarti, 618, 619
　eosinophilic gastroenteritis, 625
　epiploic foramen hernia, 611
　granulomatous enteritis, 620, 624
　ileal impaction, 623
　inguinal hernia, 612, 613, 684
　intussusception, 613, 614
　lactase deficiency, 622
　malabsorption, 607, 609

malassimilation, 607
maldigestion, 607
Meckel's diverticulum, 608
mesenteric hernia, 611, 612
mesodiverticular band, 608, 609
neoplasia, 621, 622
obstruction, 490-498, 606
Parascaris equorum, 617, 618, 621
pedunculated lipoma, 615, 616
protein-losing enteropathy, 607, 608
protozoans, 618, 619
proximal enteritis, 626, 627
roundworms, 442, 617, 618, 621
stricture, 610, 611
Strongyloides westeri, 616
tapeworms, 618
thread worms, 616
umbilical hernia, 613, 683, 684
viral enteritis, 619, 620
volvulus, 614, 615
intoxication, see toxicity
intraabdominal hemorrhage, 667-669
intracarotid injection, 774
intradermal testing, **1579, 1580**
intubation, nasogastric, 475, 516
intussusception, 613, 614, 632, 663
iodism, **1683**
iris, cysts, **1125**
　prolapse, **1120**
iron deficiency, **1809**
irradiation, tumor, **1639-1642**
isoerythrolysis, neonatal, **1804, 1805**

J

jaundice, 692, 693
joints, anesthesia, **1168-1170**
　angular deformities, **1298-1307,**
　　1399-1401, 1420, 1421, 1435, 1436
　arthritis, **1281-1288**
　arthrodesis, **1253-1258**
　arthrography, **1175**
　borreliosis, **1292, 1293**
　capped elbow, **1446**
　capped hock, **1471**
　capped knee, **1433**
　carpal joint infection, **1434**
　coxofemoral luxation, **1504, 1505**
　degenerative joint disease, **1216-1220,**
　　1258-1261, 1378, 1379, 1402-1405,
　　1438-1440, 1476
　distal interphalangeal flexural
　　deformity, **1366-1369**
　distal interphalangeal joint infection,
　　1345, 1346
　distal interphalangeal joint luxation,
　　1375, 1376
　distal tarsal luxation, **1470**
　elbow joint infection, **1447**
　fetlock joint infection, **1395, 1396**
　flexural deformities, **1307, 1308,**
　　1366-1369, 1397-1399, 1436-1438
　hip joint infection, **1505, 1506**
　hip luxation, **1504, 1505**
　hock joint infection, **1477, 1478**
　hygroma, **1433, 1446, 1471**
　lumbar arthritis, **1515**
　Lyme disease, **1292, 1293**
　olecranon bursitis, **1446**
　patellar luxation, **1488, 1489**
　polysynovitis, **1292**
　proximal interphalangeal degenerative
　　joint disease, **1378, 1379**
　proximal interphalangeal joint infection,
　　1377

(J continued)

shoe boil, **1446**
stifle joint infection, **1493, 1494**
synovial fluid analysis, **1168-1170,
1221, 1222, 1284**
temporomandibular luxation, **1464**
trauma, **1220-1223, 1610**
villonodular synovitis, **1392-1394, 1403**
wounds, **1610**
jugular, pulse, 173-175
thrombophlebitis, 293-295
junctional mechanobullous disease, **1706**

K

keloid, **1661**
keratitis, **1110, 1114, 1115, 1117**
keratoma, hoof, **1332, 1333**
keratosis, cannon, **1713**
linear, **1712**
solar, **1694**
kidney, amyloidosis, **1556**
azotemia, **1545, 1546**
biopsy, **1543**
calculi, **1550**
diabetes insipidus, **1557**
examination, **1539-1545**
failure, **1545, 1547-1549**
glomerulonephritis, **1550-1552**
hydronephrosis, **1556**
hypoplasia, **1549**
infection, **1546, 1547**
Klossiella equi, **1552**
Micronema deletrix, **1552**
neoplasia, **1555**
nephritis, **1550**
toxicity, **1553-1555**
tubular acidosis, **1556, 1557**
uremia, **1546**
Klossiella equi, **1552**
kunkers, **1669, 1670**
kyphosis, **1508**

L

lacerations, **1585, 1591-1596**
lactase deficiency, 622
lactation tetany, **1326, 1327**
lameness, see musculoskeletal system
laminectomy, 820-822
laminitis, **1354-1366, 1843**
lampus, 547
laparoscopy, 489
laparotomy, 489, 519-520
large colon, see colon, large
larynx, 411-424
arytenoid chondritis, 412-414
epiglottic entrapment, 421-424
hemiplegia, 414-421
palatopharyngeal arch displacement,
411, 412
lasalocid poisoning, 762
laser therapy, **1278-1280**
lathyrism, 831
lavage, wound, **1596**
lead poisoning, 790
leeches, **1669, 1670**
lens, cataracts, **1125-1128**
luxation, **1126**
Leptospira, ocular, **1121-1124**
lethal white syndrome, 532, **1716**
leucaenosis, **1683**
leukemia, **1798, 1800, 1815-1819**
leukoderma, **1717**
leukoencephalomalacia, 777, 778

leukotrichia, hyperesthetic, **1717**
reticulated, **1716**
spotted, **1716**
libido, **849, 883, 884**
lice infestation, **1692**
lighting, artificial, **866, 999**
lightning strike, 743
lipoma, pedunculated, 615, 616, 662, 666
listeriosis, 754
liver, 692-702
biliary atresia, 698
biopsy, 696
cholelithiasis, 701
clotting disorder, **1842**
enzymes, serum, 694
examination, 696
hepatic encephalopathy, 693, 775, 776
hepatitis, acute, 700, 701
hepatopathy, toxic, 699
jaundice, 692, 693
mycotoxicosis, 700
pyrrolizidine toxicity, 699
signs of disease, 692-697
Theiler's disease, 700, 701
treatment, 697, 698
Tyzzer's disease, 698
lockjaw, 782, 785-788
locoweed poisoning, 795, 796, **1784**
lordosis, **1507**
louse infestation, **1692**
lumbar arthritis, **1515**
lumbar fractures, **1515**
lumps, 27, 28
lungs, 429-456
aspiration pneumonia, 431, 432
bleeders, 451-454
Bordetella bronchiseptica, 438
chronic obstructive pulmonary disease,
443-449
coccidioidomycosis, 451
Dictyocaulus arnfieldi, 442, 443
exercise-induced pulmonary
hemorrhage, 451-454
foal pneumonia, 386, 441, 454, 455
glanders, 440, 441
granulomatous pneumonia, 449-451
hypoxemia, foals, 455, 456
lungworms, 442, 443
meconium aspiration, 430
melioidosis, 439, 440
neonatal respiratory distress syndrome,
429, 430
neoplasia, 451
Parascaris equorum, 442
persistent pulmonary hypertension, 430
Pneumocystis carinii, 441, 442
Rhodococcus equi, 436-438
silicate pneumonoconiosis, 449
smoke inhalation, 431
strangles, 434, 435
Streptococcus equi, 434 435
Streptococcus pneumoniae, 435, 436
Streptococcus zooepidemicus, 433, 434
summer pasture-associated pulmonary
disease, 449
tuberculosis, 450
lungworms, 442, 443
lupus erythematosus, discoid, **1717**
systemic, **1713**
Lyme disease, **1292, 1293**
lymphangitis, epizootic, **1672, 1843,
1844**
ulcerative, **1666**
lymphocytosis, **1813**
lymphopenia, **1813**

lymphosarcoma, 334, 463, 537, 621,
1662, 1797-1799, 1845

M

mal de caderas, **1802**
malabsorption, 607, 609
malassimilation, 607
maladjustment syndrome, neonatal,
764, 765
maldigestion, 607
malformation, 28, 29
mandible, cysts, 563,
deformities, 391, 561
fractures, **1461-1464**
mange, chorioptic, **1693**
demodectic, **1680, 1681**
psoroptic, **1693**
sarcoptic, **1692. 1693**
mastocytoma, **1662**
maxilla, deformities, 391
fractures, **1461-1464**
maxillary sinus, see sinuses, paranasal
Meckel's diverticulum, 608
meconium aspiration, 430
impaction, 659, 660
median nerve paralysis, 828
mediastinal abscess, 462
medical records, 64, 70-78
megaesophagus, 581, 582
melanoma, malignant, **1660, 1661**
melioidosis, 439, 440
meningitis, foals, 754-756
meningoencephalomyelitis, verminous,
759-761
mercury poisoning, 762, **1683**
mesodiverticular band, 608, 609
metacarpus, angular deformities, **1420,
1421**
bowed tendons, **1416, 1417**
bucked shins, **1410-1413**
exostoses, **1414-1416**
inferior check desmitis, **1417, 1418**
osteomyelitis, **1419, 1420**
polydactylism, **1405, 1406**
second, fourth metacarpal/metatarsal
fractures, **1413, 1414**
splint bone fractures, **1413, 1414**
"splints," **1414-1416**
stress fractures, **1410-1413**
suspensory desmitis, **1418, 1419**
tendinitis, **1416, 1417**
tendon lacerations, **1416**
third metacarpal/metatarsal fractures,
1406-1410
metaldehyde poisoning, 777
metatarsus, see metacarpus
metritis, contagious equine, **922, 923,
938**
metritis-laminitis-septicemia complex,
1015
Micronema deletrix, **1552**
microphthalmia, **1094**
midbrain syndrome, 783
moldy corn poisoning, 777, 778
molluscum contagiosum, **1701**
monensin poisoning, 762
monocytosis, **1813**
moonblindness, **1121-1124**
Morgagni, cyst, **969**
mosquito bites, **1649, 1650**
motor oil toxicity, **1708, 1709**
mouth, see oral cavity
multiple myeloma, **1800, 1819**
murmurs, cardiac, 220-228

(M continued)

murrina de caderas, 1802
muscle, azoturia, 327, 1321-1324
  back muscle strain, 1508
  biopsy, 1163
  clostridial myonecrosis, 1324, 1325
  Colorado strangles, 1325, 1326, 1665
  Corynbacterium pseudotuberculosis,
    abscesses, 1325, 1326
  cramping, 1328, 1329
  diaphragmatic flutter, 1327
  electromyography, 1162
  examination, 1160-1163
  extensor carpi radialis rupture, 1431
  gastrocnemius rupture, 1488
  hyperkalemic periodic paralysis, 1318,
    1319
  hypocalcemia, 1326
  injury, response, 1223, 1224
  malignant hyperthermia, 1327, 1328
  myotonia, 1317, 1318
  nutritional myodegeneration, 1329,
    1330
  ossifying myopathy, 1324
  pectoral abscesses, 1325, 1326
  pigeon breast, 1325, 1326, 1665
  postanesthetic myoneuropathy,
    117-119, 1319-1321
  rhabdomyolysis, exertional, 327,
    1321-1324
  serratus ventralis rupture, 1456
  thumps, 1327
  tying up, 327, 1321-1324
  white muscle disease, 1329, 1330
musculocutaneous nerve paralysis, 828
musculoskeletal system, 1143-1518
  accessory carpal bone fracture, 1429
  acetabular fractures, 1502, 1503
  Achilles tendon rupture, 1488
  amputation, limb, 1253
  angular deformities, 1298-1307,
    1397-1399, 1420, 1435, 1436, 1478,
    1479
  arthritis, 1281-1288
  arthrodesis, 1253-1258
  arthrography, 1175
  azoturia, 327, 1321-1324
  back muscle strain, 1508
  back problems, 1154-1160, 1507-1518
  bicipital bursitis, 1457
  biopsy, muscle, 1163
  bog spavin, 1476
  bone cysts, 1402, 1459, 1494-1499
  bone spavin, 1474-1476
  borreliosis, 1292, 1293
  bowed tendons, 1416, 1417
  brachygnathia, 561, 1460
  bucked shins, 1410-1413
  canker, 1371, 1372
  capped elbow, 1446
  capped hock, 1471
  capped knee, 1433
  carpal canal syndrome, 1430, 1431
  carpal fractures, 1420-1430
  carpal joint infection, 1434
  carpus, 1421-1440
  casts, 1229-1234
  cervical vertebral malformation, 807-822
  clostridial myonecrosis, 1324, 1325
  collateral cartilage necrosis, 1339
  collateral cartilage ossification, 1340
  Colorado strangles, 1325, 1326, 1665
  common digital extensor tendon
    rupture, 1432
  contracted heels, 1371
  coxofemoral luxation, 1504, 1505
  cramping, muscle, 1328, 1329

cunean bursitis, 1474
curb, 1474
deep digital flexor tendon rupture,
  1338, 1339
deep digital flexor tenosynovitis, 1476
degenerative joint disease, 1216-1220,
  1258-1261, 1378, 1379, 1402-1405,
  1438-1440, 1476
diaphragmatic flutter, 1327
distal interphalangeal joint infection,
  1345, 1346
distal interphalangeal flexural
  deformity, 1366-1369
distal interphalangeal osteochondrosis,
  1369
distal phalanx fracture, 1335-1338
distal sesamoidean desmitis, 1394
distal sesamoidean ligament rupture,
  1394
elbow, 1440-1450
elbow, joint infections, 1447
electromyography, 1162
enzymes, serum, 1161, 1162
epidural anesthesia, 1168
examination, 1143-1200
exostoses, 1281, 1414-1416, 1449
extensor carpi radialis muscle rupture,
  1431
facial fractures, 1464-1466
femoral fractures, 1499-1502
fetlock, 1379-1405
fetlock joint infection, 1395, 1396
fetlock luxation, 1391, 1392
first aid, fractures, 1224-1229
flexural deformities, 1307, 1308,
  1399-1401, 1435, 1436
fluoride toxicosis, 1293-1296
foot, 1331-1372
founder, see laminitis
fracture management, 1200-1215
gait evaluation, 732-734, 1151, 1152,
  1194-1200
gastrocnemius rupture, 1488
hip joint infection, 1505, 1506
hip luxation, 1504, 1505
hock, 1467-1482
hoof, 1331-1372
humeral fractures, 1450, 1451, 1454
hunters' bumps, 1157, 1515
hydrotherapy, 1273
hygroma, 1433, 1446, 1471
hyperkalemic periodic paralysis, 1318,
  1319
hypertrophic osteopathy, 1316
hypocalcemia, 1326
implants, bone, 1236-1242
inferior check desmitis, 1417, 1418
infraspinatus bursitis, 1457
intrasynovial anesthesia, 1166-1168
joint anesthesia, 1166-1168
joint trauma, 1220-1223
keratoma, 1332, 1333
kyphosis, 1508
lameness, 26, 27, 261, 262
laminitis, 1354-1366, 1843
laser therapy, cold, 1278-1280
local anesthesia, 1163-1168
long toe, 1342, 1343
lordosis, 1507
lumbar arthritis, 1515
lumbar fractures, 1515
Lyme disease, 1292, 1293
malalignment, dorsal spinous processes,
  1511, 1512
mandibular fractures, 1461-1464
maxillary fractures, 1461-1464

metacarpus, 1405-1421
metatarsus, 1405-1421
middle phalanx fractures, 1372-1375
muscle, diseases, 1317-1331
muscle, examination, 1160-1163
muscle, injury, 1223, 1224
myotonia, 1317, 1318
navicular disease, 1346-1354
nerve blocks, 1163-1168
nerve stimulation, transcutaneous,
  1274-1276
nuclear imaging, 743, 1185-1191
nutritional imbalances, 1296-1298,
  1301
nutritional myodegeneration, 1329,
  1330
occipitoatlantoaxial malformation, 797,
  798
olecranon bursitis, 1446
osselets, 1403
ossifying myopathy, 1324
osteochondritis dissecans, see
  osteochondrosis
osteochondroma, 1449
osteochondrosis, 1308-1316, 1369,
  1378, 1401, 1402, 1438, 1447, 1448,
  1458, 1480, 1481, 1494
osteomyelitis, 804, 805, 1289-1292,
  1419, 1420
osteopetrosis, 1281
osteotomy, 1248-1253
overriding spinous processes, 1510,
  1511
parrot mouth, 561, 1460
pastern, 1372-1379
pastern joint osteochondrosis, 1378
patella, upward fixation, 1491, 1492
patellar chondromalacia, 1491
patellar fracture, 1489-1491
patellar luxation, 1488, 1489
pectoral abscesses, 1325, 1326, 1665
pedal osteitis, 1340, 1341
pelvic fractures, 1503, 1504
pelvis, 1502-1506
periorbital fractures, 1466, 1467
peroneus tertius rupture, 1487, 1488
physical therapy, 1269-1274, 1513
physitis, 1315, 1316
pins, bone, 1241
plantar desmitis, 1474
plates, bone, 1238-1241
pododermatitis, 1344, 1345
polydactylism, 1405, 1406
polysynovitis, 1292
postanesthetic myopathy, 117-119,
  1319-1321
proximal interphalangeal degenerative
  joint disease, 1378, 1379
proximal interphalangeal joint
  infection, 1377
proximal interphalangeal joint luxation,
  1375, 1376
proximal phalanx fractures, 1379-1385
proximal sesamoid fractures, 1385-1391
quittor, 1339
radial fractures, 1440-1442
radiography, 1170-1178
regional anesthesia, 1163-1168
rhabdomyolysis, exertional, 327,
  1321-1324
ringbone, 1370, 1378
round ligament rupture, 1505
sacral fractures, 823
sacralization, 1507
sacroiliac injury, 1516-1518
Salter-Harris fracture types, 1213-1215

(M continued)

scapular fractures, 1452-1454
scapulohumeral instability, **1454, 1455**
scintigraphy, 743, **1185-1191**
scoliosis, **1507**
screws, **1236-1238**
second, fourth metacarpal/metatarsal
  fractures, **1413, 1414**
serratus ventralis muscle rupture, **1456**
sesamoiditis, **1404, 1405**
sheared heels, **1341, 1342**
shoe boil, **1446**
shoeing, **1264-1269**
shoulder, **1451-1460**
shoulder joint infection, **1457**
shoulder luxation, **1455, 1456**
shoulder slip, **1454, 1455**
sidebone, **1340**
sinography, **1176**
sole bruising, **1333-1335**
spine, 797, 798, 804, 805, 807-822, 823,
  1507-1518
splint application, **1225-1235**
splint bone fractures, **1413, 1414**
"splints," **1414-1416**
spondylosis deformans, **1511**
stifle, **1488-1499**
stifle, joint infections, **1493, 1494**
stress fractures, metacarpal/metatarsal,
  1413, 1414
stringhalt, 830-832, **1481, 1482**
subsolar abscess, **1343, 1344**
superficial digital flexor tendon
  luxation, **1473**
supraglenoid fractures, **1452-1454**
supraspinous ligament injury, **1508**
suspensory desmitis, **1418, 1419**
synostosis, **1507**
synovial fluid analysis, **1168-1170,**
  1221, 1222, 1284
tarsal fractures, **1468-1470**
tarsal luxation, **1470**
tarsitis, **1474-1476**
tarsocrural synovitis, **1477, 1478**
tarsus, **1467-1482**
temporomandibular luxation, **1464**
tendinitis, **1416, 1417**
tendons, injury, **1215, 1216, 1263,**
  1264, 1338, 1339, 1376, 1377, 1416,
  1417, 1432, 1471-1474
tenosynovitis, **1396, 1397, 1476**
thermography, 743, **1191-1194**
third metacarpal/metatarsal fractures,
  1406-1410
thoracolumbar fractures, **1509**
thoroughpin, **1476**
thrush, **1344, 1345**
thumps, **1327**
tibial fractures, **1482-1487**
treadmill exercise, **1273**
trochanteric bursa infection, **1502**
tying up, 327, **1321-1324**
ulnar fractures, **1442-1446**
ultrasonography, **1178-1185**
ultrasound, therapeutic, **1276-1278**
underrun heels, **1342, 1343**
villonodular synovitis, **1392-1394, 1403**
wall cracks, **1331**
white muscle disease, **1329, 1330**
wobbler syndrome, 807-822
wry nose, 391, **1460, 1461**
myasthenia, postanesthetic, 120, 835
mycetoma, **1668**
mycobacteriosis, **1655**
mycoses, systemic, **1672, 1673**
mycotoxicosis, 700, 764
myelitis, verminous, 759-761

myelodysplasia, 798, 799
myeloencephalitis, herpesvirus-1,
  751-753
myeloencephalitis, protozoal, 756-759
myeloencephalopathy, degenerative,
  806, 807
myelography, 742
myeloma, plasma-cell, **1800, 1819**
myeloproliferative disorders, **1800,**
  1815-1819
myiasis, **1675, 1676**
myocardial fibrosis, 324-327
myocardial hypertrophy, 329
myocarditis, 320, 321
myopathy, exertional, 327, **1321-1324**
  nutritional, **1329, 1330**
  ossifying, **1324**
  postanesthetic, 117-119
  pressure, 119
myospherulosis, **1677**
myotonia, **1317, 1318**

N

nagana, **1802**
narcolepsy, 791
nasal discharge, 29, 30
nasal septum, 390, 396
nasolacrimal lavage, **1093**
nasolacrimal punctum, absence, **1105**
nasolacrimal system, obstruction, **1106**
natural service, **869, 1034**
navicular disease, **1346-1354**
Near Eastern equine encephalitis, 744
nebulization, 374, 375
necropsy, 123-137
neonatal isoerythrolysis, **1804, 1805**
neonatal maladjustment syndrome, 764,
  765
neonatal respiratory distress syndrome,
  429, 430
neonates, see foals
neoplasia, adenoma, pituitary, **1718,**
  1740-1745
  alimentary, 536-538
  blood, **1797-1800**
  bladder, **1561**
  cryotherapy, **1635-1637**
  esophageal, 593
  eye, 1097, 1102, 1109, 1117, 1118,
    1125
  fibroma, **1663**
  fibrosarcoma, **1663**
  granulosa-cell tumor, **1025**
  hemolymphatic, **1797-1800**
  hyperthermia, **1637, 1638**
  intestinal, 621, 622
  keloid, **1661**
  keratoma, **1332, 1333**
  kidney, **1555**
  leukemia, **1798, 1800, 1815-1819**
  Leydig-cell tumor, **905**
  lipoma, pedunculated, 615, 616, 662, 666
  lung, 451
  lymphosarcoma, 334, 463, 537, 621,
    1662, 1797-1799, 1845
  mandible, **1467**
  mastocytoma, **1662**
  maxilla, **1467**
  melanoma, **1660, 1661**
  myeloma, multiple, **1800, 1819**
  nasopharynx, 395
  nervous system, 778, 779
  oral cavity, 395, 548
  oropharyngeal, 395

osteochondroma, **1449**
  ovary, **1025-1027**
  pancreas, 703, **1749**
  paranasal sinus, 395
  penis, **935**
  peritoneum, 681
  pituitary, **1718, 1740-1745**
  plasma-cell myeloma, **1800, 1819**
  prepuce, **938**
  radiotherapy, **1639-1642**
  renal, **1555**
  salivary gland, 572
  scrotum, **894**
  seminoma, **904**
  Sertoli-cell tumor, **903, 905**
  skin, **1630-1642**
  squamous-cell carcinoma, 536, 593, 603,
    1561, 1659, 1660
  stomach, 536, 603
  teratoma, **904, 905**
  testes, **903-905**
  transitional-cell carcinoma, **1561**
  uterus, **1036**
nephritis, **1550**
nephropathy, pigment, **1553**
nerve blocks, see anesthesia
nerve stimulation, transcutaneous,
  1274-1276
nervous system, 723-835
  arthrogryposis, 822
  ataxia, 733
  bacterial meningoencephalomyelitis,
    754-756
  Birdsville indigo poisoning, 806
  blind staggers, 762
  Borna disease, 743
  borreliosis, 761
  botulism, 782, 832
  bracken fern poisoning, 805, 806
  brain-heart syndrome, 743
  cauda equina disorders, 823-826
  cauda equina neuritis, 824, 825
  cerebellar abiotrophy, 793, 794
  cerebellar disorders, 793, 794
  cerebellar hypoplasia, 793
  cerebral abscess, 774, 775
  cervical vertebral malformation, 807-822
  chlorinated hydrocarbon poisoning, 762
  cholesteatoma, 780, 781
  cholesterol granuloma, 780, 781
  contracted foal syndrome, 822
  convulsions, 770, 779, 780
  coprophagia, 766
  cranial nerves, 725-731
  cribbing, 766
  cryptococcosis, 756
  CSF analysis, 739-742
  Dallis grass poisoning, 795
  darling pea toxicity, 795, 796
  dysphagia, 781, 782
  electroencephalography, 743
  electromyelography, 742
  encephalomyelitis, 744-749
  epilepsy, 779, 780
  equine degenerative
    myeloencephalopathy, 806, 807
  equine infectious anemia, 754
  equine protozoal myeloencephalitis,
    756-759
  examination, 723-743
  facial nerve injury, 784
  femoral nerve injury, 828, 829
  gait evaluation, 732-734
  Gomen disease, 796
  grove poisoning, 765
  guttural pouch diseases, 788, 789

(N continued)

Halicephalobus deletrix, 760
head-shaking, 767
head trauma, 771-774
hepatoencephalopathy, 693, 775, 776
herpesvirus myeloencephalitis, 751-753
horsetail poisoning, 805, 806
hydrocephalus, 771
hypermetria, 733
Hypoderma, 760, 761
hypoglossal nerve,
hypoglycemia, 776
hypometria, 733
hypoxemia, 776, 777
inner ear syndrome, 783
intoxications, 761-765, 777
intracarotid injection, 774
laryngeal hemiplegia, 414-421
lasalocid poisoning, 762
lathyrism, 831
lead poisoning, 790
leukoencephalomalacia, 777, 778
lightning strike, 743
listeriosis, 754
lockjaw, 782, 785-788
locoism, 795, 796
Lyme disease, 761
median nerve injury, 828
medullary disease,
meningitis, foals, 754-756
mercury poisoning, 762
metaldehyde poisoning, 777
midbrain syndrome, 783
moldy corn poisoning, 777, 778
monensin poisoning, 762
musculocutaneous nerve injury, 828
mycotoxicosis, 764
myelodysplasia, 798, 799
myelography, 742
narcolepsy, 791
Near Eastern equine encephalitis, 744
neonatal maladjustment syndrome, 764,
    765
neoplasia, 778, 779
nerve stimulation, transcutaneous,
    1274-1276
nigropallidal encephalomalacia, 789, 790
obturator paralysis, 830
occipitoatlantoaxial malformation, 797,
    798
optic nerve injury, 782
organophosphate poisoning, 762
otitis interna, 794, 795
peripheral nerve injury, 826-830
peroneal nerve paralysis, 119, 829
plant poisoning, 762, 763, 789, 795, 805,
    806, 831
postanesthetic myasthenia, 120, 835
postanesthetic myelopathy, 822, 823
postfoaling paralysis, 830
protozoal myeloencephalitis, 756-759
rabies, 749-751
radial nerve injury, 827
Russian knapweed poisoning, 789, 790
ryegrass staggers, 795
sacral fractures, 823
sciatic nerve injury, 830
scintigraphy, 743
seizures, 770, 779, 780
selenium poisoning, 762
self-mutilation, 769
Setaria, 760, 761
shivering, 830-832
snail bait poisoning, 777
snakebite, 764
sorghum poisoning, 825, 826
spinal cord disorders, 797-823

spinal cord infarction, 803
spinal injury, 799-803
stall-walking, 766
stringhalt, 830-832
Strongylus vulgaris, 759-761
suprascapular nerve injury, 826, 827
sweeney, 826, 827
tail injuries, 824
temporohyoid osteoarthropathy, 791
tetanus, 782, 785-788
thermography, 743
tibial nerve injury, 829
tick paralysis, 764
tremors, 769
trypanosomiasis, 761
ulnar nerve injury, 828
urea poisoning, 762
verminous meningoencephalomyelitis,
    759-761
vertebral osteomyelitis, 804, 805
vestibular disorders, 792-796
vices, 765-769
water intoxication, 777
weakness, 732
wobbler syndrome, 807-822
yellow star thistle poisoning, 789, 790
neutropenia, **1811**
neutrophilia, **1809-1811**
night blindness, **1129-1131**
nigropallidal encephalomalacia, 789, 790
nocardiosis, **1666, 1667**
nodular granuloma, **1651**
nonsteroidal antiinflammatory toxicity,
    535, 536, 602, 603
nuclear imaging, 743, **1185-1191**
nutrition, 152-158
    bone disorders, **1296-1298, 1301**
    disorders, 152
    embryonic loss, **1066**
    feed evaluation, 153, 154
    food allergy, **1653**
    hyperalimentation, 507-510
    hypoallergenic diets, **1581**
    iron eficiency, **1809**
    myodegeneration, **1329, 1330**
    myopathy, 321
    pasture, 153, 154
    protein bumps, **1651, 1652**
    ration evaluation, 157, 158
    sick horses, 507-510
    stallions, 865
    water consumption, **1540**
    weight loss, 46-48
nyctalopia, **1129-1131**

O

obstruction, intestinal, 490-498
obdurator paralysis, 830
occipitoatlantoaxial malformation, 797,
    798
ocular system, see eye
olecranon bursitis, **1446**
oligodontia, 564
oligospermia, **942, 943**
omphalitis, 687, **1564, 1565**
onchocerciasis, **938, 1102, 1107, 1115,
    1121-1124, 1687-1690**
onion poisoning, **1807**
ophthalmia, periodic, **1121-1124**
ophthalmology, see eye
optic nerve, hypoplasia, **1132**
    injury, 782, **1133**
    neuritis, **1133**
    neuropathy, proliferative, **1133**

oral cavity, 543-548
    anatomy, 543
    cleft palate, 544-546
    examination, 543
    foreign bodies, 546, 547
    lampus, 547
    neoplasia, 548
    stomatitis, 547, **1707**
    surgery, 543, 544
orbital cellulitis, **1096**
organochlorine poisoning, 762
organophosphate poisoning, 762
osselets, **1403**
ossifying myopathy, **1324**
osteochondrosis, **1308-1316**
    distal interphalangeal, **1369**
    elbow, **1447, 1448**
    fetlock, **1401, 1402**
    hock, **1480, 1481**
    pastern, **1378**
    shoulder, **1458**
    stifle, **1494**
osteopathy, hypertrophic, **1316, 1317**
osteochondritis dissecans, see
    osteochondrosis
osteochondroma, **1449**
osteomyelitis, 804, 805, **1289-1292,
    1419, 1420**
osteopetrosis, **1281**
osteotomy, **1248-1253**
ovaries, abscess, **1025**
    anestrus, **1028**
    cysts, **1025**
    diestrual ovulation, **1028**
    diestrus, prolonged, **1027**
    diseases, **1022-1028**
    gonadal dysgenesis, **1024**
    granulosa-cell tumor, **1025**
    hematoma, **1024**
    Morgagni, cyst, **969**
    neoplasia, **1025-1027**
    ovariectomy, **1022-1024**
    ovulation, induction, **998-1001**
    ovulatory failure, **1028**
    rectal palpation, **952-954**
    ultrasonography, **969**
overriding spinous processes, **1510,
    1511**
oviducts, **1028, 1029**
ovulation, diestrual, **1028**
    failure, **1028**
    induction, **998-1001**
Oxyuris equi, **1575, 1691, 1692**

P

pain control, 81-86, 409-502, 516
palate, cleft, 544-546
palatopharyngeal arch displacement,
    411, 412
palpation, rectal, 70, 476-479, 516,
    952-954, 1539
pancreas, 702-704
pancreatitis, 703, 704, **1749**
panniculitis, **1677**
panophthalmitis, **1125**
papillomatosis, **1105, 1656**
papular dermatosis, **1654**
paracentesis, ocular, **1086**
parafilariasis, **1676**
paranasal sinuses, see sinuses,
    paranasal
paraphimosis, **920-922**
Parascaris equorum, 442, 617, 618, 621
parasitism, see endoparasites or
    ectoparasites

(P continued)

parasystole, 252-254
paroxysmal atrial fibrillation, 246
parrot mouth, 561, **1460**
parturition, **994-998**
  cesarean section, **1020-1022**
  dystocia, **1015-1022**
  gastrointestinal complications, **1014**
  induction, **997, 998**
  management, **1010-1012**
  postpartum hemorrhage, 285, **1014**
pastern, dermatitis, **1711, 1712**
  grease heel, **1711, 1712**
  middle phalanx fractures, **1372-1375**
  osteochondrosis, **1378**
  proximal interphalangeal degenerative
    joint disease, **1378, 1379**
  proximal interphalangeal joint infection,
    1377
  proximal interphalangeal joint luxation
    1375, 1376
  scratches, **1711, 1712**
  tendon lacerations, **1376, 1377**
pasture management, 153, 154
patella, chondromalacia, **1491**
  fracture, **1489-1491**
  luxation, **1488, 1489**
  upward fixation, **1491, 1492**
patent urachus, **1563**
pectoral abscesses, **1325, 1326**
pedal osteitis, **1340, 1341**
pediatrics, see foals
pediculosis, **1692**
Pelodera dermatitis, **1709**
pelvic fracture, **1503, 1504**
pelvis, see hip
pemphigoid, bullous, **1708**
pemphigus, ocular, **1108**
pemphigus foliaceus, **1701, 1702**
penis, **920-935**
  agenesis, **927**
  amputation, **925-927**
  bacterial colonization, **933, 934**
  balanitis, **934**
  Bolz operation, **924, 925**
  coital exanthema, **931, 932**
  contagious equine metritis, **932, 933**
  erection, 863-865, **884, 885**
  examination, **920**
  habronemiasis, **934, 935**
  hematoma, **929, 930**
  lacerations, **927, 928**
  necrosis, **928, 929**
  neoplasia, **935**
  paralysis, **922-924**
  paraphimosis, **920-922**
  phallectomy, **925-927**
  phallopexy, **924, 925**
  phimosis, **920, 935, 936**
  priapism, **922-924**
  smegma accumulation, **930, 931**
  stallion ring, **928, 929**
  summer sores, **934, 935**
  suspensory ligament rupture, **929**
  Taylorella equigenitalis, **932, 933,**
    1034-1036
pentachlorophenol toxicity, **1708, 1709**
performance problems, 33, 34
pericardiocentesis, 332, 333
pericarditis, 330-333
perineum, laceration, 667, **1049-1057**
periodic ophthalmia, **1121-1124**
periodontal disease, 567
periorbital fractures, **1466, 1467**
periorchitis, **911**
periostitis, alveolar, 567
peritoneal fluid, see abdominocentesis

peritonitis, 670-674, **881**
peroneus tertius rupture, **1487, 1488**
peroneal nerve paralysis, 119, 829
persistent ductus arteriosus, 278, 279
persistent foramen ovale, 319, 320
persistent right aortic arch, 279
persistent truncus arteriosus, 279, 280
phallectomy, **925-927**
phallopexy, **924, 925**
pharmacology, see drugs
pharynx, collapse, 401
  foreign bodies, 399
  lymphoid hyperplasia, 399, 400
  soft palate displacement, 400, 401
  trauma, 399
phenothiazine toxicity, **1807**
phimosis, **920, 935, 936**
phonocardiography, 208, 209
photosensitization, **1705, 1706, 1710**
phthisis bulbi, **1096**
phycomycosis, 394, **1613**
physical restraint, 55-63
physical therapy, **1269-1274, 1513**
physitis, **1315, 1316**
piedra, **1680**
pigeon breast, **1325, 1326, 1665**
pinky syndrome, **1716**
pins, bone, **1241**
pinworms, **1575, 1691**
piroplasmosis, **1765, 1806**
pituitary adenoma, **1718, 1740-1745**
placenta, **1058-1063**
  abortion, twinning, **1059, 1060**
  hydramnios, **1063**
  hydroallantois, **1063**
  hydrops amnii, **1063**
  hypoplastic villi, **1060**
  placentitis, **1061**
  postabortion examination, **1067**
  premature separation, **1061**
  retained, **1061-1063**
placenta, retained, **1061-1063**
placentitis, **1061**
plant poisoning, acorn, **1555**
  Amsinckia intermedia, 699
  Birdsville indigo, 806
  blind staggers, 762
  bracken fern, 805, 806
  Dallis grass, 795
  darling pea, 795, 796
  hairy vetch, **1680**
  horsetail, 805, 806
  lathyrism, 831
  Lathyrus hirsutus, 831
  locoweed, 796, 796, **1784**
  moldy corn, 777, 778
  oak, **1555**
  onion, **1807**
  pyrrolizidine, 699, **1555**
  Quercus, **1555**
  red maple leaf, **1806**
  Russian knapweed, 789, 790
  ryegrass, 795
  Senecio spp, 699
  Sorghum, 825, 826, **1561**
  Sudan grass, 825, 826, **1561**
  sweet clover, **1838**
  yellow star thistle, 789, 790
plantar desmitis, **1474**
plasma-cell myeloma, **1800, 1819**
plasma transfusion, **1793, 1794**
plastic surgery, **1600**
plate, bone compression, **1238-1241**
platelets, evaluation, **1764**
  thrombocytopenia, **1832-1835**
Pneumocystis carinii, 441, 442

pneumonia, foal, 386, 441, 454, 455
  granulomatous, 449-451
pneumothorax, 457, 458
pododermatitis, **1344, 1345**
poisoning, see toxicity
poll evil, **1667**
polycythemia, **1808, 1819**
polydactylism, **1405, 1406**
polyodontia, heterotopic, 562, **1654**
polysynovitis, **1292**
postanesthetic myasthenia, 120, 835
postanesthetic myelopathy, 822, 823
postanesthetic myopathy, 117-119,
  1319-1321
postfoaling paralysis, 830
postmortem examination, 123-137
postpartum hemorrhage, 285, **1014**
posthioplasty, **936, 937**
posthitis, **937**
Potomac horse fever, 651-653, **1765**
pregnancy, cesarean section, **1020-1022**
  detection, hormonal, **979-982**
  detection, ultrasonographic, **969-974**
  dystocia, **1015-1022**
  foaling, **994-998**
  parturition, **994-998**
  physiology, **988-994**
  tests, **979-982**
  twins, **971, 1012, 1013**
premature atrial contractions, 247, 248
premature ventricular contractions, 251
prepubic tendon rupture, 690-692
prepuce, **935-939**
prepurchase examination, 16-19, 70-78
pressure sores, **1721**
priapism, **922-924**
prolapse, rectal, 666, 667
  uterine, **1033**
prostaglandins, **1001**
prostheses, limb, **1253**
protein bumps, **1651, 1652**
protein-losing enteropathy, 607, 608,
  1828-1831
protozoal encephalomyelitis, 756-759
proud flesh, see granulation tissue
pruritus, 38, 39, 666, **1685-1694**
pruritus ani, 666
pseudohermaphroditism, **889**
psoroptic mange, **1693**
puberty, **862**
pulmonic atresia, 280
pulmonic stenosis, 313, 314
pulse, evaluation, 176-179
punctures, **1586, 1607, 1608, 1610**
purchase examination, 16-19, 70-78
purpura hemorrhagica, **1710, 1836**
pyelonephritis, **1552**
pyloric stenosis, 599, 600, 602
pyometra, **1036**
pyrrolizidine alkaloid intoxication, 699,
  1555
pythiosis, 394, **1613, 1669-1671**

Q

quittor, **1339**

R

rabies, 749-751
radial fractures, **1440-1442**
radial paralysis, 827
radiation therapy, **1639-1642**
rain scald, **1694-1696**

(R continued)

records, medical, 64, 70-78
rectovestibular fistula, 667, **1049-1057**
recumbency, 35, 36
recurrent uveitis, **1121-1124**
red blood cells, see hemolymphatic
  system
rectum, 663-667
  atresia ani, 664
  examination, 70, 476-479, 516,
    952-954, 1539
  lacerations, 664-666
  prolapse, 666, 667
  pruritus ani, 666
  rectovaginal laceration, 667
  stenosis, 666
  strangulation, 666
red maple leaf toxicity, **1806**
reefing operation, **936, 937**
reference intervals, blood, **1774**
renal, see kidney
reproductive system, mare, **949-1071**
  abortion, **1059, 1060, 1066-1071**
  anestrus, **1028**
  artificial lighting, **999**
  biopsy, **960-963**
  cervix, diseases, **1037-1039**
  cesarean section, **1020-1022**
  coital exanthema, **1058, 1706, 1707**
  contagious equine metritis, **1034-1036**
  culture, **958-960**
  cysts, ovarian, **1025**
  cytologic examination, **957, 958**
  diestrual ovulation, **1028**
  diestrus, prolonged, **1027**
  dystocia, **1015-1022**
  embryonic loss, **1063-1066**
  endometrial cups, **993**
  endometrial fibrosis, **1036, 1037, 1065**
  endometritis, **1029-1033, 1036, 1065**
  estrous cycle, **982-988**
  estrus synchronization, **1003**
  examination, **949-979**
  fetal mummification, **1071**
  foaling, **994-998**
  gonadal dysgenesis, **1024**
  hormonal therapy, **998-1004**
  hydramnios, **1063**
  hydroallantois, **1063**
  intrauterine therapy, **1004-1008**
  lactation tetany, **1326, 1327**
  management, **1008**
  metritis-laminitis-septicemia complex,
    1015
  Morgagni, cyst, **969**
  neoplasia, **1025-1027, 1036**
  ovariectomy, **1022-1024**
  ovaries, diseases, **1022-1024**
  oviducts, **1028, 1029**
  ovulation induction, **998-1001**
  ovulatory failure, **1028**
  parturition, **994-998**
  perineal laceration, **1049-1057**
  placenta, diseases, **1058-1063**
  placentitis, **1061**
  postabortion fetal examination, **1067**
  postpartum hemorrhage, 285, **1014**
  postpartum paralysis, 830
  pregnancy, physiology, **988-994**
  pregnancy tests, **979-982**
  prolapse, uterine, **1033**
  prostaglandin therapy, **1001**
  pyometra, **1036**
  rectal palpation, **952-954**
  rectovestibular fistula, **1049-1057**
  retained placenta, **1061-1063**
  rupture, uterine, **1033**

  salpingitis, **1029, 1065**
  teasing, **1009**
  therapeutic abortion, **1069**
  torsion, uterine, **1032**
  twins, **971, 1012, 1013, 1059, 1060**
  ultrasonography, **963-978**
  umbilical cord torsion, **1069**
  uterus, diseases, **1029-1037**
  vagina, diseases, **1039-1058**
  vaginitis, **1057**
  vaginoscopy, **954-956**
reproductive system, stallion, **847-943**
  accessory genital glands, **916-918**
  aggression, **887, 888**
  anatomy, **856-861**
  artificial insemination, **870, 871**
  artificial lighting, **866**
  artificial vagina, **871-873**
  azoospermia, **942, 943**
  bacteriospermia, **941**
  balanitis, **934**
  biopsy, testicular, **856, 907**
  breeding soundness examination,
    847-856, 866
  bulbourethral gland, **916, 917**
  castration, **877-883**
  champignon, **881**
  chromosomal analysis, **856**
  circumcision, **936, 937**
  coital exanthema, **1058, 1706, 1707**
  contagious equine metritis, **922, 923,
    938**
  cultures, **850**
  dourine, **851, 892, 920, 938**
  ejaculation, **863-865, 885-887, 940**
  endoscopy, **855**
  epididymis, **908-910**
  epididymitis, **909**
  erection, **863-865, 884, 885**
  examination, **847-856**
  exercise, **865**
  funiculitis, **881, 914**
  hemospermia, **939**
  hermaphroditism, **889**
  hormonal analysis, **856**
  hydrocele, **881, 911**
  immunization, **865**
  infections, **849-851**
  infertility, 25, 26
  intersexuality, **889, 900**
  inguinal hernia, 612, 613, 684, 685,
    911-914
  libido, **849, 883, 884**
  management, **865-871**
  natural service, **869, 1034**
  neoplasia, **894, 903-905, 935, 1938**
  nutrition, **865**
  oligospermia, **942, 943**
  paraphimosis, **920-922**
  penis, diseases, **920-935**
  periorchitis, **911**
  phallopexy, **925-927**
  phimosis, **920, 935, 936**
  posthioplasty, **936, 937**
  posthitis, **937**
  prepuce, diseases, **935-939**
  priapism, **922-924**
  pseudohermaphroditism, **889**
  puberty, **862**
  reefing operation, **936, 937**
  scrotum, diseases, **888-894**
  semen collection, **852, 871-875**
  semen evaluation, **852-855**
  semen preservation, **875, 876, 939**
  semen transport, **876, 939**
  sex reversal syndrome, **889**

  sexual behavior dysfunction, **883-888**
  smegma accumulation, **930, 931**
  spermatic cord thrombosis, **915, 916**
  spermatic cord torsion, **914, 915**
  spermatogenesis, **862**
  spermatozoa, abnormal, **941, 942**
  sperm granuloma, **909**
  spermiostasis, **909, 910**
  stallion book, **867-869**
  stallion ring, **928, 929**
  Taylorella equigenitalis, **922, 923, 938,
    1034-1036**
  testes, diseases, **894-908**
  testicular descent, **861, 862, 895**
  tunica vaginalis, **910-914**
  ultrasonography, **855**
  urethra, diseases, **918-920**
  urethritis, **919, 920**
  urospermia, **940, 941**
  variocele, **915**
  venereal diseases, **849-851, 1034, 1058,
    1706**
  vesicular gland, **916, 917**
respiratory system, 353-463
  adenovirus infection, 385
  African horse sickness, 378-380
  alar folds, redundant, 391, 392
  arytenoid chondritis, 412-414
  arytenoidectomy, 412-414
  Aspergillus, 394, 408-410
  aspiration pneumonia, 431, 432
  atheroma, 395, 396
  bleeders, 451-454
  Bordetella bronchiseptica, 438
  bronchoalveolar lavage, 359
  bronchodilator therapy, 375-377
  chronic obstructive pulmonary disease,
    443-449
  coccidioidomycosis, 394, 451
  Corynebacterium equi, 436-438
  coughing, 13, 14
  cryptococcosis, 394
  Dictyocaulus arnfieldi, 442, 443
  disease in foals, 356, 360, 361, 377, 378,
    386, 429, 430, 441, 454-458
  dyspnea, 36, 37
  empyema, 392-394, 406-408
  endoscopy, 357
  epiglottic entrapment, 421-424
  epistaxis, 451-454
  ethmoid hematoma, 397
  examination, 353-361
  exercise-induced pulmonary
  foal pneumonia, 386, 441, 454, 455
  follicular cysts, paranasal sinus, 396
  glanders, 440, 441
  granulomatous pneumonia, 449-451
  guttural pouch, 402-411
  heaves, 443-449
  hemothorax, 458
  herpesvirus infections, 382-384
  hydrothorax, 458
  hypoxemia, foals, 455, 456
  influenza, 380-382
  inhalation therapy, 374, 375
  laryngeal hemiplegia, 414-421
  larynx, 411-424
  lung biopsy, 359, 360
  lungworms, 442, 443
  meconium aspiration, 430
  mediastinal abscess, 462
  melioidosis, 439, 440
  nasal amyloidosis, 395
  nasal polyps, 397, 398
  nasal septum, deformation, 396
  nebulization, 374, 375

(R continued)

neonatal respiratory distress syndrome, 429, 430
neoplasia, 395, 451, 463
noise, 36, 37
oxygen therapy, 372
palatopharyngeal arch displacement, 411, 412
Parascaris equorum, 442
paranasal sinus cyst, 396
paranasal sinuses, 386-390, 392, 394
persistent pulmonary hypertension, 430
pharyngeal collapse, 401
pharyngeal cysts, 398, 399
pharyngeal lymphoid hyperplasia, 399, 400
pharyngitis, 399, 400
phycomycosis, 394
physiology, 362-372
pleuritis, 459-462
Pneumocystis carinii, 441, 442
pneumonia, foal, 386, 441, 454, 455
pneumothorax, 457, 458
radiography, 357
rhinitis, 392
rhinopneumonitis, 382-384
Rhinosporidium seeberi, 394
rhinovirus infection, 385, 386
Rhodococcus equi, 436-438
silicate pneumoconiosis, 449
sinusitis, 392-394
smoke inhalation, 431
soft palate displacement, 400, 401
sounds, 36, 37
summer pasture-associated pulmonary disease, 449
strangles, 434, 435
Streptococcus equi, 434, 435
Streptococcus pneumoniae, 435, 436
Streptococcus zooepidemicus, 433, 434
surgery, 390
thoracentesis, 359
trachea, 424-429
tracheal collapse, 427, 428
tracheal stenosis, 428
tracheostomy, 372-374, 424, 425
transtracheal aspiration, 358, 359
tuberculosis, 450
ultrasonography, 357, 358
viral arteritis, 384, 385
restraint, chemical, 81-120
physical, 55-63
retained placenta, 1061-1063
retinal detachment, **1131, 1132**
rhabditic dermatitis, **1709**
rhabdomyolysis, exertional, 327, **1321-1324**
rhinitis, 392
rhinopneumonitis, 382-384
Rhinosporidium seeberi, 394
rhinovirus infection, 385, 386
Rhodococcus equi, 436-438
ringbone, **1370, 1378**
ringworm, **1698-1700**
round ligament rupture, **1505**
roundworms, 617, 618, 621
rupture, uterine, **1033**
Russian knapweed poisoning, 789, 790
ryegrass staggers, 795

S

sacral fractures, 823
sacralization, **1507**
sacroiliac injury, **1516-1518**

salivary glands, 570-572
calculi, 571
neoplasia, 572
salivation, excessive, 37, 38
sialoadenitis, 572
wounds, 571
salmonellosis, 120, 483, 643-647, **1812**
salpingitis, **1029, 1065**
Salter-Harris fracture types, **1213-1215**
sarcoid, **1103-1105, 1633, 1657-1659, 1714**
sarcoidosis, generalized, **1714**
sarcoptic mange, **1692, 1693**
scapular fractures, **1452-1454**
scapulohumeral instability, **1454, 1455**
scapulohumeral luxation, **1455, 1456**
screwworm myiasis, **1675**
sciatic nerve paralysis, 830
scintigraphy, 743, **1185-1191**
scoliosis, **1507**
scratches, **1711, 1712**
screws, bone, **1236-1238**
scrotum, 888-894
dermatitis, **892, 893**
edema, **892, 894**
habronemiasis, **894**
infection, **893**
melanoma, **894**
sarcoid, **894**
summer sores, **894**
trauma, **890-892**
seborrhea, **1714-1716**
second-intention healing, **1594-1596**
sedatives, 81-86, 93-97
seizures, 770, 779, 780
selenium poisoning, 762, **1681-1683**
semen, artificial vagina, 871-873
azoospermia, **942, 943**
bacteriospermia, **941**
collection, 852, 871-875
ejaculation, 863-865, 885-887, **940**
evaluation, 852-855
hemospermia, **939**
oligospermia, **942, 943**
preservation, 875, 876, **939**
spermatozoa, abnormal, **941, 942**
transport, 876, **939**
urospermia, **940, 941**
septicemia, 159-161, **1812**
serologic evaluation, **1764, 1765**
Sertoli-cell tumor, **903, 905**
sesamoid bone fractures, **1385-1391**
sesamoiditis, **1404, 1405**
sesamoidean desmitis, **1394**
sesamoidean ligament rupture, **1394**
Setaria, 760, 761
sex reversal syndrome, **889**
sexual behavior dysfunction, 883-888
shampoos, **1643**
shear mouth, 562
sheared heels, **1341, 1342**
shedding, abnormal, **1719**
shivering, 830-832
shock, 161, 162
shoe boil, **1446**
shoeing, **1264-1269**
shoulder, **1451-1460**
anesthesia, **1452**
bicipital bursitis, **1456, 1457**
cyst-like lesions, **1459**
humeral fractures, **1454**
infraspinatus bursitis, **1457**
joint infection, **1457**
luxation, **1455, 1456**
osteochondritis dissecans, **1458**
osteochondrosis, **1458**

scapular fractures, **1452-1454**
scapulohumeral instability, **1454, 1455**
serratus ventralis muscle rupture, **1456**
shoulder slip, **1454, 1455**
supraglenoid tubercle fracture, **1452-1454**
shoulder slip, **1454, 1455**
sidebone, **1340**
silicate pneumonoconiosis, 449
Simulium, **1690, 1691**
sinoatrial block, 234-236
sinography, **1176**
sinus arrhythmia, 233, 234
sinuses, paranasal, cysts, 396
ethmoid hematoma, 397
examination, 386-390
neoplasia, 395
sinusitis, 392-394
sinusitis, 392-394
skin, **1569-1722**
abrasions, **1584, 1590**
actinomycosis, **1666, 1667**
alopecia, **1683-1694**
amyloidosis, **1663**
anagen defluxion, **1683**
anatomy, **1569-1572**
angioedema, **1679**
anhidrosis, 42, 43, **1683, 1684**
antiinflammatories, **1645, 1646**
antifungals, **1645, 1647**
antimicrobials, **1602, 1603, 1645-1647**
antiparasitics, **1644, 1645, 1647**
antipruritics, **1645, 1646**
aplasia cutis, **1720**
Arabian fading syndrome, **1716**
arsenic poisoning, **1714**
astringents, **1644**
atopy, **1653**
aural plaques, **1720**
axillary nodular necrosis, **1664**
avulsions, **1586**
bandaging, **1603, 1604**
bee stings, **1678**
besnoitiosis, **1713**
biopsy, **1577, 1578**
black flies, **1690, 1691**
blastomycosis, **1672, 1673**
blowflies, **1676**
botryomycosis, **1665**
bullous pemphigoid, **1708**
burns, **1625-1630**
bursitis, bacterial, **1667**
calcinosis circumscripta, **1664**
calluses, **1721**
candidiasis, **1706**
cellulitis, **1608, 1609, 1677, 1678**
chorioptic mange, **1693**
chromomycosis, **1671**
Claviceps purpurea, **1711**
closure, **1592, 1593, 1598-1600**
coccidioidomycosis, 394, 451, **1673**
coital exanthema, **1058, 1706, 1707**
contact dermatitis, **1702, 1703**
contact hypersensitivity, **1704**
contusions, **1585, 1590**
corynebacterial abscesses, **1325, 1326, 1665**
corynebacterial folliculitis, **1697**
cryotherapy, **1635-1637**
cryptococcosis, 394, 756, **1673**
Culicoides hypersensitivity, **1685-1687**
cultures, **1575, 1576**
curly coat, **1718, 1741**
cutaneous vasculitis, **1710**
cytologic examination, **1578**
debridement, **1597, 1598**

(S continued)

decubital ulcers, **1721**
demodectic mange, **1680, 1681**
dentigerous cyst, 562, **1654**
dermatophilosis, **1575, 1694-1696**
dermatophytosis, **1698-1700**
dermographism, **1652**
dermoid cysts, **1654**
discoid lupus erythematosus, **1717**
dracunculiasis, **1676**
drainage, wound, **1600-1602**
drug eruption, **1653**
ear hematoma, **1655**
ear tick infestation, **1650, 1719**
endocrine function tests, **1581**
eosinophilic dermatitis, **1713**
eosinophilic granuloma, **1651**
epitheliogenesis imperfecta, **1720**
epizootic lymphangitis, **1672**
ergotism, **1711**
erythema multiforme, **1653**
examination, **1569-1581**
face flies, **1722**
farcy, **1667**
fibroma, **1663**
fire ant stings, **1704**
fistulous withers, **1667**
fly bites, **1649**
food allergy, **1653**
foreign bodies, **1648**
frostbite, **1709**
fungal granulomas, **1668-1673**
gasterophiliasis, **1676**
girth galls, **1664**
glanders, 440, 441, **1667**
gold therapy, **1647**
grafting, **1613-1625**
granulation tissue, **1594, 1595,**
    1604-1607, 1676
grease heel, **1711, 1712**
habronemiasis, 601, 602, **894, 934, 935,**
    1101, 1613, 1673-1675
hair follicle dystrophy, **1680**
hair loss, **1683-1694**
hairy vetch toxicosis, **1680**
healing, **1587-1590**
hematidrosis, **1722**
hematoma, **929, 930, 1585, 1591, 1655**
histoplasmosis, **1673**
hives, **1651, 1652**
horn flies, **1690**
horse pox, **1701**
hyperelastosis cutis, **1720, 1721**
hyperesthetic leukotrichia, **1717**
hyperhidrosis, 42, 43, **1722**
hyperthermia, **1637, 1638**
hypertrichosis, **1719**
hypoallergenic diets, **1581**
hypodermiasis, **1655**
hypothyroidism, **1648, 1681**
immunologic tests, **1581**
incisions, **1585, 1591-1596**
intertrigo, **1704**
intradermal skin tests, **1579, 1580**
iodism, **1683**
junctional mechanobullous disease,
    1706
keloid, **1661**
keratosis, **1694, 1712, 1713**
kunkers, **1669**
lavage, wound, **1596**
leeches, **1669, 1670**
lethal white syndrome, 532, **1716**
leucaenosis, **1683**
leukoderma, **1717**
leukotrichia, **1716, 1717**
louse infestation, **1692**

lumps, 27, 28
lymphosarcoma, **1662**
mast-cell tumor, **1662**
mastocytoma, **1662**
melanoma, **1660, 1661**
mercury toxicosis, 762, **1683**
molluscum contagiosum, **1701**
mosquito bites, **1649, 1650**
mycetoma, **1668**
mycobacteriosis, **1655**
myiasis, **1675, 1676**
myospherulosis, **1677**
neoplasia, **1630-1642**
nocardiosis, **1666, 1667**
nodular granuloma, **1651**
onchocerciasis, **938, 1102, 1107, 1115,**
    1121-1124, 1687-1690
Oxyuris equi, **1575, 1691, 1692**
panniculitis, **1677**
papillomatosis, **1105, 1106**
papular dermatosis, **1654**
parafilariasis, **1676**
pastern dermatitis, **1711, 1712**
pediculosis, **1692**
Pelodera dermatitis, **1709**
pemphigus foliaceus, **1701, 1702**
pentachlorophenol toxicosis, **1708,**
    1709
photoactivated vasculitis, **1710**
photosensitization, **1705, 1706**
phycomycosis,
piedra, **1680**
pigeon breast, **1325, 1326, 1665**
pinky syndrome, **1716**
pinworms, **1575, 1691**
pituitary adenoma, **1718, 1740-1745**
plastic surgery, **1600**
polyodontia, heterotopic, **1654**
poll evil, **1667**
postanesthetic reactions, 119, 120
pressure sores, **1721**
protein bumps, **1651, 1652**
proud flesh, **1594, 1595, 1604-1607,**
    1676
pruritus, 38, 39, 666, **1685-1694**
psoroptic mange, **1693**
psoroptic otitis, **1719**
punctures, **1586, 1607, 1608, 1610**
purpura hemorrhagica, **1710, 1836**
pythiosis, **1613, 1669-1671**
radiotherapy, **1639-1642**
rain scald, **1694-1696**
reticulated leukotrichia, **1716**
rhabditic dermatitis, **1709**
ringworm, **1698-1700**
sarcoid, **1103-1105, 1633, 1657-1659**
sarcoidosis, generalized, **1714**
sarcoptic mange, **1692, 1693**
scrapings, **1574**
scratches, **1711, 1712**
screwworms, **1675**
seborrhea, **1714-1716**
second-intention healing, **1594-1596**
selenium toxicosis, **1681-1683**
shampoos, **1643**
shedding, abnormal, **1719**
spider bites, **1679**
sporotrichosis, **1671, 1672**
spotted leukotrichia, **1716**
squamous-cell carcinoma, **1659, 1660**
stachybotryotoxicosis, **1708**
staphylococcal folliculitis, **1696, 1697**
streptothricosis, **1694-1696**
subcutaneous emphysema, **1677**
summer sores, 601, 602, **894, 934, 935,**
    938, 1101, 1613, 1673-1675

sunburn, **1703**
suturing, **1598-1600**
swellings, 43-45
systemic lupus erythematosus, **1713**
systemic mycosis, **1672, 1673**
telogen effluvium, **1683**
teratoma, 562, **1654**
therapy, **1581-1583**
tick bites, 764, **1650, 1719**
tick paralysis, 764
topical therapy, **1642-1645**
trichorrhexis nodosa, **1680**
trombiculid mite infestation, **1694**
tumors, **1630-1642, 1657-1663**
ulcerative lymphangitis, **1666**
urticaria, **1651, 1652**
vaccinia, **1701**
vesicular stomatitis, **1707**
viral papular dermatitis, **1700**
vitiligo, **1716**
warbles, **1655**
warts, **1105, 1106**
Wood's lamp examination, **1575**
wounds, 48, 49, **1584-1613**
zygomycosis, **1668, 1669**
slap test, 731
slit-lamp examination, **1087**
small colon, see colon, small
small intestines, see intestines
smegma accumulation, **930, 931**
smoke inhalation, 431
smooth mouth, 566
snail bait poisoning, 777
snakebite, 764
soft palate displacement, 400, 401
sole bruising, hoof, **1333-1335**
sorghum poisoning, 825, 826
soundness examination, 16-19, 70-78
sounds, heart, 182-186, 220-228
    intestinal, 516, 539, 540
    respiratory, 36, 37
sow mouth, 561
spavin, bog, **1476**
    bone, **1474-1476**
sperm granuloma, **909**
spermatic cord, thrombosis, **914, 915**
    torsion, **914, 915**
spermatogenesis, **862**
spermatozoa, abnormal, **941, 942**
spermiostasis, **909, 910**
spider bites, **1679**
spinal cord disorders, **797-823**
    infarction, **803**
    injury, **799-803**
spine, cervical vertebral malformation,
    807-822
    hunters' bumps, **1157, 1515**
    kyphosis, **1508**
    lordosis, **1507**
    lumbar arthritis, **1515**
    lumbar fractures, **1515**
    malalignment, lumbar spinous
        processes, **1511, 1512**
    muscle strain, **1508**
    occipitoatlantoaxial malformation, 797,
        798
    overriding spinous processes, **1510,**
        1511
    sacral fractures, **823**
    sacralization, **1507**
    sacroiliac injury, **1516-1518**
    scoliosis, **1507**
    spondylosis deformans, **1511**
    supraspinous ligament injury, **1508**
    synostosis, **1507**
    thoracolumbar fractures, **1509**

Page numbers in **boldface type** are located in Volume II.

(S continued)

vertebral osteomyelitis, 804, 805
wobbler syndrome, 807-822
spleen, **1844-1846**
abscess, **1845**
lymphosarcoma, **1845**
puncture, **1845**
rupture, **1845**
splenomegaly, **1845**
splint application, **1225-1235**
splint bone fractures, **1413, 1414**
"splints," **1414-1416**
spondylosis deformans, **1511**
sporotrichosis, **1671, 1672**
squamous-cell carcinoma, 536, 593, 603, **1561, 1659, 1660**
stable flies, **1649**
stachybotryotoxicosis, **1708**
stallion, see also reproductive system, stallion
book, **867-869**
examination, **847-856,** 866
exercise, **865**
immunization, **865**
infertility, 25, 26
management, **865-871**
nutrition, **865**
ring, **928, 929**
stall-walking, 766
stapling, intestinal, 527-530
step mouth, 566
stifle, joint infection, **1493, 1494**
meniscal tears, **1492, 1493**
osteochondrosis, **1494**
patellar chondromalacia, **1491**
patellar fracture, **1489-1491**
patellar luxation, **1488, 1489**
patellar upward fixation, **1491, 1492**
stomach, 593-606
anatomy, 593, 594
dilatation, 600
examination, 596, 597
gastritis, 604
gastroscopy, 597
impaction, 600
neoplasia, 603
nonsteroidal antiinflammatory toxicity, 602, 603
parasitism, 601, 602
pyloric stenosis, 599, 600, 602
radiography, 597
rupture, 600, 601
surgery, 598, 599
ulcers, 605, 606
stomatitis, 547, **1707**
strangles, 434, 435, 674-677
abdominal abscesses, 674-677
Colorado, **1325, 1326, 1665**
strangulation, bowel, 490-498
Streptococcus equi, 434, 435, 674-677
abdominal abscesses, 674-677
Streptococcus pneumoniae, 435, 436
Streptococcus zooepidemicus, 433, 434, 674-677, **1034, 1667**
streptothricosis, **1694-1696**
stringhalt, 830-832, **1481, 1482**
Strongyloides westeri, 616
Strongylus vulgaris, anthelmintic therapy, 510, 511
bowel infarction, 496, 538
diarrhea, 649, 650
verminous arteritis, 679-681
verminous meningoencephalomyelitis, 759-761
subconjunctival injection, **1088, 1089**
subpalpebral lavage, **1092**
subsolar abscess, **1343, 1344**

sudden death, 40-42, 260, 261
summer pasture-associated pulmonary disease, 449
summer sores, see habronemiasis
sunburn, **1703**
supraglenoid tubercle fracture, **1452-1454**
suprascapular paralysis, 826, 827
supraspinous ligament injury, **1508**
surgery, amputation, limb, **1253**
amputation, penis, **925-927**
anastomosis, bowel, 523-530
angular deformities, **1302-1307**
arthrodesis, **1253-1258**
Bolz operation, **924, 925**
Caslick's operation, **1040**
castration, **877-883**
cecum, 630, 631
cervical fusion, 817-820
cervical vertebral malformation, 817-822
cesarean section, **1020-1022**
circumcision, **936, 937**
colon, 637-640
cribbing, 767, 768
cryptorchid, **898-900**
cystotomy, **1562**
debridement, **1597, 1598**
epiglottis, 422-424
esophagus, 577-593
fracture fixation, **1235-1243**
grafts, bone, **1243-1246**
guttural pouches, 402-404
herniorrhaphy, inguinal, **913,** 914
joints, **1261-1263**
laminectomy, 820-822
laparotomy, 489, 518-520
larynx, 417-421
limb amputation, **1253**
Moh's tumor excision, **1631**
nasal septum, 390
nephrectomy, **1549**
nephrotomy, **1549**
oral cavity, 543, 544
osteotomy, **1248-1253**
ovariectomy, **1022-1024**
penile amputation, **925-927**
penis, **923-927**
perineal laceration, **1050-1057**
perineal reconstruction, **1041, 1042**
phallectomy, **925-927**
phallopexy, **924, 925**
plastic, **1600**
posthioplasty, **936, 937**
preputial resection, **936, 937**
rectovestibular fistula, **1050-1057**
rectum, 664-666
reefing operation, **936, 937**
stapling, bowel, 527-530
stomach, 598, 599
suturing, wounds, **1598-1600**
tendons, **1263**
trachea, 372-374, 424-426
tumor excision, **1632-1635**
urethral extension, **1045-1049**
urethrostomy, **1563**
urine pooling, **1045-1049**
vestibuloplasty, **1041, 1042**
wobbler, 817-822
wound closure, **1598-1600**
surra, **1801, 1802**
suspensory desmitis, **1418, 1419**
suturing, wound, **1598-1600**
sweating abnormalities, 42, 43, **1683, 1684, 1722**
sweeney, 826, 827

sweet clover poisoning, **1838**
swellings, 43-45
syncope, 260, 261
synchysis scintillans, **1128**
synostosis, **1507**
synovial fluid analysis, **1168-1170, 1221, 1222, 1284**
synovitis, villonodular, **1392-1394, 1403**

T

tachycardia, 229
ventricular, 251, 252
tail injuries, 824
tapeworms, 618
tarsal joint infection, **1477, 1478**
tarsitis, **1474-1476**
tarsocrural synovitis, **1476**
tarsus, see hock
Taylorella equigenitalis, **922, 923, 938, 1034-1036**
tear system, **1093, 1105, 1106**
teasing, mares, **1009**
teeth, 550-570
absence, 564
age determination, 553
anatomy, 552
caries, 567-569
decay, 567-569
deciduous, 566
dentigerous cysts, 562, **1564**
eruption, 550-552, 563, 564
examination, 553-556
extraction, 557-561
floating, 556, 557
oligodontia, 564
periodontal disease, 567
periostitis, alveolar, 567
points, 565
polyodontia, heterotopic, 562, **1564**
smooth mouth, 566
step mouth, 566
supernumerary, 562
wave mouth, 565
wolf teeth, 557, 564
telogen effluvium, **1683**
temporohyoid osteoarthropathy, 791
temporomandibular luxation, **1464**
tendinitis, **1416, 1417**
tendons, Achilles tendon rupture, **1488**
bowed tendons, **1416, 1417**
carpal canal syndrome, **1430, 1431**
common digital extensor rupture, **1432**
cunean tendinitis, **1474**
deep digital flexor rupture, **1338, 1339**
deep digital flexor tenosynovitis, **1476**
extensor tendon laceration, **1471-1473**
injury, response, **1215, 1216**
injury, treatment, **1263, 1264**
lacerations, **1376, 1377, 1416, 1471-1473**
peroneus tertius rupture, **1488**
stringhalt, 830-832, **1481, 1482**
tendinitis, **1416, 1417**
tenosynovitis, **1396, 1397, 1476**
tenesmus, 39, 40
tenosynovitis, **1396, 1397, 1476**
teratoma, 562, **1654**
testes, **894-908**
agenesis, **894**
anabolic steroids, **903**
castration, **877-883**
cryptorchidism, **895-900**
degeneration, **906-908**
ectopic, **900**

heat injury, 901
hematoma, 901
hypoplasia, 905, 906
irradiation, 901
lacerations, 901
Leydig-cell tumor, 905
neoplasia, 903-905
orchitis, 902, 903
seminoma, 904
Sertoli-cell tumor, 903, 905
teratoma, 904
thermoregulation, 863
tetanus, 782, 785-788
tetralogy of Fallot, 280, 281
Theiler's disease, 700, 701
Thelazia conjunctivitis, 1107
thermography, 743, 1191-1194
therapy, 139-158
anthelmintics, 510, 511
antifungals, 1645, 1647
antiinflammatories, 145-150, 1645, 1646
antimicrobials, 142-145, 511-513, 1087-1089, 1602, 1603, 1645-1647
antiparasitics, 1644, 1645, 1647
antipruritics, 1645, 1646
antipyretics, 145-150
astringents, 1644
back problems, 1512-1518
bandaging, 1603, 1604
blood diseases, 1791-1794
blood transfusion, 1791-1793, 1805, 1808
bronchodilator, 375-377
burns, 1625-1630
corneal, 1109, 1110
corticosteroids, 149, 150, 1089
cryotherapy, 1635-1637
diabetes mellitus, 1749
digitalization, 276, 277
dimethylsulfoxide, 148, 149
drainage, wound, 1600-1602
electrolyte, 139-142
first aid, fractures, 1224-1229
fluid, 139-142
gastrointestinal diseases, 499-514
gold therapy, 1647
hormonal, 998-1004
hydrotherapy, 1273
hyperthermia, 1637, 1638
immunotherapy, 1638, 1639, 1647, 1648
inhalation, 374, 375
insulin, 1749
irradiation, tumor, 1639-1642
laser therapy, 1278-1280, 1514
lavage, wound, 1596
liver disease, 697
manipulative therapy, 1514
nasolacrimal lavage, 1093
natural medicine, 1514
nerve stimulation, transcutaneous, 1274-1276
nonsteroidal antiinflammatories, 145-148, 1090
oxygen, 372
physical therapy, 1269-1274, 1513
plasma transfusion, 1793, 1794
plastic surgery, 1600
radiotherapy, tumor, 1639-1642
shampoos, 1643
shoeing, 1264-1269
skin disease, 1581-1583, 1602, 1603, 1635-1637, 1642-1648
subconjunctival injection, 1088, 1089
subpalpebral lavage, 1092

suturing, 1548-1600
systemic, 1645-1648
thoracolumbar problems, 1512-1518
topical, 1642-1645
transfaunation, 511
treadmill exercise, 1273
ultrasound, therapeutic, 1276-1278
wounds, 1590-1612
thoracentesis, 359
thoracolumbar fractures, 1509
thoroughpin, 1476
thread worms, 616
thrombocytes, see platelets
thrombocytopenia, 1832-1835
thromboembolism, parasitic, 287-293
thrombophlebitis, jugular, 293-295
thrombosis, aortoiliac, 287-291
spermatic cord, 915, 916
thrush, 1344, 1345
thumps, 1327
thyroid gland diseases, 1745-1748
tibial fractures, 1482-1487
tibial nerve paralysis, 829
tick infestation, 764, 1650, 1719
tick paralysis, 764
toe, long, 1342, 1343
tonometry, ocular, 1085, 1087
torsion, uterine, 1032
toxicity, abortion, 1071
acorn, 1555
aminoglycoside, 1553
amphotericin B, 1555
aplastic anemia, 1795
arsenic, 1714
Birdsville indigo, 806
blind staggers, 762
blister beetle, 324, 483, 533-535, 655, 656, 920, 1555, 1561
bracken fern, 805, 806
cantharidin, 324, 483, 533-535, 655, 656, 920, 1555, 1561
chlorinated hydrocarbon, 762
Dallis grass, 795
darling pea, 795, 796
drugs, anemia, 1795
fluoride, 1293-1296
grove poisoning, 765
hairy vetch, 1680
heavy metal, 1553
horsetail, 805, 806
iodism, 1683
ionophore, 321-324
lasolocid, 762
lathyrism, 831
lead, 790
leucaenosis, 1683
leukoencephalomalacia, 777, 778
locoweed, 795, 796, 1784
mercury, 762, 1553, 1683
metaldehyde, 777
moldy corn, 777, 778
monensin, 762
motor oil, 1708
mycotoxicosis, 700, 764, 1708
nonsteroidal antiinflammatory, 535, 536, 602, 603, 1554
onion, 1807
organophosphate, 762
pentachlorophenol, 1708
phenothiazine, 1807
plant poisoning, 699, 762, 763, 789, 795, 805, 806, 831, 1555, 1561, 1680
pyrrolizidine, 699, 1555
red maple leaf, 1806
Russian knapweed, 789, 790
ryegrass staggers, 795

selenium, 762, 1681-1683
snail bait, 777
snakebite, 764
Sorghum, 825, 826, 1561
stachybotryotoxicosis, 1708
Sudan grass, 825, 826, 1561
urea, 762
vitamin D, 1554
vitamin K$_3$, 1554
warfarin, 1837, 1888
water intoxication, 777
yellow star thistle, 789, 790
trachea, 424-429
anastomosis, 425, 426
aspiration, 358, 359
collapse, 427, 428
foreign bodies, 426, 427
granulomas, 428
stenosis, 428
tracheostomy, 372-374, 424, 425
trauma, 426
tracheostomy, 372-374, 424, 425
tranquilizers, 81-86, 93-97
transfaunation, 511
transfloration, 511
transfusions, 1791-1794, 1805, 1808
transtracheal aspiration, 358, 359
trauma, cranial, 771-774
ocular, 1095
spinal, 799-803
treadmill exercise, 1273
tremors, 769
trichiasis, 1100
trichorrhexis nodosa, 1680
Trichostrongylus axei, 601, 602
tricuspid atresia, 299-301
trochanteric bursa infection, 1502
trombiculosis, 1694
trypanosomiasis, 761, 851, 892, 920, 1800-1802
tuberculosis, 450
tumor, see neoplasia
tunica vaginalis, 910-914
twins, 971, 1012, 1013, 1059, 1060
tying up, 327, 1321-1324
typhlitis, 629
Tyzzer's disease, 698

U

ulcers, corneal, 1111, 1113, 1114
decubital, 1721
gastric, 605, 606
ulnar fractures, 1442-1446
ulnar nerve paralysis, 828
ultrasound therapy, 1276-1278
umbilical cord, hematoma, 1564
hernia, 613, 683, 684
infection, 687, 1564, 1565
torsion, 1069
umbilical hernia, 613, 683, 684
underrun heels, 1342, 1343
urachus, abscess, 1564, 1565
patent, 1563
ruptured, 1564
urea poisoning, 762
uremia, 1546
ureteral rupture, 1558
ureterolithiasis, 1558
urethra, diseases, 918-920
urethritis, 919, 920
urinalysis, 45, 46, 1540, 1739
urinary bladder, see bladder
urinary system, 1539-1565
aminoglycoside toxicity, 1553

(U continued)

amyloidosis, **1556**
azotemia, **1545, 1546**
biopsy, kidney, **1543**
bladder, diseases, **1558-1563**
bladder paralysis, **1561**
cystic calculi, **1562, 1563**
diabetes insipidus, **1557**
ectopic ureters, **1558**
electrolyte excretion, **1541**
enzymes, urine, **1541**
examination, **1539-1545**
glomerulonephritis, **1550-1552**
heavy metal poisoning, **1553**
hydronephrosis, **1556**
infection, **1546, 1547**
Klossiella equi, **1552**
Micronema deletrix, **1552**
neoplasia, **1555, 1561**
nephritis, **1550**
nonsteroidal antiinflammatory toxicity, **1554**
patent urachus, **1563**
peritoneal fluid analysis, **1541**
pigment nephropathy, **1553**
plant poisoning, **1555, 1561**
pyelonephritis, **1552**
radiography, **1542**
renal calculi, **1550**
renal hypoplasia, **1549**
renal tubular acidosis, **1556, 1557**
ruptured urachus, **1564**
serum chemistry, **1540**
tenemus, 39, 40
ultrasonography, **1542**
umbilical hematoma, **1564**
urachal abscess, **1564, 1565**
uremia, **1546**
ureteral rupture, **1558**
ureterolithiasis, **1558**
urethra, diseases, **918-920**
urethritis, **919, 920**
urinalysis, 45, 46, **1540**
urination, abnormal, 45, 46, **1545**
urine output, **1540**
uroperitoneum, 678, 679, **1541**
urospermia, **940, 941**
vasopressin challenge, **1544**
vitamin D toxicity, **1554**
vitamin K$_3$ toxicity, **1554**
water consumption, **1540**
water deprivation test, **1544**
urination, abnormal, 45, 46, **1545**
urine, output, **1540**
urolithiasis, **1550, 1558, 1562, 1563**
uroperitoneum, 678, 679, **1541**
urospermia, **940, 941**
urticaria, **1651, 1652**
uterus, artery rupture, 285, **1014**
biopsy, **960-963**
cesarean section, **1020-1022**
contagious equine metritis, **922, 923, 938, 1034-1036**
culture, **958-960**
cysts, **977, 1037**
cytologic examination, **957, 958**
diseases, **1029-1037**
dystocia, **1015-1022**
endometrial fibrosis, **1036, 1037, 1065**
endometrial hypoplasia, **1032**
endometritis, **1029-1032, 1033, 1036, 1065**
evacuation, **1031**
fiberoptic examination, **978**

fluid accumulation, **975-977, 1031**
intrauterine therapy, **1004-1008**
metritis-laminitis-septicemia complex, **1015**
neoplasia, **1036**
parturition, **994-998**
postpartum hemorrhage, 285, **1014**
pregnancy, **988-994**
pregnancy tests, **979-982**
prolapse, **1033**
pyometra, **1036**
rectal palpation, **952-954**
rupture, **1033**
torsion, **1032**
ultrasonography, **963, 969-978**
uveitis, **1120-1124**
uveitis, phacoanaphylactic, **1127**

V

vaccinia, **1701**
vagina, **1039-1058**
  Caslick's operation, **1041**
  cystic Gartner's ducts, **1040**
  lacerations, **1040-1045**
  persistent hymen, **1040**
  pseudohermaphroditism, **1040**
  rupture, **1042-1045**
  urine pooling, **1045-1049**
  vaginitis, **1057**
  varicose veins, **1040**
  vesicovaginal reflux, **1045-1049**
varicocele, **915**
vasculitis, 281, **1835, 1836**
  cutaneous, **1710**
  photoactivated, **1710**
vasopressin challenge, **1544**
vectorcardiography, 191-196
veins, diseases, 291-295
  arteriovenous mastomosis, 292
  rupture, 291, 292
  thrombophlebitis, jugular, 293-295
  thrombosis, 292, 293
venereal diseases, **849-851, 1034, 1058, 1706, 1707**
Venezuelan equine encephalomyelitis, 744-749
ventilation, mechanical, 114-116
ventricular arrhythmias, 249-255
ventricular fibrillation, 254
ventricular septal defect, 315-319
ventricular tachycardia, 251, 252
verminous arteritis, 679-681
verminous meningoencephalomyelitis, 759-761
vertebral malformation, cervical, 807-822
vertebral osteomyelitis, 804, 805
vesicular gland, **916, 917**
vesicular stomatitis, **1707**
vestibular disorders, 792-796
vices, 765-769
villonodular synovitis, **1392-1394, 1403**
viral abortion, **1069, 1070**
viral arteritis, 384, 385, **918, 1678, 1836**
viral papular dermatitis, **1700**
vitamin D toxicity, **1554**
vitamin K$_3$ toxicity, **1554**
vitiligo, **1716**
vitreous body, abscesses, **1127**
  floaters, **1127, 1128**
  vitritis, **1127**

volvulus, small colon, 662

W

wandering pacemaker, 234
warbles, **1655**
warfarin poisoning, **1837, 1838**
warts, **1105, 1656**
water intoxication, 777
water consumption, **1540**
wave mouth, 565
weakness, 732
weight loss, 46-48
Western equine encephalomyelitis, 744-749
white blood cells, see hemolymphatic system
white muscle disease, **1329, 1330**
wobbler syndrome, 807-822
wolf teeth, 557, 564
Wolff-Parkinson-White syndrome, 248, 249
Wood's lamp examination, **1575**
worms, see endoparasites
wounds, 48, 49, **1584-1613**
  abdominal, 669, 670, **1611**
  abrasions, **1584, 1590**
  antimicrobial therapy, **1602, 1603**
  avulsions, **1586**
  axilla, **1609**
  bandaging, **1603, 1604**
  burns, **1625-1630**
  closure, **1592, 1593, 1598-1600**
  complications, **1612, 1613**
  contusions, **1585, 1590**
  debridement, **1597, 1598**
  dehiscence, 685-689
  drainage, **1600-1602**
  evisceration, **882, 1611**
  granulation tissue, **1594, 1595, 1604-1607**
  groin, **1609**
  healing, **1587-1590, 1594-1596**
  hematomas, **929, 930, 1585, 1591**
  incisions, **1585, 1591-1596**
  lacerations, **1585, 1591-1596**
  lavage, **1596**
  open, **1585, 1591-1612**
  plastic surgery, **1600**
  punctures, **1586, 1607, 1608, 1610**
  second-intention healing, **1594-1596**
  skin grafting, **1613-1625**
  suturing, **1598-1600**
  treatment, **1590-1600**
  types, **1584-1587**
wry nose, **391, 1460, 1461**

X

xylose absorption test, 485

Y

yellow star thistle poisoning, 789, 790

Z

zygomycosis, **1668, 1669**

This page is intentionally left blank.